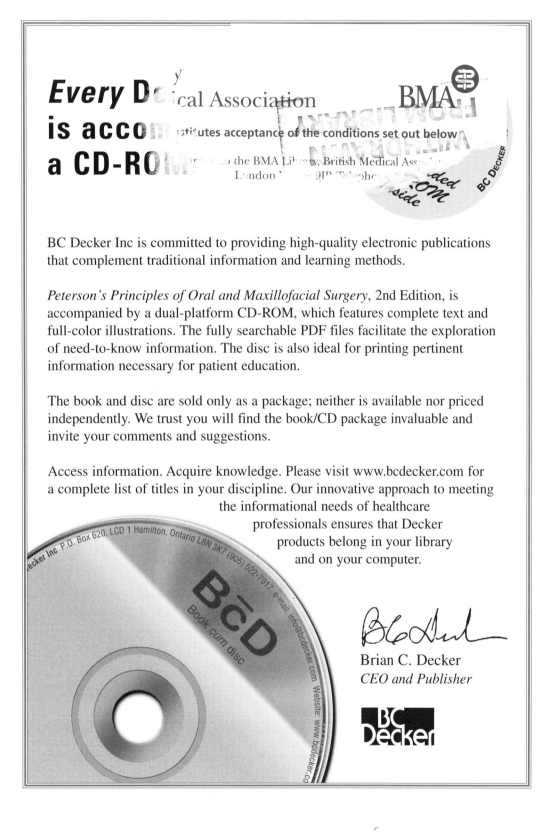

BC Decker Inc is committed to providing high-quality electronic publications that complement traditional information and learning methods.

Peterson's Principles of Oral and Maxillofacial Surgery, 2nd Edition, is accompanied by a dual-platform CD-ROM, which features complete text and full-color illustrations. The fully searchable PDF files facilitate the exploration of need-to-know information. The disc is also ideal for printing pertinent information necessary for patient education.

The book and disc are sold only as a package; neither is available nor priced independently. We trust you will find the book/CD package invaluable and invite your comments and suggestions.

Access information. Acquire knowledge. Please visit www.bcdecker.com for a complete list of titles in your discipline. Our innovative approach to meeting the informational needs of healthcare professionals ensures that Decker products belong in your library and on your computer.

Brian C. Decker
CEO and Publisher

BC Decker

PETERSON'S

PRINCIPLES OF

ORAL AND MAXILLOFACIAL SURGERY

Second Edition

Volume 2

Michael Miloro

Editor

G. E. Ghali • Peter E. Larsen • Peter D. Waite

Associate Editors

2004

BC Decker Inc

Hamilton • London

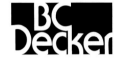

BC Decker Inc

P.O. Box 620, L.C.D. 1
Hamilton, Ontario L8N 3K7
Tel: 905-522-7017; 800-568-7281
Fax: 905-522-7839; 888-311-4987
E-mail: info@bcdecker.com
www.bcdecker.com

04 05 06 07 / FP / 9 8 7 6 5 4 3 2 1

ISBN 1-55009-234-0
Printed in Canada
Illustrations by Paulette Dennis, Andrée Jenks, and Kevin Millar.

Sales and Distribution

United States
BC Decker Inc
P.O. Box 785
Lewiston, NY 14092-0785
Tel: 905-522-7017; 800-568-7281
Fax: 905-522-7839; 888-311-4987
E-mail: info@bcdecker.com
www.bcdecker.com

Canada
BC Decker Inc
20 Hughson Street South
P.O. Box 620, LCD 1
Hamilton, Ontario L8N 3K7
Tel: 905-522-7017; 800-568-7281
Fax: 905-522-7839; 888-311-4987
E-mail: info@bcdecker.com
www.bcdecker.com

Foreign Rights
John Scott & Company
International Publishers' Agency
P.O. Box 878
Kimberton, PA 19442
Tel: 610-827-1640
Fax: 610-827-1671
E-mail: jsco@voicenet.com

Japan
Igaku-Shoin Ltd.
Foreign Publications Department
3-24-17 Hongo
Bunkyo-ku, Tokyo, Japan 113-8719
Tel: 3 3817 5680
Fax: 3 3815 6776
E-mail: fd@igaku-shoin.co.jp

UK, Europe, Scandinavia, Middle East
Elsevier Science
Customer Service Department
Foots Cray High Street
Sidcup, Kent
DA14 5HP, UK
Tel: 44 (0) 208 308 5760
Fax: 44 (0) 181 308 5702
E-mail: cservice@harcourt.com

Singapore, Malaysia,Thailand, Philippines, Indonesia, Vietnam, Pacific Rim, Korea
Elsevier Science Asia
583 Orchard Road
#09/01, Forum
Singapore 238884
Tel: 65-737-3593
Fax: 65-753-2145

Australia, New Zealand
Elsevier Science Australia
Customer Service Department
STM Division
Locked Bag 16
St. Peters, New South Wales, 2044
Australia
Tel: 61 02 9517-8999
Fax: 61 02 9517-2249
E-mail: stmp@harcourt.com.au
www.harcourt.com.au

Mexico and Central America
ETM SA de CV
Calle de Tula 59
Colonia Condesa
06140 Mexico DF, Mexico
Tel: 52-5-5553-6657
Fax: 52-5-5211-8468
E-mail: editoresdetextosmex@prodigy.net.mx

Brazil
Tecmedd
Av. Maurílio Biagi, 2850
City Ribeirão Preto – SP – CEP: 14021-000
Tel: 0800 992236
Fax: (16) 3993-9000
E-mail: tecmedd@tecmedd.com.br

India, Bangladesh, Pakistan, Sri Lanka
Elsevier Health Sciences Division
Customer Service Department
17A/1, Main Ring Road
Lajpat Nagar IV
New Delhi – 110024, India
Tel: 91 11 2644 7160-64
Fax: 91 11 2644 7156
E-mail: esindia@vsnl.net

DEDICATIONS

To Beth and Macy, my two reasons for being, for your love and support. To Pete, my teacher, for making me a better surgeon and person.

Michael Miloro

To my wife, Hope, for being my best friend and the love of my life. To my parents, Elias and Linda, and my brother Fred, for their support, inspiration, devotion, and love.

G. E. Ghali

To my wife, Patty, and my sons, Michael, Matthew, and Mark. You are the most important people in my life, yet always understand and are patient with my absence. To my father who inspired me to enter medicine. Lastly, to my former and current residents who teach me every day.

Peter Larsen

To my wife, Sallie, and my children, Allison, Eric, and Jon. To my father who inspired my interest in oral and maxillofacial surgery and to my residents who have continued to teach me.

Peter Waite

CONTENTS

†Deceased

v

PREFACE

The Second Edition of *Peterson's Principles of Oral and Maxillofacial Surgery*, reflects the efforts of many people made in a very short period of time. The time from the decision to undertake a second edition until publication release totaled less than 2 years. This is a monumental accomplishment considering the current state of affairs in the specialty of oral and maxillofacial surgery and the difficulties in pursuing scholarly activity, even for the academic practitioner. Although it is certainly not a simple task to assemble an author list as extensive as the one in this text, it was perhaps made easier because editors and authors were inspired by feelings of tribute to Larry Peterson to deliver on short notice.

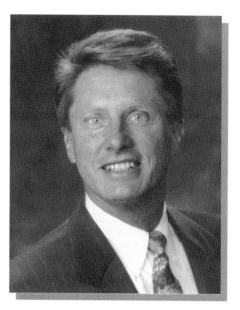

When Larry Peterson decided to publish the first edition of this book over a decade ago, he recognized the need in our specialty for a comprehensive and complete reference textbook in oral and maxillofacial surgery that was practical and readable. Oral and maxillofacial surgery encompasses an ever-expanding range of diverse topics that makes it unique among the medical and dental specialties. There was no concise textbook that dealt with the full scope of the specialty that was available for residents and surgeons to use as a reference for clinical practice. The textbook *Contemporary Oral and Maxillofacial Surgery* appropriately covers the requisite information for the dental student and general dental practitioner, but *Peterson's Principles of Oral and Maxillofacial Surgery* provides an organized and systematic approach to the specialty for residents and clinicians practicing full-scope oral and maxillofacial surgery. The first edition of this text was the only reference of its kind. It is now continued with the second edition, which is unique in many respects, among them the inclusion of contributions from more than 100 oral surgeons and other dental and medical specialists, 500 pieces of original artwork, and a CD-ROM.

The clear purpose of this textbook is to provide a concise, authoritative, easy-to-read, currently referenced, contemporary survey of the specialty of oral and maxillofacial surgery that contains the information that a competent surgeon should possess and understand. Although some of the information may be outside of the scope of the individual practitioner, the material contained in this text is definitely within the scope of the specialty. This textbook should be considered a reference for the oral and maxillofacial surgeon during residency and into clinical practice. It will be an excellent resource for examination preparation purposes as well; in fact, the first edition was adopted in some European countries as a required textbook for oral surgery board certification.

As with the first edition, the authors, primarily oral and maxillofacial surgeons, were chosen because of their broad experience and expertise in each specific area of the specialty. The contributions from these national and international authors certainly reflect their knowledge and specialization. Whenever appropriate, each chapter attempts to review etiology, diagnosis, patient assessment, treatment plan development, surgical and nonsurgical treatment options, and recognition and management of complications. The information contained in this textbook is based upon a thorough evaluation of the current literature, as well as clinical expertise, and is free from commercial and personal bias. If additional information is required, references have been provided so that other specialty textbooks may be consulted. Considering the rapid advancements and developments in the fields of medicine and surgery, a nearly constant survey of the current published literature is required to maintain a working knowledge of the standards of diagnosis and treatment. Future editions of this text will reflect these changes in clinical practice.

This text would not have been possible without the help and support of many people, including Ghali, Pete, and Peter; the outstanding authors who contributed their practice-defining knowledge; and the group at BC Decker Inc, including Catherine Travelle, Susan Cooper, and Paula Presutti, who sent a seemingly endless number of e-mails in an attempt to ensure deadlines were met. Certainly a debt of gratitude is owed to Brian Decker for his vision, dedication, and commitment to publish this textbook.

Peterson's Principles of Oral and Maxillofacial Surgery is *the* authoritative textbook for the specialty of oral and maxillofacial surgery.

MICHAEL MILORO, DMD, MD

ENCOMIUM

Dr. Larry J. ("Pete") Peterson is easily the smartest person I have ever known, and I do not mean with regard to medicine and surgery alone. Pete certainly forgot more information in his life than most people ever know. He made everyone around him want to be better than they were, and he helped them to reach their potential. *Peterson's Principles of Oral and Maxillofacial Surgery,* Second Edition, is dedicated to this man. Unfortunately, the majority of readers will never have had the opportunity to meet him and to experience his imposing presence. The fact that this book will continue to educate many surgeons for years to come would have pleased him very much since his greatest passion in life was, perhaps, teaching.

Pete obtained his doctor of dental surgery degree at the University of Missouri, Kansas City, in 1968. He completed his training in oral and maxillofacial surgery at Georgetown University, where he also received his masters of science degree. Pete served on the faculty at the Medical College of Georgia and, subsequently, at the University of Connecticut as the director of Oral and Maxillofacial Surgery Residency Training. However, he is best known for his academic accomplishments at Ohio State University, where he served as chairman of Oral and Maxillofacial Surgery, Pathology, and Anesthesiology from 1982 through 1999. To experience the full range of our specialty, Pete entered private practice in 1999 and continued in that area until his death on August 7, 2002.

Pete's professional and personal accomplishments and his contributions to our specialty are innumerable. In 1993 Pete assumed the role of editor-in-chief of *Oral Surgery, Oral Medicine, Oral Pathology, Oral Radiology and Endodontics,* upon the retirement of Dr. Robert Shira. Pete demanded excellence in the manuscript submissions and maintained high standards for this journal during his tenure. Pete also edited *Contemporary Oral and Maxillofacial Surgery,* which, like its predecessor from his mentor Dr. Gustav O. Kruger, defined dental undergraduate education in oral and maxillofacial surgery nationwide. Pete's dedication to education was further demonstrated in his role as chair of the American Association of Oral and Maxillofacial Surgeons Committee on Residency Education and Training. He lectured and published extensively both nationally and internationally, with a particular emphasis on the topics of odontogenic infections and dental implantology, and his contributions to the literature are many and varied.

Pete was a loving husband and father and enjoyed life to the fullest at each and every opportunity. To Pete, life was a journey. The answer to any problem was inconsequential; the long arduous path from question to answer was the only purpose for the question in the first place. Dr. Peter Larsen and I had the privilege of working closely with Pete and experiencing his talents and benefiting from his wisdom and guidance at Ohio State University for several years. We had the unique opportunity to observe Pete in and out of the hospital—the phrase "work hard, play hard" epitomizes the Peterson philosophy. Peter Larsen remembered Pete at his funeral; here is a portion of that eulogy:

When I tried to decide what to say about this amazing man, I started by making a list. What I discovered was a man of what I like to call "wonderful contradiction."

Pete was perhaps one of the most successful men I have known, yet he would have listed his Eagle Scout Award as being more important than many of the prestigious professional honors he received.

He was our most vigorous critic and yet our strongest advocate.

He was the teacher of teachers but also the perpetual student.

He was not an OSU alumnus but bled scarlet and gray.

He demanded hard work but taught me that it isn't really work if you love what you do.

He was a teacher who, when honored, thanked his students for teaching him.

Although surrounded by personal success, he found the greatest satisfaction in the success of others.

He was our boss but was more comfortable as our partner in a raft on the New River.

He would argue with you, not to get you to agree, but to get you to disagree and defend.

He trained many to reach great financial success but placed the reward gained by teaching higher than any financial reward.

He had much of which to boast and be proud, but instead practiced humility.

He was perhaps the smartest man I have ever known but was always first to admit when you had a good idea, and was gracious enough not to point out that he had thought of it himself, perhaps even years prior.

I never heard him speak on a topic when I was not totally impressed with the insight and knowledge he seemed to have, but he was often more content listening to what others had to say.

He was more interested in finding the truth than about being right himself.

He was 15 years older than me but looked younger.

He would often tell residents, much to their dismay, I might add, that it is not the answer that is important, but the question.

Many of his accomplishments could easily be ranked on a 1-to-10 scale as a "10." Yet, I can still hear him say, "There is no such thing as a '10.'"

He had the same enthusiasm for a giant rope swing as he did for a new operation.

He knew more than many of the speakers at the lectures he attended, but he always took notes.

He built what is perhaps the best Oral and Maxillofacial Surgery Department in the country, but, for me, his finest hour as our leader was when he tenderly took care of Vicki, Arden Hegtvedt's wife, when Arden died.

He was a man most deserving of a long and wonderful life, yet we are here today because this wonderful life has been tragically cut short.

If, as said by William James, "the greatest use of life is to spend it for something that will outlast it," then Pete spent his life well. For, as I look around, I see scores of us who owe so much of what we are to this one life well spent.

Pete died too young, and he will be missed, but through this textbook his teachings will continue.

Michael Miloro, DMD, MD

CONTRIBUTORS

Ronald M. Achong, DMD, MD
Department of Oral and Maxillofacial Surgery
Louisiana State University School of Dentistry
New Orleans, Louisiana

Marc B. Ackerman, DMD
Private Practice
Orthodontics
Bryn Mawr, Pennsylvania

C. Moody Alexander, DDS, MS
Department of Orthodontics
Baylor College of Dentistry, Texas A&M
    University System
Dallas, Texas

Carl M. Allen, DDS, MSD
Section of Oral and Maxillofacial Surgery,
    Pathology, and Dental Anesthesiology
The Ohio State University, College of Dentistry
Columbus, Ohio

Brian Alpert, DDS, FACD
Department of Surgical and Hospital Dentistry
University of Louisville School of Dentistry
Louisville, Kentucky

Meredith August, DMD, MD
Department of Oral and Maxillofacial Surgery
Harvard University
Boston, Massachusetts

Jonathan S. Bailey, DMD, MD
Department of Surgery
University of Illinois College of Medicine at
    Urbana-Champaign
Urbana, Illinois

Robert A. Bays, DDS
Department of Surgery
Emory University School of Medicine
Atlanta, Georgia

Jeffrey D. Bennett, DMD
Department of Oral Surgery and Hospital
    Dentistry
Indiana University School of Dentistry
Indianapolis, Indiana

Charles N. Bertolami, DDS, D.Med.Sc.
Department of Oral and Maxillofacial Surgery
University of California
San Francisco, California

Norman J. Betts, DDS, MS
Department of Oral and Maxillofacial Surgery
University of Michigan School of Dentistry
Ann Arbor, Michigan

Remy H. Blanchaert Jr, MD, DDS
Department of Oral and Maxillofacial Surgery
Kansas City Schools of Dentistry and Medicine
University of Missouri
Kansas City, Missouri

Michael S. Block, DMD
Department of Oral and Maxillofacial Surgery
Louisiana State University School of Dentistry
New Orleans, Louisiana

Dale S. Bloomquist, DDS, MS
Department of Oral and Maxillofacial Surgery
University of Washington School of Dentistry
Seattle, Washington

Kevin J. Butterfield, DDS, MD
Department of Oral and Maxillofacial Surgery
University of Connecticut
Farmington, Connecticut

Eric R. Carlson, DMD, MD
Department of Oral and Maxillofacial Surgery
University of Tennessee Graduate School of
    Medicine
Knoxville, Tennessee

Guillermo E. Chacon, DDS
Department of Oral and Maxillofacial Surgery
The Ohio State University Medical Center
Columbus, Ohio

Rakesh K. Chandra, MD
Department of Otolaryngology-Head and
    Neck Surgery
University of Tennessee Health Science Center
Memphis, Tennessee

M. Scott Connor, DDS, MD
Department of Oral and Maxillofacial Surgery
Louisiana State University Health Sciences
    Center
Shreveport, Louisiana

Bernard J. Costello, DMD, MD
Department of Oral and Maxillofacial Surgery
University of Pittsburgh
Pittsburgh, Pennsylvania

Larry L. Cunningham Jr, DDS, MD
Department of Oral Health Science
University of Kentucky, College of Dentistry
Lexington, Kentucky

Angelo Cuzalina, MD, DDS
Department of Oral and Maxillofacial Surgery
University of Oklahoma Health Science Center
Oklahoma City, Oklahoma

Jeffrey B. Dembo, DDS, MS
Department of Oral Health Science
University of Kentucky College of Dentistry
Lexington, Kentucky

Eric J. Dierks, DMD, MD
Department of Oral and Maxillofacial Surgery
Oregon Health Sciences University
Portland, Oregon

David N. Duddleston, MD
Department of Medicine
University of Mississippi Medical Center
Jackson, Mississippi

Sean P. Edwards, DDS, MD
Department of Oral and Maxillofacial Surgery
University of Michigan School of Dentistry
Ann Arbor, Michigan

Edward Ellis III, DDS, MS
Department of Surgery
University of Texas Southwestern Medical
    Center
Dallas, Texas

Bruce N. Epker, DDS, MSD, PhD
Aesthetic Facial Surgery Center
Weatherford, Texas

T. William Evans, DDS, MD, FACS
Department of Oral and Maxillofacial Surgery
The Ohio State University
Columbus, Ohio;
Department of Oral and Maxillofacial Surgery
University of Michigan
Ann Arbor, Michigan

Michael W. Finkelstein, DDS, MS
Department of Oral Pathology, Radiology, and
    Medicine
University of Iowa, College of Dentistry
Iowa City, Iowa

Mark C. Fletcher, DMD, MD
Department of Oral and Maxillofacial Surgery
University of Connecticut School of Dental
    Medicine
Farmington, Connecticut

Thomas R. Flynn, DMD
Department of Oral and Maxillofacial Surgery
Harvard School of Dental Medicine
Boston, Massachusetts

M. Cynthia Fukami, DMD, MS
Section of Pediatric Dentistry
The Ohio State University, College of Dentistry
Columbus, Ohio

Steven I. Ganzberg, DMD, MS
Section of Oral and Maxillofacial Surgery,
    Pathology, and Anesthesiology
The Ohio State University, College of Dentistry
Columbus, Ohio

G. E. Ghali, DDS, MD, FACS
Department of Oral and Maxillofacial Surgery
Louisiana State University Health Sciences
    Center
Shreveport, Louisiana

Robert Glickman, DMD
Department of Oral and Maxillofacial Surgery
New York University College of Dentistry
New York, New York

Michael S. Goldwasser, DDS, MD
Department of Surgery
University of Illinois College of Medicine at
    Urbana-Champaign
Urbana, Illinois

Steven G. Gollehon, DDS, MD
Department of Oral and Maxillofacial Surgery
Louisiana State University Health Sciences
    Center
New Orleans, Louisiana

Joao Roberto Goncalves, DDS, PhD
Departmento de Clínica Infantil
Faculdade de Odontologia de Araraquara-UNESP
Araraquara, Sao Paolo
Brazil

Reginald E. Gowans, DDS
Department of Oral and Maxillofacial Surgery
Charles R. Drew University of Medicine
    and Science
Los Angeles, California

Richard H. Haug, DDS
Division of Oral and Maxillofacial Surgery
University of Kentucky College of Dentistry
Lexington, Kentucky

Leslie B. Heffez, DMD, MS, FRCD
Department of Oral and Maxillofacial Surgery
University of Illinois, College of Dentistry
Chicago, Illinois

Joseph I. Helman, DMD
Department of Oral and Maxillofacial Surgery
University of Michigan
Ann Arbor, Michigan

Alan S. Herford, DDS, MD
Department of Oral and Maxillofacial Surgery
Loma Linda University School of Dentistry
Loma Linda, California

Jon D. Holmes, DMD, MD, FACS
Department of Oral and Maxillofacial Surgery
University of Alabama
Birmingham, Alabama

**James R. Hupp, DMD, MD, JD, MBA, FACS,
    FACD**
Departments of Oral and Maxillofacial Surgery,
Otolaryngology, and Surgery
University of Mississippi Medical Center School
    of Dentistry
Jackson, Mississippi

Heidi L. Jarecki, MD
Department of Ophthalmology and Visual
    Sciences
University of Wisconsin School of Medicine
Madison, Wisconsin

Ole T. Jensen, DDS, MS
University of Colorado School of Dentistry
Denver, Colorado

Milan J. Jugan, DMD
Dental Department
Naval Medical Center
San Diego, California

Leonard B. Kaban, DMD, MD
Department of Oral and Maxillofacial Surgery
Harvard University
Boston, Massachusetts

John R. Kalmar, DMD, PhD
Section of Oral Surgery, Oral Pathology, and
    Dental Anesthesia
The Ohio State University, College of Dentistry
Columbus, Ohio

Vasiliki Karlis, DMD, MD
Department of Oral and Maxillofacial Surgery
New York University College of Dentistry
New York, New York

David W. Kennedy, MD, FACS, FRCSI
University of Pennsylvania School of Medicine
Philadelphia, Pennsylvania

James Koehler, DDS, MD
Department of Oral and Maxillofacial Surgery
University of Alabama
Birmingham, Alabama

George M. Kushner, DMD, MD
Department of Surgical and Hospital Dentistry
University of Louisville
Louisville, Kentucky

Peter E. Larsen, DDS
Department of Oral and Maxillofacial Surgery
The Ohio State University, College of Dentistry
Columbus, Ohio

Richard D. Leathers, DDS
Department of Oral and Maxillofacial Surgery
Charles R. Drew University of Medicine and
    Science
Los Angeles, California

Jessica J. Lee, DDS
Department of Oral and Maxillofacial Surgery
University of Washington School of Dentistry
Seattle, Washington

Bradley N. Lemke, MD
Department of Ophthalmology and Visual
    Sciences
University of Wisconsin School of Medicine
Madison, Wisconsin

Stuart E. Lieblich, DMD
Department of Oral and Maxillofacial Surgery
University of Connecticut School of Dental
    Medicine
Farmington, Connecticut

Patrick J. Louis, DDS, MD
Department of Oral and Maxillofacial Surgery
University of Alabama
Birmingham, Alabama

Mark J. Lucarelli, MD
Department of Ophthalmology and Visual
    Sciences
University of Wisconsin School of Medicine
Madison, Wisconsin

Stephen B. Milam, DDS, PhD, FACD
Department of Oral and Maxillofacial Surgery
University of Texas Health Science Center
San Antonio, Texas

Michael Miloro, DMD, MD
Department of Oral and Maxillofacial Surgery
The Nebraska Medical Center
Omaha, Nebraska

Dale J. Misiek, DMD
Department of Oral and Maxillofacial Surgery
Louisiana State University Health Sciences
    Center
New Orleans, Louisiana

Gary D. Monheit, MD
Departments of Dermatology and Ophthalmology
University of Alabama
Birmingham, Alabama

Jeffrey J. Moses, DDS, FACD, FICD, FAACS
Department of Dentistry
University of California
Los Angeles, California

Gregory M. Ness, DDS
Department of Oral and Maxillofacial Surgery
The Ohio State University, College of Dentistry
Columbus, Ohio

Mark W. Ochs, DMD, MD
Department of Oral and Maxillofacial Surgery
University of Pittsburgh School of Dental
    Medicine
Pittsburgh, Pennsylvania

Robert. A. Ord, MD, DDS, MS, FRCS, FACS
Department of Oral and Maxillofacial Surgery
University of Maryland
Baltimore, Maryland

Todd G. Owsley, DDS, MD
Carolina Surgical Arts, PA
Greensboro, North Carolina

Stephen M. Parel, DDS, FACD, FICD
Department of Oral and Maxillofacial Surgery
Baylor College of Dentistry, Texas A&M
    University System
Dallas, Texas

Alex E. Pazoki, MD, DDS
Department of Oral and Maxillofacial Surgery
University of Maryland
Baltimore, Maryland

Vincent J. Perciaccante, DDS
Department of Surgery
Emory University School of Medicine
Atlanta, Georgia

Larry J. Peterson, DDS, MS[†]
Department of Oral and Maxillofacial Surgery
The Ohio State University, College of Dentistry
Columbus, Ohio

Joseph F. Piecuch, DMD, MD
Department of Oral and Maxillofacial Surgery
University of Connecticut School of Dental
    Medicine
Farmington, Connecticut

Michael A. Pikos, DDS
Department of Oral and Maxillofacial Surgery
University of Miami School of Medicine
Miami, Florida

M. Anthony Pogrel, DDS, MD, FRCS, FACS
Department of Oral and Maxillofacial Surgery
University of California
San Francisco, California

Jeffrey C. Posnick, DMD, MD, FRCS(C), FACS
Departments of Surgery and Pediatrics
Georgetown University Medical Center
Washington, District of Columbia

Michael P. Powers, DDS, MS
Department of Oral and Maxillofacial Surgery
Case Western Reserve University School of
    Dental Medicine
Cleveland, Ohio

Ramon L. Ruiz, DMD, MD
Departments of Oral and Maxillofacial Surgery
    and Pediatrics
University of North Carolina
Chapel Hill, North Carolina

Thomas J. Salinas, DDS
Department of Otolaryngology
University of Nebraska Medical Center
Omaha, Nebraska

Noah A. Sandler, DMD, MD
Department of Diagnostic and Surgical Sciences
University of Minnesota
Minneapolis, Minnesota

David M. Sarver, DMD, MS
Department of Orthodontics
University of North Carolina
Chapel Hill, North Carolina

Michael S. Scherer, DDS, MD
Department of Oral and Maxillofacial Surgery
Case Western Reserve University School of
    Dental Medicine
Cleveland, Ohio

Sterling R. Schow, DMD
Department of Oral and Maxillofacial Surgery
Baylor College of Dentistry, Texas A&M
    University System
Dallas, Texas

Anthony G. Sclar, DMD
Department of Surgery
University of Miami School of Medicine
Miami, Florida

Vivek Shetty, DDS, Dr.Med.Dent.
Department of Oral and Maxillofacial Surgery
University of California
Los Angeles, California

James W. Sikes Jr, DMD, MD
Department of Oral and Maxillofacial Surgery
Louisiana State University Health Sciences
    Center
Shreveport, Louisiana

Massimo Simion, DDS
Department of Periodontology
University of Milan
Milan, Italy

Douglas P. Sinn, DDS
Department of Surgery
University of Texas Southwestern Medical
    Center
Dallas, Texas

Daniel B. Spagnoli, DDS, PhD
Department of Oral and Maxillofacial Surgery
Louisiana State University Health Sciences
    Center
New Orleans, Louisiana

Peter M. Spalding, DDS, MS, MS
Department of Growth and Development
University of Nebraska Medical Center College
    of Dentistry
Lincoln, Nebraska

Eber L. L. Stevao, DDS, PhD
Department of Oral and Maxillofacial Surgery
Baylor College of Dentistry, Texas A&M University System
Dallas, Texas

[†]Deceased

Suzanne U. Stucki-McCormick, MS, DDS
Pacific Center for Jaw and Facial Surgery
Encinitas, California

B. D. Tiner, DDS, MD
Department of Oral and Maxillofacial Surgery
University of Texas Health Science Center
San Antonio, Texas

Paul S. Tiwana, DDS, MD, MS
Department of Oral and Maxillofacial Surgery
University of North Carolina
Chapel Hill, North Carolina

Yan Trokel, MD, DDS
Department of Oral and Maxillofacial Surgery
University of Texas Southwestern Medical Center
Dallas, Texas

Maria J. Troulis, DDS, MSc
Department of Oral and Maxillofacial Surgery
Harvard University
Boston, Massachusetts

Timothy A. Turvey, DDS
Department of Oral and Maxillofacial Surgery
University of North Carolina
Chapel Hill, North Carolina

Scott D. Urban, DMD, MD
Department of Oral and Maxillofacial Surgery
University of Alabama
Birmingham, Alabama

Joseph E. Van Sickels, DDS
Department of Oral Health Science
University of Kentucky
Lexington, Kentucky

Tomaso Vercellotti, MD, DDS
Department of Ear, Nose, and Throat
University of Studies of Genova (Italy)
Genova, Italy

Katherine W. L. Vig, BDS, MS, D. Orth, FDS(RCS)
Department of Orthodontics
The Ohio State University, College of Dentistry
Columbus, Ohio

Steven D. Vincent, DDS, MS
Department of Oral Pathology, Radiology, and
    Medicine
University of Iowa, College of Dentistry
Iowa City, Iowa

Peter D. Waite, MPH, DDS, MD, FACD
Department of Oral and Maxillofacial Surgery
University of Alabama School of Dentistry
Birmingham, Alabama

Joel M. Weaver, DDS, PhD, FACD, FICD
Department of Anesthesiology
College of Medicine and Public Health
The Ohio State University
Columbus, Ohio

Randall M. Wilk, DDS, PhD, MD
Department of Oral and Maxillofacial Surgery
Louisiana State University Health Sciences Center
New Orleans, Louisiana

Larry M. Wolford, DMD
Department of Oral and Maxillofacial Surgery
Baylor College of Dentistry, Texas A&M
    University System
Dallas, Texas

Deborah L. Zeitler, DDS, MS
Department of Oral and Maxillofacial Surgery
University of Iowa College of Dentistry
Iowa City, Iowa

Michael F. Zide, DMD
Department of Oral and Maxillofacial Surgery
University of Texas Southwestern Medical
    School
Dallas, Texas

Part 6

Maxillofacial Reconstruction

CHAPTER 38

Local and Regional Flaps

Alan S. Herford, DDS, MD
G. E. Ghali, DDS, MD

Flap Principles

Over the past 50 years the development and application of several different flaps has led to reliable reconstruction of facial defects. Most defects can be reconstructed immediately, leading to better restoration of form and function with early rehabilitation.[1] Reconstructing facial defects can be both challenging and rewarding. Missing tissue most often results from either trauma or oncologic surgery. Commonly there is a wide range of options for repairing a given defect, including healing by secondary intention, primary closure, placement of a skin graft, or mobilization of local or regional tissue. Compared to skin grafts, local flaps often produce superior functional and esthetic results.[2–6] A great advantage of local tissue transfer is that the tissue closely resembles the missing skin in color and texture. These flaps can be rotated, advanced, or transposed into a tissue defect. Regional tissue can also be recruited to repair facial defects.

When deciding which option to use, there should be a progression from simple to complex treatments. Consideration should be given to primary closure or the use of skin grafts first, followed by local, then regional, and finally distant pedicled or microsurgical free tissue transfer. Flaps require additional incisions and tissue movement, which increase the risks of postoperative bleeding, hematoma, pain, and infection. Confirmation of tumor-free margins should be done prior to flap reconstruction if a malignant lesion has been excised.[7]

Some defects are amenable to closure with a single flap, but others require a combination of flaps for optimal results.[8] An advantage of using multiple flaps is that they can be harvested from separate esthetic units. This decreases the size of the secondary defect and may allow placement of scars between esthetic units, thus improving scar camouflage leading to better cosmesis. Often, separated repair of individual facial subunits with separate flaps provides a better cosmetic result than if a single flap is used to reconstruct the entire defect.

Flaps differ from grafts in that they maintain their blood supply as they are moved. Abundant dermal and subdermal plexus allow for predictable elevation of random cutaneous flaps. A cutaneous flap may also have its arterial supply based on a dominant artery in the subcutaneous layer. Muscular perforating arteries are important contributors to the cutaneous vascular bed. The most important variable for flap viability is not the length-to-width ratio but, rather, the perfusion pressure and vascularity at the pedicle base.[9] Because local flaps provide their own blood supply, they are particularly useful in patients with compromised recipient sites such as those that have been irradiated.

As local flaps heal, regaining of blood flow and cutaneous sensibility increases. The rate of blood flow and two-point discrimination on the surface of local flaps is statistically no different when compared with the corresponding area of the unoperated side.[10] The recovery of sensory nerve function in facial flaps is dependent on the intimacy of contact between the flap and the recipient bed and on the viability of the type of restoration.

Relaxed skin tension lines (RSTLs) result from vectors within the skin that reflect the intrinsic tension of the skin at rest. They are due to the microarchitecture of the skin and represent the directional pull on wounds. The RSTLs are generally parallel to the facial rhytids. Lines of minimal tension (rhytids) result from repeated bending of the skin from muscular contraction. A permanent crease results from the adhesions between the dermis and deeper tissues. These natural skin creases run perpendicular to the direction of muscle pull and can guide incision orientation for optimal scar camouflage and cosmesis.

The face is composed of esthetic subunits.[11,12] The areas where these subunits meet are referred to as anatomic borders. The esthetic subunit principle is based on the fact that our eyes see objects as a series of block images that are spatially organized. Scars that are located at the junction of two adjacent anatomic subunits are inconspicuous because one expects to see a delineation between these areas.

Flap Nomenclature

There are many methods described for classifying cutaneous flaps: by the arrangement of their blood supply, their configuration, location, tissue content, and method of transferring the flap.

Blood Supply

Cutaneous flaps consist of skin and subcutaneous tissue and can be characterized by their predominant arterial supply. These include random pattern, axial pattern, and pedicle flaps (Figure 38-1). Random flaps are supplied by the dermal and subdermal plexus alone and are the most common type of flap used for reconstructing facial defects. Axial pattern flaps are supplied by more dominant superficial vessels that are oriented longitudinally along the flap axis. Pedicle flaps are supplied by large named arteries that supply the skin paddle through muscular perforating vessels. Free tissue transfer refers to flaps that are harvested from a remote region and have the vascular connection reestablished at the recipient site.

Location

Another means of classification is by the region from which the tissue is mobilized. This includes local, regional, and distant flaps. Local flaps imply use of tissue adjacent to the defect, whereas regional flaps refer to those flaps recruited from different areas of the same part of the body. Distant flaps are harvested from different parts of the body.

Configuration

Flaps are often referred to by their geometric configuration. Examples of these flaps include bilobed, rhombic, and Z-plasty.

Tissue Content

The layers of tissue contained within the flap can also be used to classify a flap. *Cutaneous flap* refers to those flaps that contain the skin only. When other layers are incorporated into the flap they are classified accordingly. Examples include myocutaneous and fasciocutaneous flaps.

Method of Transfer

The most common method of classifying flaps is based on the method of transfer. Advancement flaps are mobilized along a linear axis toward the defect (Figure 38-2). Rotation flaps pivot around a point at the base of the flap (Figure 38-3). Although most flaps are moved by a combination of rotation and advancement into the defect, the major mechanism of tissue transfer is used to classify a given flap. *Transposition flap* refers to one that is mobilized toward an adjacent defect over an incomplete bridge of skin. Examples of transposition flaps include rhombic flaps and bilobed flaps (Figure 38-4). Interposition flaps differ from transposition flaps in that the incomplete bridge of adjacent skin is also elevated and mobilized. An example of an interposition flap is a Z-plasty. Interpolated flaps are those flaps that are mobilized either over or beneath a complete bridge of intact skin via a pedicle. These flaps often require a secondary surgery for pedicle division. Microvascular free tissue transfer

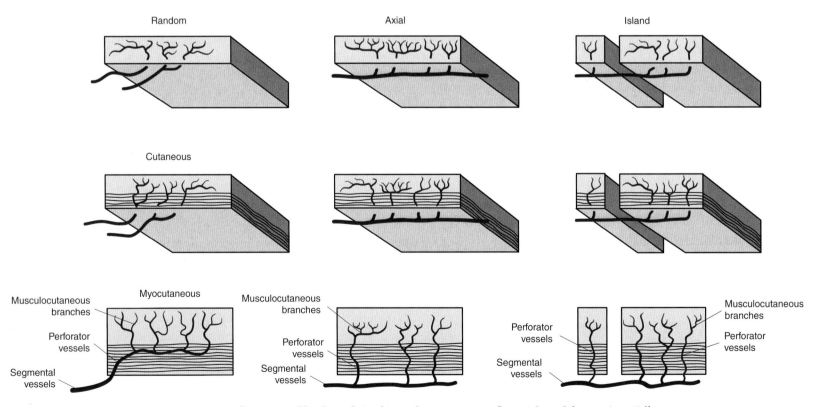

FIGURE **38-1** *Diagrammatic representation of cutaneous blood supply in skin and myocutaneous flaps. Adapted from Ariyan S.[41]*

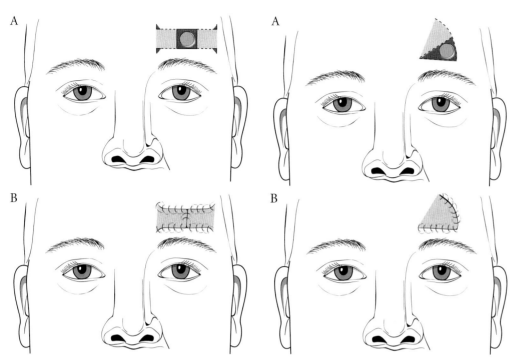

FIGURE **38-2**   A, *Double advancement flaps with Burow's triangles.* B, *Closure of the defect.*

FIGURE **38-3**   A, *Rotation flap for closure of a forehead defect.* B, *Closure of the defect.*

The secondary defect that is created as the tissue is transferred into the primary defect must be able to be closed easily. When designing a flap, it is important to avoid secondary deformities that distort important facial landmarks or affect function. Avoid obliterating critical anatomic lines that are essential for normal function and appearance.

Proper surgical technique involves gentle handling of the tissue by grasping the skin margins with skin hooks or fine-toothed tissue forceps. Avoid traumatizing the vascular supply by twisting or kinking the base of the flap. Deep pexing sutures minimize tension on the flap and eliminate dead space. Excessive tension on the flap may decrease blood flow and cause flap necrosis. Meticulous hemostasis should be achieved prior to final suturing so that a hematoma does not develop beneath the flap. It is important to

from a different part of the body relies on reanastomosis of the vascular pedicle.

Designing the Flap

There are many options for reconstructing facial defects. Often the optimal method is not readily apparent. A stepwise approach can be helpful in selecting and designing a flap. The characteristics of the defect and adjacent tissue must be analyzed. These include color, elasticity, and texture of the missing tissue. The defect size, depth, and location are evaluated as well as the availability and characteristics of adjacent or regional tissue. It is important to determine the mobility of adjacent structures and to identify those anatomic landmarks that must not be distorted. The orientation of the RSTLs and esthetic units should by analyzed closely.

Potential flap designs should be drawn on the skin surface being careful to avoid those designs that obliterate or distort anatomic landmarks. The final location of the resultant scar should be anti-cipated by previsualizing suture lines and choosing flaps that place the lines in normal creases.

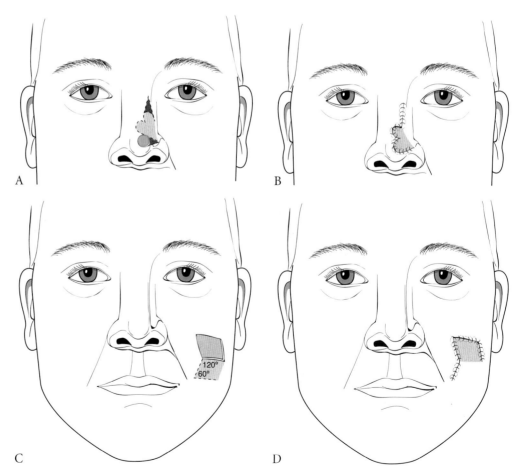

FIGURE **38-4**   A, *Bilobed flap for closure of a nasal tip defect.* B, *Closure of the defect.* C, *Rhombic flap for closure of a check defect. Note the 120 and 60˚ angles.* D, *Closure of the defect.*

adequately mobilize and extend the flap, which should be of adequate size to remain in place without tension to minimize the chance of dehiscence, scarring, or ectropion.

Types of Flaps

Local Flaps

Advancement Flaps Advancement flaps have a linear configuration and are advanced into the defect along a single vector. These flaps can be single or double. Advancement flaps are often chosen when the surrounding skin exhibits good tissue laxity and the resulting incision lines can be hidden in natural creases. Advancement flaps limit wound tension to a single vector with minimal perpendicular tension. They are often helpful in reconstructing defects involving the forehead, helical rim, lips, and cheek. In these areas advancement flaps capitalize on the natural forehead furrows without causing vertical distortion of the hairline superiorly or the eyebrow inferiorly (Figure 38-5).

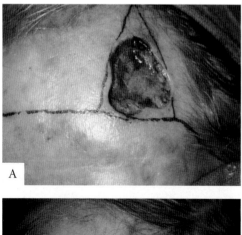

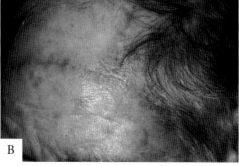

FIGURE **38-5** A, *Advancement flap for closure of forehead defect.* B, *Closure of defect with incision lines placed in natural forehead crease.*

Advancement flaps are created by parallel incisions approximately the width of the defect. Standing cutaneous deformities ("dog ears") are usually created and are managed with excision. A **Z**-plasty incision or Burow's triangle may be performed at the base of the flap, reducing the standing cutaneous deformities.

A variation of the advancement flap is the **V-Y** flap. A triangular island of tissue adjacent to the defect is isolated and attached only to the subcutaneous tissue. It relies on a subcutaneous pedicle for blood supply. As it is advanced into the defect, the secondary defect is closed primarily in a simple **V-Y** manner. These flaps are especially amenable for cheek defects along the alar facial groove and are generally avoided where there are superficial nerves because of the depth of the incisions.

Intraoral uses of advancement flaps include covering oroantral fistulas and alveolar clefts. A disadvantage of buccal advancement flaps is the decrease in vestibular sulcus depth (Figure 38-6).

Rotation Flaps Rotation flaps have a curvilinear configuration. Defects reconstructed with rotation flaps should be somewhat triangular or modified by removing normal tissue to create a triangular defect. These flaps have a large base and are usually random in their vascularity but may be axial. One or more rotation flaps are often used to reconstruct scalp defects. Because of the relative inelasticity of the scalp tissue, these flaps must be large relative to the size of the defect. Scoring of the galea is helpful in gaining additional rotation and advancement (Figure 38-7).

The axial frontonasal flap is a modified simple rotation flap with a back cut.[13–16] It is useful for closing nasal defects (Figure 38-8). The flap is based on a vascular pedicle at the level of the medial canthus. This pedicle consists of a branch of the angular artery and the supraorbital artery.

Rotated palatal flaps are helpful for closing large oroantral fistulas.[8,17] Fistulas < 5 mm in diameter usually close

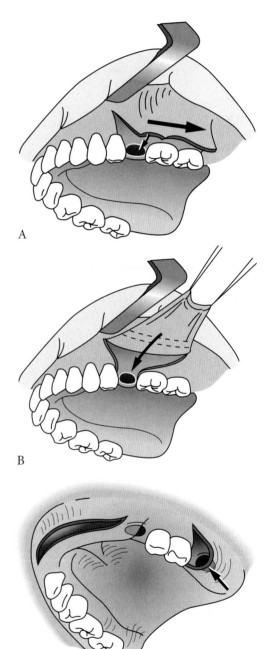

FIGURE **38-6** *Buccal advancement flaps can be used to cover an oroantral fistula.* A, *A Moczair buccal sliding trapezoidal flap is slid* (arrow) *to use the papilla of the adjacent tooth to rotate into the defect.* B, *Rehrman's buccal advancement flap uses a flap that has vertical extensions. To adequately mobilize this flap to cover the defect without tension, the periosteum must be incised* (broken line) *along its base and the flap advanced* (arrow) *over the defect.* C, *If the fistula is present along an edentulous region, a transverse flap or bipedicle flap can be used.*

Transposition Flaps These flaps are rotated and advanced over adjacent skin to close a defect. Examples of transposition flaps include rhombic flaps and bilobed flaps. These flaps are advantageous in areas where it is desired to transfer the tension away from closure of the primary defect and into the repair of the secondary defect. Transposition flaps have a straight linear axis and are usually designed so that one border of the flap is also a border of the defect. An advantage of this type of flap is that it can be developed at variable distances. Areas where these flaps are often used include the nasal tip and ala, the inferior eyelid, and the lips.

The rhombic flap is a precise geometric flap that is useful for many defects of the face.[20,21] The traditional rhombic ("Limberg") flap is designed with 60 and 120° angles and equal-length sides. The angle of the leading edge of the rhombic flap is approximately 120° but may vary. The flap is begun by extending an incision along the short axis of the defect that is equal to the length of one side of the rhombic defect. Another incision is then made at 60° to the first and of equal length (Figure 38-9). Disadvantages of the rhombic flap are the significant tension at the closure point as well as the amount of discarded tissue to transform a circular defect into a rhombus.

The bilobed flap is a transposition flap with two circular skin paddles (see Figure 38-4).[22,23] Esser is credited with the design of the bilobed flap in 1918. It

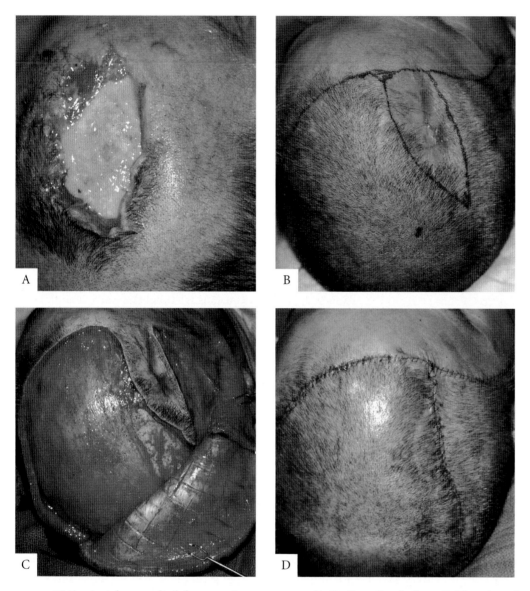

FIGURE 38-7   A, *A large scalp defect secondary to trauma.* B, *Outline of scalp flaps.* C, *Elevation of flaps with scoring of the galea.* D, *Closure of the defect.*

spontaneously.[18,19] Local flaps or grafts can be used to close larger fistulas. Two-layer closures are less prone to developing recurrence of oroantral fistulas. Approximately 75% of the palatal soft tissue can be rotated to cover adjacent defects.

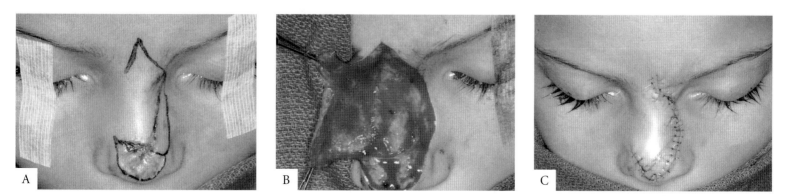

FIGURE 38-8   A, *Axial frontonasal flap for repair of a nasal defect.* B, *Elevation of the flap with thorough undermining.* C, *Closure of the defect*

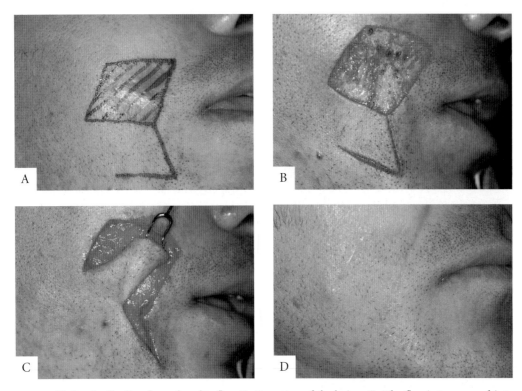

FIGURE 38-9   A, *Outline for a rhombic flap.* B, *Resection of the lesion.* C, *The flap is transposed into the defect.* D, *Postoperative result with the incisions placed in the relaxed skin tension lines.*

is useful for skin repairing of lateral nose and nasal tip defects up to 1.5 cm. The bilobed flap has a random pattern blood supply. The flap is primarily rotated around a pivot point and the paddles are transposed over an incomplete bridge of skin. The second lobe allows the transfer of tension further from the primary defect closure. The bilobed design rotates around an arc that is usually 90 to 100°. In the bilobed flap the first lobe closes the defect and the second closes the first lobe defect. The flap is designed with a pivot point approximately a radius of the defect away from the wound margin. The first lobe is usually the same size as the defect, and the second lobe is slightly smaller with a triangular apex to allow for primary closure. The axis of the second flap is roughly 90 to 100° from the primary defect and undermined widely to distribute the tension.

An advantage of the bilobed flap is that one can construct a flap at some distance from the defect with an axis that is independent of the linear axis of the

defect. A disadvantage of this flap is that it leaves a circular scar that does not blend with the existing skin creases. During healing the flap may become elevated ("pin cushioning") because of the narrow pedicle that is prone to congestion, scar tissue that impedes lymphatic drainage, and curvilinear scars that tend to bunch the flap up as they shorten.

Interpolation Flaps   Interpolation flaps contain a pedicle that must pass over or under intact intervening tissue. A disadvantage of these types of flaps is that for those passing over bridging skin, the pedicle must be detached during a second surgical procedure. Occasionally it is possible to perform a single-stage procedure by de-epithelializing the pedicle and passing it under the intervening skin. Advantages of interpolation flaps include their excellent vascularity, and also their skin color and texture match.

The forehead flap (median and para-median) is a commonly used interpolation flap and remains the workhorse flap for

large nasal defects.[24–27] It is a robust and dependable flap. The forehead flap is primarily based on the supratrochlear vessel, is relatively narrow, and uses a skin paddle from the forehead region. The flap is supplied by a rich anastomosis between the supratrochlear and angular arteries. Because of the marked vascularity, it is possible to incorporate cartilage or tissue grafts for nasal reconstruction. The forehead flap has abundant tissue available, allowing resurfacing of the entire nasal unit with a single flap and provides a good texture and color match to the native nose.

The technique for elevating the forehead flap is straightforward. The flap can be designed directly in the midline or in a paramidline location. A template of the defect is used to outline the flap. Elevation of the flap proceeds in either a subgaleal or subcutaneous plane. The pedicle is always elevated in such a way as to incorporate the frontalis muscle. The width of the pedicle is usually 1.0 to 1.5 cm, which allows for easy rotation of the pedicle. Prior to inset the skin paddle is selectively thinned to match the native skin thickness. The pedicle is divided approximately 3 weeks later, with the base of the pedicle inset into the glabellar area to reestablish brow symmetry. The incision, and resulting scar, is perpendicular to the RSTLs but tends to heal well (Figure 38-10).

The nasolabial flap (melolabial) is useful for reconstructing defects involving the oral cavity and those involving the lower third of the nose (Figure 38-11).[28–31] It can be used as an interpolation flap with either a single or staged technique. The flap is supplied by the angular artery, intraorbital artery, and infratrochlear artery and can be based either superiorly or inferiorly. The area of recruitment for nasal reconstruction is in closer proximity to the primary defect than is the forehead flap. A disadvantage of the nasolabial flap is that there is a limited amount of tissue available, and asymmetry can occur along the

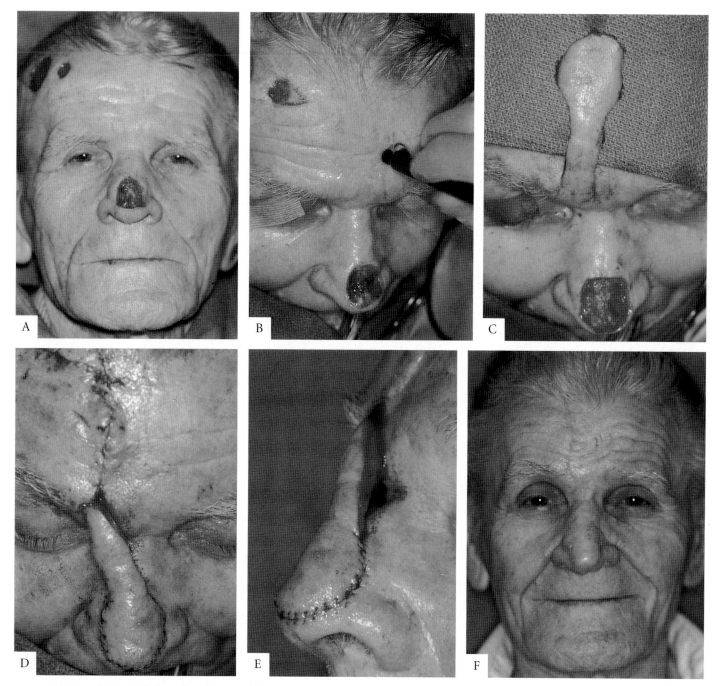

FIGURE **38-10** A, *Nasal defect after excision of squamous cell carcinoma lesion.* B, *Use of Doppler ultrasonography to locate the supratrochlear artery.* C, *The forehead flap has been elevated.* D, *The flap is turned 180° and sutured into place.* E, *The pedicle is divided 2 to 3 weeks later.* F, *Postoperative result*

nasolabial flap folds. When the pedicle is divided, the defect can be closed primarily by placing the scar in the nasal facial junction and the nasolabial flap fold.

The lip-switch flap (Abbe) can be taken from either lip, but it is most commonly switched from the lower to the upper lip.[32–34] This flap can be used to reconstruct as much as one-third of the upper lip. The lower lip can supply a flap of one-quarter of its length, and the Abbe flap offers immediate replacement of total lip anatomy (Figure 38-12). The labial artery supplies the flap and should be maintained with a small cuff of subcutaneous tissue and muscle surrounding the vascular pedicle. The pedicle is divided after approximately 2 to 3 weeks.

Tongue flaps are excellent flaps for intraoral reconstruction. They use adjacent tissue, have an excellent blood supply, and are associated with minimal morbidity. The tongue has excellent axial and collateral circulation, with the lingual artery providing the main blood supply. Up to one-half of the tongue can be rotated for tissue coverage without compromising speech,

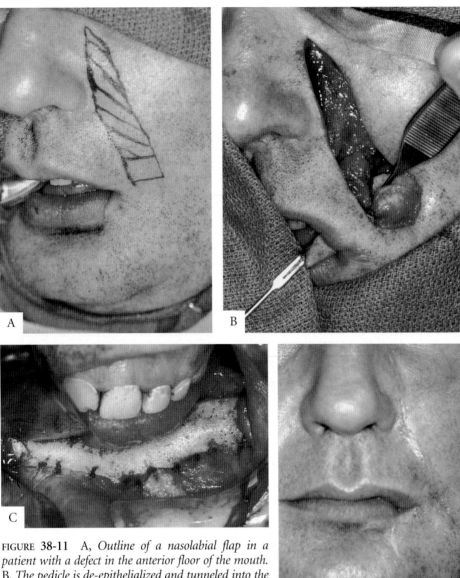

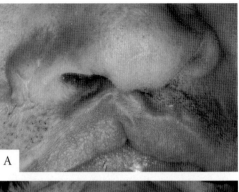

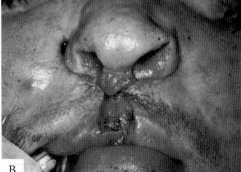

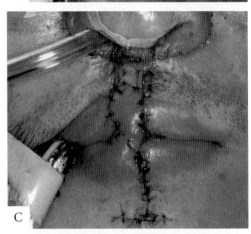

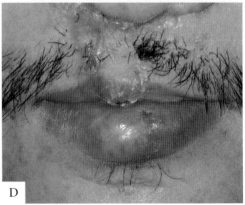

FIGURE 38-11 A, *Outline of a nasolabial flap in a patient with a defect in the anterior floor of the mouth. B, The pedicle is de-epithelialized and tunneled into the mouth. C, The flap is sutured into place to restore the missing soft tissue. D, The incision has been hidden in the nasolabial fold.*

mastication, or deglutition.[35] A variety of flap designs have been described including anterior- and posterior-based tongue flaps (Figure 38-13). Some indications include repair of oral defects and fistula closure. These flaps are helpful for providing closure of large oroantral fistulas.

Regional Flaps

For large facial defects, local flaps may not provide sufficient tissue to adequately restore the missing tissue. In these cases consideration should be given to using a regional flap.[36,37] Regional flaps are defined as those that are located near a defect but are not in the immediate proximity. They are frequently harvested from the neck, chest, or axilla and can provide coverage of large surface areas on the face. Selection of a specific regional flap depends on the size and location of the defect and also on the intrinsic properties of the flap. Advantages of regional flaps include the large amount of soft tissue and skin available. Disadvantages of these types of flaps include poor color and texture match, excessive bulkiness of the flap, and donor site morbidity.

FIGURE 38-12 A, *Patient with a traumatic lip deformity with avulsion of a portion of his upper lip. B, Reapproximation of the orbicularis oris muscles and perialar advancement flaps to reestablish upper lip length. C, An Abbe flap is used to restore the missing philtrum. D, Postoperative result.*

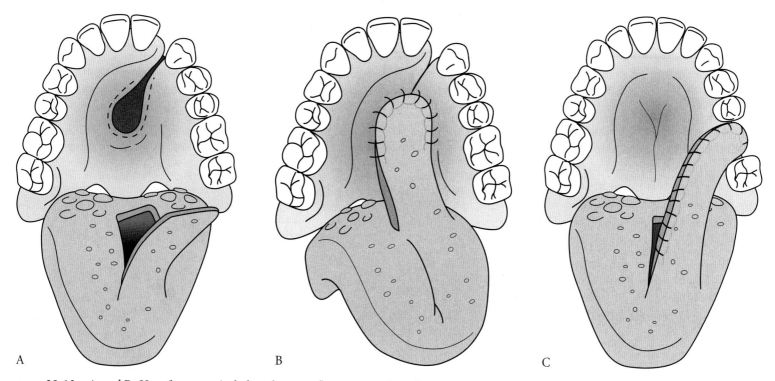

FIGURE **38-13**   A *and B, Use of an anteriorly based tongue flap to cover the soft tissue deficit resulting from an alveolar cleft. C, This type of flap is also useful for closing large oroantral fistulas..*

Pectoralis Major Myocutaneous Flap

The pectoralis major myocutaneous flap remains a workhorse of reconstructive surgery.[38–40] The flap was introduced by Ariyan[41] and has provided a reliable method of soft tissue reconstruction of bone and soft tissue defects of the mandible and maxilla. The pectoralis major myocutaneous flap can be rotated around a pivot point 180° and is supplied by two separate blood supplies (Figure 38-14). The thoracoacromial artery arises from the second portion of the axillary artery and forms four branches as it penetrates the fascia. The pectoral branch is the major artery that supplies the pectoralis major myocutaneous flap. The position of the vascular pedicle can be approximated by drawing a line from the shoulder point to the xiphoid. The pectoral branch descends at a right angle from the middle of the clavicle until it meets this line. Branches of the internal mammary artery supply the medial portion of the muscle and skin over the sternum. The flap provides good coverage

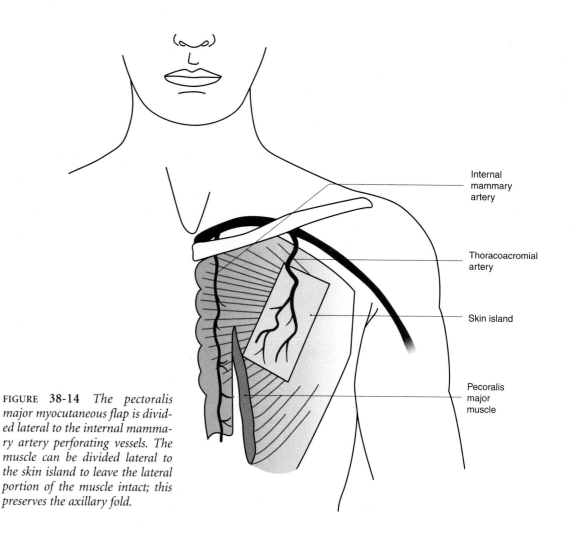

FIGURE **38-14** *The pectoralis major myocutaneous flap is divided lateral to the internal mammary artery perforating vessels. The muscle can be divided lateral to the skin island to leave the lateral portion of the muscle intact; this preserves the axillary fold.*

Internal mammary artery

Thoracoacromial artery

Skin island

Pecoralis major muscle

for the carotid artery when combined with a neck dissection.

Deltopectoral Flap The introduction of the deltopectoral flap by Bakamjian and colleagues represented a significant improvement for reconstructing large ablative resections for head and neck cancer.[42–44] Currently it is used as an alternative to the pectoralis major myocutaneous flap for soft tissue reconstruction of the mandible and maxilla. This flap is composed of fascia, subcutaneous tissue, and skin but does not contain muscle (Figure 38-15). Perforators from the internal mammary artery provide vascular supply to the flap. The secondary defect is covered with a skin graft.

Temporalis Flap The temporalis flap was introduced by Golovine in 1898 and remains useful for covering intraoral defects (Figure 38-16).[45–48] The outer portion of the muscle is invested by the deep temporal fascia. This fascia is supplied by the middle temporal vessel, which originates just below the zygomatic arch. The temporalis muscle is supplied by both the anterior and posterior deep temporal arteries, which arise from the second portion of

the internal maxillary artery. This dual blood supply allows for splitting of the muscle into anterior and posterior flaps.

When elevating the muscle, it is important to remain on the deep temporal fascia beneath the superficial temporal fascia to avoid damage to the frontal branch of the facial nerve. Elevation of

the inferior portion of the flap is performed in a subperiosteal plane to avoid damage to the deep temporal arteries, which lie on the undersurface of the muscle. An osteotomy of the zygomatic arch is often helpful to facilitate placement of the muscle into the mouth. The arch can be put back into place and secured with

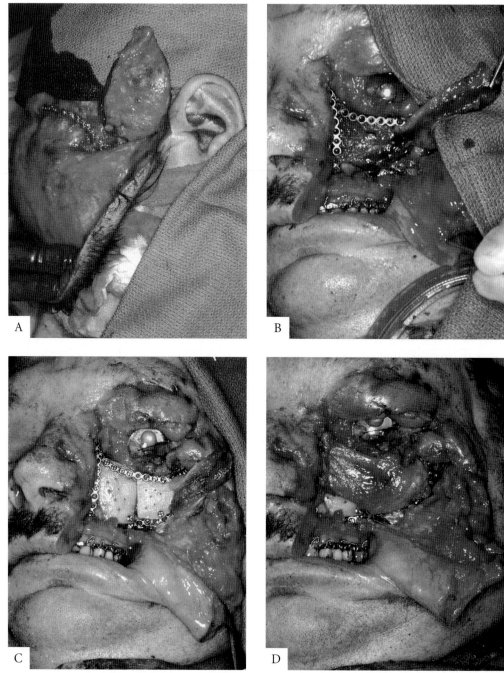

FIGURE 38-16 *A, Temporalis muscle flap for repair of a midface defect caused from a shotgun wound. B, The temporalis muscle is divided, and the posterior portion is sutured into place. C, Cranial bone is used to restore the missing tissue. D, The anterior portion of the temporalis flap is sutured into place to "sandwich" the bone grafts.*

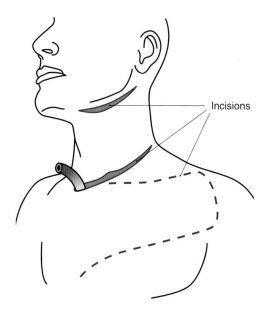

FIGURE 38-15 *Incisions for a deltopectoral flap.*

enters the muscle below the mastoid tip and supplies the superior portion of the muscle. The superior thyroid artery supplies the middle portion, and the thyrocervical trunk supplies the inferior third of the muscle.

The muscle is elevated over the deep cervical fascia superior to the carotid sheath. It is recommended to maintain two of the three vessels when elevating the flap to enhance the viability of the flap. The spinal accessory nerve enters the deep portion of the muscle approximately at the carotid bifurcation and should be preserved to prevent denervation atrophy of the muscle (Figure 38-17). Advantages of the sternocleidomastoid flap include its close proximity to the defect and minimal donor site defect (Figures 38-18 and 38-19).

Trapezius Myocutaneous Flap The trapezius myocutaneous flap is supplied by three arteries, allowing several flaps to be used. The main vessel supplying the trapezius muscle is the transverse cervical artery, which is a branch of the thyrocervical trunk. The upper portion of the muscle is supplied by the occipital artery. The trapezius myocutaneous flap is a ready source of skin of uniform thickness without excessive

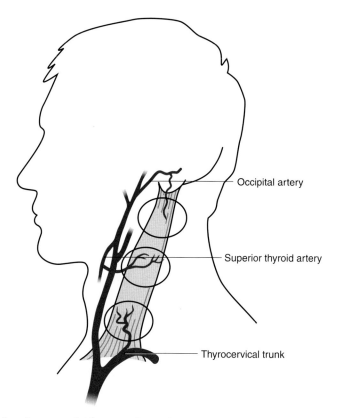

FIGURE **38-17** *Blood to the sternocleidomastoid muscle is supplied through three arteries.*

- Occipital artery
- Superior thyroid artery
- Thyrocervical trunk

plates and screws. A disadvantage of the temporalis flap is the minimal cosmetic deformity of hollowing in the temporal region; this can be corrected with autogenous or alloplastic materials and can be minimized by using either an anterior or a posterior flap.

Sternocleidomastoid Flap First described by Jinau in 1909 for facial reanimation, the sternocleidomastoid flap was repopularized by Owens.[49–55] The muscle is invested by the deep cervical fascia and is supplied by three arteries. The dominant vessel is the occipital artery, which

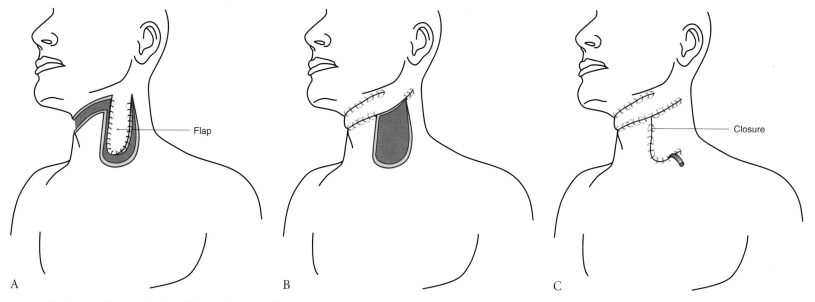

A | B | C

FIGURE **38-18** A, *Superiorly based flap with skin pedicle.* B, *Transposition of the flap.* C, *Closure of the donor defect.*

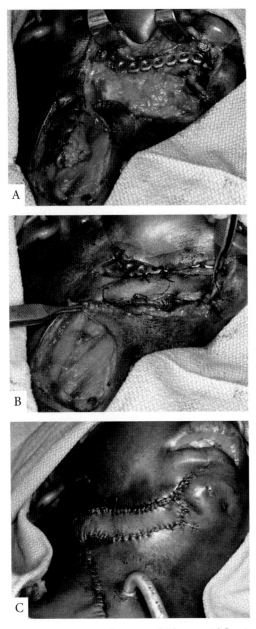

FIGURE 38-19   *A, The sternocleidomastoid flap is elevated with a superior base. B, The flap is rotated in place to provide soft-tissue coverage over the reconstruction plate. C, The flap is sutured into place and the donor site closed primarily.*

muscle bulk.[56] The main disadvantage is the limited rotation and the short pedicle.

Latissimus Dorsi Myocutaneous Flap
Quillen and colleagues first described the use of the latissimus dorsi myocutaneous flap for head and neck reconstruction in 1978.[57,58] The flap is not commonly used for head and neck reconstruction unless other flaps are unavailable or there are very large defects requiring coverage. The muscle is supplied by the thoracodorsal artery, which is the dominant vessel, and also by four to six perforators from the posterior intercostals and lumbar vessels. The main advantage of the latissimus dorsi flap is the large amount of skin provided. The main disadvantages are the need to reposition the patient during the operation and morbidity from the donor site.

Complications

Postoperative complications can be minimized with careful preoperative planning of flap design and by early recognition of problems.[59] A medical history can be used to identify patients with risk factors involving small vessels. These risk factors include smoking, diabetes, hypertension, previous radiation, and preexisting scars.[60,61] Complications may be reversible or irreversible. Early recognition and treatment can minimize complications and prevent them from becoming irreversible. Two main unwanted outcomes are flap failure and unacceptable cosmetic results.

Flap survival depends on early recognition of flap compromise. Ischemia is defined as an inadequacy of perfusion in providing tissue needs. Signs of arterial ischemia include a pale and cool flap that does not blanch with pressure and typically does not bleed with a pinprick. Flaps are somewhat ischemic initially because the original tissue perfusion has been compromised by flap elevation. Most tissue can survive on 10% of its average blood flow.[59] Whether the flap will undergo necrosis depends on patient-related and surgery-related factors that influence the risk of necrosis in facial flaps. Smoking is associated with an increased risk of flap failure. The deleterious effects of smoking on flap survival include hypoxemia and vasoconstriction. Patients should be advised to quit smoking during the perioperative period.

Common causes of bleeding in facial reconstruction with local flaps include inadequate hemostasis and drug-induced coagulopathy. Hematoma formation should be identified and decompressed within 24 hours.[62] Decompression can be accomplished with aspiration using a 22-gauge needle or by taking out one or two sutures and applying gentle compression on the flap. Hematoma formation may diminish tissue perfusion and can lead to ischemia or necrosis by inducing vasospasm, stretching the subdermal plexus, or separating the flap from its recipient bed. Patients should be questioned carefully about the use of medications that affect coagulation such as acetylsalicylic acid, nonsteroidal anti-inflammatory drugs, and vitamin E. If possible, these medications should be avoided for 2 weeks prior to and 1 week after surgery.

Congestion is the most common vascular problem associated with facial flaps. Signs of a congested flap include warmth, edema, and a purple color that blanches with pressure then immediately refills. A pinprick will cause release of dark venous blood. Venous congestion can lead to arterial compromise and flap necrosis. Management of congested flaps may include temporarily releasing sutures to allow decompression at the flap edges or possible impingement involving the flap pedicle. Tight bandages around the flap pedicle should be removed. Medicinal leeches (*Hirudo medicinalis*) may be useful in decompressing congested flaps.[63,64] Saliva from the leech contains an anticoagulant and a vasodilator that facilitate continued oozing from the site even up to 6 hours after they detach.

Hyperbaric oxygen (HBO) has been shown to be beneficial in improving the vascularity of marginal tissues.[65] Prophylactic HBO therapy in cutaneous flap surgery in the irradiated tissue bed may be particularly helpful to combat the hypoxia and hypocellularity. HBO is beneficial in treating both venous congestion and arterial ischemia by creating a local arterial vasoconstriction through the rise in arterial oxygen content, which reduces the amount of inflow. The tissue oxygen levels continue to rise owing to the improved diffusion even though there is vasoconstriction and a reduction in vascular perfusion. The flap can maintain viability while continued neovascularization occurs. Other options include the use of heparin and dipyridamole to help increase the survival of an ischemic flap.[66]

Infection can complicate flap healing.[67] The postoperative infection rate for clean wounds in facial surgery is as low as 2.8%, with higher rates in facial reconstruction with local flaps.[68] Tissue oxygenation is an important factor in prevention of wound infection and is closely related to blood supply. Infections involving local flaps may result in flap failure or poor cosmetic outcome secondary to wound dehiscence and scarring.

Conclusion

A variety of facial flaps are available to the reconstructive surgeon for repairing facial defects. The goal of flap surgery is to restore form, function, and esthetics. There are many advantages to using local and regional flaps, which can lead to optimal esthetic results.

References

1. Schliephake H, Furrert K, Schneller T. Prospective study of the quality of life of cancer patients after intraoral tumor surgery. J Oral Maxillofac Surg 1996;54:664–9.
2. Kruger E. Reconstruction of bone and soft tissue in extensive facial defects. J Oral Maxillofac Surg 1982;40:714–20.
3. Summers BK, Siegle RJ. Facial cutaneous reconstructive surgery: general aesthetic principles. J Am Acad Dermatol 1993;29:669–81.
4. Baker SR. Resurfacing flaps in reconstructive rhinoplasty. Aesthetic Plast Surg 2002;26:17-23.
5. Baker SR. Local cutaneous flaps. Otolaryngol Clin North Am 1994;27:139–59.
6. Baker SR. Regional flaps in facial reconstruction. Otolaryngol Clin North Am 1990;23:925–46.
7. Escobar V, Zide MF. Delayed repair of skin cancer defects. J Oral Maxillofac Surg 1999;57:271–9.
8. Ducic Y, Herford AS. The use of palatal island flaps as an adjunct to microvascular free tissue transfer for reconstruction of complex oromandibular defects. Laryngoscope 2001;111:1666–9.
9. Milton S. Pedicled skin-flaps: the fallacy of the length:width ratio. Br J Surg 1970;57:502-8.
10. Schliephake H, Schmelzeisen R, Neukam FW. Long-term results of blood flow and cutaneous sensibility of flaps used for the reconstruction of facial soft tissues. J Oral Maxillofac Surg 1994;52:1247–52.
11. Gonzalez-Ulloa M. Restoration of the face covering by means of selected skin in regional aesthetic units. Br J Plast Surg 1956;9:212–21.
12. Burget GC, Menick FJ. The subunit principle in nasal reconstruction. Plast Reconstr Surg 1985;76:239–47.
13. Rieger RA. A local flap for repair of the nasal tip. Plast Reconstr Surg 1967;40:147–9.
14. Marchac D, Toth B. The axial frontonasal flap revisited. Plast Reconstr Surg 1985;76:686–94.
15. Haneke E. Surgical treatment of defects on the tip of the nose. Dermatol Surg 1998;24:711–7.
16. Herford AS, Zide MF. Reconstruction of superficial skin cancer defects of the nose. J Oral Maxillofac Surg 2001;59:760–7.
17. Millard DR. The island flap in cleft palate surgery. Surg Gynecol Obstet 1963;116:197–8.
18. Liposky RB. Immediate repair of the oroantral communication: a preventative dental procedure. J Am Dent Assoc 1981;103:727-9
19. Yih WY, Merrill RG, Howerton DW. Secondary closure of oroantral and oronasal fistulas: a modification of existing techniques. J Oral Maxillofac Surg 1988;46: 357–64.
20. Limberg AA. Planimetrie und Stereometrie der Hautplastik. Jena, Germany: Fischer Verlag; 1967.
21. Borges AF. Choosing the correct Limberg flap. Plast Reconstr Surg 1978;62:542–5.
22. Zitelli JA. The bilobed flap for nasal reconstruction. Arch Dermatol 1989;125:957–9.
23. Iida N, Ohsumi N, Tonegawa M, et al. Simple method of designing a bilobed flap. Plast Reconstr Surg 1999;104:495–9.
24. Shumrick KA, Smith TL. The anatomic basis for the design of forehead flaps in nasal reconstruction. Arch Otolaryngol Head Neck Surg 1992;118:373–9.
25. Burget GC, Medick FJ, editors. The paramedian forehead flap. In: Aesthetic reconstruction of the nose. St. Louis: Mosby; 1994. p. 57–92.
26. Burget GC. Aesthetic restoration of the nose. Clin Plast Surg 1985;12:463–80.
27. McCarthy JG, Lorenc ZP, Cutting C, et al. The median forehead flap revisited: the blood supply. Plast Reconstr Surg 1985;76:866–9.
28. Ducic Y, Burye M. Nasolabial flap reconstruction of oral cavity defects: a report of 18 cases. J Oral Maxillofac Surg 2000;59:1104–8.
29. Kakinuma H, Iwasawa U, Honjoh M, Koura T. A composite nasolabial flap for an entire ala reconstruction. Dermatol Surg 2002;28:237–40.
30. Maurer P, Eckert AW, Schubert J. Functional rehabilitation following resection of the floor of the mouth: the nasolabial flap revisited. J Craniomaxillofac Surg 2002;30:369–72.
31. Lazaridis N, Zouloumis L, Venetis G, et al. The inferiorly and superiorly based nasolabial flap for reconstruction of moderate-sized oronasal defects. J Oral Maxillofac Surg 1998;56:1255–9.
32. Zide MF, Fuselier C. The partial-thickness cross-lip flap for correction of postoncologic surgical defects. J Oral Maxillofac Surg 2001;59:760–7.
33. Yih WY, Howerton DW. A regional approach to reconstruction of the upper lip. J Oral Maxillofac Surg 1997;55:383–9.
34. Schulte DL, Sherris DA, Kasperbaurer JL. The anatomical basis of the Abbe flap. Laryngoscope 2001;111:382–6.
35. Massengill R, Pickrell K, Mladick R. Lingual flaps: effect on speech articulation and physiology. Ann Otol Rhinol Laryngol 1970;l79:853–7.
36. Motamedi MH, Behnia H. Experience with regional flaps in the comprehensive treatment of maxillofacial soft-tissue injuries in war victims. J Craniomaxillofac Surg 1999;27:256–65.
37. Blackwell KE, Buchbinder D, Biller HF, Urken ML. Reconstruction of massive defects in the head and neck: the role of simultaneous distant and regional flaps. Head Neck 1997;19:620–8.
38. Ariyan S. The pectoralis major myocutaneous flap. A versatile flap for reconstruction in the head and neck. Plast Reconstr Surg 1979;63:73-81.
39. Ariyan S. Further experiences with the pectoralis major myocutaneous flap for the immediate repair of defects from excisions of head and neck cancers. Plast Reconstr Surg 1979;65:605-12.
40. Marx RE, Smith BR. An improved technique for development of the pectoralis major myocutaneous flap. J Oral Maxillofac Surg 1990;48:1168–80.
41. Ariyan S. Pectoralis major, sternomastoid, and other musculocutaneous flaps for head and neck reconstruction. Clin Plast Surg 1980;7(1): 89-109.

42. Bakamjian VY. Total reconstruction of phyarynx with medially based deltopectoral skin flap. NY State J Med 1968;68:2771–8.

43. Sasaki K, Nozaki M, Honda T, et al. Deltopectoral skin flap as a free skin flap revisited: further refinement in flap design, fabrication and clinical usage. Plast Reconstr Surg 2001;107:1134–41.

44. Lazaridis N, Tilaverdis I, Dalambiras S, et al. The fasciocutaneous cervicopectoral rotation flap for lower cheek reconstruction: report of three cases. J Oral Maxillofac Surg 1997;55:1166–71.

45. Golovine SS. Procede de cloture plastique de l'orbite après l'exenteration. Arch Ophthal 1898;18:679.

46. Alonso del Hoyo J, Fernandez Sanroman J, Gil-Diez JL, et al. The temporalis muscle flap: an evaluation and review of 38 cases. J Oral Maxillofac Surg 1994;52:143–7.

47. Burggasser G, Happak W, Gruber H, Freilinger G. The temporalis: blood supply and innervation. Plast Reconstr Surg 2002;109:1862–9.

48. Abubaker AO, Abouzgia MB. The temporalis muscle flap in reconstruction of intraoral defects: an appraisal of the technique. Oral Surg Oral Med Oral Pathol Oral Radiol Endod 2002;94:24–30.

49. Jinau A. Die Chirurgishe behanolung der facialislachmung. Dtsch ZF Chin 1909; 102:377–81.

50. Owens NA. A compound neck pedicle designed for the repair of massive facial defects. Plast Reconstr Surg 1955;15:369–89.

51. Zhao YF, Zhang WF, Ahao JH. Reconstruction of intraoral defects after cancer surgery using cervical pedicle flaps. J Oral Maxillofac Surg 2001;59:1142–6.

52. Ariyan S. Further experience with the sternocleidomastoid myocutaneous flap. Plast Reconstr Surg 2003;111:381–2.

53. Kerawala CJ, McAloney N, Stassen LF. Prospective randomized trial of the benefits of a sternocleidomastoid flap after superficial parotidectomy. Br J Oral Maxillofac Surg 2002;40:468–72.

54. Kierner AC, Zelenka I, Gstoettner W. The sternocleidomastoid flap—its indications and limitations. Laryngoscope 2001;111:2201–4.

55. Marx RE, McDonald DK. The sternocleidomastoid muscle as a muscular or myocutaneous flap for oral and facial reconstruction. J Oral Maxillofac Surg 1985; 43:155–62.

56. Papadopoulos O, Tsakoniatis N, Georgiou P, Christopoulos A. Head and neck soft-tissue reconstruction using the vertical trapezius musculocutaneous flap. Ann Plast Surg 1999;42:457–8.

57. Quillen CG, Shearing JG, Georgiade NG. Use of the latissimus dorsi myocutaneous island flap for reconstruction in the head and neck area. Plast Reconstr Surg 1978;62:113–7.

58. Posnick JC, McCraw JB, Magee W Jr. Use of a latissimus dorsi myocutaneous flap for closure of an orocutaneous fistula of the cheek. J Oral Maxillofac Surg 1988;46:224–8.

59. Vural E, Key JM. Complications, salvage, and enhancement of local flaps in facial reconstruction. Otolaryngol Clin North Am 2001;34:39–51.

60. Goldminz D, Bennett RG. Cigarette smoking and flap and full-thickness graft necrosis. Arch Dermatol 1991;127:1012–5.

61. Kinsella JB, Rassekh CH, Wassmuth ZD, et al. Smoking increases facial skin flap complications. Ann Otol Rhinol Laryngol 1999; 108:139–42.

62. Mulliken JB, Healey NA. Pathogenesis of skin flap necrosis from an underlying hematoma. Plast Reconstr Surg 1979;63:540–5.

63. Utley DS, Koch RJ, Goode RL. The failing flap in facial plastic and reconstructive surgery: role of the medicinal leech. Laryngoscope 1998;108:1129–35.

64. Dabb RW, Malone JM, Leverett LC. The use of medicinal leeches in the salvage of flaps with venous congestion. Ann Plast Surg 1992;29:250–6.

65. Zamboni WA, Roth AC, Russell RC, et al. The effect of hyperbaric oxygen on reperfusion of ischemic axial skin flaps: a laser Doppler analysis. Ann Plast Surg 1992;28:339–41.

66. Kerrigan CL, Daniel RK. Pharmacologic treatment of the failing skin. Plast Reconstr Surg 1982;70:541–8.

67. Bumpous JM, Johnson JT. The infected wound and its management. Otolaryngol Clin North Am 1995;28:987–1001.

68. Sylaidis P, Wood S, Murray DS. Postoperative infection following clean facial surgery. Ann Plast Surg 1997;39:342–6.

CHAPTER 39

Bony Reconstruction of the Jaws

Randall M. Wilk, DDS, PhD, MD

Overview and Goals

Bony reconstruction of the jaws represents one of the most daunting tasks presenting to the oral and maxillofacial surgeon. The demands of reconstruction of the mandible and maxilla represent challenges for the following reasons. The requirements for success follow a strict criterion for occlusion of the dentition and oral rehabilitation. Minor malpositionings result in occlusal problems that are both perceptible to the patient and provide a formidable task to the restorative dentist. Major malpositions may make oral rehabilitation near impossible. The functional loads to be carried on the bone can challenge both hardware and the reconstituted mandible and maxilla. The environment of the oral cavity can be hostile for adequate healing and regeneration. Indigenous flora of the oral cavity is one of the most diverse in the human body, and the bacterial load can be considerable. When pathogenic flora is present, as is not uncommon in the compromised host, healing can be further challenging. The bones themselves represent complex morphologies, curved shapes, and complex relationships with adjacent structures. Reproducing these parameters adds to the complexity of the task. The jaws by virtue of their prominent placement on the exposed face impart considerable esthetic requirements. Unlike other parts of the body, which are hidden by clothing, the face is rarely concealed.

The goals of reconstruction under the aforementioned conditions are to provide morphology and position of the bone in relation to its opposing jaw, provide adequate height and width of bone, restore continuity of the mandible and maxilla, and provide facial contour and support for soft tissue structures. While these concepts may seem straightforward, surgeons have struggled for centuries to achieve them and success is often elusive. Various success rates have been described for bony reconstruction of the jaws, but criteria have usually been incomplete and rates uninspiring.

The factors leading to the lack of adequate bone development or loss of bone in the first place have a role in the types and methods used to begin a reconstruction. Ablative loss of both bone and associated soft tissue from treatment of neoplastic or other pathologic processes represent a far different task from loss of bone from trauma or infection. Other modulating factors include the presence of systemic diseases, exposure to therapeutic doses of ionizing radiation, or failure of development of normal bony structures. Success rates in irradiated jaws are typically lower by significant amounts, and rates of complications have been reported as high as 81.3%.[1] Complete graft loss in 30% of irradiated patients undergoing bone grafting to the jaws and an additional 50% of patients experiencing partial graft loss after reconstructive procedures have been reported.[2] Use of hyperbaric oxygen therapy and microvascular reconstruction has improved these rates.[3,4]

Bony reconstruction begins with assessing the bone to be reconstructed. The location, size, and relationship to the other structures are the prime factors in planning a reconstruction. A large defect of the angle region is managed differently than a small defect in the same region. A defect in the alveolus of the maxilla is managed differently than a similar-size defect in the hard palate. Defects in areas that are opposed by natural dentition are managed differently that those that are in areas that have little functional consequence.

Anatomic Considerations in Reconstruction of the Jaws

Anatomically the mandible can be divided into four broad regions (Figure 39-1) with somewhat indistinct boundaries: condylar portion, ramus, body, and alveolus. Several subsets or overlapping areas have been described. The coronoid region can be considered as part of the ramus, the angle region encompasses both part of the ramus and body, and the symphysis is the anterior part of the body. Each of the areas presents unique characteristics, and the decision to reconstruct or repair certain areas is dependent on the goals to be achieved.

The condylar region is critical to the masticatory functions of the jaws and overall movements of the mandible. In the

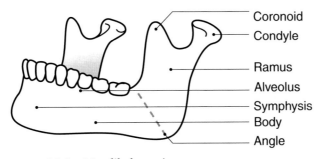

FIGURE 39-1 *Mandibular regions.*

young and growing patient there are implications for growth of the jaw. The relationship of this area with the temporal bone and the interarticular disk is beyond the scope of this chapter. Anatomic features of the condylar region are the muscular attachments and morphologic support of facial height. The lateral pterygoid muscle attaches to the condylar region and provides for translatory movement of the mandible and its excursive movements. When reconstructing large or entire portions of the condyle with grafts, failure of reattachment of the lateral pterygoid muscles will result in impairment or loss of these functions. The condylar region contributes to the posterior vertical height of the mandible. Loss of the condylar region or insufficient reconstruction results in reduced height with resulting malocclusion and esthetic contour deficiencies. Not only does the reconstructed condyle need to have adequate bulk and form, but it also needs to be placed in appropriate relationship to the temporomandibular joint fossa.

The ramus area participates in masticatory function as the site of attachment of the major muscles of mastication. The masseter, medial pterygoid, and temporalis muscles all attach here and provide the major input for developing bite force. These muscles also serve as a potent blood supply for the reconstructed bone and serve as an excellent recipient bed. The ramus region provides bulk, facial contour, and continuity between major segments of the mandible. Damage or loss of bone structure in this area can lead to decreased posterior mandibular height with resulting malocclusion, facial contour defects, and decreased masticatory function. The major sensory nerve of the mandible enters this area and is prone to injury during reconstructive efforts. The coronoid process is considered part of the ramus, and its loss can be considered to be trivial. There are no good reasons to reconstruct a coronoid process. As in other parts of the mandible, the relationship of the coronoid process to the surrounding bones is critical. Malpositioning of the coronoid process can impede opening of the jaw owing to interferences with the zygoma and zygomatic arch.

The body of the mandible is probably the most complex area of the mandible to reconstruct for several reasons. It has a complex curved shape that makes reconstruction difficult, it is along the lever of the mandible and has the highest loads placed on it, it contains a sensory nerve that is prone to injury, and it is the site of attachment of a complex array of muscles. The mylohyoid, geniohyoid, digastric, mentalis, buccinator, and tongue musculature all have attachment to this part of the bone. Their presence helps to serve as an excellent recipient bed, but the forces they exert on the bone present problems in reconstruction and maintaining the contour of the bone. In the anterior region the muscle attachments serve a vital function in maintaining airway patency through attachment of the tongue musculature and support of the hyoid complex. The body of the mandible supports the alveolus and tooth-bearing structures, and it has a critical relationship to the opposing jaw.

The alveolus of the mandible is the site of the functional component of the mandible, the dental occlusion. This portion of the mandible is dependent on the position of the mandibular body for its relationship to the maxillary arch. The alveoli need proper height and width to subserve the functions of the dentition. In the maxilla the alveolus is in relationship to the maxillary sinus and nasal cavity, and this relationship alters reconstructive efforts. In the anterior portion of the jaws this alveolar component is essential to maintaining position of the overlying soft tissue, especially the lips. Loss in this area or inadequate reconstruction can lead to both functional and esthetic deficiencies.

The maxilla, or upper jaw (Figure 39-2), is a complex bone comprising the bulk of the midface. It has relationships with the opposing mandible, the orbital complex, paranasal sinuses, zygoma, and nasal cavity. The palate forms the roof of the mouth and serves to partition the oral and nasal cavities. Incomplete reconstruction of the palate leads to hypernasal speech and regurgitation of the oral cavity contents, unless obturated. The paucity and quality of soft tissue surrounding this region makes bony reconstruction especially difficult. At the posterior aspect of the maxilla, a complex array of muscles attaches and subserves the functions of the

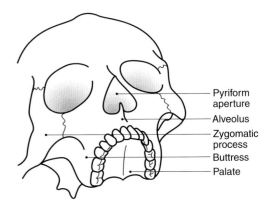

FIGURE 39-2 *Maxillary regions.*

soft palate. These attachments are involved not only in speech and swallowing but also in eustachian tube function. In the alveolar portion of the maxilla, the relationship to the maxillary sinus is an often-confounding factor in reconstruction. Highly pneumatized sinuses provide little support for grafting procedures. In the anterior region of the maxilla, support for nasal and orbital structures is required for maintaining nasal airway support and facial contour and esthetics for the nose.

Defects of the Mandible

Defects of the mandible can involve single subsets of the mandible, several segments, or the entire mandible. Marginal defects involve loss of the mandibular bone with the inferior and posterior portions left intact. In marginal defects the continuity of the mandible is intact, and reconstructive efforts are focused on maintaining bulk and contour. Segmental defects involve loss of mandibular bone and either the posterior or inferior border and confer a continuity defect of the mandible. Descriptions of the size of the defect are usually expressed in centimeters, measured at the inferior border. This measurement will serve as a guide in estimating the amount of bone necessary to reconstruct the defect. Segmental defects can cause a wide variety of reconstructive challenges, depending on their anatomic location. Small lateral continuity defects are surprisingly well tolerated, and following ablative procedures, it was not unusual to defer or omit reconstructive techniques. Segmental defects of the anterior mandible, however, are not well tolerated because of unfavorable anatomic and biomechanical features. Maintenance of tongue position and interramal width are severely compromised with large anterior segmental defects. The defects need to be interpreted not only in terms of their relationship to the rest of the mandible but also in relation to the opposing maxillary structures, both dental and nondental.

Identifying and categorizing defects of the mandible in terms of both size and extent represent the first step in bony reconstruction of the lower jaw.

Defects of the Maxilla

Defects of the maxilla can be divided into those that disrupt partitioning of cavities and those that represent inadequate bulk or position of bone in one of the subsets. Partitioning disruptions need to be evaluated in terms of both size and location. Small defects in the bone interfering with partitioning can be managed by soft tissue procedures only and may not necessarily need to undergo bony reconstruction. Larger defects in bone interfering with partitioning can be successfully obturated by maxillofacial prostheses and, similarly, may not need bony reconstruction. Many reconstructive options exist for these types of defects. The demands of occlusal restoration or stability of the upper jaw represent the majority of needs for bony reconstruction. Positioning of the upper jaw segments can be managed through orthognathic surgery, which is not the focus of this chapter. With defects in the alveolar portion of the jaws, evaluation of adequate bone in terms of height, width, and relationship to bone in the opposing mandible is the critical first step in reconstruction of the upper jaw.

Limitation of Bony Reconstruction

Bony reconstruction of the jaws depends largely on the amount of soft tissue available. Soft tissue coverage and recipient bed nourishment need to be addressed prior to any bony reconstruction. The soft tissue evaluation and management should precede any efforts at bony reconstruction. The limitations of bony reconstruction lie largely in the imagination and skills of the practitioner. Host limitations relate to the existing soft tissue envelope in terms of both bulk and blood supply and systemic factors in the patient. Identification of all

factors influencing outcome will be a critical step in determining choice of best methods for bony reconstruction.

Bone Biology

The hallmark of reconstruction of the jaws is the grafting of bone into sites of loss or need. Bone, unlike most other tissues of the body, heals not by formation of scar tissue but by regeneration of bone. Advances in the understanding of bone physiology, immunologic concepts, and technology have made successful reconstruction of the jaws possible and somewhat predictable. The success of jaw reconstruction today is several times what it was only three decades ago. Bone reconstruction on a physiologic level is accomplished by combinations of three processes: osteogenesis, osteoconduction, and osteoinduction. Osteogenesis is the formation of new bone from osteocompetent cells. Osteoconduction is the formation of new bone along a scaffold from the host's osteocompetent cells. Osteoinduction is the formation of new bone from the differentiation and stimulation of mesenchymal cells by the bone-inductive proteins.

The understanding of the basic biologic processes in bone has blossomed over the past thirty years. Key discoveries in the bioactive molecules began with the findings of Urist and Strates relating to the bone morphogenetic proteins (BMPs).[5,6] BMP is not a single protein but a family of proteins belonging to the transforming growth factor-β superfamily (TGF-β). At least 13 BMPs have been identified (BMP-1 does not belong to the TGF-β superfamily). The ones that are of clinical interest and are involved in human bone metabolism are BMP-2, BMP-4, and BMP-7 (also called osteogenic protein 1 [OP-1]).[7] As with most biologic systems, antagonists to these molecules exist for biologic regulation.[7–14] These antagonists called noggin, chordin, gremlin, dan, and cerberus are proteins that bind to BMPs and thus govern cartilage and skeletal morphogenesis.[15]

BMPs 2, 4, and 7 have effects on stem cells and osteoblast precursor cells to convert them to mineralizing osteoblasts. BMPs bind and initiate a cell signal through a transmembrane receptor complex and generate an intracellular response involving Smad proteins that promotes osteoblast differentiation. The Smad proteins function as inducible transcriptional activators associated with a component that binds deoxyribonucleic acid (DNA) when they enter the osteoblast nucleus. Research into the specific genes activated is an active area of work and definitive elucidation of the mechanisms is ongoing.

Bone Grafting Biology

Axhausen initially described the repair of bone and divided it into two phases.[16] The first phase consists of cellular proliferation and production of osteoid in a disorganized fashion. The second phase is characterized by resorption of the osteoid and replacement by more organized lamellar bone. During the first phase of bone regeneration the transplanted cells within the graft proliferate and form new osteoid over the course of a few weeks. The amount of bone regeneration is dependent on the amount of bone cells that survive the transplantation procedure. These cells' survival is integrally related to the nourishment from the recipient bed. For the first 3 to 5 days diffusion by plasmatic circulation is the source of nutrients; by day 5, capillary ingrowth from the surrounding soft tissue and bone edges penetrate the graft.[17]

Free grafts of bone can be either cancellous, cortical, or corticocancellous blocks (Table 39-1). Within a graft, cancellous bone revascularizes sooner than cor-

ticocancellous or cortical block grafts. Endosteal osteoblasts proliferate and form osteoid on the surface of cancellous bone trabeculae.[18] Those cells within the trabeculae may die as a result of their encasement in mineralized matrix and impaired diffusion through it. Osteocytes within their lacunae appear to survive if they are less than 0.3 mm from the surface.[19] In cortical grafts, revascularization is much slower because the process follows preexisting haversian systems from the periphery into the interior.[20] A histologic difference in cortical grafts is the initiation of osteoclastic rather than osteoblastic activity. The osteoclasts will enlarge the haversian systems peripherally, then centrally. The haversian systems of a cortical graft will undergo significant resorption before osteoblastic activity will fill in the resorbed areas. The process of osteoclastic resorption followed by osteoblastic deposition is termed "creeping substitution." New bone may be deposited throughout the graft, leaving areas of necrotic bone covered by viable bone. The necrotic bone areas may persist indefinitely.[20] The osteoid from the transplanted cells and from the endosteum fuse in a process called consolidation.

A second phase of bone growth follows the initial consolidation and begins at about 2 weeks. Fibroblasts and other mesenchymal cells differentiate into osteoclasts and begin a resorption of the osteoid. This differentiation of cells is accomplished by BMPs found in the transplanted bone. New bone is laid down in a more orderly fashion. The two-phase theory of bone healing applies to all types of autogenous grafts. In summary: (1) cancellous grafts are revascularized more rapidly than cortical grafts, (2) cancellous bone incorporates by an appositional phase followed by a resorptive phase but cortical grafts incorporate by a resorptive phase followed by an appositional phase, and (3) cancellous grafts tend to repair completely whereas cortical grafts remain a mixture of necrotic and viable bone.

Table 39-2   Bone Grafts
Autogenous grafts: free grafts, composite grafts
Homologous grafts (allografts)
Heterogeneous grafts (xenografts)

Bone grafts improve in their mechanical properties over time. Cancellous bone grafts tend to be strengthened over time with the addition of new bone. As the necrotic cores are replaced, the strength of the bone returns to normal. Cortical grafts have a different time course and actually undergo a weakening of the bone during the osteoclastic phase. Cortical grafts have been shown to be 40 to 50% weaker than normal bone from 6 weeks to 6 months following transplantation, a period in which the porosity of the graft increases approximately 15%.[21] After 1 to 2 years the mechanical strength becomes equal to normal bone.

Other sources of bone are available for grafting, but none has surpassed autogenous grafts (Table 39-2). Grafts can be either homologous grafts (Table 39-3) (allografts) or heterografts (xenografts). The ability to obtain grafted bone without donor site morbidity to the patient has been a longtime goal of reconstructive surgeons. Autogenous bone grafts have been shown to be superior to allogeneic bone, xenogeneic bone, bone substitutes, and alloplasts in terms of the function, form, and adaptability.[22] The superiority is due to the transfer of a greater number and density of osteocompetent cells.[23] Homologous grafts, also known as allografts or allogeneic grafts come from another person. Allogeneic grafts are genetically dissimilar and to avoid tissue rejection

Table 39-1   Free Autogenous Grafts
Cancellous
Cortical
Corticocancellous

Table 39-3   Allografts
Undemineralized
Partially demineralized
Totally demineralized

phenomena must be rendered nonantigenic. These grafts serve a purpose merely as a scaffold for reconstruction and do not transfer osteocompetent cells. Grafts of the mandible can be used in conjunction with an autogenous cancellous graft with the allogeneic bone used as a scaffolding with desired contour, size, and shape.[24] There are many methods for rendering an allograft less antigenic including boiling, deproteinizing, merthiolating, freezing, freeze-drying, irradiating, and dry heating. The most common method used is freeze-drying (lyophilization). The major source of antigenicity in allografts is the cellular elements of bone. Boiling, drying, or chemically treating the bone will kill the cells but has a deleterious effect on coagulation of organic elements, reducing or eliminating their inductive effects and making their removal by host cellular processes difficult.[25] Heat in excess of 80°C destroys the biologic properties of the bone matrix.[26]

Allograft materials have been used in several jaw reconstructive procedures, but their volume and lack of osteocompetent cells make their use limited.[27–30]

Alloplastic graft materials include hydroxylapatite crystals, bioactive glasses, calcium sulfate, beta tricalcium phosphate, and biphasic calcium phosphate.[31–33] Hydroxylapatites are the most commonly used alloplasts. Porous nonresorbable hydroxylapatite found in coral has been used but with only limited success. New bone can grow into the pores, but the nonresorbable coral matrix shields the new bone from stress and prevents it from maturing as well as might be desired.

Bone Morphogenetic Proteins

BMPs are an attractive restorative material. Although technically a graft, this material derives its ultimate effect by bone formation in the host. The role of BMPs in reconstruction of the jaws, indications for and limitations of their use, and the ideal carrier to deliver the material have yet to be defined.[34–37] The safety of BMPs has been studied extensively in orthopedic applications, with most of the studies having been conducted with grafting to the spine and reported in the orthopedic literature.[38–40] With a goal to increase the available bone for placement of endosseous implants in the maxilla, BMPs have been placed into the maxillary sinus with collagen sponges as a carrier to induce new bone formation.[41,42] With a similar goal in mind BMP-7 has been placed in fresh extraction sites prior to the placement of dental implants in dogs showing greater amount, density, and degree of remodeling of bone.[43] They have been placed in alveolar ridges with a resorbable collagen sponge as a carrier; however, safety and feasibility was assessed in only one study.[44,45] They have also been placed with a poly(α-hydroxy acid) carrier into alveolar cleft defects in dogs with equivocal results.[46] Large mandibular defects (3 cm segmental) in animal studies have been reconstituted with BMPs.[47–49] Only two human BMP studies have been published.[42,50]

Autogenous Bone Grafting Sites

Intraoral Bone Grafts

Grafts that can be obtained from a local or regional site are attractive in that they are easily obtained, often in the same surgical field (Figure 39-3). They are, however, usually limited in size, quality, or cancellous bone content. Intraoral donor sites include the symphysis (chin), ramus, mandibular inferior border, mandibular body, coronoid process, and zygoma.[51–64] Limited amount of bone is available from these sites, and the amount of cancellous bone is sparse.

For harvesting of grafts from the chin either an intrasulcular or vestibular incision can be made. The periosteum and mentalis muscle are stripped from the chin region, and osteotomies are performed on the buccal surface beginning below the apices of the teeth. Alternatively a trephine can be used to obtain the graft. The midline is usually left intact, and grafts can be harvested from the right and left sides simultaneously if necessary; graft volumes of 1 to 3 cc have been reported.[3] A mild pressure dressing is applied to the chin region for 5 days. Temporary paresthesia of the chin has been reported in at least 43% of cases.[65]

For harvesting of ramal grafts, several incisions can be used. In the edentulous patient a crestal incision is used extending posteriorly to the ascending ramus at the level of the occlusal plane. With healthy natural teeth, an intrasulcular incision is used, extending it posteriorly to the ascending ramus. When prosthetic crowns are present, consideration should be given to a submarginal incision along the mucogingival line, again extending to the ascending ramus. Following any of these incisions, a full thickness mucoperiosteal flap is developed along the lateral aspect of the mandible, exposing the lateral ramus of the mandible. A rectangular block of cortical bone up to 4 mm in thickness, up to 3.5 cm in anteroposterior dimension, and up to 1 cm superoinferiorly can be harvested. The medialmost osteotomy cut is lateral to the teeth and 4 to 6 mm medial to the external oblique line. The osteotomies can be cut with burs, saws, or a small diamond wheel (especially useful for the inferiormost cut). Using osteotomes and chisels the block can be

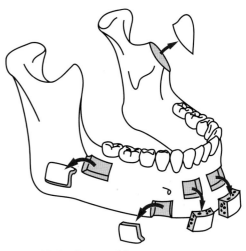

FIGURE 39-3 *Intraoral bone graft donor sites.*

removed. Alternatively, trephines can be used to obtain bone. Morbidity from this procedure includes fracture of the mandible, lingual or inferior nerve neurosensory disturbance, bleeding, and incision dehiscence, although these events are considered rare.[66]

Cranial Bone Grafts

Cranial bone is a time-honored site for obtaining bone for grafting. Initially described for use in facial reconstruction by Tessier and refined by Jackson and colleagues, the technique can yield considerable amounts of cortical bone but limited amounts of cancellous bone.[67,68] There is an age-dependent relationship of the development of diploic space in the calvarial bones: 80% of children have a diploic space by the age of 3 years, and when present it is less than 50% of its adult thickness.[69] The grafts can be harvested from either the inner or outer cortical tables and the procedure is well tolerated by patients. Fearon looked at postharvest magnetic resonance imaging (MRI) of the brain in 20 patients and did not detect any abnormalities, even though 3 of the patients had a full thickness breach.[70] The thickness of the bone should be at least 6.0 mm to consider in situ harvesting. Koenig and colleagues recommend not performing in situ bone graft harvesting from this site prior to 9 years of age.[69] Selection of the side of the head to use should be in the nondominant hemisphere. Grafts from the areas of the parietal bone are the most useful; although harvest from the frontal or occipital regions has been described, the temporal region should be avoided. The incision through the scalp for obtaining the graft can be either coronal (full or partial) or sagittal (Figure 39-4). The dissection of the scalp flap should proceed in the subgaleal plane, and then the pericranium of the calvaria should be incised sharply. The area of the graft is marked out with a bur staying at least 2 cm from the sagittal suture to avoid overlying the sagittal sinus

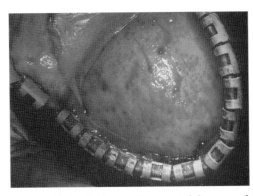

FIGURE **39-4** *Exposure for cranial bone graft harvest.*

or arachnoid granulations. The graft donor site should also be chosen to avoid other sutures.

For harvest of small areas of bone, a single block can be obtained (Figure 39-5). A bur is used to make initial cuts through the outer cortex of the calvaria. One side is beveled to allow insertion of a curved osteotome in a plane parallel to the outer surface and at the diploic level. For larger block grafts (Figure 39-6) it is advisable to bevel two or more sides to avoid inadvertent perforation of the inner cortex. When larger amounts of graft are needed it may be safer to harvest the bone as several strips, rather than a single block (Figure 39-7). Once the graft has been harvested the donor bed is checked to assure integrity of the inner cortex, and a piece of gelatin foam is placed over the site. The periosteum is reapproximated and the scalp closed in layers, with the galea being

reapproximated. The skin can be closed with either staples or sutures.

For grafts from the inner table of the skull (internal table of calvaria), a formal craniotomy is performed and the bone flap is handled ex vivo (Figure 39-8). The graft is obtained from the inner cortex, and the flap is replaced after resuspending the dura then fixated.

In a series of 212 in situ cranial bone graft harvests, Zins and colleagues noted a 0.5% incidence of dural tear and a 2.4% incidence of dural exposure without tear.[71] No infections, seromas, or bleeding were encountered in his series. In a large series of 12,672 cranial bone graft harvests, the total complications comprised only 0.18%.[72] Inadvertent exposure of the dura (not reported as a complication) occurred in 11%.

Costochondral Grafts

Grafts from the rib are useful in that they contain both bony and cartilaginous tissues. The cartilaginous component is useful for providing an articular surface for the temporomandibular joint and for providing a growth center in growing patients. This source of bone, however, is limited by the size, curvature, and strength of the rib. For reconstructing the temporomandibular joint the contralateral rib usually has the more favorable contours. Ribs from either side can be harvested, but most surgeons prefer to use the right side over the left side

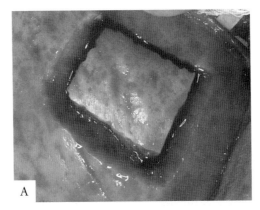
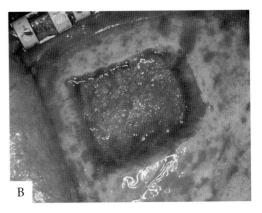

FIGURE **39-5** A *and* B, *Harvest of small cranial bone graft.*

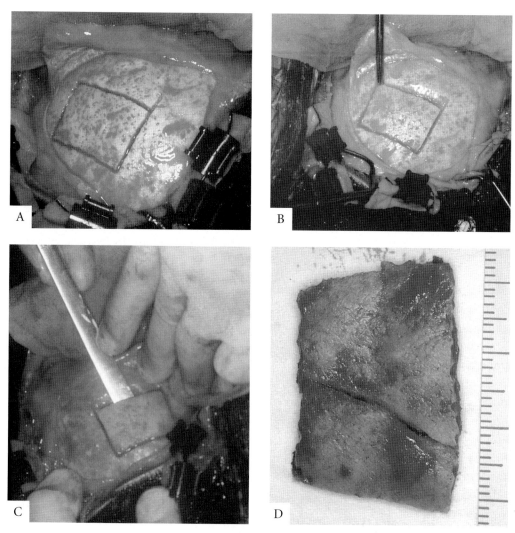

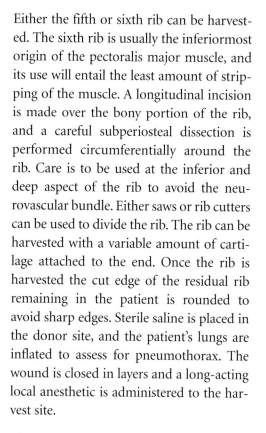

Either the fifth or sixth rib can be harvested. The sixth rib is usually the inferiormost origin of the pectoralis major muscle, and its use will entail the least amount of stripping of the muscle. A longitudinal incision is made over the bony portion of the rib, and a careful subperiosteal dissection is performed circumferentially around the rib. Care is to be used at the inferior and deep aspect of the rib to avoid the neurovascular bundle. Either saws or rib cutters can be used to divide the rib. The rib can be harvested with a variable amount of cartilage attached to the end. Once the rib is harvested the cut edge of the residual rib remaining in the patient is rounded to avoid sharp edges. Sterile saline is placed in the donor site, and the patient's lungs are inflated to assess for pneumothorax. The wound is closed in layers and a long-acting local anesthetic is administered to the harvest site.

Iliac Crest Bone Grafts

The ilium is the most preferred donor site for bone grafting. Grafts may be obtained from either the anterior or posterior portions of the bone. It contains the greatest absolute cancellous bone volume and has the highest cancellous-to-cortical bone ratio. Greater amounts of bone can be obtained from the posterior ilium. From a single side, the maximum amount of obtainable bone approaches 50 cc. From the posterior ilium, the maximum obtainable bone approaches 90 cc. Documented

FIGURE 39-6   A *to* D, *Harvest of a larger cranial bone block graft.*

because of the position of the heart. An incision is used that corresponds to the submammary crease (Figure 39-9). This incision is well hidden in women and is a minor concern in men. The incision will

usually overlie the sixth rib. A curvilinear incision is used and the skin is incised sharply; sharp dissection is used to enter the plane overlying the ribs from the costochondral junction to the midaxillary line.

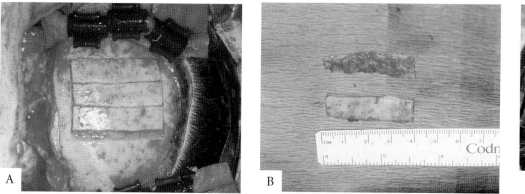

FIGURE 39-7   A *to* C, *Harvest of several cranial strip grafts.*

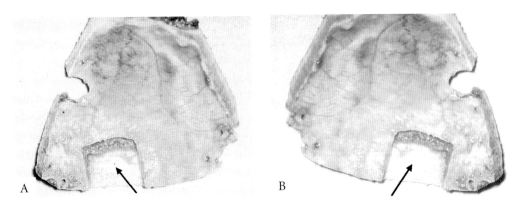

FIGURE 39-8   A *and* B, *Inner table cranial bone graft* (arrow).

donor site complications include hematoma, seroma, nerve and arterial injuries, gait disturbances, fractures of the iliac wing, peritoneal perforation, infection, sacroiliac instability, and pain. Major complications have been reported to be less common (0.7–25%) than minor ones (1.8–15.4%). The reported prevalence of complications following anterior or posterior iliac crest bone grafting has varied.[73]

Harvest of the anterior iliac crest bone graft begins with site selection. Harvesting of the graft from the ipsilateral or contralateral side from the recipient site is largely determined by positioning of the patient relative to the rest of the operating room team. A separate field is used to avoid contamination of donor and recipient sites, and the contralateral side is usually preferred. The anatomic landmarks of the anterior superior iliac crest and relative position of nerve structures are marked (Figure 39-10). The nerve branches that are most at risk are the lateral cutaneous branch of the subcostal nerve (T12) and the lateral cutaneous branch of the iliohy-pogastric nerve (L1). The lateral femoral cutaneous nerve is located anterior and medial to the anterosuperior iliac tubercle; careful delineation of landmarks will avoid damage to this nerve. Anesthesia or paresthesia of the skin following harvesting of iliac crest bone grafts has ranged from 8 to 38% of patients.[73–78] The skin overlying the iliac crest is gently pulled superiorly and medially to allow the incision to rest in a position inferior and lateral to the prominence of the bone. The resultant scar should be in a position where it is not rubbed or chafed afterward by a belt or clothing (Figure 39-11A). The incision is made parallel to the crest of the iliac bone and approximately 2 cm posterior to the anterosuperior iliac tubercle. A 3 cm incision is usually adequate to gain access to the iliac bone. The skin is incised sharply down to the subcutaneous fat. Using electrocautery, the subcutaneous tissue is incised down to the fascia overlying the fascia lata and external oblique muscles. An incision is made along the crest of the bone down to and through the periosteum. This incision can usually be made with minimal cutting into the muscle fibers. Once the incision is made through the periosteum, the subperiosteal dissection can proceed onto the medial or lateral surfaces of the ilium, depending on the approach used and the need for a multilaminar graft. In the anteromedial approach the subperiosteal dissection continues onto the medial side of the bone (Figure 39-11B). Care is taken not to strip muscle from the lateral surface of the ilium. Keeping the tendons of the tensor fascia lata attached to the ilium minimizes gait disturbances and pain. Acute ambulation difficulty has been reported in as many as 50% of patients immediately following iliac crest bone harvest, with long-term ambulation difficulty ranging from 3 to 12.7%.[75,78,79] A Bennett retractor is helpful to protect the iliacus muscle and peritoneal contents.

In the anterolateral approach, the periosteum is stripped from the lateral

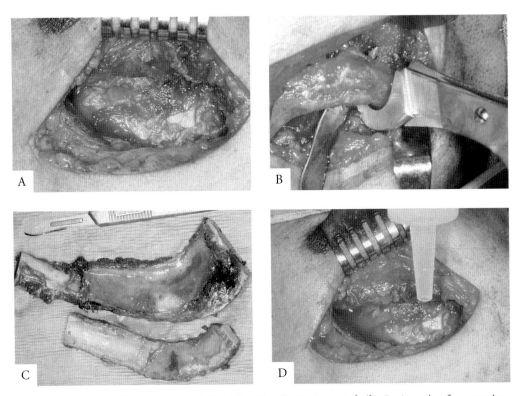

FIGURE 39-9   A, *Incisions for access.* B, *Dividing the rib.* C, *Harvested ribs.* D, *Assessing for entry into the pleural space.*

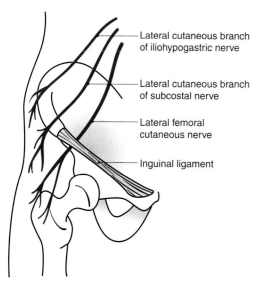

FIGURE **39-10** *Diagram of nerves. Adapted from Lew D, Hinkle RM. Bony reconstruction of the jaws. In: Peterson LJ, Indresano AT, Marciano RD, Roser SM. Principles of oral and maxillofacial surgery. Vol. 2. Philadelphia: J.B. Lippincott Company; 1992. p. 923.*

surface of the ilium for easier access but at a cost of increased incidence of gait disturbance. Once the ilium is exposed by any approach, the bone can be harvested as a corticocancellous block graft, a cortical graft,

or a cancellous graft (Figure 39-11C–F). The size of the graft is outlined, and using saws, osteotomes, or a bur, osteotomies are performed. The cancellous graft can be harvested with curettes, gouges, or trephines.[74,79–82] Hemostasis is obtained with the use of gelatin foam or other hemostatic agents if necessary. Use of drains at the donor sites of either posterior or anterior approaches is not indicated; and no difference has been shown in wound healing.[83] Injection of a long-acting local anesthetic agent into the overlying soft tissue provides some comfort in the immediate postoperative period.[84]

Harvest of the posterior iliac crest is another well-documented source for bone.[85–88] Patient positioning in the supine position for most maxillofacial procedures involves a patient repositioning when posterior iliac crest bone is harvested. Larger amounts of bone available from this approach may make it worthwhile to consider this option. The patient is positioned in the prone position with a small amount of flexion and placement of a hip roll. The

landmarks identified are the spinous processes of the vertebra and the posterosuperior iliac crest and spine. A 5 cm curvilinear incision is made through the skin overlying the iliac crest. Nerves at risk are the superior and middle cluneal nerves (L1 to S3). Using sharp and blunt dissection through the subcutaneous tissues, the posterosuperior crest is identified and the fascia divided between the abdominal and gluteal muscles. A subperiosteal dissection proceeds, and the tissue is reflected laterally. Care is used to avoid the sacroiliac ligaments. Bone can be harvested as a corticocancellous block graft, a cortical graft, or a cancellous graft similar to the approach to the iliac crest. Complication rates for posterior iliac crest bone harvest are, in general, lower than those for anterior harvest.[73–77,79]

Tibial Bone Graft

The tibial metaphysis is another important source of autogenous bone. O'Keefe and colleagues reported the first large series (230 cases) using the tibia as a donor site.[89] They found adequate bone for grafting

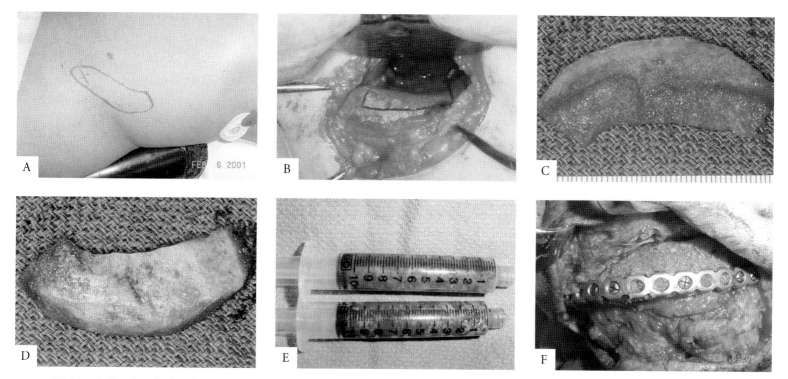

FIGURE **39-11** A, *Landmarks for obtaining graft.* B, *Osteotomies for harvest.* C, *Corticocancellous grafts.* D, *Cortical surface of graft.* E, *Cancellous graft.* F, *Cancellous graft applied.*

and a low incidence (1.3%) of complications, none of which were long-term. The tibial region heals exceptionally well, but radiographic findings in the donor site may persist indefinitely.[90] The use of this site is relatively contraindicated in growing patients because of the risk of disturbance to a growth center site, although its use has been reported in the repair of alveolar clefts.[91] Catone and colleagues described the use of tibial bone in maxillofacial surgery and was able to obtain up to 42 mL of uncompressed cancellous bone per site.[92] Bone from the tibial site was successfully used to graft mandibular nonunions, in orthognathic surgery, as a sinus augmentation, and in mandibular reconstruction. Comparison of tibial grafts against iliac crest grafts in secondary alveolar clefts shows similar bone densities at 6 months.[91]

The graft is usually harvested with the patient in the supine position, although the graft can be harvested with the patient in the prone position.[89] A 3 cm longitudinal and slightly angled incision (Figure 39-12) is made through the skin overlying Gerdy's tubercle. Gerdy's tubercle is a prominence of bone on the anterior surface of the proximal end of the tibia located lateral to the tibial tuberosity. It is the distalmost insertion of the iliotibial tract. Sharp dissection is used to obtain a supraperiosteal dissec-

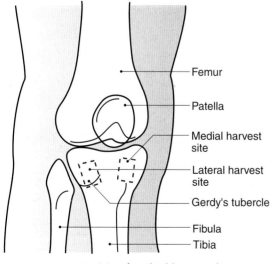

FIGURE **39-12**   *Incision for tibial bone graft.*

Femur
Patella
Medial harvest site
Lateral harvest site
Gerdy's tubercle
Fibula
Tibia

tion overlying and inferior to Gerdy's tubercle. The dissection should be medial to the tibialis anterior muscle and lateral to the patellar ligament. If a cortical graft is desired, the dissection can proceed in a subperiosteal plane, exposing Gerdy's tubercle.[89] If no cortical bone is required, an osteoperiosteal flap can be created by incising through the periosteum in a "U" shape, leaving periosteum attached to the cortex.[92] A cortical window is made with burs, saws, or osteotomes measuring 1 cm by 1 cm. The window should incorporate the crest of the tubercle at the superior portion of the window. The crest represents a simple and reliable landmark to avoid the articular surface of the tibia and the joint space. It is recommended to keep at least a 2 cm distance from the articular surface of the tibia to avoid damage.[93] A medial approach to the tibia has also been advocated that avoids the insertion of the iliotibial tract and several other anatomic landmarks.[94,95] In the medial approach, the landmarks are two lines: one vertical line drawn through the patella and tibial tuberosity and the other perpendicular to the first, through the tibial tuberosity. It is recommended that an oblique skin incision be made centered over a point 15 mm superior to the horizontal line and 15 mm medial to the vertical line.[95] Dissection continues through the periosteum overlying the bone underneath the incision. A bone window is made to provide access to the cancellous bone. Regardless of the approach (medial vs lateral) used, once the window has been removed or elevated, the cancellous bone can be harvested with curettes. Equal amounts of bone are available from either lateral or medial approaches.[95] For larger volumes of grafts, bilateral grafting can be done, with some possible impairment to early ambulation. No attempt is made to fill the metaphyseal dead space, and no drains are used. The wound is closed in layers. If smaller amounts of bone are needed (< 15 cc), the procedure can continue through a small stab incision and with use

of a trephine or curettes.[92,96] van Damme reported up to 40 cc of cancellous bone obtained through this method.[96]

Microvascular Free Flaps

Many microvascular free flaps have been described for reconstruction of the mandible and maxilla, including the fibula, iliac crest, and scapula. Free microvascular flaps have the advantage of having their own blood supply independent of the local tissue bed, and they behave as a microvascular transfer of tissue, except where they interface with the existing recipient bone. In areas of poor vascular supply they have superiority over other bone grafts. Additionally they may be transferred as composite grafts including soft tissue components. A detailed discussion of microvascular free flap reconstruction is presented in Chapter 40, "Microvascular Free Tissue Transfer."

Platelet-Rich Plasma

With the advent of blood factor fractionation in hematology and the search for hemostatic agents, interest has increased in platelet-rich plasma (PRP) fractions. PRP is a volume of autologous plasma that has a platelet concentration higher than normal. In general, PRP contains $> 1 \times 10^6$ platelets/μL. In clinical practice, PRP is applied to the site of a bone graft to deliver a high concentration of growth factors from platelets.[97] Once the PRP-containing high concentrations of fibrinogen and platelets are mixed with thrombin and calcium, a gel is formed resulting in the release of growth factors from the platelet (α) granules. Within 10 minutes the platelets secrete 70% of their stored growth factors and close to 100% within the first hour.[98] The platelets then synthesize additional amounts of growth factors for about 8 days until they are depleted and die. The precise content and concentration of growth factor has yet to be fully elucidated. The α-granules of platelets release at least seven growth factors, including platelet-derived growth factor, TGF-β, platelet-derived epidermal growth factor, platelet-derived angiogenesis factor, insulin-like growth factor-1, and platelet factor-4.[99] There is a complex interplay between the growth factors that depends on their concentration, local microenvironment, and interactions with other molecules. Many of these growth factors can have effects that are in opposite directions depending on the context of expression.[100] The PRP constellation of growth factors allows the complex interplay of these agents to be exploited to better advantage than relying on a single growth factor agent.

PRP is an autologous preparation; therefore, the risk of disease transmission from its use should theoretically be nil. There has been some concern about the antigenicity of the bovine thrombin used, although this has not been a problem in maxillofacial applications.[101] It is believed that some of the antigenicity attributed to thrombin results from contamination from bovine factor V in the thrombin preparation. Another gelling agent, ITA, has been used in place of bovine thrombin but its constituents are proprietary and unknown.[102]

There are several systems for preparing PRP (Figure 39-13) ranging from the simple to the complex, from those that require whole units of blood to those that require only 50 mL. The most complex are the general-purpose cell separators that are widely used by blood banks and hospitals. Using a plasmapheresis technique, 450 mL of whole blood is drawn off into a collection bag containing an anticoagulant, usually citrate phosphate dextrose. Other anticoagulants are available; anticoagulant citrate dextrose-A is also used and may be preferred.[98] Edetic acid is avoided since it fragments the platelets.[102] The preparation is then centrifuged first at high speed to separate the plasma from the red cells and the buffy coat. The centrifuge is then slowed down and run for a period of time to further separate the PRP and the platelet-poor plasma (PPP). Approxi-

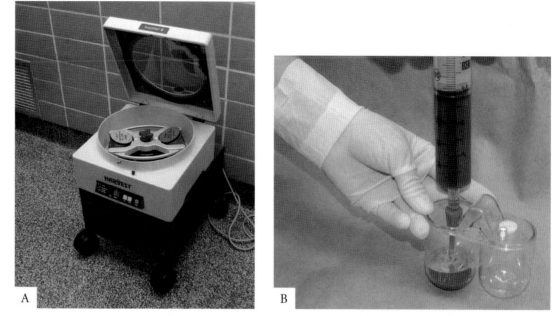

FIGURE 39-13   A, *Machine for harvest of platelet-rich plasma.* B, *Fractionated sample containing platelet-rich plasma.*

mately 30 cc of PRP can be obtained from the sample in about 30 minutes. Platelet counts of 0.5 to $1.0 \times 10^6/\mu L$ can usually be attained with this method. It is recommended that the PRP be used within 6 hours of being procured. Once developed, PRP is stable and remains sterile in the anticoagulated state for 8 hours.[98]

In a quest to achieve a concentrated delivery of platelets at a reasonable cost, several systems were developed that use smaller procurements of whole blood, are faster, produce more concentrated product, and are less expensive.[97,102,103] Two of the units that are currently approved by the US Food and Drug Administration are the Harvest SmartPRep Platelet Concentrate System and the 3i Platelet Concentrate Collection System. These systems both use tailored centrifuge containers to manipulate the blood cells to achieve the separation and sequestration of platelets. They both have long and short spin cycles. Average platelet counts of 1.4 to $1.8 \times 10^6/\mu L$ are obtained in a 5 mL sample.[99] Run times for the preparation are usually 15 to 20 minutes.

Once the PRP has been prepared, the coagulation process is initiated using a mixture of 100 US units of topical bovine

thrombin (TBT) powder suspended in 10 mL sterile saline and 10% calcium chloride. In a 10 cc syringe, 6 mL of PRP is mixed with 1 mL of 10% $CaCl_2$, 1 mL TBT, and 1 mL air for mixing. The mixture is applied to the bone grafts in a layered fashion. Some of the newer systems have special syringe tips that combine the constituents from several syringes simultaneously. Once applied, the mixture sets in a matter of minutes.

There is a paucity of strong clinical data to support many of the claims being made for PRP in the jaws; only one prospective trial is published.[104] The majority of the publications are case series or case reports. Marx and coworkers evaluated the effect of PRP on bone graft reconstructions of mandibular continuity defects 5 cm or greater, showing a maturity index of about twice actual maturity at 2 and 4 months.[97] In a case series of 15 patients, PRP has been added to freeze-dried demineralized bone to augment the maxillary sinus and alveolar ridge.[105] The authors posit that use of PRP may allow for earlier implant placement and loading, but this conclusion will require further study to be supported. In another cases, 24 maxillary sinuses were augmented with a combination of PRP and deproteinized bovine bone along with simultaneous insertion of endosseous implants.[104] In three of these cases bone density measurements made at 4 months showed increased density compared with the surrounding native bone. Only preliminary data are available to date on the histologic evaluation of the PRP-augmented sinuses.[106,107] A case report of use of PRP with autogenous bone and a titanium mesh for a large anterior maxillary defect has also been described.[108] Fourier and fractal analysis of radiographs of maxillary alveolar ridge repair using PRP and inorganic bovine bone showed trabecular patterns of the regenerated bone similar to but lower in complexity than the native bone, which the authors attributed to the PRP.[109]

Hyperbaric Oxygen Therapy

After success with treating osteoradionecrosis of the mandible with hyperbaric oxygen therapy, the modality was applied to patients undergoing mandibular reconstruction.[110] Applying fairly stringent success criteria, a rate of 94% was reported. Hyperbaric oxygen therapy consists of breathing 100% O_2 at 2.4 atm for 90 minutes, commonly referred to as a dive. Protocols for reconstructive procedures differ from those used to treat osteoradionecrosis and consist of 20 dives preoperatively and 10 dives postoperatively.

The mechanisms by which hyperbaric oxygen thereapy exerts its effects are biochemical, cellular, and physiologic.[111] During a dive, arterial oxygen tensions in excess of 2,000 mm Hg, and tissue oxygen tensions of almost 400 mm Hg have been attained. Physiologically at 2.4 atm, oxygen not only saturates the available hemoglobin but dissolves in the plasma to more than 10 times the amount at sea level (0.3 mL/dL). Tissue irradiated beyond 5,000 cGy exhibits hypoxia, hypovascularity, and hypocellularity. This predisposes the tissue to infection and poor wound healing in addition to making it a poor donor bed for a bone

graft. Hypoxia inhibits and decreases the neutrophil-mediated killing of bacteria by free radicals. Tissue PO_2 levels in irradiated patients have been documented as low as 5 mm Hg and often range between 5 and 15 mm Hg. During hyperbaric oxygen therapy the tissue PO_2 rises to between 100 and 250 mm Hg but falls to baseline within 10 minutes following a dive in the initial period of therapy. Improved collagen formation and fibroblast proliferation occur when the tissue oxygen tension is raised over 20 to 30 mm Hg.[112] Capillary proliferation occurs along collagen laid down following hyperbaric oxygen exposure. As this neovascularization spreads, tissue oxygenation improves between 20 and 35 mm Hg in the hours after treatment. The improvement plateaus after 10 to 20 dives; dives beyond this time do not marginally improve the host bed.

Complications of hyperbaric oxygen therapy include reversible myopia; barotrauma to the middle ear, lungs, teeth, and sinuses from rapid pressure changes; seizures (self-limited and causing no permanent damage); claustrophobia; reversible tracheobronchial symptoms (chest tightness, substernal burning sensation, and cough). No evidence of a tumorigenic effect of hyperbaric oxygen has been found to date.[113]

Reconstruction of the Mandible

Reconstruction of the mandible can occur immediately at the conclusion of an ablative procedure of the jaw (primary reconstruction); delayed (secondary), after an appropriate time of primary soft tissue healing; or, in the case of developmental or gradually acquired defects, at the time of recognition of the need for reconstruction. The first step in reconstruction is to classify the defect determined by its size, location, and functional or cosmetic impairment. The size of the defect in three dimensions will define the magnitude of the reconstruction. Small defects of the alveolus may require limited bone grafting, while larger defects may require more extensive or

staged procedures. Some defects may not necessarily be restored to the original size and bulk of the missing part. Loss of a significant portion of a ramus may be adequately managed by providing continuity from the condyle to the body of the mandible without restoring a coronoid process or several centimeters of anteroposterior width. The bulk of the bone need only be enough to provide for adequate strength to manage the functional loads. Location is important as some defects may not need to be restored, such as the very posterior of the body of the mandible (distal to the first or second molar) where no plan is made for restoration of the dental occlusion of the mandible or opposing dental arch. The functional deficits that exist and those that are to be addressed play a role in the choice of reconstruction.

Once the area of bony defect has been defined and the assessment of how much bone to reconstruct has been determined, attention should be directed to how to best achieve these goals. The available soft tissue in terms of quantity and quality is paramount in choosing a reconstructive method. Indeed the soft tissue will determine to a large extent the available options. If the soft tissue is adequate in both of these parameters, the options will be many. If, however, the soft tissue is inadequate in size or bulk, efforts will need to be made to provide adequate soft tissue before undergoing bony reconstruction. This can be accomplished by introducing more soft tissue through local flaps, pedicled flaps, or microvascular free flaps. Composite flaps are an option for simultaneous hard and soft tissue reconstruction. Techniques such as distraction osteogenesis can provide increased bone and soft tissue simultaneously like the composite grafts. If the quantity of soft tissue is adequate but the quality of the soft tissue is poor, the reconstruction will be compromised or the options limited. Tissue that has been irradiated or has extensive scarring will provide a poor host bed for any grafting procedures. Adjunctive procedures such as hyperbaric oxygen therapy or soft tissue flaps may be necessary to provide an adequate donor bed.

The functional and esthetic requirements will dictate the goal to be accomplished; multiple-stage procedures are the norm rather than the exception.

Reconstruction of the Maxilla

The same general parameters in approaching the mandibular reconstruction are operative in the maxilla. Identification of the goals of reconstruction will dictate the course of reconstruction to take. Once the goal has been delineated, attention is first given to the soft tissue envelope to support bony reconstruction of the maxilla. Appropriate grafting procedures are undertaken, and provision is made for interim prosthetics. The following cases illustrate specific points of consideration in reconstruction of the areas of the jaws.

Case Example 1: Reconstruction of Large Traumatic Mandibular Defect

The patient is a 17-year-old man who suffered a gunshot wound to the anterior mandible with loss of both hard and soft tissue (Figure 39-14). The maxilla was unaffected. The first step in this case is to define the defect in terms of both hard and soft tissue and decide on a strategy for reconstruction. As this is a contaminated

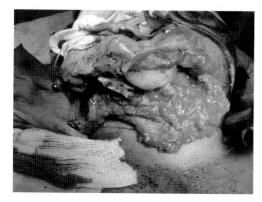

FIGURE **39-14**   *Gunshot wound to mandible.*

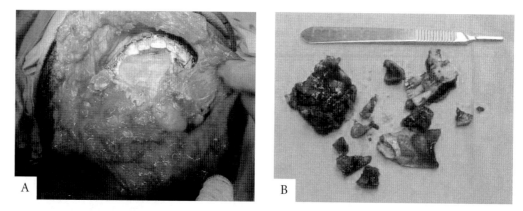

FIGURE **39-15**   A *and* B, *Débridement of nonviable hard and soft tissues.*

wound with ill-defined areas of vital hard and soft tissue, delayed reconstruction is the preferred option. Débridement of free bone fragments and grossly nonperfused soft tissue will enhance the rapidity of primary healing (Figure 39-15). Once the débridement is complete, the bone components are aligned using available dental landmarks (Figure 39-16) and soft tissue components are reapproximated (Figure 39-17). To aid the ease of reconstruction, anatomic relations are maintained and stabilized with fixation devices (Figure 39-18) to preserve interramal width. At this time a more accurate assessment of soft tissue and bone deficits can be appreciated in three dimensions. There is a segmental mandibular defect with inadequate soft tissues and an opposing dental arch. The functional requirements for reconstruction include (1) restoration of continuity of the mandible, (2) adequate bone height and width to allow restoration of the occlusion, and (3) restoration of mandibular morphology for esthetic and functional requirements. Because of the avulsive nature of the defect, the soft tissue is inadequate in terms of quality and quantity. A period of weeks to months may be required for the soft tissues to mature and heal. Before bony reconstruction can begin, soft tissue must be brought in to provide for an adequate recipient bed for grafting and restoration of contours. In this otherwise healthy individual, autogenous grafting will most effectively supply the adequate bulk and form necessary to achieve the goals. A pedicled myocutaneous graft (pectoralis major) with a skin paddle will provide the blood supply to nourish the graft and to provide adequate bulk of skin in the chin region. The residual bilateral condyle-ramal complexes will be stabilized with a titanium reconstruction plate (Figure 39-19). An appropriately sized skin paddle will restore

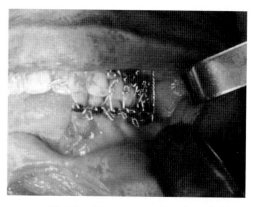

FIGURE **39-16**   *Alignment using dental landmarks.*

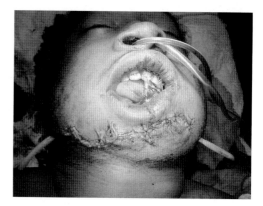

FIGURE **39-17**   *Reapproximation of skin and mucosa.*

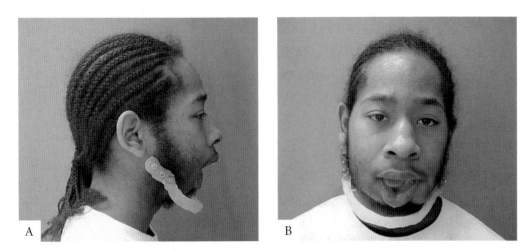

FIGURE **39-18** A *and* B, *Stabilization with external fixator.*

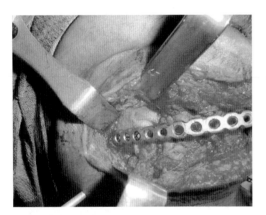

FIGURE **39-19** *Stabilization of mandible with titanium reconstruction plate.*

the missing skin over the chin (Figure 39-20). The muscle is positioned to restore bulk to the region and to approximate the area of the future bone graft. The soft tis-

sues are then allowed to heal over several weeks prior to definitive bone grafting (see Figure 39-20D). Both allografts and autografts will be used, with a cadaveric mandibular crib (Figure 39-21) secured to the reconstruction plate used to maintain the proper morphology of the mandible. A cancellous marrow graft is obtained to provide adequate bulk (Figure 39-22). Restoration of the contours and functionality of the mandible results at the completion of the reconstruction (Figure 39-23).

Case Example 2: Delayed Reconstruction of an Ablative Defect of the Mandible

A swelling with associated radiolucency of the mandible is noted (Figure 39-24). Both

the medial and lateral cortices have been destroyed in the area of the lesion. Because of the location and size of the defect, reconstruction of the defect is indicated to restore bulk and strength of the residual mandible following treatment. After adequate soft tissue healing, an anterior iliac crest cancellous bone graft is obtained and placed in the defect (see Figure 39-24B). One year following reconstruction, the bone graft has matured with a normal trabecular pattern. The graft is maintained and the bone is adequate for oral rehabilitation 2 years after grafting (see Figure 39-24E).

Case Example 3: Reconstruction of the Anterior Maxilla

A 37-year-old man had undergone avulsive trauma to the anterior maxilla during a motor vehicle accident. The residual defect was from the loss of anterior maxillary teeth and a large portion of the alveolus (Figure 39-25A). Dental models were obtained, and a diagnostic wax-up was prepared to assess the ideal position of the restored teeth. The bony reconstructive effort is therefore guided by the prosthetic plan so that adequate bulk and position of the grafted bone can be assured. The defect in the upper jaw consisted of inadequate bone in terms of height and width and inadequate soft tissues. No oral–nasal cavity partitioning defect existed. A wide pedicled flap is raised

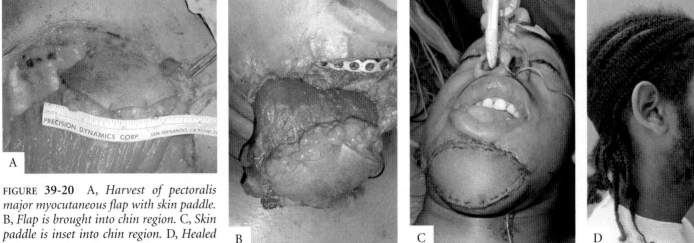

FIGURE **39-20** A, *Harvest of pectoralis major myocutaneous flap with skin paddle.* B, *Flap is brought into chin region.* C, *Skin paddle is inset into chin region.* D, *Healed soft tissue prior to bone grafting.*

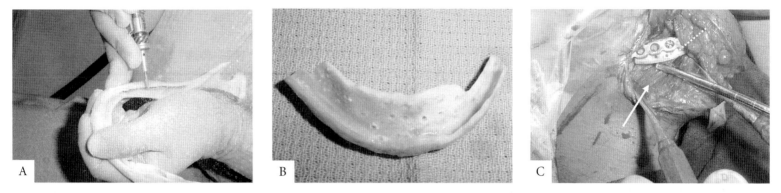

FIGURE 39-21   A, *A freeze-dried allogeneic cadaver mandible is obtained and hollowed out.* B, *Useful section of the crib is perforated.* C, *The crib is secured to the plate* (arrow) *with the pectoralis major muscle* (arrow) *nourishing the bone graft.*

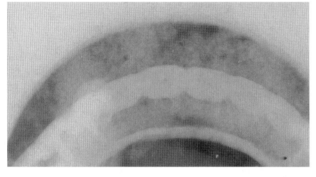

FIGURE 39-22   *Occlusal radiograph in the area of the graft.*

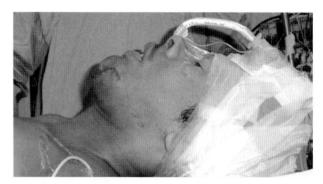

FIGURE 39-23   *Restoration of contour of chin.*

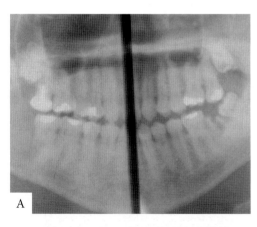

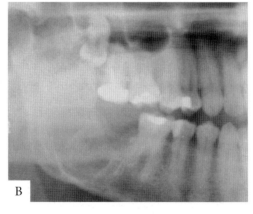

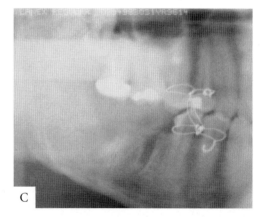

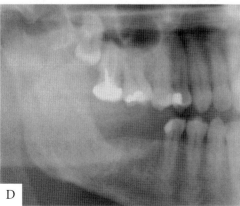

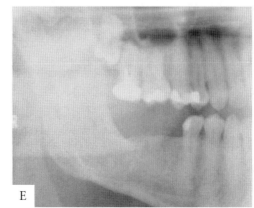

FIGURE 39-24   *Radiographs illustrating delayed reconstruction of an ablative defect of the mandible:* A, *prebiopsy;* B, *immediately postgraft;* C, *2 weeks postgraft;* D, *1 year postgraft;* E, *2 years postgraft.*

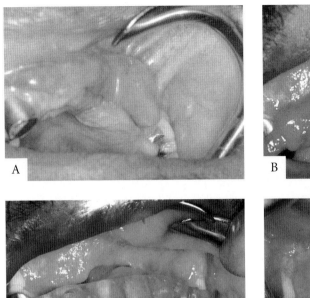

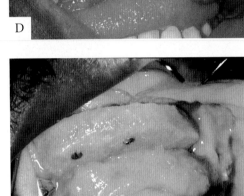

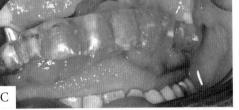

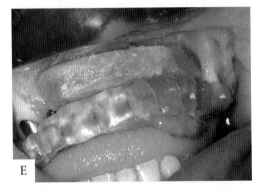

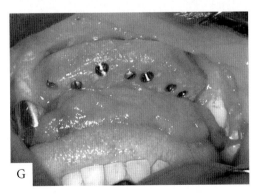

FIGURE **39-25**   A, *Defect in anterior maxilla.* B, *Flap elevated to expose bony defect.* C, *Stent with outline of occlusal scheme.* D, *Bone wax applied to create template for graft.* E, *Bone contoured and placed in relation to stent.* F, *Bone graft secured with titanium screws.* G, *Endosseous implants placed.*

(Figure 39-25B) to expose the bony defect, and a stent prepared from the diagnostic wax-up is used to assess the bony defect more accurately (Figure 39-25C). Sterile bone wax is used to prepare a template for the graft dimensions (Figure 39-25D). A corticocancellous graft is obtained from the anterior iliac crest, contoured from the template and secured with titanium screws (Figure 39-25E and F). Using the stent as a guide, endosseous root-form implants are placed in the graft (Figure 39-25G).

References

1. Adamo AK, Szal RL. Timing, results, and complications of mandibular reconstructive surgery: report of 32 cases. J Oral Surg 1979;37:755–60.
2. Obwegesser HL, Sailer HF. Experience with intraoral resection and immediate reconstruction in cases of radio-osteomyelitis of the mandible. J Maxillofac Surg 1978; 6:257–66.
3. Marx RE, Ames JR. The use of hyperbaric oxygen therapy in bony reconstruction of the irradiated and tissue deficient patient. J Oral Maxillofac Surg 1982;40:412–20.
4. Hidalgo DA. Fibula free flap: a new method of mandibular reconstruction. Plast Reconstr Surg 1989;84:71–9.
5. Urist MR. Bone: formation by autoinduction. Science 1965;150:893–9.
6. Urist MR, Strates BS. Bone morphogenetic protein. J Dent Res 1971;50:1392–406.
7. Schmitt JM, Hwang K, Winn SR, Hollinger JO. Bone morphogenetic proteins: an update on basic biology and clinical relevance. J Orthopedic Res 1999;17:269–78.
8. Wozney JM. Overview of bone morphogenetic proteins. Spine 2002;27:52–8.
9. Wozney JM, Rosen V. Bone morphogenetic protein and bone morphogenetic protein gene family in bone formation and repair. Clin Orthop Rel Res 1998;346:26–37.
10. Ebara S, Nakayama K. Mechanism for the action of bone morphogenetic protein and regulation of their activity. Spine 2002; 27:S10–5.
11. Lieberman JR, Daluiski A, Einhorn TA. The role of growth factors in the repair of bone. J Bone Joint Surg 2002;84A:1032–44.
12. Reddi AH. Bone morphogenetic proteins: from basic science to clinical application. J Bone Joint Surg 2001;83:S1–5.
13. Sakou T. Bone morphogenetic proteins: from basic science to clinical approaches. Bone 1998;22:591–603.
14. Ten Dijke P, Fu J, Schaap P, Roelen AJ. Signal transduction of bone morphogenetic proteins in osteoblast differentiation. J Bone Joint Surg 2003;85A:34–8.
15. Brunet LJ, McMahon JA, McMahon AP, Harland RM. Noggin, cartilage morphogenesis and joint formation in the mammalian skeleton. Science 1998;280:1455–7.
16. Axhausen W. The osteogenic phases of regeneration of bone, a historical and experimental study. J Bone Joint Surg 1956;38:593–601.
17. Gray JC, Elves MW. Early osteogenesis in compact bone isografts: a quantitative study of the different graft cells. Calcif Tissue Int 1979;29:225–37.

18. Bassett, CAL, Creighton DK, Stinchfield FE. Contributions of endostium, cortex, and soft tissue to osteogenesis. Surg Gynecol Obstet 1961;112:145–52.

19. Heslop BK, Zeiss IM, Nisbet NW. Studies on transference of bone. A comparison of autologous and homologous transplants with reference to osteocyte survival, osteogenesis, and host reaction. Br J Exp Pathol 1960;41:269–72.

20. Enneking WF, Burchardt H, Puhl JJ, et al. Physical and biological aspects of repair in dog cortical-bone transplants. J Bone Joint Surg 1975;57:237–52.

21. Enneking WF, Eady JL, Burchard H. Autogenous cortical bone grafts in the construction of segmental skeletal defects. J Bone Joint Surg 1980;62:1039–58.

22. Habal MB, Reddi AR. Bone grafts and bone induction substitutes. Clin Plast Surg 1994;21:525–42.

23. Friedenstein AJ, Piatetzky-Shapiro II, Petrakova KV. Osteogenesis in transplants of bone marrow cells. J Embr Exp Morph 1966;16:381–90.

24. Marx RE, Kline SN, Johnson RP, et al. The use of freeze-dried allogeneic bone in oral and maxillofacial surgery. J Oral Surg 1981;39:264–74.

25. Williams G. Experiences with boiled cadaveric cancellous bone from fractures of long bones. J Bone Joint Surg 1964;46:398–403.

26. Dubuc FL, Urist MR. The accessibility of the bone induction principle in surface decalcified bone implants. Clin Orthop 1967;55:217–23.

27. Callan DP, Salkeld SL, Scarborough N. Histologic analysis of implant sites after grafting with demineralized bone matrix putty and sheets. Implant Dent 2000;9:36–44.

28. Feuille F, Knapp CI, Brunsvold MA, Mellonig JT. Clinical and histologic evaluation of bone-replacement grafts in the treatment of localized alveolar ridge defects. Part 1: mineralized freeze dried bone allograft. Int J Periodontics Restorative Dent 2003;23:29–35.

29. Merkx MAW, Maltha JC, Stoelinga PJW. Assessment of the value of anorganic bone additives in sinus floor augmentation: a review of clinical reports. Int J Oral Maxillofac Surg 2003;32:1–6.

30. Artzi Z, Dayan D, Alpern Y, Nemcovsky CE. Vertical ridge augmentation using xenogenic material supported by a configured titanium mesh: clinicopathologic and histochemical study. Int J Oral Maxillofac Implants 2003;18:440–6.

31. Schepers E, Declerq M, Ducheyne P, Kempeneers R. Bioactive glass particulate material as a filler for bone lesions. J Oral Rehab 1991;18:439–52.

32. Knapp CI, Feuille F, Cochran DL, Mellonig JT. Clinical and histologic evaluation of bone-replacement grafts in the treatment of localized alveolar ridge defects. Part 2: bioactive glass particulate. Int J Periodontics Restorative Dent 2003;23:129–37.

33. Wiltfang J, Schlegel KA, Schultze-Mosgau S, et al. Sinus floor augmentation with β-tricalciumphosphate (β-TCP): does platelet-rich plasma promote its osseous integration and degradation? Clin Oral Impl Res 2003;14:213–8.

34. Boyne PJ. Animal studies of the application of rhBMP-2 in maxillofacial reconstruction. Bone 1996;19:S83–92.

35. Einhorn TA. Clinical applications of recombinant human BMPs: early experience and future development. J Bone Joint Surg 2003;85A:82–8.

36. Boyne PJ, Shabahang S. An evaluation of bone induction delivery materials in conjunction with root form implant placement. Int J Periodontics Restorative Dent 2001;21:333–43.

37. Seeherman H, Wozney J, Li R. Bone morphogenetic protein delivery systems. Spine 2002;27:S16–23.

38. Poynton AR, Lane JM. Safety profile for the clinical use of bone morphogenetic proteins in the spine. Spine 2002;27:S40–8.

39. Valentin-Opran A, Wozney J, Csimma C, et al. Clinical evaluation of recombinant human bone morphogenetic protein-2. Clin Orthop and Rel Res 2002;395:110–20.

40. Sandhu HS, Khan SN. Recombinant human bone morphogenetic protein-2: use in spinal fusion applications. J Bone Joint Surg 2003;85A:89–95.

41. Nevins M, Kirker-Head C, Nevins M, et al. Bone formation in the goat maxillary sinus induced by absorbable collagen sponge implants impregnated with recombinant human bone morphogenetic protein-2. Int J Periodont Res Dent 1996;16:9–19.

42. Boyne PJ, Marx RE, Nevins M, et al. A feasibility study evaluating rhBMP-2/absorbable collagen sponge for maxillary sinus augmentation. Int J Periodont Restor Dent 1997;17:11–25.

43. Cook SD, Salkeld SL, Rueger DC. Evaluation of recombinant human osteogenic protein (rhOP-1) placed with dental implants in fresh extraction sites. J Oral Implantol 1995;21:281–9.

44. Howell TH, Fiorellini J, Jones A, et al. A feasibility study evaluating rhBMP-2/absorbable collagen sponge device for local alveolar ridge augmentation. Int J Periodontics Restorative Dent 1997;17:124–39.

45. Wikesjo UME, Sorensen RG, Kinoshita A, Wozney JM. RhBMP-2/αBSM induces significant vertical alveolar ridge augmentation and dental implant osseointegration. Clin Impl Dent Rel Res 2002;4:174–82.

46. Mayer M, Hollinger J, Ron E, Wozney J. Maxillary alveolar cleft repair in dogs using recombinant human bone morphogenetic protein-2 and a polymer carrier. Plast Reconstr Surg 1996;98:247–59.

47. Toriumi DM, Kotler HS, Luxenberg DP, et al. Mandibular reconstruction with a recombinant bone-inducing factor: functional, histologic and biomechanical evaluation. Arch Otolaryngol Head Neck Surg 1991;117:1101–12.

48. Yudell RM, Block MS. Bone gap healing in the dog using rhBMP-2. J Oral Maxillofac Surg 2000;58:761–6.

49. Terheyden H, Knak C, Jepsen, et al. Mandibular reconstruction with a prefabricated vascularized bone graft using recombinant human osteogenic protein-1: an experimental study in miniature pigs. Int J Oral Maxillofac Surg 2001;30:373–9.

50. Philippart P, Brasseur M, Hoyaux D, Pochet R. Human recombinant tissue factor, platelet-rich plasma, and tetracycline induce a high-quality human bone graft: a 5-year study. Int J Oral Maxillofac Implants 2003;18:411–6.

51. Zeiter DJ, Ries WL, Sanders JJ. The use of a bone block graft from the chin for alveolar ridge augmentation. Int J Periodontics Restorative Dent 2000;20:619–27.

52. Cranin AN, Katzap M, Demirdjan E, Ley J. Autogenous bone ridge augmentation using the mandibular symphysis as a donor. J Oral Implantol 2001;27:43–7.

53. Balaji SM. Management of deficient anterior maxillary alveolus with mandibular parasymphyseal bone graft for implants. Implant Dent 2002;11:363–9.

54. Matsumoto MA, Filho HN, Francischone CE, Consolaro A. Microscopic analysis of reconstructed maxillary alveolar ridges using autogenous bone grafts from the chin and iliac crest. Int J Oral Maxillofac Implants 2002;17:507–16.

55. Kaufman E, Wang PD. Localized vertical maxillary ridge augmentation using symphyseal bone cores: a technique and case report. Int J Oral Maxillofac Implants 2003;18:293–8.

56. Misch CM. Comparison of intraoral donor sites for onlay grafting prior to implant placement. Int J Oral Maxillofac Implants 1997;12:767–76.

57. Pikos MA. Block autografts for localized ridge augmentation: part II the posterior mandible. Implant Dent 2000;9:67–74.

58. Misch CM. Use of the mandibular ramus as a

donor site for onlay bone grafting. 2000;26:42–9.

59. Sethi A, Kraus T. Ridge augmentation using mandibular block bone grafts: preliminary results of an ongoing prospective study. Int J Oral Maxillofac Implants 2001;16:378–88.

60. Proussaefs P, Lozada J, Kleinman A, Rohrer MD. The use of ramus autogenous block grafts for vertical alveolar ridge augmentation and implant placement: a pilot study. Int J Oral Maxillofac Implants 2002;17:238–48.

61. Capelli M. Autogenous bone graft from the mandibular ramus: a technique for bone augmentation. Int J Periodontics Restorative Dent 2003;23:277–85.

62. Cotter CJ, Maher A, Gallagher C, Sleeman D. Mandibular lower border: donor site of choice for alveolar grafting. Br J Oral Maillofac Surg 2002;40:429–32.

63. Li KK, Schwartz HC. Mandibular body bone in facial plastic and reconstructive surgery. Laryngoscope 1996;106:504–6.

64. Kainulainen VT, Sandor GKB, Oikarinen KS, Clokie CM. Zygomatic bone: an additional donor site for alveolar bone reconstruction. Technical note. Int J Oral Maxillofac Implants 2002;17:723–8.

65. Ragheobar GM, Louwerse C, Kalk WWI, Vissink A. Morbidity of chin bone harvesting. Clin Oral Impl Res 2001;12:503–7.

66. Nkenke E, Radespiel-Troger M, Wiltfang J, et al. Morbidity of harvesting of retromolar bone grafts: a prospective study. Clin Oral Impl Res 2002;13:514–21.

67. Tessier P. Autogenous bone grafts taken from the calvarium for facial and cranial applications. Clin Plast Surg 1982;9:531–9.

68. Jackson IT, Pellet C, Smith JM. The skull as a bone graft donor site. Ann Plast Surg 1983;11:527–34.

69. Koenig WJ, Donovan JM, Pensler JM. Cranial bone grafting in children. Plast Reconstr Surg 1995;95:1–4.

70. Fearon JA. A magnetic resonance imaging investigation of potential subclinical complications after in situ cranial bone graft harvest. Plast Reconstr Surg 2000;105:1935–9.

71. Zins JE, Weinzweig N, Hahn J. A simple failsafe method for the harvesting of cranial bone. Plast Reconstr Surg 1995;96:1444–7.

72. Klein RM, Wolfe SA. Complications associated with the harvesting of cranial bone grafts. Plast Reconstr Surg 1995;95:5–13.

73. Ahlmann E, Patzakis M, Roidis N, et al. Comparison of anterior and posterior iliac crest bone harvest in terms of harvest site morbidity and functional outcomes. J Bone Joint Surg 2002;84:716–20.

74. Marx RE, Morales MJ. Morbidity from bone harvest in major jaw reconstruction: a randomized trial comparing the lateral anterior and posterior approaches to the ilium. J Oral Maxillofac Surg 1988;48:196–203.

75. Kurz LT, Garfin SR, Booth RE. Harvesting autogenous iliac crest bone grafts: a review of complications. Spine 1989;14:1324–31.

76. Banwart JC, Asher MA, Hassanein RS. Iliac crest bone graft donor site morbidity: a statistical evaluation. Spine 1995;20:1055–60.

77. Arrington ED, Smith WJ, Chambers HG, et al. Complications of iliac crest bone graft harvesting. Clin Orthop 1996;329:300–9.

78. Silber JS, Anderson DG, Daffner SD, et al. Donor site morbidity after anterior iliac crest bone harvest for single level anterior cervical discectomy and fusion. Spine 2003;28:134–9.

79. Burstein FD, Simms C, Cohen SR, et al. Iliac crest bone graft harvesting techniques: a comparison. Plast Reconstr Surg 2000;105:34–9.

80. Sandor GKB, Rittenberg BN, Clokie CML, Caminiti MK. Clinical success in harvesting autogenous bone using a minimally invasive trephine. J Oral Maxillofac Surg 2003;61:164–8.

81. Westrich GH, Geller DS, O'Malley MJ, et al. Anterior iliac crest harvesting using the corticocancellous reamer system. J Orthop Trauma 2001;15:500–6.

82. Caminiti MF, Sandor GK, Carmichael RP. Quantification of bone harvested from the iliac crest using a power-driven trephine. J Oral Maxillofac Surg 1999;57:801–5.

83. Sasso RC, Williams JI, Dimasi N, Meyer PR. Postoperative drains at the donor sites of iliac crest bone grafts. A prospective randomized study of the morbidity at the donor site in patients who have had a traumatic injury to the spine. J Bone Joint Surg 1998;80:631–5.

84. Puri R, Moskovich R, Gusmorino P, Shott S. Bupivacaine for postoperative pain relief at the iliac crest bone graft harvest site. Am J Orthop 2000;29:443–6.

85. Albee FH. Evolution of bone graft surgery. Am J Surg 1944;63:421–36.

86. Dick IL. Iliac bone transplantation. J Bone Joint Surg 1946;18:1–14.

87. Bloomquist DS, Feldman GR. The posterior ilium as a donor site for maxillofacial bone grafting. J Maxillofac Surg 1980;8:60–4.

88. Robertson PA, Wray AC. Natural history of posterior iliac crest bone graft donation for spinal surgery. Spine 2001;26:1473–6.

89. O'Keefe RM, Riemer BL, Butterfield SL. Harvesting of autogenous cancellous bone grafts from the proximal tibial metaphysis. J Orthop Trauma 1991;5:469–74.

90. Daffner RH. Case report 592. Skeletal Radiol 1990;19:73–5.

91. Sivarajasingam V, Fell G, Morse M, Shepherd JP. Secondary bone grafting of alveolar clefts: a densitometric comparison of iliac crest and tibial bone grafts. Cleft Palate Craniofac J 2001;38:11–4.

92. Catone GA, Reimer BL, McNeir D, Ray R. Tibial autogenous cancellous bone as an alternative donor site in maxillofacial surgery: a preliminary report. J Oral Maxillofac Surg 1992;50:1258–63.

93. Meeder PJ, Eggers C. Techniques for obtaining autogenous bone graft. Injury 1994;25:A5–16.

94. Jakse N, Seibert FJ, Lorenzoni M, et al. A modified technique of harvesting tibial cancellous bone and its use for sinus grafting. Clin Oral Implants Res 2001;12:488–94.

95. Herford AS, King BJ, Audia F, Bector J. Medial approach for tibial bone graft: anatomic study and clinical technique. J Oral Maxillofac Surg 2003;61:358–63.

96. van Damme PA, Merkx MA. A modification of the tibial bone graft harvesting technique. Int J Oral Maxillofac Surg 1996;25:346–8.

97. Marx RE, Carlson ER, Eichstaedt SR, et al. Platelet-rich plasma: growth factor enhancement for bone grafts. Oral Surg Oral Med Oral Path Oral Radiol Endol 1998;85:638–46.

98. Marx RE. Platelet-rich plasma (PRP): what is PRP and what is not PRP. Implant Dent 2001;10:225–8.

99. Sanchez AR, Sheridan PJ, Kupp LI. Is platelet rich plasma the perfect enhancement factor? A current review. Int J Oral Maxillofac Implants 2003;18:93–103.

100. Schmitz JP, Hollinger JO. The biology of platelet rich plasma. J Oral Maxillofac Surg 2001;29:1119–20.

101. Marx RE, Morales MJ. Morbidity from bone harvest in major jaw reconstruction: a randomized trial comparing the lateral anterior and posterior approaches to the ilium. J Oral Maxillofac Surg 1988;48:196–203.

102. Landesberg R, Roy M, Glickman RS. Quantification of growth factor levels using a simplified method of platelet-rich plasma gel preparation. J Oral Maxillofac Surg 2000;58:297–300.

103. Sonnleitner D, Huemer P, Sullivan DY. A simplified technique for producing platelet-rich plasma and platelet concentrate for intraoral bone grafting techniques: a technical note. Int J Oral Maxillofac Implants. 2000;15:879–82.

104. Rodriguez A, Anastassov GE, Lee H, et al. Maxillary sinus augmentation with deproteinated bovine bone and platelet rich plasma with simultaneous insertion of endosseous implants. J Oral Maxillofac Surg 2003;61:157–63.

105. Kassolis JD, Rosen PS, Reynolds MA. Alveolar ridge and sinus augmentation utilizing platelet-rich plasma in combination with freeze-dried bone allograft: case series. J Periodontol 2000;71:1654–61.

106. Danesh-Meyer MJ, Filstein MR, Shanaman R. Histological evaluation of sinus augmentation using platelet rich plasma (PRP) a: a case series. J Int Acad Periodontol 2001;3:48–56.

107. Lozada JL, Caplanis N, Proussaefs P, et al. Platelet-rich plasma application in sinus graft surgery: part 1—background and processing techniques. J Oral Implant 2001; 27:38–42.

108. Thor A. Reconstruction of the anterior maxilla with platelet gel, autogenous bone, and titanium mesh: a case report. Clin Implant Dent Rel Res 2002;4:150–5.

109. Wojtowicz A, Chaberek S, Kryst L, et al. Fourier and fractal analysis of maxillary alveolar ridge repair using platelet rich plasma (PRP) and inorganic bovine bone. Int J Oral Maxillofac Surg 2003;32:84–6.

110. Marx RE. Ames JR. The use of hyperbaric oxygen therapy in bony reconstruction of the irradiated and tissue-deficient patient. J Oral Maxillofac Surg 1982;40:412–20.

111. Tibbles PM, Edelsberg JS. Hyperbaric oxygen therapy. N Engl J Med 1996;334:1642–8.

112. Hunt TK, Pai MP. The effects of varying ambient oxygen tensions on wound metabolism and collagen synthesis. Surg Gynecol Obstet 1972;135:561–7.

113. Kindwall EP. Hyperbaric oxygen's effect on radiation necrosis. Clin Plast Surg 1993; 20:473–83.

CHAPTER 40

Microvascular Free Tissue Transfer

Joseph I. Helman, DMD
Remy H. Blanchaert Jr, MD, DDS

Reconstruction of the maxillofacial region has been a challenge due to the significant complexity of function and esthetics. The introduction of free tissue transfer to the armamentarium of available techniques has facilitated this task, and therefore allowed for a better quality of life for our patients. Following the description of the history of free flaps in this chapter, the surgical techniques are reviewed and discussed along with the most common specific donor sites: the radial forearm flap, the free fibula flap, and the iliac crest with the deep circumflex iliac vessels.

History of the Surgical Microscope

The development of microsurgical free tissue transfer resulted in a dramatic evolution in head and neck reconstruction, allowing for a significant increase in the available choices of anatomic and functional rehabilitation. There is no doubt that the availabilities of surgical loupes and intraoperative microscopes have been the facilitating factors to performing microvascular and microneurosurgical anastomoses.

In 1590 Dutch opticians Zacharias and Hans Janssen aligned two lenses within a sliding tube, thereby inventing the microscope. Galileo Galilei independently developed the same device a decade later by inverting his "tubum opticum" or telescope.

From the sixteenth to the nineteenth centuries many technical advances were made, including the mathematical formulas of Ernst Abbe who predicted and standardized optical qualities, allowing Zeiss to mass produce high-quality microscopes. Operating spectacles were introduced in the 1860s and surgical loupes were used for the first time in surgery by the German physician Saemisch in 1876. The first surgical microscope was built by Dr. Carl Nylen, a Swedish otolaryngologist who used it for the first time in the operating theater in 1921.[1]

History of Free Tissue Transfer for Head and Neck Reconstruction

Early attempts to achieve free tissue transfer resulted in few successes. Carrel first reported free vascularized transfer of intestine into the cervical region of experimental animals in 1907.[2] In the late 1950s and early 1960s Jacobson and Suarez performed successful anastomosis of carotid arteries in dogs and rabbits with a 100% patency rate.[3] When Jacobson presented the outcome of his research at a national meeting, a leading surgeon at a prestigious institution stated in front of the audience, "This is very nice work, but it is simply ridiculous to bring a microscope into the operating room."[1] During the 1960s the art of microsurgery was promoted by neurosurgeons and plastic surgeons with encouraging results.

New flaps were designed for reconstruction of the head and neck based on the ability to transfer distant tissues and provide immediate viability through a vascular anastomosis.

In 1975 Taylor and colleagues described the free fibula flap, while Hidalgo applied the technique for mandibular reconstruction in 1989.[4,5] In 1981 Yang developed the radial forearm flap, while Soutar and colleagues popularized the technique for intraoral reconstruction with and without the addition of a portion of the radius in the mid-1980s.[6–8] In 1978 Taylor described the transfer of the iliac crest as an osteomyocutaneous flap based on the blood supply from the circumflex artery and vein.[9,10]

Free flaps became popular in the head and neck region due to the ability to transfer vascularized bone and soft tissue in one stage at the time of the resection, with predictable high success rates. It is also obvious that they increased the choices of tissue availability, as well as pliability, texture, color, etc, in the quest to achieve an ideal reconstruction and a functional rehabilitation of the patient.

Principles of Microvascular Anastomosis

Instrumentation

The microsurgery instruments require the following specifications:

1. Their weight must not exceed 15 to 20 g. Titanium instruments usually have less weight.

2. They must be at least 10 cm long so that they lie loosely in the hand.

3. The closing pressure of some instruments such as forceps or scissors should lie between 50 and 60 g. Tremor increases with higher closing pressure.

4. The vascular clamps must exert an evenly distributed pressure over the whole length of the jaw of the clamp. The jaws must lie parallel with each other.

5. Microscissors should have an opening of less than 4 mm. They can be either straight or curved, but it is imperative that they cut tissue in a clean fashion in order to reduce the risk of a thrombosis in a vascular anastomosis or the formation of a neuroma in a crushed nerve.

6. Watchmaker forceps are extremely useful, either straight or angled. They can be used as needle holders as long as there is no need to exert a significant force on the needle, in which case a microneedle holder would be the instrument of choice.

7. Microsurgical bipolar coagulation allows for concentrated coagulation between the two ends of the forceps, avoiding unnecessary devitalization of tissues.

8. Microscope and/or loupes. Surgical microscopes were developed by Zeiss in the early days and presently there are several similar microscopes manufactured by other companies. A magnification of 10× is usually enough for anastomosis. The zoom allows for regulation from a magnification of 10× while performing the anastomosis, to a lower magnification (4× to 6×) while the suture is being knotted.[11]

Anastomosis Technique

The suture (usually 9-0) is passed at a distance from the margin of the vessel similar to that of the thickness of the wall. It is recommended to apply a counterforce while passing the needle through the vessel by holding the forceps open inside the lumen (Figures 40-1A and B) instead of grasping the vessel wall which may damage the edge of the vascular structure (Figure 40-1C). After the suture has passed through both ends of the vessel, a small "tail" of 2 to 3 mm is left in order that the knot can be performed while seeing the suture end within the field of the surgical microscope (Figures 40-1D and E).

After the first suture is placed the second suture is usually placed 180° from the first. The third suture is placed in between the first and the second, and two more interrupted sutures are placed on the same side. After finishing one side the vascular clamps are turned to expose the other side of the anastomosis. The sutures should always be at the same distance as the edges of the vessel as well as the same distance between each one of the sutures (Figure 40-2).

When the vascular anastomosis cannot be performed "end-to-end" due to very significant differences in the diameter of the lumen, an "end-to-side" anastomosis is a viable alternative (Figure 40-3). An oval excision of the wall of the large-diameter artery is performed, and the sutures are executed in a similar fashion as explained in the end-to-end anastomosis.

Radial Forearm Free Flap

Many types of free flaps have been used in head and neck reconstruction. The radial forearm flap is perhaps the most commonly used soft tissue microvascular flap for intraoral and oropharyngeal defects. It has gained wide acceptance because of its reliability, adaptability, ease of harvest, and the thin pliable nature of the flap. The flap allows restoration of the complex three-dimensional anatomy inherent in oral and oropharyngeal defects. This is demonstrated by the commonplace reconstruction of combined tongue and floor-of-mouth defects. Folding the flap on itself to simultaneously reconstruct the tongue and floor of mouth creates redundancy and allows the residual tongue to retain outstanding mobility (Figure 40-4).

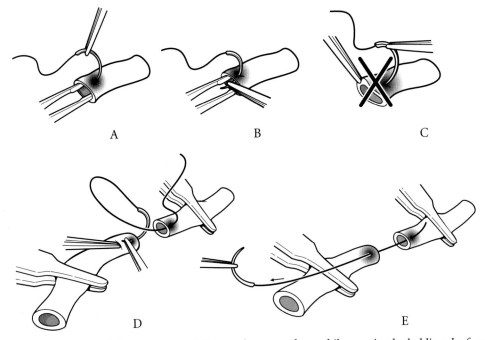

FIGURE 40-1 *A and B, It is recommended to apply counterforce while suturing by holding the forceps open inside the lumen. C, Grasping the vessel with the forceps may damage the edge of the vessel. While passing the needle the motion should be circular, following the needle shape in order to avoid a tear of the vascular structure. D and E, A small "tail" of 2 to 3 mm should be left at the end of the suture to perform the knot within the microscope surgical field. Adapted from Medhorn HM and Muller GH.[11]*

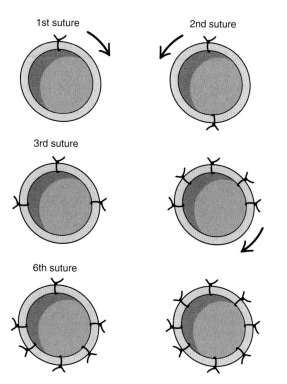

1st suture   2nd suture

3rd suture

6th suture

FIGURE **40-2** *The first and second sutures are performed 180° from each other. The third suture is placed between the first two while holding the vessel on both sides with the tails of the first and second sutures. After interrupted sutures are placed on one side of the vessel, the microvascular clamps are turned to expose the other side of the anastomosis and proceed in a similar fashion as on the first side. Adapted from Medhorn HM and Muller GH.[11]*

tive mandibular reconstruction using the osteocutaneous radial forearm flap and dental implants.[16] The volume and height of the bone compare poorly to those of other flaps. The fibula and deep circumflex iliac artery flap appear to have the most suitable bone stock to facilitate dental implant–based mandibular rehabilitation and are therefore more popular when bone is necessary.[17]

Refinement and adaptation of the radial forearm flap continued throughout the early 1990s. Urken and colleagues reported on the use of the neurofasciocutaneous radial forearm flap in head and neck reconstruction.[18] This report included a means of monitoring buried or poorly accessible flaps that could be facilitated by the inclusion of a skin paddle on the proximal fascial/subcutaneous element of the flap. Protection of the flap vessels and augmentation of the contour deformity created by neck dissection are additional advantages of this modification.[19,20] The literature abounds with descriptions of suitable adaptations of the radial forearm flap to specific sites within the head and neck. Urken and Biller published a

Clinically the skin paddle of the radial forearm flap often takes on an appearance similar to that of oral mucosa following its transfer to the oral cavity. This change in appearance has been shown to be reactive in nature and does not represent true metaplasia.[12]

Development

The history of the spread of understanding of the flap is interesting. Soutar and colleagues reported and referenced the introduction of the flap to German surgeons visiting China in 1980.[7] Subsequently these surgeons published in the German language literature on the use of the radial forearm as a donor site for the creation of neurofasciocutaneous and osteocutaneous flaps in neck and in hand reconstructions.

Soutar and colleagues reported the use of the radial forearm flap in primary mandibular reconstruction in 1983.[7] Corrigan and O'Neill published a report of the cases outlining the technique of osteocutaneous flap harvest and transfer, and included a description of complications encountered.[13] The most devastating of these complications is distal radius frac-

ture, which results in significant deformity. Vaughan documented extensive experience with 120 radial forearm flaps, praising the adaptability and applicability of the flap in head and neck reconstruction.[14,15] Published reports have demonstrated it to be possible to perform defini-

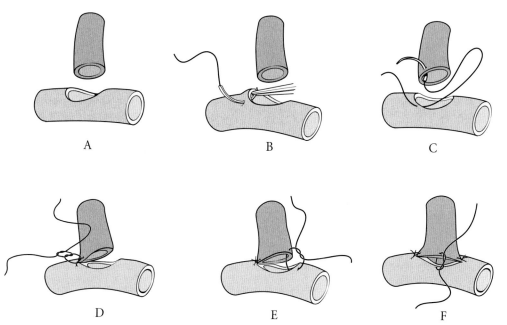

A   B   C

D   E   F

FIGURE **40-3**   A–F, *The end-to-side anastomosis is performed after excision of an oval segment of the "side" donor vessel. The sequence of suturing is similar to the technique described in Figure 40-2. Adapted from Medhorn HM and Muller GH.[11]*

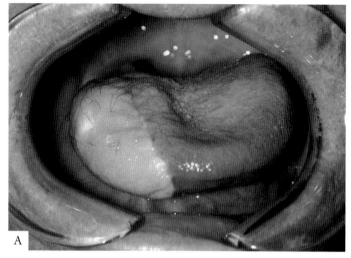

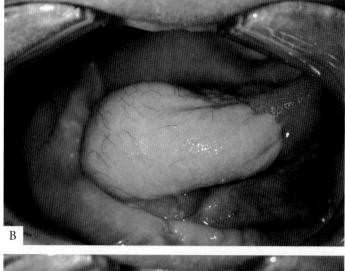

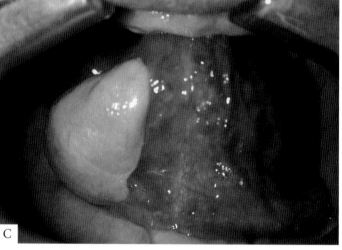

FIGURE **40-4** *Clinical photos taken at a 3-month follow-up examination illustrating the excellent mobility achieved following right partial glossectomy and free radial forearm flap (FRFF) reconstruction. This degree of mobility is common and is the primary reason for the minimal alteration in function following hemiglossectomy reconstruction with the FRFF. A, Unlimited protrusion of the tongue. B, Excellent lateral motion of the tongue is clearly demonstrated. C, Elevation of the tongue tip is unimpaired.*

description of a bilobed neurofasciocutaneous flap for hemiglossectomy defects that allows preservation of residual tongue function.[21] Oromandibular reconstruction has been reported using the free radial forearm flap alone or in combination with a fibula free flap.[7,13,22,23] Lower lip reconstruction has been described wherein the palmaris longus tendon provides support and suspension to the flap.[24,25] Simultaneous lip and cheek, full-thickness cheek, and soft palate reconstruction have also been described.[24–28] Oral cavity and pharyngoesophageal reconstruction with the radial forearm flap has advantages over other reconstructive modalities, demonstrating good functional outcomes.[29,30] Reconstruction of facial defects (forehead, nasal) has also been described as an appropriate use of the radial forearm flap.[31,32]

Extreme uses of the flap include reports of the creation of hybrid flaps, wherein the cephalic vein remains pedicled for use in cases with inadequate venous outflow and the simultaneous use of bilateral flaps.[33,34]

Throughout the development of the free radial forearm flap, reinnervation of the flap has received considerable attention. Many authors have discussed the role of sensory reinnervation in functional outcomes in oral cavity and oropharynx reconstruction.[17,18,21,35,36] Recall that some of the earliest descriptions of the use of the flap were neurofasciocutaneous flaps.[7] The neurofasciocutaneous radial forearm flap is typically designed to include only the median antebrachial cutaneous nerve (see Figure 40-6). Sensory nerve mapping accomplished by cadaveric microdissection and selective nerve block technique

in 8 forearms of 4 human subjects has revealed that much of the skin territory harvested with the flap is supplied by either the lateral antebrachial cutaneous nerve or the superficial radial sensory nerve.[37] This brings into question the means by which the radial forearm flap achieves reinnervation. Many authors have postulated that reinnervation occurs by ingrowth of nerve fibers from the recipient bed and peripheral or adjacent tissues.[27,36,38–41] Close and colleagues compared spontaneous sensory recovery in myocutaneous pectoralis major flaps and radial forearm fasciocutaneous flaps and found the forearm flaps to exhibit significantly better sensation.[35] This supports the idea that the characteristics of both the flap and the recipient bed influence the sensory recovery within non-reinnervated soft tissue flaps. Netscher and colleagues studied 12 patients who underwent free radial forearm flap reconstruction of the tongue and floor of mouth.[39] Seven patients received reinnervated flaps and 5 received flaps without intentional neural anastomosis. Improved sensory recovery in the patients who received reinnervated flaps was documented, but no statistically significant difference in function could be found.

Santamaria and colleagues reported objectively evaluated sensory recovery in reinnervated flaps to be near normal when neural anastomosis was accomplished to the lingual or inferior alveolar nerve.[36] Sensation was found to be poor if the anastomosis was carried out to other recipient nerves (posterior auricular nerve, cervical plexus, hypoglossal nerve). The study also found the recovery of sensation to be significantly diminished in patients who received postoperative radiotherapy. In summary the decision to perform the radial forearm flap as a neurofasciocutaneous flap must be made on a case-by-case basis dependant on the defect characteristics and location, recipient bed, and the ability to accomplish anastomosis to the lingual or inferior alveolar nerve.

Anatomic Considerations

Blood Supply The arterial blood supply of the radial forearm fasciocutaneous flap is based on perforators of the radial artery. The fascial plexus supplied by these perforators supplies the skin of nearly the entire forearm. There are discrete groups of these perforators. The most clinically relevant is the small number of perforators at the site where the flexor carpi radialis and brachioradialis muscles overlap. One particularly relevant implication of this is the ability to develop multiple skin flap elements based on a single vascular pedicle without the requirement of preservation of the entire fascial element.[42,43] The bone element of the flap is supplied by branches of the radi-

al artery within the lateral intramuscular septum. Branches that form a longitudinal plexus within the periosteum pass through the insertion of this fascia.[44]

The venous drainage of the radial forearm flap occurs through the interconnecting superficial (cephalic vein) and deep (venae comitantes) systems. Thoma and colleagues published an excellent description of the variation on the pattern of venous drainage identified in 40 clinical cases.[22] Five distinct patterns were described. The type I pattern, found 20% of the time, exhibits wide communication of an anastomosing vein of the venae comitantes and the cephalic vein, which split to separate cephalic median and basilic median veins. The type II pattern existed 43% of the time and was similar to type I, with the exception that no division of the fusion of vessels occurred. The type III pattern, seen 18% of the time, displayed an anastomosis of the paired venae comitantes that remained separate from the cephalic vein. The type IV pattern occurred 5% of the time and exhibited no fusion of the venae comitantes of near equal size. Although pattern V, seen 15% of the time, also exhibited no fusion of the two systems, there was clearly a dominant venae comitantes.[45] Thoma and colleagues made a strong recommendation for completing multiple venous anastomoses. Their view appears to be common in early free flap and replant experiences. However, a single venous anastomosis has been shown to be adequate in the more recent literature. Futran and Stack compared outcomes and operating time in 43 consecutive radial forearm flaps.[46] Two anastomoses were performed in 16 patients and one anastomosis was performed in 23 patients. They reported no difference in flap survival and no flaps were re-explored for venous complications. Twenty-one to 36 minutes less surgical time was documented in cases in which a single venous anastomosis was completed. Surgeon preference and individual patient and flap

characteristics determine the most appropriate vein for anastomosis. Clearly in cases with a superficial venous system compromised by trauma or extensive venipuncture, the deep system (venae comitantes) must be used. The reliability of the deep system has been well documented.[47] Netscher and colleagues used dye injection to study the venous drainage system.[48] They found that careful mapping of the cephalic vein was necessary to ensure its capture within the flap, occasionally necessitating localization of the flap skin paddle over a portion of the dorsum of the forearm. Venae comitantes vessel diameters were found to be less than 2 mm in several specimens. The study also concluded that selection of the site for venous anastomosis significantly alters the vessel diameter. In order to obtain the greatest diameter, the confluence of the venae comitantes must be identified. This may result in venous pedicle redundancy and kinking. The superficial venous drainage system exhibits a larger diameter throughout its entire length and is significantly easier to elevate, and its separation from the arterial pedicle increases options for recipient vein selection with acceptable vessel geometry.

Vascular Abnormalities Preoperative evaluation of the arterial supply to the hand is required prior to harvest of the free radial forearm flap. This is traditionally accomplished by an Allen's test. Accurate performance of the test involves exsanguination of the hand by clenching and releasing the fist multiple times while both the radial and ulnar arteries are compressed. Return of color to the blanched thenar eminence and thumb following release of the ulnar artery confirms adequate communication between the superficial (ulnar) and deep (radial) palmar arches. Thus harvest of the flap would not compromise the blood supply to the hand. A single published report of acute ischemia to the hand following radial forearm flap harvest despite a "normal" Allen's test initiated further investigation into forearm vascular anatomy.[49] The subjective nature of the Allen's test has led to the use of adjunctive clinical aids such as Doppler and pulse oximetry to ensure adequate perfusion of the thumb with radial artery occlusion. In their description of a method for preoperative vascular assessment, Nukols and colleagues reported the use of an "objective Allen's test" in a clinical series of 65 patients.[50] Twenty-five patients were thought to have inadequate flow by subjective testing, 18 of whom were found to have acceptable flow by objective testing. The authors concluded that objective testing was more reliable in identifying potential problem donor sites. Color flow duplex assessment of 18 patients revealed 5 with unilateral or bilateral arteriopathy. This finding impacted the site selection of the radial forearm harvest or resulted in the use of alternate reconstructive modalities in those 5 cases.[51] Interestingly, color flow duplex quantifications of the flow rates in the upper extremities of 11 patients preoperatively and 4 to 5 months postoperatively revealed overall increased flow rates (mean 162 mL/min to 215 mL/min). The increased flow resulted from dramatic increases in blood flow through the anterior and posterior interosseous arteries. In fact the anterior interosseous artery was found to take on a flow rate (33% of the total) that was nearly equal to that of the radial artery before flap harvest (39%).[51,52]

Many authors have published case reports of vascular abnormalities of the radial artery.[39,53–57] Funk and colleagues published a review of the literature on forearm vascular anomalies that included clinical correlation based on 52 patients.[58] The paper described six types of anomalies, the most common of these being a high origin (proximal to the antecubital fossa) of the radial artery occurring in approximately 15% of all upper extremities. The majority of radial arteries in these patients originate from the brachial artery,

but 10 to 25% were reported to arise directly from the axillary artery. This anomaly poses no problem for safe radial forearm flap harvest. The second most common anomaly reported was a superficial ulnar artery. The superficial location of the ulnar artery places the vessel at risk in flaps involving the entire volar surface of the forearm. Surgeons are strongly encouraged to palpate the entire antecubital fossa and volar forearm in order to rule out this anomaly. The abnormal vessel course is typically best palpated overlying the flexor carpi muscle. The superficial ulnar artery anomaly reported in 2.5% of upper extremities should prompt the surgeon to preferentially use other sites for flap harvest because of the risk incurred in selection of such a donor site. The flap can be done safely with this anomaly if the flap is positioned more to the radial side of the ventral forearm. Distal takeoff of the radial artery has been reported once. No risk of vascular insufficiency is incurred with this anomaly, and there is no reason to believe it could be identified prior to flap elevation. The other anomalies reported result in significant risk of vascular insufficiency to the hand in the case of radial artery flap harvest and should be easily identified on the basis of abnormal Allen's tests (Figure 40-5).

Complications In general, patients with head and neck defects tend to be less than ideal surgical candidates because of medical comorbidities. Comorbidities are common and are related to advanced age, alcohol abuse, and tobacco abuse. Complications can occur at the operative sites directly or they may be medically related. Singh and colleagues analyzed a cohort of 200 consecutive patients with head and neck defects who had undergone free tissue transfer, to determine factors that influence both surgical site and medical complication rates.[59] Successful free tissue transfer was accomplished in 98% of cases. Complications occurred in 56 cases (28%) with 21 (10.5%)

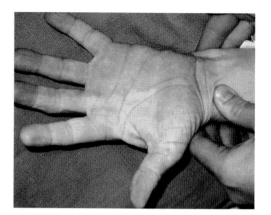

FIGURE 40-5 *An abnormal Allen's test. Note the clearly delineated vascular territory of the ulnar artery.*

patients developing multiple complications. Using univariate analysis, statistically significant factors that increased the risk of complication included prior radiation therapy, anesthesia time >10 hours, and advanced Charlson comorbidity grade. However, after multivariate analysis only advanced Charlson grade proved significant. Prior radiation therapy appeared to have no significant effect on flap survival, as reported in other studies, although significant alteration in technique including vein grafting may be required.[60,61] Surgical time has also been shown to correlate significantly with increased rates of surgical site infection, which is the most common factor in late vascular compromise of free tissue transfers through direct effect on the vascular pedicle.[62,63]

The free radial forearm flap is a very reliable reconstruction. The international microvascular research group published a multi-institutional prospective study of 493 free flaps.[64] In a subgroup of the report, 84 free radial forearm flaps exhibited a thrombosis rate of 8.3% and a flap failure rate of 3.6%, indicating a significant role for flap monitoring and flap salvage surgery in head and neck reconstruction.

Monitoring of the radial forearm flap is required in order to identify early compromise of the flap vasculature. Conventional techniques of monitoring have been shown to be adequate for this purpose. These techniques include visual inspection for color, capillary refill assessment, Doppler probe assessment, and needlestick test. Flap design for deep or buried flaps in which direct observation is not possible should include either a monitor skin paddle that can be directly evaluated or an implantable Doppler probe.[20,65] An extensive review of 750 consecutive microvascular flaps demonstrated a re-exploration rate of 8.5% and a flap loss rate of 2.3%.[65] The majority of those flaps salvaged were re-explored at < 48 hours due to observed changes in the parameters monitored. Late re-exploration at > 72 hours was most commonly the result of wound infection causing compromise of the vascular pedicle by pressure or thrombosis. Late re-exploration is associated with high rates of flap loss.

Several assessments of donor site morbidity of the radial forearm flap harvest have been carried out.[66–70] Complete or partial failure of split thickness skin graft at the donor site is the most common complication encountered. This can lead to flexor tendon exposure and prolonged healing. Many methods have been devised to decrease the incidence of this complication including coverage of the defect with rotation/advancement flaps, preoperative tissue expansion and primary closure, full-thickness grafting, suprafascial dissection, and the use of vacuum-assisted wound care.[71–79]

A devastating complication of osteocutaneous radial forearm flap harvest is postoperative radius fracture. Prophylactic plating is strongly recommended when bone is included in the flap.[80,81] Selection of an alternative donor site seems a more prudent alternative provided that one is available. Overall, with the exception of cases in which a radius fracture occurs, donor site function, though objectively altered, is subjectively insignificant.[62,66,68]

Flap Technique

Simultaneous clinical evaluation of the tumor defect site by both the ablative and reconstructive surgeons is particularly useful in design of the radial forearm flap and allows planning for the most appropriate vessel geometry. Careful examination of the proposed donor site is required to verify the patency of the superficial venous system and to document the arterial anatomy of the hand. An Allen's test is mandatory and should be supplemented with Doppler or pulse oximetry whenever the examination is inconclusive. Palpation of the entire forearm to determine the vascular anatomy should be done without a tourniquet (arterial assessment) and with the use of a venipuncture tourniquet and dependant positioning of the upper extremity (venous anatomy).

Preliminary planning is supplemented by the intraoperative examination of both the resection specimen and the defect site. Occasionally modifications are required due to extension of the planned resection to achieve tumor margins or due to vascular insufficiency identified in access flaps following a lip split–mandibulotomy procedure. Accurate determinations of the pedicle length required allow further tailoring of the flap harvest to the specifics of the defect site. This facilitates flap harvest because the surgeon need not dissect the entire available vascular pedicle length. This also facilitates the anastomosis procedure because the surgeon can skeletonize the region of the pedicle at which the anastomosis will be completed during a non-ischemic period.

The donor site is prepared for surgery by removing hair in the surgical field with clippers. The radial artery is outlined along its length with a surgical marker. A venipuncture tourniquet is applied to distend the veins and the superficial venous system is outlined with a surgical marker. A preliminary outline of the flap is then marked on the wrist that will be refined following the completion of the resection and identification of the most appropriate recipient vessels. For most cases a fasciosubcutaneous segment of the flap proximal to the skin paddle can be included to optimize the blood supply, resist vessel kinking, and protect the vascular pedicle. The surgical site is prepared with a chlorhexidine surgical scrub and isolated using extremity drapes. A standard armboard is sufficient for support of the extremity throughout surgery. Care is taken to ensure absolute isolation of the arm from the head and neck field. Cross-contamination has been implicated in causing suppurative tenosynovitis resulting in a frozen hand.[82]

Upon completion of the resection or refining of the defect site, the neck is carefully explored to identify likely recipient vessels. The selected vessels should be checked for patency, presence of atherosclerosis, and intimal injury. Loupe magnification facilitates this process. Although any suitable vessel can be used as a recipient vessel, the facial artery and common facial vein are most commonly selected as recipient vessels in intraoral reconstruction. Because these vessels lie central in the lateral neck, less alteration of the flap vessel geometry occurs on extreme head movement when these vessels are used. The reader is reminded of the transverse cervical artery (a branch of the thyrocervical trunk) because of its similar diameter to the radial artery. Because of the position of the transverse cervical artery low in the neck, it is commonly available and in good condition following prior selective neck dissection or radiotherapy. Although the available pedicle length allows for use of neck vessels, when performing an upper facial reconstruction the superficial temporal artery and vein or the facial artery and vein are often used.

Daily aspirin therapy to decrease platelet aggregation is initiated on the evening of surgery and continued for 6 weeks. Flap harvest is accomplished following exsanguination of the upper extremity and inflation of a tourniquet to 250 mm Hg. Tourniquet control facilitates the flap harvest by maximizing visualization. This creates an excellent environment for teaching the microvascular flap harvest technique. Enough cannot be said about the crucial role that gentle tissue/vessel handling plays in the ultimate viability of the microvascular transfer. The distal flap is elevated first, requiring ligation of the distal radial artery and cephalic vein. A subfascial plane of dissection allows capture of all available communications between the elements of the vascular supply of the flap without significantly increased morbidity (Figure 40-6).

The superficial radial nerve is resected to avoid violation of the fascial compartment. This can be used as a free nerve graft of 4 to 6 cm length if needed. The sensory defect is limited to the dorsal portion of the thumb and index finger. We have found that skin graft placement over a preserved dorsal radial nerve provides insufficient protection. Severe pain can result from stimulation of the nerve by a sleeve or wristwatch.

Continued dissection around the circumference of the designed flap is accomplished deep to fascia laterally and deep to the dermis proximally. Skin flaps are then elevated proximally coincident with the

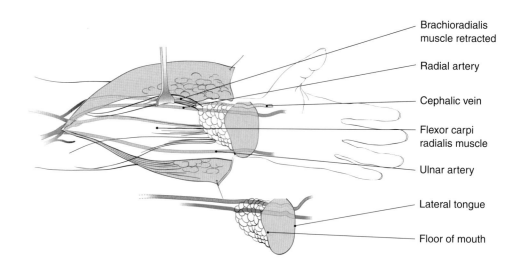

FIGURE **40-7**   *The harvest of the flap. Note the retraction of the brachioradialis muscle required to dissect the radial artery.*

volume of the planned fasciosubcutaneous element of the flap. Proximal to this the cephalic vein and antebrachial cutaneous nerve are isolated. Proximal dissection of the arterial vascular pedicle requires the separation of the fascia joining the flexor carpi radialis and brachioradialis muscles and the lateral retraction of these muscles (Figure 40-7).

The venae comitantes are dissected from the radial artery for a few centimeters either side of the planned arterial

anastomosis and are preserved. Where one of the venae comitantes is clearly dominant, only this vessel is preserved. Numerous interconnections exist between these two vessels and careful dissection is required to achieve their separation. With the vascularity assured the flap is then elevated distal to proximal. This requires identification and ligation of deep branches of the radial artery. We prefer to use titanium vessel clips to accomplish this. These facilitate rapid flap harvest and are excellent markers of the pedicle position in the event that the neck must be explored at a later date. After completion of the flap harvest, the tourniquet is released. Careful examination of the flap during this reperfusion interval should be accomplished to ensure absolute hemostasis because access following inset and reanastomosis will be limited. The surgeon should examine the hand for adequate perfusion. Tourniquet time less than 45 minutes is the norm following familiarity with the flap harvest. This can be significantly less with increased surgical experience.

The vascular pedicle is then transected following a suitable period of reperfusion (30 minutes on average). The flap vessels should be occluded with appropriately sized microvascular clamps during completion of the inset. The flap is then transferred

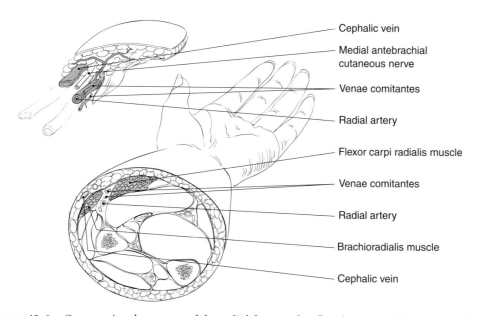

FIGURE **40-6**   *Cross-sectional anatomy of the radial forearm free flap donor site. The harvested flap demonstrates subfascial dissection of the flexor compartment. Adapted from Urken ML.[99]*

to the defect site. Care must be taken to avoid rotation or kinking of the flap vessels, particularly when the flap must be passed through a tunnel to the defect site. Insetting should be accomplished completely prior to microvascular anastomosis to allow accurate determination of the vascular pedicle geometry. Meticulous closure with gentle eversion to achieve a watertight seal is necessary because of the deleterious effects of saliva on the flap vessels. Care is taken to achieve a flap vessel–recipient vessel geometry that contains only slight curves to prevent vessel kinking. We prefer end-to-end interrupted sutured anastomoses with the vessels secured in Acland frame clamps. The artery is approximated first because the recipient artery is generally deeper than the venous structures. Heparinized saline (500 U/100 cc NS) is used to irrigate during the anastomosis. Papavarine is occasionally used if arterial spasm is noted. It should be recognized that gentle handling is the best defense against spasm. Following the release of the approximator clamps, the flap should be carefully evaluated. Evaluation of color and capillary refill is generally adequate for flap monitoring. In situations wherein this is difficult or the status of the flap is unclear, pricking the flap with a 25-gauge needle confirms flap perfusion. Color and character of the bleeding are important. A venous-compromised flap will bleed dark blood that does not clot as well as serous fluid.

Closed-suction drains are used in the neck with care taken to prevent them being displaced onto the vascular pedicle. The proximal skin flaps at the donor site are approximated over a closed-suction drain. The distal skin elements are sutured to the muscle to fixate them. A split-thickness skin graft is placed over the donor site defect and secured. A compressive dressing and volar splint or vacuum-assisted closure dressing are applied. These remain in place for 5 days. Active and passive range-of-motion exercises are initiated at 2 weeks post flap harvest.

The free radial forearm fasciocutaneous flap is extremely useful in head and neck reconstruction. The flap's reliability, adaptability, ease of harvest, and the similar character of the thin pliable skin to the lining tissues of the oral cavity make its use commonplace in modern maxillofacial reconstruction.

Free Fibula Flap

Anatomic Considerations

The fibula is ideal for large bony defects since it offers up to 25 cm of vascularized cortical bone. If we view the fibula in a cross section, we can identify a triangular shape established by three borders. The anterior border is the area of attachment of the anterior intermuscular septum, and the interosseous or medial border is the point of attachment of the interosseous membrane that binds the fibula to the tibia. The posterior intermuscular septum attaches to the posterior border (Figure 40-8).

In the proximal aspect the fibula articulates with the tibia and the knee joint, whereas in the distal aspect it articulates with the tibia and the talus.

Above the knee the popliteal artery divides into the anterior and posterior tibial arteries. Distal to the knee the posterior

tibial artery has a collateral branch, the peroneal artery. The blood supply to the fibula is delivered through perforators originating in the peroneal artery which is usually between 2 and 4 mm in diameter. The venae comitantes provide the venous drainage; these are paired vessels that run along the artery (Figure 40-9).

A significant limitation of the free fibula flap is the common presence of peripheral vascular disease in the lower extremities. In population-based studies that evaluated the incidence of arterial disease in the lower extremity in patients older than 55 years, the parameter was an ankle-brachial index lower than 0.9.[83] The value was obtained by dividing the systolic blood pressure measured at the ankle by that obtained at the brachial artery. A Danish study that included 700 individuals aged 60 years showed a prevalence of lower extremity arterial disease of 16% in men and 13% in women.[84] A similar study from Edinburgh showed an overall incidence of 17%.[83]

Unfortunately the same risk factors (age and tobacco) are a common denominator for head and neck cancer patients as well as patients with peripheral vascular disease; therefore, it is indicated to perform either a conventional angiography or

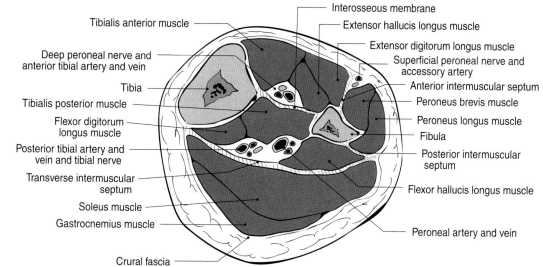

FIGURE **40-8** *Cross-sectional view of the tibia and fibula with the surrounding anatomic structures. Adapted from Serafin D.[93]*

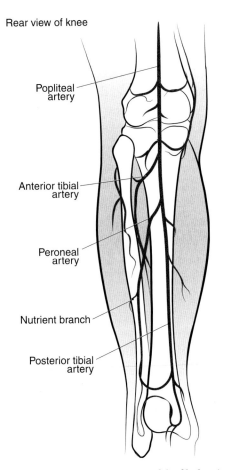

Rear view of knee

Popliteal artery

Anterior tibial artery

Peroneal artery

Nutrient branch

Posterior tibial artery

FIGURE **40-9**   *Vascular anatomy of the fibula, view from a posterior view of the leg. Adapted from O'Leary MJ et al.*[88]

a magnetic resonance angiography to establish the safety of harvesting the flap.

In a recent retrospective study Smith and colleagues reviewed 17 potential free fibula flap candidates (34 legs) evaluated by both a color flow Doppler (CDF) and angiography. Sixteen legs were normal by both studies, 18 legs showed abnormal CFD study results, and the angiogram revealed anatomy that was considered to represent a high risk for fibula flap harvest in 16 legs and considered safe in the other 2 legs.[85]

The free fibula flap can be raised with or without a skin paddle. The skin paddle had a poor prognosis, based on the original series by Hidalgo who harvested the attached skin based on septocutaneous perforators.[5] Schusterman and colleagues later performed an anatomic study that showed more soleus musculocutaneous

perforators than septal perforators.[86] Furthermore the clinical success of the skin paddle is above 90% when the musculocutaneous perforators are incorporated in the flap, whereas the viability of the skin is only 33% when the flap is based on septal branches.

Neurosensory potential to the skin paddle was described by Hayden and colleagues by incorporating the lateral cutaneous nerve of the calf (LCNC) and/or the sural communicating nerve (SCN) in order to restore intraoral sensation by anastomosis of the lingual nerve to the LCNC and/or the inferior alveolar nerve to the SCN.[87,88]

Flap Technique

The patient is placed in the supine position, the hip and the knee are slightly flexed, and a pneumatic tourniquet is placed in the proximal aspect of the leg. A line is drawn from the lateral malleolus to the fibular head. If a skin paddle is included, it should be centered more posteriorly than the axis of the fibula in order to include both the septocutaneous and the musculocutaneous perforators.

The dissection is carried down to the crural fascia that is incised. The dissection continues through the anterior border of the peroneal muscles while maintaining a cuff of 2 to 3 mm of muscle surrounding the bone. The extensor digitorum longus and the extensor hallucis longus are elevated anteriorly, exposing the interosseous septum that connects between the fibula and the tibia. The peroneal vessels and the anterior tibial vessels are located posterior to the interosseous septum; therefore, careful dissection with fine dissecting scissors should be performed in order to avoid damage to the vascular structures or to the deep peroneal nerve. At this stage, two horizontal incisions are performed in the proximal and distal aspects of the fibula where the osteotomy is being planned. The bony cuts are performed with a Gigli, a reciprocating, or an oscillating saw while the medial aspect is protected with a malleable

retractor. The peroneal vessels are ligated in their distal aspect and the vascular pedicle is carefully dissected superiorly until the branching of the peroneal artery from the posterior tibial is identified. The flexor hallucis longus muscle and part of the soleus muscle are included in the flap, especially if a skin paddle is planned (Figure 40-10).

It is recommended to perform the osteotomies to shape the fibula while pedicled to the proximal vessels in order to minimize the ischemia time as well as preparation of the vessels in the recipient site before ligation of the proximal aspect of the peroneal artery.

The skin defect in the leg can be closed primarily or through the addition of a split-thickness skin graft.

An example of the application of this technique is as follows:

A patient presented with a large mass in the anterior aspect of the mandible with an obvious clinical deformity due to significant buccal expansion of the buccal cortical bone, with a progressive growth during the 3 years previous to his clinical evaluation (Figure 40-11). Panoramic radiography showed a multilocular lesion extending from tooth no. 21 to tooth no. 31 (Figure 40-12).

A histopathologic diagnosis of ameloblastoma was obtained through an incisional biopsy of the lesion. A magnetic resonance angiogram was obtained which showed a normal vascular pattern in both lower extremities. A segmental resection of the lesion was performed along with the mental and inferior alveolar nerves (Figure 40-13).

The defect was immediately reconstructed with a free fibula flap without the need for a skin paddle since residual mucosa was available for primary closure. Two osteotomies were performed in the fibula to allow for appropriate contour, resulting in three bony segments that were fixated to the recipient mandible by means of a reconstruction plate (Figure 40-14). A postoperative panoramic radiograph was obtained

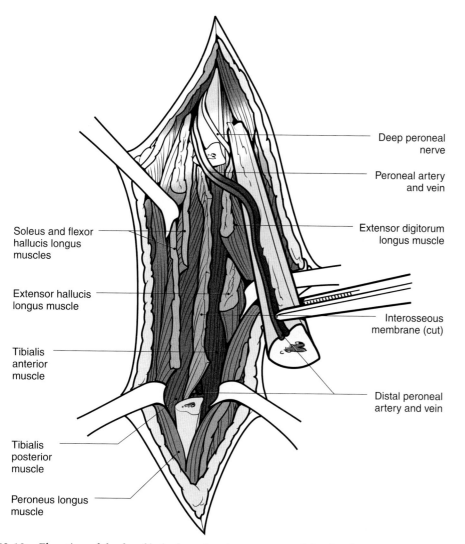

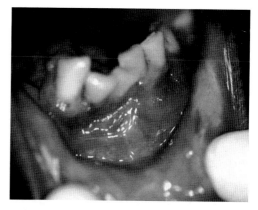

FIGURE **40-11** *Clinical aspect of a patient with buccal expansion of the mandible due to a large ameloblastoma.*

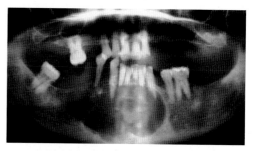

FIGURE **40-12** *Radiographic view of the patient in Figure 40-11 with a large ameloblastoma of the mandible.*

FIGURE **40-10** *Elevation of the free fibula flap after the osteotomy of the distal and proximal attachments. The ligation of the feeding vessels is obvious in the distal aspect of the flap, while the proximal blood supply is maintained until the osteotomies are performed. Adapted from Serafin D.* [93]

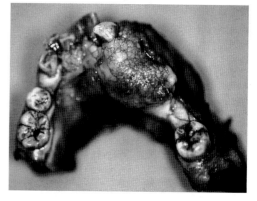

FIGURE **40-13** *Mandibular specimen after surgical resection of the ameloblastoma.*

which showed good continuity of the bony segments (Figure 40-15). In a previous retrospective study it was reported that radiographic bony healing was achieved in 93% of osteotomy sites of free fibula flaps.[89]

The amount of bone available in free flaps in order to place osseointegrated implants has been investigated in an anatomic study in 28 cadavers evaluating the most commonly employed donor sites.[90] Implantability was established based on measurements of height, width, and cross-sectional area. The results showed that the iliac crest was the most implantable donor site (83%), followed by the scapula (78%), the fibula (67%), and the radius (21%).[90]

A retrospective analysis of patients treated with a free fibular flap for mandibular reconstruction was performed by Disa and colleagues evaluating the long-term bone mass of the fibula.[89] Only patients with at least 24 months of follow-up were included in the study. The comparative measurements of fibular height revealed that central segments underwent a mean decrease in height by 4%, body segments decreased by 7%, and ramus segments decreased by 5%. The findings were not affected by the site of reconstruction, patient age, length of follow-up, adjuvant radiation therapy, or placement of osseointegrated implants.

Morbidity following Free Fibula Flaps

A retrospective analysis of donor site morbidity was performed by Shindo and colleagues on 53 consecutive patients who underwent fibula osteocutaneous free tissue transfer.[91] Donor site wound complications occurred in 15 patients, 4 of whom (8%) had extensive wound breakdown,

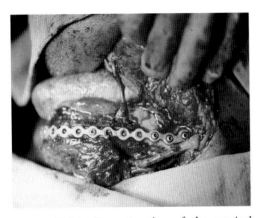

FIGURE **40-14** *Reconstruction of the surgical defect with a free fibula flap. The structures located superior to the reconstruction plate are the spared inferior alveolar and mental nerves. The vascular structures below the screws and the reconstruction plate at the level of the angle of the mandible are the peroneal vessels after microanastomosis to the facial vessels.*

muscle necrosis, and/or exposure of tendon and/or bone, whereas the other 11 patients (21%) had only minor wound complications limited to superficial skin slough.

Shindo and colleagues recommended avoiding skin closure under tension since the group with the higher complication rate had primary closure of the donor site.[91] Other reported complications have included weakness of great toe dorsiflexion, reduced spring action of the donor leg, ankle stiffness, and in a few cases, ankle instability. Despite the mentioned deficits, all patients were able to resume daily and recreational activities.[92]

Iliac Crest Osteomyocutaneous Free Flap

Anatomic Considerations

The blood supply to the osteomyocutaneous iliac crest flap is based on the deep circumflex iliac artery (DCIA) and vein. The DCIA takes origin from the external iliac artery or femoral artery in the region of the inguinal canal (42% below the inguinal ligament from the femoral artery, 41% behind the inguinal ligament from the external iliac artery, and 17% above the inguinal ligament from the external iliac artery).[93]

The artery courses a distance of about 5 to 7 cm between its origin and the anterior superior iliac spine, following thereon the inner aspect of the iliac crest. The DCIA provides an ascending branch that perforates through the transversus abdominis muscle giving blood supply to the transversus as well as the internal and external oblique muscles (Figure 40-16).

Through its pathway the artery provides multiple perforators to the bone, muscle, and overlying skin. The deep circumflex iliac vein follows the arterial course.

The lateral femoral cutaneous nerve crosses the DCIA near the anterior superior iliac spine. The nerve should be dissected, retracted, and protected during the harvesting of the vascular pedicle and the flap.

Flap Technique

The skin paddle is designed by drawing a line from the femoral artery to the inferior angle of the scapula. The skin paddle is then designed with an axis on the abovementioned line and centered on the iliac crest, including the myocutaneous perforators which enter the skin along the inner aspect of the crest.

The external oblique muscle (with the attached overlying skin) is incised, leaving a cuff of about 3 cm of muscle attached to the inner aspect of the iliac crest. If a significant portion of the internal oblique muscle has to be harvested in order to cover soft tissue defects in the oropharyngeal region, then the muscle is divided in a horizontal fash-

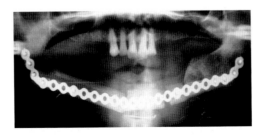

FIGURE **40-15** *Radiographic view of the reconstructed mandible with a free fibula flap.*

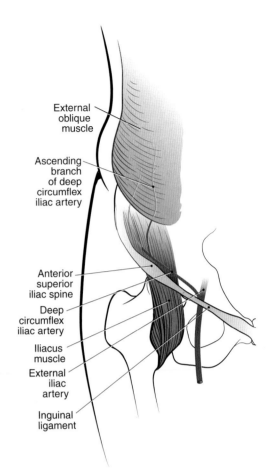

FIGURE **40-16** *Anatomy of the deep circumflex iliac artery (DCIA). Adapted from Strauch B, Yu HL, editors. Atlas of microvascular surgery. New York: Thieme Medical Publisher Inc.; 1993. p. 142–58.*

ion below the costal margin, and the dissection is initiated in the superior, medial, and lateral aspects while incorporating the ascending branch of the DCIA. After identifying the ascending branch of the DCIA in the inner aspect of the internal oblique muscle, the deep circumflex iliac vessels are dissected proximally. The transversus abdominis muscle is incised parallel to the crest, leaving a cuff of about 3 cm attached to the inner aspect of the crest.

The peritoneum is then retracted medially and the iliacus muscle is identified. The transversalis fascia fuses with the iliacus fascia, and the deep circumflex vessels consistently travel lateral to this fascial fusion. A 1 to 2 cm incision is performed medial to the insertion of the iliacus fascia down to the periosteum.

The lateral or lower aspect of the skin paddle is incised, proceeding through the deep fascia of the thigh and the gluteus muscle, detaching them from the periosteum of the lateral aspect of the iliac crest until achieving the desired bone depth (Figure 40-17).

When both the medial and lateral cortices are exposed, the osteotomy is performed.

If additional osteotomies are necessary in order to contour the bone, it is recommended to proceed while the tissue is still pedicled to the feeding deep circumflex vessels.

After the flap is harvested the muscles are approximated in layers to prevent the potential complication of herniation of the abdominal contents. The transversalis fascia and transverse abdominis muscle are sutured to the iliacus fascia and the iliacus muscle. The fascia lata and the gluteus are sutured to the external oblique muscle. The inguinal ligament should be reattached if it had been divided.

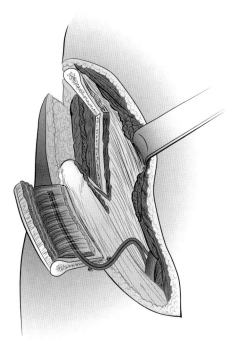

FIGURE **40-17** *Harvesting of a full-thickness iliac crest bone flap. Adapted from Strauch B, Yu HL, editors. Atlas of microvascular surgery. New York: Thieme Medical Publisher Inc.; 1993. p. 142–58.*

In most cases the inner aspect of the iliac crest is sufficient to reconstruct a mandibular defect, having the advantages of a less deforming defect and avoiding the lateral dissection of the gluteus medius muscles (Figure 40-18).

Morbidity following Iliac Crest Free Flaps

Rogers and colleagues analyzed the associated morbidity and the quality of life of patients who had undergone harvesting of either a deep circumflex iliac or a fibula free flap.[94] They used the University of Washington Quality of Life questionnaire, which showed no statistical differences between the patients in their activity, anxiety, mood, pain, recreation, or shoulder function. Rogers reported that the patients reconstructed with free fibula flaps had lower scores for swallowing and taste. On the other hand, for maxillectomy defects, they preferred the deep circumflex iliac flap over the fibula free flap, the latter being almost exclusively used for mandibular continuity defects. The known incidence of inguinal hernia was about 10% for patients who underwent free iliac flap harvesting.

Overall the conclusion is that both flaps are viable options for complex reconstructive needs in the head and neck regions requiring bone and soft tissue coverage. Donor site morbidity should be presented to the patient with emphasis on the potential impact on their quality of life.

Discussion

The iliac crest provides a significant segment of bone that may reach 4 cm in height and 11 cm in length. The dimensions of the flap may allow for a reconstruction of a hemimandibulectomy or anterior mandibular defect.

There are two significant advantages to the iliac crest/internal oblique free flap: (1) the amount of bone available for potential reconstruction with osseointegrated implants; and (2) the availability of

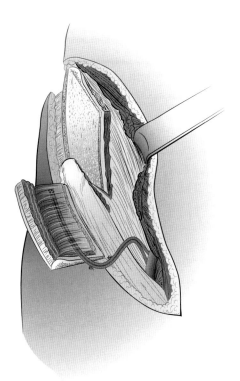

FIGURE **40-18** *Harvesting of a split-thickness iliac crest bone flap. Adapted from Strauch B, Yu HL, editors. Atlas of microvascular surgery. New York: Thieme Medical Publisher Inc.; 1993. p. 142–58.*

a thin and broad muscle that can be left to heal by secondary epithelization intraorally. Brown and colleagues developed the concept of reconstruction of the maxillary alveolus with the iliac crest while the palate was reconstructed with the muscle.[95,96]

The disadvantage of the flap is the relatively short vascular pedicle and the potential for herniation of the abdominal contents.

Versatility of Free Tissue Transfer

The flaps described in the current chapter are the most commonly used in head and neck reconstruction. The ability to transfer vascularized tissues allows for a significant variety of options.

The rectus abdominis free flap has been used mostly for base of skull reconstruction and tongue reconstruction. It is based on two vascular pedicles: the deep superior epigastric vessels, which are a continuation of the mammary vessels; and the deep inferior epigastric vessels, which are branches of the external iliac artery. The deep inferior epigastric vessels have a larger diameter and a longer vascular pedicle which makes them the preferred choice for anastomosis to the recipient vessels with very high reliability and success.[97]

The free scapular flap has been used for mandibular and maxillary reconstructions. The flap can be elevated together with the latissimus dorsi muscle, adding a large amount of soft tissue to large and complex defects of the maxillofacial region. The vascular supply to the scapular bone is provided by the scapular vessels, whereas the blood supply to the latissimus dorsi muscle is provided by the thoracodorsal vessels.

Urken and colleagues have described this combination of flaps as the subscapular system and specified some of its unique features[98]:

- Long length and large caliber of the vascular pedicle
- Abundant surface area of thin skin that can be transferred
- Separation between the soft tissue and bony flaps which provides freedom for three-dimensional insetting
- The potential to combine the latissimus dorsi and the serratus anterior muscles with overlying skin and adjacent segments of rib

Other flaps have been used for oropharyngeal reconstruction, including free omentum for oral lining, gracilis muscle free flaps with the anterior obturator nerve for facial reanimation, and lateral thigh or lateral arm free flaps for pharyngeal reconstruction. Even free temporoparietal fascial flaps have been used based on the superficial temporal vessels for intraoral lining or combined with the overlying skin or underlying bone.

When the reconstructive options are maximized, the selection of the donor site may resemble most accurately the functional needs of the recipient site.

References

1. Kriss TC, Kriss VM. History of the operating microscope: from magnifying glass to microneurosurgery. Neurosurgery 1998; 42:899–907.
2. Carrel A. The surgery of blood vessels. Johns Hopkins Hosp Bull 1907;19:18–28.
3. Jacobson JH, Suarez EL. Microsurgery in anastomosis of small vessels. Surg Forum 1960;11:243–5.
4. Taylor GI, Miller GDH, Ham FJ. The free vascularized bone graft: a free vascularized bone graft. Plast Reconstr Surg 1975; 55:533–44.
5. Hidalgo DA. Free fibula flap: a new method of mandibular reconstruction. Plast Reconstr Surg 1989;84:71–9.
6. Yang G, Chen B, Gao Y, et al. Forearm free skin graft transplantation. Nat Med J China 1981;61:139.
7. Soutar DS, Scheker LR, Tanner NSB, McGregor IA. The radial forearm flap: a versatile method for intraoral reconstruction. Br J Plast Surg 1983;36:1–8.
8. Soutar DS, McGregor IA. The radial forearm flap in intraoral reconstruction: the experience of 60 consecutive cases. Plast Reconstr Surg 1986;78:1–8.
9. Taylor GI, Watson N. One-stage repair of compound leg defects with free, revascularized flaps of groin skin and iliac bone. Plast Reconstr Surg 1978;61:494–506.
10. Taylor GI. Reconstruction of the mandible with free composite iliac bone grafts. Ann Plast Surg 1982;9:361–76.
11. Mehdorn HM, Muller GH. Microsurgical exercises. New York: Thieme Medical Publishers Inc.; 1989. p. 1–16.
12. Badran D, Soutar DS, Robertson AG, et al. Behavior of radial forearm skin flaps transplanted into the oral cavity. Clin Anat 1998;11:379–89.
13. Corrigan AM, O'Neill TJ. The use of the compound radial forearm flap in oro-mandibular reconstruction. Br J Oral Maxillofac Surg 1986;24:86–95.
14. Vaughan ED. The radial forearm free flap in orofacial reconstruction. A personal experience in 120 consecutive cases. J Craniomaxillofac Surg 1990;18:2–7.
15. Vaughan ED. The radial forearm flap in orofacial reconstruction. Int J Oral Maxillofac Surg 1994;23:194–204.
16. Martin IC, Cawood JL, Vaughan ED, Barnard N. Endosseous implants in the irradiated composite radial forearm free flap. Int J Oral Maxillofac Surg 1992;21:266–70.
17. Frodel JL, Funk GF, Capper DT, et al. Osseointegrated implants: a comparative study of bone thickness in four vascularized bone flaps. Plast Reconstr Surg 1993;92:449–55.
18. Urken ML, Weinberg H, Vickery C, Biller HF. The neurofasciocutaneous radial forearm flap in head and neck reconstruction: a preliminary report. Laryngoscope 1990; 100:161–73.
19. Moscoso JF, Urken ML. Radial forearm flaps. Otolaryngol Clin North Am 1994; 27:1119–40.
20. Urken ML, Futran N, Moscoso JF, Biller HF. A modified design of the buried radial forearm flap in oral cavity and pharyngeal reconstruction. Arch Otolaryngol Head Neck Surg 1994;120:1233–9.
21. Urken ML, Biller HF. A new bilobed design for the sensate radial forearm flap to preserve tongue mobility following significant glossectomy. Arch Otolaryngol Head Neck Surg 1994;120:26–31.
22. Thoma A, Khadaroo R, Grigenas O, et al. Oromandibular reconstruction with the radial-forearm osteocutaneous flap: experience with 60 consecutive cases. Plast Reconstr Surg 1999;104:368–78.
23. Serletti JM, Coniglio JU, Tavin E, Bakamjian VY. Simultaneous transfer of free fibula and radial forearm flaps for complex oromandibular reconstruction. J Reconstr Microsurg 1998;14:297–303.
24. Sadove RC, Luce EA, McGrath PC. Reconstruction of the lower lip and chin with the composite radial forearm-palmaris longus free flap. Plast Reconstr Surg 1991;88:209–14.
25. Serletti JM, Tavin E, Moran SL, Coniglio JU. Total lower lip reconstruction with a sensate composite radial forearm-palmaris longus free flap and a tongue flap. Plast Reconstr Surg 1997;99:559–61.
26. Furuta S, Sakaguchi Y, Iwasawa M, et al. Reconstruction of the lips, oral commissure, and full-thickness cheek with a composite radial forearm palmaris longus free flap. Ann Plast Surg 1994;33:544–7.
27. Savant DN, Patel SG, Deshmukh SP, et al. Folded free radial forearm flap for reconstruction of full-thickness defects of the cheek. Head Neck 1995;17:293–6.
28. Brown JS, Zuydam AC, Jones DC, et al. Functional outcome in soft palate reconstruction using a radial forearm free flap in conjunction with a superiorly based pharyngeal flap. Head Neck 1997;19: 524–34.
29. Anthony JP, Singer MI, Mathes SJ. Pharyngoesophageal reconstruction using the tubed free radial forearm flap. Clin Plast Surg 1994;21:137–47.
30. Jacobson MC, Franssen E, Fliss DM, et al. Free

forearm flap in oral reconstruction. Functional outcome. Arch Otolaryngol Head Neck Surg 1995;121:959–64.

31. Baird W, Wornom I, Culbertson J. Forehead reconstruction with a modified radial forearm flap: a case report. J Reconstr Microsurg 1988;4:363–7.

32. Santamaria E, Grandos M, Barrera-Franco JL. Radial forearm free tissue transfer for head and neck reconstruction: versatility and reliability of a single donor site. Microsurgery 2000;20:195–201.

33. To EW, Wang JC. Radial forearm free flap: hybrid version. Plast Reconstr Surg 1999;104:1066–9.

34. Kirn DS, Finical SJ, Kenady DE. Bilateral radial forearm free flaps for oral cavity reconstruction. J Reconstr Microsurg 1998; 14:551–3.

35. Close L, Truelson J, Milledge R, Schweitzer C. Sensory recovery in noninnervated flaps used for oral cavity and oropharyngeal reconstruction. Arch Otolaryngol Head Neck Surg 1995;121:967–72.

36. Santamaria E, Wei F, Chen I, Chuang D. Sensation recovery on innervated radial forearm flap for hemiglossectomy reconstruction by using different recipient nerves. Plast Reconstr Surg 1999; 103:450–7.

37. Boutros S, Yuksel E, Weinfield AB, et al. Neural anatomy of the radial forearm flap. Ann Plast Surg 2000;44:375–80.

38. Lvoff G, O'Brien CJ, Cope C, Lee KK. Sensory recovery in noninnervated radial forearm free flaps in oral and oropharyngeal reconstruction. Arch Otolaryngol Head Neck Surg 1998;124:1206–8.

39. Netscher D, Armenta AH, Meade RA, Alford EL. Sensory recovery of innervated and non-innervated radial forearm free flaps: functional implications. J Reconstr Microsurg 2000;16:179–85.

40. Shindo ML, Sinha UK, Rice DH. Sensory recovery in noninnervated free flaps for head and neck reconstruction. Laryngoscope 1995;105:1290–3.

41. Vriens JP, Acosta R, Soutar DS, Webster MH. Recovery of sensation in the radial forearm free flap in oral reconstruction. Plast Reconstr Surg 1996;98:649–56.

42. Timmons MJ. The vascular basis of the radial forearm flap. Plast Reconstr Surg 1986;77:80–92.

43. Yousif NJ, Ye Z, Grunert BK, et al. Analysis of the distribution of cutaneous perforators in cutaneous flaps. Plast Reconstr Surg 1998;101:72–84.

44. Cormack G, Duncan MJ, Lamberty B. The blood supply of the bone component of the compound osteocutaneous radial artery forearm flap – an anatomical study. Br J Plast Surg 1986;39:173–5.

45. Thoma A, Archibald S, Jackson S, Young JEM. Surgical patterns of venous drainage of the free forearm flap in head and neck reconstruction. Plast Reconstr Surg 1994;93:54–9.

46. Futran ND, Stack BC. Single versus dual venous drainage of the radial forearm flap. Am J Otolaryngol 1996;17:112–7.

47. Demirkan F, Wei FC, Lutz BS, et al. Reliability of the venae comitantes in venous drainage of the free radial forearm flaps. Plast Reconstr Surg 1998;102:1544–52.

48. Netscher DT, Sharma S, Alford EL, et al. Superficial versus deep: options in venous drainage of the radial forearm free flap. Ann Plast Surg 1999;36:536–41.

49. Jones BM, O'Brien CJ. Acute ischemia of the hand resulting from elevation of a radial forearm flap. Br J Plast Surg 1985;38:396–7.

50. Nukols DA, Tsu TT, Toby EB, Girod DA. Preoperative evaluation of the radial forearm free flap with the objective Allen's test. Otolaryngol Head Neck Surg 2000;123:553–7.

51. Ciria-Llorens G, Gomez-Cia T, Talegon-Melendez A. Analysis of flow changes in forearm arteries after raising the radial forearm flap: a prospective study using colour duplex imaging. Br J Plast Surg 1999;52:440–4.

52. Talegon-Melendez A, Ciria-Llorens G, Gomez-Cia T, Mayo-Iscar A. Flow changes in forearm arteries after elevating the radial forearm flap: prospective study using color duplex imaging. J Ultrasound Med 1999; 18:553–8.

53. Fatah MF, Nancarrow JD, Murray DS. Raising the radial artery forearm flap: the superficial ulnar artery "trap." Br J Plast Surg 1985;38:394–5.

54. Madares A, McGibbon IC. Anatomic variation in the blood supply of the radial forearm flap. J Reconstr Microsurg 1993;9:277–9.

55. Mordick TG. Vascular variation of the radial forearm flap: a case report. J Reconstr Microsurg 1995; 11:345–6.

56. Porter CJ, Mellow CG. Anatomically aberrant forearm arteries: an absent radial artery with co-dominant median and ulnar arteries. Br J Plast Surg 2001;54:727–8.

57. Saski K, Nozaki M, Aiba H, Isono N. A rare variant of the radial artery: clinical considerations in raising a radial forearm flap. Br J Plast Surg 2000;53:445–7.

58. Funk GF, Valentino J, McCulloch TM, et al. Anomalies of forearm vascular anatomy encountered during elevation of the radial forearm flap. Head Neck 1995;17:284–92.

59. Singh B, Cordiero PG, Santamaria E, et al. Factors associated with complications in microvascular reconstruction of head and neck defects. Plast Reconstr Surg 1999; 103:403–11.

60. Kiener JL, Hoffman WY, Mathes SJ. Influence of radiotherapy on microvascular reconstruction in the head and neck region. Am J Surg 1991;162:404–7.

61. Mulholland S, Boyd JB, McCabe S, et al. Recipient vessels in head and neck microsurgery: radiation effect and vessel access. Plast Reconstr Surg 1993; 92:628–32.

62. Blanchaert RH. Identification, management, and prevention of infections after head and neck surgery. In: Topazian RG, Goldberg MH, Hupp JR, editors. Oral and maxillofacial infections. 4th ed. Philadelphia: W.B. Saunders; 2002. p. 399–409.

63. Cole RR, Robbins KT, Cohen JL, Wolf PF. A predictive model for wound sepsis in oncologic surgery of the head and neck. Otolaryngol Head Neck Surg 1987;96:165–71.

64. Khouri PK, Cooley BC, Kunselman AR, et al. A prospective study of microvascular free-flap surgery and outcome. Plast Reconstr Surg 1998;102:711–21.

65. Disa JJ, Cordiero PG, Hidalgo DA. Efficacy of conventional monitoring techniques in free tissue transfer: an 11 year experience in 750 consecutive cases. Plast Reconstr Surg 1999;104:97–101.

66. Brown MT, Cheney ML, Gliklich RL, et al. Assessment of functional morbidity in the radial forearm free flap donor site. Arch Otolaryngol Head Neck Surg 1996; 122:991–4.

67. Brown MT, Couch ME, Huchton DM. Assessment of donor-site functional morbidity from radial forearm fasciocutaneous free flap harvest. Arch Otolaryngol Head Neck Surg 1999;125:1371–4.

68. Richardson D, Fisher SE, Vaughan ED, Brown JS. Radial forearm flap donor-site morbidity: a prospective study. Plast Reconstr Surg 1997;99:109–15.

69. Timmons MJ, Missotten FE, Poole MD, Davies DM. Complications of radial forearm flap donor sites. Br J Plast Surg 1986;39:176–8.

70. Toschka H, Feifel H, Erli HJ, et al. Aesthetic and functional results of harvesting radial forearm flap, especially with regard to hand function. Int J Oral Maxillofac Surg 201;30:42–8.

71. Akyurek M, Safak T. Direct closure of radial forearm free-flap donor sites by double opposing rhomboid transposition flaps: case report. J Reconstr Microsurg 2002; 18:33–6.

72. Avery CM, Pereira J, Brown AE. Suprafascial dissection of the radial forearm flap and donor site morbidity. Int J Oral Maxillofac Surg 2001;30:37–41.

73. Bardsley AF, Soutar DS, Elliot D, Batchelor AG. Reducing morbidity in the radial forearm flap donor site. Plast Reconstr Surg 1990;86:287–92.

74. Berge SJ, Wiese KG, von Lenden JJ, et al. Tissue expansion using osmotically active hydrogel systems for direct closure of the donor defect of the radial forearm flap. Plast Reconstr Surg 2001;108:1–5.

75. Chang SC, Miller G, Halbert CF, et al. Limiting donor site morbidity by suprafascial dissection of the radial forearm flap. Microsurgery 1996;17:136–40.

76. Fenton OM, Roberts JO. Improving the donor site of the radial forearm flap. Br J Plast Surg 1985;38:504–5.

77. McGregor AD. The free radial forearm flap – the management of the secondary defect. Br J Plast Surg 1987;40:83–5.

78. Samis AJ, Davidson JS. Skin-stretching device for intraoperative primary closure of radial forearm donor site. Plast Reconstr Surg 2000;105:698–702.

79. Sleeman D, Carton AT, Stassen LF. Closure of radial forearm free flap defect using full-thickness skin from the anterior abdominal wall. Br J Oral Maxillofac Surg 1994; 32:54–5.

80. Nunez VA, Pike J, Avery C, et al. Prophylactic plating of the donor site of osteocutaneous radial forearm flaps. Br J Oral Maxillofac Surg 1999;37:210–2.

81. Werle AH, Tsue TT, Toby EB, Girod DA. Osteocutaneous radial forearm free flap: its use without significant donor site morbidity. Otolaryngol Head Neck Surg 2000;123:711–7.

82. Hallock GG. Complications of free-flap donor site from a community hospital perspective. J Reconstr Microsurg 1991;7:331–4.

83. Fowkes FGR, Housley E, Cawood EM, et al. Edinburgh Artery Study: prevalence of asymptomatic and symptomatic peripheral arterial disease in the general population. Int J Epidemiol 1991;20:384–92.

84. Reunanen A, Takkunen H, Aromaa A. Prevalence of intermittent claudication and its effect on mortality. Acta Med Scand 1982;211:249–56.

85. Smith RB, Thomas RD, Funk GF. Fibula free flaps: the role of angiography in patients with abnormal results on preoperative color flow Doppler studies. Arch Otolaryngol Head Neck Surg 2003; 129:712–5.

86. Schusterman MA, Reece GP, Miller MJ, et al. The osteocutaneous free fibula flap: is the skin flap reliable? Plast Reconstr Surg 1992;90:787–93.

87. Hayden RE. The neurocutaneous free fibula flap [abstract]. Third International Conference on Head and Neck Cancer, San Francisco, 1992 Jul 27. American Head and Neck Society.

88. O'Leary MJ, Martin PJ, Hayden RE. The neurocutaneous free fibula flap in mandibular reconstruction. Otolaryngol Clin North Am 1994;27:1081–96.

89. Disa JJ, Winters RM, Hidalgo DA. Long term evaluation of bone mass in free fibula flap mandible reconstruction. Am J Surg 1997;174:503–6.

90. Moscoso JF, Keller J, Gender E, et al. Vascularized bone flaps in oromandibular reconstruction. A comparative study of bone stock from various donor sites to assess suitability for endosseous dental implants. Arch Otolaryngol Head Neck Surg 1994;120:36–43.

91. Shindo M, Fong B, Fung G, et al. The fibula osteocutaneous flap in head and neck reconstruction: a critical evaluation of donor site morbidity. Arch Otolaryngol Head Neck Surg 2000;126:1467–72.

92. Anthony JP, Rawnsley JD, Benhaim P, et al. Donor leg morbidity and function after fibula free flap mandible reconstruction. Plast Reconstr Surg 1995;20:146–52.

93. Serafin D. Atlas of microsurgical composite tissue transplantation. Philadelphia: W.B. Saunders Co.; 1996. p. 525–35.

94. Rogers SN, Lakshmiah SR, Narayan B, et al. A comparison of the long term morbidity following deep circumflex iliac and fibula free flaps for reconstruction following head and neck cancer. Plast Reconst Surg 2003; 112:1517–25.

95. Brown JS, Jones DC, Summerwill A, et al. Vascularized iliac crest with internal oblique muscle for immediate reconstruction after maxillectomy. Br J Oral Maxillofac Surg 2002;40:183–90.

96. Brown JS. Deep circumflex iliac artery free flap with internal oblique muscle as a new method of immediate reconstruction of maxillectomy defect. Head Neck 1996;18(5):412–21.

97. Urken ML, Turk J, Weinberg H, et al. The rectus abdominis free flap in head and neck reconstruction. Arch Otolaryngol Head Neck Surg 1991;117:857–66.

98. Urken ML, Cheney ML, Sullivan MJ, Biller HF. Subscapular system. In: Urken ML, Cherney ML, Sullivan MJ, Biller HF, editors. Atlas of regional and free flaps for head and neck reconstruction. New York (NY): Raven Press; 1995. p. 213–6.

99. Urken ML. Radial forearm. In: Urken ML, Cheney ML, Sullivan MJ, Biller HF, editors. Atlas of regional and free flaps for head and neck reconstruction. New York (NY): Raven Press; 1995. p. 152.

CHAPTER 41

Microneurosurgery

Michael Miloro, DMD, MD

Injuries to the terminal branches of the trigeminal nerve may occur commonly following a variety of routine oral and maxillofacial surgical procedures, and the overwhelming majority of these injuries undergo spontaneous recovery without treatment. Third molar surgery is responsible for most of the injuries to both the inferior alveolar and lingual nerves. The reported incidence of nerve injury varies in the literature, but generally both temporary and permanent paresthesia must be considered. Nerve injury may occur following mandibular and maxillary orthognathic surgery, maxillofacial trauma, dental implant placement, endodontic therapy, facial fractures, and treatment of pathology. The anatomy of the trigeminal nerve system is unique since it carries, in some branches, both general sensory information and special (eg, taste) sensation. Injury to a nerve may result in neuroma formation, which can manifest in a variety of clinical signs and symptoms. Nerve injuries are classified by two popular classification schemes, which are based on the likelihood of an injured nerve recovering spontaneously. A basic understanding of nerve terminology (Appendix) and normal neural wound healing is essential to most appropriately manage clinical situations.

The initial evaluation of patients with nerve injuries must proceed in an orderly fashion, with several levels of testing to determine most accurately the degree of individual nerve injury. A standardized clinical neurosensory test (CNT) may be employed for most patients; however, some advanced testing is available for special circumstances. A variety of nonsurgical and pharmacologic treatments are available for the patient with nerve injury. For most patients with dysesthesia, pharmacologic therapy is the mainstay of treatment.

Once the decision is made to proceed with microneurosurgery, a sequence of surgical steps must be followed meticulously. Specific surgical techniques depend on which specific nerve is involved, as well as the extent of the injury. In general, microneurosurgical repair of a trigeminal nerve injury involves neurolysis and preparation of the nerve stumps to perform neurorrhaphy. The deleterious effects of tension on a nerve repair site have been well documented, so the inability to perform a primary tension-free repair warrants consideration for an autogenous nerve graft or another option for nerve gap management such as conduit repair. Following microneurosurgery, postoperative sensory reeducation may play a role in the regenerative process. The overall success rates of microneurosurgical repair of the trigeminal nerve vary considerably; however, an important factor in determining success is the length of time from injury to repair since this impacts on the degree of ganglion cell death, wallerian degeneration, and cortical somatosensory reorganization. The American Association of Oral and Maxillofacial Surgeons Clinical Interest Group on Maxillofacial Neurologic Disorders has promulgated certain treatment time recommendations for the patient who sustains a trigeminal nerve injury.[1]

The field of microneurosurgery is in its infancy. As more surgeons become familiar with the diagnosis and management of patients with trigeminal nerve injuries, more laboratory, radiologic, and clinical information will become available to guide therapy. Also, residency programs will become more capable of training residents in the principles and practice of microneurosurgery and will thus foster access to this aspect of specialty care throughout the country and abroad.

Demographics

Trigeminal nerve injuries result from a variety of routine oral and maxillofacial surgical procedures, such as third molar odontectomy, management of facial trauma, orthognathic surgery, endosseous dental implant placement, salivary duct and gland surgery, treatment of benign and malignant lesions of the head and neck, preprosthetic surgery, and endodontic and periradicular surgery. Complications of third molar removal are responsible for the majority of nerve injuries.[2] These can occur during any phase of third molar surgery, including local anesthetic injection, incision and flap design, the use of a high-speed drill for bone removal or tooth sectioning, elevation of the tooth with trauma to the lingual soft tissues, socket curettage with exposed neurovascular tissue, removal of remnants of an assumed "dental follicle" that may contain neural or vascular tissue, the use of medicaments in the extraction site to aid healing or prevent alveolar osteitis (eg, tetracycline-containing compounds[3,4]), and the placement of sutures. The efficacy of lingual nerve retraction during lower third molar surgery has shown that although the incidence of temporary lingual nerve paresthesia is increased owing to a slight stretching or manipulation (6.4% with retraction vs 0.6% without retraction), the difference in long-term dysfunction is not significant (0.6% with retraction vs 0.2% without retraction).[5] Other studies have indicated a temporary paresthesia rate of approximately 10 to 15% with lingual nerve retraction and protection, with a permanent rate of < 1%.

The incidence of trigeminal nerve injury may be estimated based on a review of the available literature. Overall the incidence of inferior alveolar nerve (IAN) injury from third molar surgery is 0.41 to 7.5% and from sagittal split osteotomy is 0.025 to 84.6%, whereas the lingual nerve is affected 0.06 to 11.5% of the time following third molar removal. However, the more important clinical distinction is to differentiate temporary from permanent paresthesia rates. For sagittal split osteotomies, temporary inferior alveolar paresthesia may be as high as 80 to 100%, but permanent rates are < 1 to 5%. For third molar surgery, both inferior alveolar and lingual nerve temporary paresthesias range from 2 to 6% each, whereas permanent rates are approximately 25% of the temporary rates, or 0.5 to 2% overall. Many risk factors for nerve injury during third molar surgery have been reported and include advanced patient age, female sex (recent animal studies indicate that

gender may play a role in spontaneous neurosensory recovery following injury), depth of impaction, mesiodistal angulation of the tooth (distoangular), lingual angulation of the tooth, integrity of the lingual cortex, the need for tooth sectioning, removal of bone distal to the third molar, and surgeon experience. Certainly the risk of an IAN injury may be influenced by so-called Rood radiographic predictors of potential tooth proximity to the inferior alveolar canal.[6] These seven radiographic predictors on panoramic radiograph may indicate the potential for increased risk of injury to the IAN, and they are listed in Table 41-1. In cases with a high index of suspicion of nerve injury (eg, deep impaction, advanced age), intentional coronectomy with close observation should be considered.[7] As opposed to the relatively consistent course of the IAN, the lingual nerve position is variable; and it is injured less often than the IAN following third molar surgery.[8-12] The position of the lingual nerve has been documented clinically,[13] in cadaveric dissections,[14,15] and radiologically.[16] On average, in the third molar region, the lingual nerve lies 2.5 mm medial to the lingual plate of the mandible and 2.5 mm inferior to the lingual crest. The lingual nerve may be in direct contact with the lingual plate in 25% of cases (Kisselbach and Chamberlain reported 62%[13]) and may lie above the lingual crest in 10 to 15% of cases (Kisselbach and Chamberlain reported 17.6%[13]) based on an undisturbed radiographic assessment of the nerve.

Mandibular blocks may result in inferior alveolar and lingual nerve injuries; however, the incidence is unknown owing to unreported cases. An estimated 1 in 100,000 to 1 in 500,000 blocks result in paresthesia. Perhaps the largest study of its kind, Harn and Durham's study of 9,587 mandibular blocks showed a 3.62% incidence of temporary paresthesia and a 1.8% incidence of long-term paresthesia lasting > 1 year.[17] Several theories have

been proposed to explain the mechanism of injury. Direct neural trauma is unlikely owing to abundant interfascicular neural components resulting in separation of the fascicles by a needle or suture without direct neural disruption.[18] The resultant edema may be responsible for the transient paresthesia that resolves spontaneously. Local anesthetic toxicity may be responsible for prolonged paresthesia following a mandibular block, especially if the solution is deposited within the confines of the epineurium. Recent reports indicate that prilocaine and articaine may be associated with an increased risk of long-term paresthesia compared with other local anesthetic solutions, but further investigation is warranted.[19-21] The third potential mechanism of injury involves the formation of an epineurial hematoma. The epineurium and perineurium contain a vast plexus of vessels that nurture the neural elements, and a needle may cause disruption of one or more vessels. The localized bleeding most certainly tamponades itself owing to the surrounding epineurium, and the pressure may impinge on select groups of fascicles contained within the nerve. The resultant clinical signs and symptoms of localized paresthesia, not involving the entire distribution of the inferior alveolar/ mental nerve, nicely match the expected histologic situation, making this theory plausible. Also, lymphatic drainage of the localized hematoma over the few days to weeks

Table 41-1   Rood's Radiographic Predictors of Potential Tooth Proximity to the Inferior Alveolar Canal
1. Darkening of the root
2. Deflection of the root
3. Narrowing of the root
4. Dark and bifid root apex
5. Interruption of the white line of the canal
6. Diversion of the canal
7. Narrowing of the canal
Adapted from Rood JP and Shehab AAN.[6]

following surgery coincides with the clinical resolution of symptoms in most cases. The final theory is that of the needle-barb mechanism of injury.[22] During a mandibular block injection, the needle may be advanced to the medial ramus where a small barb may form at the needle tip. On withdrawal, if the needle has passed through or in the vicinity of the lingual nerve or IAN, fascicular disruption may occur with potentially long-standing clinical consequences. Recent trends in our clinical understanding of injection-related nerve injuries are the following:

- These injuries are difficult to predict and prevent
- The classic electric-shock sensation is reported uncommonly by patients who sustain these injuries
- Injection injuries are more likely to result in dysesthesia than are other causes of nerve injuries
- There may be a nonanatomic distribution of nerve involvement (including the second and third divisions of the trigeminal nerve)
- Injection injuries occur more commonly in females
- The lingual nerve, which is stretched more upon mouth opening than is the IAN, is more commonly affected
- The majority of cases resolve within 8 weeks, and if paresthesia persists for > 8 weeks, then only one-third of those injuries resolve spontaneously

Microneurosurgery is a poor option for patients with injection-related nerve injuries because surgical access is difficult; therefore, most cases are managed with pharmacologic therapy. One of the difficulties for microneurosurgeons is differentiating a mandibular block injury from a third molar injury to the IAN. On rare occasions the third molar site of the IAN has been explored and found to be normal, with the assumption that the injury occurred as a result of injection rather than extraction.[23]

It is well known that orthognathic surgery may result in nerve injury. The IAN is affected more often than is the lingual nerve, and rarely the facial nerve may be affected (0.67% with sagittal split osteotomy in one study[24]). Certainly much is known about the risks of IAN injury associated with sagittal split osteotomy, as well as screw overpenetration injury to the lingual nerve.[25,26] Unfortunately, the reported incidence of immediate and long-term neurosensory deficit varies considerably (from < 5% to > 90%) owing to poorly controlled factors inherent in the study designs, such as individual operator variability and surgeon experience, lack of standardization of neurosensory testing, lack of control sites for normal cutaneous facial sensibility, and variation in the periods of neurosensory testing. Several studies have examined the specific parameters of neurosensory recovery after bilateral sagittal split osteotomy by using objective and subjective assessment.[27] One study found a 39% incidence of neurosensory dysfunction following sagittal ramus surgery,[28] and others have shown < 15% dysfunction at 6 months.[29] Although the incidence of nerve dysfunction varies, there are well-known risk factors for nerve injury, including the following[30]: patient age[31]; increased length of the surgical procedure; proximal or distal segment fracture ("bad splits"); concomitant third molar removal; concomitant genioplasty procedures; compression during fixation; inadvertent use of chisels; nerve entrapment in the proximal segment; nerve manipulation in the area of the osteotomy and, perhaps more significantly, in the lingual region during medial dissection (based on intraoperative recordings of IAN somatosensory evoked potentials)[32]; the location of the inferior alveolar canal close to the inferior border; low corpus height and retrognathism (IAN closer to buccal cortex)[33]; and frank nerve transection during surgery. Unfortunately, long-term neurosensory dysfunction following

orthognathic surgery is not generally amenable to surgical correction. However, most patients tolerate the paresthesia well following correction of a significant dentofacial deformity. Two caveats are that patients tolerate mild paresthesia following major surgery well (with informed consent) and that the magnitude of neurosensory dysfunction decreases as the time from injury increases. This certainly applies to orthognathic nerve injuries.

Maxillofacial trauma may result in injury to any of the terminal branches of the trigeminal nerve. Mandible fractures that violate the IAN canal result in temporary or permanent paresthesia. Treatment of mandible fractures with inadvertent placement of screws may cause iatrogenic nerve injury. In general, reduction of the fracture aids in realigning the natural conduit (ie, the IAN canal) that will help to guide spontaneous neurosensory recovery even with a transection injury.

Also, the presence and/or treatment of oral pathologic lesions may result in nerve injury. The use of Carnoy's solution (ferric chloride 0.1 g/mL, absolute alcohol 6 mL, chloroform 3 mL, glacial acetic acid 1 mL) following treatment of pathology has been shown to have a critical exposure time in an animal model of 5 minutes, after which time there may be long-term irreversible neural injury.[34,35] Following a resection procedure, consideration should be given to immediate or delayed neural reconstruction using autogenous nerve grafts.

Although preprosthetic surgery is performed less frequently today than in the past, procedures such as torus mandibularis reduction and vestibuloplasty place the terminal branches of the mental nerve and infraorbital nerve at risk of injury. Surgical repair of small terminal nerve fibers is difficult and often results in scarring and a poor chance of neurosensory recovery. The maxilla and mandible are excellent sources of autogenous bone grafts; however, they are not without potential morbidity. The majority of patients who undergo genial bone graft harvest complain of desensitiza-tion of the mandibular anterior teeth. Depending on the specific technique employed for posterior mandibular ramus grafting, the IAN may be at risk of iatro-genic injury. Mandibular endodontic ther-apy and periapical surgery may result in an injury to the IAN, depending on the prox-imity of the root apex to the canal. Some endodontic filling materials may be neuro-toxic, and to prevent irreversible paresthe-sia that in many cases results in dysesthesia, consideration should be given to prompt exploration and débridement of medica-ments that have permeated through the root apex and are in direct contact with the nerve. Distraction osteogenesis of the mandible has been shown to induce tran-sient changes in neuronal conduction without significant long-term nerve dys-function.[36,37] On a clinical level, a younger patient would certainly tolerate a "stretch-type" of injury to the nerve well. Recent data indicate that with a corticotomy and distraction rates of 1 mm/d neural changes are unlikely but that rates greater than this may be deleterious to nerve function; how-ever, more studies are necessary.[38]

Finally, implant-related injuries to the IAN are common (30–40%) and problem-atic to manage appropriately. Unfortu-nately there is a lack of data regarding appropriate patient assessment and man-agement, with a lack of consensus on treatment protocols. In the posterior mandible the likely cause of nerve damage is that the initial pilot (depth) drill pene-trates the superior cortex of the canal and violates the IAN vein (or artery, which is less likely). This results in some bleeding that, on placement of the implant, tam-ponades itself. The resultant increased pressure in the closed environment creates a compartment syndrome, with harmful effects on neurosensory function. This type of injury commonly results in long-term unpleasant altered sensation (dyses-thesia) rather than simple decreased sen-sation (hypoesthesia). The recognition

postoperatively that the patient has pares-thesia and that the implant is within the confines of the canal warrant the clinician to consider removal of the implant, with or without immediate replacement with a shorter implant. If, however, the injury was due to a compartment syndrome effect, then implant removal without replacement may be prudent. For patients with persistent paresthesia, referral to a microneurosurgeon may be warranted. The procedure of IAN repositioning (lat-eralization and transpositioning) is an option that theoretically would induce a "controlled" injury to the nerve and pro-tect it during implant preparation. With lateral decortication of the mandible and nerve exposure, a compartment syndrome is not possible. Despite the potential advantages of nerve repositioning, there is a high incidence of long-term paresthesia ranging from 0 to 77%, with a mean of approximately 30 to 40%.[39] With appro-priate surgeon experience, proper patient selection, and informed consent, this pro-cedure remains a viable option in posteri-or mandibular reconstruction.

Trigeminal Nerve Anatomy and Physiology

A brief review of the trigeminal nerve is necessary to understand clinical diagnosis and management. The trigeminal nerve (Figure 41-1) is composed of a mesoneuri-um that suspends the nerve within the surrounding tissues and is continuous with the outer epineurium that defines and surrounds the nerve trunk. The epineurium contains a vast plexus of ves-sels called the vasa nervorum, as well as lymphatic channels. The epineurium is divided into outer and inner epineuriums, and the inner layer is composed of a loose connective tissue sheath with longitudinal collagen bundles that protect against com-pressive and stretching forces imposed on the nerve. Individual fascicles are defined by the perineurium, which is a continua-tion of the pia-arachnoid layer of the cen-

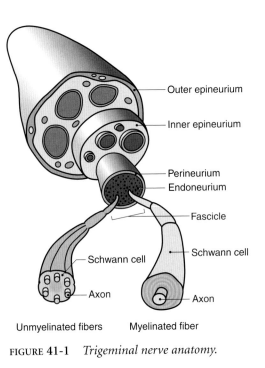

FIGURE **41-1**   *Trigeminal nerve anatomy.*

tral nervous system. It functions to pro-vide structural support and act as a diffu-sion barrier, similar to the blood-brain barrier that prevents the transport of cer-tain molecules. The individual nerve fibers and Schwann cells are surrounded by the endoneurium, which is composed of colla-gen, fibroblasts, and capillaries. There are three types of neural fascicular patterns: monofascicular (one large fascicle), oligo-fascicular (2–10 fascicles), and polyfascic-ular (> 10 fascicles) (Figure 41-2). The inferior alveolar and lingual nerves are polyfascicular in nature. Polyfascicular nerves have abundant interfascicular con-nective tissue—the importance of which is that needle penetrations rarely cause direct neural trauma and that nerve repair with realignment of the fascicles is chal-lenging. The nerve is composed of a func-tional unit with differing fiber types that transmit a variety of information (Table 41-2). The A alpha fibers are the largest myelinated fibers with the fastest conduc-tion velocity; they mediate position and fine touch through muscle spindle affer-ents and skeletal muscle efferents. The A beta fibers mediate proprioception. The smallest myelinated fibers are the A delta

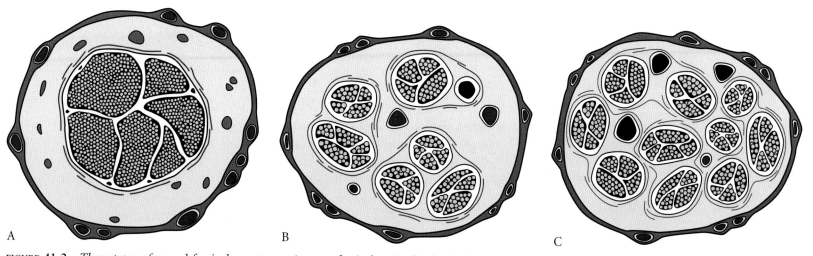

FIGURE **41-2** *Three types of neural fascicular patterns:* A, *monofascicular;* B, *oligofascicular;* C, *polyfascicular. Adapted from Lundborg G. The nerve trunk. In: Lundborg G, editor. Nerve injury and repair. New York: Churchill Livingston; 1998. p. 198.*

fibers that carry pain ("first" or "fast" pain) and temperature information. The smaller-diameter and slower-conducting unmyelinated C fibers mediate "second" or "slow" pain and temperature sensations. The Schwann cells surround both myelinated (one Schwann cell per nerve fiber) and unmyelinated (one Schwann cell per several nerve fibers) nerves, and they play a major role in nerve survival and regeneration following injury. Although the myelin sheath may not survive a nerve injury, the Schwann cells do, and they provide a supportive role in the production of neurotrophic and neurotropic factors (such as nerve growth factor) that enhance neural recovery. The nodes of Ranvier are the 0.3 to 2.0 μm unmyelinated segments between the myelin sheaths that are responsible for the diffusion of certain ions that cause nerve depolarization and repolarization

and the saltatory conduction of a nerve impulse along the nerve.

Following nerve injury many changes occur, but the basic process of nerve healing involves both degeneration and regeneration (Figure 41-3).[40,41] The nerve cell body responds with an increased metabolic phase with a heightened production of ribonucleic acid and breakdown of Nissl's substance for export from the cell body. At the site of injury, there is edema and particulate cellular debris. In addition, there is a proliferation of phagocytes, and macrophages begin to clean the area. Within days there are axonal sprouts that extend from the proximal nerve stump. Each axon may have as many as 50 collateral sprouts. There is proliferation and a high level of activity of Schwann cells as well. These begin to lay down new myelin for the arrival of the new axons. Addition-

ally, nerve growth factors are produced that influence the direction of sprouting and guide the new axons into the newly

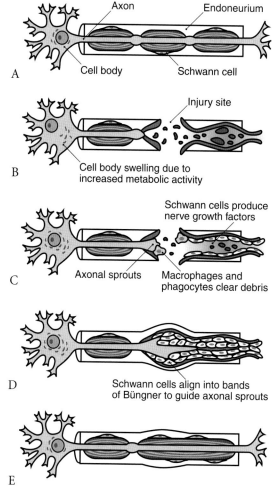

FIGURE **41-3** A *to* E, *Neural wound-healing mechanisms.*

Table 41-2	Trigeminal Nerve Fibers		
Fiber	Size (μ)	Conduction Velocity (m/s)	Function
A alpha (myelin)	12–20	70–120	Position, fine touch
A beta (myelin)	6.0–12	35–170	Proprioception
A delta (thin myelin)	1.0–6.0	2.5–3.5	Superficial (first) pain, temperature
C (unmyelinated)	0.5–1.0	0.7–1.5	Deep (second) pain, temperature

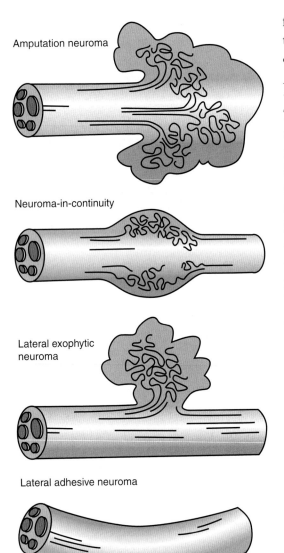

FIGURE **41-4** *Neuroma types: amputation neuroma, neuroma-in-continuity, lateral exophytic neuroma, lateral adhesive neuroma.*

formed myelin sheaths, known as the bands of Büngner. In the event that all of these interrelated processes occur appropriately, then spontaneous neural regeneration occurs. In the event that one or more of the reparative processes fail, there may be neuroma formation. A neuroma is simply a disorganized mass of collagen fibers and randomly oriented small nerve fascicles (sprouts). Neuromas are classified by gross morphology into the following types (Figure 41-4): amputation (stump) neuroma, neuroma-in-continuity (central or

fusiform neuroma), and lateral neuromas that are either lateral exophytic neuromas or lateral adhesive neuromas.

Nerve Injury Classification

There are two acceptable classification schemes used to describe the histologic changes that occur following nerve injury. Seddon described a three-stage classification system in 1943,[42] and Sunderland revised and further subclassified nerve injuries into five grades in 1951 (Figure 41-5 and Table 41-3).[43] A neurapraxia (Seddon) or first-degree (Sunderland) injury is characterized as a conduction block from transient anoxia owing to acute epineurial/endoneurial vascular interruption resulting from mild nerve

manipulation (traction or compression), with rapid and complete recovery of sensation and no axonal degeneration. Damage is confined to within the endoneurium. Sunderland further subdivides first-degree injuries into types I, II, and III. Type I results from mild nerve manipulation with rapid (hours) return of sensation when neural blood flow is restored. Type II is due to moderate traction or compression with the formation of transudate or exudate fluid and intrafascicular edema, with return of sensation following edema resolution (days). Type III injuries result from more severe nerve manipulation that may result in segmental demyelination, with recovery within days to weeks. An axonotmesis (Seddon) corre-

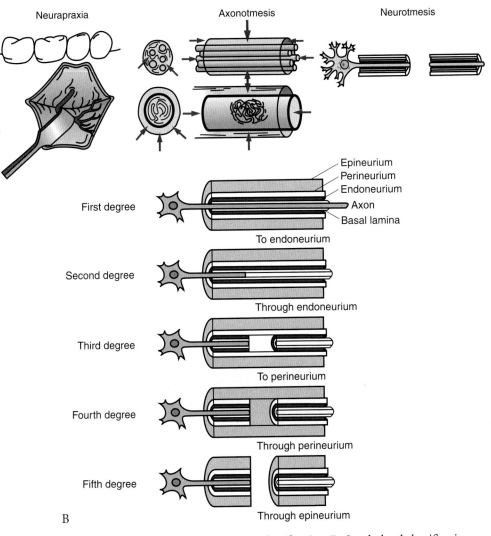

FIGURE **41-5** *Nerve injury classifications: A, Seddon classification; B, Sunderland classification.*

Table 41-3	Nerve Injury Classifications: Seddon versus Sunderland		
Seddon	*Sunderland*	*Histology*	*Outcomes*
Neurapraxia	First degree	No axonal damage, no demyelination, no neuroma	Loss of sensation, rapid recovery (days to weeks), no microneurosurgery
Axonotmesis	Second, third, and fourth degrees	More axonal damage, demyelination, possible neuroma	Loss of sensation, slow incomplete recovery (weeks to months), possible microneurosurgery
Neurotmesis	Fifth degree	Severe axonal damage, epineurial discontinuity, neuroma formation	Loss of sensation, spontaneous recovery unlikely, microneurosurgery

sponds to second-, third-, and fourth-degree (Sunderland) injuries, with the difference being the degree of axonal damage. Second-degree injuries are due again to traction or compression that results in ischemia, intrafascicular edema, or demyelination. This damage extends through and includes the endoneurium with no significant axonal disorganization. Recovery is slow and may take weeks to months, and it may not be complete. Third-degree injuries continue the spectrum of more advanced injury owing to more significant neural trauma with variable degrees of intrafascicular architectural disruption and damage extending to the perineurium. Recovery is variable; it may take months and be incomplete. Fourth-degree injuries result in damage to the entire fascicle that extends through the perineurium to the epineurium, but the epineurium remains intact. There is axonal, endoneurial, and perineurial damage with disorganization of the fascicles. Spontaneous recovery is unlikely, but minimal improvement may occur in 6 to 12 months. Finally, neurotmesis (Seddon) and fifth-degree (Sunderland) injuries result from complete or near complete transection of the nerve with epineurial discontinuity and likely neuroma formation. Spontaneous neurosensory recovery is unlikely. For completeness, in 1988 Dellon and Mackinnon described a sixth-degree injury, which recognizes that many nerve injuries exhibit features of different degrees of injury according to Sunderland (Table 40-4).[44] The Seddon and Sunderland classification schemes attempt to correlate histologic changes with clinical outcome (see Table 41-3).

Clinical Neurosensory Testing

The patient who sustains an injury to the trigeminal nerve may present with a variety of signs and symptoms. These may be divided into nonpainful anesthesia, hypoesthesia, hyperesthesia, or painful anesthesia (anesthesia dolorosa), hypoesthesia, or hyperesthesia (allodynia—pain from a nonpainful stimulus—or hyperpathia—increased pain owing to a painful or nonpainful stimulus). The history usually indicates the etiologic event, and the chief complaint may include the following descriptive terms: numbness, itchy, crawling, stretched, drooling, painful, tingling, tickling, pulling, burning, stinging, pins and needles, hot sensation, cold sensation, inability to feel food on lip, inability to taste, inability to shave, inability to smile, and loss of consortium. The history of present illness should be explored in depth with a description of the onset and progression of symptoms, change in symptoms, treatment received and response, aggravating and alleviating factors, and present symptoms.

The McGill Pain Questionnaire (MPQ) may be used to assess pain and altered sensation, and it is a useful tool for monitoring progression of neurosensory recovery. The MPQ uses three classes of descriptive words to assess the level of dysfunction and interference with activity: sensory class (temporal, spatial, thermal, punctate, incisive, constrictive, traction pressure), affective class (tension, fear, autonomic properties, punishment), and evaluative class (patient perception). Perhaps the simplest and most reliable measure of subjective patient assessment is the use of a visual analog scale. Generally, this is a 10 cm five-degree scale, with a degree marked every 2.5 cm (Figure 41-6). This is a useful tool for monitoring subjective improvement. It must be remembered that subjective and objective nerve testings are

Table 41-4	Sunderland Grade and Recovery Patterns		
Degree of Injury	*Recovery Pattern*	*Rate of Recovery*	*Treatment*
First degree	Complete	Fast (days to weeks)	None
Second degree	Complete	Slow (weeks)	None
Third degree	Variable	Slow (weeks to months)	Possible nerve exploration
Fourth degree	None	Unlikely recovery	Microneurosurgery
Fifth degree	None	No recovery	Microneurosurgery
Sixth degree*	Varies†	Varies†	Varies†

*Sixth-degree injury data from Dellon AL and Mackinnon SE[44]
†Depending on specific injury pattern.

Please indicate with an "X" on each of the two lines your perception of your current level of sensation.

Right	1 Complete absence of sensation	2 Almost no sensation	3 Reduced sensation	4 Almost normal sensation	5 Fully normal sensation
Left	1 Complete absence of sensation	2 Almost no sensation	3 Reduced sensation	4 Almost normal sensation	5 Fully normal sensation

FIGURE 41-6   *Visual analog scale.*

rarely at the same level. For example, in one study of nerve testing following sagittal split osteotomy, the subjective neurosensory deficit was 26.0%, whereas the objective tests revealed an 89.5% deficit.[45] Treatment planning decisions must be based on an assessment of both the subjective and objective testing results. Also, a radiographic assessment may reveal prior radiographic predictors of root proximity to the canal, retained root fragments, distal bone removal, or the presence of foreign bodies in extraction sites.

Clinical examination begins with inspection of the oral cavity, which may show signs of self-induced trauma, a lingually placed third molar incision scar, or atrophic changes of the tongue fungiform papillae.[46] Palpation may induce a Tinel's sign, which is a provocative test of regenerating nerve sprouts that it is performed by light palpation over the area of suspected injury. This maneuver elicits a distal referred "tingling" sensation at the target site. This sign is thought to indicate small-diameter fiber recovery; however, it is poorly correlated with functional recovery and is often confused with neuroma formation. To perform the CNT appropriately, the patient should be seated comfortably in a quiet room, and the specific testing procedures should be explained clearly to the patient, with confirmation that there is an understanding of what the patient is being asked to do and what possible responses are acceptable. The specific tests are performed with the patient's eyes closed, and the contralateral uninjured side serves as the control, when appropriate.

The CNT is performed at three levels: A, B, and C (Table 41-5).[47] The CNT involves a dropout algorithm that attempts to correlate the results of the test with the level of nerve injury (Figure 41-7). If the results of level A testing are normal, then the CNT is terminated and the patient is considered normal; this would correspond to a Sunderland first-degree injury. An abnormal result at level A indicates the need to proceed to level B testing. If the results of level B testing are normal, then the patient is considered mildly impaired (Sunderland second-degree injury). If level B results are abnormal, then level C testing is performed. If level C results are normal, then the patient is moderately impaired (Sunderland third-degree injury). If level C results are abnormal, then the patient is considered severely impaired (Sunderland fourth-degree injury). If the patient's test results are abnormal at levels A, B, and C and there is no response to any noxious stimulus, the patient is considered completely impaired (Sunderland fifth-degree injury). Level A testing includes brush-stroke directional and static two-point discriminations. These tests assess function of the larger myelinated A alpha and beta fibers. These fibers are the most sensitive to compression and traction injuries; therefore, the CNT is terminated if level A is normal. Brush-stroke directional discrimination is performed with a fine sable or camel hair brush. The brush is stroked gently across the area of involvement at a constant rate, and the patient is asked to indicate the direction of movement (ie, to the left or right) and the correct number of patient statements out of 10 is recorded. Two-point discrimination is performed in a static fashion (vs a moving two-point discrimination) and with blunt tips to avoid A delta and C fiber stimulation. This test can be performed with any device that is capable of allowing the distance between two points to be measured consistently (eg, a Boley gauge). The closest distance (in millimeters) at which the patient can consistently discern the two points is recorded. At level B testing, contact detection is performed with Semmes-Weinstein monofilaments or von Frey hairs, which, again, assess the A beta fiber integrity and function. These devices are acrylic resin or plastic transparent/translucent rods with nylon filaments of varying diameters. The stiffness of each filament determines the force necessary to deflect or bend the filament. The narrowest diameter filament that requires the least amount of force to deflect that is detected consistently is recorded. At level C testing, pinprick nociception and thermal discrimination assess the smaller A delta and C fibers, which are most resistant to injury. Pinprick nociception may be performed simply with a 30-gauge needle; however, a pressure sensitive device is more appropriate. Thermal discrimination may be performed with suprathreshold methods using ice or ethyl chloride or hot water on a cotton swab, but other options are

Table 41-5   Clinical Neurosensory Testing
Subjective assessment: visual analog scale
Objective assessment
Level A: static two-point discrimination, brush-stroke directional discrimination
Level B: contact detection
Level C: pinprick nociception, thermal discrimination

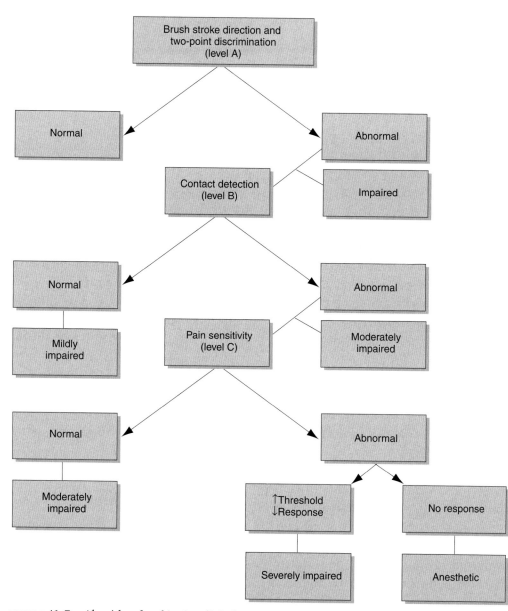

FIGURE 41-7   *Algorithm for objective clinical neurosensory test.*

injury may not report any taste alteration subjectively but may test abnormally with different solutions. The complex sense of taste is mediated not only by the chorda tympani branch of the facial nerve but also through feedback mechanisms in the nasopharynx, oropharynx, and hypopharynx, as well as the nucleus tractus solitarius in the brainstem.[49] Regarding lingual nerve repair, objective and subjective neurosensory recovery also is inconsistent.[50]

Diagnostic nerve blocks can be a useful component of the patient evaluation when dysesthesia or unpleasant sensations predominate the clinical scenario. The primary purpose of the diagnostic block is to localize the source of pain and determine the prognosis for recovery following either pharmacologic or surgical therapy. The preferred local anesthetic solution is of a low concentration (eg, 0.25% lidocaine) to selectively block the smaller A delta and C fibers while not affecting the larger myelinated fibers. If the low concentration fails to relieve the pain, a higher concentration is used in the same location. Diagnostic blocks begin peripherally and proceed centrally with constant reassessment of the area of involvement both objectively and subjectively. If patients present with symptoms consistent with sympathetically mediated pain or causalgia, a stellate ganglion block may be performed. These symptoms indicate a problem not amenable to peripheral microneurosurgery. Other pain syndromes that generally are not relieved with diagnostic nerve blocks include anesthesia dolorosa and deafferentation pain; these also are not managed surgically but, rather, pharmacologically.

Nonsurgical Treatment

Pharmacologic management of peripheral nerve injuries is reserved for patients who present with unpleasant abnormal sensations or dysesthesia. In the majority of cases, pharmacologic treatment should be managed with a consultation from an experienced individual such as a neurologist or

available. Minnesota thermal disks made of copper, stainless steel, glass, and polyvinyl chloride can be used.

Although the tests employed in the CNT are considered objective tests, they are, in reality, subjective since they require a patient response. There are few purely objective tests of nerve function available, and these include trigeminal somatosensory evoked potentials and magnetic source imaging.[48] Unfortunately, these tests are not readily available and are not considered a part of the routine assessment of a nerve-injured patient. Also, there is little data on the trigeminal nerve

and the patterns of responses based on specific injuries.

Finally, taste can be assessed by a variety of means, but generally it is performed as either whole-mouth or localized testing. Solutions such as 1 M sodium chloride (salt), 1 M sucrose (sweet), 0.4 M acetic acid (sour), and 0.1 M quinine (bitter) may be used. There are many difficulties with taste assessment in the patient with a lingual nerve injury. The perception of taste alteration is extremely variable and has little correlation with the degree of lingual nerve injury. For example, a patient with a fourth- or fifth-degree lingual nerve

Table 41-6	Systemic Pharmacologic Agents

Local anesthetics
Corticosteroids
Nonsteroidal anti-inflammatory agents
Antidepressants
Narcotic analgesics
Anticonvulsants
Muscle relaxants
Benzodiazepines
Antisympathetic agents

facial pain specialist. Many systemic (Table 41-6) and topical (Table 41-7) medications are available.[51] Whereas the systemic drugs may have significant side effects, topical agents offer the advantages of little systemic absorption, possibly only minor irritation (which can be relieved with a period of abstinence), and over-the-counter availability in many cases. There are also many combinations of topical agents that can be used, such as a eutectic mixture of local anesthetics (EMLA) that contains 2.5% lidocaine and 2.5% prilocaine. Many of the topical agents are prepared in a pleuronic lecithin organogel base. For most oral surgeons long-term pharmacologic management is not part of their routine practice, so the prompt referral to a microneurosurgeon or neurologist may offer the best chance for long-term success. Consideration may be given to a trial of a topical

agent such as capsaicin cream 0.025% tid and/or a systemic medication with few side effects, such as baclofen 10 mg tid or gabapentin 100 mg tid.

Some oral surgeons manage perioperative paresthesia following third molar removal or implant placement with a short course of corticosteroid therapy in an attempt to decrease perineural edema. Although there is little evidence to suggest that systemic steroids actually provide any effect, the use of steroids when a nerve injury occurs, indicates that the surgeon has recognized a problem and has taken an action to improve outcome, which is advantageous when considering medicolegal involvement issues.

Perhaps the most important consideration should be prompt referral, when indicated, to a specialist for pharmacologic or surgical management of the patient with a nerve injury. The indications for referral include but are not limited to those listed in Table 41-8.

In the past, prior to consideration of surgical management, a variety of neuroablative techniques have been used to manage painful neuropathies. Some of these include radiofrequency thermal neurolysis, cryoneurolysis, and alcohol and glycerol injections at the site of injury as well as at the gasserian ganglion. Based on the complications and recurrence rates of dysesthesia, caution should be employed when

Table 41-8	Microneurosurgeon Referral Indications

Observed nerve transection
Complete postoperative anesthesia
Persistent paresthesia (lack of improvement in symptoms) at 4 wk
Presence or development of dysesthesia

considering these options.[52,53] The use of a low-level laser (gallium-aluminumarsenide, wavelength 820 nm) has promise in the area of neural healing. Several studies have shown improvement in objective and subjective neurosensory recoveries with the use of laser therapy in some of the more difficult cases, such as long-standing injuries, orthognathic IAN paresthesia, and prolonged dysesthesia unresponsive to pharmacologic or surgical therapy.[54–56] However, the current limited availability of the low-level laser and the lack of approval by the US Food and Drug Administration preclude its routine use for patients with nerve injuries.

Treatment Algorithms

The decision to proceed with microneurosurgery must be made following a careful patient assessment over a defined period of time. The dilemma is that sufficient time must be given to allow for spontaneous neurosensory recovery but that prompt surgical intervention may afford the best chance for recovery. Time is a critical issue for three main reasons. First, at the site of injury, distal nerve degeneration (wallerian degeneration—named for Augustus Waller in 1892) occurs owing to the interruption of axonal transport. This progressive loss of neural tissue may compromise future repair attempts. Second, at the nerve cell bodies there is ganglion cell death that occurs early following injury.[57] Third, as the time from nerve injury increases, there is a higher likelihood that central cortical changes may occur, and these would make peripheral repair ineffective.[58] As a result, if 30 to 50% of gan-

Table 41-7	Topical Medications	
Category	Example	
Topical anesthetics	5% viscous lidocaine gel; 20% benzocaine gel; 2.5% lidocaine with 2.5% prilocaine	
Neuropeptides	Capsaicin cream (0.025% or 0.075%)	
Nonsteroidal anti-inflammatory drugs	Ketoprofen 10–20% PLO base; diclofenac 10–20% PLO base	
Sympathomimetics	Clonidine 0.01% PLO base or patch	
N-methyl-D-aspartate blocking agents	Ketamine 0.5% PLO base	
Anticonvulsants	Carbamazepine 2% PLO base	
Tricyclic antidepressants	Amitriptyline 2% PLO base	
Antispasmodics	Baclofen 2% PLO base	

PLO = pleuronic lecithin organogel.

glion cells have undergone necrosis, the best possible success rate from surgical repair may also be 30 to 50%.

Microneurosurgery is indicated for persistent paresthesia that fails to improve over successive examinations. This includes both subjective and objective assessments. Surgery is not indicated if there is continued improvement at each subsequent assessment. The current recommendations are to consider surgery for the lingual nerve within 1 to 3 months following the injury, and for the IAN within 3 to 6 months following the injury (Figure 41-8). The rationale for the difference in time is that the IAN lies within a bony canal that can guide spontaneous regeneration, so more time is allotted for that process, whereas a lingual nerve injured within soft tissue does not have a "physiologic conduit" to guide regeneration. In general, the oral surgeon should have follow-up examinations with the patient over a period of approximately 4 weeks. If there is persistent paresthesia or a worsening of symptoms, referral should be made to a microneurosurgical specialist.

For an unobserved nerve injury, the plan should be to continue neurosensory testing for 1 month and then to refer for surgery in the 1- to 3-month (lingual nerve) or 3- to 6-month (IAN) time periods. For an observed nerve injury, treatment should focus on the specific etiology. For a suspected traction injury (Sunderland first-, second-, and third-degree injuries), the patient should be tested for 1 month for signs of expected spontaneous recovery. In the case of nerve compression, immediate decompression should be considered. This includes removal of a root displaced into the IAN canal, removal or replacement when there is evidence of implant impingement within the confines

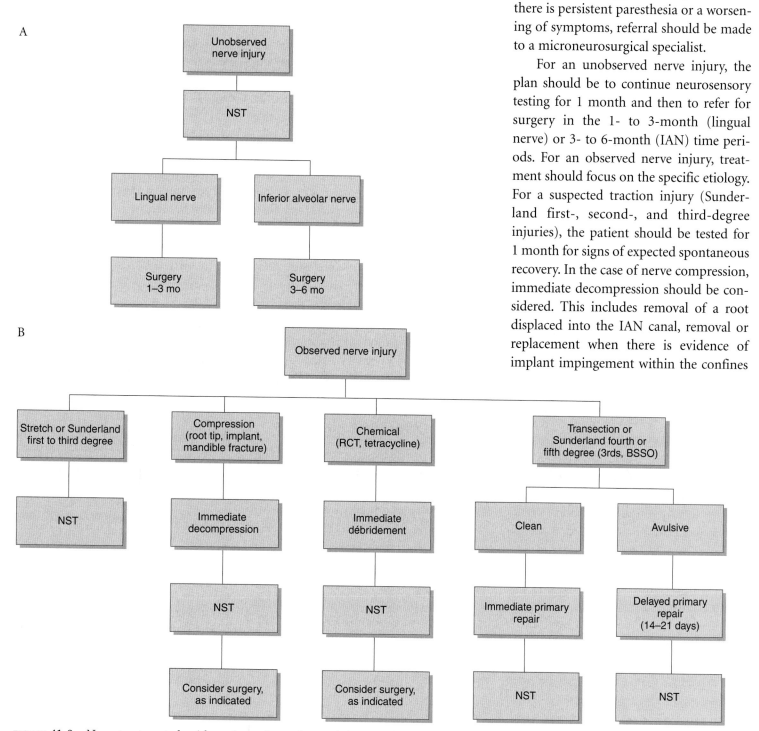

FIGURE **41-8**   *Nerve treatment algorithms: A, unobserved nerve injury; B, observed nerve injury. BSSO = bilateral sagittal split osteotomy; NST = neurosensory testing; RCT = root canal therapy.*

of the IAN canal, or reduction and alignment of a displaced posterior mandible fracture including the IAN canal. Neurosensory testing should be performed following decompression, and microneurosurgery should be considered as indicated. Chemical injuries should be débrided promptly. For observed transection injuries (Sunderland fourth- or fifth-degree injuries), an immediate primary repair may be performed for a clean transection injury (eg, scalpel transection). For an avulsive injury (eg, lingual nerve entangled in a bur), consideration is given to a delayed primary repair performed at 3 weeks following the injury. This allows time for the proximal and distal nerve stumps to define the degree of injury, and to determine whether the surrounding environment is conducive to nerve surgery, when there are high levels of neurotropic and neurotrophic factors. After surgery, patients should be followed up with repeat neurosensory testing.

The success rates of microneurosurgical reconstruction following nerve injury are variable in the literature. This is due to many factors including the lack of standardization with the following[59]: age, the etiology of injury, the time of delay from injury to repair, specific surgical techniques used, the length of the nerve gap, the method of neurosensory examination, the use of normative values for control sites, follow-up period variability, and criteria to define success (Table 41-9). A global review of the literature might indicate a success rate of 30 to 50% following microneurosurgery, including direct and gap repairs. In general, direct repair is preferred over gap repair (eg, using an autogenous nerve graft) and has higher reported success rates.[60] Perhaps the largest study to date indicates an overall "success" rate of 76.2% in 521 patients.[61] The success criteria were defined as light touch detected > 80% of the time and a 30% decrease in postoperative pain level. The study results suggested some important trends in outcome.

Hypoesthetic injuries improved better following microneurosurgery than did hyperesthetic injuries, the lingual nerve recovered better than did the IAN overall, and there was a decrease in success associated with a delay of > 6 months. A recent report of 51 microneurosurgical reconstructions (direct and gap repairs) found that 10 patients subjectively reported good improvement, 18 patients some improvement, 22 patients no improvement, and 1 patient reported feeling worse following surgery.[62] This indicates that 55% of patients showed some improvement. In another study of 53 surgical patients, with a mean follow-up of 13 months, light touch improved from 0 to 51% and pinprick nociception improved from 34 to 77%. Patients also experienced improved taste and an increased number of fungiform papillae, and there was a decrease in incidence of accidental tongue biting. Interestingly, there was no correlation of success with delay from time of injury to repair. No patient became completely normal, and there was no reduction in dysesthesia; however, most patients considered the surgery worthwhile. There is certainly a need for standardization in all aspects of evaluation and management of microneurosurgical patients.

Surgical Treatment

Microneurosurgical reconstruction involves a sequence of surgical procedures including exposure, dissection, assessment, manipulation, and repair. Many of the techniques of trigeminal nerve repair follow those of hand surgery and use similar instruments. In general, surgical loupe magnification (×3.5 magnification) is adequate. An operating microscope (×12 magnification) is cumbersome and difficult to use with a transoral exposure, although it may be more useful with a transfacial approach.

Exposure

Surgical access to the lingual or IAN may be accomplished transfacially or transoral-

ly. The transfacial approach affords wide exposure and access; however, it necessitates a facial incision with subsequent scar formation. The intraoral approach provides a more difficult surgical access and requires more diligence in microsurgery in the posterior regions of the oral cavity, but it avoids a facial incision. The decision regarding surgical access depends on an individual patient's anatomy, the site of nerve injury, planned surgical procedures, patient preference, and surgeon's skill and experience.

External Neurolysis

Microdissection of the nerve once exposed involves liberation of the nerve from the surrounding tissues to facilitate inspection. For the lingual nerve this procedure may involve the release of the nerve from a lateral adhesive neuroma in the area of the lingual plate in the third molar region, whereas for the IAN a corticotomy is generally required for external neurolysis. Sev-

Table 41-9 Classification of Sensory Recovery	
Grade (Stage)	*Recovery of Sensibility*
S0	No recovery
S1	Recovery of deep cutaneous pain
S1+	Recovery of some superficial pain
S2	Return of some superficial pain and tactile sensation
S2+	S2 with over-response
S3*	Return of some superficial pain and tactile sensation without over-response; two-point discrimination > 15 mm
S3+	S3 with good stimulus localization; two-point discrimination = 7–15 mm
S4	Complete recovery, S3+; two-point discrimination = 2–6 mm

*S3 score indicates significant clinical recovery (Wyrick JD, Stern PJ. Secondary nerve reconstruction. Hand Clin 1992;8:587).
Adapted from Mackinnon SE. Surgical management of the peripheral nerve gap. Clin Plast Surg 1989;16:587.

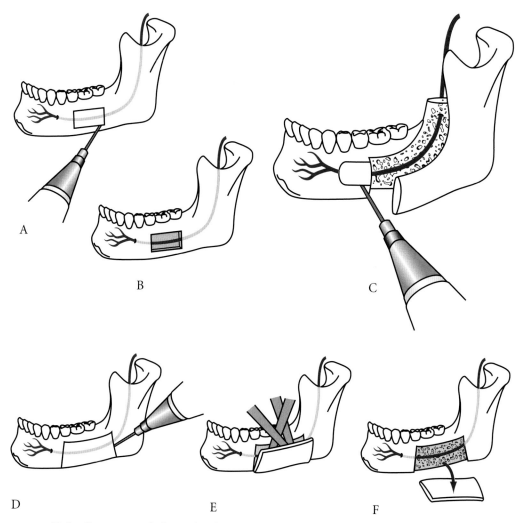

FIGURE **41-9** *Exposure techniques for the IAN: A, Lateral decortication of the mandible; B, with exposure of the inferior alveolar neurovascular bundle. C, Sagittal ramus osteotomy with anterior extension via lateral decortication to the mental foramen. D, Lateral mandibular decortication. E, Bone removal with chisels. F, Wide exposure of the neurovascular bundle.*

eral techniques have been described for lateral decortication in the area of the third molar for IAN exposure, and these range from a simple nerve transpositioning to a modified buccal corticotomy or a unilateral sagittal split ramus osteotomy (Figure 41-9).[63] The location of the injury and the surgeon's preference frequently dictate the specific approach used. The lingual nerve is usually exposed via a modified incision used for third molar surgery with a sulcular lingual extension (Figure 41-10). For the infraorbital nerve, external neurolysis may be performed secondary to reduction and fixation of a displaced zygomatico-maxillary complex fracture impinging on the neurovascular bundle at the infraorbital foramen. It has been suggested that external neurolysis may provide definitive treatment for a nerve injury if the nerve compression is < 25% of the normal diameter, if the paresthesia is of short duration (< 6 mo), and if there is no evidence of neuroma formation.[64]

Internal Neurolysis

The term *internal neurolysis* refers to surgical manipulations within the epineurium to prepare the nerve for repair. Sophisticated maneuvers may compromise repair by unnecessary removal of tissue and

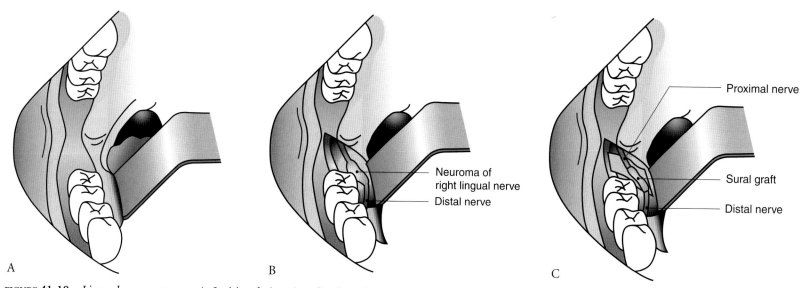

FIGURE **41-10** *Lingual nerve exposure. A, Incision design via a distobuccal extension and lingual gingival sulcus approach. B, Right lingual nerve exposure with neuroma. C, Right lingual nerve repair with an interpositional nerve graft.*

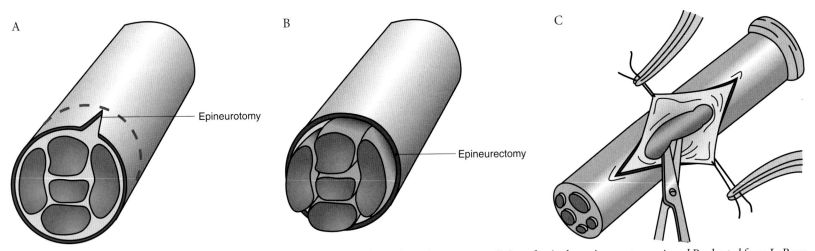

FIGURE **41-11**   *Internal neurolysis: A, epifascicular epineurotomy; B, epifascicular epineurectomy; C, interfascicular epineurectomy. A and B adapted from LaBanc JP. Reconstructive microneurosurgery of the trigeminal nerve. In: Peterson LJ, Indresano AT, Marciani RD, Roser SM. Principles of oral and maxillofacial surgery. Vol 2. Philadelphia: J.B. Lippincott Company; 1992. p. 1067.*

induction of cicatrix formation owing to excessive manipulation. Several types of internal neurolysis have been described, including epifascicular epineurotomy, epifascicular epineurectomy, and interfascicular epineurectomy (Figure 41-11). The first two prepare the epineurium for repair; any interfascicular surgery may cause further fascicular disruption and scarring. Extensive internal neurolysis procedures should be used with caution.

Nerve Stump Preparation

Perhaps the most critical portion of the surgical procedure involves the inspection of the proximal and distal nerve stumps via magnification. The preparation of the nerve stumps follows exposure; there may already be an existing discontinuity from a transection injury. When a neuroma is present, meticulous excision is required (Figure 41-12). It must be recognized that with any neuroma, the clinical appearance of neuronal edema or atrophy is less than the internal fascicular changes (see Figure 41-12A). Failure to resect enough nerve tissue to reach normal fascicles results in a failure of neurosensory recovery. Once the nerve is divided, if necessary, into proximal and distal stumps, care must be taken to resect small (1 mm) portions of the nerve trunk in both directions (see Figure

41-12B) until healthy glistening white mushrooming fascicles are seen to herniate through the edges of the epineurium (see Figure 41-12C).

Approximation

The trigeminal nerve is similar to other peripheral nerves in that it does not tolerate tension well; therefore, tension-free closure is mandatory.[65] The deleterious effects of tension result from vascular compromise and subsequent fibrosis at the nerve repair site. Approximation is the act of

bringing the nerve stumps into contact and assessing the degree of tension that is present. At the time of approximation a decision must be made regarding whether to use an interpositional graft. In general, mobilization with primary epineurial repair is possible for lingual nerve gaps < 10 mm and for IAN gaps < 5 mm.

Coaptation

Coaptation is the process of aligning the proximal and distal nerve stumps into the premorbid cross-sectional fascicular ori-

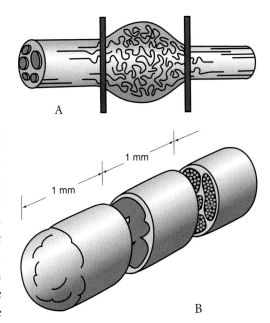

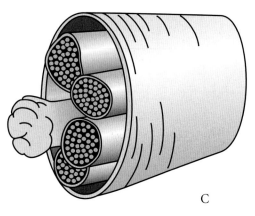

FIGURE **41-12** *Nerve stump preparation. A, Neuroma; resection at the "clinical margin" of the neuroma fails to complete nerve preparation. B, Neuroma resection in 1 mm increments. C, Mushrooming fascicle.*

entation. This is a difficult maneuver with a polyfascicular nerve that has undergone any degree of distal nerve changes in diameter or fascicular pattern. This step is usually not performed painstakingly in trigeminal nerve repair because of the complex polyfascicular pattern.

Neurorrhaphy

Neurorrhaphy is the act of nerve suturing for both direct and gap repairs. The trigeminal nerve is repaired using epineurial sutures, not perineurial sutures (Figure 41-13). Generally, an 8-0 monofilament nonresorbable nylon suture is chosen since a resorbable material would invoke inflammation and disturb the area of anticipated neural healing. At least two sutures are used per anastomosis site to prevent rotation, but not more than three or four sutures should be used per anastomosis. The first suture is placed on the medial side of the anastomosis since it is more difficult to access. The epineurium is pierced with the needle 0.5 to 1.0 mm from the edge of the nerve. The second suture is placed 180° from the first suture, and then an assessment is made regarding the need for more sutures.

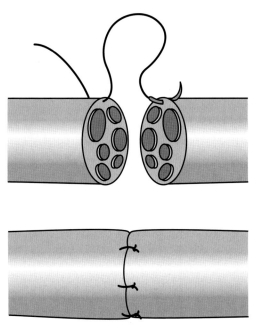

FIGURE 41-13 *Direct epineurial neurorrhaphy.*

Table 41-10	Size of Donor Nerve Grafts Relative to Injured Nerve		
	Donor Nerve		
Injured Nerve	*Sural* *(2.1 mm)*	*Greater Auricular* *(1.5 mm)*	*Greater Auricular* *Cable (3.0 mm)*
Inferior alveolar (2.4 mm)	88%	63%	125%
Lingual (3.2 mm)	66%	47%	94%
Adapted from Brammer JP and Epker BN.[68]			

Nerve Grafts

When neurorrhaphy is not possible without tension and a nerve gap exists, an interpositional graft must be considered for indirect neurorrhaphy.[66] The options for autogenous nerve grafting include but are not limited to the sural nerve, the greater auricular nerve, and possibly the medial antebrachial cutaneous nerve.[67] The sural nerve is the preferred nerve for grafting since it most appropriately matches the nerve diameter and the fascicular number and pattern of the trigeminal nerve (Table 41-10).[68] The area of the nerve superior to the lateral malleolus exhibits less branching than at or below the lateral malleolus. The sural nerve, or medial sural cutaneous nerve, is a branch of the sacral plexus (S1, S2) and supplies sensory information to the posterior lower extremity and the dorsolateral foot. Sural grafts up to 20 cm in length are possible, and patients tolerate the donor site deficit well.[69] The greater auricular nerve is a poor choice for trigeminal repair. As a branch of the cervical plexus (C1, C2), the greater auricular nerve supplies sensation to the pre- and postauricular regions, the lower third of the ear, and the skin overlying the posteroinferior border at the angle of the mandible. Patients are generally not amenable to sacrificing one facial region for another. Additionally, the small diameter of the nerve makes it useful only when used as a cable graft (Figure 41-14). The sole advantage of a greater auricular graft over a sural graft is in situations when it can be harvested via the same incision for another procedure, such as the repair of an

extraoral mandibular fracture or management of pathology. The basic premise with graft repair is that the graft supplies the Schwann cells and growth factors necessary to support and encourage axonal sprouting through the graft toward the target site.

Entubulation Techniques

In an attempt to avoid donor site morbidity, a variety of entubulation techniques have been proposed to create conduits during nerve regeneration (Figure 41-15). These conduits involve both autogenous and alloplastic materials (Table 41-11). The autogenous options include vein,[70–72] collagen,[73,74] and muscle grafts.[75] Alloplastic

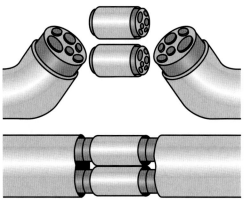

FIGURE 41-14 *Greater auricular nerve cable graft.*

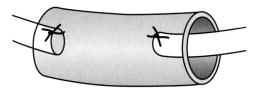

FIGURE 41-15 *Entubulation (conduit) nerve repair.*

Table 41-11 Materials for Entubulation (Conduit) Repair

Autogenous materials
  Collagen
  Muscle
  Fascia
  Vein
Alloplastic materials
  Polyglycolic acid
  Polyester
  Polytetrafluoroethylene (PTFE)
  Expanded PTFE
  Silicone, polymeric silicone

materials include polyglycolic acid,[76] polymeric silicone,[77] and expanded polytetrafluoroethylene.[78–81] It appears that the use of these alloplastic materials has a high success in the animal model but poor clinical outcomes. Further investigation is warranted as new materials are developed.

Postsurgical Management

In the majority of cases, patients experience a variable period of complete anesthesia following nerve repair. In general, nerve regeneration progresses at approximately 1 mm/d (about 3 cm/mo) from the cell body to the target site. For example, with a direct IAN repair, the approximate distance from the trigeminal ganglion to the lower lip and chin is 10 cm; therefore, complete nerve regeneration takes about 100 days or 12 weeks following repair. With graft repair the time frame is lengthened owing to slowed regeneration through the graft site, but recovery is variable. A poor outcome following microneurosurgery may preclude future surgical options; therefore, the best chance for microneurosurgical success is at the first (and most likely, the last) surgical intervention.

Medicolegal Issues

Oral and maxillofacial surgeons currently practice during a time of "malpractice crisis," and nerve injuries secondary to third molar removal account for a large propor-

tion of the complaints.[82] Based on the information contained in this chapter and recent trends in malpractice, all oral and maxillofacial surgeons should have a minimum of understanding of the diagnosis and management of nerve injuries according to the so-called legal parameters of care.[83] These are summarized as follows:

- Spontaneous sensory recovery occurs in most but not all patients. It is difficult to predict early, it may not be "complete," and it may not be to the patient's satisfaction. Nerves in soft tissue (lingual nerve) have a lower rate of spontaneous regeneration than do those in bony canals (IAN)
- All nerve injuries should be documented and evaluated with a history, examination, and neurosensory testing (objective and subjective). The injury should be classified (Seddon or Sunderland). In cases of observed or known nerve injury, prompt referral for microsurgery provides the best opportunity for sensory recovery
- Repeat examinations at frequent intervals may be necessary. Patients should be followed up for at least 1 month. Complete recovery in 1 month indicates neurapraxia, and no further treatment is indicated. Neurosensory dysfunction that lasts > 1 month indicates a higher-grade injury with uncertain spontaneous neurosensory recovery. Microneurosurgical consultation should be considered
- Nerve injuries that show improvement (objective and/or subjective) may be followed up expectantly. Once improvement stops for a period of time, it usually does not begin again
- Most nerve injuries resolve within 3 to 9 months, but *only* if improvement begins prior to 3 months. Patients who are anesthetic at 3 months usually do not achieve significant neurosensory recovery. Prompt microsurgery is usually indicated

- Patients with partial sensory loss and/or painful sensations *that they find unacceptable* should be considered for microsurgery if objective and subjective findings have not improved or returned to normal by 4 months. Microsurgical delay decreases the chance of success because progressive distal nerve degeneration and/or the development of a central pain syndrome occur
- Some painful neuropathies may be managed nonsurgically under the supervision of a microneurosurgeon or other experienced individual (eg, neurologist)
- Angry uninformed patients with nerve injuries are less likely to improve with any treatment, surgical or nonsurgical. A discussion regarding options and the risk of nerve injury should be provided so that the patient can give informed consent. Local anesthetic injections carry a risk of nerve injury
- Early surgical intervention (ie, at 3–4 mo) is *more likely* to produce neurosensory improvement than is late intervention. Surgery delayed beyond 12 months is seriously compromised by distal nerve degeneration and the development of chronic pain syndromes
- Surgery is *more likely* to improve responses to objective sensory testing and/or to reduce functional impairment than it is to reduce pain or subjective feelings of numbness

References

1. American Association of Oral and Maxillofacial Surgeons. Parameters and pathways: clinical practice guidelines for oral and maxillofacial surgery (AAOMS ParPath 01), Version 3.0. J Oral Maxillofac Surg 2001;59 Suppl.
2. Pogrel MA, Thamby S. The etiology of altered sensation in the inferior alveolar, lingual, and mental nerve as a result of dental treatment. J Calif Dent J 1999;27:531, 534–8.
3. Zuniga JR, Leist JC. Topical tetracycline-induced neuritis: a case report. J Oral Maxillofac Surg 1995;53:196.
4. Leist JC, Zuniga JR. Experimental topical

tetracycline-induced neuritis in the rat. J Oral Maxillofac Surg 1995;53:427.

5. Pichler JW, Beirne OR. Lingual flap retraction and prevention of lingual nerve damage associated with third molar surgery: a systematic review of the literature. Oral Surg Oral Med Oral Pathol Oral Radiol Endod 2001;91:395.

6. Rood JP, Shehab AAN. The radiological prediction of inferior alveolar nerve injury during third molar surgery. Br J Oral Maxillofac Surg 1990;28:20.

7. Pogrel MA, Lee JS, Muff DF. Coronectomy in lower third molar removal. J Oral Maxillofac Surg 2003;61 Suppl 1:25.

8. Alling CC. Dysesthesia of the lingual and inferior alveolar nerves following third molar surgery. J Oral Maxillofac Surg 1986;44:454.

9. Gulicher D, Gerlach KL. Sensory impairment of the lingual and inferior alveolar nerves following removal of impacted third molars. Int J Oral Maxillofac Surg 2001; 30:306.

10. Carmichael FA, McGowan DA. Incidence of nerve damage following third molar removal: a West Scotland Oral Surgery Research Group study. Br J Oral Maxillofac Surg 1992;30:78.

11. Valmaseda-Castellon E, Berini-Aytes L, Gay-Escoda C. Lingual nerve damage after third lower molar surgical extraction. Oral Surg Oral Med Oral Pathol Oral Radiol Endod 2000;90:567.

12. Valmaseda-Castellon E, Berini-Aytes L, Gay-Escoda C. Inferior alveolar nerve damage after lower third molar surgical extraction: a prospective study of 1117 surgical extractions. Oral Surg Oral Med Oral Pathol Oral Radiol Endod 2001;92:377.

13. Kisselbach JE, Chamberlain JG. Clinical and anatomic observations on the relationship of the lingual nerve to the mandibular third molar region. J Oral Maxillofac Surg 1984; 42:565.

14. Pogrel MA, Renaut A, Schmidt B, Ammar A. The relationship of the lingual nerve to the mandibular third molar region: an anatomic study. J Oral Maxillofac Surg 1995; 53:1178.

15. Holzle FW, Wolff KD. Anatomic position of the lingual nerve in the mandibular third molar region with special consideration of an atrophied mandibular crest: an anatomical study. Int J Oral Maxillofac Surg 2001; 30:333.

16. Miloro M, Halkias LE, Slone HW, Chakeres DW. Assessment of the lingual nerve in the third molar region using magnetic resonance imaging. J Oral Maxillofac Surg 1997;55:134.

17. Harn SD, Durham TM. Incidence of lingual nerve trauma and postinjection complications in conventional mandibular block anesthesia. J Am Dent Assoc 1990;121:519.

18. Pogrel MA, Bryan J, Regezi J. Nerve damage associated with inferior alveolar nerve blocks. J Am Dent Assoc 1995;126:1150.

19. Pogrel MA, Thamby S. Permanent nerve involvement resulting from inferior alveolar nerve blocks. J Am Dent Assoc 2000; 131:901.

20. Pogrel MA, Schmidt BL, Sambajon V, et al. Lingual nerve damage due to inferior alveolar nerve blocks: a possible explanation. J Am Dent Assoc 2003;134:195.

21. Van Eeden SP, Patel MF. Letter: prolonged paraesthesia following inferior alveolar nerve block using articaine. Br J Oral Maxillofac Surg 2002;40:519.

22. Stacy GC, Hajjar G. Barbed needle and inexplicable paresthesias and trismus after dental regional anesthesia. Oral Surg Oral Med Oral Pathol 1994;77:585.

23. Pogrel MA, Schmidt BL. Trigeminal nerve chemical neurotrauma from injectable materials. Oral Maxillofac Surg Clin North Am 2001;13:247.

24. Behrman S. Complications of sagittal osteotomy of the mandibular ramus. J Oral Surg 1972;35:554.

25. Hegdvedt AK, Zuniga JR. Lingual nerve injury as a complication of sagittal ramus osteotomy. J Oral Maxillofac Surg 1990;48:647.

26. Schow SR, Triplett RG, Solomon JM. Lingual nerve injury associated with overpenetration of bicortical screws used for rigid fixation of a bilateral sagittal split osteotomy. J Oral Maxillofac Surg 1996;54:1451.

27. August M, Marchena J, Donady J, Kaban L. Neurosensory deficit and functional impairment after sagittal ramus osteotomy: a long-term follow-up study. J Oral Maxillofac Surg 1998;56:1231.

28. Westermark A, Bystedt H, von Konow L. Inferior alveolar nerve function after mandibular osteotomies. Br J Oral Maxillofac Surg 1998;36:425.

29. Karas ND, Boyd SB, Sinn DP. Recovery of neurosensory function following orthognathic surgery. J Oral Maxillofac Surg 1990;48:124.

30. Teerijoki-Oksa T, Jaaskelainen SK, Forssell K, et al. Risk factors of nerve injury during mandibular sagittal split osteotomy. Int J Oral Maxillofac Surg 2001;31:33.

31. Nishioka GJ, Zysset MK, van Sickels JE. Neurosensory disturbance with rigid fixation of the bilateral sagittal split osteotomy. J Oral Maxillofac Surg 1987;45:20.

32. Jones DL, Wolford LM. Intraoperative record-

ing of trigeminal evoked potentials during orthognathic surgery. Int J Adult Orthodon Orthognath Surg 1990;5:167.

33. Hallikainen D, Iizuka T, Lindqvist C. Cross-sectional tomography in evaluation of patients undergoing sagittal split osteotomy. J Oral Maxillofac Surg 1992;50:1269.

34. Frerich B, Cornelius C-P, Wietholter H. Critical time of exposure of the rabbit inferior alveolar nerve to Carnoy's solution. J Oral Maxillofac Surg 1994;52:599.

35. Loescher AR, Robinson PP. The effect of surgical medicaments on peripheral nerve function. Br J Oral Maxillofac Surg 1998;36:327.

36. Block MS, Daire J, Stover J, Matthews M. Changes in the inferior alveolar nerve following mandibular lengthening in the dog using distraction osteogenesis. J Oral Maxillofac Surg 1993;51:652.

37. Hu J, Zou S, Tang Z, et al. Response of Schwann cells in the inferior alveolar nerve to distraction osteogenesis: an ultrastructural and immunohistochemical study. Int J Oral Maxillofac Surg 2003;32:318.

38. Hu J, Tang Z, Wang D, Buckley MJ. Changes in the inferior alveolar nerve after mandibular lengthening with different rates of distraction. J Oral Maxillofac Surg 2001;59:1041.

39. Louis P. Inferior alveolar nerve transposition for endosseous implant placement: a preliminary report. Oral Maxillofac Surg Clin North Am 2001;13:265.

40. Zuniga JR. Normal response to nerve injury: histology and psychophysics of degeneration and regeneration. Oral Maxillofac Surg Clin North Am 1992;4:323.

41. Muller HW, Stoll G. Nerve injury and regeneration: basic insights and therapeutic interventions. Curr Opin Neurol 1998;11:557.

42. Seddon JJ. Three types of nerve injury. Brain 1943; 66:237.

43. Sunderland S. A classification of peripheral nerve injuries produced by loss of function. Brain 1951;74:491.

44. Dellon AL, Mackinnon SE. Basic scientific and clinical applications of peripheral nerve regeneration. Surg Annu 1988;20:59.

45. Coglan KM, Irvine GH. Neurological damage after sagittal split osteotomy. Int J Oral Maxillofac Surg 1986;15:369.

46. Zuniga JR, Cheng N, Miller I, Phillips C. Regeneration of taste receptors and recovery of taste after lingual nerve repair. J Oral Maxillofac Surg 1994;52 Suppl 2:128.

47. Zuniga JR, Meyer RA, Gregg JM, et al. The accuracy of clinical neurosensory testing for nerve injury diagnosis. J Oral Maxillofac Surg 1998;56:2.

48. McDonald AR, Roberts TPL, Rowley HA,

Pogrel MA. Noninvasive somatosensory monitoring of the injured inferior alveolar nerve using magnetic source imaging. J Oral Maxillofac Surg 1996;54:1968.

49. Scrivani SJ, Moses M, Donoff, RB, Kaban LB. Taste perception after lingual nerve repair. J Oral Maxillofac Surg 2000;58:3.

50. Hillerup S, Hjorting-Hansen E, Reumert T. Repair of the lingual nerve after iatrogenic injury: a follow-up study of return of sensation and taste. J Oral Maxillofac Surg 1994;52:1028.

51. Padilla M, Clark GT, Merrill RL. Topical medications for orofacial neuropathic pain: a review. J Am Dent Assoc 2000;131:184.

52. Gregg JM, Small EW. Surgical management of trigeminal pain with radiofrequency lesions of peripheral nerves. J Oral Maxillofac Surg 1986;44:122.

53. Fardy MJ, Patton DW. Complications associated with peripheral alcohol injections in the management of trigeminal neuralgia. Br J Oral Maxillofac Surg 1994;32:387.

54. Khullar S, Emami B, Westermark A, Haanes H. Effect of low-level laser treatment on neurosensory deficits subsequent to sagittal ramus osteotomy. Oral Surg Oral Med Oral Pathol Oral Radiol Endod 1996;82:132.

55. Khullar S, Brodin E, Barkvoll B, Haanes H. Preliminary study of low-level laser treatment of long-standing sensory aberrations of the inferior alveolar nerve. J Oral Maxillofac Surg 1996;54:2.

56. Miloro M, Repasky M. Low-level laser effect on neurosensory recovery after sagittal ramus osteotomy. Oral Surg Oral Med Oral Pathol Oral Radiol Endod 2000;89:12.

57. Zuniga JR. Trigeminal ganglion cell response to mental nerve section and repair in the rat. J Oral Maxillofac Surg 1999;57:427.

58. Pons TP. Massive cortical reorganization after sensory deafferentation in adult macaques. Science 1991; 252:1159.

59. Dodson TB, Kaban LB. Recommendations for management of trigeminal nerve defects based on a critical appraisal of the literature. J Oral Maxillofac Surg 1997;55:1380.

60. Smith KG, Roninson PP. An experimental study of three methods of lingual nerve defect repair. J Oral Maxillofac Surg 1995; 53:1052.

61. LaBanc JP, Gregg JM. Trigeminal nerve injuries: basic problems, historical perspectives, early successes, and remaining challenges. Oral Maxillofac Surg Clin North Am 1992;4:277.

62. Pogrel MA. The results of microneurosurgery of the inferior alveolar and lingual nerve. J Oral Maxillofac Surg 2002;60:485.

63. Miloro M. Surgical access for inferior alveolar nerve repair. J Oral Maxillofac Surg 1995;53:1224.

64. Joshi A, Rood JP. External neurolysis of the lingual nerve. Int J Oral Maxillofac Surg 2002; 31:40.

65. Millesi H, Terzis JK. Nomenclature in peripheral nerve surgery. Clin Plast Surg 1984;11:3.

66. Eppley BL, Snyders RV. Microanatomic analysis of the trigeminal nerve and potential nerve graft donor sites. J Oral Maxillofac Surg 1991;49:612.

67. McCormick SU, Buchbinder D. Microanatomic analysis of the medial antebrachial cutaneous nerve as a potential donor nerve in maxillofacial grafting. J Oral Maxillofac Surg 1994;52:1022.

68. Brammar JP, Epker BN. Anatomic-histologic survey of the sural nerve: implications for inferior alveolar nerve grafting. J Oral Maxillofac Surg 1988;46:111.

69. Miloro M. Subjective outcomes following sural nerve harvest. J Oral Maxillofac Surg 2002;60 Suppl 1:75.

70. Miloro M. Inferior alveolar nerve regeneration through an autogenous vein graft. J Oral Maxillofac Surg 1996;54:65.

71. Pogrel MA, Maghen A. The use of autogenous vein grafts for inferior alveolar and lingual nerve reconstruction. J Oral Maxillofac Surg 2001;59:985.

72. Miloro M. Discussion: the use of autogenous vein grafts for inferior alveolar and lingual nerve reconstruction. J Oral Maxillofac Surg 2001;59:988.

73. Kitahara AK, Suzuki Y, Qi P. Facial nerve repair using a collagen conduit in cats. Scand J Plast Reconstr Surg Hand Surg 1999; 33:187.

74. Eppley BL, Delfino JJ. Collagen tube repair of the mandibular nerve: a preliminary investigation in the rat. J Oral Maxillofac Surg 1996;46:41.

75. DeFranzo AJ, Morykwas MJ, LaRosse JR. Autologous denatured muscle as a nerve graft. J Reconstr Microsurg 1994;10:145.

76. Mackinnon SE, Dellon AL. Clinical nerve reconstruction with a bioabsorbable polyglycolic acid tube. Plast Reconstr Surg 1990;85:419.

77. Eppley BL, Snyders RV, Winkelmann T. Efficacy of nerve growth factor in regeneration of the mandibular nerve: a preliminary report. J Oral Maxillofac Surg 1991;49:61.

78. Miloro M, Macy J. Expanded polytetrafluoroethylene entubulation of the rabbit inferior alveolar nerve. Oral Surg Oral Med Oral Pathol 2000;89:292–8.

79. Miloro M, Halkias L, Mallery S, et al. Low level laser effect on neural regeneration in Gore-Tex tubes. Oral Surg Oral Med Oral Pathol Oral Radiol Endod 2002;93:27–34.

80. Pitta MC, Wolford LM, Mehra P, Hopkin J. Use of Gore-Tex tubing as a conduit for inferior alveolar and lingual nerve repair: experience with 6 cases. J Oral Maxillofac Surg 2001;59:493.

81. Pogrel MA, McDonald AR, Kaban LB. Gore-tex tubing as a conduit for repair of lingual and inferior alveolar nerve continuity defects: a preliminary report. J Oral Maxillofac Surg 1998;56:319.

82. Lydiatt DD. Litigation and the lingual nerve. J Oral Maxillofac Surg 2003;61:197.

83. Deegan AE. The numbing truth. Monitor 1998;9:1.

APPENDIX   Nerve Terminology Review*

allodynia: Pain due to a stimulus that does not normally provoke pain.

analgesia: Absence of pain in the presence of stimulation that would normally be painful.

anesthesia: Absence of any sensation in the presence of stimulation that would normally be painful or nonpainful.

anesthesia dolorosa: Pain in an area or region that is anesthetic.

atypical neuralgia: A pain syndrome that is not typical of classic nontraumatic trigeminal neuralgia.

axonotmesis (Seddon) or second- sthrough fourth-degree injuries (Sunderland): Nerve injury characterized by axonal injury with subsequent degeneration and regeneration.

causalgia: Burning pain, allodynia, and hyperpathia after a partial injury of a nerve.

central pain: Pain associated with a primary central nervous system lesion (spinal cord or brain trauma, vascular lesions, tumors).

chemoreceptor: A peripheral nerve receptor that is responsive to chemicals, including catecholamines.

deafferentation pain: Pain occurring in a region of partial or complete traumatic nerve injury in which there is interruption of afferent impulses by destruction of the afferent pathway or other mechanism.

dysesthesia: An abnormal sensation, either spontaneous or evoked, that is unpleasant. All dysesthesias are a type of paresthesia but not all paresthesias are dysesthesias.

endoneurium: A connective tissue sheath surrounding individual nerve fibers and their Schwann cells.

epineurium: A loose connective tissue sheath that encases the entire nerve trunk.

fascicle: A bundle of nerve fibers encased by the perineurium.

hyperalgesia: An increased response to a stimulus that is normally painful.

hyperesthesia: An increased sensitivity to stimulation, excluding the special senses (ie, seeing, hearing, taste, and smell).

hyperpathia: A painful syndrome characterized by increased reaction to a stimulus, especially a repetitive stimulus. The threshold is increased as well.

hypoalgesia: Diminished pain in response to a normally painful stimulus.

hypoesthesia: Decreased sensitivity to stimulation, excluding the special senses (ie, seeing, hearing, taste, and smell).

mechanoreceptor: A peripheral nerve receptor preferentially activated by physical deformation from pressure and associated with large sensory axons.

mesoneurium: A connective tissue sheath, analogous to the mesentery of the intestine, that suspends the nerve trunk within soft tissue.

monofascicular pattern: Characteristic cross-section of a nerve containing one large fascicle.

neuralgia: Pain in the distribution of a nerve or nerves.

neurapraxia (Seddon) or first-degree injury (Sunderland): Nerve injury characterized by a conduction block, with rapid and virtually complete return of sensation or function and no axonal degeneration.

neuritis: A special case of neuropathy now reserved for inflammatory processes affecting nerves.

neurolysis: The surgical separation of adhesions from an injured peripheral nerve.

neuroma: An anatomically disorganized mass of collagen and nerve fascicles, and a functionally abnormal region of a peripheral nerve resulting from a failed regeneration following injury.

neuropathy: A disturbance of function or a pathologic change in a nerve.

neurotization: Axonal invasion of the distal nerve trunk.

neurotmesis (Seddon) or fifth-degree injury (Sunderland): Nerve injury characterized by severe disruption of the connective tissue components of the nerve trunk, with compromised sensory and functional recovery. Third-degree injury: Characterized by axonal damage and a breach of the endoneurial sheath, resulting in intrafascicular disorganization. The perineurium and epineurium remain intact. The mechanism is typically traction or compression. Fourth-degree injury: Characterized by disruption of the axon, endoneurium, and perineurium, resulting in severe fascicular disorganization. The epineurium remains intact. Possible mechanisms include traction, compression, injection injury, and chemical injury. Fifth-degree injury: Characterized by complete disruption of the nerve trunk with considerable tissue loss. Possible mechanisms include laceration, avulsion, and chemical injury.

nociceptor: A receptor preferentially sensitive to a noxious stimulus or to a stimulus that would become noxious if prolonged.

oligofascicular pattern: Characteristic cross-section of a nerve containing 2 to 10 rather large fascicles.

paresthesia: An abnormal sensation, either spontaneous or evoked, that is not unpleasant. A global term used to encompass all types of nerve injuries.

perineurium: A thick connective tissue sheath surrounding fascicles.

polyfascicular pattern: Characteristic cross-section of a nerve containing > 10 fascicles of different sizes, with a prevalence of small fascicles.

protopathia: The inability to distinguish between two different modes of sensation, such as a painful and nonpainful pinprick.

sympathetically mediated pain: A general term that refers to a family of related disorders including causalgia, reflex sympathetic dystrophy, minor causalgia, Sudeck's atrophy, and postherpetic neuralgia, which may be sympathetically maintained.

synesthesia: A sensation felt in one part of the body when another part is stimulated.

wallerian degeneration: The distal degeneration of the axon and its myelin sheath following injury.

*Adapted from LaBanc JP, Gregg JM. Glossary. Trigeminal nerve injury: diagnosis and management. Oral Maxillofac Surg Clin North Am 1992;4:563.

CHAPTER 42

Cleft Lip and Palate: Comprehensive Treatment Planning and Primary Repair

Bernard J. Costello, DMD, MD
Ramon L. Ruiz, DMD, MD

The comprehensive treatment of cleft lip and palate deformities requires thoughtful consideration of the anatomic complexities of the deformity and the delicate balance between intervention and growth. Comprehensive and coordinated care from infancy through adolescence is essential in order to achieve an ideal outcome, and surgeons with formal training and experience in all of the phases of care must be actively involved in the planning and treatment.[1–3] Specific goals of surgical care for children born with cleft lip and palate include the following:

- Normalized esthetic appearance of the lip and nose
- Intact primary and secondary palate
- Normal speech, language, and hearing
- Nasal airway patency
- Class I occlusion with normal masticatory function
- Good dental and periodontal health
- Normal psychosocial development

Successful management of the child born with a cleft lip and palate requires coordinated care provided by a number of different specialties including oral/maxillofacial surgery, otolaryngology, genetics/dysmorphology, speech/language pathology, orthodontics, prosthodontics, and others.[4] In most cases care of patients with congenital clefts has become a subspecialty area of clinical practice within these different professions. In addition to surgery for cleft repair, treatment plans routinely involve multiple treatment interventions to achieve the above-stated goals. Because care is provided over the entire course of the child's development, long-term follow-up is critical under the care of these different health care providers. The formation of interdisciplinary cleft palate teams has served two key objectives of successful cleft care: (1) coordinated care provided by all of the necessary disciplines, and (2) continuity of care with close interval follow-up of the patient throughout periods of active growth and ongoing stages of reconstruction. The best outcomes are achieved when the team's care is centered on the patient, family, and community rather than a particular surgeon, specialty, or hospital. The idea of having an objective team that does not revolve around the desires of one particular individual or discipline is sometimes impeded by competitive interactions between surgical specialties. Historic battles over surgical domains between surgical specialties and economic factors contribute to these conflicts and negatively affect the work of the team. Healthy team dynamic and optimal patient care are achieved when all members are active participants, when team protocols and referral patterns are equitable and based on the surgeons' formal training and experience instead of specialty identity, and when the needs of the child are placed above the needs of the team.

This chapter presents an overview of the concepts for reconstruction of the cleft lip and palate deformity. The surgical reconstruction of clefts requires that the surgeon undertaking this important work maintain a cognitive understanding of the complex malformation itself, the varied operative techniques employed, facial growth considerations, and the psychosocial health of the patient and family. The objectives of this chapter will be to present the overall staged reconstructive approach for repair of cleft lip and palate from infancy through the time of skeletal maturity, as well as a focused discussion of the specific surgical procedures involved in primary cleft lip and palate repair. Secondary revision procedures, bone graft reconstruction of the cleft maxilla, and orthognathic surgery for cleft-related dysmorphology are discussed in Chapter 43, "Reconstruction of the Alveolar Cleft," Chapter 44, "Reconstruction of Cleft Lip and Palate: Secondary Procedures," and Chapter 61, "Orthognathic Surgery in the Patient with Cleft Palate."

History of Cleft Lip and Palate Repair

The history of cleft lip and palate care has always been closely linked to dentistry and oral and maxillofacial surgery. The birth and roots of what is now the American Cleft Palate-Craniofacial Association are strongly rooted in dentistry.

The first documented cleft lip repair was performed in AD 390 on a patient who later became the Governor General of several regions in China, although nothing is known about the actual surgeon.[5,6] Jehan Yperman is believed to have been the first to describe unilateral and bilateral cleft lip repair.[6,7] The first diagrammatic representation of cleft lip repair and cleft palate obturator use is credited to Ambrose Pare in the fourteenth century.[6,8] Much later the first documented successful cleft palate repair was performed by a dentist, Le Monnier, in 1766 in Paris.[6,9] The concepts of cleft lip and palate repair have evolved from straight line repairs to a variety of techniques using various cutbacks, triangles, and Z-plasties.[6–14] During the 1950s, Asensio, an oral and maxillofacial surgeon from Guatemala, developed a novel technique for cleft lip repair, which involved the rotation of the philtral segment inferiorly and advancement of the lateral segment medially using a quadrangular flap. Although he used this approach in Guatemala throughout the 1950s, he did not report it until much later.[15,16] Ralph Millard of Miami described his classic rotational-advancement technique in the mid-1950s, and his concepts changed cleft repair forever.[17,18] Millard is credited with perhaps the most important technical development related to cleft lip

repair, and today the majority of surgeons use his original technique or some close modification of it.

In the mid-nineteenth century, Hullihen, recognized as the father of American oral and maxillofacial surgery, published a treatise on comprehensive care of cleft lip and palate deformities.[19] Another pioneer, Truman Brophy, was the professor of oral surgery and dean of the Chicago College of Dentistry and contributed greatly to the care of many patients with clefts. Brophy published a text detailing his experiences with the management of various malformations of the mouth and their surgical repairs including the details of cleft repair.[20] One of his pupils was Chalmers Lyons who started a residency program in oral surgery at the University of Michigan in 1917.[20] Lyons developed the largest cleft practice in America and contributed extensively to the literature.[20]

Many of the concepts related to interdisciplinary care with a cleft palate team care were introduced by Robert Ivy, an oral and maxillofacial surgeon who later became dually qualified in plastic surgery.[20] Robert Ivy trained both in dentistry and medicine at the University of Pennsylvania. After his training in dentistry, Ivy further developed his interests in maxillofacial surgery as an assistant to his uncle, Matthew Cryer, who was a professor in oral surgery at the University of Pennsylvania. Robert Ivy became interested in clefts during his training as the first dental intern at Philadelphia General Hospital at the University of Pennsylvania. His interests in maxillofacial injury led him to serve in France in World War I as an assistant to Vilray Blair. After the war Ivy and Blair's collaboration resulted in two landmark publications by Ivy, *Essentials of Oral Surgery* and *Fractures of the Jaws*. Through work with his state representatives in Harrisburg, Pennsylvania, he was able to start the very first cleft palate clinics in Lancaster, Pittsburgh, Philadelphia, Erie, and Scranton that provided interdisciplinary

care to children for cleft lip and palate deformities. When Reed Dingman put forth a resolution of the American Society of Maxillofacial Surgeons condemning oral and maxillofacial surgeons practicing in the hospital setting, Ivy resigned his membership and sent a letter of protest to the organization that he helped build in support of his dental colleagues.[20]

In the 1950s the concept of primary or early bone grafting of the cleft maxillary defect was introduced by Schmid.[21] Although the concept was initially met with enthusiasm from a number of surgeons, primary bone grafting was eventually abandoned due to unfavorable outcomes. During the decades that followed, the negative skeletal, dental, and growth-related consequences of primary bone grafting became better understood.[22,23] During the early 1970s oral and maxillofacial surgeons Boyne and Sands were the first to publish their favorable outcomes using autogenous particulate bone grafts for reconstruction of the cleft maxilla/alveolus later in childhood during the mixed dentition rather than earlier in life.[24] Although their work and results represented a landmark discovery in the field of cleft reconstruction, cleft palate teams were slow to integrate his approach into their treatment protocols because of the negative associations that lingered following the days of primary bone grafting. Today their principles of secondary bone grafting represent the standard approach for almost all of the world's cleft centers.[24,25]

Orthognathic reconstruction of the patient with cleft deformities has been discussed by many authors.[26–36] Early techniques limited some surgeons' options to procedures centered on mandibular setback.[37] During the 1970s the use of total maxillary osteotomy was pioneered by Bell.[38] His novel ideas provided oral and maxillofacial surgeons with an understanding of the biologic basis for maxillary osteotomy, described the vascular supply that allowed the procedures to be performed safely, and as a result incorporated the Le Fort I osteotomy into modern-day practice.[38] Since that time a number of technical refinements have been described for use of the Le Fort I osteotomy specifically in the cleft patient. Much of this work has been done by two of Bell's former pupils, Fonseca and Turvey, who went on to make substantial contributions to the skeletal reconstruction of patients with clefts.[39] Another dual qualified oral and maxillofacial surgeon, Posnick, has published the most complete descriptions of surgical technique modifications for patients undergoing midfacial advancement in the absence of prior bone graft reconstruction and his extensive experiences with the long-term stability of midfacial advancement after correction of various types of cleft deformities with orthognathic techniques.[26–30] Distraction osteogenesis has gained recent popularity for correction of midfacial hypoplasia but has yet to show significant advantages over traditional techniques for the majority of patients.[32,33,40–42]

Comprehensive and coordinated care has become more prevalent across the world, involving many different types of specialty care for children with clefts. Posnick has provided the most comprehensive, succinct, and evidenced-based discussions on the topic of cleft lip and palate reconstruction from infancy through adolescence.[26] These efforts as well as craniofacial training programs associated with oral and maxillofacial surgery have helped to solidify the role of oral and maxillofacial surgery in the comprehensive care of patients with clefts.

Embryology

To understand the goals of lip and palate repair from an anatomic standpoint the cleft surgeon must have an appreciation for the failure of embryogenesis that results in clefting. There are critical points in the development of the fetus when the fusion of various prominences creates continuity and form to the lip, nose, and palate. Anomalies occur when the normal developmental process is disturbed between these components. Each of these prominences is made up of ectomesenchyme derived from neural crest tissue of the mesencephalon and rhombencephalon. Mesoderm is also present within these prominences as mesenchymal tissue. The prescribed destiny of each of these cells and tissues is controlled by various genes to alter the migration, development, and apoptosis and form the normal facial tissues of the fetus. At the molecular level there are many interdependent factors such as signal transduction, mechanical stress, and growth factor production that affect the development of these tissues. Currently only portions of this complex interplay of growth, development, and apoptosis are clear.

At approximately 6 weeks of human embryologic development the median nasal prominence fuses with the lateral nasal prominences and maxillary prominences to form the base of the nose, nostrils, and upper lip. The confluence of these anterior components becomes the primary palate. When this mechanism fails, clefts of the lips and/or maxilla occur. At approximately 8 weeks the palatal shelves elevate and fuse with the septum to form the intact secondary palate. When one palatal shelf fails to fuse with the other components, then a unilateral cleft of the secondary palate occurs. If both of the palatal shelves fail to fuse with each other and the midline septum, then a bilateral cleft of the palate occurs.

Fusion occurs when programmed cell death (apoptosis) occurs at the edges of the palatal shelves. The ectodermal component disintegrates and the mesenchyme fuses to form the intact palate. Soon after this the anterior primary palate fuses with the secondary palate and ossification occurs. At any point, if failure of fusion occurs with any of the above components, a cleft will occur of the primary and/or secondary palates. Clefts may be complete or incomplete based on the degree of this failure of fusion.

Genetics and Etiology

Clefts of the upper lip and palate are the most common major congenital craniofacial abnormality and are present in approximately 1 in 700 live births.[43] Although inheritance may play a role, cleft lip and palate is not considered a single-gene disease. Instead clefts are thought to be of a multifactorial etiology with a number of potential contributing factors. These factors may include chemical exposures, radiation, maternal hypoxia, teratogenic drugs, nutritional deficiencies, physical obstruction, or genetic influences. One prevailing theory relates the process of clefting as a threshold in which multiple factors come together to raise the individual above a threshold at which time the mechanism of fusion fails.[44,45] Recently multiple genes have been implicated in the etiology of clefting.[46–48] Some of these genes include the *MSX*, *LHX*, *goosecoid*, and *DLX* genes. Additional disturbances in growth factors or their receptors that may be involved in the failure of fusion include fibroblast growth factor, transforming growth factor-β, platelet-derived growth factor, and epidermal growth factor.

Clefts of the lip occur more commonly in males than in females.[49] In addition left-sided cleft lips are more common than right-sided cleft lips, and unilateral cleft lips are more common than the bilateral cleft of the lip.[50] Bilateral clefts of the lip are most often associated with clefting of both the primary and secondary palates. Cleft palate alone is seen in approximately 1 in 2,000 live births and this incidence is similar in all racial groups.[51] Significant differences in the prevalence of clefts exist when specific ethnic/racial populations are examined. For example, African Americans have a birth prevalence that is less common than the total population, but Asians tend to have a higher prevalence.

In the majority of cases unilateral cleft lip and palate is an isolated nonsyndromic birth defect that is not associated with any other major anomalies.[43,52,53] By comparison a much greater proportion of patients with an isolated cleft palate will have an associated syndrome or sequence.[43,53] Some of the more common syndromes seen in this group include Stickler's, Van der Woude's, or DiGeorge syndromes. It is important to identify the diagnosis early, as functional issues may arise early in life and go unnoticed. For example, patients with an isolated cleft palate should be evaluated early by an experienced pediatric ophthalmologist to evaluate the possibility of Stickler's syndrome. Patients with Stickler's syndrome may have ocular abnormalities that lead to retinal detachment. In an otherwise healthy-appearing child these findings may be difficult to diagnose and so early visual loss may go unnoticed. In many cases long-term genetics follow-up is necessary to make a definitive diagnosis and to provide genetic counseling.

The chances of a recurrence of clefting within a family are dependent on many factors, including family history, severity, gender, degree of relationship to the affected individual, and the expression of a syndrome. Predicting the inheritance patterns of families who have a history of cleft lip and/or palate can be complicated. A skilled geneticist/dysmorphologist is best equipped to make these determinations based on pedigree analysis and genetic testing. Since most clefts are sporadic the chances of a family having another child with a cleft after having a child with a unilateral cleft lip and palate in which there was no family history of clefting is approximately 2 to 4%. The chances are higher if additional family history is present or if the cleft is bilateral.[54,55] The nature of any genetic influence will have an effect on the presence of a cleft. Such is the case in patients with autosomal dominant syndromes such as Stickler syndrome where 50% of the children may express the syndrome if one of the parents carries the altered gene.

Classification

The typical classification system used clinically to describe standard clefts of the lip and palate is based on careful anatomic description. Clefts can be unilateral or bilateral; microform, incomplete, or complete; and may involve the lip, nose, primary palate, and/or secondary palates (Figure 42-1). The presentation of clefts is extremely variable, and the individual repairs are custom-tailored to achieve the best symmetry and balance. More severe facial clefting is most commonly described using Tessier's orbitocentric system of numbering (Figure 42-2).[56] Other systems exist that are based on embryologic fusion planes, but these are cumbersome to use in routine clinical practice.[57]

Prenatal Counseling

Recent advances in ultrasound imaging have revolutionized prenatal care and maternal-fetal medicine. Currently ultrasound images of clefts of the lip can be visualized as early as 16 weeks.[58–60] Diagnostic images of the palate are more difficult to acquire, making the correct prenatal diagnosis of a cleft palate less predictable. Palatal structures may be visualized using sagittal and coronal views, but this currently requires the very latest technology and a skilled ultrasonographer with experience performing this type of study.

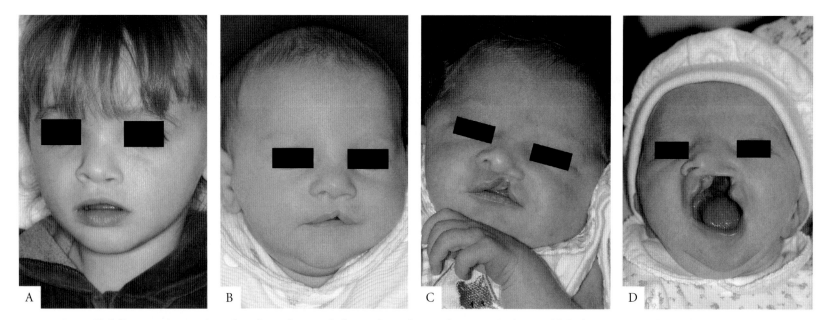

FIGURE 42-1   *Cleft lips come in a variety of configurations, such that each repair must be customized to establish the most normal morphology. A, Microform left unilateral cleft lip only, not requiring primary repair. B, Minor left incomplete unilateral cleft lip only. C, Left incomplete unilateral cleft lip and palate with a Simonart's band. D, Wide left complete unilateral cleft lip and palate.*

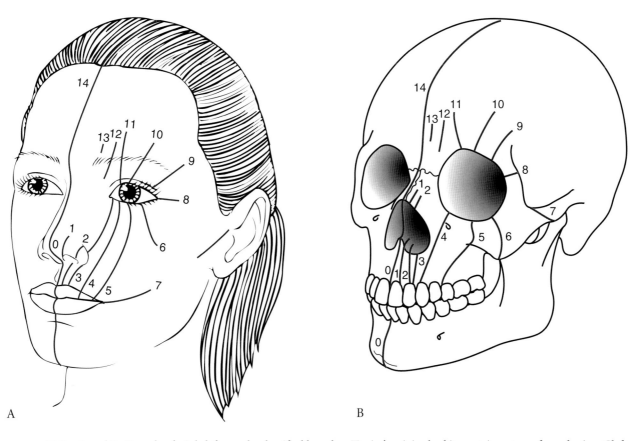

FIGURE 42-2   A and B, *Complex facial clefts can be classified based on Tessier's original orbitocentric system of numbering. Clefts may involve all tissue planes including skin, mucosa, bone, teeth, muscle, brain, peripheral nerve, and other specialized tissues.*

When the diagnosis of cleft lip is made during pregnancy the family can then be referred to an experienced surgeon for a prenatal discussion. A prenatal consultation provides an excellent opportunity to explain the diagnosis, review the different stages of cleft lip and palate reconstruction that may be necessary, and prepare the parents for practical considerations such as feeding of a child with a cleft palate. This gives the family the opportunity to ask questions, calm fears, and learn about feeding techniques that will be important during the first week of life for their baby. Parents are empowered with this new knowledge, and the preparations made during a prenatal consultation allow them to anticipate the delivery of their baby with a greater comfort level regarding the necessary care of the child during the early postnatal period. The family is then referred to a cleft and craniofacial team in order to undergo a more thorough interdisciplinary approach.

Critical to this process is consultation with a geneticist/dysmorphologist to further discuss the issues associated with the birth and the possibility of other associated deformities. Additional testing may be warranted to evaluate the possibility of associated deformities, syndromes, or sequences that could affect the birthing process. Exceptionally skilled ultrasonographers can visualize airway development and other abnormalities that may require early intervention with fetal surgery, exit procedures, extracorporeal membrane oxygenation, or surgical airway management (tracheotomy) at the time of delivery.

In some medical centers fetal diagnosis and treatment teams are in place to deal with issues associated with various deformities diagnosed in the prenatal period. These teams foster a cohesive environment where information is exchanged through consultation. Much like in the environment of a cleft and craniofacial team, families can get the best information available to consider their child's treatment decisions using an interdisciplinary care model that is patient (mother and fetus), family, and community oriented.

Feeding Concerns

Children born with isolated cleft lip can feed quite well and even have the opportunity to breastfeed in most instances. However, infants with cleft palate can have difficulty feeding due to the inability to form an adequate seal between the tongue and palate for creation of sufficient negative pressure to suck fluid from a bottle. Nasal regurgitation and inefficient handling of secretions and foodstuffs may also be observed during early development. Specialized nipples and bottles are necessary to improve feeding immediately after birth. The most useful devices combine oversized nipples with reservoir spaces and large openings, a squeezable bottle to push fluid into the nipple assembly, and a one-way valve that allows the bolus of fluid to pass from the bottle to the nipple only in order to minimize the amount of work the child must perform to feed. These include a variety of nipples with reservoirs that collect a variable volume of liquid that can be expressed more easily when sucking is inefficient or not possible. Bottles that can be squeezed to allow for manual flow of liquid to the infant are helpful for improving feeding. No single bottle and nipple combination tends to work better than another, but trials with a variety of types using different techniques are helpful in optimizing feeding early in life. Close attention to weight gain is necessary for these children. Generally, in 24 hours each infant should have approximately 2 to 3 ounces of milk for each pound of weight. Feeding sessions should last no longer than 35 minutes as longer sessions are fatiguing and burn more calories than the baby can consume. Infants should be weighed at least weekly using the same scale, preferably at their pediatrician's office.

The subject of breast-feeding an infant with a cleft palate is controversial, with some practitioners encouraging the practice and others strongly opposed to it. There are clear advantages to breast-feeding a newborn, including passive immunologic contribution of the mother to the child in the form of secretory immunoglobulin A and an experience that enhances bonding between the mother and child during such a critical period.[61,62] At the same time the infant's inability to create negative oral pressure will often make successful nursing difficult, if not impossible. It is relatively common to encounter an exclusively breast-fed infant with severe dehydration and failure to thrive secondary to these difficulties. This is especially a concern in infants that have a wide cleft of the secondary palate, where breast-feeding may not be possible. The authors' approach with regard to breast-feeding in the presence of a cleft palate is

to use a combined protocol that includes intermittent feeding with the use of a specialized bottle (as described above) and attempts at nursing. Breast milk may be pumped for use with the specialized nipple and bottle that will provide the nutritional and immunologic benefits desired. This also allows the parents to keep a more quantitative record of how many ounces have been ingested over the course of the day since this is normally difficult with breast-feeding alone. At the same time the mother and baby are not deprived of an opportunity to incorporate breast-feeding into the daily regimen. This approach obviously requires rigorous documentation of the child's weight, consultation with a lactation consultant and infant feeding specialist, and frequent follow-up evaluations through the surgeon and/or pediatrician.

Treatment Planning and Timing: Overview

The timing of cleft lip and palate repair is controversial. Despite a number of meaningful advancements in the care of patients with cleft lip and palate, a lack of consensus exists regarding the timing and specific techniques used during each stage of cleft reconstruction. Surgeons must continue to carefully balance the functional needs, esthetic concerns, and the issue of ongoing growth when deciding how and when to intervene. In no other type of surgical problem is the issue of early surgery's effect on growth more apparent than in the treatment of cleft lip and palate deformities. The decision to surgically manipulate the tissues of the growing child should not be made lightly and should take into account the possible growth restriction that can occur with early surgery. Nevertheless many patients with congenital deformities will benefit from surgical intervention based on functional or psychosocial reasons. Understanding the growth and development of the craniofacial skeleton is critical to the treatment

planning process.[33] In many cases waiting for a greater degree of growth to occur is advantageous unless compelling functional or esthetic issues are present that can not or should not wait.

Due to many different treatment philosophies the timing of treatment interventions is considerably variable amongst cleft centers. Therefore, it is difficult to produce a timing regimen that everyone agrees on. Each stage of surgical reconstruction and the suggested timing based on the patient's age are presented in Table 42-1. Special considerations may alter the sequencing or timing of the various procedures based on individual functional or esthetic needs.

Cleft lip repair is generally undertaken at some point after 10 weeks of age. One advantage of waiting until the child is 10 to 12 weeks of age is that it allows a complete medical evaluation of the patient so that any associated congenital defects affecting other organ systems (eg, cardiac or renal anomalies) may be uncovered. The surgical procedure itself may be easier when the child is slightly larger and the anatomic landmarks more prominent and well defined. Historically the anesthetic risk-related data suggested that the safest time period for surgery in this population of infants could be outlined simply by using the "rule of 10's." This referred to the idea of delaying lip repair until the child was at least 10 weeks old, 10 pounds in weight, and with a minimum hemoglobin value of 10 dL/mg.[63,64] Today more sophisticated pediatric techniques, advances in intraoperative monitoring, and improved anesthetic agents have all resulted in the ability to provide safe general anesthesia much earlier in life.[65] Despite the ability to provide safe anesthesia earlier in life, there is no measurable benefit to performing lip repair prior to 3 months of age.[64,66,67] Some surgeons have advocated that lip repair be carried out in the first days of infancy based on the idea of capitalizing on early "fetal-like" healing. Unfortunately these hoped-for benefits have not been

Table 42-1 Staged Reconstruction of Cleft Lip and Palate Deformities	
Procedure	*Timing*
Cleft lip repair	After 10 weeks
Cleft palate repair	9–18 months
Pharyngeal flap or pharyngoplasty	3–5 years or later based on speech development
Maxillary/alveolar reconstruction with bone grafting	6–9 years based on dental development
Cleft orthognathic surgery	14–16 years in girls, 16–18 years in boys
Cleft rhinoplasty	After age 5 years but preferably at skeletal maturity; after orthognathic surgery when possible
Cleft lip revision	Anytime once initial remodeling and scar maturation is complete but best performed after age 5 years

observed, and problems with excessive scarring and less favorable outcomes have been encountered instead.[68–70] Children may have more scarring at this early age, and their tissues are smaller and more difficult to manipulate. Consequently the esthetic outcomes may be worse if surgery is performed at an earlier age, and since there are no clear benefits to earlier repair the recommendations for repair stand at approximately 3 months of age.

Cleft palate repair is usually performed at approximately 9 to 18 months of age. In deciding the timing of repair the surgeon must consider the delicate balance between facial growth restriction after early surgery and speech development that requires an intact palate. Most children will require an intact palate to produce certain speech sounds by 18 months of age. If developmental delay is present and speech will not likely develop until later, then the repair can be delayed further. There is little evidence to suggest any benefit to palate repair prior to 9 months of age.[71–73] Repairs prior to this time are associated with a much higher incidence of maxillary hypoplasia later in life and show no improvements in speech. For these reasons most surgeons will perform primary palate repair at approximately 9 to 12 months of age.

As the child continues to develop, approximately 20% of children will have inadequate closure of the velopharyngeal mechanism (velopharyngeal insufficiency or VPI), and this may produce hypernasal speech.[74] These children are usually diagnosed at 3 to 5 years of age when a detailed speech examination can be obtained by a skilled speech pathologist familiar with clefts. When VPI is shown to be consistent and due to a definable anatomic defect, surgery is often helpful in correcting this problem. A pharyngeal flap or sphincter pharyngoplasty may be used to treat VPI, with the goal of improving closure between the oral and nasal cavities and reducing nasal air escape during the production of certain sounds. The details of assessment, diagnosis, and treatment of VPI associated with cleft palate are discussed in Chapter 44, "Reconstruction of Cleft Lip and Palate: Secondary Procedures." Approximately 75% of patients with any type of cleft will present with clefting of the maxilla and alveolus.[24–26] Bone graft reconstruction of this site is performed during the mixed dentition prior to the eruption of the permanent canine and/or the permanent lateral incisor. The timing of this procedure is based on dental development and not chronologic age. Based on work by Boyne and Sands, most surgeons reconstruct this area during the mixed dentition prior to eruption of the permanent canine. Earlier reconstruction of this area has been associated with a high degree of maxillary

growth restriction requiring orthognathic correction later in life in a much higher percentage of patients.[22,24] The gold standard for reconstruction in this area is autogenous bone from the anterior iliac crest. Cranial bone, rib, tibia, symphysis of the mandible, zygoma, and allogeneic bone have all been studied, but none have been shown to be appreciably better than the iliac crest.[26,75,76]

Orthognathic reconstruction of maxillary and mandibular discrepancies is performed at 14 to 18 years of age based on individual growth characteristics.[26–36,38] This is done in conjunction with orthodontics prior to and after surgery. However, in some cases of severe maxillary hypoplasia, early Le Fort I osteotomy may be performed to optimize facial esthetics and occlusion with the supposition that revision osteotomies will likely be necessary. These early osteotomies may complicate later treatment. Early orthognathic correction is reserved for the most severe dysmorphology, and in most cases the authors prefer standard orthognathic techniques.[31–33] Attempts at using distraction osteogenesis have been associated with a higher complication rate than with standard orthognathic techniques.[32,42,77] Orthognathic correction of the deformities associated with cleft lip and palate defects is discussed in Chapter 61, "Orthognathic Surgery in the Patient with Cleft Palate."

As with the timing of other interventions, lip and nasal revision is best reserved until after the majority of growth is complete. Most of the lip and nasal growth is complete after age 5 years. Lip revision can be considered prior to school age at about 5 years of age. However, this may be performed earlier if the deformity is severe. Nasal revision is performed after age 5 years as most of the nasal growth is also complete by this time. If orthognathic reconstruction is likely, then rhinoplasty is usually best performed after orthognathic surgery as maxillary advancement improves many characteristics of nasal support. However, when nasal deformity is particularly severe, rhinoplasty can be considered earlier even if orthognathic surgery is expected. Multiple early revisions of the lip or nose should be avoided so that excess scarring does not potentially impair ongoing growth. Secondary revisions of cleft lip and palate deformities are discussed in Chapter 44, "Reconstruction of Cleft Lip and Palate: Secondary Procedures."

Cleft Lip and Palate Repair

Presurgical Taping and Presurgical Orthopedics

Facial taping with elastic devices is used for application of selective external pressure and may allow for improvement of lip and nasal position prior to the lip repair procedure. In the authors' opinions these techniques often have greater impact in cases of wide bilateral cleft lip and palate where manipulation of the premaxillary segment may make primary repair technically easier. Although one of the basic surgical tenets of wound repair is to close wounds under minimal tension, attempts at improving the arrangement of the segments using taping methods have not shown a measurable improvement.[78–80]

Some surgeons prefer presurgical orthopedic (PSO) appliances rather than lip taping to achieve the same goals.[81,82] PSO appliances are composed of a custom-made acrylic base plate that provides improved anchorage in the molding of lip, nasal, and alveolar structures during the presurgical phase of treatment (Figure 42-3). Although the use of appliances probably makes for an easier surgical repair, there has been a lack of clinical evidence to demonstrate that there is any measurable improvement in esthetics of the nose or lip, dental arch relationship, tooth survival, or occlusion. Studies have looked at the dental arch relationship outcomes in patients who have infant presurgical orthopedic devices, and no improvement in dental arch relationship was seen.[83,84] Addition-

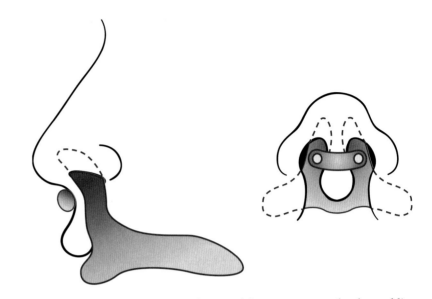

FIGURE 42-3 *Frontal and lateral views of the Grayson nasoalveolar molding appliance showing the nasal projections that help to theoretically mold the nasal cartilages and maxillary segments into a more appropriate configuration prior to repair.*

ally no long-term improvement in speech outcome has be demonstrated in patients who had PSOs.[85] Furthermore concerns regarding potential negative consequences with these types of appliances have been raised.[86] PSOs also add significant cost and time to treatment early in the child's life. Many appliances require a general anesthetic for the initial impression used to fabricate the device. Frequent appointments are necessary for monitoring of the anatomic changes and periodic appliance adjustment.

The Latham appliance was popular for expanding and aligning the maxillary segments of the patient with a cleft palate.[87] It is a pin-retained device that is inserted into the palate with acrylic extensions onto the alveolar ridges. A screw mechanism is then used to manipulate the segments as desired. The Latham appliance has been shown to be associated with significant growth restriction of the midface when used in infancy to approximate the segments prior to definitive repair.[86] Children who have had Latham appliances have been shown to have significant midfacial growth restriction in adolescence 100% of the time whereas children who have not had the

Latham appliance have midface hypoplasia 25 to 35% of the time.[42,80,86]

The nasoalveolar molding appliance has become popular with some surgeons in attempts to manipulate the segments without pin retention prior to lip and nose repair (see Figure 42-3). The appliance popularized by Grayson is adjustable by removing or adding acrylic and manipulating protrusive elements that attempt to mold the nasal cartilages. This device attempts to align the alveolar segments, lip structures, and nasal cartilages to optimize repair. Unfortunately the hoped-for advantages of this appliance have not been realized. Additionally no long-term data are available regarding growth in the craniofacial skeleton after using this protocol. The limited short-term data that are available cannot be extrapolated to determine the ultimate outcome on growth, function, or esthetics. Some surgeons use gingivoperiosteoplasty in conjunction with the PSO, using limited flaps to close the alveolus cleft during the primary repair of the lip or palate. Many surgeons who use this appliance in conjunction with their primary lip repairs will perform a gingivoperiosteoplasty in attempts to have bone form at the alveolus. This is more easily performed with the segments aligned in close proximity as the flaps are small.[82] Experiences with similar techniques in the 1960s involving primary bone grafting were poor with respect to growth.[22,23] Additionally there has been no convincing long-term objective data showing improvement in either lip or nose esthetics.

In their current state of technical refinement there is no evidence that any of the PSOs offer an improved outcome with respect to esthetics, function, or growth in patients with cleft lip and palate. Coupled with the fact that appliances are time-consuming and have a high cost of fabrication and utilization, it is difficult to advocate their uniform use. As with other interventions considered for patients with clefts, costly and unproven interventions should be avoided, although they may prove to be helpful in some select cases.[88] Hopefully, long-term data will be forthcoming and positive to help determine which patients may benefit from PSO appliance treatment.

Lip Adhesion

Some surgeons attempt to surgically approximate the segments of the cleft lip prior to definitive lip repair in an attempt to achieve a better relationship of both the lip structures and the dental arches.[89–91] This is achieved by advancing small flaps of tissue across the cleft site. While some surgeons advocate the use of this technique in wide bilateral clefts, it is rarely performed in unilateral cases. When used, the lip adhesion is usually completed at 3 months of age. In most cases this will convert a wide complete cleft into a wide incomplete cleft as the scar will eventually be excised from the cleft site recreating a similar wide deformity. The definitive lip repair is then completed 3 to 9 months later by excising the scar and reapproximating the remaining lip structures. Furthermore at the second procedure there is usually less supple tissue to work with

when performing the definitive repair due to scarring. As with most endeavors in cleft surgery, repeated early interventions tend to complicate later refinements due to excessive scarring. In general adequate mobilization of the flaps in one stage will make tension-free skin closure possible in almost every case without the need for taping, presurgical orthopedic appliances, and/or lip adhesion.

Unilateral Cleft Lip Repair

Clefts of the lip and nose that are unilateral present with a high degree of variability, and thus each repair design is unique (see Figure 42-1).[26,92] The repair technique preferred by the authors for cleft lip and nasal deformities is shown in Figures 42-4 and 42-5 and is usually performed after 10 weeks of age.[17,18,26,63] The basic premise of the repair is to create a three-layered closure of skin, muscle, and mucosa that approximates normal tissue and excises hypoplastic tissue at the cleft margins. Critical in the process is the reconstruction of the orbicularis oris musculature into a continuous sphincter. The Millard rotation-advancement technique has the advantage of allowing for each of the incision lines to fall within the natural contours of the lip and nose. This is an advantage because it is difficult to achieve "mirror image" symmetry in the unilateral cleft lip and nose with the normal side immediately adjacent to the surgical site. A Z-plasty technique such as the Randall-Tennison repair may not achieve this level of symmetry because the Z-shaped scar is directly adjacent to the linear nonclefted philtrum (Figure 42-6). Achieving symmetry is more difficult when the rotation portion of the cleft is short in comparison to the advancement segment.

Primary nasal reconstruction may be considered at the time of lip repair to reposition the displaced lower lateral cartilages and alar tissues. Several techniques are advocated, and considerable variation exists with respect to the exact nasal reconstruc-

tion performed by each surgeon.[93,94] The primary nasal repair may be achieved by releasing the alar base, augmenting the area with allogeneic subdermal grafts, or even a formal open rhinoplasty. Since lip repair is done at such an early point in growth and development, the authors prefer minimal surgical dissection due to the effects of scarring on the subsequent growth of these tissues. McComb described a technique that has become popular, consisting of dissecting the lower lateral cartilages free from the alar base and the surrounding attachments through an alar crease incision.[93,95–97] This allows the nose to be bolstered and/or stented from within the nostril to improve symmetry.

Bilateral Lip Repair

Bilateral cleft lip repair can be one of the most challenging technical procedures performed in children with clefts. The lack of quality tissue present and the widely displaced segments are major challenges to achieving exceptional results, but superior technique and adequate mobilization of the tissue flaps usually yields excellent esthetic results (Figures 42-7–42-10). Additionally the columella may be quite short in length, and the premaxillary segment may be significantly rotated. Adequate mobilization of the segments and attention to the details of only using appropriately developed tissue will yield excellent results even in the face of significant asymmetry.

Some surgeons have used aggressive techniques to surgically lengthen the columella and preserve hypoplastic tissue using banked fork flaps.[98,99] Early and aggressive tissue flaps in the nostril and columella areas do not look natural after significant growth has occurred and result in abnormal tissue contours. While surgical attempts at lengthening the columella may look good initially, they frequently look abnormally long and excessively angular later in life (Figure 42-11). Revision of these iatrogenic deformities is difficult

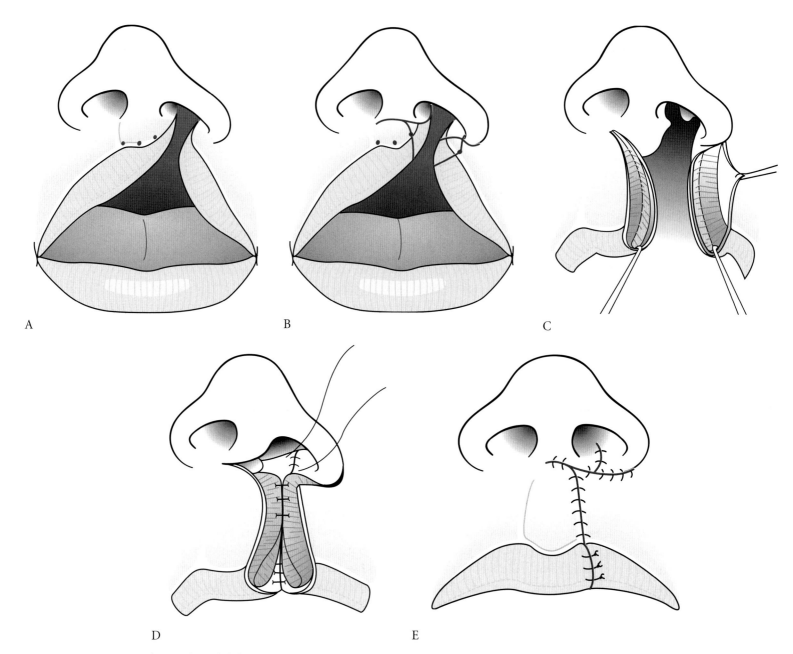

A

B

C

D

E

FIGURE 42-4 A, *A complete unilateral cleft of the lip is shown highlighting the hypoplastic tissue in the cleft site that is not used in the reconstruction. Note the nasal deformities that are typical in the unilateral cleft, including displaced lower lateral nasal cartilages, deviated anterior septum, and nasal floor clefting. B, The typical markings for the authors' preferred repair are shown highlighting the need to excise the hypoplastic tissue and approximate good vermilion and white roll tissue for the repair. C, Once the hypoplastic tissue has been excised, the three layers of tissue are dissected (skin, muscle, and mucosa). It is important to completely free the orbicularis oris from its abnormal insertions on the anterior nasal spine area and lateral alar base. Nasal flaps are also incorporated into the dissection to repair the nasal floor (not shown). D, The orbicularis oris muscle is approximated with multiple interrupted sutures, and the vermilion border/white roll complex is reconstructed. The nasal floor and mucosal flaps are approximated. E, The lateral flap is advanced and the medial segment is rotated downward to create a healing scarline that will resemble the natural philtral column on the opposite side. The incision lines are hidden in natural contours and folds of the nose and lip.*

and some of the contour irregularities will not be able to be revised adequately. Usually if the hypoplastic tissue is excised and incisions within the medial nasal base and columella are avoided, the long-term esthetic results are excellent.

The authors prefer a primary nasal reconstruction that can be performed in a similar fashion to the unilateral technique described by McComb.[100] This allows for release and repositioning of the lower lateral cartilages and alar base on both sides

without aggressive degloving of the entire nasal complex. Other open rhinoplasty techniques have been suggested using either direct incision on the nasal tip or through prolabial unwinding techniques.[100–103] As with most early maneuvers

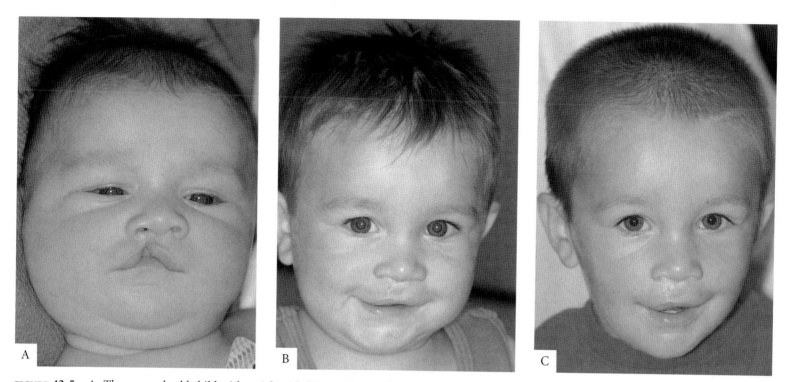

FIGURE 42-5   A, *Three-month-old child with a right-sided incomplete unilateral cleft lip. Note the short philtrum near the midline that must be rotated downward to avoid notching and to improve symmetry. B, Nine-month-old boy after the rotation-advancement repair of his cleft lip and nasal deformities. C, The same child in B 2½ years after his cleft lip and nasal repairs.*

aggressive rhinoplasty at this time may incur early scarring that affects the growth potential of the surrounding tissues, making revision more difficult and long-term esthetics less than ideal.

Cleft Palate Repair

The term *primary palate* is used to describe the anatomic structures anterior to the incisive foramen (eg, the alveolar ridge, maxilla, piriform rim). The term *secondary palate* refers to those structures posterior to the incisive foramen. Therefore, when surgeons refer to the initial or "primary" cleft palate repair, they are actually describing the closure of the secondary palate structures that include the hard palate, soft palate, and uvula. The structures of the embryologic primary palate are reconstructed later in childhood during the cleft maxillary/alveolar bone graft procedure.

There are two main goals of cleft palate repair during infancy: (1) the water-tight closure of the entire oronasal communication involving the hard and soft palate; and

(2) the anatomic repair of the musculature within the soft palate that is critical for normal creation of speech. The soft palate, or velum, is part of the complex coupling and decoupling of the oral and nasal cavities involved in the production of speech. When a cleft of the soft palate is present there are abnormal muscle insertions located at the posterior edge of the hard palate. Surgery must not simply be aimed at closing the palatal defect but rather at the release of abnormal muscle insertions. Muscle continuity with correct orientation should be established so that the velum may serve as a dynamic structure.

The exact timing of repair of a palate cleft is controversial. Generally the velum must be closed prior to the development of speech sounds that require an intact palate. On average this level of speech production is observed by about 18 months of age in the normally developing child. If the repair is completed after this time, compensatory speech articulations may result. Repair completed prior to this time allows

for the intact velum to close effectively, appropriately separating the nasopharynx from the oropharynx during certain speech sounds.[104–107]

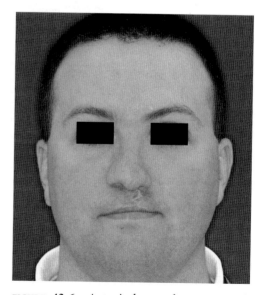

FIGURE 42-6   *A typical scar that may result from a Z-type lengthening repair. Although the length and symmetry of the lip is good, an unnatural contour can occur due to the Z shape of the closure.*

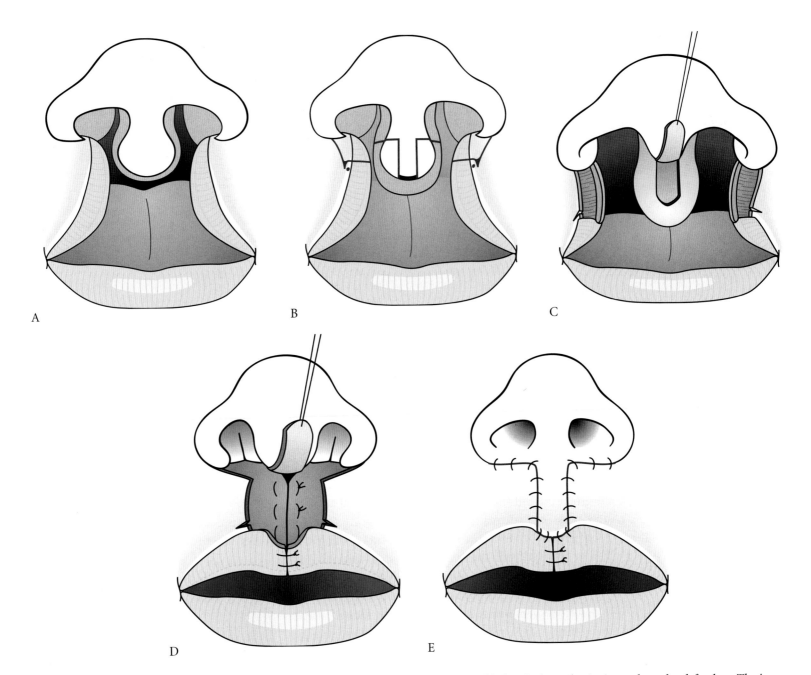

FIGURE 42-7 *A, The bilateral cleft of the lip and maxilla shown here is complete and highlights the hypoplastic tissue along the cleft edges. The importance of the nasal deformity is evident in the shorter columella and disrupted nasal complexes. B, Markings of the authors' preferred repair are shown with an emphasis on excision of hypoplastic tissue and approximating more normal tissue with the advancement flaps. C, A new philtrum is created by excising the lateral hypoplastic tissue and elevating the philtrum superiorly. Additionally the lateral advancement flaps are dissected into three distinct layers (skin, muscle, and mucosa). Nasal floor reconstruction is also performed. D, The orbicularis oris musculature is approximated in the midline with multiple interrupted and/or mattress sutures. This is a critical step in the total reconstruction of the functional lip. There is no musculature present in the premaxillary segment, and this must be brought to the midline from each lateral advancement flap. The nasal floor flaps are sutured at this time as well. The new vermillion border is reconstructed in the midline with good white-roll tissue advanced from the lateral flaps. E, The final approximation of the skin and mucosal tissues is performed leaving the healing incision lines in natural contours of the lip and nose.*

In patients with cleft palate, concerns for normal speech development are frequently balanced with the known biologic consequences of surgery during infancy; namely, the problem of surgery during the growth phase resulting in maxillary growth restriction.[33,72,73,108] When repair of the palate is performed between 9 and 18 months of age, the incidence of associated growth restriction affecting the maxillary development is approximately 25%.[31,33,109–111] If repair is carried out earlier than 9 months of age, then severe growth restriction requiring future orthognathic surgery is seen with greater frequency.[22,26,31,33,109,112–114] At the

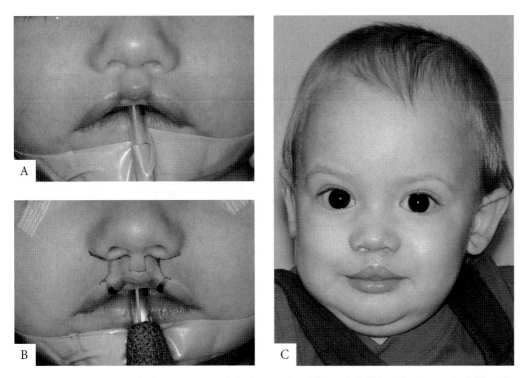

FIGURE 42-8   A, *Presurgical appearance of the incomplete bilateral cleft lip of a 3-month-old boy. B, Surgical markings for excision of the hypoplastic tissue and the planned creation of a new philtrum. Advancement flaps from the lateral lip segments bring good white-roll to the midline via small cutbacks. C, The same child at 1 year of age after the repair of his bilateral cleft lip.*

lowed by closure of the hard palate later in infancy. The idea is that timely repair of the soft palate, which is critical for speech, is accomplished while hard palate repair with mucoperiosteal stripping is delayed until growth is further along.[117,118] Although this technique is not advocated by the majority of surgeons, some surgeons may feel that repairing the hard palate portion later may offer the advantages of less growth restriction, easier repair of larger clefts, and less chance for fistula formation. No convincing data exist to favor this approach over a single-stage repair, but the practice is continued by some centers where anecdotal evidence suggests that there may be some benefit. In contrast most North American speech and language pathologists prefer closure of the palate as a single operation.[117]

Cleft palate reconstruction requires the mobilization of multilayered flaps to reconstruct the defect due to the failure of fusion of the palatal shelves. Generally when the initial palate closure is performed, this refers to closure of the tissues posterior to the incisive foramen. This is done in a layered fashion by first closing the nasal mucosa and then the oral mucosa. Since the main function of the palate is to close the

same time proceeding with palatoplasty prior to 9 months of age is not associated with any increased benefit in terms of speech development so the result is an increase in growth-related problems with an absence of any functional benefit.[115,116] Using only the chronologic age it seems that carrying out the operation during the 9 to 18 months timeline best balances the need to address functional concerns such as speech development with the potential negative impact on growth. To date no case-controlled rigorous clinical trial has examined what is likely the most critical factor in dictating the exact timing of cleft repair—the individual child's true language age. In cases where significant developmental delay is present surgery should be delayed since speech formation is not yet an issue and there is a likely benefit in terms of growth of the maxilla. Delaying palatal closure is relevant in situations where the cleft palate is associated with other complex medical conditions, neurodevelopmental delay, complex craniofacial anomalies, and/or the presence of a tracheotomy.

Another approach used to balance speech issues with growth-related concerns is to stage the closure of the secondary palate with two operations. Generally this involves the repair of the soft palate early in life as an initial step, fol-

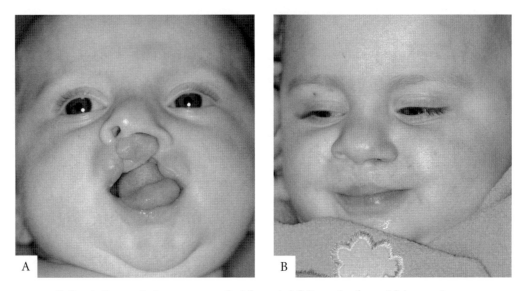

FIGURE 42-9   A, *Presurgical appearance of a bilateral cleft lip and palate with impressive asymmetry and rotation of the premaxillary segment. Note the significant nasal asymmetry and bunching of the orbicularis oris laterally. B, The same child at 14 months of age.*

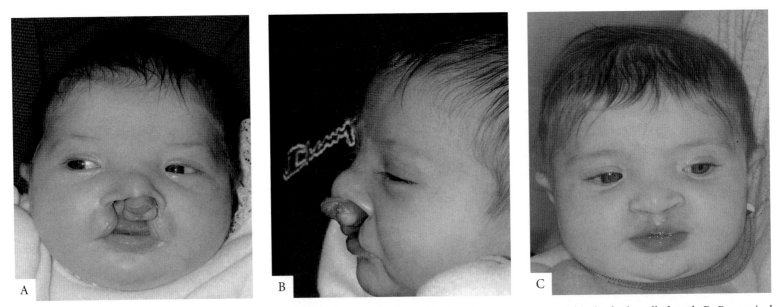

FIGURE 42-10   A, *Presurgical frontal view of a wide bilateral cleft lip and palate with significant asymmetry and lack of columella length. B, Presurgical left lateral view of a wide bilateral cleft lip and palate with a protrusive premaxillary segment. Note the short columella length. C, The same child at 10 months of age after repair of her bilateral cleft lip and palate. No presurgical taping or orthopedic appliances were used.*

space between the nasopharynx and oropharynx during certain speech sounds, the surgeon must also reconstruct the musculature of the velopharyngeal mechanism. The musculature of the levator palatini is abnormally inserted on the posterior aspect of the hard palate and therefore must be disinserted and reconstructed in the midline.[26,119] Therefore, the soft palate is closed in three layers by approximating the nasal mucosa, levator musculature, and the oral mucosa. The hard palate portion is closed in two layers using nasal mucosa flaps and then oral mucosa flaps. Both the hard and soft palate repairs must be done in a tension-free manner to avoid wound breakdown and fistula formation. Adequate mobilization of the flaps during the dissection is essential to achieve tension-free closure. At times some surgeons may elect to incorporate vomer flaps into the repair if there is difficulty in mobilizing the lateral flaps to the midline.

Many techniques have been described for repair of the palate.[120–127] The Bardach two-flap palatoplasty uses two large full-thickness flaps that are mobilized with

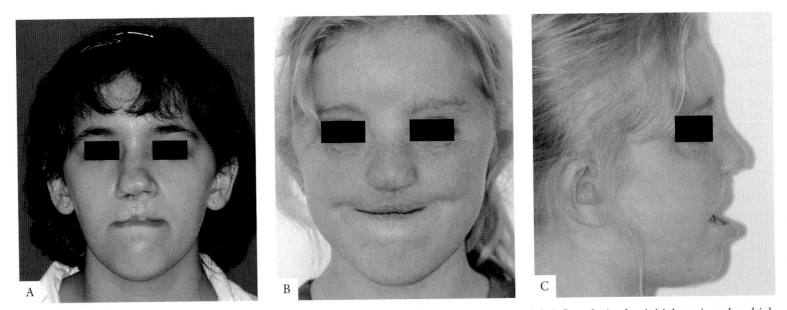

FIGURE 42-11   A, *Frontal view of a teenage girl who had undergone columella lengthening and banked fork flaps during her initial repair and multiple attempts at secondary rhinoplasty by another surgeon prior to orthognathic surgery. B, Frontal view of a patient who underwent columella lengthening and banked fork flaps during her initial repair. C, Lateral view of the patient from B with a columella that is curved upwards and abnormally angular.*

layered dissection and brought to the midline for closure (Figure 42-12).[26,120] This technique preserves the palatal neurovascular bundle as well as a lateral pedicle for adequate blood supply. The von Langenbeck technique is similar to the Bardach palatoplasty but preserves an anterior pedicle for increased blood supply to the flaps.[26,121] This technique is also successful in achieving a layered closure but may be more diffi-cult when suturing the nasal mucosa near the anteriorly based pedicle attachments. The authors do not favor push-back techniques as they may incur more palatal scarring, restrict growth, and do not show a measurable benefit in speech.

Another common technique is the Furlow double-opposing **Z** plasty, which attempts to lengthen the palate by taking advantage of a **Z**-plasty technique on both the nasal mucosa and the oral mucosa (Figure 42-13).[26,124–127] This technique can be effective at closing the palate but has been reported by some to have a higher rate of fistula formation at the junction of the soft and hard palates where theoretical lengthening of the soft palate may compromise the closure.[26,128–133] No benefit has been convincingly demonstrated with any particular repair technique when one looks at dental arch form, speech outcome, feeding, or any other functional variable. At this point in our understanding surgeons often consider their own experiences and training when repairing clefts, since definitive data suggesting that one repair is preferable over another are lacking.

In very wide clefts some surgeons will advocate the consideration of a pharyngeal flap at the primary palatoplasty procedure to assist in closure since revision palatoplasty is sometimes unsuccessful in eradicating fistulas. Those who use this technique usually perform it in extremely wide clefts and do so very selectively. This allows the central portion of the closure to be filled with posterior pharyngeal wall tissue making the closure of the nasal and palatal mucosa easier. Patients with Pierre Robin syndrome or Treacher Collins syndrome may have exceptionally wide clefts that are difficult to close with no tension, and this technique may be considered. The drawbacks of using a pharyngeal flap during the repair of the palate include a significantly increased risk for complications such as bleeding, snoring, obstructive sleep apnea, or hyponasality. The details of pharyngeal flap surgery and revision palatoplasty techniques are discussed in Chapter 44, "Reconstruction of Cleft Lip and Palate: Secondary Procedures."

Complex Facial Clefting

Clefting of the facial structures other than the typical nasolabial region is rare and often presents difficult challenges to the reconstructive cleft surgeon. Therefore it is important to consider referring patients

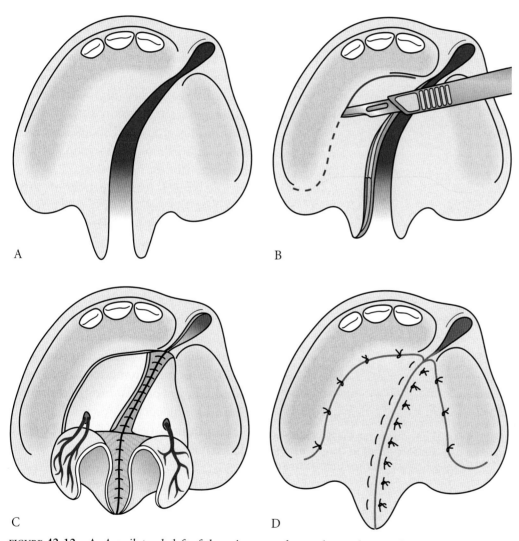

A

B

C

D

FIGURE 42-12 *A, A unilateral cleft of the primary and secondary palates is shown with the typical involvement from the anterior vestibule to the uvula. B, The Bardach palatoplasty technique requires two large full-thickness mucoperiosteal flaps to be elevated from each palate shelf. The anterior portion (anterior to the incisive foramen) of the cleft is not reconstructed until the mixed dentition stage. C, A layered closure is performed in the Bardach palatoplasty by reapproximating the nasal mucosa. The muscle bellies of the levator palatini are elevated off of their abnormal insertions on the posterior palate. They are then reapproximated in the midline to create a dynamic functional sling for speech purposes. D, Once the nasal mucosa and musculature of the soft palate are approximated, the oral mucosa is closed in the midline. The lateral releasing incisions are quite easily closed primarily due to the length gained from the depth of the palate. In rare cases, in very wide clefts a portion of the lateral incisions may remain open and granulate by secondary intention.*

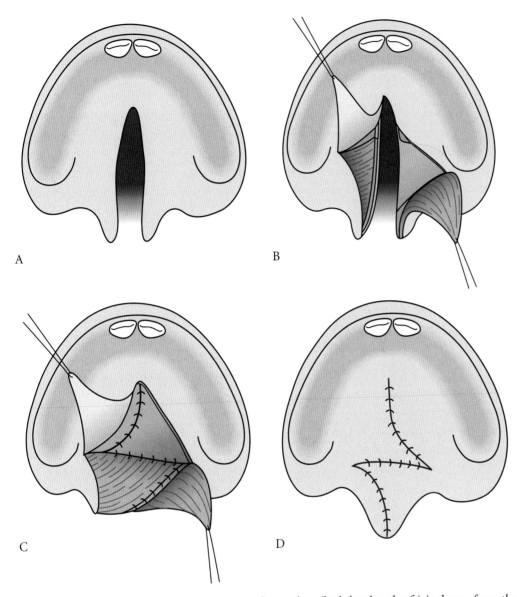

A

B

C

D

FIGURE 42-13   A, *A complete cleft of the secondary palate (both hard and soft) is shown from the incisive foramen to the uvula. B, The Furlow double-opposing* Z*-plasty technique requires that separate* Z*-plasty flaps be developed on the oral and then nasal side. Note the cutbacks creating the nasal side flaps highlighted in* blue. *C, The flaps are then transposed to theoretically lengthen the soft palate. A nasal side closure is completed in the standard fashion anterior to the junction of the hard and soft palate. Generally this junction is the highest area of tension and can be difficult to close. This contributes to the higher fistula rate in this type of repair. D, The oral side flaps are then transposed and closed in a similar fashion completing the palate closure.*

gene disease. Many complex facial clefts involve the orbit, and the classification system most often used is orbitocentric in design (see Figure 42-2). Paul Tessier described a numbering system for facial clefting phenomena to make description and surgical planning more easily discussed.[56] Other systems exist but have a more cumbersome nomenclature.[57]

Primary repair of severe facial clefts is often more difficult than even the most difficult standard bilateral clefts.[134–136] While mobilization of the lip and nose structures is rather straightforward, the closure of clefts in the orbital region can be challenging due to the lack of eyelid and adjacent tissue for advancement and/or rotation. Revision surgery is the norm in this group and should include a skilled ophthalmologic surgeon early in the process for the best results.

The staged reconstruction of these types of severe facial clefts is similar to the more common cleft lip and palate protocols. However, several functional issues are present in patients with complex facial clefting that require more immediate attention. For example, patients with large Tessier no. 7 clefts may have problems with retaining foodstuffs in their oral cavities due to the discontinuity of the orbicularis oris (Figure 42-14). This may prompt early repair and reestablishment of the orbicularis oris musculature for functional concerns.

For those patients with orbital clefts a skilled pediatric ophthalmologist should evaluate the child early to avoid severe corneal abrasion and desiccation. Immediate lubrication of the globes is necessary to prevent severe irreversible corneal damage until eyelid structures can be mobilized to cover the globe adequately. Early after birth tarsorrhaphy stitches can be used to gain adequate closure of the lids for corneal protection. Ignoring the need for eye protection may result in severe corneal scarring that may cause blindness and prompt consideration for corneal transplantation. Corneal transplants in infants

with complex facial clefting to surgeons with experience in this particular area. Comprehensive interdisciplinary care is mandatory to achieve the best results including involvement of neurosurgery, ophthalmology, orthodontics, speech pathology, and other members of the craniofacial team. Some interventions such as eye lubrication may be necessary within hours after birth, and accurate pre-

natal diagnosis of severe facial clefting is helpful in planning for early care.

The etiology of the various facial clefts may be related to failure of embryologic fusion, physical obstruction in fetal life, association with an encephalocele or tumor, amniotic bands, or other anatomic disruptions during fetal life.[55] The vast majority of complex facial clefts are sporadic events and not related to a single

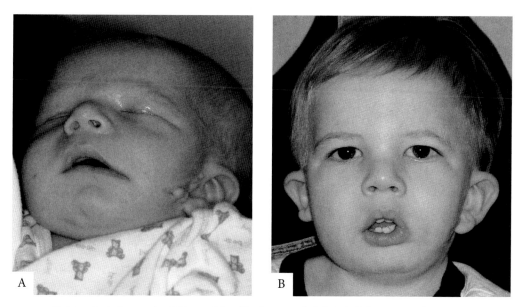

FIGURE 42-14   A, *A 2-month-old boy with a Tessier no. 7 left facial cleft associated with craniofacial microsomia (Kaban type IIb), congenital ear anomalies, a lateral tongue cleft, and a left-sided epibulbar dermoid.* B, *The same child at 8 months after the primary repair.*

are often not successful but are possible in patients with severe orbitofacial clefts. Another concern is the support of the globes at the orbit floor that may be involved in some facial clefts. The timing of orbital reconstruction is dependent on the functional needs of the cleft area in each patient. These are just some of the concerns present in complex facial clefting, and a customized treatment plan must be formulated for each patient.

Outcome Assessment

Decision-making in cleft care should be based on evidenced-based research and a critical look at outcomes. Unfortunately there is little evidenced-based research available to guide clinicians through the many treatment protocols for cleft care.[113] Although the clinical experience of the surgeon certainly has value, this must be integrated with a constant review of evidence-based research. Typically enthusiasm by a surgeon or a particular group of surgeons regarding a specific intervention because of personal experiences may help popularize that intervention but with little outcome data to support its use. Too frequently the long-term results are not forthcoming, and

the treatment regimen may still persist. Unfortunately some of the treatment regimens used today are based on the poor outcomes and mishaps of previous surgeons rather than regimens chosen as a consequence of published evidence of the actual success of a particular treatment.

Additionally the pressures of a costly health care system have made treatment decision questions even harder to investigate.[88] A need to understand the outcome differences between treatment philosophies will be critical to help determine which protocols will be most beneficial to the patient without extending valuable health care resources on unproven or ineffective methods. For this reason among many others, the need to discard unproven and unnecessary interventions has never been greater. Outcomes studies based on functional results such as appearance, facial growth, occlusion, patient satisfaction, and psychosocial development are all critical in this process. Surgeons involved in the care of patients with clefts must critically review the literature on a regular basis and not be tempted by poorly evaluated techniques popularized by clinical reports.

Conclusions

The comprehensive care of patients with clefts requires an interdisciplinary approach that demands precise surgical execution of the various procedures necessary to correct cleft deformities, as well as frequent long-term follow-up. Clinicians experienced in the comprehensive interdisciplinary care of patients with clefts are best equipped to deal with these concerns. The treatment of patients with cleft and craniofacial deformities should be free of bias and should demand team care that is patient, family, and community oriented. Only in this fashion can the overall treatment be optimally successful. This type of care maximizes the patient's ability to grow into adulthood and succeed in life without focusing on their deformity.

References

1. Adams GR. The effects of physical attractiveness on the socialization process. In: Lucker GW, Ribbens KA, McNamara JA, editors. Psychological aspects of facial form. Craniofacial growth series monograph no. 11. Ann Arbor: University of Michigan Press; 1981. p. 25–47.
2. Kapp K. Self concept of the cleft lip and or palate child. Cleft Palate J 1979;16:171.
3. Kapp-Simon KA. Psychological interventions for the adolescent with cleft lip and palate. Cleft Palate Craniofac J 1995;32:104–8.
4. American Cleft Palate-Craniofacial Association. Parameters for the evaluation and treatment of patients with cleft lip/palate or other craniofacial anomalies. Cleft Palate Craniofac J 1993;30 Suppl 1:4.
5. Boo-Chai K. An ancient Chinese text on a cleft lip. Plast Reconstr Surg 1966;38:89.
6. Rogers BO. Harelip repair in colonial America: a review of 18th century and earlier surgical techniques. Plast Reconstr Surg 1964;34:142.
7. Bushe G. An essay on the operation for cleft palate. New York (NY): William Jackson; 1835.
8. Pare A. Dix Livres de la Chirurgie. Paris: Iean le Royer; 1564. p. 211.
9. LeMesurier AB. Method of cutting and suturing lip in complete unilateral cleft lip. Plast Reconstr Surg 1949;4:1.
10. Veau V. Operative treatment of complete double harelip. Ann Surg (Paris) 1922;76:143.
11. Tennison CW. The repair of unilateral cleft lip

by the stencil method. Plast Reconstr Surg 1952;9:115.

12. Skoog T. A design for the repair of unilateral cleft lip. Am J Surg 1958;95:223.

13. Brauer RO. Repair of unilateral cleft lip. Triangular flap repairs. Clin Plast Surg 1985;12:595.

14. Randall P. Long-term results with the triangular flap technique for unilateral cleft lip repair. In: Bardach J, Morris H, editors. Multidisciplinary management of cleft lip and palate. Philadelphia (PA): W.B. Saunders; 1990. p. 173.

15. Asensio OE. Labioleporino y paladar heindido. Acta Odontol Venez 1971;3:229–42.

16. Asensio OE. A variation of the rotation-advancement operation for repair of wide unilateral cleft lips. Plast Reconstr Surg 1974;53:167–73.

17. Millard DR. Cleft craft. Vol 1. Boston (MA): Little Brown; 1976. p. 165–73.

18. Millard DR. A primary camouflage of the unilateral harelip. In: Transactions of the international congress of plastic surgeons. Baltimore (MD): Williams & Wilkins; 1957. p. 160–6.

19. Hullihen SP. A treatise on hare-lip and its treatment. Baltimore (MD): Woods and Crane; 1844.

20. The building of a specialty: oral and maxillofacial surgery in the United States 1918–1998. J Oral Maxillofac Surg. 1998;7 Suppl 56.

21. Schmid E. Die Annaherung der Kieferstumpfe bei Lippen-Kiefer-Gaumenspalten: Ihre schadlichen Folgen und Vermeidung. Fortschr Kiefer Gesichtschir 1955;1:37.

22. Pruzansky S. Presurgical orthopaedics and bone grafting for infants with cleft lip and palate: a dissent. Cleft Palate J 1964;1:164.

23. Robertson NR, Jolleys A. Effects of early bone grafting in complete clefts of the lip and palate. Plast Reconstr Surg 1968;42:414–21.

24. Boyne PJ, Sands NR. Secondary bone grafting of residual alveolar and palatal clefts. J Oral Surg 1972;30:87–92.

25. Millard DR. Cleft craft: the evolution of its surgery. Alveolar and palatal deformities. Vol 3. Boston (MA): Little Brown; 1980.

26. Posnick JC. The staging of cleft lip and palate reconstruction: infancy through adolescence. In: Posnick JC, editor. Craniofacial and maxillofacial surgery in children and young adults. Philadelphia (PA): W.B. Saunders; 2000. p. 785–826.

27. Posnick JC, Tompson B. Cleft-orthognathic surgery. Complications and long-term results. Plast Reconstr Surg 1995;96:255.

28. Posnick JC. Cleft-orthognathic surgery: the unilateral cleft lip and palate deformity. In: Posnick JC, editor. Craniofacial and maxillofacial surgery in children and young

adults. Philadelphia (PA): W.B. Saunders; 2000. p. 860–907.

29. Posnick JC. Cleft-orthognathic surgery: the bilateral cleft lip and palate deformity. In: Posnick JC, editor. Craniofacial and maxillofacial surgery in children and young adults. Philadelphia (PA): W.B. Saunders; 2000. p. 908–50.

30. Posnick JC. Cleft-orthognathic surgery: the isolated palate deformity. In:Posnick JC, editor. Craniofacial and maxillofacial surgery in children and young adults. Philadelphia (PA): W.B. Saunders; 2000. p. 951–78.

31. Ruiz RL, Costello BJ, Turvey T. Orthognathic surgery in the cleft patient. In: Ogle O, editor. Oral and maxillofacial surgery clinics of North America: secondary cleft surgery. Philadelphia (PA): W.B. Saunders; 2002. p. 491–507.

32. Costello BJ, Ruiz RL. The role of distraction osteogenesis in orthognathic surgery of the cleft patient. Selected Readings Oral Maxillofac Surg 2002;10(3):1–27.

33. Costello BJ, Shand J, Ruiz RL. Craniofacial and orthognathic surgery in the growing patient. Selected Readings Oral Maxillofacial Surg 2003;11(5):1–20.

34. Braun TW, Sotereanos GC. Orthognathic and secondary cleft reconstruction of adolescent patients with cleft palate. J Oral Surg 1980;38:425–34.

35. Kiehn CL, DesPrez JD, Brown F. Maxillary osteotomy for late correction of occlusion and appearance in cleft lip and palate patients. Plast Reconstr Surg 1968;42:203–7.

36. Westbrook MT, West RA, McNeill RW. Simultaneous maxillary advancement and closure of bilateral alveolar clefts and oronasal fistulas. J Oral Maxillofac Surg 1983;41:257–60.

37. Georgiade NG. Mandibular osteotomy for the correction of facial disproportion in the cleft lip and palate patient. Symposium on management of cleft lip and palate and associated deformities. Am Plast Reconstr Surg 1974;8:238.

38. Bell WH. Le Fort I osteotomy for correction of maxillary deformities. J Oral Surg 1975; 33:412–26.

39. Fonseca RJ, Turvey TA, Wolford LM. Orthognathic surgery in the cleft patient. In: Fonseca RJ, Baker SJ, Wolford LM, editors. Oral and maxillofacial surgery. Philadelphia (PA): W.B. Saunders; 2000. p. 87–146.

40. Polley JW, Figueroa AA, Charbel FT, et al. Monoblock craniomaxillofacial distraction osteogenesis in a newborn with severe craniofacial synostosis: a preliminary report. J Craniofac Surg 1995;6:421–3.

41. Polley JW, Figueroa AA. Rigid external distraction: its application in cleft maxillary deformities. Plast Reconstr Surg 1998;102:1360–72.

42. Posnick JC, Ruiz RL. Management of secondary orofacial cleft deformities [discussion]. In: Goldwyn RM, Cohen MN, editors. The unfavorable result in plastic surgery: avoidance and treatment. 3rd ed. Philadelphia (PA): Lippincott Williams & Wilkins; 2000.

43. Tolarova MM, Cervenka J. Classification and birth prevalence of orofacial clefts. Am J Med Genet 1998;75: 126–37.

44. Tolarova M. Etiology of clefts of lip and/or palate: 23 years of genetic follow-up in 3660 individual cases. In: Pfeifer G, editor. Craniofacial abnormalities and clefts of the lip, alveolus, and palate. Stuttgart: Thieme; 1991.

45. Gundlach KKH, Abou Tara N, von Kreybig T. Tierexperimentelle Ergebnisse zur Entstehung und Pravention von Geischtsspalten und anderen kraniofazialen Anomalien. Fortschr Kieferorthop 1986;47:356–61.

46. Prescott NJ, Lees MM, Winter RM, Malcolm S. Identification of susceptibility loci for non-syndromic cleft lip with or without cleft palate in a two stage genome scan of affected sib pairs. Hum Genet 2000;106:345–50.

47. Suzuki K, Hu D, Bustos T, et al. Mutations of PVRL1 encoding a cell-cell adhesion molecule/herpesvirus receptor, in cleft lip/ palate-ectodermal dysplasia. Nat Genet 2000;25:427–30.

48. Van den Boogaard MJ, Dorland M, Beemer FA, van Amstel HKP. MSX1 mutation is associated with orofacial clefting and tooth agenesis in humans. Nat Genet 2000;24:342–3.

49. Oliver-Padilla G, Martinez-Gonzales V. Cleft lip and palate in Puerto Rico: a 33 year study. Cleft Palate J 1986;23:48–57.

50. Lettieri J. Human malformations and related anomalies. In: Stevenson RE, Hall JG, Goodman RM, editors. New York (NY): Oxford University Press; 1993. p. 367–81.

51. Wyszynski DF, Beaty TH, Maestri NE. Genetics of non-syndromic and syndromic oral clefts revisited. Cleft Palate Craniofac J 1996;33:16406–17.

52. Saal HM. Syndromes and malformations associated with cleft lip with or without cleft palate. Am J Hum Genet 1998;64:A118.

53. Jones MC. Etiology of facial clefts: prospective evaluation of 428 patients. Cleft Palate J 1988;25:16–20.

54. Gorlin R, Cohen MJ, Levin L. Syndromes of the head and neck. 4th ed. New York (NY): Oxford University Press; 2003.

55. Cohen MM. Etiology and pathogenesis of

orofacial clefting. Cleft lip and palate: a physiological approach, Oral Maxillofac Clin North Am 2000;12:379–97.

56. Tessier P. Anatomical classification of facial, cranio-facial, and latero-facial clefts. J Maxillofac Surg 1976;4:69–92.

57. Van der Meulen J, Mazzola B, Vermey-Keers, et al. A morphogenetic classification of craniofacial malformations. Plast Reconstr Surg 1983;71:560.

58. Pretorius DH, House M, Nelson TR, Hollenbach KA. Evaluation of normal and abnormal lips in fetuses: comparison between three- and two-dimensional sonography. Am J Roentgenol 1995;165:1233–7.

59. Pretorius DH, Nelson TR. Fetal face visualization using three-dimensional ultrasonography. J Ultrasound Med 1995;14:349–56.

60. Shaikh D, Mercer NS, Sohan K, et al.Prenatal diagnosis of cleft lip and palate. Br J Plast Surg 2001;54:288–9.

61. Lawrence RA. Breastfeeding: benefits, risks, and alternatives. Curr Opin Obstet Gynecol 2000;12:519–24.

62. Hamosh M, Peterson JA, Henderson TR, et al. Protective function of human milk: the milk fat globule. Semin Perinatol 1999;23:242–9.

63. Thompson JE. An artistic and mathematically accurate method of repairing the defect in cases of harelip. Surg Gynecol Obstet 1912;14:498.

64. Marsh JL. Craniofacial surgery: the experiment on the experiment of nature. Cleft Palate Craniofac J 1996;33:1.

65. Van Boven MJ, Pendeville PE, Veyckemans F, et al. Neonatal cleft lip repair: the anesthesiologist's point of view. Cleft Palate Craniofac J 1993;30:574-7.

66. Eaton AC, Marsh JL, Pigram TK. Does reduced hospital stay affect morbidity and mortality rates following cleft lip and palate repair in infancy? Plast Reconstr Surg 1994;94:916–18.

67. Field TM, Vega-Lahr N. Early interactions between infants with craniofacial anomalies and their mothers. Infant Behav Dev 1984;7:527.

68. Estes JM, Whitby DJ, Lorenz HP, et al. Endoscopic creation and repair of fetal cleft lip. Plast Reconstr Surg 1992;90:743–6.

69. Hallock GG. Endoscopic creation and repair of fetal cleft lip [discussion]. Plast Reconstr Surg 1992;90:747.

70. Hedrick MH, Rice HE, Vander Wall KJ, et al. Delayed in utero repair of surgically created fetal cleft lip and palate. Plast Reconstr Surg 1996;97:906–7.

71. Dorf DS, Curtin JW. Early cleft palate repair and speech outcome. Plast Reconstr Surg 1982;70:74–81.

72. Dorf DS, Curtin JW. Early cleft palate repair and speech outcome: a ten year experience. In: Bardach J, Morris HL. Multidisciplinary management of cleft lip and palate. Philadelphia (PA): W.B. Saunders; 1990. p. 341–8.

73. Copeland M. The effect of very early palatal repair on speech. Br J Plast Surg 1990; 43:676.

74. Costello BJ, Ruiz RL, Turvey T. Surgical management of velopharyngeal insufficiency in the cleft patient. In: Oral and maxillofacial surgery clinics of North America: secondary cleft surgery. Philadelphia (PA): W.B. Saunders; 2002. p. 539–51.

75. Sadove AM, Nelson CL, Eppley BL, et al. An evaluation of calvarial and iliac donor sites in alveolar cleft grafting. Cleft Palate J 1990;27:225–8.

76. Sindet-Pedersen S, Enemark H. Reconstruction of alveolar clefts with mandibular or iliac crest bone graft: a comparative study. J Oral Maxillofac Surg 1990;48:554–8.

77. Lo LJ, Hung KF, Chen YR. Blindness as a complication of LeFort I osteotomy for maxillary disimpaction. Plast Reconstr Surg 2002;109:688–98.

78. Poole R, Farnworth TK. Preoperative lip taping in the cleft lip. Ann Plast Surg 1994; 32:243–9.

79. Shaw WC, Semb G. Current approaches to the orthodontic management of cleft lip and palate. J R Soc Med 1990;83:30–3.

80. Ross RB, MacNamera MC. Effect of presurgical infant orthopedics on facial esthetics in complete bilateral cleft lip and palate. Cleft Palate Craniofac J 1994;31: 68–73.

81. Grayson BH, Cutting CB, Wood R. Preoperative columella lengthening in bilateral cleft lip and palate. Plast Reconstr Surg 1993;92:1422–3.

82. Grayson BH, Santiago PE, Brecht LE, et al. Presurgical nasoalveolar molding in infants with cleft lip and palate. Cleft Palate Craniofac J 1999;36:486–98.

83. Prahl C, Kuijpers-Jagman AM, Van'tHof MA, et al. A randomized prospective clinical trial of the effect of infant orthopedics in unilateral cleft lip and palate: prevention of collapse of the alveolar segments (Dutchcleft). Cleft Palate Craniofac J 2003;40:337–42.

84. Chan KT, Hayes C, Shusterman S, et al. The effects of active infant orthopedics on occlusal relationships in unilateral complete cleft lip and palate. Cleft Palate Craniofac J 2003;40:511–7.

85. Konst EM, Rietveld T, Peters HFM, et al. Language skills of young children with unilateral cleft lip and palate following infant orthopedics: a randomized clinical trial. Cleft Palate Craniofac J 2003;40:356–62.

86. Berkowitz S. The comparison of treatment results in complete cleft lip/palate using conservative approach vs. Millard-Latham PSOT procedure. Semin Orthod 1996;2:169.

87. Georgiade NG, Latham RA. Maxillary arch alignment in the bilateral cleft lip and palate infant, using the pinned coaxial screw appliance. Plast Reconstr Surg 1975; 56:52–60.

88. Strauss RP. Health policy and craniofacial care: issues in resource allocation. Cleft Palate Craniofac J 1994;31:78–80.

89. Randall P, Graham WP. Lip adhesion in the repair of bilateral cleft lip. In: Grabb WC, Rosenstein SW, Bzoch KR, editors. Cleft lip and palate. Boston (MA): Little Brown; 1971.

90. Millard DR. A preliminary adhesion. In: Cleft craft, Vol 1: the unilateral deformity. Boston (MA): Little Brown; 1976.

91. Vander Woude DL, Mulliken JB. Effect of lip adhesion on labial height in two-stage repair of unilateral complete cleft lip. Plast Reconstr Surg 1997;100:567–72.

92. Mulliken JB, Pensler JM, Kozakewich HPW. The anatomy of cupid's bow in normal and cleft lip. Plast Reconstr Surg 1993;92:395–403.

93. McComb H. Primary correction of unilateral cleft lip nasal deformity: a 10 year review. Plast Reconstr Surg 1985;75:791–9.

94. Horswell BB, Pospisil OA. Nasal symmetry after primary cleft lip repair: comparison between Delaire cheilorhinoplasty and modified rotation-advancement. J Oral Maxillofac Surg 1995;53:1025–30.

95. Schendel SA. Nasal symmetry after primary cleft lip repair: comparison between Delaire cheilorhinoplasty and modified rotation-advancement [discussion]. J Oral Maxillofac Surg 1995;53:1031.

96. Trier WC. Bilateral complete cleft lip and nasal deformity: an anthropometric analysis of staged to synchronous repair [discussion]. Plast Reconstr Surg 1995;96:24.

97. Takato T, Yonehara Y, Mori Y, et al. Early correction of the nose in unilateral cleft lip patients using an open method: a 10-year review. J Oral Maxillofac Surg 1995;53:28–33.

98. Millard DR. Columella lengthening by a forked flap. Plast Reconstr Surg 1958;22:454.

99. Cronin TD. Lengthening the columella by use of skin from nasal floor and alae. Plast Reconstr Surg 1958;21:417.

100. McComb H. Primary repair of the bilateral cleft lip nose: a 15-year review and a new treatment plan. Plast Reconstr Surg 1990;86:882–9.

101. Mulliken JB. Bilateral complete cleft lip and

nasal deformity: an anthropometric analysis of staged to synchronous repair. Plast Reconstr Surg 1995;96:9–23.

102. Trott JA, Mohan NA. A preliminary report on one-stage open tip rhinoplasty at the time of lip repair in bilateral cleft lip and palate. The Alo Setar experience. Br J Plast Surg 1993;46:215–22.

103. Cutting C, Grayson B. The prolabial unwinding flap method for one-stage repair of bilateral cleft lip, nose and alveolus. Plast Reconstr Surg 1993;91:37–47.

104. Maher W. Distribution of palatal and other arteries in cleft and non-cleft human palates. Cleft Palate J 1977;14:1–12.

105. Ross RB, Johnston MC. Cleft lip and palate. Baltimore (MD). William & Wilkins; 1972.

106. Broomhead I. The nerve supply of the soft palate. Br J Plast Surg 1957;10:81.

107. Riski JE, DeLong E. Articulation development in children with cleft lip/palate. Cleft Palate J 1984;21:57–64.

108. Devlin HB. Audit and the quality of clinical care. Ann R Coll Surg Engl 1990;72 Suppl 1:3–14.

109. Trotman CA, Ross RB. Craniofacial growth in bilateral cleft lip and palate: ages six years to adulthood. Cleft Palate Craniofac J 1993;30:261–73.

110. Bishara SE. Cephalometric evaluation of facial growth in operated and unoperated individuals with isolated clefts of the palate. Cleft Palate J 1973;10:239–46.

111. Bardach J, Kelly KM, Salyer KE. Relationship between the sequence of lip and palate repair and maxillary growth. An experimental study in beagles. Plast Reconstr Surg 1994;93:269–78.

112. Semb G. A study of facial growth in patients with bilateral cleft lip and palate treated by the Oslo CLP team. Cleft Palate Craniofac J 1991;28:22–48.

113. Shaw WC, Asher-McDade C, Brattstrom V, et al. A six-center international study of treatment outcome in patients with clefts of the lip and palate. Part 5. General discussion and conclusions. Cleft Palate Craniofac J 1992;29:413–8.

114. Canaday JW, Thompson SA, Colburn A. Craniofacial growth after iatrogenic cleft palate repair in a fetal ovine model. Cleft Palate Craniofac J 1997;34:69–72.

115. Peterson-Falzone SJ. Speech outcomes in adolescents with cleft lip and palate. Cleft Palate Craniofac J 1995;32:125–8.

116. Dalston RM. Timing of cleft palate repair: a speech pathologist's viewpoint. In: Lehman JA, editor. Problems of plastic surgery in cleft palate surgery. Philadelphia (PA): J.B. Lippincott; 1992. p. 30–8.

117. Witzel MA, Salyer KE, Ross RB. Delayed hard palate closure: the philosophy revisited. Cleft Palate J 1984;21:263–9.

118. Schweckendiek W. Primary veloplasty: long-term results without maxillary deformity. A twenty-five year report. Cleft Palate J 1991;15:268–74.

119. Kriens O. Fundamental anatomic findings for an intravelar veloplasty. Cleft Palate Journal 1970;7:27–36.

120. Bardach J, Nosal P: Geometry of the two-flap palatoplasty. In: Bardach J, Salyer K, editors. Surgical techniques in cleft lip and palate. 2nd ed. St. Louis (MO): Mosby-Year Book; 1991.

121. Von Langenbeck B. Operation der angeborenen totalen spaltung des harten gaumens nach einer neuen methode. Dtsch Klin 1861;8:231.

122. Wardill WFM. Cleft palate: results of operation for cleft palate. Br J Plast Surg 1928;16:127.

123. Wardill WFM. The technique of operation for cleft palate. Br J Surg 1937;25:117.

124. Furlow LT. Cleft palate repair by double opposing Z-plasty. Plast Reconstr Surg 1986;78:724–38.

125. Furlow LT. Bilateral buccal flaps with double opposing Z-plasty for wider palatal clefts [discussion]. Plast Reconstr Surg 1997;100:1144–5.

126. Randall P, LaRossa D, Solomon M, Cohen M. Experience with the Furlow double-reversing Z-plasty for cleft palate repair. Plast Reconstr Surg 1986;77:569–76.

127. Horswell BB, Castiglione CL, Poole AE, et al. The double-reversing z-plasty in primary palatoplasty: operative experience and early results. J Oral Maxillofac Surg 1993; 51:145–9.

128. Reid DA. Fistulae in the hard palate following cleft palate surgery. Br J Plast Surg 1986; 77:569.

129. Abyholm FE. Palatal fistulae following cleft palate surgery. Scand J Plast Reconstr Surg 1979;13:295–300.

130. Cohen SR, Kalinowski J, La Rossa D, et al. Cleft palate fistulas: a multivariate statistical analysis of prevalence, etiology, and surgical management. Plast Reconstr Surg 1991; 87:1041–7.

131. Emory RE, Clay RP, Bite U, et al. Fistula formation and repair after palatal closure: an institutional perspective. Plast Reconstr Surg 1997;99:1535–8.

132. Rintala AE. Surgical closure of palatal fistulae: follow-up of 84 personally treated cases. Scand J Plast Reconstr Surg Hand Surg 1980;14:235–8.

133. Schultz RC. Management and timing of cleft palate fistula repair. Plast Reconstr Surg 1986;78:739–47.

134. Tessier P. Colobomas: vertical and oblique complete facial clefts. Panminerva Med 1969;11:95–101.

135. Kawamoto HK. The kaleidoscopic world of rare craniofacial clefts: order out of chaos (Tessier Classification). Clin Plast Surg 1976;3:529–72.

136. Posnick JC. Rare craniofacial clefts: evaluation and treatment In: Posnick JC, editor. Craniofacial and maxillofacial surgery in children and young adults. Philadelphia (PA): W.B. Saunders; 2000. p. 487–502.

CHAPTER 43

Reconstruction of the Alveolar Cleft

Peter E. Larsen, DDS

In the management of patients with cleft lip and cleft palate, the decision regarding alveolar cleft grafting is one of the most controversial. Is grafting of the residual alveolar defect indicated? If so, at what age is it most appropriate, what material is most ideal, and should adjunctive procedures such as orthodontic expansion be used before or after grafting? Lastly, what are appropriate measures of success? This chapter reviews what is known, discusses these controversies, and provides a rationale for the approach to the residual alveolar cleft defect.

Rationale for Grafting

Although some authors have advocated nongrafting techniques[1] or prosthodontic approaches, the general consensus is that achieving continuity between the cleft alveolar segments has significant advantages, regardless of how and when this is accomplished. Potential advantages include the following[2]:

1. Grafting achieves stability of the arch and prevents collapse of the alveolar segments. This provides improved orthodontic stability
2. Grafting preserves the health of the dentition. Grafting provides room for the canine and lateral incisors to erupt into the arch into stable alveolar bone and maintains bony support of teeth adjacent to the cleft[3,4]

3. Grafting restores continuity not only of the alveolus, but also of the maxilla at the piriform rim. This supports the ala and provides improved stability and support for the nose. This may have a direct esthetic benefit and may also prove to be of long-term benefit when formal rhinoplasty procedures are performed[3]
4. Palatal and nasolabial fistulas are often present even following palatoplasty. Grafting of the alveolar defect provides an opportunity for the surgeon to address the residual oronasal fistula. This may have potential benefit for both hygiene and speech. Many cleft patients present with chronic upper respiratory and sinus disease, which may be related to reflux into the nasal cavity and sinus. There is some evidence that the residual fistula, whether labial or palatal can have an effect on speech articulation and nasality. There is evidence that closure of the fistula and grafting the cleft defect can improve nasal emission and nasality[5]

Measuring Outcomes

Prior to discussing the controversies associated with reconstruction of the residual alveolar cleft, it is important to accept some consistent measure of successful outcome. Most reports rely on descriptive data. This makes comparison

of different approaches difficult. To evaluate bone graft success, Bergland and colleagues described a semiquantitative approach that divided grafts into four types based on alveolar crest height.[6] While this is effective, it has been suggested that occlusal alveolar bone height does not adequately measure success.[7] Support of the ala and opportunity for successful tooth movement into the site or placement of an endosseous implant also requires apical bone formation. A modification of the Bergland scale that measures both occlusal and basal bone height may be a better tool for evaluating graft success. Although the Bergland scale and modifications of it rely on a two-dimensional radiograph to evaluate bone fill within a three-dimensional cleft, studies show good correlation between bone volume as predicted by these two-dimensional radiographs and that shown on three-dimensional computed tomography scans.[8]

Timing of the Graft

Perhaps the most controversial topic in managing the alveolar cleft is when grafting should be performed. In the traditional literature, terminology is not consistent. Outcome measures for various approaches are also defined inconsistently, which makes comparison difficult. Here, alveolar grafting will be grouped according to timing as defined below (Table 43-1).

Table 43-1   Timing of Alveolar Bone Grafting
< 2 Years of Age: Primary Grafting
After lip repair Before palate repair
≥ 2 Years of Age: Secondary Grafting

Age in years
  2–5:   Early secondary
  6–12: Mixed dentition secondary (after central incisor eruption and before the canine erupts)
  6–8:   Early mixed dentition
  9–12: Late mixed dentition
  > 12: Late secondary grafting

Primary Grafting

Some define primary alveolar bone grafting as that which is performed simultaneously with lip repair.[9] Others have stated that any grafting that is performed at less than 2 years of age is considered primary grafting. Still others have defined primary grafting as grafting that is performed before the palate is repaired.[10,11]

Primary grafting performed at the time of lip repair has failed to result in acceptable outcome. Long-term studies show abnormal maxillary development with maxillary retrognathia, concave profile, and increased frequency of crossbite compared with patients without grafts.[12,13]

Primary grafting performed after the closure of the lip and before the closure of the palate has proven successful in a limited number of centers when a very specific protocol is followed.[10,11] A prosthesis is placed before the lip is closed to mold the alveolar segments into close proximity. The lip is then closed, and this further aids in molding the segments. The segments must be in close proximity with good arch form before an onlay rib graft is placed across the labial surface of the cleft in a subperiosteal tunnel that is developed by limited dissection.

Advocates of this approach have not experienced problems with altered facial growth and malocclusion, most likely the result of the limited dissection used in these cases. They have reported improved occlusion and graft success in these patients, compared with patients grafted at other ages.[14] It is still difficult to wholeheartedly endorse this approach. Several additional anesthetics and surgeries are needed at a young age. This technique may not be possible in all patients, such as those with isolated alveolar clefts without palatal clefting or those patients in whom segments cannot be orthopedically aligned. In one center, because of these limitations, nearly one-half of patients could not be treated with primary grafting.[10] Outcomes may also not be as good as with other approaches. In one study,[15] there was an increased incidence of malformation of permanent lateral incisors in the primary graft group and decreased success of the graft, with only 41% of primary grafts (54% if pregrafting orthopedics was included) resulting in adequate bone height when measured with a Bergland scale. This was compared with 73% success of those sites grafted in the mixed dentition stage (after eruption of the permanent central incisors and before eruption of the maxillary canine).

Early Secondary Grafting

Grafting after the child reaches 2 years of age and before 6 years is considered early secondary grafting. The literature does not support early secondary grafting.

Secondary Grafting During the Mixed Dentition (after Eruption of the Maxillary Central Incisors and before Eruption of the Canine)

Alveolar reconstruction with grafting during the eruption of the permanent dentition may be best for various reasons. Rationale for grafting and for timing of grafting during this time period include the following:

1. There is minimal maxillary growth after age 6 to 7 years, and the effect of grafting at this time will result in minimal to no alteration of facial growth[16,17]

2. Cooperation with orthodontic and perioperative care is predictable. General anesthesia is not required for routine orthodontic procedures such as expansion

3. The donor site for graft harvest is of acceptable volume for predictable grafting with autogenous bone

4. Bone volume may be improved by eruption of the tooth into the newly grafted bone[18]

5. Grafting during this phase allows placement of the graft before eruption of permanent teeth into the cleft site, which achieves one of the primary goals of grafting — to enhance the health of teeth in and adjacent to the alveolar cleft

The landmark papers by Boyne and Sands established that grafting in the mixed dentition achieves many of the goals of reconstruction of the cleft alveolus.[19,20] The ideal patient is between the ages of 8 and 12 years with a maxillary canine root that is one-half to two-thirds developed. This timing is supported by several well-documented studies.[6,21–25] However, some authors have suggested that earlier grafting should be considered as a means of preserving the lateral incisor as well.[12,26,27] These authors have suggested that grafting be considered as early as 6 years of age. There is some evidence that grafting between the ages of 6 and 8 years, in addition to achieving the expected goal of preserving the canine, can preserve the lateral incisor as well, but this remains controversial. Despite clear indications that grafting in the mixed dentition is preferable to either primary, early secondary, or late secondary grafting, it is not entirely clear whether this grafting should be performed early (age 6–8 years) or late (age 8–12 years). Various individual factors should be evaluated when determining the ideal time for grafting during the mixed dentition (Table 43-2).

Table 43-2   Factors Contributing to Timing of Grafting During the Mixed Dentition
Dental age vs chronologic age
Presence of the lateral incisor
Position of the lateral incisor
Degree of rotation/angulation of the central incisor
Trauma/mobility of premaxillary segment (bilateral clefts)
Social issues
Size of the patient and of the cleft
Occlusion
Need for adjunctive procedures
Dynamic of the team

Dental Versus Chronologic Age Many outcomes of grafting are related to preserving health of the dentition adjacent to and erupting into the cleft site. It makes sense that the timing of the graft be determined on the basis of dental rather than chronologic age. When the maxillary central incisors begin to erupt, regardless of chronologic age, the patient should be evaluated for grafting, taking into consideration the other factors discussed below. In some patients this may be much earlier than the traditionally recommended age for evaluation.

Presence of the Lateral Incisor Many proponents of earlier mixed dentition grafting advocate this timing because of the opportunity to salvage the lateral incisor.[12,24,26] During the evaluation, attention should be directed to the presence of the lateral incisor and to whether this tooth appears to be normally formed. The incidence of congenitally missing permanent lateral incisors within the alveolar cleft is between 35 and 60%.[15,28] If a lateral incisor is present and appears to be well formed, earlier grafting may be beneficial. Even if the tooth is not perfectly formed, it may still be beneficial to attempt to preserve it. The grafted alveolus will often thin to the point that alveolar width is not adequate for definitive reconstruction

with an endosseous implant without additional grafting.[29] Retaining the lateral incisor will maintain bone width and perhaps eliminate the need for yet another graft at the time of implant placement.

Position of the Lateral Incisor If the lateral incisor is mesial to the cleft it often has adequate space for eruption. However, if the lateral incisor is located in the posterior segment, earlier grafting may be necessary to preserve the lateral incisor.[9] In one review, 36% of patients with cleft lip and alveolus had missing lateral incisors. Of the 64% who had lateral incisors, 90% of the lateral incisors were located distal to the cleft. In the same series of patients, 57% of those with cleft lip and palate had missing lateral incisors, and of the remaining 43%, 86% of the lateral incisors were located distal to the cleft.[28] Therefore, a significant number of patients may benefit from earlier grafting to preserve the lateral incisor (Figure 43-1).

Rotation of the Central Incisor The maxillary permanent central incisor will often erupt in a rotated and angled position (Figure 43-2). This reflects the morphology of the underlying bone. In extreme cases, the crowding of the two incisors can preclude normal oral hygiene methods, and this can lead to decay of the central incisor. The patient or parent may also be concerned with the position of the incisors for social reasons. If a decision is made to rotate these teeth into alignment, it may be necessary to graft the alveolar defect prior to this orthodontic tooth movement.[30] Failure to consider the morphology of the bone on the distal surface of the erupted central incisor can result in bone loss and periodontal defects as a result of orthodontic tooth movement. Since the incisor teeth erupt around age 6 years, the surgeon may choose to graft at an earlier age so that orthodontic movement of the incisors can be accomplished.

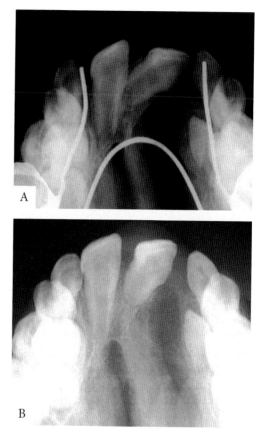

FIGURE 43-1   A, *Occlusal radiograph shows lateral incisor distal to the cleft.* B, *Grafting which was done at age 7 years to facilitate eruption of the lateral incisor.*

Social Issues The window for mixed dentition grafting is large (age 6–12 years). This is also during a period of tremendous social development for the patient. If a graft is necessary, the timing of surgery should respect the social and educational development of the child. Slightly earlier grafting, when it may cause less interference with education or other important opportunities for social development, may be preferable to grafting at an exact stage of dental development.

Size of the Patient and of the Cleft Petite patients with large cleft defects are challenging. Adequate closure of the defect may be difficult, and harvesting an adequate amount of graft material may be challenging as well. This is particularly true for large bilateral cleft defects. In these patients, the lateral incisor is often absent, the oronasal communication is often quite

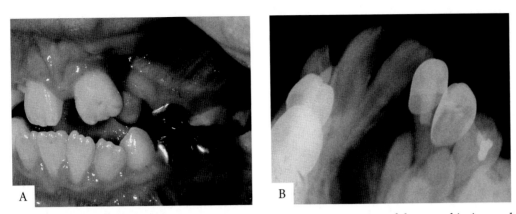

FIGURE 43-2   A, *Photograph of a typical unilateral cleft. There is rotation of the central incisor and angulation of the crown toward the cleft. This maintains bone support for the root of the tooth. B, Occlusal radiograph shows that the cleft defect is larger than it appears clinically and support for the incisor root is provided by only a thin margin of bone.*

large, and the premaxilla is frequently in less than ideal position. In these large defects, later grafting is often better, to wait for growth of the patient and orthodontic alignment of the cleft segments.

Need for Other Procedures   Patients are often evaluated for velopharyngeal incompetence, minor esthetic revision of the nose or the lip, and pressure-equalizing tubes for otitis media. It is reasonable to coordinate the timing of surgery for the alveolar cleft with other procedures that may be necessary. If velopharyngeal flap surgery is planned during the mixed dentition phase, it should take precedence over the alveolar graft. Improved speech is more important to the child's development than achieving continuity of the alveolus. Alveolar grafting would be compromised if performed simultaneously with velopharyngeal flap surgery, and in these patients, it is appropriate to delay the graft until the velopharyngeal flap surgery is accomplished and speech therapy re-instituted. Minor soft tissue, nasal, and lip revision are often desired by the patient and parents. These can be accomplished with alveolar grafting. The grafting process can distort the nose and soft tissue; these soft tissue procedures should be performed first with alveolar grafting undertaken in the same setting and with care not to disrupt the esthetic procedures already done.

Dynamic of the Team   Cleft management should always involve a multidisciplinary team, with the wide expertise to develop a proper treatment plan. Difficulties may arise when the priorities of one specialty compete with those of another. If the surgical team is faced with an orthodontic provider who feels strongly that it is appropriate to align the maxillary central incisors as soon as they erupt, it will be necessary for the alveolar defect to be grafted earlier to prevent compromise of osseous support for the central incisors. Some orthodontists and surgeons believe that palatal expansion is necessary prior to grafting. These teams may find that it is more appropriate to graft patients at a later age, as it may take months to achieve the desired expansion prior to the graft.

Secondary Grafting after Eruption of the Permanent Canine (Late Secondary Grafting)

Late secondary grafting has received some support; however, data show that when all the goals of alveolar reconstruction are considered it has a less than acceptable outcome. Patients older than 12 years of age who undergo grafting have been reported to have decreased success when evaluated using the Bergland scale,[6,15,25,27,31,32] loss of osseous support of teeth adjacent to the cleft,[18] and increased morbidity.[27] There is less

opportunity to salvage the lateral incisor, and there is a delay in correction of the orthodontic condition. This delayed grafting does allow for increased options with regard to donor site for graft material, as harvest of the mandibular symphysis becomes possible. Such grafts are difficult in the mixed dentition stage, where it is difficult to obtain adequate bone without damaging unerupted teeth.

Source of Bone Graft

The selection of the ideal grafting material is somewhat dependent on the timing of the graft. In primary bone grafting, the rib is the only site for adequate quantity of bone with acceptable morbidity. In the mixed dentition stage, the rib is not as appropriate as other sites such as the calvaria or iliac crest. These options would also be possible sources for bone for late secondary grafting, as well as grafts from the mandibular symphysis and possibly the tibia.

As the data suggest that grafting during the mixed dentition is ideal, discussion will focus on comparing various sources of graft material for this group of patients. The advantages and disadvantages of various potential sources of bone are outlined in Table 43-3.

Iliac Crest

Potential advantages of the iliac crest bone graft include low morbidity and high volume of viable osteoblastic cells (cancellous bone); two teams may work simultaneously, and this procedure is well accepted by the patient.

Bone can be harvested from the iliac crest through various approaches. Some have suggested that a lateral approach is appropriate in the growing patient.[33] This procedure disrupts the iliotibial tract and has a higher incidence of gait disturbance and postoperative pain.[34] In theory it may be appropriate to avoid the anterior crest, which does not complete its growth until after age 20 years.[34] However, the carti-

Site	Advantage	Disadvantage	Considerations
Ilium	Large quantity cancellous bone, two teams	Mild transient gait disturbance	All clefts, particularly large and bilateral clefts
Calvaria	Minimal postoperative discomfort, incision hidden, low morbidity	Limited cancellous/diploic bone, increased operative time	Unilateral clefts, lower success
Mandibular symphysis	Same operative field, rapid procurement, minimal pain	Limited bone	Older children with small defects
Rib	Two teams	Poor source cancellous bone, postoperative pain, visible scar, risk of pneumothorax	Not recommend except for primary grafting
Proximal tibia	Abundant cancellous bone, easy procedure, mild postoperative pain, two teams	—	Not recommend in patients that have not completed growth

Table 43-3 Comparison of Graft Sources

Adapted from Ochs MW.[49]

laginous cap overlying the crest is reduced in thickness to about 1 cm by age 9 years. Damage to the crest at this time could lead to disturbance in growth and cosmetic deformity of the crest; however, splitting the crest longitudinally, which allows access to the underlying cancellous marrow, has been used for harvest of bone in this age-group with no reported growth alteration and less postoperative gait disturbance than with the lateral subcrestal approach.[35,36]

Calvarial Bone

Calvarial bone has been recommended by some as an alternative to iliac crest grafting.[37,38] Some authors have concerns about the potential for success when calvaria is used as a graft source.[39,40] This may be related to the technique of harvest. Bone grafts consisting of diploic bone have been shown to be more successful than those grafts harvested using a high-speed rotary device to shave off primarily cortical bone from the surface of the calvaria.[40] However, even when harvesting calvarial bone in such a way as to maximize diploic bone, results may not be as good as with iliac crest bone. In one study where primarily diploic bone was carefully harvested from the calvaria, the results were still less successful (80% graft success) than with tra-

ditional iliac crest bone (93% graft success).[41] It is likely that either source is effective as long as primarily diploic bone is used. This limitation may render calvaria as a less useful source for large clefts and bilateral clefts.

Calvarial grafts may have decreased morbidity compared with iliac crest harvest. There is less postoperative pain and no gait disturbance. Other potential advantages include decreased surgery time. Cranial bone grafts can be harvested more quickly than iliac crest grafts. If a single team is performing surgery, this may be significant. However, it is not possible to harvest the cranial graft simultaneously with the alveolar cleft repair; grafting from the iliac crest if two teams are used can decrease overall operating time compared with calvarial grafting. Lastly, the incision for graft harvest is hidden in the hairline, which may have a cosmetic advantage.

Grafting from the calvaria has potential disadvantages. There is a perceived increased risk by patients and their families, although several studies show that the morbidity of bone harvest from the calvaria is minimal.[34] As mentioned previously, the volume of diploic bone is limited, making this less predictable for large or bilateral clefts.

Allogeneic Bone and Bone Substitutes

In an effort to eliminate the morbidity and time necessary to harvest bone from any autogenous site, some authors have evaluated allogeneic bone as a potential source of graft material. Studies have shown that allogeneic bone can be used successfully to graft secondary alveolar cleft defects and that results can be compared favorably with those achieved with autogenous bone.[42] However, the demands of bone healing in the alveolar defect where there is potential communication between the graft and the nasal and oral cavity may make this less predictable in large cleft defects or bilateral clefts. In general, bone healing with autogenous bone is biologically different than with allogeneic bone. Autogenous bone grafts initiate an angioblastic response early in the healing process, and some of the transplanted cells remain viable, resulting in a more rapid formation of new bone. In contrast, allogeneic bone grafts demonstrate slower revascularization, as there are no viable cells transferred with the graft.[42,43] There is also a theoretical risk of disease transmission from allogeneic sources of bone. Mathematically the risk is quite small but may be of concern to patients and families.

Preliminary work suggests that bone morphogenic proteins and other tissue-derived growth factors could be useful in eliminating the need for autogenous bone harvest in this patient population; however, there are insufficient outcome data and availability of these products commercially to make them the material of choice.

In summary, autogenous bone harvested from either the iliac crest or calvaria remains the most predictable technique for cleft reconstruction. The iliac crest has some potential advantage over the calvarial graft; however, this certainly depends on technique and surgeon preference.

Pre- versus Postsurgical Orthodontics

Controversy exists regarding the use of orthopedic expansion of the cleft segments and the relationship between expansion and grafting. This issue has not been entirely settled. Most authors prefer presurgical expansion, citing easier expansion because of less resistance, improved access to the cleft for closure of the nasal floor, better postoperative hygiene, and less chance of reopening the oronasal fistula.[23,24] Presurgical expansion may also allow orthopedic movement of the premaxillary segment in the bilateral cleft patient, which can eliminate traumatic occlusion that can negatively impact graft success. Proponents of

expansion following grafting cite advantages of improved bone consolidation when the graft is placed under a dynamic load during healing, a smaller soft tissue defect to close, less difficulty procuring an adequate volume of bone, and a narrower defect, which will regenerate bone more quickly.[26] Both approaches have been used in conjunction with autogenous grafting in the mixed dentition stage with success.[9]

In practice, both approaches are valid, and the decision should be based on individual clinical presentation.[31] Small unilateral clefts with collapse of the arch may be easier to graft with some presurgical expansion. In these cases, such expansion may not increase the size of the defect appreciably, and better alignment of the segments can improve hygiene of the teeth adjacent to the cleft and improve access (Figure 43-3). In these cases, the end point of presurgical expansion is improved arch form, not necessarily resolution of crossbite. Bilateral clefts with collapse of the lateral segments may also benefit from presurgical expansion. Expanding the lateral segments may allow the premaxilla, which is often anteriorly positioned, to be brought back into better relation with the arch, improving arch form, and, in some cases, eliminating traumatic occlusion (Figure 43-4). If this is not done prior to grafting, it may be difficult to

obtain ideal arch continuity, and positioning of the segments after grafting may be difficult. In patients with reasonable arch form, good alignment of the segments, and dental development corresponding to ideal timing for grafting, it makes little sense to delay grafting in order to expand preoperatively, even in the presence of a buccal crossbite. These crossbites may be related only to the anterior-posterior discrepancy, and even if they are truly representative of transverse deficiency, they can be treated easily with expansion following the graft. These clefts can be expanded without opening the oronasal fistula or having a negative effect on the graft.

Not only is there controversy regarding pre- versus postsurgical expansion, there are also two schools of thought regarding orthodontic movement of the erupted teeth adjacent to the cleft. Some authors suggest that aligning the teeth adjacent to the cleft produces better hygiene and an improved result.[23] However, orthodontic movement of teeth adjacent to the cleft is not typically desired.[44] Orthodontic movement of teeth adjacent to the cleft prior to grafting increases the risk of moving these teeth into the cleft site, compromising osseous support. Studies have directly correlated the success of grafting with the presence of adequate bone on the distal surface of the central incisor preoperatively.[45] These defects cannot subsequently be

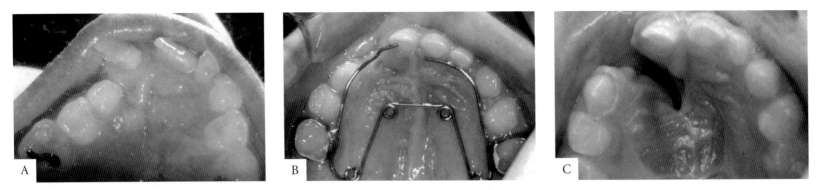

FIGURE 43-3   A, *Occlusal photograph of a typical unilateral cleft. There is rotation of the central incisors and collapse of the lesser segment. Expansion of the lesser segment will bring the arch into better form and facilitate grafting without widening the cleft. B, Similar cleft that has been expanded. C, This cleft is already wide without any expansion. It would not be appropriate to expand this cleft before grafting even if a crossbite is present.*

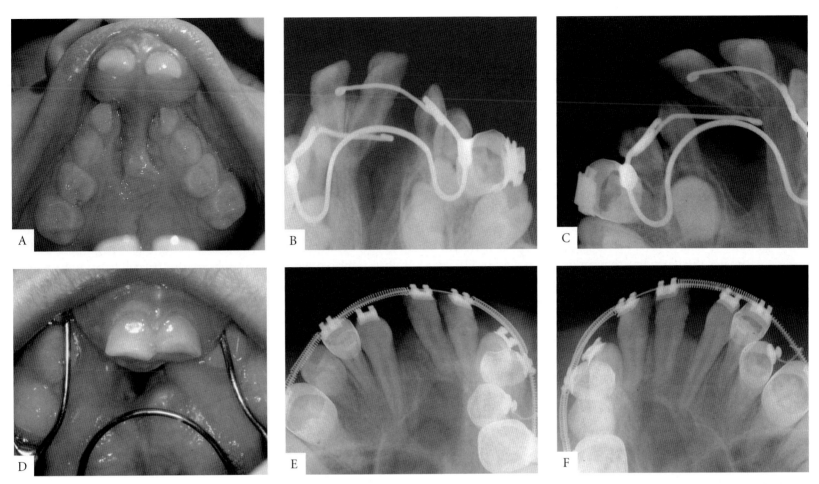

FIGURE 43-4 A, *Occlusal photograph of bilateral cleft with collapse of the lateral segments and protrusion of the premaxilla. B and C, Right and left oblique occlusal radiographs show the cleft defect. D, Expansion of the bilateral cleft allows the premaxilla to move posteriorly and improves arch form and alignment of the segments. E and F, Occlusal radiographs of the same patient following grafting with eruption of the canine.*

grafted as the bone graft will not adhere to the tooth surface. The central incisor adjacent to the cleft site is usually rotated and angled with the crown tipped toward the cleft. This rotation and angulation decreases the mesial-distal dimension of the tooth and allows for the best bony support of the tooth (see Figure 43-2). Orthodontic forces of rotation and tipping will have the undesirable effect of increasing the mesial-distal dimension, encroaching on the bony support at the cemento-enamel junction of the tooth. Orthodontic root torque to correct the angulation of the tooth will have the undesired effect of pushing the apical portion of the root toward the cleft site. The underlying osseous cleft is frequently much larger than the overlying soft tissue defect may indicate, giving a false sense of securi-

ty to the orthodontist who may want to move these teeth in the absence of a graft (Figure 43-5).

Surgical Technique for Grafting the Cleft Alveolus

The ideal technique will meet the following criteria:

1. Predictable closure of the nasal floor produces a watertight barrier between the graft and the nasal cavity
2. There is access to closure of residual palatal and labial fistula
3. Keratinized attached tissue is maintained around the teeth adjacent to the cleft and in the site where the yet unerupted lateral incisor and canine will erupt

4. Mobilization of tissue is adequate to close large defects without tension, when such defects are present

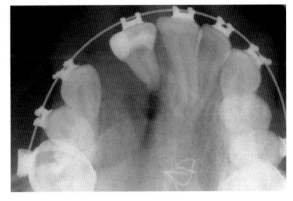

FIGURE 43-5 *Occlusal radiograph of a patient that had orthodontic rotation of the maxillary central incisor adjacent to the cleft prior to grafting the defect. There is loss of bone on the distal surface of the root to the apex. The tooth required removal.*

5. The vestibule is not shortened, and scarring is not excessive

Given these requirements, the technique most often used employs advancing buccal gingival and palatal flaps. This approach has some disadvantages, including the following:

1. Difficulty obtaining closure in large bilateral clefts, which heal by secondary intention of full-thickness wounds created by the advancement

2. A four-corner suture line that approximates the flaps directly overlying the graft, which may lead to dehiscence

3. The possibility that elevating large full thickness mucoperiosteal flaps leads to growth alteration in young patients. However, when compared with finger flaps and trapezoidal flaps, which can shorten the vestibule and place nonkeratinized tissue around the dentition, this approach remains the best

The procedure can be broken down as follows. The first step requires development

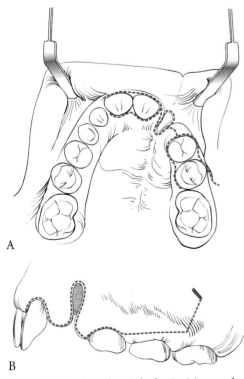

FIGURE **43-6** A and B, *Sulcular incision used to develop sliding flaps for closure over the graft. Adapted from Hall HD and Posnick JC.* [23]

of full-thickness mucoperiosteal buccal flaps (Figure 43-6). Some authors may recommend papilla preservation. When grafting is done in the mixed dentition, especially if early, this is not necessary as the papilla will regenerate. Palatal flaps are then developed, incorporating whatever residual palatal defect may be present to allow for closure of the residual palatal fistula. Some diagrams show this incision being made from a palatal approach. This may be possible in wide clefts but in practice is more easily accomplished by starting reflection of the palatal flaps from a sulcular incision that is placed on the palatal side of the dentition followed by reflection of full-thickness palatal flaps toward the palatal defect. The palatal flaps can then be separated from the nasal tissue along the cleft margin by sharp dissection with scissors from the anterior extending posteriorly as the flaps are elevated (Figure 43-7A). In this manner, the maximum palatal soft tissue is preserved for closure, while assuring adequate nasal mucosa to obtain a watertight nasal closure. Once the buccal and palatal flaps have been developed, access is readily obtained to the nasal mucosa, which is then reflected and sutured, burying the knots to obtain a watertight nasal closure (Figure 43-7B and C). Most schematic diagrams of cleft closure show this portion of the procedure being performed from the palatal aspect. However, it is generally most readily accomplished in narrow clefts from the anterior through the cleft defect. Once the nasal mucosa is closed, the palatal defect is closed by first closing the palatal flaps, converting the cleft palate into a single flap (Figure 43-7D). The graft material is then placed into the cleft from the anterior, making certain to fill all voids completely to the piriform rim. Graft material can be condensed using an orthodontic band pusher or periosteal elevator (Figure 43-7E). It is helpful to place a malleable retractor to protect the nasal floor as the bone is packed into place. Finally, the labial flaps can be advanced, and they are sutured to each other and then to the palatal flap producing the

classic four-corner closure over the crest of the ridge (Figure 43-7F and G). In most cases, the sliding flaps will be advanced one papilla on either side of the cleft, or, in some cases, only a single papilla advancement from the posterior segment is necessary. It may be necessary to perform a small back cut or to release or score the periosteum to obtain a tension-free closure. It is best to use a resorbable monofilament suture.

A palatal stent can be used to stabilize the cleft and protect the soft tissue closure. This may compromise hygiene and blood supply to the palatal flaps and, in most cases, is not required for success. In the bilateral cleft, if there is a traumatic occlusion to the anterior maxillary dentition, a mandibular bite plane is helpful to open the bite and prevent mobility of the premaxilla.

It is appropriate to use intraoperative antibiotics. Previous studies show that graft success and incidence of infection are not improved by the use of postoperative antibiotics. [46] Some surgeons feel more comfortable with a 1-week course of antibiotics, particularly when the soft tissue closure is questionable.

The postoperative diet should be limited to full liquids for approximately 5 days. This can be advanced to a soft mechanical diet. However, it is critical that the patient refrain from incising food with the anterior dentition; rather the patient should cut food into small pieces and masticate primarily on the posterior teeth. In bilateral cases, this is particularly important as any trauma to the premaxilla will cause mobility of the segment leading to graft failure. Radiographic evidence of graft consolidation should be visible within 8 weeks. The surgeon should confirm successful consolidation of the graft prior to any orthodontic manipulation of the teeth adjacent to the cleft.

Overview

This chapter has outlined historic benefits of grafting, discussed many of the controversies, and provided data on the benefits and disadvantages of several approaches.

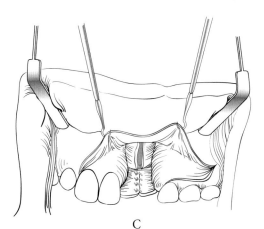

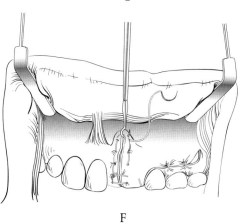

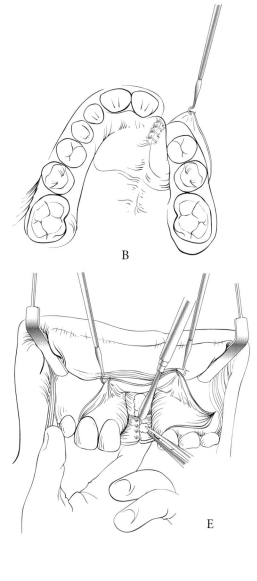

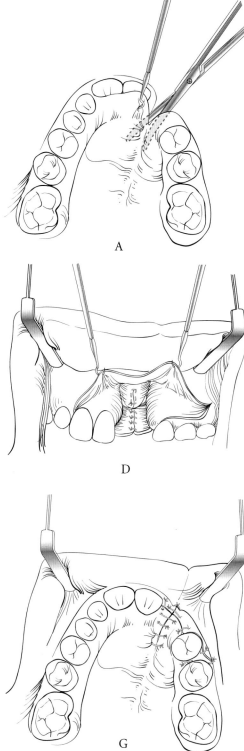

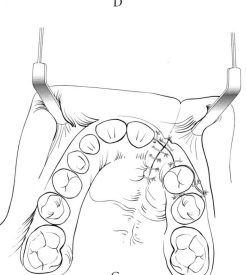

FIGURE 43-7 A, *Palatal flaps are developed sharply with scissors. This also separates the nasal mucosa from the palatal tissue. B, Palatal closure. This can be done before or after the nasal mucosa is closed. C, Nasal mucosal flaps are reflected from the bony walls of the cleft. D, Nasal flaps are approximated with sutures burying the knots when possible. E, Bone is packed into the defect with a periosteal elevator or orthodontic band pusher. Digital pressure against the palatal flap facilitates packing and protects the palatal closure. F and G, The labial flaps are advanced toward each other and closed. This provides attached keratinized tissue. Exposed areas distally where the flaps have been advanced are left to granulate. Adapted from Hall HD and Posnick JC. [23]*

The following is a stepwise approach to managing the alveolar cleft from one perspective.

1. At age 5 to 6 years an orthodontic evaluation is performed. The ability of the patient to cooperate with ortho-

dontic treatment is assessed, the arch is evaluated for collapse, and erupted supernumerary teeth in the area of the cleft are identified. Radiographic examination should include a panoramic film as well as an intraoral view that allows detailed evaluation of

the cleft site. Periapical films can be used for this, but a lateral oblique occlusal film is best. An occlusal film is placed in the standard position while directing the beam obliquely to the midline along the long axis of the cleft (Figure 43-8)

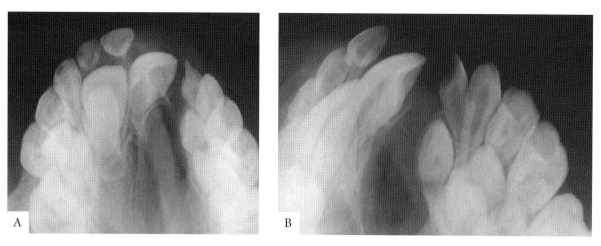

FIGURE **43-8** A, *Traditional maxillary occlusal radiograph. The cleft is identifiable, but overlap of the bone makes it difficult to determine the size of the defect and relationship of the teeth to the defect. B, Oblique occlusal radiograph is exposed by directing the beam obliquely to the midline, along the long axis of the cleft. Note that the morphology of the cleft is better identified, as is the relationship of unerupted teeth to the defect.*

2. If erupted supernumerary teeth are identified in the area of the cleft, these are extracted now or, at a minimum, 8 weeks before the graft (Figure 43-9A)
3. Orthodontic expansion is performed if there are specific goals that can be met prior to grafting. These would include decreasing traumatic occlusion to the premaxillary segment in bilateral cleft patients and correcting arch collapse that will compromise grafting. No attempt is made to correct the crossbite at this stage, and there is no attempt to orthodontically correct rotation of the permanent central incisor (see Figure 43-9A)

4. The alveolar cleft is grafted when the patient is between 6 and 8 years of age. Two teams perform the surgery with graft harvest from the iliac crest simultaneous with the cleft closure
5. The graft is evaluated with a lateral oblique occlusal radiograph 3 months following surgery (Figure 43-9B)
6. Final orthodontic expansion is performed if indicated, and permanent incisor teeth are then rotated into proper alignment

7. Conventional orthodontic treatment is performed at a more traditional age, following eruption of the remaining permanent dentition. Patients are periodically monitored for eruption of the canine in the cleft. Some authors have indicated that in 30 to 73% of patients, eruption of the canine into the alveolar graft requires surgical uncovering of the tooth or uncovering and orthodontic assistance.[12,47,48] Others have reported that nearly all of these teeth can be expected to erupt without surgical intervention[24] (Figure 43-9C).

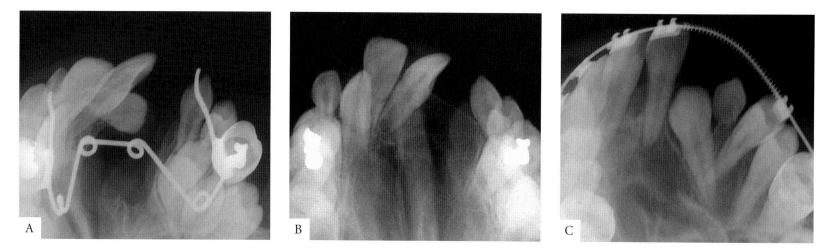

FIGURE **43-9** A, *The cleft has been expanded. The canine is in position to begin eruption. There is a supernumerary/malformed lateral incisor erupting horizontally into the cleft. B, The supernumerary tooth has been removed. The defect was grafted 2 months following extraction and the film shows good bone consolidation. C, The maxillary canine can be seen erupting into the graft.*

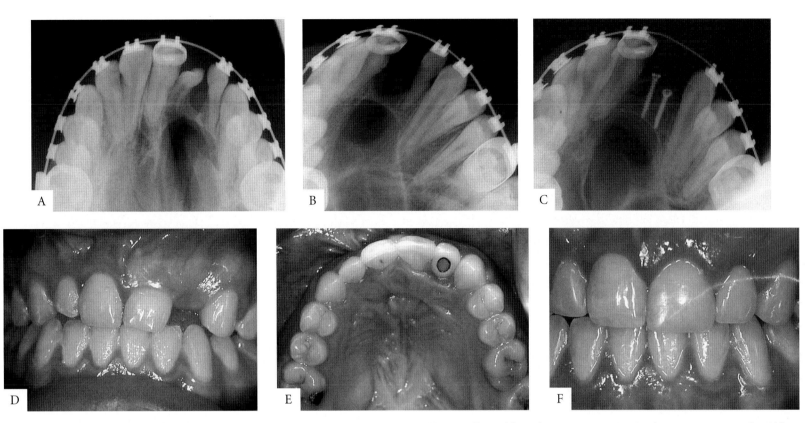

FIGURE 43-10 A, *Occlusal radiograph shows thin bridge of bone with inadequate height. A malformed lateral incisor was maintained to preserve as much width as possible.* B, *The tooth was removed.* C, *After 2 months of healing, an onlay bone graft was placed.* D, *Clinical view after grafting.* E *and* F, *View following placement of the implant and reconstruction.*

If uncovering is necessary, techniques to preserve attached tissue are used as would be appropriate for impacted canines in noncleft patients

8. Missing lateral incisors are managed with space development and implant placement, as opposed to canine substitution. This is accomplished following definitive orthodontic treatment and orthognathic surgery if indicated, after maxillary growth is complete. Even when bone height is adequate and teeth adjacent to the graft have good support, the graft undergoes resorption resulting in a narrow ridge. This is not unlike the bone resorption found with congenitally absent lateral incisors in noncleft patients. Successful implant restoration is possible, but further grafting is likely needed before adequate labial-palatal width is available for implant placement[30] (Figure 43-10). Attention to soft and hard tissue is critical in these patients to achieve esthetic results

Conclusion

Restoration of the cleft alveolus and maxilla by grafting is a critical part of the overall management of the patient with cleft palate. A systematic approach can improve predictability. This is best accomplished during the mixed dentition stage. Adjunctive expansion may be accomplished before or after grafting, depending on the needs of the patient.

References

1. Santiago PE, Grayson BH, Cutting CB, et al. Reduced need for alveolar bone grafting by pre-surgical orthopedics and primary gingivoperiosteoplasty. Cleft Palate Craniofac J 1998;35:77–80.
2. Horswell BB, Henderson JM. Secondary osteoplasty of the alveolar cleft defect. J Oral Maxillofac Surg 2003;61:1082–90.
3. Kalaaji A, Lilja J, Friede H. Bone grafting at the stage of mixed and permanent dentition in patients with clefts of the lip and primary palate. Plast Reconst Surg 1994;93:690–6.
4. Teja A, Persson R, Omnell ML. Periodontal status of teeth adjacent to nongrafted unilateral alveolar clefts. Cleft Palate Craniofac J 1992;29:357–62.
5. Bureau S, Penko M, McFadden L. Speech outcome after closure of oronasal fistulas with bone grafts. J Oral Maxillofac Surg 2001;59:1408–13.
6. Bergland O, Semb G, Abyholm RD. Elimination of the residual alveolar cleft by secondary bone grafting and subsequent orthodontic treatment. Cleft Palate J 1986;23:175–205.
7. Hynes PJ, Earley MJ. Assessment of secondary alveolar bone grafting using a modification of the Bergland grading system. Br J Plast Surg 2003;56:630–6.
8. Dado DV, Rosenstein SW, Adler ME, Kernahan DA. Long term assessment of early alveolar bone grafts using three-dimensional computer assisted tomography: a pilot study. Plast Reconst Surg 1997;99:1840–5.
9. Vig KWL, Turvey TA, Fonseca RJ. Orthodontic and surgical considerations in bone grafting in the cleft maxilla and palate. In: Turvey TA, Vig KWL, Fonseca RJ, editors. Facial

clefts and craniosynostosis: principles of management. Philadelphia: WB Saunders; 1996. p. 396.

10. Eppley B. Alveolar cleft bone grafting (part 1): Primary bone grafting. J Oral Maxillofac Surg 1996;54:74–82.

11. Rosenstein SW. Early bone grafting of alveolar cleft deformities. J Oral Maxillofac Surg 2003;61:1078–81.

12. Kwon JK, Waite DE, Stickel FR, Chisholm T. The management of alveolar cleft defects. J Am Dent Assoc 1981;102:848–53.

13. Robertson NRE, Jolleys A. An 11 year follow up of the effects of early bone grafting in infants born with complete clefts of the lip and palate. Br J Plast Surg 1983;36:438–43.

14. Helms JA, Speidel M, Denis KL. Effect of timing on long-term clinical success of alveolar cleft bone grafts. Am J Orthod Dentofacial Orthop 1987; 92:232–40.

15. Brattstrom V, McWilliam J. The influence of bone grafting age on dental abnormalities and alveolar bone height in patients with unilateral cleft lip and palate. Eur J Orthod 1989;11:351–8.

16. Daskalogiannakis J, Ross RB. Effect of alveolar bone grafting in the mixed dentition on maxillary growth in complete unilateral cleft lip and palate patients. Cleft Palate Craniofacial J 1997;34:455–8.

17. Witsenburg B. The reconstruction of anterior residual bone defects in patients with cleft lip, alveolus and palate: a review. J Maxillofac Surg 1985;13:197–208.

18. Dempf R, Teltzrow T, Kramer FJ, Hausamen JE. Alveolar bone grafting in patients with complete clefts: a comparative study between secondary and tertiary bone grafting. Cleft Palate Craniofac J 2002; 39:18–25.

19. Boyne PJ, Sands NR. Combined orthodontics-surgical management of residual palato-alveolar cleft defects. Am J Orthod 1976; 70:20–37.

20. Boyne PJ, Sands NR. Secondary bone grafting of residual alveolar and palatal clefts. J Oral Surg 1972;30:87–92.

21. Abyholm RE, Bergland E, Semb G. Secondary bone grafting of alveolar clefts. Scand J Plast Reconstr Surg 1981;15:127–40.

22. Broude D, Waite DE. Secondary closure of alveolar defects. Oral Surg 1974;37:829.

23. Hall HD, Posnick JC. Early results of secondary bone grafts in 106 alveolar clefts. J Oral Maxillofac Surg 1983;41:289–94.

24. Turvey TA, Vig K, Moriarty J. Delayed bone grafting in the cleft maxilla and palate: a multidisciplinary analysis. Am J Orthod 1984;86:244–56.

25. Yi-Lin J, James DR, Mars M. Bilateral alveolar bone grafting: a report of 55 consecutively treated patients. Eur J Orthod 1998; 20:299–307.

26. Boyne PJ. Bone grafting in the osseous reconstruction of alveolar and palatal clefts. Oral Maxillofac Clin North Am 1991;3:589–97.

27. Hall HD, Werther JR. Conventional alveolar cleft bone grafting. Oral Maxillofac Clin North Am 1991; 3:609–16.

28. Suzuki A, Watanabe M, Nakano M, Takahama Y. Maxillary lateral incisors of subjects with cleft lip and or palate: part 2. Cleft Palate Craniofac J 1992; 29:380–4.

29. Kearns G, Perrott DH, Sharma A, et al. Placement of endosseous implants in grafted alveolar clefts. Cleft Palate Craniofac J 1997;34:520–5.

30. Vig KWL. Alveolar bone grafts: the surgical/orthodontic management of the cleft maxilla. Ann Acad Med Singapore 1999;28:721–7.

31. Enemark H, Sindet-Pedersen S, Bundgaard M. Long-term results after secondary bone grafting of alveolar clefts. J Oral Maxillofac Surg 1987;45:913–8.

32. Paulin G, Astrand P, Rosenquist JB, Bartholdson L. Intermediate bone grafting of alveolar clefts. J Craniomaxillofac Surg 1988; 16:2–7.

33. Crockford DA, Converse JM. The ilium as a source of bone grafts in children. Plast Reconstr Surg 1972;50:270–4.

34. Larsen PE. Sources of autogenous bone grafts in pediatric patients. Oral Maxillofac Clin North Am 1994;6:137–52.

35. Rudman RA. Prospective evaluation of morbidity associated with iliac crest harvest for alveolar cleft grafting. J Oral Maxillofac Surg 1997;55:219–23.

36. Wolfe SA, Kawamoto HK. Taking the iliac bone graft. J Bone Joint Surg 1978;60:411.

37. Harsha BC, Turvey TA, Powers SK. Use of autogenous cranial bone grafts in maxillofacial surgery. J Oral Maxillofac Surg 1986; 44:11–5.

38. Turvey TA. Donor site for alveolar cleft bone grafts (letter). J Oral Maxillofac Surg 1997; 45:834.

39. Jackson IT, Helden G, Marx R. Skull bone grafts in maxillofacial and craniofacial surgery. J Oral Maxillofac Surg 1986; 44:949–56.

40. Kortebein MJ, Nelson CL, Sadove MA. Retrospective analysis of 135 secondary alveolar cleft grafts using iliac or calvarial bone. J Oral Maxillofac Surg 1991;49:493–8.

41. Sadove MA, Nelson CL, Epply BL, Nguyen B. An evaluation of calvearial and iliac donor sitres in alveolar cleft grafting. Cleft Palate Craniofac J 1990;27:225–9.

42. Maxson BB, Baxter SD, Vig KWL, Fonseca RJ. Allogeneic bone for secondary alveolar cleft osteoplasty. J Oral Maxillofac Surg 1990; 48:933–41.

43. Marx RE, Miller RI, Ehler WJ, et al. A comparison of particulate allogeneic and particulate autogenous bone grafts into maxillary alveolar clefts in dogs. J Oral Maxillofac Surg 1984;42:3–9.

44. Vig KWL, D'orth RCS, Turvey TA. Orthodontic-surgical interaction in the management of cleft lip and palate. Clin Plast Surg 1985;12:735–48.

45. Aurouze C, Moller KT, Bevis RR, et al. The presurgical status of the alveolar cleft and success of secondary bone grafting. Cleft Palate Craniofac J 2000;37:179–84.

46. Larsen PE, Myers G, Beck MF. Morbidity of alveolar cleft grafting in the early mixed dentition (<8years). J Oral Maxillofac Surg 1997; 55(Suppl 3):127.

47. Eldeeb M, Messer LB, Lehnert MW, et al. Canine eruption into grafted bone in maxillary alveolar cleft defects. Cleft Palate J 1988;19:9–16.

48. Enemark H, Sindet-Pedersen S, Bundgaard M, Simonsen EK. Combined orthodontic-surgical treatment of alveolar clefts. Ann Plast Surg 1988;21:127–33.

49. Ochs MW. Alveolar cleft bone grafting (part 2): secondary bone grafting. J Oral Maxillofac Surg 1996; 54:83–8.

CHAPTER 44

Reconstruction of Cleft Lip and Palate: Secondary Procedures

Ramon L. Ruiz, DMD, MD
Bernard J. Costello, DMD, MD

A congenital cleft of the lip and palate represents a complex malformation involving the hard and soft tissues of the face. Children born with cleft lip and palate face several unique functional and esthetic challenges requiring a combined (interdisciplinary) treatment approach in order to obtain an ideal outcome relative to speech, occlusion, facial appearance, and individual self-esteem. This successful reconstruction routinely requires multiple phases of surgical intervention. Because treatment is carried out during periods of growth, the benefit-risk ratio of any planned surgical procedure must be carefully considered in order to provide the maximum benefit to the patient.[1,2] Surgeons caring for these children must maintain a firm cognitive understanding of the three-dimensional anatomy of the cleft lip and palate malformation and the complex interplay that exists between the surgical procedures and ongoing facial growth.

The various surgical procedures involved in staged reconstruction of cleft lip and palate have been described extensively in the literature and are presented in Chapters 42, "Cleft Lip and Palate: Comprehensive Treatment Planning and Primary Repair," Chapter 43, "Reconstruction of the Alveolar Cleft," and Chapter 61, "Orthognathic Surgery in the Patient with Cleft Palate."[3–6] In addition, the American Cleft Palate–Craniofacial Association (ACPCA) has developed parameters of care in order to facilitate the coordinated interdisciplinary treatment of individuals affected with cleft lip and palate deformities.[7] The ACPCA document summarizes a management protocol that is centered around thoughtful timing of specific interventions based on the patient's dental, skeletal, speech, and psychological development. The general staged approach to cleft lip and palate reconstruction from infancy through adolescence is presented in Table 44-1. Contemporary management protocols involve several phases of surgery during infancy (cleft lip repair and palate closure) and early childhood (bone graft reconstruction of the cleft maxilla and alveolus) that are considered required operations in all cases of complete unilateral or bilateral cleft lip and palate. In addition to those primary stages of repair, several children will go on to require additional procedures for correction of secondary problems. Secondary reconstruction of cleft lip and palate may involve

Table 44-1 Stages of Cleft Lip and Palate Reconstruction: Infancy through Adolescence		
Surgical Treatment	*Age*	*Timing Considerations*
Cleft lip repair*	10 to 12 weeks	
Cleft palate repair*	9 to 18 months	Exact timing of repair is based on child's speech/language age
Secondary palate surgery for VPI	3 to 5 years	
Bone graft reconstruction of cleft maxilla/alveolus*	6 to 9 years	Based on dental development
Orthognathic surgery	14 to 16 years for females, 16 to 18 years for males	
Dental implant placement	16 to 18 years	
Lip/nasal revision	After age 5 years	Varies widely depending on clinical findings and psychosocial concerns. Definitive nasal surgery usually delayed until adolescence.
*Reconstruction stage is required for all patients with complete cleft lip and palate. VPI = velopharyngeal insufficiency.		

surgery for treatment of velopharyngeal dysfunction, bone graft reconstruction of bony clefts of the maxilla, correction of residual skeletal disproportion with malocclusion, closure of palatal fistulas, normalization of lip and nasal form, and prosthetic rehabilitation of the cleft dental gap. Although the indications for each of the primary and secondary surgical undertakings are different and the decision-making processes may vary, one cannot view each of these procedures as isolated events. This chapter reviews the different phases of secondary cleft lip and palate reconstruction that may be required after primary cleft lip and palate repair with the purpose of providing an organized description of the contemporary philosophy and rationale for surgical interventions and specific timing.

Fistula Closure

Background

When a child is born with a cleft palate, there is an abnormal communication between the oral and nasal cavities. One of the principles essential to successful surgical repair involves the separation of oral and nasal side soft tissues from each other and then reconstruction of those distinct tissue layers to establish separate nasal floor and oral mucosal linings. The result is closure of the hard palate in two layers (nasal mucosa and oral mucosa) and closure of the soft palate in three layers (nasal side, levator musculature, and oral side mucosa).

Residual abnormal oronasal communications, or "fistulas," following the initial repair are relatively frequent problems that require subsequent surgical procedures in patients with cleft palate. Before addressing the specific management approach to residual fistulas, one must define the clinical situation based on the patient's age, previous surgical history, and the exact location of the fistula. Another important consideration is the extent to which the cleft defect involves the primary and secondary palates. The primary palate comprises the anatom-

ic structures anterior to the incisive foramen (alveolus, maxilla, piriform, lip). The secondary palate comprises the anatomic structures between the incisive foramen and the uvula. Using this terminology, a complete cleft of the primary and secondary palates would involve the maxilla, alveolus, hard palate, and soft palate. An isolated cleft palate involving the hard and soft palate (without affecting the alveolar ridge) would be described as a complete cleft of the secondary palate while a cleft involving only the soft palate (and not the hard palate or alveolus) is described as an incomplete cleft of the secondary palate.

Even when a child is born with a complete cleft palate (ie, affecting the primary and secondary palate), the primary repair involves closure of the secondary palate only—those structures from the incisive foramen to the uvula. The goals of cleft palate repair during infancy are twofold: first, to establish complete watertight closure of the secondary palate for separation of the oral and nasal cavities and, second, to repair the levator musculature in order to allow for normal speech formation. Repair of the skeletal maxillary/alveolar cleft defect and its associated oronasal communication are not generally undertaken at this stage. Many surgeons consider this alveolar defect part of the original cleft deformity that has been purposely left unrepaired instead of a true "fistula." Definitive repair of the anterior alveolar or nasolabial fistula is instead incorporated into the bone graft reconstruction performed during midchildhood based on the child's dental development.[5,6,8,9] Bone graft reconstruction of the cleft defect is presented in greater detail in Chapter 43, "Reconstruction of the Alveolar Cleft."

Ideally, a child with a complete cleft palate will undergo palate repair during infancy with successful closure of the hard and soft (or secondary) palates and then bone graft reconstruction of the maxilla/alveolus (or primary palate) with closure of any residual nasolabial fistula

during childhood. Unfortunately, residual palatal fistulas are frequently encountered after the initial palate repair. The risk of fistula formation seems to be closely associated with the size of the original cleft defect.[10,11] The type of repair used by the surgeon may also affect the fistula rate. Recent reports indicate that a two-flap palatoplasty technique is associated with the lowest rate (3.4%) of palatal fistula formation.[12] Another frequently employed technique, the Furlow double opposing Z-plasty, is associated with a higher incidence of oronasal fistula.[5] This difference in the rate of fistula occurrence is probably more noticeable when the cleft defect being repaired is very wide. The most common location for development of a residual palatal fistula following cleft palate repair is the junction of the hard and soft palates followed by the anterior hard palate and incisive foramen region.[5,6,11,13] The incidence of palatal fistula following single-stage palatoplasty varies greatly, with the reported rates as high as 50%.[11]

Indications for Fistula Repair and Timing of Surgery

Most fistulas are noted early on in the postsurgical period following palate repair and are the direct result of local wound breakdown owing to tension or vascular compromise. Another time period when a palatal fistula may be encountered is during Phase I (pre-bone graft) orthodontic treatment, especially if maxillary expansion has been undertaken. There is disagreement about the causal relationship of orthodontic expansion and development of a palatal fistula. However, most experienced cleft surgeons believe that fistula defects discovered during maxillary expansion are preexisting oronasal communications and are not actually caused by the orthodontic treatment. Small fistulas present since infancy can be hidden within a narrow palate by collapsed maxillary segments and then uncovered as the maxillary arch form is expanded by orthodontic or orthopedic means.

The recommended timing of fistula closure may vary significantly and remains a controversial topic. Some surgeons and cleft teams may advocate relatively aggressive management with early closure of any fistula present after the initial palate repair. We prefer to take a more long-range view of these problems and delay surgery for several years whenever possible.

In infants, the closure of a small (1 to 4 mm), nonfunctional fistula can generally be deferred until later in childhood. In such cases, fistula repair may be incorporated into any future necessary procedures such as pharyngeal surgery for velopharyngeal insufficiency or bone graft reconstruction of the cleft maxilla and alveolus as long as there are no functional speech or feeding-related concerns. When a larger (> 5 mm) fistula is present, there is a greater likelihood that functional concerns will be encountered, such as nasal air escape which impacts speech, nasal reflux of food and liquids, and hygiene-related difficulties. In clinical situations where significant functional problems exist, earlier closure of the persistent fistula is indicated. As part of the decision-making process, surgeons must weigh the benefits of fistula repair against the negative effects of a second palatal surgery involving stripping of mucoperiosteum on subsequent maxillary growth. Another consideration in planning the exact timing of fistula closure is the type of repair technique being used for the repair. Attempts to close a fistula with local flaps or repeat palatoplasty may be undertaken during infancy and early childhood. On the other hand, in cases in which the use of a regional (eg, tongue) flap is required, the child must be old enough to cooperate with the perioperative regimen.

Operative Techniques for Closure of Palatal Fistulas

The repair of residual palatal fistulas following cleft palate repair has been described using several different techniques.[5,10,14–16] Current operations used

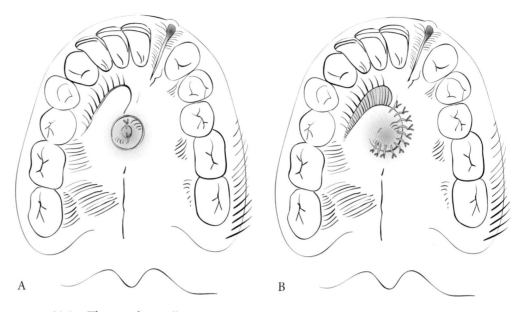

FIGURE 44-1   *The use of a small, rotational flap for closure of a residual palatal fistula. This type of repair has a high failure rate. A, Turnover flaps are used to establish a nasal side closure and a palatal mucosal flap is outlined. B, Random pattern, full-thickness mucoperiosteal flap is elevated and mobilized for coverage of defect.*

for fistula repair include local palatal flaps, modifications of the von Langenbeck and two-flap palatoplasty techniques, palatoplasty with incorporation of a pharyngeal flap, and the use of a tongue flap. Other regional flaps, including the tongue, buccal mucosa, buccinator myomucosal, temporalis muscle, and vascularized tissue transfer are less frequently used but have been described.[14,17–21]

One of the most frequently described procedures for closure of residual fistulas is the use of local soft tissue flaps created within the palatal mucosa and rotated over the defect for closure (Figure 44-1). The components of this approach are the creation of turnover flaps around the defect for nasal side closure, elevation of a palatal finger flap, and rotation of the flap for coverage of the defect. A significant area of exposed bone is left at the donor site, and this is allowed to heal by secondary intention. Unfortunately, this type of repair is useful only for very small palatal defects and is associated with a relatively high failure rate.[14] Small rotational flaps within palatal tissues that contain extensive scarring from prior surgical procedures are difficult to

mobilize without residual tension and may have diminished blood supply resulting in a less-than-ideal healing capacity and a greater chance of wound breakdown.

Our preferred approach to residual palatal fistulas involves the modification of one of the primary palate repair techniques, namely the Bardach or von Langenbeck procedures.[5,22] These approaches allow adequate coverage of even large defects with the use of bulky soft tissue flaps, a layered repair of the nasal and oral sides, and a tension-free line of closure (Figures 44-2 and 44-3). In addition, the amount of bone that is left exposed after the repair is minimal to none. This is because the vertical depth of the palatal vault translates into soft tissue extension medially, and so the result is palatal soft tissue flaps that adequately cover the underlying bone with a layer of dead space between the palatal shelves and the oral mucosa lining. The Bardach (two-flap) palatoplasty is our preferred operation in cases where the fistula defect is 5 mm or larger. The primary advantage of this approach is the ability to raise large soft tissue flaps, which can be mobilized easily and allow for easy visualization and closure of

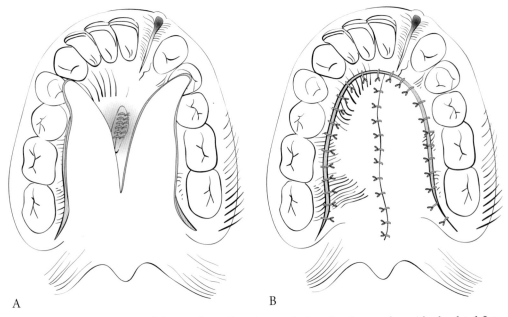

A   B

FIGURE **44-2**   *Modification of the two-flap palatoplasty technique for closure of a residual palatal fistula. A, Two large mucoperiosteal flaps are developed with dissection extended to a point posterior of the fistula defect. The nasal mucosa is repaired as a separate layer. B, Closure of the oral side. The midline is closed first using multiple interrupted sutures, and then the lateral incisions are reapproximated.*

the nasal mucosa. By comparison, one of the theoretical advantages of the von Langenbeck procedure is the creation of bipedicled flaps that maintain anterior and posterior blood supplies. While the anterior pedicles do provide additional perfusion, they also result in less freely movable flaps with limited access and visualization of the nasal side tissues. For this reason, we use the von Langenbeck technique only for relatively small defects within the hard palate.

In situations where there is a much larger (> 1.5 cm) defect, successful closure may dictate that the surgeon recruit additional soft tissue using a regional flap. Fistula defects within the posterior hard palate or soft palate may be addressed with the use of a modified palatoplasty procedure as described above in combination with a superiorly based pharyngeal flap. After the palatal flaps are developed and the nasal side dissection is complete, a pharyngeal flap is harvested. The pharyngeal flap soft tissue is then incorporated into the nasal side closure of the area where the fistula was present. Using this technique, a substantial amount of additional soft tissue can be recruited for tension-free repair of a large palatal defect. When the fistula is located within the anterior two-thirds of the hard palate, the procedure of choice for recruitment of additional soft tissue is the anteriorly based dorsal tongue flap (Figure 44-4). First, nasal side closure of the palatal defect is performed using turnover flaps with multiple interrupted sutures. Next, this technique calls for development of an anteriorly based tongue flap that is approximately 5 cm in length by one- to two-thirds the width of the tongue. The tongue flap is elevated along the underlying musculature and then inset using multiple mattress sutures for closure of the oral side. The recipient bed within the tongue is closed primarily. After the initial surgery, the tongue flap is allowed to heal for approximately 2 weeks. At that time, the patient is returned to the operating room. Nasal fiber-optic intubation is indicated for the second procedure since the tongue is still sutured to the palate, restricting normal visualization of the airway. The flap is sectioned and the stump at the donor site is freshened and inset into the tongue. The use of laterally and posteriorly based tongue flaps has also been

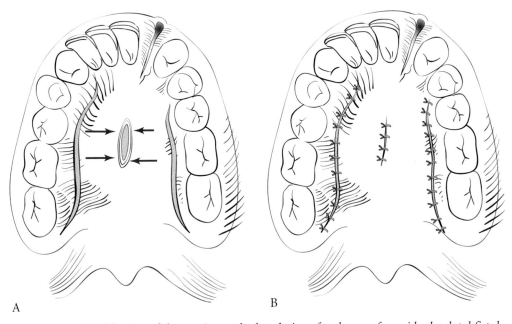

A   B

FIGURE **44-3**   *Modification of the von Langenbeck technique for closure of a residual palatal fistula. A, Incisions are created at the fistula defect along the junction of oral and nasal mucosa, and laterally in order to develop palatal flaps. Care is taken to maintain anterior soft tissue attachment for improved blood supply. This may make flap mobilization and visualization of the defect difficult. B, The nasal side is closed first, and then oral side closure is accomplished with interrupted sutures.*

presented in the cleft literature.[23,24] In our opinion, however, an anteriorly based flap is better tolerated by most patients and allows for the greatest degree of tongue mobility with less risk of tearing the flap from its palatal insertion.

Secondary Cleft Palate Surgery for Management of Velopharyngeal Dysfunction

Background

The secondary palate is composed of a hard (bony) palate anteriorly and a soft palate or "velum" posteriorly. Within the soft palate, the levator veli palatini muscle forms a dynamic sling that elevates the velum toward the posterior pharyngeal wall during the production of certain sounds. Other muscle groups within the velum, the tonsillar pillar region,[1] and pharyngeal walls also impact resonance quality during speech formation (Table 44-2). The combination of the soft palate and pharyngeal wall musculature jointly form what is described as the velopharyngeal (VP) mechanism (Figure 44-5A). The VP mechanism functions as a sphincter valve in order to regulate airflow between the oral and nasal cavities and create a combination of orally based and nasally based sounds.

Children born with a cleft palate have, by definition, a malformation that dramatically impacts the anatomic components of the VP mechanism. Specifically, clefting of the secondary palate causes division of the musculature of the velum into separate muscle bellies with abnormal insertions along the posterior edge of the hard palate (Figure 44-5B). The initial palatoplasty is not carried out simply for closure of the palatal defect (oronasal communication) itself, but is aimed also at addressing these underlying anatomic discrepancies involving the musculature. During surgery for palatal closure, care must be taken to sharply separate the muscles off of the palatal shelves, realign them, and establish continuity in order to create

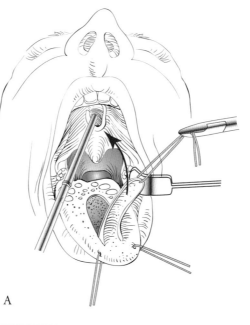

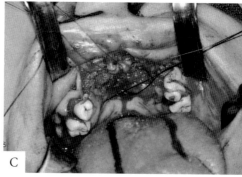

FIGURE **44-4** *Use of an anteriorly based dorsal tongue flap for repair of a large fistula within the anterior hard palate. A, Diagram of palatal defect and elevation of anteriorly based tongue flap. Turnover flaps are first used to create a nasal side repair and then the tongue flap is developed. The width of the flap may be as wide as two-thirds the width of the tongue and approximately 4 to 6 cm in length. B, The donor site is closed using multiple interrupted sutures and the tongue flap is inset and sutured to the palatal mucosa surrounding the defect. C and D, Intraoperative views of tongue flap harvest and inset. A and B adapted from Posnick JC. Cleft-orthognathic surgery: the isolated cleft palate deformity. In: Posnick JC, Rose A, Ross A, editors. Craniofacial and maxillofacial surgery in children and young adults. 1st ed. Philadelphia (PA): W.B. Saunders; 2000. p. 957–8.*

a functional palatal-levator muscle sling. Some describe this primary repair of the palatal musculature as "intravelar veloplasty," a component of the cleft palate closure. Although this description helps to articulate the importance of addressing the levator muscle, it may confuse some clinicians by suggesting that muscle repair or intravelar veloplasty is a separate procedure. Irrespective of the type of cleft palate

Table 44-2	Muscle Groups Contributing to the Velopharyngeal Mechanism		
Muscle	*Insertion*	*Origin*	*Function*
Uvulus muscle	Mucous membrane of soft palate	Palatal aponeurosis	Velar extension
Tensor veli palatini	Soft and hard palates	Medial pterygoid plate	Opens auditory tube
Salpingopharyngeous	Palatopharyngeal aponeurosis	Torus tubarius	Motion of the lateral walls
Superior constrictor	Medial pharyngeal raphe	Velum; medial pterygoid plate	Posterior and lateral wall sphinctering
Levator veli palatini	Soft palate	Temporal bone	Elevation of the velum
Palatopharyngeous	Soft palate aponeurosis	Pharyngeal wall	Adduction of posterior pillars; sphinctering of velum
Palatoglossus	Tongue	Soft palate	Retracts tongue; antagonistic to the levator during speech

repair technique employed (von Langenbeck, Bardach, Furlow, etc), meticulous release of abnormal muscle insertions and velar muscle reconstruction must be incorporated as a critical element of the surgical procedure.

Most children who undergo successful cleft palate repair during infancy (9 to 18 months) will go on to develop speech that is normal or to demonstrate minor speech abnormalities that are amenable to treatment with speech therapy. In a smaller segment of this patient population, however, the velopharyngeal mechanism will not demonstrate normal function despite surgical closure of the palate.[25] "Velopharyngeal insufficiency" (VPI) is defined as inadequate closure of the nasopharyngeal airway port during speech production. The exact etiology of VPI following successful cleft palate repair is a complex problem that remains difficult to completely define. Inadequate surgical repair of the musculature is one cause of VPI, but even muscles that have been appropriately realigned and reconstituted may fail to heal normally or function properly because of congenital defects with their innervation. The role of postsurgical scarring and its impact on muscle function and palatal motion is poorly understood. When using a Furlow double opposing Z-plasty procedure for the initial palate repair, the theoretical advantages include better realignment of the palatal muscles and lengthening of the soft palate, but these benefits may be negatively balanced by a velum that demonstrates less motion or elevation owing to the additional scarring associated with two separate sets of Z-plasty incisions. In addition, it must be considered that the repaired cleft palate is

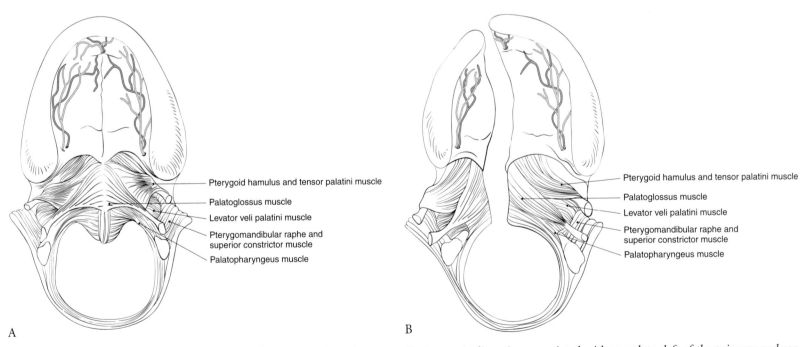

FIGURE 44-5   *Anatomy of the velopharyngeal mechanism. A, Normal anatomy. B, Anatomic distortions associated with complete cleft of the primary and secondary palate. Note abnormal insertions of levator veli palatini muscle along the posterior edge of the hard palate.*

only one factor contributing to VP function, and other abnormalities related to oropharyngeal morphology, lateral and posterior pharyngeal wall motion, and nasal airway dynamics may all contribute to VP dysfunction. Certainly, these other structures may also play a role in compensating for the palatal deformity. For example, a short, scarred soft palate that does not elevate very well may be compensated for by the recruitment and hypertrophy of muscular tissue within the posterior pharyngeal wall ("activation of Passavant's ridge").[26–28]

The audible nasal air escape with resultant hypernasal speech that is associated with VPI is perhaps the most debilitating consequence of the cleft palate malformation. Approximately 20% of children with VPI following palatoplasty will go on to require management involving additional palatal surgery.[25] Left untreated, nasal air escape-related resonance problems will lead to other speech abnormalities, namely, abnormal compensatory articulations. Warren's elegant aerodynamic demands theory provides the best explanation of what occurs with severe VPI.[29] His theory states that nasal air escape owing to inadequate VP closure will cause the patient to articulate pressure consonants at the level of the larynx or pharynx instead of within the oral cavity. These abnormal, compensatory, misarticulations further complicate problems with speech formation and decrease speech intelligibility in patients with cleft palate–related VPI.

Indications for Surgery and Timing

Following the initial cleft palate repair, periodic evaluations are critical in order to assess the speech and language development of each child. Typically, this involves a standardized screening examination performed by a speech and language pathologist as part of an annual visit to the cleft palate team. In patients with speech problems such as VPI, more detailed studies including the use of videofluoroscopy and nasopharyngoscopy may be indicated. Videofluoroscopy studies are used to radiographically examine the upper airway with the aid of an oral contrast material. These techniques allow dynamic testing of the VP mechanism with views of the musculature in action. In addition, details of the upper airway anatomy including residual palatal fistulas can be visualized and their contribution to speech dysfunction evaluated during the study. For a videofluoroscopy study to be of diagnostic value, it must include multiple views of the VP mechanism and a speech pathologist must be present in order to administer verbal testing in the radiology suite. Nasopharyngoscopy using a small, flexible, fiber-optic endoscope is routinely used for the evaluation of patients with VPI. Nasopharyngoscopy allows for direct visualization of the upper airway and specifically the VP mechanism from the nasopharynx. This technique avoids the radiation exposure associated with videofluoroscopy but requires preparation of the nose with a topical anesthetic, skillful maneuvering of the scope, and a compliant patient. Once the endoscope is inserted, observations of palatal function, airway morphology, and pharyngeal wall motion are made while the patient is verbally tested by the speech pathologist.[5] The opportunity for direct visualization of the VP mechanism in action during speech formation provides information that is critical to clinical decision-making related to secondary palatal surgery in cases of confirmed or suspected VPI.

Secondary palatal surgery in young children is indicated when VPI causes hypernasal speech on a consistent basis and is related to the anatomical problem.[30–32] The exact timing of surgery for VPI remains controversial, however, with recommendations ranging from 2.5 to 5 years of age. In children 2.5 to 4 years of age, obtaining enough diagnostic information to make a definitive decision regarding treatment is often difficult. In such a young age group, variables such as the child's language and articulation development and a lack of compliance during the speech evaluation compromise the diagnostic accuracy of preoperative assessments.[33–35] By the time a child reaches 5 years of age, compliance with nasopharyngoscopy is better, and there is enough language development to allow for a more thorough perceptual speech evaluation. These factors allow for more definitive conclusions regarding the status of VP function or dysfunction in the child with a repaired cleft palate. One final salient point is that decisions regarding the advisability of surgery for VPI must be made only through close collaboration with an experienced speech and language pathologist. The decision to go forward with additional surgery for VPI simply is not an isolated surgical judgment.

The problem of VPI with hypernasal speech may also be encountered later in life in patients that require orthognathic surgery for correction of cleft-related maxillary deficiency. As discussed in Chapter 61, "Orthognathic Surgery in the Patient with Cleft Palate," approximately 25% of patients who have undergone cleft palate repair during infancy will require additional surgery for correction of midfacial deficiency during adolescence when they are nearing skeletal maturity.[36] This usually involves midfacial advancement at the Le Fort I level with or without mandibular surgery in order to normalize skeletal position, correct malocclusion, and improve facial form. Large advancements of the maxilla in patients with a repaired cleft palate may worsen preexisting VPI or may be the cause of new-onset VPI.[37–39] A minority of patients with borderline VP closure preoperatively will develop hypernasal speech even after relatively small degrees of maxillary forward displacement. Since predicting exactly how each patient will respond to maxillary advancement is difficult, formal speech assessment and detailed counseling of the patient and family regarding the possibility of developing postoperative VPI is recommended prior to undertaking any cleft orthognathic surgery involving maxillary advancement. Fortunately, most patients who develop VPI following maxillary advancement will recover adequate VP closure without the need for additional palatal surgery. In a study by Turvey and Frost, pressure-flow studies were used to examine VP function after maxillary advancement in patients with repaired cleft palate.[40] In their study group of patients with adequate VP closure before surgery, the VP apparatus demonstrated three different responses following midfacial advancement: (1) adequate VP closure after surgery, (2) deterioration with inadequate VP function after surgery followed by a gradual improvement and recovery of normal closure over a 6-month period, and (3) inadequate VP closure after surgery without improvement necessitating pharyngeal flap surgery. When maxillary advancement does result in clinically significant VPI, additional corrective surgery should be delayed at least 6 months. In most cases, postoperative neuromuscular adaptation allows the VP mechanism to recover, and the patient returns to a baseline level of function with resolution of hypernasal speech without the need for additional operative intervention.

Operative Techniques

Contemporary surgical management of VPI generally involves the use of either of two types of procedures: (1) the superiorly based pharyngeal flap, and (2) the sphincter pharyngoplasty. The use of autogenous and alloplastic implants for augmentation of the posterior pharyngeal wall has been described, but is not a commonly used procedure. More recently, some surgeons have advocated the use of a second palatoplasty operation as an attempt at palatal lengthening in the patient with VPI; however, limited data exist to support this as a preferred technique.

The superiorly based pharyngeal flap remains the standard approach for surgical management of VPI after palate repair.

The procedure was initially described by Schoenborn in 1876.[41–43] Surgical maneuvers are directed at recruiting tissue by developing a superiorly based soft tissue flap from the posterior pharyngeal wall (Figure 44-6). The soft palate is then divided along midsagittal plane from the junction of the hard and soft palate to the uvula and the flap from the posterior pharyngeal wall is inset within the nasal layer of the soft palate. As a result, a large nasopharyngeal opening which cannot be completely closed by the patient's VP mechanism is converted into two (right and left) lateral pharyngeal ports. Closure of these ports is easier for the patient to accomplish as long as adequate lateral pharyngeal wall motion is present. When randomly applied to patients with VPI, the superiorly based pharyngeal flap procedure is effective 80% of the time.[44] When the flap is applied using careful preoperative objective evaluations, success rates as high as 95 to 97% have been reported.[45,46] Shprintzen and colleagues have advocated custom tailoring of the pharyngeal flap width and position based on the particular characteristics of each patient as seen on nasopharyngoscopy.[44,47] The high overall success rate and the flexibility to design the dimensions and position of the flap itself are advantages of the superiorly based pharyngeal flap procedure. The disadvantages of the pharyngeal flap procedure are primarily related to the possibility of severe nasal obstruction resulting in mucous trapping and postoperative obstructive sleep apnea.

Inferiorly based pharyngeal flaps for management of VPI are rarely used. Previous reports have documented increased morbidity without better speech outcomes associated with inferiorly based flaps.[48] In addition, inferiorly based flaps tend to cause downward pull on the soft palate following healing and contracture of the flap. The result may be a tethered palate with decreased ability to elevate during the formation of speech sounds.

The dynamic sphincter pharyngoplasty is another option for the surgical management of VPI. This procedure was described by Hynes in 1951 and modified by several other authors.[49–54] The operative procedure involves the creation of two superiorly based myomucosal flaps created within each posterior tonsillar pillar (Figure 44-7). Each flap is elevated with care taken to include as much of the palatopharyngeal muscle as possible. The flaps are then attached and inset within a horizontal incision made high on the posterior pharyngeal wall. The goal of this procedure is the creation of a single nasopharyngeal port (instead of the two ports of the superiorly based pharyngeal flap) that has a contractile ridge posteriorly to improve VP valve function. The main advantage of the sphincter pharyngoplasty over the superiorly based flap is a lower rate of complications related to nasal airway obstruction as described above.[55–57] Despite this advantage, there is no evidence that pharyngoplasty procedures achieve superior outcomes in the resolution of VPI. Also, the use of a sphincter pharyngoplasty technique may be associated with increased scarring along the tonsillar pillar region.

In the past, augmentation of the posterior pharyngeal wall has been attempted in order to facilitate closure of the nasal airway. Various autogenous and alloplastic materials have been used including local tissue, rib cartilage, injections of Teflon, silicon, Silastic, Proplast, and collagen.[58,59] Improvement in speech after augmentation of the posterior pharyngeal wall is unpredictable. Problems with migration or extrusion of the implanted material and an increased rate of infection added to the problems with these techniques. For these reasons, pharyngeal wall implants are rarely used.

Some surgeons advocate the use of a revisional palatoplasty instead of a pharyngeal flap or pharyngoplasty procedure in the management of patients with VPI after

established. The clinician also must consider the disadvantages of this type of surgical procedure and weigh them against potential benefits. The double opposing Z-plasty procedure requires a more aggressive dismantling of the palate than what is required during a conventional pharyngeal flap procedure. The result may be a slightly longer palate, but one with more extensive scarring and less physiologic movement. Another consideration is the significantly higher rate of fistula formation associated with this type of repair.

Complications Related to Surgical Procedures for VPI

Surgery involving airway structures is always associated with the potential for complications related to postoperative hemorrhage and edema. As a result, patients who undergo attachment of a pharyngeal flap require admission to the surgical intensive care unit with continuous airway monitoring during the first 24 hours following surgery. This type of setting permits the rapid recognition and prompt management of complications that may result in airway compromise. Of all the procedures related to cleft care, the pharyngeal flap and sphincteroplasty operations carry the greatest risk for early airway compromise. Airway loss and compromise are not common but require immediate management when they are encountered in order to avoid life-threatening consequences.

Long-term postoperative complications related to the superiorly based pharyngeal flap are frequently associated with problems related to increased airway resistance. Insertion of a pharyngeal flap will decrease the size of the nasopharyngeal airway, facilitate VP closure, decrease nasal air escape, and make speech more intelligible. At the same time, however, the procedure may create a pathologic level of upper airway obstruction that leads to new problems. In several cases, patients who have undergone pharyngeal flap surgery

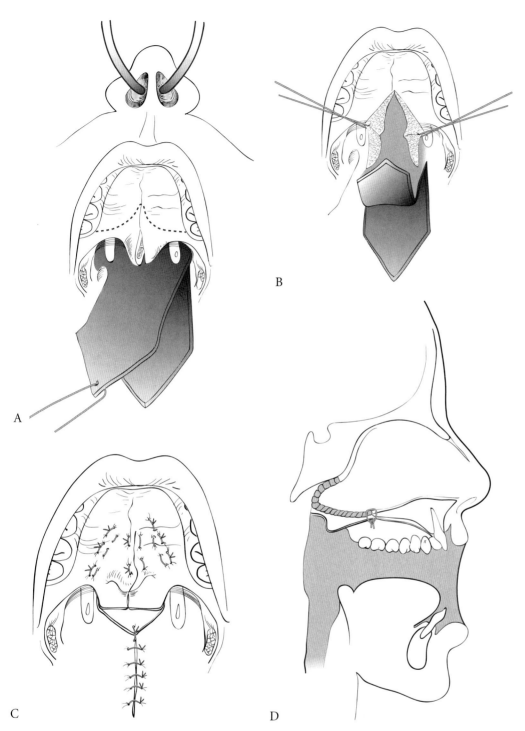

FIGURE 44-6 *Illustration of superiorly based pharyngeal flap operative procedure. A, Creation of superiorly based flap of posterior pharyngeal wall soft tissues. The pharyngeal flap is developed and elevated off of the prevertebral fascia. Soft palate is divided with a midline incision from the uvula to the junction of the hard and soft palates. B, Soft palate oral, nasal, and muscle layer dissection in preparation for flap inset. Nasopharyngeal airways are placed in order to help size each lateral pharyngeal port. C, The flap is sutured into the nasal side of the soft palate before the nasal side is repaired and the oral mucosa and underlying musculature are repaired. D, Sagittal view demonstrating appropriate vertical level of flap inset.*

cleft palate repair in infancy.[60] Specifically, a Furlow double opposing Z-plasty palatoplasty is carried out in order to lengthen the soft palate and facilitate VP closure. Unfortunately, the anticipated benefits of these second palatoplasties have never been

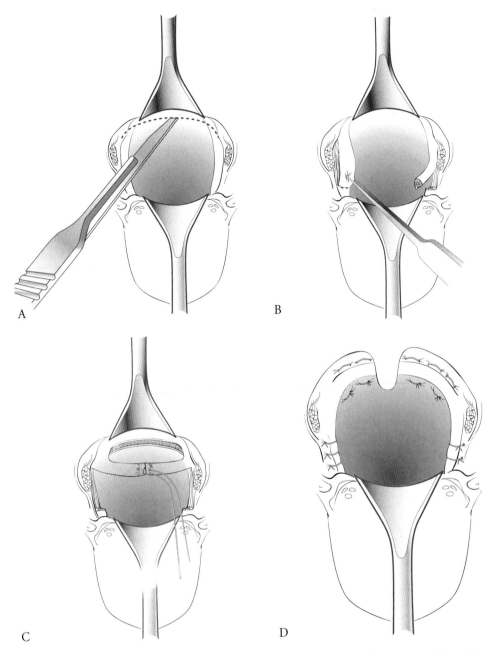

FIGURE 44-7   *Sphincteroplasty procedure. A, Incision of the posterior pharyngeal wall and the posterior tonsillar pillars. B, Elevation of bilateral myomucosal flaps within the tonsillar pillars. Care is taken to include palatopharyngeous muscle. C, The mobilized flaps are then sutured to each other at the midline. D, Closure is then achieved by insetting the joined flaps within the posterior pharyngeal wall incision. The donor site of each flap is also closed with interrupted sutures.*

start snoring. Snoring itself does not represent any significant pathophysiology but may concern parents or significant others who observe the patient during sleep. When the degree of upper airway resistance is more severe, the result may be postoperative obstructive sleep apnea (OSA). OSA is a cessation of breathing during sleep secondary to upper airway obstruction that disrupts the sleep cycle, compromises effective oxygenation, and may cause behavioral changes and daytime somnolence in affected individuals. Left untreated, OSA is associated with severe cardiac and pulmonary consequences. When OSA is suspected in a child who has previously undergone a pharyngeal flap procedure, a formal work-up including nasopharyngoscopy and sleep study (polysomnography) is indicated. Care should be taken to evaluate the entire airway in order to determine the level of the obstruction. Surgeons may initially assume that the airway obstruction is related to the flap only to discover that a more severe problem exists somewhere else in the upper airway tract. Often, a thorough clinical evaluation yields abnormal findings that contribute to the problem of OSA at multiple levels of the upper airway. Because of the complexity of these clinical problems, the decision to modify or take down a pharyngeal flap in a child with OSA must be made only after discussions between the surgeon, airway expert (eg, pediatric otolaryngologist or pediatric pulmonologist), and speech and language pathologist. Interestingly, many patients who have had pharyngeal flap placement during their childhood will tolerate surgical division of the flap without a recurrence of severe VPI or hypernasal speech. On the rare occasion when VPI does recur following flap take-down, interval treatment with a prosthetic device such as a palatal lift appliance for at least 6 months should be considered prior to embarking on any further airway surgery.

Management of the Submucous Cleft Palate

A submucous cleft palate is another form of the congenital cleft palate malformation in which the overlying mucosal layer is intact, but the underlying soft palate musculature is divided. As described by Calnan, the classic clinical findings with a submucous cleft palate are a triad of bifid uvula, hard palate bony notch, and separation along the median raphe of the soft palate especially during elevation of the velum.[61]

When a submucous cleft palate is present, the levator muscle is clefted and abnormally inserts into the posterior edge of the hard palate. The primary functional concern related to submucous cleft palate is the possibility that the patient will develop VPI and resultant hypernasal speech as encountered in other cleft palate patients. Despite this concern, the majority of patients with a submucous cleft palate will not require surgical intervention. In fact, 44% of patients will actually remain completely asymptomatic until childhood.[62]

As described above, the bifid uvula is often the most easily detected feature of the submucous cleft palate triad of clinical findings. However, a bifid uvula may also be observed in the absence of any other features of submucous clefting (eg, notched hard palate, velar separation, hypernasality). In fact, the incidence of bifid uvula is approximately 1:80 while the incidence of submucous cleft palate is 1:280.[63] Previous investigation has suggested a connection between the isolated finding of a bifid uvula and VP dysfunction when otherwise asymptomatic patients were evaluated using a nasopharyngoscopic protocol.[64] As a result, the clinical finding of an isolated bifid uvula may be considered an indicator of increased risk for VPI in a patient who is to undergo adenoidectomy. This underscores the value of a thorough clinical examination before any of these surgical procedures are undertaken and the importance of presurgical speech evaluation and family counseling regarding the potential risks of postsurgical VPI.

A certain proportion of children will present with an occult submucous cleft palate. The occult submucous cleft palate does not have any of the classic triad of physical findings. In most cases, the reason for consultation is VPI-related speech difficulties that have been noted during childhood speech development or that have arisen following a surgical intervention (eg, adenoidectomy). In our experience, the proportion of children with occult submucous cleft palate approaches 10% and preoperative diagnosis is often difficult. Prior reports have attempted to describe characteristic facial features, cephalometric findings, and voice studies

that can assist in the presumptive diagnosis of submucous cleft palate.[65]

The vast majority of patients with a submucous cleft palate will require either no treatment or speech therapy only. Surgical intervention is not undertaken simply because the diagnosis of submucous cleft palate has been made. The speech of these individuals is closely monitored during childhood with interval speech evaluations, and surgery is reserved for only those cases where VPI is diagnosed and not amenable to speech therapy. The type of specific surgical procedure used to manage submucous cleft-related VPI varies depending on the preference of the surgeon and speech pathologist. Several early procedures emphasized exploration of the soft palate through a limited midline incision with repair of the levator muscle. Contemporary methods primarily involve the use of a standard palatoplasty (two-flap, pushback, or Furlow) and repair of the velar musculature, with or without a simultaneous pharyngeal flap procedure.

Bone Graft Reconstruction of the Cleft Maxilla and Palate

Approximately 75% of all orofacial clefts will involve the maxilla.[5] Despite successful lip repair and closure of the hard and soft palate during infancy, a residual nasolabial fistula and bony cleft defect that involves the alveolar ridge, maxilla, and piriform rim will remain. These residual deformities are addressed by secondary bone grafting performed during middle childhood (6 to 9 years of age). The objectives of bone graft reconstruction of the cleft maxilla are to establish adequate bony matrix for eruption of the permanent cuspid tooth, close any residual alveolar fistula communication, establish bony continuity of the maxillary ridge, and improve the underlying bony support of the nasal base. In the case of bilateral cleft lip and palate, an added benefit of bone graft reconstruction is the stabilization of the previously mobile premaxilla segment.

The details of bone graft reconstruction of the cleft maxilla are discussed in greater detail in Chapter 43, "Reconstruction of the Alveolar Cleft."

Orthognathic Surgery for Correction of Midfacial Deficiency

Patients who have undergone cleft palate repair during infancy will often exhibit some degree of maxillary growth restriction. This disproportionate jaw growth is the biological consequence of prior surgical intervention and is not related to the congenital cleft deformity. Previous authors have reported a 25% incidence of maxillary hypoplasia that is severe enough to produce a clinically significant dentofacial deformity with negative effects on speech and occlusion.[5,6,17,36] The successful correction of these secondary skeletal deformities frequently requires treatment protocols that include orthognathic surgery in conjunction with the final phase of orthodontic treatment. Simultaneous bone grafting is used for contouring the dysmorphic skeletal structures. The use of orthognathic techniques to correct residual skeletal problems in the patient with cleft lip and palate is discussed in greater detail in Chapter 61, "Orthognathic Surgery in the Patient with Cleft Palate."

Revisional Surgery for Cleft Lip and Nasal Deformities

Reconstruction of the Cleft Nasal Deformity

Congenital clefts that involve the lip, nose, and underlying skeletal structure will cause a complex three-dimensional deformity of the nasal complex that affects both form and function.[66,67] In the case of a complete unilateral cleft, the typical nasal deformity is characterized by splaying of the alar base, inferior displacement of the alar rim, deviation of the nasal tip, and irregularity of the caudal nasal septum. Abnormal fibrous insertions exist between the lateral crus of the lower lateral cartilage and the lateral piriform rim on the cleft side. At the time of the initial lip repair procedure, maneuvers for primary nasal reconstruction include dissection along the lower lateral cartilage in order to separate the overlying skin from the cartilage and sharp release of the fibrous insertions along the piriform rim so that the nostril can be repositioned appropriately. Despite effective primary cleft lip and nasal repair during infancy, most patients will demonstrate enough residual nasal dysmorphology that secondary nasal surgery for correction of the cleft-associated malformation or improvement in nasal airflow will be required later in life.

The timing of cleft nasal revisional surgery also remains controversial. Some surgeons take a more aggressive approach and undertake extensive nasal reconstruction during early childhood. Our philosophy is to delay the definitive cleft rhinoplasty until the nasal complex is close to mature size. If the patient's reconstructive treatment plan also requires maxillary advancement, then nasal surgery should be delayed until approximately 6 months following the orthognathic procedure. This allows for a more predictable outcome and long-lasting improvement in nasal function and facial esthetics. Early surgery is reserved for individuals with severe airway or nasal airflow problems or children that have the potential to experience psychosocial consequences such as teasing at school. When possible, early nasal surgery should be timed after the bone graft reconstruction of the maxilla so that a stable bony foundation along the piriform rim and nasal base exists first.

Secondary cleft-nasal reconstruction will often require dorsal reduction, lower lateral cartilage sculpting, cartilage grafting, and nasal osteotomies. Cartilage grafting is a critical component of the final nasal reconstruction and is used for augmentation of the dysmorphic lower lateral cartilage and improvement of nasal tip projection[5,68,69] (T.J. Tejera, DMD, MD,

personal communication, November 2003). Several different donor sites may be used including auricular cartilage, nasal septum, and rib cartilage. Ear cartilage is most useful in situations where augmentation of hypoplastic cleft-side lower lateral cartilage is required. Septal cartilage is most easily accessible and provides an excellent scaffold for repositioning of the lower lateral cartilages and improvement of nasal tip symmetry and projection. Unfortunately, patients may present for definitive nasal reconstruction having undergone previous septal cartilage harvest and not have sufficient quantity for a second septal cartilage graft. In these cases, the use of costochondral cartilage is another excellent option. Rib cartilage provides adequate amounts of graft material, but requires a distant donor surgical site. We have found this type of cartilage graft to provide excellent strength for straightening the nasal tip and alar complex. These techniques are best carried out through an open rhinoplasty approach.[5] A transcolumellar splitting incision is combined with marginal incisions in order to provide wide access and direct visualization of the nasal dorsum, upper and lower lateral cartilages, and nasal septum.

A similar rationale is applied when considering the timing of secondary nasal reconstruction in the bilateral cleft lip patient, but the specific dysmorphology addressed is somewhat different. Generally, nasal asymmetry is less problematic, and the dysmorphology is characterized by deficient columellar length. Previous literature has focused on the secondary lengthening of the columella through the use of banked forked flaps or columellar lengthening using soft tissue flaps from the floor of the nose and alar flaps.[70,71] Unfortunately, these types of surgical procedures often result in a distorted columellar-labial angle, excessive "railroad" scars that extend onto the nasal tip, and additional distortion of the broad nasal tip. We find that the approach described by Posnick

using septal cartilage strut grafts attached to the caudal nasal septum and lower lateral cartilages yields the most natural-looking results.[5,6] The objective is correction of the underlying cartilaginous anatomy with stretching of the overlying soft tissue envelope, instead of direct surgical manipulation of the columellar skin.

Secondary Surgery for Cleft Lip Scar Revision

Even when the initial cleft lip repair procedure is considered to be successful, the vast majority of children will go on to require an additional operation for lip revision at some point in their lifetime.[4,72] Although revisional procedures are often viewed as optional phases of cleft lip reconstruction, surgeons must advise families of this likelihood.

As a child grows, the hard and soft tissues of the maxillofacial complex grow and change, and the repaired lip is affected. Ongoing growth often makes it difficult to predict which children will need additional lip surgery. A child's lip may initially look satisfactory and over time demonstrate unfavorable changes necessitating revision. On the other hand, favorable changes may occur during the healing process that actually improve the appearance of the repaired cleft lip. At approximately 8 to 10 weeks following surgery, significant lip contracture may be seen during the fibroblastic phase of healing. The result is vertical shortening of the repaired cleft side that will seemingly require further surgery. If the same child is reevaluated 6 months later, after additional wound maturation, they may demonstrate perfectly acceptable lip esthetics and not be considered a candidate for revision.

Ideally, only one lip scar revision is undertaken, when the child is between the ages of 5 and 15 years. The procedure is staged for as late in childhood as possible. When a severe deformity persists or psychosocial concerns exist, lip revision may be carried out earlier in life before the child becomes school aged.

The surgical objectives of cleft lip revision include excision of residual scar, reapproximation of key anatomic landmarks such as the vermilion-cutaneous junction and vermilion-mucosal junction, and leveling of vertical lip lengths (philtral columns). Critical to an acceptable outcome is the meticulous repair of the orbicularis oris muscle as a distinct layer. The cleft surgeon must dissect and repair all layers (skin or vermilion, muscle, oral mucosa) in order to establish improved lip form and normalize lip function and animation (Figure 44-8). Often this requires complete take-down of the lip and recreation of a full-thickness defect.

Comprehensive Dental and Prosthetic Rehabilitation

In patients with a cleft of the primary palate (maxilla and alveolus), three possibilities exist with regard to the status of the permanent lateral incisor: (1) the lateral is present and erupts normally, (2) the lateral is congenitally missing, or (3) the lateral is present, but is dysmorphic and not a restorable tooth. When the lateral incisor is this dysmorphic, extraction is usually required prior to or at the time of bone graft reconstruction.

In those cases where a lateral incisor is not present, management of the residual dental gap will eventually be required. Treatment options include the placement of a three-unit fixed prosthesis, replacement of the missing tooth with an endosseous dental implant, or orthodontic substitution of the ipsilateral cuspid tooth for the lateral incisor.

In contemporary practice, the use of a three-unit bridge for replacement of a congenitally missing incisor is generally avoided, especially in young patients. This prosthetic option has several disadvantages: it usually requires preparation of two otherwise perfectly healthy teeth (central and cuspid), hygiene is more difficult around the pontic, and even in the best of circumstances the prosthetic restoration will require replacement several times during the patient's lifetime.

Over the course of the past two decades, the use of titanium dental implants has revolutionized the prosthetic rehabilitation of patients with missing teeth. This technology has also been applied to patients born with cleft lip and palate (Figure 44-9).[73–75] The use of an implant-supported crown provides a natural-looking restoration with excellent long-term viability and obviates the need for instrumentation of the surrounding teeth. When a dental implant is being considered, pertinent treatment-planning concerns include the maintenance of adequate space for the implant and restoration and the quantity of alveolar bone available for placement of the titanium fixture. Our preferred approach involves the preservation of approximately 7 mm of interdental space in order to allow for placement of a 3.5 mm dental implant. In most patients who have undergone previous successful bone grafting, the vertical dimension of the alveolar ridge seems to be well maintained until the time of implant placement. Facial-palatal width of the ridge, however, may be more problematic, and a significant number of cleft patients may require some additional minor bone grafting approximately 3 to 4 months prior to implant surgery. In most cases, the width of the alveolus can be nicely augmented with bone harvested from the mandibular symphysis or ramus region. Implant placement requires that the patient be at or near skeletal maturity.

Another option for management of the cleft dental gap when the lateral incisor is not present is the use of orthodontic therapy in order to substitute the missing lateral incisor with the ipsilateral cuspid tooth. Interestingly, this maneuver frequently results in very acceptable dental esthetics even if prosthetic modification of the cuspid is not undertaken. Like the use of a dental implant, this treatment option also obviates the need for preparation of the adjacent healthy tooth structure. In most cases, the substitution option also eliminates the need for any prosthetic component at all. Another advantage of this treatment option is that it may be undertaken at a younger age than the other prosthetic options. Limiting factors

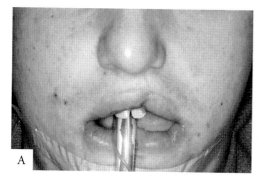

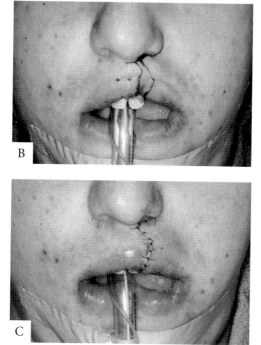

FIGURE **44-8** A to C, *Unilateral cleft lip revision. Pre- and immediate postoperative photographs of a patient undergoing revision of a unilateral cleft lip. The full-thickness cleft defect is recreated with care taken to reconstitute the orbicularis oris muscle. The hypertrophic scar was excised and anatomic landmarks including the vermilion border, white roll, wet-dry line, and nasal sill are reapproximated.*

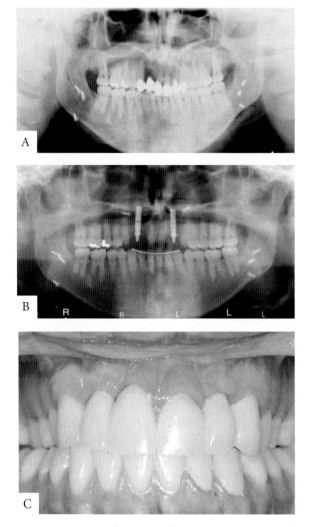

FIGURE **44-9** *Prosthetic rehabilitation of a 27-year-old patient with previously unrepaired bilateral maxillary alveolar clefts. She had undergone primary lip and palate repair during infancy but never underwent bone graft reconstruction. Treatment consisted of bone graft reconstruction of the bony clefts using autogenous corticocancellous bone graft obtained from the anterior iliac crest followed by dental implant placement 6 months later. A, Preoperative panoramic radiograph reveals large bilateral bony cleft defects. B, Panoramic radiograph following bone graft reconstruction and implant placement. C, Temporary prosthetic restoration. Implant placement was performed as a single-stage procedure with construction of temporary bilateral three-unit bridges.*

related to this option are primarily related to issues of orthodontic anchorage.

Summary

Orofacial clefts are complex malformations that affect the three-dimensional anatomy of the maxillofacial hard and soft tissues and have profound functional and esthetic consequences. Successful reconstruction of these defects involves multiple stages of surgical intervention. Primary surgery is centered on initial closure of the lip and palatal defects. Secondary surgical procedures are then carried out in order to close residual oronasal communication, address VPI, reconstruct the bony maxillary cleft, normalize maxillary skeletal position and occlusion, improve lip and nasal esthetics and function, and facilitate the dental prosthetic rehabilitation of the patient. Because multiple, separate surgical interventions are carried out during active growth, thoughtful timing of each stage of reconstruction is critical in order to maximize the benefit for the patient and mitigate the potentially negative biologic consequences related to growth. Surgeons must maintain a thorough understanding of the anatomy, the intricacies of the cleft malformation, and the underlying patterns of growth and development of the craniomaxillofacial region.

References

1. Leonard BJ, Brust JD, Abrahams G, et al. Self concept of children and adolescents with cleft lip and/or palate. Cleft Palate Craniofac J 1991;28:347.

2. Strauss RP. Health policy and craniofacial care: issues in resource allocation. Cleft Palate Craniofac J 1994;31:78.

3. Bergstrom LV. Congenital and acquired deafness in clefting and craniofacial syndromes. Cleft Palate J 1978;15:254.

4. Cohen SR, Corrigan M, Wilmot J, et al. Cumulative operative procedures in patients aged 14 years and older with unilateral or bilateral cleft lip and palate. Plast Reconstr Surg 1995;96:267.

5. Posnick JC. The staging of cleft lip and palate reconstruction: infancy through adolescence. In: Posnick JC. Craniofacial and maxillofacial surgery in children and young adults. Philadelphia (PA): W.B. Saunders; 2000.

6. Posnick JC, Ruiz RL. Stages of cleft lip and palate reconstruction: infancy through adolescence. In: Wyszynski DF, editor. Cleft lip and palate: from origin to treatment. New York; Oxford University Press; 2002.

7. American Cleft Palate–Craniofacial Association. Parameters for the evaluation and treatment of patients with cleft lip/palate or other craniofacial anomalies. Cleft Palate Craniofac J 1993;30(Suppl 1):4.

8. Abyholm FE, Bergland O, Semb G. Secondary bone grafting of alveolar clefts. Scand J Reconstr Surg 1981;15:127.

9. Turvey TA, Vig K, Moriarty J, et al. Delayed bone grafting in the cleft maxilla and palate: a retrospective multidisciplinary analysis. Am J Orthod 1984;86:244.

10. Cohen SR, Kalinowski J, LaRossa D, Randall P. Cleft palate fistulas: a multivariate statistical analysis of prevalence, etiology, and surgical management. Plast Reconstr Surg 1991;87:1041.

11. Ogle OE. The management of oronasal fistulas in the cleft palate patient. Oral Maxillofacial Surg Clin North Am 2002;14:553–62.

12. Wilhelmi BJ, Appelt EA, Hill L, Blackwell SJ. Palatal fistulas: rare with the two-flap palatoplasty repair. Plast Reconstr Surg 2001;107:315–8.

13. Stal S, Spira M. Secondary reconstructive procedures for patients with clefts. In: Serafin D, Georgiade NG, editors. Pediatric plastic surgery. St Louis (MO): C.V. Mosby; 1984.

14. Lehman JA. Closure of palatal fistulas. Op Tech Plast Surg 1995;2:255–62.

15. Schendel SA. Secondary cleft surgery. Select Read Oral Maxillofac Surg 1992;3(6): 1–27.

16. Posnick JC. Cleft orthognathic surgery: the isolated cleft palate deformity. In: Posnick JC. Craniofacial and maxillofacial surgery in children and young adults. Philadelphia (PA): W.B. Saunders; 2000.

17. Turvey TA, Vig KWL, Fonseca RJ. Maxillary advancement and contouring in the presence of cleft lip and palate. In: Turvey TA, Vig KWL, Fonseca RA, editors. Facial clefts and craniosynostosis: principles and management. Philadelphia (PA): W.B. Saunders; 1996.

18. Posnick JC, Ruiz RL. Invited discussion. Repair of large anterior palatal fistulas using thin tongue flaps: long-term follow-up of 10 patients. Ann Plast Surg 2000;45:115–7.

19. Bozola AR, Ribeiro-Garcia ERB. Partial buccinator myomucosal flap, posteriorly based. Op Tech Plast Surg 1995;2:263–9.

20. Ninkovic M, Hubli EH, Schwabegger A, Anderl H. Free flap closure of recurrent palatal fistula in the cleft lip and palate patient. J Craniofac Surg 1997;8:491–5.

21. Posnick JC. The treatment of secondary and residual dentofacial deformities in the cleft patient. Surgical and orthodontic treatment. Clin Plast Surg 1997;24:583–97.

22. Bardach J. Two-flap palatoplasty: Bardach's technique. Op Tech Plast Surg 1995; 2:211–4.

23. Johnson PA, Banks P, Brown AE. Use of the posteriorly-based lateral tongue flap in the repair of palatal fistula. Int J Oral Maxillofac Surg 1992;23:6–9.

24. Kinnebrew MC, Malloy RB. Posteriorly based, lateral lingual flaps for alveolar cleft bone graft coverage. J Oral Maxillofac Surg 1983;41:555–61.

25. Costello BJ, Ruiz RL, Turvey TA. Velopharyngeal insufficiency in patients with cleft palate. Oral Maxillofac Surg Clin 2002;14:539–51.

26. Glaser ER, Skolnick ML, McWilliams BJ, Shprintzen RJ. The dynamics of Passavant's ridge in subjects with and without velophyngeal insufficiency. A multiview videofluoroscopic study. Cleft Palate Journal 1979;16:24–33.

27. Passavant G. On the closure of the pharynx in speech. Archiv Heilk 1863;3:305.

28. Passavant G. On the closure of pharynx in speech. Virchows Arch 1869;46:1.

29. Warren DW. Compensatory speech behaviors in cleft palate: a regulation/control phenomenon. Cleft Palate J 1986;23:251–60.

30. Henningsson G, Isberg A. Velopharyngeal movements in patients alternating between oral and glottal articulation: a clinical and cineradiographical study. Cleft Palate J 1986;23:1.

31. Isberg A, Henningsson G. Influence of palatal fistula on velopharyngeal movements: a cineradiographic study. Plast Reconstr Surg 1987;79:525.

32. Lohmander-Agerskov A, Dotevall H, Lith A, et al. Speech and velopharyngeal function in children with an open residual cleft in the hard palate, and the influence of temporary covering. Cleft Palate Craniofac J 1996;33:324.

33. Shprintzen RJ, Bardach J. The use of information obtained from speech and instrumental evaluations in treatment planning for velopharyngeal insufficiency. In: Cleft palate speech management: a multidisciplinary approach. St Louis (MO): Mosby Year Book; 1995. p. 257.

34. Golding-Kushner KJ, Argamaso RV, Cotton RT, et al. Standardization for the reporting of nasopharyngoscopy and multi-view videofluroscopy: a report from an international working group. Cleft Palate J 1990;27:337.

35. Warren DW, Dalston RM, Mayo R. Hypernasality and velopharyngeal impairment. Cleft Palate Craniofac J 1994;31:257.

36. Turvey TA, Ruiz RL, Costello BJ. Surgical correction of midface deficiency in the cleft lip and palate malformation. Oral Maxillofac Surg Clin 2002;14:491–507.

37. Fonseca RJ, Turvey TA, Wolford LM. Orthognathic surgery in the cleft patient. In: Fonseca RJ, Baker SJ, Wolford LM, editors. Oral and maxillofacial surgery. Philadelphia (PA): W.B. Saunders Co; 2000. p 87–146.

38. Posnick JC, Tompson B. Cleft-orthognathic surgery: complications and long-term results. Plast Reconstr Surg 1995;96:255–66.

39. Posnick JC, Ruiz RL. Discussion of management of secondary orofacial cleft deformities. In: Goldwyn RM, Cohen MM, editors. The unfavorable result in plastic surgery: avoidance and treatment. 3rd ed. Philadelphia (PA): Lippincott, Williams and Wilkins; 2000.

40. Turvey TA, Frost D. Maxillary advancement and velopharyngeal function in the presence of cleft palate. Abstract of presentations at the 38th annual meeting of the American Cleft Palate Association, Lancaster, Pennsylavania, May 1980.

41. Bernstein L. Treatment of velopharyngeal incompetence. Arch Otolaryngol 1967;85:67–74.

42. Rosseli S. Divisione palatine 3 sua aura chirurgico. Alu Congr Internaz Stomatal 1935-36;391–92.

43. Schoenborn D. Uber eine neue Methode der Staphylorraphies. Arch Klin Chirurgie 1876;19:528.

44. Shprintzen RJ. The use of multiview videofluoroscopy and flexible fiberoptic nasopharyngoscopy as a predictor of success with pharyngeal flap surgery. In: Ellis F, Flack E, editors. Diagnosis and treatment of palatoglossal malfunction. London: College of Speech Therapists; 1979. p 6–14.

45. Argamaso RV, Levandowski G, Golding-Kushner KJ, et al. Treatment of asymmetric velopharyngeal insufficiency with skewed pharyngeal flap. Cleft Palate Craniofac J 1994;31:287.

46. Shprintzen RJ, Lewin ML, Croft CB, et al. A comprehensive study of pharyngeal flap surgery: tailor–made flaps. Cleft Palate J 1979;16:46.

47. Shprintzen RJ, McCall GN, Skolnick ML, Lencione RM. Selective movement of the lateral aspects of the pharyngeal walls during velopharyngeal closure for speech, blowing, and whistling in normals. Cleft Palate J 1975;12:51–8.

48. Randall P, Whitaker LA, Noone RB, Jones WD. The case for the inferiorly based pharyngeal flap. Cleft Palate Craniofac J 1978;15:262–5.

49. Hynes W. Pharyngoplasty by muscle transplantation. Br J Plast Surg 1951;3:128.

50. Hynes W. The results of pharyngoplasty by muscle transplantation in "failed cleft palate" cases, with special reference to the influence of the pharynx on voice production. Ann R Coll Surg Engl 1953;13:17.

51. Orticochea M. Physiopathology of the dynamic muscular sphincter of the pharynx. Plast Reconstr Surg 1997;100:1918–23.

52. Orticochea M. Constriction of a dynamic muscle sphincter in cleft palates. Plast Reconstr Surg 1968;41:323–7.

53. Jackson I, Silverton JS. The sphincter pharyngoplasty as a secondary procedure in cleft palates. Plast Reconstr Surg 1983;71:180.

54. Jackson IT. Sphincter pharyngoplasty. Clin Plast Surg 1985;12:711–7.

55. Guilleminault C, Stoohs R. Chronic snoring and obstructive sleep apnea syndrome in children. Lung 1990;168:912.

56. Sirois M, Caouette–Laberge L, Spier S, et al. Sleep apnea following a pharyngeal flap: a feared complication. Plast Reconstr Surg 1994;93:943.

57. Ysunza A, Garcia–Velasco M, Garcia–Garcia M, et al. Obstructive sleep apnea secondary to surgery for velopharyngeal insufficiency. Cleft Palate Craniofac J 1993;30:387.

58. Bluestone, CD, Musgrave RH, McWilliams BJ. Teflon injection pharyngoplasty—status 1968. Laryngoscope 1968;78:558–64.

59. Smith JK, McCabe DF. Teflon injection in the nasopharynx to improve velopharyngeal closure. Ann Otol Rhinol Laryngol 1977;86:559–86.

60. Chen PK, Wu JT, Chen YR, Noordhoff MS. Correction of secondary velopharyngeal insufficiency in cleft palate patients with the Furlow palatoplasty. Plast Reconstr Surg 1994;94:933.

61. Calnan J. Submucous cleft palate. Br J Plast Surg 1954;6:264–82.

62. McWilliams BJ. Submucous clefts of the palate: how likely are they to be symptomatic? Cleft Palate J 1991;28:247–8.

63. Paradise JL. Tonsillectomy and adenoidectomy. In: Bluestone CD, Stool SE, Alper CU, et al, editors. Pediatric otolaryngology. Philadelphia (PA): W.B. Saunders Co.; 2003. p. 1218.

64. Shprintzen RJ, Schwartz RH, Daniller A, Hoch L. Morphologic significance of bifid uvula. Pediatrics 1985;75:553–61.

65. Kaplan EN. The occult submucous cleft palate. Cleft Palate J 1975;12:356–68.

66. McComb H. The nasal deformity in clefts. In: Kernahan DA, Rosenstein SW, editors. Cleft lip and palate: a system of management. Baltimore (MD): Williams and Wilkins; 1990. p. 68–73.

67. Horswell BB, Pospisil OA. Nasal symmetry after primary cleft lip repair: comparison between Delaire cheilorhinoplasty and modified rotation-advancement. J Oral Maxillofac Surg 1995;53:1025.

68. Gubiscla W. How to obtain symmetries in a unilaterally cleft nose. Eur J Plast Surg 1990;13:241.

69. Takato T, Yonehara Y, Mori Y, et al. Correction of the nose in unilateral cleft lip patients using an open method: a 10-year review. J Oral Maxillofac Surg 1995;53:28.

70. Millard DR. Bilateral cleft lip and a primary forked flap: a preliminary report. Plast Reconstr Surg 1967;30:50.

71. Cronin TD. Lengthening columella by use of skin from nasal floor and alae. Plast Reconstr Surg 1958;21:417.

72. Harper DC. Children's attitudes to physical differences among youth from Western and non-Western cultures. Cleft Palate Craniofac J 1995;32:114.

73. Laine J, Vahatalo K, Peltola J, et al. Rehabilitation of patients with congenital unrepaired cleft palate defects using free iliac crest bone grafts and dental implants. Int J Oral Maxillofac Implants 2002;17:573–80.

74. Fukuda M, Takahashi T, Yamaguchi T, et al. Dental rehabilitation using endosseous implants and orthognathic surgery in patients with cleft lip and palate: report of two cases. J Oral Rehabil 2000; 27:546–51.

75. Jensen J, Sindet-Pedersen S, Enemark H. Reconstruction of residual alveolar cleft defects with one-stage mandibular bone grafts and osseointegrated implants. J Oral Maxillofac Surg 1998;56:460–6.

CHAPTER 45

Nonsyndromic Craniosynostosis

G. E. Ghali, DDS, MD
Douglas P. Sinn, DDS

In its basic form craniosynostosis represents premature suture fusion. It occurs in approximately 1 per 1,000 live births in the United States. Craniosynostosis may be classified as nonsyndromic or syndromic. Most forms of craniosynostosis are isolated and not associated with any other conditions and are therefore nonsyndromic. Syndromic craniosynostosis will be covered in another chapter. The pathogenesis of craniosynostosis is complex and probably multifactorial. Moss theorized that craniosynostosis such as seen in Apert and Crouzon syndromes results from abnormal tensile forces transmitted to the dura from an anomalous cranial base through key ligamentous attachments.[1] This hypothesis fails to explain craniosynostosis in patients with a normal cranial base configuration. The cause of craniosynostosis may be postulated to be the result of either primary suture abnormalities, sufficient extremes of forces that overcome the underlying expansive forces of the brain, inadequate intrinsic growth forces of the brain, or various genetic and environmental factors.[2] Cranial vault growth achieves approximately 80% of the adult size at birth and definitive size by 2.5 to 3 years of age.[3] The existence of the six major sutural regions allows for head expansion as well as transvaginal head deformation.[4] Recall that posterior fontanelle closure (3 –6 mo) generally precedes anterior fontanelle closure (9 – 12 mo).

Functional Considerations

The major functional problems associated with craniosynostosis are intracranial hypertension, visual impairment, limitation of brain growth, and neuropsychiatric disorders.[5] In general the functional problems increase as the number of sutures involved increases.[5] These functional abnormalities are gradual in their development, difficult to detect, and often irreversible in nature.

Intracranial Hypertension

Intracranial hypertension is defined as a pressure of greater than 15 mm Hg. Studies by Marchac and Renier have demonstrated a 13% incidence of intracranial hypertension with single suture stenosis and up to a 42% incidence in multisuture-stenosed children.[6] The clinical symptoms of intracranial hypertension include headaches, irritability, and difficulty sleeping. The radiographic signs may include cortical thinning or a lückenschädel (hammered metal) appearance of the inner table of the skull; these clinical and radiographic signs are relatively late developments. If intracranial hypertension goes untreated, it affects brain function; if persistent this may necessitate early operative intervention during the first few months of life. Intracranial hypertension most likely affects those with the greatest disparity between brain growth and intracranial capacity and may occur in as many as 42% of untreated children with more than one suture affected. Currently intracranial volume is measured using computed tomography (CT) scans, a noninvasive method appropriate for use in children with craniosynostosis. It might be possible to identify individuals who are at a greater risk for developing intracranial hypertension and would benefit the most from early surgery.

Visual Impairment

Intracranial hypertension, if left untreated, may lead to papilledema, typically acute. After chronic intracranial hypertension, eventually optic atrophy develops, which results in complete or partial blindness. Some forms of craniosynostosis may involve orbital hypertelorism and may lead to compromised visual acuity and restricted binocular vision.

Limitation of Brain Growth

Brain volume in the normal child almost triples during the first year of life. By 2 years of age the cranial capacity is four times that at birth. If brain growth is to proceed unhindered, open sutures at the level of the cranial vault and base must spread during phases of rapid growth for marginal ossification.

In craniosynostosis, premature suture fusion is combined with continuing brain growth. Depending on the number and location of prematurely fused sutures and the timing of closure, the growth potential of the brain may be limited. Surgical intervention can provide suture release and reshaping to restore a more normal intracranial volume. In general this does not completely reverse craniosynostosis, and diminished volume is often the end result.

Neuropsychiatric Disorders

Neuropsychiatric disorders are believed to be secondary to cerebral compression. Disorders range from mild behavioral disturbances to overt mental retardation. Several studies have shown that children with craniosynostosis and associated neuropsychiatric disorders often improve after cranial vault reconstruction.

Diagnosis

One should suspect craniosynostosis in any infant with an abnormal head shape. Definitive diagnosis is based on clinical and radiographic evaluations. The clinical evaluation involves the palpation of the skull for any movement, ridging, and presence of the anterior and posterior fontanelles. Quantitative measurements of the superior orbital rims, relative to the most anterior aspect of the cornea, also may help in planning treatment for superior orbital rim advancements.

The radiographic evaluation of craniosynostosis is used to define quantitatively aberrant anatomy, plan surgical procedures, and, most importantly, provide a means to demonstrate to the parents the difference between stenosed and nonstenosed sutures. Conventional skull radiographs, such as plain skull films and lateral cephalograms, are inexpensive and widely available. The preoperative assessment of patients with suspected or known craniosynostosis is based on these conventional radiographs. Most cases of synostosis can be demonstrated on plain skull films. Normal or patent cranial sutures manifest as a line. The absence of a radiolucent line in the normal anatomic position of a suture may suggest craniosynostosis.

Currently, CT scans provide improved hard tissue imaging. The definition of these elements of the bony facial structures on high-resolution CT images with or without three-dimensional reconstruction is unmatched by other imaging techniques (Figure 45-1). The development of CT scanning, particularly three-dimensional reformatting, and the maturation of readily available means of craniofacial surgery have led to a close dependence on CT scanning for preoperative surgical planning. CT scanning also has been used to document surgical changes in vivo and to follow developments longitudinally.[7–18]

Classification

The classification of craniosynostosis is based on the shape of the skull, which usually reflects the underlying prematurely fused suture or sutures.[19,20] The major cranial vault sutures that may be involved include the left and right coronal, metopic, sagittal, and lambdoid sutures.

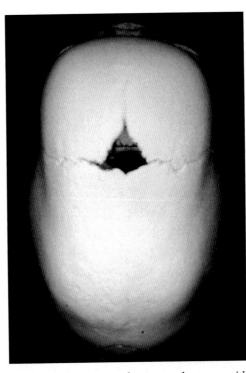

FIGURE **45-1** *Computed tomography scan with three-dimensional reconstruction. Patency of metopic and coronal sutures as well as anterior fontanelle; premature fusion of sagittal suture. Reproduced with permission from Ghali GE et al.[46] p. 3.*

Unilateral Coronal Synostosis

Unilateral coronal synostosis results in flatness on the ipsilateral side of the forehead and supraorbital ridge region. The head is inherently asymmetric in shape with a flattened or retropositioned forehead on the ipsilateral side, especially when viewed from the top (Figure 45-2). The term for this deformity is "anterior plagiocephaly." One should rule out infant molding or positional plagiocephaly and congenital torticollis as other possible diagnoses. Premature fusion of the unilateral

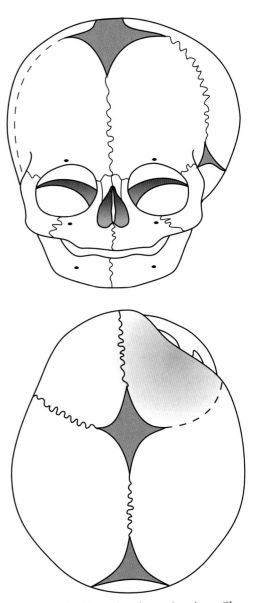

FIGURE **45-2** *Frontal and superior views. Characteristic right anterior plagiocephaly. Adapted from Ghali GE et al.[46] p. 4.*

coronal suture represents 20% of the isolated or nonsyndromic cases of synostosis in the United States. Characteristic morphologic features occur on the ipsilateral side. The frontal bone is flat, and the supraorbital ridge and lateral orbital rim are recessed (Figure 45-3). The orbit is shallow, and the anterior cranial base is short in the anteroposterior dimension. The root of the nose may be constricted and deviated to the affected side (Figure 45-4). The ipsilateral zygoma and infraorbital rim also may be flat and recessed.

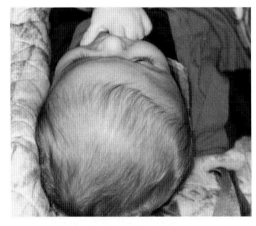

FIGURE **45-3** *Superior view. Recessed frontal bone, supraorbital ridge, and lateral orbital rim on patient's right side. Reproduced with permission from Ghali GE et al.[46] p. 5.*

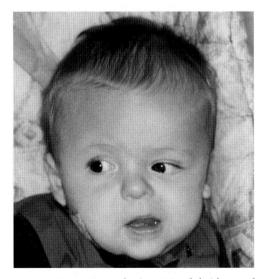

FIGURE **45-4** *Frontal view. Nasal bridge and root deviation to the affected (right) side characteristic in plagiocephaly. Reproduced with permission from Ghali GE et al.[46] p. 5.*

Bilateral Coronal Synostosis

Bilateral coronal synostosis is the most common cranial vault suture synostosis pattern associated with Apert and Crouzon syndromes. Bilateral coronal synostosis results in recession of the supraorbital ridges, which causes the overlying eyebrows to sit posterior to the corneas. In addition to the recessed supraorbital bone, the forehead appears to be lower and there is sagittal shortening of the skull (Figure 45-5). The term for this cranial vault deformity is "brachycephaly." The anterior cranial base is short in the anteroposterior dimension and wide transversely. The

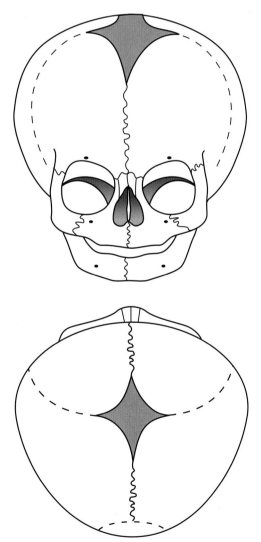

FIGURE **45-5** *Frontal and superior views. Characteristic brachycephaly. Adapted from Ghali GE et al.[46] p. 4.*

overlying cranial vault is high in the superior-inferior dimension, with anterior bulging of the upper forehead that results from compensatory growth of the patent metopic suture (Figure 45-6). The orbits are also shallow (exorbitism), with the eyes bulging (exophthalmus) and abnormally separated (orbital hypertelorism). Brachycephaly represents 20% of the isolated craniosynostosis cases in the United States and is the most common syndrome-associated synostosis.

Metopic Synostosis

Metopic synostosis usually occurs in isolation and results in a triangular shape to the skull (Figure 45-7). The term for this cranial vault deformity is "trigonocephaly." The associated cranial vault deformity consists of relative hypotelorism, an elevated supraorbital ridge medially, and posterior-inferior recession of the lateral orbital rims and lateral aspect of the supraorbital ridges. Palpation often reveals a prominent midline keel in the region of the metopic suture. (Figure 45-8). The bitemporal width is decreased, which results in an

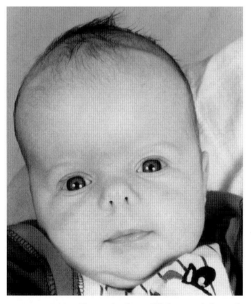

FIGURE **45-6** *Frontal view. High cranial vault and transverse widening characteristic of brachycephaly. Note visible ridging in the bicoronal suture region. Reproduced with permission from Ghali GE et al.[46] p. 7.*

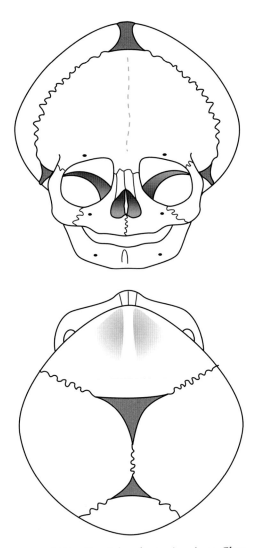

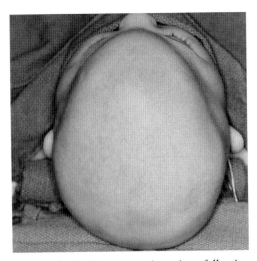

FIGURE **45-7** *Frontal and superior views. Characteristic trigonocephaly. Adapted from Ghali GE et al.[46] p. 8.*

FIGURE **45-8** *Intraoperative view following shaving of the head demonstrates prominent midline ridging. Reproduced with permission from Ghali GE et al.[46] p. 9.*

abnormal anterior cranial vault shape and decreased anterior cranial vault volume. The overlying forehead is sloped posteriorly to approximately the level of the coronal sutures. Trigonocephaly represents 10% of the nonsyndromic craniosynostosis cases in the United States.

Sagittal Synostosis

Sagittal synostosis, the most common form, is rarely associated with increased intracranial pressure. The skull typically has anteroposterior elongation with a compensatory transverse narrowing (Figure 45-9). The term for this cranial vault deformity is "scaphocephaly." The deformity consists of an elongated anteroposterior dimension and a narrow transverse dimension to the cranial vault (Figure 45-10). Usually, the midface and anterior cranial vault sutures are not affected. Scaphocephaly represents 50% of all single-suture craniosynostosis cases in the United States.

Unilateral Lambdoid Synostosis

Unilateral lambdoid synostosis results in flatness of the affected ipsilateral parieto-occipital region. The location of the ear canal and external ear are more posterior and inferior on the ipsilateral side compared with the contralateral side. This configuration is more noticeable when the patient is examined from the superior view and is relatively inconspicuous from the frontal or profile views. The term for this cranial vault deformity is "posterior plagiocephaly." One should rule out infant molding and congenital torticollis (Figure 45-11). With positional (or deformational) plagiocephaly, the ipsilateral ear and forehead are positioned anteriorly, and the ear is not inferiorly displaced as it is with true unilateral lambdoid fusion. The use of head-molding helmet therapy has received renewed interest in the past decade as the preferred treatment of children with positional head shape abnor-

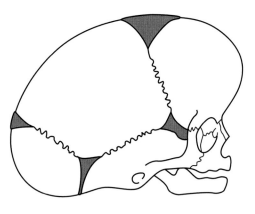

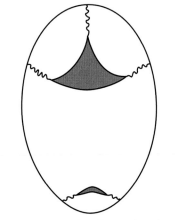

FIGURE **45-9** *Lateral and superior views. Characteristic scaphocephaly. Adapted from Ghali GE et al.[46] p. 10.*

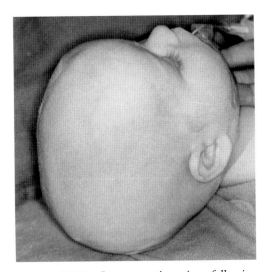

FIGURE **45-10** *Intraoperative view following shaving of the head demonstrates prominent sagittal suture ridging associated with scaphocephaly. Reproduced with permission from Ghali GE et al.[46] p. 11.*

malities.[21] The overall incidence of true unilateral lambdoid synostosis is less than 3% of all isolated synostosis cases in the United States.

Principles of Management

Multidisciplinary Team Approach

The multidisciplinary team approach was developed in response to the failures that commonly occurred when various aspects of care were not coordinated and when the relationships among coexisting problems were not known.[3,22] The objectives of this approach are diagnosis, formulation, and execution of treatment plans and longitudinal follow-up for patients with craniofacial deformities; the team should meet at least monthly for regular outpatient evaluations. Transcripts of these evaluations are forwarded with recommendations to primary care providers and appropriate agencies. Children under the age of 5 years are usually evaluated annually, whereas children over 5 years of age are seen every other year. The frequency of evaluation varies with the stability of the deformity and its consequences.

The craniofacial team should consist of a pediatric anesthesiologist, a pediatric ophthalmologist, a surgeon, an audiologist, a maxillofacial prosthodontist, an orthodontist, a psychologist, a geneticist, an otolaryngologist, a pediatrician, social workers, a speech pathologist, and a nurse.[23–27] All these team members have integral roles at various times in the child's development.[28,29]

Current Surgical Approach

The goals of craniosynostosis suture release are twofold. The first goal is to allow the brain to grow and expand without restriction. The second goal is to establish a more normal contour to the forehead, supraorbital ridges, and skull.[30–32] In most cases, an intracranial approach is used for cranial vault and orbital osteotomies, with reshaping and advancement of bony segments for ideal age-appropriate bony morphology. When planning the time and type of surgical

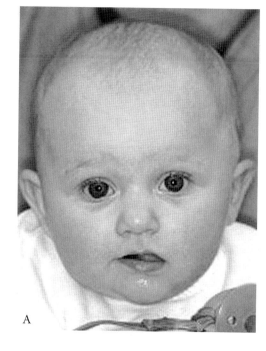

A

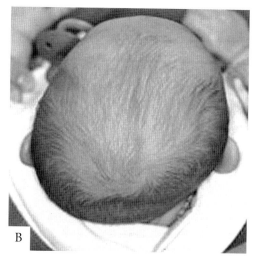

B

FIGURE **45-11** *Frontal (A) and superior (B) views of a child with positional plagiocephaly. Radiographic and clinical examination demonstrated no evidence of craniosynostosis; note asymmetry of external ear position.*

intervention, one must consider the functions, future growth, and the development of the craniofacial skeleton and the maintenance of normal body image. Simple craniosynostosis can be managed successfully with frontocranial remodeling.

Although the timing of craniosynostosis repair remains controversial and individualized, we prefer early surgical repair between the ages of 4 and 8 months.[33–35] Early surgical repair allows for rapid frontal lobe growth, which supports the forehead and supraorbital ridge advancement. At this age, the cranium is highly malleable and therefore easier to contour; a positive effect on facial growth may be achieved and future deformities may be lessened. Also during this period of rapid growth, residual bony defects heal more rapidly. In severe forms of craniosynostosis, additional revision of the cranial vault and orbit is necessary during infancy or early childhood to increase intracranial volume further, which allows for continued brain growth and avoids or reduces the likelihood of intracranial hypertension.

A craniotomy is performed by a pediatric neurosurgeon to remove the deformed section of cranium and provide access for osteotomies to be performed in the cranial base. The skeletal segments are reshaped and replaced into a new position. Although many of the following examples of surgical repair depict transosseous wiring and titanium plating, the current trend includes the use of resorbable plates and screws. These plates, which are composed of polylactic and polyglycolic acid, are completely resorbed by hydrolysis within 9 to 14 months while maintaining tensile strength for initial stabilization.[36–38] As a result, growth restrictions are minimized, as is the potential for transcranial migration.

Surgical Considerations

Unilateral Coronal Synostosis

Multiple surgical approaches for the correction of unilateral coronal synostosis (Figures 45-12 and 45-13) have been described.[39–41] Good long-term results are obtained when treatment of coronal synostosis includes suture release along with cranial vault and orbital osteotomies for reshaping and advancement in infancy. At the Louisiana State University Health Sciences Center in Shreveport, unilateral orbital rim advancement and

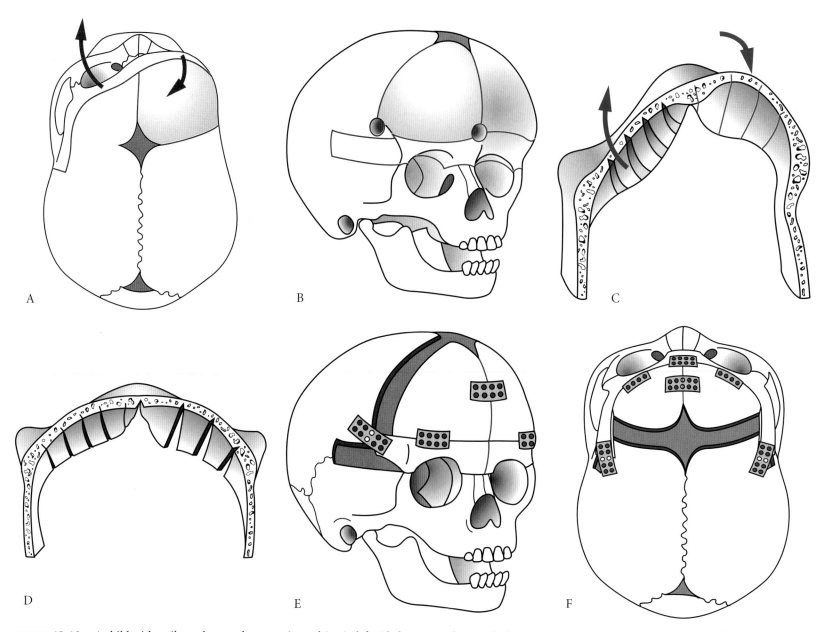

FIGURE **45-12** *A child with unilateral coronal synostosis resulting in left-sided anterior plagiocephaly. A, Asymmetric forehead and orbit viewed from above. Note marked left supraorbital retrusion and right forehead and cranial vault bulging. B, Bur holes prepared for bifrontal craniotomy at the level of the supraorbital region, allowing a 1 cm fronto-orbital unit (bandeau), which extends into the temporal fossa via tongue-in-groove (tenon) extensions. Note that the degree of extension into the lateral and inferior orbital rims is variable based on esthetics. C, The removed bandeau is contoured bilaterally via removal of wedges from the left orbital roof and scoring the right orbital roof. D, The bandeau is reshaped to achieve symmetry by bending the left side and straightening the right side. E and F, Stabilization of forehead and bandeau achieved via resorbable plates and screws. Adapted from Ghali GE et al.[46] p. 14–15.*

frontal bone reshaping are ideally performed at 6 to 8 months of age. Other centers have reported good results when treatment is provided between the ages of 2.5 and 3 years. To achieve optimal symmetry, we prefer to use a bilateral surgical approach. Symmetry of the cranial vault and orbit must be achieved during surgery, because results generally do not improve over time. Stabilization is achieved by using direct intraosseous wires or resorbable plates and screws.

Bilateral Coronal Synostosis

The treatment of bilateral coronal synostosis (Figures 45-14 and 45-15) requires suture release and simultaneous bilateral orbital rim and frontal bone advancements.[42,43] Surgery is performed when the patient is between 6 and 8 months of age. Other centers have reported good results with children treated between the ages of 2.5 and 3 years of age. The osteotomies for the bilateral orbital rim advancement are made superior to the nasofrontal and frontozygomatic sutures and extend to the squamous portion of the temporal bone. Stabilization is achieved with direct transosseous wires or resorbable plates and screws. The more normalized shape provides the needed increase

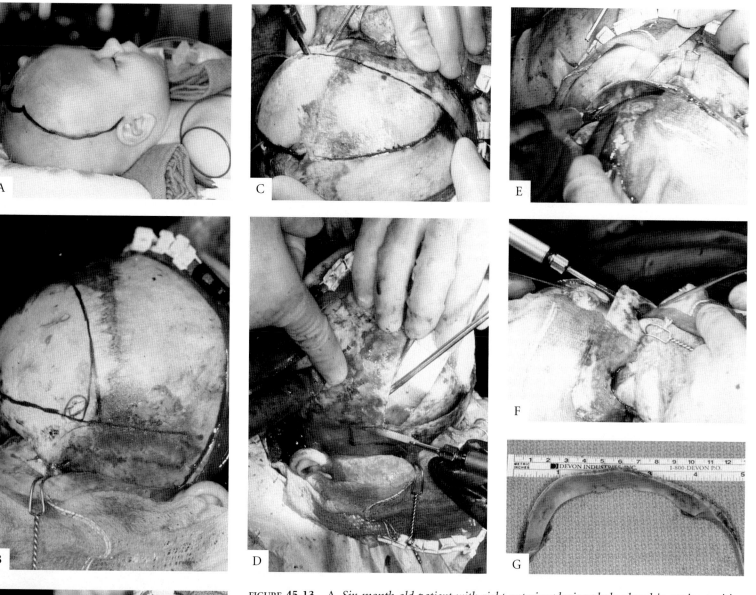

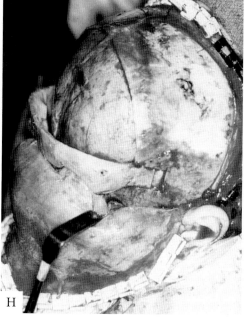

FIGURE 45-13   A, *Six-month-old patient with right anterior plagiocephaly placed in supine position and head secured in a Mayfield headrest. A coronal incision is used and the anterior scalp flap is elevated subperiosteally along with the temporalis muscle. Extension may be carried pre- or postauricular as needed. B, Subperiosteal dissection is achieved bilaterally circumferentially in the periorbital, lateral canthal, lateral orbital, and zygomatic buttresses. Care is taken to maintain the integrity of the medial canthal ligaments. Posterior scalp flap is dissected subperiosteally to between the coronal and lambdoid sutures. Area of proposed bifrontal craniotomy and bur holes are marked. C, Neurosurgeon performs bifrontal craniotomy using Midas Rex drill. D, Frontal and temporal lobes of the brain are gently repositioned to perform upper orbital and temporal osteotomies through the skull base. Reciprocating saw is used to perform bilateral tongue-in-groove extensions from external approach to the level of pterion. E, Attention is turned to the anterior skull base osteotomy and the saw is directed internally across the skull base anterior to the olfactory bulbs while retracting the frontal lobe. F, In addition to frontal lobe retraction, the orbital contents must be protected via retraction at this time. The level of the osteotomy at the lateral orbital rim is customized as needed from as high as the frontozygomatic suture to as low as the lateral aspect of the orbital floor into the inferior orbital fissure. G, Bandeau has been removed and asymmetry noted prior to reshaping. H, Left oblique view following remodeling and recontouring of the bandeau but prior to frontal bone placement. Resorbable plates and screws are used for fixation.*
(CONTINUED ON NEXT PAGE)

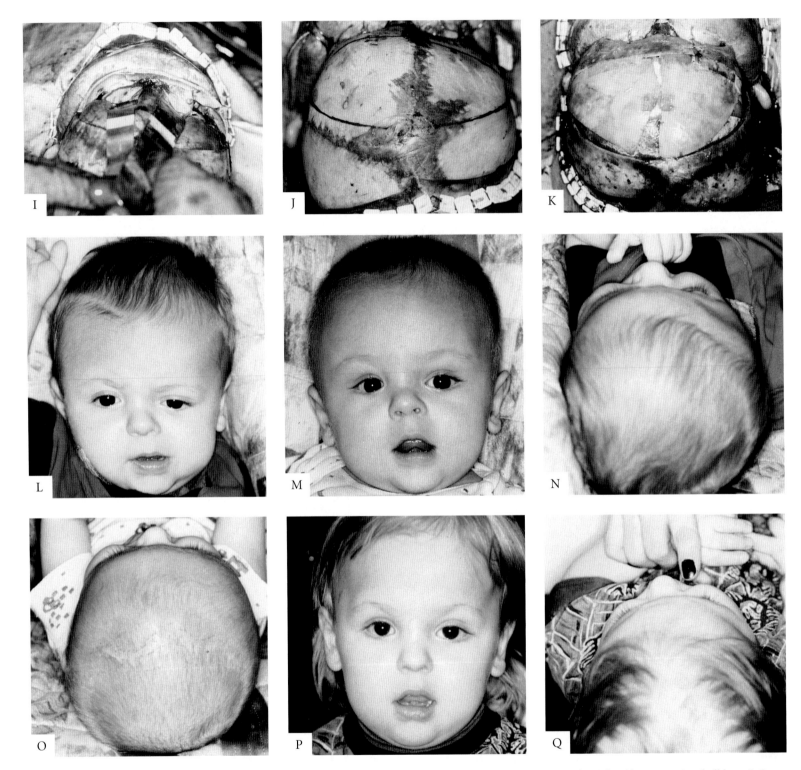

FIGURE 45-13 (CONTINUED) I, *Retraction of bifrontal lobes demonstrates differential degree of advancement on the right side at anterior skull base. J, Superior view of anterior cranial vault prior to reshaping. K, Superior view of anterior cranial vault after osteotomies, reshaping, and resorbable plate and screw fixation of the bone segments. Barrel-staving cuts may be made in the temporal and parietal bones as needed for reshaping purposes. L, A 6-month-old boy with right unilateral plagiocephaly. He underwent anterior cranial vault and bilateral superior orbital rim osteotomies with reshaping and advancement by the procedure described. Preoperative frontal view is shown. M, Frontal view 6 weeks after reconstruction. N, Preoperative superior view. O, Superior view 6 weeks after reconstruction. P, Frontal view 2 years after reconstruction. Q, Superior view 2 years after reconstruction. Reproduced with permission from Ghali GE et al.[46] p. 16–24.*

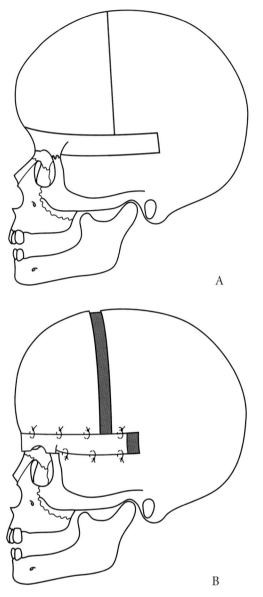

FIGURE 45-14 *Brachycephaly before and after anterior cranial vault and bilateral superior orbital rim osteotomies, reshaping, and advancements. A, Site of osteotomies as indicated. Dissection and osteotomies are similar to that previously described for plagiocephaly repair. B, After osteotomies, reshaping, and fixation of bandeau and frontal plates. Adapted from Ghali GE et al.[46] p. 25.*

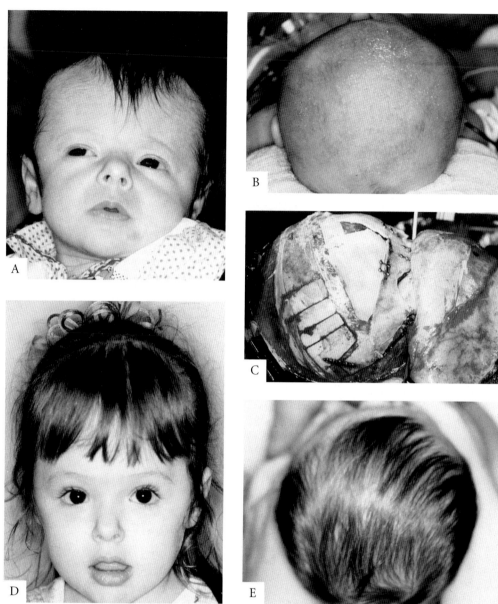

FIGURE 45-15 *A female infant born with bilateral coronal synostosis and apparent normal growth of her midface. She underwent anterior cranial vault and bilateral superior orbital rim osteotomies with reshaping at 6 months of age as previously described. A, Frontal view soon after birth. B, Superior view preoperatively at 6 months of age. C, Intraoperative lateral view of anterior cranial vault and orbits after osteotomies, reshaping, and fixation of segments. D, Frontal view at 3 years of age. E, Superior view at 1 year of age. Reproduced with permission from Ghali GE et al.[46] p. 25–7.*

in intracranial volume within the anterior cranial vault.

Metopic Synostosis

Surgical treatment of metopic synostosis (Figures 45-16 and 45-17) involves metopic suture release, simultaneous bilateral orbital rim advancements, and lateral widening via frontal bone advancement. These procedures are usually performed at 6 to 8 months of age. Orbital hypotelorism is corrected by splitting the supraorbital ridge unit vertically in the midline and placing autogenous cranial bone grafts to increase the intraorbital distance. Stabilization is achieved with direct transosseous wires or resorbable microplate fixation. The microplate fixation is usually placed at the inner surface of the cranial bone. The abnormally shaped bone that has been removed is cut into sections of appropriate shape for the new forehead configuration. The anterior cranial base, anterior cranial vault, and orbit are given a more esthetic shape, and the volume of the anterior cranial vault is increased, which

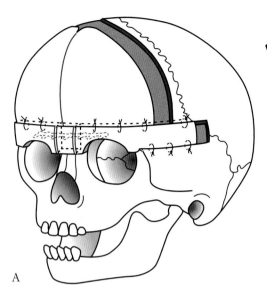

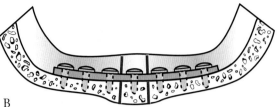

B

FIGURE **45-16** *Trigonocephaly repair after anterior cranial vault and superior orbital rim osteotomies. For the most part, the surgical approach is similar to that previously described for anterior cranial vault and superior orbital rim osteotomies and reshaping. A, As part of the reshaping, the bandeau is often split vertically at the midline and an interpositional autogenous cranial bone graft placed to correct hypotelorism. B, Resorbable forms of fixation lend themselves to internal plating of the bandeau as shown. Adapted from Ghali GE et al.*[46] *p. 28.*

A

allows the brain adequate space. Autogenous bone may be taken from the posterior cranium, when required, to enhance frontal reconstruction.

Sagittal Synostosis

Historically, when premature closure of a sagittal suture (Figures 45-18 and 45-19) was recognized in early infancy, most neurosur-

geons believed that simple release of the sagittal suture through a strip craniectomy without simultaneous skull reshaping was adequate treatment.[4,36,44,45] Our results using this technique have been less than favorable, and a residual cranial vault deformity usually results. If improvements in cranial vault shape are to be achieved, most cases require a formal total cranial vault reshaping at the age of 4 to 8 months. Variations in the degree of the scaphocephalic deformity are common, depending on the extent of sagittal suture stenosis. When the posterior half is fused, the patient is treated in the prone position with the posterior two-thirds of the cranial vault reshaped. When the anterior half is fused, the patient is treated in the supine position with the anterior two-thirds of the cranial vault reshaped, with or without superior orbital rim reshaping. When the entire suture is fused, a combination of

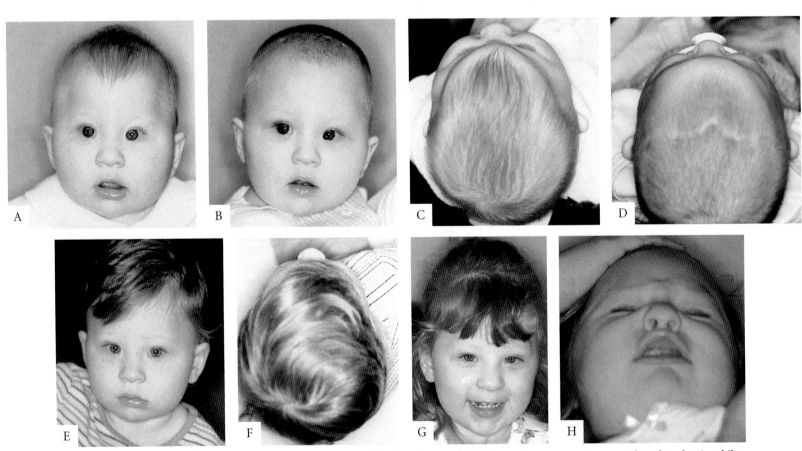

FIGURE **45-17** *A 10-month-old girl with metopic synostosis resulting in trigonocephaly. She underwent anterior cranial vault reshaping, bilateral superior orbital rim advancements, and bitemporal widening via barrel-staving osteotomies. A, Frontal view before surgery. B, Frontal view after reconstruction. C, Superior view before surgery. D, Superior view after reconstruction. E, Frontal view at 2 years of age. F, Superior view at 2 years of age. G, Frontal view at 4 years of age. H, Inferior view at 4 years of age.* (CONTINUED ON NEXT PAGE)

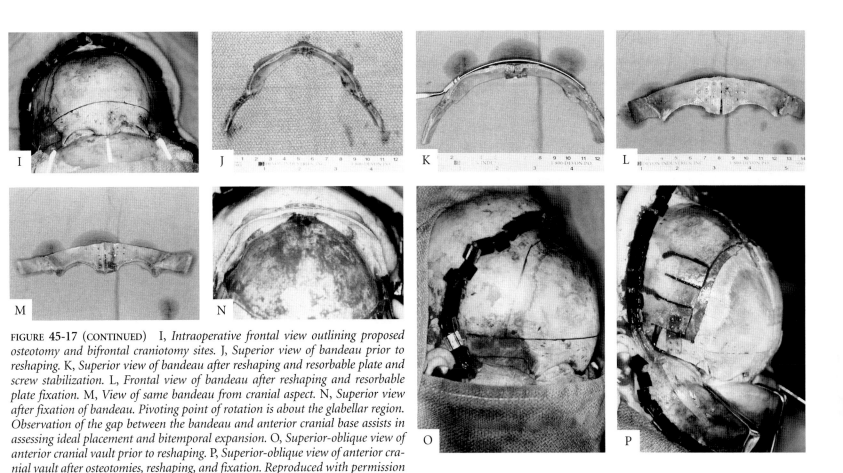

FIGURE 45-17 (CONTINUED) I, *Intraoperative frontal view outlining proposed osteotomy and bifrontal craniotomy sites. J, Superior view of bandeau prior to reshaping. K, Superior view of bandeau after reshaping and resorbable plate and screw stabilization. L, Frontal view of bandeau after reshaping and resorbable plate fixation. M, View of same bandeau from cranial aspect. N, Superior view after fixation of bandeau. Pivoting point of rotation is about the glabellar region. Observation of the gap between the bandeau and anterior cranial base assists in assessing ideal placement and bitemporal expansion. O, Superior-oblique view of anterior cranial vault prior to reshaping. P, Superior-oblique view of anterior cranial vault after osteotomies, reshaping, and fixation. Reproduced with permission from Ghali GE et al.[46] p. 28–34.*

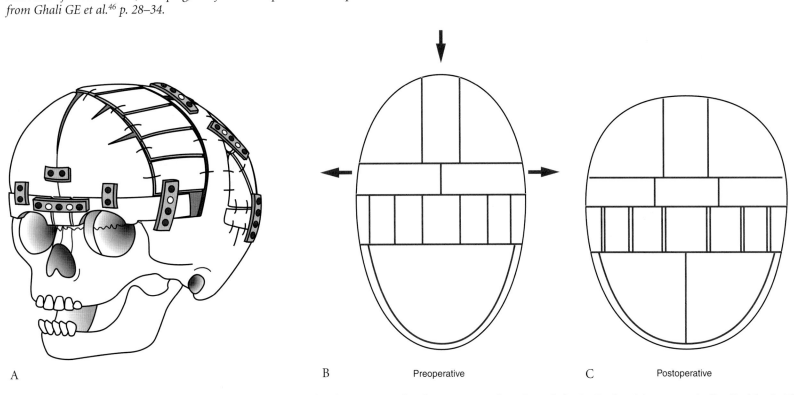

A	B		C	
	Preoperative		Postoperative	

FIGURE 45-18 *A child after total cranial vault and upper orbital osteotomies for the treatment of scaphocephaly. A, Forehead is symmetrically tilted back. The occiput is symmetrically tilted forward. The anterior-posterior dimension is thereby shortened and secured via resorbable plates and screws. Barrel-stave cuts are made laterally to widen the transverse dimension or the squamous portion of the temporal plates as osteotomized, interchanged, and stabilized with resorbable plates and screws. Superior view preoperatively (B) and postoperatively (C). Total cranial vault reshaping as well as orbital rim alteration is accomplished to increase the biparietal width and decrease the frontal and occipital prominences. Adapted from Ghali GE et al.[46] p. 35.*

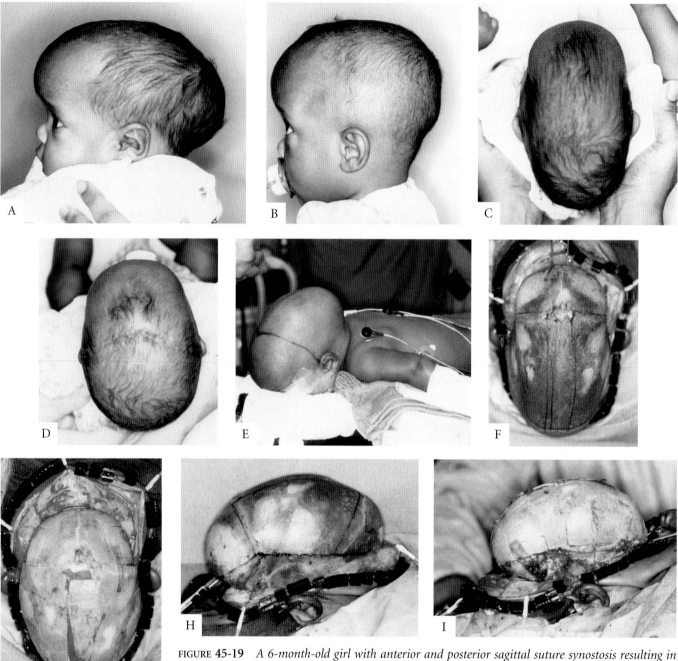

FIGURE 45-19 *A 6-month-old girl with anterior and posterior sagittal suture synostosis resulting in scaphocephaly. She underwent total cranial vault reshaping without the need for any orbital osteotomies. A prone position was used throughout the procedure. A, Lateral view before surgery. B, Lateral view after reconstruction. C, Superior view before surgery. D, Superior view after reconstruction. E, Prone positioning is necessary and requires careful protection of both the airway and globes. F, Intraoperative superior view of proposed osteotomy sites for total cranial vault reshaping. G, Intraoperative superior view of the osteotomies, reshaping, and resorbable plate fixation. H, Intraoperative left lateral view prior to reshaping. I, Intraoperative left lateral view after osteotomies, reshaping, and resorbable plate fixation. Reproduced with permission from Ghali GE et al.[46] p. 36–40.*

both approaches may be necessary. Unless a significant concomitant supraorbital deformity exists, we prefer to treat full sagittal suture stenosis (anterior and posterior) at one operative setting in the prone position via a total cranial vault reshaping. For older children (older than 1 year) or children with a need for upper orbital reconstruction, we prefer the supine position at one operative setting or, rarely, in two stages, with posterior reconstruction preceding anterior and orbital reconstruction by 4 to 6 months. Other centers have reported good results when routinely staging full sagittal synostosis.

Unilateral Lambdoid Synostosis

Many surgeons consider simple strip craniectomy of the involved suture or partial craniectomy of the region to be adequate treatment. More extensive vault craniectomy and reshaping are generally necessary. If improvements in cranial vault shape are required after 10 to 12 months of age, formal posterior cranial vault reshaping is performed.

Summary

In approximately 1 in 1,000 live births in the United States, an infant has some variant of a craniofacial deformity. If cleft lip and palate deformities are included, the incidence is even greater. Surgical management of these patients has been advocated to occur from the first few weeks after birth until well into the second decade. Many of these patients require multiple, staged procedures that involve movements of the bone and soft tissue from both the intracranial and extracranial approaches. The surgical approach to most of these congenital deformities was radically changed by techniques introduced to the United States by Paul Tessier of France in 1967. From his imaginative intracranial and extracranial approaches, numerous advances have been made that facilitate the biodegradable plating systems, which have improved the management of these complex craniomaxillofacial deformities.

References

1. Moss ML. The pathogenesis of premature cranial synostosis in man. Acta Anat (Basel) 1959;37:351.

2. Zeiger JS, Beaty TH, Hetmanski JB, et al. Genetic and environmental risk factors for sagittal craniosynostosis. J Craniofac Surg 2002;13:602–6.

3. Brodsky L, Ritter-Schmidt DH, Holt L. Craniofacial anomalies: an inter-disciplinary approach. St. Louis (MO): Mosby Yearbook; 1989.

4. Graham JM, de Saxe M, Smith DW. Sagittal craniosynostosis: fetal head constraint as one possible cause. J Pediatr 1979;95:747–50.

5. Magge SN, Westerveid M, Pruzinsky T, Persing JA. Long-term neuropsychologic effects of sagittal craniosynostosis on child development. J Craniofac Surg 2002;13:99–104.

6. Marchac D, Renier D. Treatment of craniosynostosis in infancy. Clin Plast Surg 1987; 14:61–72.

7. Cutting C, Grayson B, Bookstein F, et al. Computer-aided planning and evaluation of facial and orthognathic surgery. Clin Plast Surg 1986;13:449–62.

8. Gault D, Brunelle F, Renier D, Marchac D. The calculation of intracranial volume using CT scans. Childs Nerv Syst 1988;4:271–3.

9. Lo LJ. Craniofacial computer-assisted surgical planning and simulation. Clin Plast Surg 1994;21:501–16.

10. Marsh JL, Gado M. The longitudinal orbital CT projection: a versatile image for orbital assessment. Plast Reconstr Surg 1983;71:308–17.

11. Marsh JL, Vannier MW. Computer-assisted imaging in the diagnosis, management and study of dysmorphic patients. In: Vig KWL, Burdi AR, editors. Craniofacial morphogenesis and dysmorphogenesis. Ann Arbor: University of Michigan Press; 1988. p. 109–26.

12. Marsh JL, Vannier MW. The "third" dimension in craniofacial surgery. Plast Reconstr Surg 1983;71:759–67.

13. Marsh JL, Vannier MW. Three-dimensional surface imaging from CT scans for the study of craniofacial dysmorphology. J Craniofac Genet Dev Biol 1989;9:61–75.

14. Marsh JL, Vannier MW, Stevens WG, et al. Computerized imaging for soft tissue and osseous reconstruction in the head and neck. Clin Plast Surg 1985;12:279–91.

15. Marsh JL, Vannier MW, Bresina S, Hemmer KM. Application of computer graphics in craniofacial surgery. Clin Plast Surg 1986;13:441–8.

16. Posnick JC, Bite U, Nakamo P. Comparison of direct and indirect intra-cranial volume measurements. In: Proceedings of the 6th International Congress on Cleft Palate and Related Craniofacial Anomalies. June 15–18, 1989.

17. Posnick JC. Indirect intracranial volume measurements using CT scans: clinical applications for craniosynostosis. Plast Reconstr Surg 1992;89:34–45.

18. Vannier MW, Marsh JL, Warren JO. Three dimension CT reconstruction images for craniofacial surgical planning and evaluation. Radiology 1984;150:179–84.

19. Longacre JJ, Destafano GA, Holmstrand K. The early versus the late reconstruction of congenital hypoplasia of the facial skeleton and skull. Plast Reconstr Surg 1961;27:489–504.

20. Oakes WJ. Craniosynostosis. In: Serafin D, Geargiade NG, editors. Pediatric plastic surgery. St. Louis (MO): C.V. Mosby Co.; 1984. p. 404–39.

21. Seymour-Dempsey K, Baumgartner JE, Teichgraeber JF, et al. Molding helmet therapy in the management of sagittal synostosis. J Craniofac Surg 2002;13:631–35.

22. Sinn DP, Ghali GE, Ortega M. Major craniofacial surgery. In: Levin DL, Morriss FC, editors. Essentials of pediatric intensive care. New York: Churchill-Livingstone; 1997. p. 636–43.

23. Arndt EM, Travis F, Lefebvre A, Munro IR. Psychological adjustment of 20 patients with Treacher Collins syndrome before and after reconstructive surgery. Br J Plast Surg 1987;40:605–9.

24. Barden RC, Ford ME, Jensen AG, et al. Effects of craniofacial deformity in infancy on the quality of mother-infant interaction. Child Dev 1989;60:819–24.

25. Barden RC, Ford ME, Wilhelm W, et al. The physical attractiveness of facially deformed patients before and after craniofacial surgery. Plast Reconstr Surg 1988;82:229–35.

26. Barden RC, Ford ME, Wilhelm W, et al. Emotional and behavioral reactions to facially deformed patients before and after craniofacial surgery. Plast Reconstr Surg 1988; 82:409–18.

27. Lafebvre A, Travis F, Arndt EM, Munro IR. A psychiatric profile before and after reconstructive surgery in children with Apert's syndrome. Br J Plast Surg 1986;39:510–3.

28. Arnaud E, Meneses P, Lajeunie E, et al. Postoperative mental and morphological outcome for nonsyndromic brachycephaly. J Craniofac Surg 2002;110:6–12.

29. Warschausky S, Kay JB, Buchman S, et al. Health-related quality of life in children with craniofacial anomalies. J Craniofac Surg 2002;110:409–14.

30. Marchac D. Forehead remolding for craniosynostosis. In: Converse JM, McCarthy JG, Wood-Smith D, editors. Symposium on diagnosis and treatment of craniofacial anomalies. St. Louis (MO): C.V. Mosby Co.; 1979. p. 323.

31. Edgerton MT, Jane JA, Berry FA, et al. The feasibility of craniofacial osteotomies in infants and young children. Scand J Plast Reconstr Surg 1974;8:164–8.

32. Edgerton MT, Jane JA, Berry FA. Craniofacial osteotomies and reconstruction in infants and young children. Plast Reconstr Surg 1974;54:13–27.

33. McCarthy JG, Epstein F, Sadove M, et al. Early surgery for craniofacial synostosis: an 8-

year experience. Plast Reconstr Surg 1984; 73:521–33.

34. Whitaker LA, Barlett SP, Schut L, Bruce D. Craniosynostosis: an analysis of the timing, treatment and complication in 164 patients. Plast Reconstr Surg 1987;80:195–212.

35. Whitaker LA, Schut L, Kerr LP. Early surgery for isolated craniofacial dysostosis. Plast Reconstr Surg 1977;60:575–81.

36. Cohen SR, Holmes RE. Immediate cranial vault reconstruction with bioresorbable plates following endoscopically assisted sagittal synostectomy. J Craniofac Surg 2002;13:578–84.

37. Pietrzak WS. Critical concepts of absorbable internal fixation. J Craniofac Surg 2000; 11:335–41.

38. Pietrzak WS, Kumar M, Eppley BL. The influence of temperature on the degradation rate of lactosorb copolymer. J Craniofac Surg 2003;14:176–83.

39. Jane JA, Park TS, Zide BM, et al. Alternative techniques in the treatment of unilateral coronal synostosis. J Neurosurg 1984; 61:550–6.

40. Mohr G, Hoffman HJ, Munro IR, et al. Surgical management of unilateral and bilateral coronal craniosynostosis: 21 years of experience. Neurosurgery 1978;2:83–92.

41. Persing JA, Babler WJ, Jane JA, Duckworth PF. Experimental unilateral coronal synostosis in rabbits. Plast Reconstr Surg 1986;77:369–77.

42. Hoffman HJ, Mohr G. Lateral canthal advancement of the supraorbital margins: a new corrective technique in the treatment of coronal synostosis. J Neurosurg 1976;45:376–81.

43. Marchac D, Renier D, Jones BM. Experience with the "floating forehead." Br J Plast Surg 1988;41:1–15.

44. Shillito J, Matson DD. Craniosynostosis: a review of 519 surgical patients. Pediatrics 1968;41:819–53.

45. Weinzweig J, Baker SB, Whitaker LA, et al. Delayed cranial vault reconstruction for sagittal synostosis in older children: an algorithm for tailoring the reconstructive approach to the craniofacial deformity. J Craniofac Surg 2002;110:397–408.

46. Ghali GE, Sinn DP, Tantipasawasin S. Management of nonsyndromic craniosynostosis. Atlas Oral Maxillofac Surg Clin N Am 2002;10:1–41.

CHAPTER 46

Craniofacial Dysostosis Syndromes: Staging of Reconstruction

Jeffrey C. Posnick, DMD, MD
Ramon L. Ruiz, DMD, MD
Paul S. Tiwana, DDS, MD, MS

Cranial sutures are a form of bone articulation in which the margins of the bones are connected by a thin layer of fibrous tissue. The cranial vault is composed of six major sutural areas and several minor sutures, which serve two critical functions during the postnatal period. Initially, the sutures allow head deformation during vaginal delivery as part of the birthing process. Later, during an infant's postnatal development, cranial vault sutures facilitate head expansion to accommodate propulsive brain growth.[1] Only small amounts of pressure (5 mm Hg) from the growing brain are required to stimulate bone deposition at the margins of a cranial bone.[2,3] Under normal conditions, the brain volume will triple within the first year of life, and by age 2 years, the cranial capacity is four times that at birth.[4] Under normal circumstances, closure of the cranial vault sutures occurs earlier than closure of the membranous facial bone sutures, which often remain patent until adulthood.

The term *craniosynostosis* is defined as a premature fusion of a cranial vault suture. With rare exception, this is an intrauterine event. A more accurate description of craniosynostosis may be a *congenital absence* of the cranial vault sutures. The result is

fusion of the bones adjacent to the suture and arrested sutural growth of the adjacent bones. The classic theory known as Virchow's law states that premature fusion of a cranial vault suture results in limited development of the skull perpendicular to the fused suture and a compensatory "overgrowth" through the sutures that remain open.[5] The result is a dysmorphology with characteristics depending on the sutures affected, and potential neurologic consequences related to underlying brain compression. Most forms of craniosynostosis represent random, nonsyndromic malformations limited to the cranial vault and orbital regions. Management typically requires a combined neurosurgical and craniofacial approach for release of the involved suture and reshaping of the dysmorphic skeletal components. For additional discussion of the treatment of nonsyndromic craniosynostosis, see Chapter 45, "Nonsyndromic Craniosynostosis." Craniofacial dysostosis is the term applied to syndromal forms of craniosynostosis. These disorders are characterized by sutural involvement that not only includes the cranial vault but also extends into the skull base and midfacial skeletal structures. Craniofacial dysostosis syndromes have been

described by Carpenter, Apert, Crouzon, Saethre-Chotzen, and Pfeiffer.[6] Although the cranial vault and cranial base are thought to be the regions of primary involvement, there is also significant impact on midfacial growth and development.[7,8] In addition to cranial vault dysmorphology, patients with these inherited conditions exhibit a characteristic "total midface" deficiency that is syndrome specific and must be addressed as part of the staged reconstructive approach.

Functional Considerations

Brain Growth and Intracranial Pressure

If the rapid brain growth that normally occurs during infancy is to proceed unhindered, the cranial vault and base sutures must remain open and expand during phases of rapid growth, resulting in marginal ossification. In craniosynostosis, premature fusion of sutures causes limited and abnormal skeletal expansion in the presence of continued brain growth. Depending on the number and location of prematurely fused sutures, the growth of the brain may be restricted.[2,9–11] In addition, abnormal cranial vault and midfacial morphology occurs as determined by

Virchow's law. If surgical release of the affected sutures and reshaping to restore a more normal intracranial volume and configuration are not performed, decreased cognitive and behavioral function is likely to be the end result.

Elevated intracranial pressure (ICP) is the most serious functional problem associated with premature suture fusion. A "beaten-copper" appearance along the inner table of the cranial vault seen on a plain radiograph or the loss of brain cisternae as observed on a computed tomography (CT) scan may suggest elevated ICP,[12] but these are considered soft radiographic findings.

Intracranial hypertension can be established invasively by means of a burhole craniotomy used to place either an epidural or intraparenchymal pressure sensor. Increased ICP is most likely to affect patients with great disparity between brain growth and intracranial capacity and may occur in as many as 42% of untreated children in whom more than one suture is affected.[2,10,13] Unfortunately, there is no absolute agreement on what levels of ICP are normal at any given age in infancy and early childhood.

The clinical signs and symptoms related to elevated ICP may have a slow onset and be difficult to recognize in the pediatric population. Although standardized CT scans allow for indirect measurement of intracranial volume, it is not yet possible to use these studies to make judgments as to who requires craniotomy for decompression.[14,15] Careful neurosurgical and pediatric ophthalmologic evaluation are critical components of the data gathering required to formulate a definitive treatment plan in a patient with craniosynostosis.

Vision

Untreated craniosynostosis with elevated ICP will cause papilledema and eventual optic nerve atrophy, resulting in partial or complete blindness. If the orbits are shallow (exorbitism) and the eyes are proptotic (exophthalmos), as occurs in the craniofacial dysostosis syndromes, the cornea may be exposed and abrasions or ulcerations may occur. An eyeball extending outside of a shallow orbit is also at risk of trauma. If the orbits are extremely shallow, herniation of the globe itself may occur, necessitating emergency reduction followed by tarsorrhaphies or urgent orbital decompression.

Some forms of craniofacial dysostosis result in a marked degree of orbital hypertelorism, which may compromise visual acuity and restrict binocular vision. Divergent or convergent nonparalytic strabismus or exotropia occurs frequently and should be considered during the diagnostic evaluation. This may be the result of congenital anomalies of the extraocular muscles themselves. Paralytic or nonparalytic unilateral or bilateral upper eyelid ptosis also occurs with greater frequency with craniofacial dysostosis than in the general population.

Hydrocephalus

Hydrocephalus affects as many as 10% of patients with a craniofacial dysostosis syndrome.[16–19] Although the etiology is often not clear, hydrocephalus may be secondary to a generalized cranial base stenosis with constriction of all the cranial base foramina, which impacts the patient's cerebral venous drainage and cerebrospinal fluid (CSF) flow dynamics. Hydrocephalus may be identified with the help of CT or magnetic resonance imaging (MRI) to document progressively enlarging ventricles. Difficulty exists in interpreting ventricular findings as seen on a CT scan especially when the skull and cranial base are brachycephalic. The skeletal dysmorphology seen in a child with severe cranial dysmorphology related to craniosynostosis may translate into an abnormal ventricular shape that is not necessarily related to abnormal CSF flow. Serial imaging and clinical correlation is indicated, and a great deal of clinical judgment is often required in making these assessments.

Effects of Midface Deficiency on Airway

All newborn infants are obligate nasal breathers. Many infants born with a craniofacial dysostosis syndrome have moderate to severe hypoplasia of the midface as a component of their malformation. They will have diminished nasal and nasopharyngeal spaces with resulting increased nasal airway resistance (obstruction). The affected child is thus forced to breath through the mouth. For a newborn infant to ingest food through the mouth requires sucking from a nipple to achieve negative pressure as well as an intact swallowing mechanism. The neonate with severe midface hypoplasia will experience diminished nasal airflow and be unable to accomplish this task and breathe through the nose at the same time.[20–23] Complicating this clinical picture may be an elongated and ptotic palate and enlarged tonsils and adenoids. The compromised infant expends significant energy respiring, and this may push the child into a catabolic state (negative nitrogen balance). Failure to thrive results unless either nasogastric tube feeding is instituted or a feeding gastrostomy is placed. Evaluation by a pediatrician, pediatric otolaryngologist, and feeding specialist with craniofacial experience can help distinguish minor feeding difficulties from those requiring more aggressive treatment.

Sleep apnea of either central or obstructive origin may also be present. If the apnea is found to be secondary to upper airway obstruction based on a formal sleep study, a tracheostomy may be indicated. In rare situations, "early" midface advancement is useful to improve the airway and allow for tracheostomy decannulation. Central apnea may occur from poorly treated intracranial hypertension and other contributing factors. If this is the case, the condition may improve by reducing the intracranial pressure to a normal range through cranio-orbital or posterior cranial vault decompression or expansion.

Dentition and Occlusion

The incidence of dental and oral anomalies is higher among children with craniofacial dysostosis syndromes than in the general population. In Apert syndrome in particular, the palate is high and constricted in width. The incidence of isolated cleft palate in patients with Apert syndrome approaches 30%.[13] Clefting of the secondary palate may be submucous, incomplete, or complete. Confusion has arisen over whether the oral malformations and absence of teeth that are often characteristic of these conditions are a result of congenital or iatrogenic factors (eg, injury to dental follicles associated with early midface surgery). The midfacial hypoplasia seen in the craniofacial dysostosis syndromes often results in limited maxillary alveolar bone to house a full complement of teeth. The result is severe crowding, which often requires serial extractions in order to address the problem. An Angle Class III skeletal relationship in combination with anterior open bite deformity is typical.

Hearing

Hearing deficits are more common among patients with the craniofacial dysostosis syndromes than in the general population.[24] In Crouzon syndrome, conductive hearing deficits are common, and atresia of the external auditory canals may also occur. Otitis media is more common in Apert syndrome, although the exact incidence is unknown. Middle ear disease may be related to the presence of a cleft palate that results in eustachian tube dysfunction. Congenital fixation of the stapedial footplate is also believed to be frequent. The possibility of significant hearing loss is paramount in importance and should not be overlooked because of preoccupation with other more easily appreciated craniofacial findings.

Extremity Anomalies

Apert syndrome results in joint fusion and bony and soft tissue syndactyly of the digits of all four limbs.[24] These Apert-associated extremity deformities are often symmetric. Partial or complete fusion of the shoulder, elbow, or other joints is common. Broad thumbs, broad great toes, and partial soft tissue syndactyly of the hands may be seen in Pfeiffer syndrome, but these are variable features. Preaxial polysyndactyly of the feet may also be seen in Carpenter syndrome.

Morphologic Considerations

Examination of the patient's entire craniofacial region should be meticulous and systematic. The skeleton and soft tissues are assessed in a standard way to identify all normal and abnormal anatomy. Specific findings tend to occur in particular malformations, but each patient is unique. The achievement of symmetry and normal proportions and the reconstruction of specific esthetic units are essential to forming an unobtrusive face in a child born with a craniofacial dysostosis syndrome.

Frontoforehead Esthetic Unit

The frontoforehead region is dysmorphic in an infant with craniofacial dysostosis.[25–30] Establishing normal position of the forehead is critical to overall facial symmetry and balance. The forehead may be considered as two separate esthetic components: the supraorbital ridge–lateral orbital rim region and the superior forehead (Figure 46-1A and B).[31,32] The supraorbital ridge–lateral orbital rim region includes the glabella and supraorbital rim extending inferiorly down each frontozygomatic suture toward the infraorbital rim and posteriorly along each temporoparietal region. The morphology and position of the supraorbital ridge–lateral orbital rim region is a key element of upper facial esthetics. In a normal forehead, at the level of the frontonasal suture, an angle ranging from 90 to 110° is formed by the supraor-

bital ridge and the nasal bones when viewed in profile. Additionally, the eyebrows, overlying the supraorbital ridge, should be anterior to the cornea. When the supraorbital ridge is viewed from above, the rim should arc posteriorly to achieve a gentle 90° angle at the temporal fossa with a center point of the arc at the level of each frontozygomatic suture. The superior forehead component, about 1.0 to 1.5 cm up from the supraorbital rim, should have a gentle posterior curve of about 60°, leveling out at the coronal suture region when seen in profile.

Posterior Cranial Vault Esthetic Unit

Symmetry, form, and the appropriate intracranial volume of the posterior cranial vault are closely linked. Posterior cranial vault flattening may result from either a unilateral or bilateral lambdoidal synostosis, which is rare; previous craniectomy with reossification in a dysmorphic flat shape, which is frequent; or postural molding because of repetitive sleep positioning.[33] A short anterior–posterior cephalic length may be misinterpreted as an anterior cranial vault (forehead) problem when the occipitoparietal (posterior) skull represents the primary region of the deformity. Careful examination of the entire cranial vault is essential to defining the dysmorphic region so that appropriate therapy may be carried out.

Orbitonasozygomatic Esthetic Unit

In craniofacial dysostosis syndromes, the orbitonasozygomatic regional deformity is a reflection of the cranial base malformation. For example, in Crouzon syndrome when bilateral coronal suture synostosis is combined with skull base and midfacial deficiency, the orbitonasozygomatic region will be dysmorphic and consistent with a short (anterior–posterior) and wide (transverse) anterior cranial base.[34] In Apert syndrome, the nasal bones, orbits, and zygomas, like

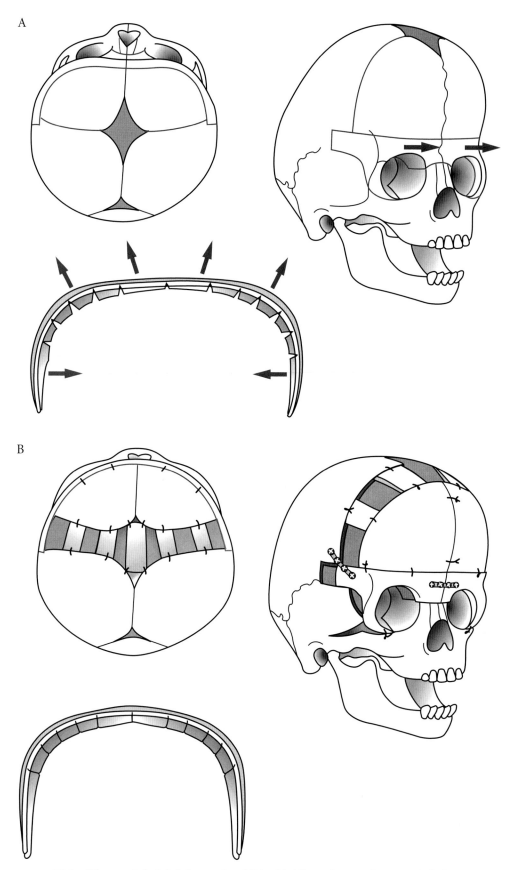

the anterior cranial base, are transversely wide and horizontally short (retruded), resulting in a shallow hyperteloric upper midface (zygomas, orbits, and nose).[34] Advancing the midface without simultaneously addressing the increased transverse width will not adequately correct the dysmorphology.[35]

Maxillary-Nasal Base Esthetic Unit

In the craniofacial dysostosis patient with midface deficiency, the upper anterior face (nasion to maxillary incisor) is vertically short, and there is a lack of horizontal anterior-posterior (A-P) projection of the midface.[36,37] These findings may be confirmed with cephalometric analysis that indicates a sella-nasion angle (SNA) below the mean value and a short upper anterior facial height (nasion to anterior nasal spine). The width of the maxilla in the dentoalveolar region is generally constricted with a high arched palate. In order to normalize the maxillonasal base region, multidirectional surgical expansion and reshaping are generally required. The maxillary lip-to-tooth relationship and occlusion are normalized through Le Fort I osteotomy and orthodontic treatment as part of the staged reconstruction.

Quantitative Assessment

A quantitative analysis of measurements taken from CT scans, surface anthropometry, cephalometric analysis, and dental casts is critical to data gathering for evaluation of craniofacial deformities.[38–43] This analysis will confirm or refute clinical impressions, aid in the treatment planning of intraoperative skeletal movements and reshaping, and provide a framework for objective assessment of immediate and long-term results. These methods of assessment rely on the measurement of linear distances, angles, and proportions based on accurate, reliable, and reproducible anatomic landmarks found to be useful for patient evaluation.

FIGURE **46-1** *The craniofacial skeleton of a child with bilateral coronal synostosis before and after anterior cranial vault and three-quarter orbital osteotomies with reshaping. A, Site of osteotomies as indicated. B, After osteotomies and reshaping and fixation of the cranio-orbital regions. Adapted from Posnick JC.[76]*

CT Scan Analysis

The use of CT scans has clarified our appreciation of the dysmorphology of a child born with a craniofacial malformation.[44,45] Accurate standardized points of reference have been identified in the cranio-orbitozygomatic skeleton based on axial CT images.[42,43] Knowledge of differential facial bone growth patterns and normal measurement values can now be used to improve diagnostic accuracy, assist in the staging of reconstruction by understanding growth vectors, and offer the option of making intraoperative measurements that correlate with the preoperative CT scan measurements and ideal dimensions. This information can effectively guide the surgeon in the reconstruction of an individual with a craniofacial malformation and also allows for accurate postoperative reassessment.

Anthropometric Surface Measurements

Cross-sectional studies of the patterns of postnatal facial growth based on anthropometric surface measurements have been carried out in growing Caucasian children.[38–41,46] This published material has proven useful in the quantitative evaluation and recognition of discrepancies in postnatal development in the head and face of patients with specific craniofacial syndromes. This is particularly useful when evaluating basic distances, angles, and proportions of the head, face, and orbits in patients affected with craniofacial dysostosis syndromes.

Cephalometric Analysis

Cephalometric radiography, first introduced by Broadbent in 1931, has been traditionally used to study the morphology and patterns of growth of the maxillofacial skeleton.[47] The large collection of normative data developed allows clinicians to monitor an individual's facial growth. The interpretation of cephalometric radiographs remains useful in the analysis of facial heights and maxillary, mandibular, and chin positions and their relationships to one another; the cranial base; and the dentition.[30,36,48,49] The lateral cephalometric radiograph offers an accurate view from the midsagittal plane if the facial skeleton being analyzed is relatively symmetric. Unfortunately, the number of anatomic landmarks that can be identified accurately in the cranio-orbitozygomatic region is limited because of the overlap of structures, which makes predictably locating these anatomic landmarks more difficult.

Surgical Management

Historic Perspectives: The Pioneers

The first recorded surgical approach to craniosynostosis was performed by Lannelongue in 1890[50] and Lane in 1892,[51] who completed strip craniectomies of the involved sutures. Their aim was to control the problem of brain compression (intracranial hypertension) within a congenitally small cranial vault.

The classic neurosurgical techniques were refined over the ensuing decades and were geared toward resecting the synostotic sutures in the hope that the "released" skull would reshape itself and continue to grow in a normal and symmetric fashion.[52] Strip craniectomy procedures were supposed to allow for creation of new suture lines at the site of the previous synostosis. With the realization that this goal was not achieved, attempts were made to surgically disassemble the involved cranial vault and then replace the pieces of calvaria as free grafts to shape the cranial vault. Problems with these methods included uncontrolled postoperative skull molding, resulting in reossification in dysmorphic configurations. In some other children, when extensive craniectomies were carried out, permanent skull defects remained.

After World War II, Gillies and Harrison reported experience with an extracranial Le Fort III osteotomy to improve the anterior projection of the midface in an adult with Crouzon syndrome.[53] The early enthusiasm for this technique later turned to discouragement when the patient's facial skeleton relapsed to its preoperative status.

In 1967, Tessier described a new (intracranial–cranial base) approach to the management of Crouzon syndrome.[54] His landmark presentation and publications were the beginning of modern craniofacial surgery.[55–63] To overcome the earlier problems encountered by Gillies and Harrison, Tessier developed an innovative basic surgical approach that included new locations for the Le Fort III osteotomy, a combined intracranial–extracranial (cranial base) approach, use of a coronal (skin) incision to expose the upper facial bones, and use of an autogenous bone graft. He also applied an external fixation device to help maintain bony stability until healing had occurred.

The concept of simultaneous suture release for craniosynostosis combined with cranial vault reshaping in infants was initially discussed by Rougerie and colleagues[64] and later refined by Hoffman and Mohr in 1976.[65] Whitaker and others proposed a more formal anterior cranial vault and orbital reshaping procedure for unilateral coronal synostosis in 1987,[66] and then Marchac and colleagues published their experience with the "floating forehead" technique for simultaneous suture release and anterior cranial vault and orbital reshaping to manage bilateral coronal synostosis in infancy.[32]

The widespread use of cranial bone as a graft option has virtually eliminated the need for rib and hip grafts when autogenous bone replacement is required in cranio-orbitozygomatic procedures. This represents another of Tessier's contributions to craniofacial surgery that has stood the test of time.

In 1968, Luhr introduced the use of small metal plates and screws to stabilize maxillofacial fractures and then osteotomies.[67] In current practice, the use of internal plate and screw fixation is the preferred form of stabilization for the three-dimensional reconstruction of multiple osteotomized bone segments and grafts. The development of resorbable plates and screws as a form of stable fixation continues to evolve as a fixation alternative, especially for use in growing bones and for immobilization of onlay bone grafts.[47] The reliability of resorbable fixation to withstand the compressive (relapse) forces after total midfacial advancement procedures and the normal loading forces of occlusion during the active bone healing phase leave it a less desirable fixation option for the craniofacial dysostosis patient.

More recently, the intraoperative placement of a distraction device as a method of achieving advancement of the midface in patients with severe forms of craniofacial hypoplasia has been added to the surgeon's armamentarium.[47] If used, distraction osteogenesis is not applied until after successful completion of standard osteotomies and disimpaction in the operating room. The distraction apparatus is either anchored to the "stable" skeleton internally or externally (through a "halo" head frame) and then to the palatal (intraoral) and infraorbital rims or zygomatic buttresses. Advancement of the "total midface" can then proceed. Once adequate (midface) advancement has been accomplished (on an outpatient basis) over a period of several weeks, the patient is generally returned to the operating room for stabilization and final reconstruction. The final reconstruction may require additional segmental osteotomies, bone grafting, or placement of plate and screw fixation. The "distraction approach" to the midface deformity is a labor-intensive, technique-specific, and relatively crude method of accomplishing horizontal advancement with difficulty in controlling the vertical dimension of the midface and without the ability to alter the transverse deformity or deficiency. In our opinion, the current level of distraction technology leaves it an adjunctive rather than primary technique. It is most useful when the midfacial hypoplasia is severe to the extent that conventional techniques cannot reliably allow the immediate (in the operating room) desired advancement and when complex vertical and transverse reconstruction is not required.

Philosophy Regarding Timing of Intervention

In considering the timing and type of intervention the experienced surgeon will take several biologic realities into account: the natural course of the malformation (ie, Is the dysmorphology associated with Crouzon syndrome progressively worsening or is it a nonprogressive craniofacial deformity?); the tendency toward growth restriction of an operated bone (esthetic unit) that has not yet reached maturity (ie, we know that operating on a palate of a child born with a cleft in infancy will cause scarring and later result in maxillary hypoplasia in a significant percentage of individuals); and the uncertain relationship between the underlying growing viscera (ie, brain or eyes) and the congenitally affected and surgically altered skeleton (ie, If the cranial vault is not surgically expanded by 1 year of life in a patient with multiple suture synostosis, will brain compression occur?).

In attempting to limit functional impairment and also achieve long-term ideal facial esthetics, an essential question the surgeon must ask is, "During the course of craniofacial development, does the operated-on facial skeletal of the child with craniofacial dysostosis tend to grow abnormally, resulting in further distortions and dysmorphology, or are the initial positive skeletal changes (achieved at operation) maintained during ongoing growth?" Unfortunately, the theory that craniofacial procedures carried out early in infancy will "unlock growth" has not been documented through the scientific method.[68–70]

Incision Placement

For exposure of the craniofacial skeleton above the Le Fort I level, the approach used is the coronal (skin) incision. This allows for a relatively camouflaged access to the anterior and posterior cranial vault, orbits, nasal dorsum, zygomas, upper maxilla, pterygoid fossa, and temporomandibular joints. For added cosmetic advantage, placement of the coronal incision more posteriorly on the scalp and with postauricular rather than preauricular extensions is useful. When exposure of the maxilla at the Le Fort I level is required, a circumvestibular maxillary intraoral incision is used. Unless complications occur that warrant unusual exposure, no other incisions are required for managing any aspect of the craniofacial dysostosis patient's reconstruction. These incisions (coronal [scalp] and maxillary [circumvestibular]) may be reopened as needed to further complete the patient's staged reconstruction.

Management of Cranial Vault Dead Space

The management of the dead space that results with cranial vault or cranial base expansion is critical to limiting complications. Dead space within the cranial vault after cranial expansion is managed by being gentle to the tissues, achieving good hemostasis, closure of tissue layers, placement of bone grafts, the stable fixation of osteotomy segments, and obliteration (of dead space) with soft tissue flaps or grafts when indicated.

Expansion of the cranial vault with forward advancement of the anterior cranial base, orbits, and midface results in both extradural (retrofrontal) dead space and a communication of the anterior fossa with the nasal cavity.[71] Dead space within the anterior cranial vault and the communication of the frontal fossa with the nasal cavity across the anterior skull base may result in hematoma formation, CSF leakage, infection, and fistula formation.[72,73] Management of this expanded space in the anterior cranial fossa following frontofacial or forehead advancement remains controversial. Relatively rapid filling of the expanded intracranial space by the frontal lobes has been documented in infants and young children when the expansion remains in a physiologic range.[71,74] This observation supports the conservative management of retrofrontal dead space in younger patients. More gradual and less complete filling is thought to occur in older children and adults. If so, this may be particularly troublesome when the anterior fossa dead space communicates directly with the nasal cavity. When possible, closing off the nasal cavity from the cranial fossa at the time of operation is preferred. Insertion of a pericranial flap can help to separate the cavities and at the same time obliterate dead space. The use of fibrin glue to seal the anterior cranial base also provides a temporary repair between the cavities, allowing time for the reepithelialization of the nasal mucosa.[75] When feasible, after midface advancement the anterior skull base is reconstructed (ie, bone grafts) to facilitate healing across the skull base to limit CSF leakage and prevent fistula formation. Until the torn nasopharyngeal mucosa heals, communication between the nasal cavity and cranial fossa is a potential for leakage (air, fluid, bacteria) and nasocranial fistula formation. To prevent this, postoperative endotracheal intubation may be extended for 3 to 5 days and bilateral nasopharyngeal airways may be placed after extubation. In addition, sinus precautions and restriction of nose blowing further limit reflux (nose to cranial fossa) of air and fluid during the postoperative period. All of these maneuvers are aimed at avoiding a pressure gradient and will facilitate sealing of the intracranial cavity from the upper aerodigestive tract. When anterior cranial vault reconstruction is performed and aerated frontal sinuses

are present, management of the sinus is by either cranialization or obliteration.

When a craniofacial dysostosis patient is to undergo intracranial volume expansion as part of the craniofacial procedure and they also require hydrocephalus management, the potential for problems increases. Complications may arise from excessive CSF drainage ("overshunting"). With overshunting there is decreased brain volume and dead space remains. Fronto-orbital advancement and cranial vault expansion procedures should be carefully staged with ventriculoperitoneal (VP) shunting procedures. Ultimately, the decision regarding the sequencing of shunting procedures is based on neurologic findings and the neurosurgeon's judgement. In a patient with a VP shunt in place before the surgery, careful neurosurgical evaluation, including CT scanning of the ventricular system, is carried out to confirm that the shunt is functioning appropriately.

Soft Tissue Management

A layered closure of the coronal incision (galea and skin) optimizes healing and limits scar widening. Resuspension of the midface periosteum to the temporalis fascia in a superior and posterior direction facilitates redraping of the soft tissues. Each lateral canthus should be adequately suspended or reattached in a superior–posterior direction to the lateral orbital rim. The use of chromic gut for closure of the scalp skin in children may be used to obviate the need for postoperative suture or staple removal.

Crouzon Syndrome

Primary Cranio-orbital Decompression: Reshaping in Infancy

The initial treatment for Crouzon syndrome generally requires bilateral coronal suture release and simultaneous anterior cranial vault and upper orbital osteotomies with reshaping and advancement (see Figure 46-1).[76–79] Our preference is to carry

this out when the child is 9 to 11 months of age unless clear signs of increased intracranial pressure are identified earlier in life (Figure 46-2). Reshaping of the upper three-quarters of the orbital rims and supraorbital ridges is geared toward decreasing the bitemporal and anterior cranial base width, with simultaneous horizontal advancement to increase the A-P dimension. This also increases the depth of the upper orbits, with some improvement of eye proptosis. The overlying forehead is then reconstructed according to morphologic needs. A degree of overcorrection is preferred at the level of the supraorbital ridge when the procedure is carried out in infancy. In our opinion, by allowing additional growth to occur (waiting until the child is 9 to 11 months old), the reconstructed cranial vault and upper orbital shape is better maintained with less need for repeat craniotomy procedures but without risking compression of the underlying brain.

The goals at this stage are to provide increased intracranial space in the anterior cranial vault for the brain; to increase the orbital volume, which allows the eyes to be positioned more normally for better protection from exposure; and to improve the morphology of the forehead and upper orbits.

A postauricular coronal (scalp) incision is made, and the anterior scalp flap is elevated along with the temporalis muscle in the subperiosteal plane. Bilateral circumferential periorbital dissection follows, with detachment of the lateral canthi, but with preservation of the medial canthi and nasolacrimal apparatus to the medial orbital walls. The subperiosteal dissection is continued down the lateral and infraorbital rims to include the anterior aspect of the maxilla and zygomatic buttress. The neurosurgeon then completes the craniotomy to remove the dysmorphic anterior cranial vault. With protection of the frontal and temporal lobes of the brain (remaining anterior to each olfactory bulb), safe direct

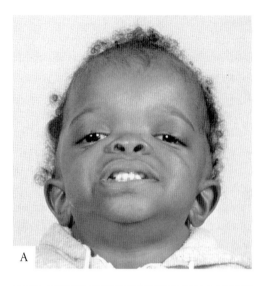

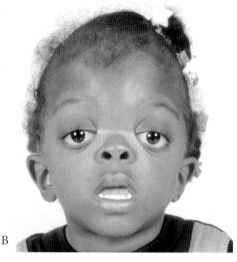

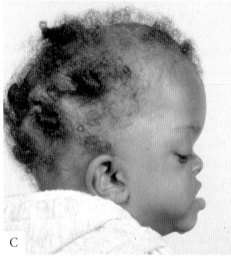

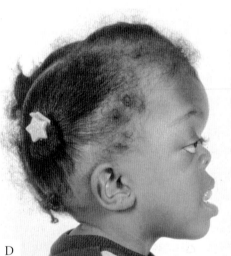

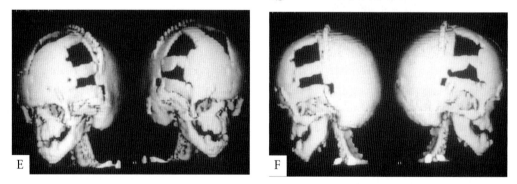

FIGURE **46-2**   *An 18-month-old girl with brachycephaly and midface deficiency with a mild degree of papilledema was referred for evaluation. She was found to have bilateral coronal synostosis and midface hypoplasia without extremity anomalies. The diagnosis of Crouzon syndrome was made. She underwent cranio-orbital reshaping (see Figure 46-1). Several months later, a ventriculoperitoneal shunt was placed for management of hydrocephalus. Further staged reconstruction will include a total midface advancement procedure later in childhood followed by orthodontic treatment and orthognathic surgery in the early teenage years. A, Frontal view before surgery. B, Frontal view at 3 years of age, 1.5 years after undergoing cranio-orbital decompression and reshaping. C, Profile view before surgery. D, Profile view at 3 years of age, 1.5 years after undergoing first-stage cranio-orbital decompression and reshaping. E and F, Three-dimensional CT scan views of craniofacial skeleton, just 1 week after cranio-orbital reshaping with advancement. Reproduced with permission from Posnick JC. Crouzon syndrome: evaluation and staging of reconstruction. In: Posnick JC, editor. Craniofacial and maxillofacial surgery in children and young adults. Philadelphia (PA): W.B. Saunders Co.; 2000. p. 275.*

visualization of the anterior cranial base and orbits is possible at the time of orbital osteotomies.

The orbital osteotomies are then completed across the orbital roof and superior aspect of the medial orbital walls, laterally through the lateral orbital walls and inferiorly just into the inferior orbital fissures. The three-quarter orbital osteotomy units, with their tenon extensions, are removed from the field. The orbital units are reshaped and reinset into a preferred position. Orbital depth is thereby increased, and global proptosis is reduced. Fixation is generally achieved with 28-gauge interosseous wires or suture at each infraorbital rim and with plates and titanium or resorbable screws at the tenon extensions and frontonasal regions.

The removed calvaria is cut into segments, which are placed individually to achieve a more normally configured anterior cranial vault. The goal of reshaping is to narrow the anterior cranial base and orbital width slightly and provide more forward projection and overall normal morphology.

Repeat Craniotomy for Additional Cranial Vault Expansion and Reshaping in Young Children

After the initial suture release, decompression, and reshaping are carried out during infancy, the child is observed clinically at intervals by the craniofacial surgeon, pediatric neurosurgeon, pediatric ophthalmologist, and developmental specialist and undergoes interval CT scanning. Should signs of increased ICP develop, urgent brain decompression with cranial vault expansion and reshaping is performed.[47] When increased ICP is suspected, the location of brain compression influences for which region of the skull further expansion and reshaping is planned.

If the brain compression is judged to be anterior, then further anterior cranial vault and upper orbital osteotomies with reshap-

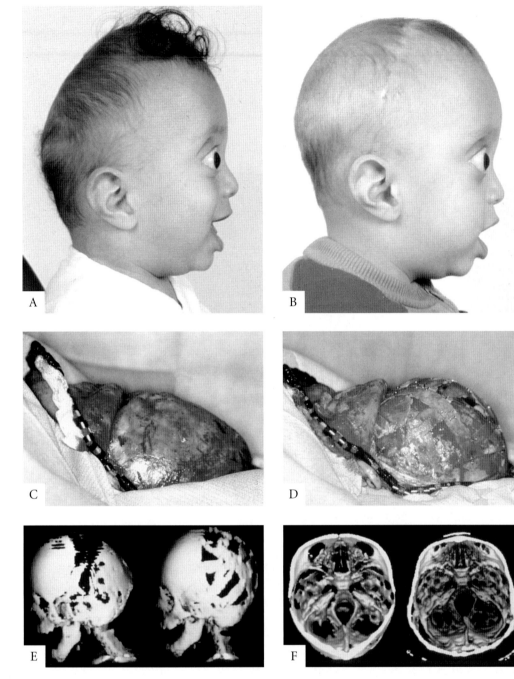

FIGURE 46-3 *A child with Crouzon syndrome is shown at 10 months of age. His deformities are characterized by mild bilateral coronal and marked bilateral lambdoid synostosis in combination with midface deficiency. He has diminished intracranial volume, resulting in brain compression. The orbits are shallow with resulting eye proptosis, and the midface is deficient with malocclusion. He is shown before and after undergoing posterior cranial vault decompression and reshaping to expand the intracranial volume. He later underwent placement of a ventriculoperitoneal shunt for management of hydrocephalus. He will require a total midface advancement (monobloc) with further anterior cranial vault reshaping after 5 years of age. This will be followed by orthognathic surgery in combination with orthodontic treatment in the teenage years. A, Profile view before surgery. B, Profile view after posterior cranial vault reconstruction. C, Intraoperative lateral view of cranial vault (patient in prone position) as seen with posterior scalp flap elevated. D, Same intraoperative view after posterior cranial vault decompression, reshaping, and fixation of bone segments with microplates and screws. E, Comparison of three-dimensional CT scan views before and after reconstruction. F, Comparison of three-dimensional CT scan views of cranial base before and after reconstruction. Reproduced with permission from Posnick JC. The craniofacial dysostosis syndromes: secondary management of craniofacial disorders. Clin Plast Surg 1997;24:429.*

ing and advancement are carried out. The technique is similar to that described previously.[47,78] If the problem is posterior compression, expansion of the posterior cranial vault, with the patient in the prone position, is required (Figure 46-3).

The "repeat" craniotomy carried out for further decompression and reshaping in the child with Crouzon syndrome is often complicated by brittle cortical bone (which lacks a diploic space and contains sharp spicules piercing the dura), the presence of previously placed fixation devices in the operative field (eg, Silastic sheeting, metal clips, stainless steel wires, plates, and screws), and convoluted thin dura compressed against (or herniated into) the inner table of the skull. All of these issues result in a greater potential for dural tears during the calvarectomy than would normally occur during the primary procedure. A greater potential for morbidity should be anticipated when re-elevating the scalp flap, dissecting the dura free of the inner table of the skull and cranial base, and then removing the cranial vault bone.

Management of "Total Midface" Deformity in Childhood

The type of osteotomies selected to manage the "total midface" deficiency or deformity and residual cranial vault dysplasia should depend on the extent and location of the presenting dysmorphology rather than on a fixed approach to the midface malformation.[47,53–57,78–84] The selection of a monobloc (with or without additional orbital segmentation), facial bipartition (with or without additional orbital segmental osteotomies), or Le Fort III osteotomy to manage the basic horizontal, transverse, and vertical orbital, and upper midface deficiencies or deformities in a patient with Crouzon syndrome depends on the patient's presenting midface and anterior cranial vault morphology. The observed dysmorphology is dependent on the original malformation, the previous procedures carried out, and the effects of ongoing growth (Figures 46-4 and 46-5).

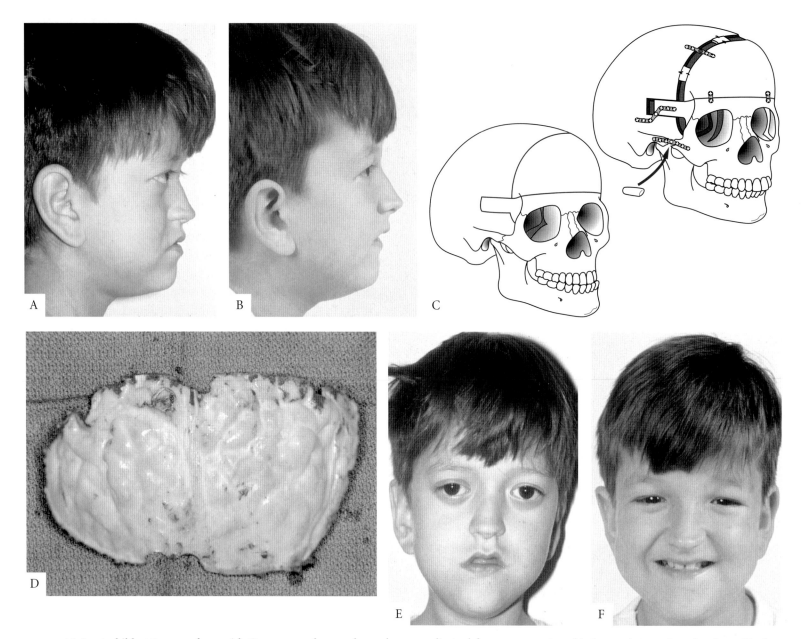

FIGURE **46-4**   *A child at 8 years of age with Crouzon syndrome who underwent a limited first-stage cranio-orbital procedure at 6 weeks of age. He then underwent anterior cranial vault and monobloc (orbits and midface) osteotomies with advancement. A, Profile view before monobloc procedure. B, Profile view after reconstruction. C, Craniofacial morphology before and after anterior cranial vault and monobloc osteotomies with advancement as carried out. Osteotomy locations indicated. Stabilization with cranial bone grafts and miniplates and screws. D, View of inner surface of frontal bones after bifrontal craniotomy. Compression of brain against inner table has resulted in resorption of the inner skull. This is an indication of long-standing increased intracranial pressure. E, Frontal view before surgery. F, Frontal view after reconstruction.* (CONTINUED ON NEXT PAGE)

When evaluating the upper and midface in a child born with Crouzon syndrome, if the supraorbital ridge is in good position when viewed from the sagittal plane (the depth of the upper orbits is adequate), the midface and forehead have a normal arc of rotation in the transverse plane (not concave), and the root of the nose is of normal width (minimal orbital hypertelorism),

there is little need to reconstruct this region (the forehead and upper orbits) any further. In such patients, the basic residual midface deformity is in the lower half of the orbits, zygomatic buttress, and maxilla. If so, the deformity may be effectively managed using an extracranial Le Fort III osteotomy.

If the supraorbital ridges, anterior cranial base, zygomas, nose, lower orbits, and

maxilla all remain deficient in the sagittal plane (horizontal retrusion), then a monobloc osteotomy is indicated (see Figures 46-4 and 46-5). In these patients, the forehead is generally flat and retruded and will also require reshaping and advancement. If upper midface hypertelorism (increased transverse width) and midface flattening (horizontal retrusion) with loss

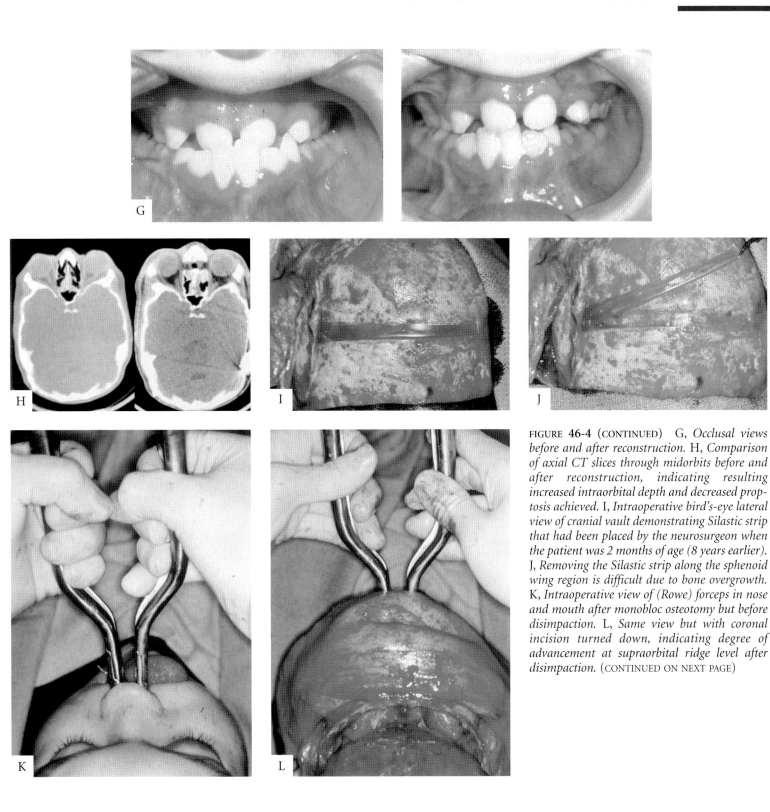

FIGURE 46-4 (CONTINUED) *G, Occlusal views before and after reconstruction. H, Comparison of axial CT slices through midorbits before and after reconstruction, indicating resulting increased intraorbital depth and decreased proptosis achieved. I, Intraoperative bird's-eye lateral view of cranial vault demonstrating Silastic strip that had been placed by the neurosurgeon when the patient was 2 months of age (8 years earlier). J, Removing the Silastic strip along the sphenoid wing region is difficult due to bone overgrowth. K, Intraoperative view of (Rowe) forceps in nose and mouth after monobloc osteotomy but before disimpaction. L, Same view but with coronal incision turned down, indicating degree of advancement at supraorbital ridge level after disimpaction.* (CONTINUED ON NEXT PAGE)

of the normal facial curvature (concave arc) are also present, then the monobloc unit is split vertically in the midline (facial bipartition), a wedge of interorbital (nasal and ethmoidal) bone is removed, and the orbits and zygomas are repositioned medially while the maxilla at the palatal level is widened. The facial bipartition is rarely required in Crouzon syndrome, but the monobloc is. When a monobloc or facial bipartition osteotomy is carried out as the "total midface" procedure, additional segmentation of the upper and lateral orbits for reconstruction may also be required to normalize the morphology of the orbital esthetic units.

For most patients, a surgeon's attempt to simultaneously adjust the orbits and idealize the occlusion using the Le Fort III, monobloc, or facial bipartition osteotomy in isolation, without completing a separate

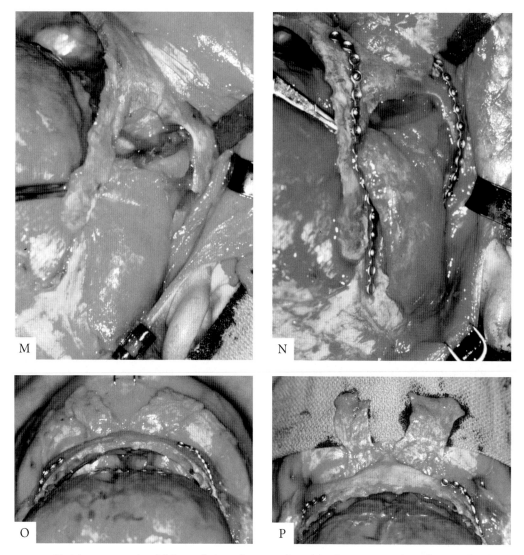

FIGURE 46-4 (CONTINUED)   *M, Lateral view of zygomatic arch and tenon extension of supraorbital rim after monobloc advancement just before miniplate fixation. N, Same view after miniplate fixation of zygomatic arch and tenon extension. O, Bird's-eye view of stabilized monobloc unit after advancement. There is increased intracranial volume (dead space) in the anterior cranial vault for brain expansion. P, Same view with elevated pericranial flaps, which will be turned in to close the opening between the nose and the anterior cranial base. A, B, D–P reproduced with permission and C adapted from Posnick JC.[98]*

Le Fort I osteotomy, is an error in judgment. The degree of horizontal deficiency observed at the orbits and maxillary dentition is rarely uniform. This further segmentation of the midface complex at the Le Fort I level is required to establish normal proportions. If a Le Fort I separation of the total midface complex is not carried out and the surgeon attempts to achieve a positive overbite and overjet at the incisor teeth, over-advancement of the orbits with enophthalmos will occur. The Le Fort I osteotomy is generally not performed at

the time of the total midface procedure. This will await skeletal maturity and then be combined with orthodontic treatment. Until then, an Angle Class III malocclusion will remain.

A major esthetic problem specific to the Le Fort III osteotomy when its indications are less than ideal is the creation of irregular step-offs in the lateral orbital rims. This will occur when even a moderate (Le Fort III) advancement is carried out. These lateral orbital step-offs are unattractive and are visible to the casual observ-

er at conversational distance. Surgical modification performed later is difficult, often with less than ideal esthetic results. Another problem with the Le Fort III osteotomy is the difficulty in judging an ideal orbital depth. A frequent result is either residual proptosis or enophthalmos. Simultaneous correction of orbital hypertelorism or correction of a midface arc-of-rotation problem is not possible with the Le Fort III procedure. Excessive lengthening of the nose, accompanied by flattening of the nasofrontal angle, will also occur if the Le Fort III osteotomy is selected when the skeletal morphology favors a monobloc or facial bipartition procedure. It is not possible to later correct the surgically created vertical elongation of the nose.

Final reconstruction, as discussed above, of the cranial vault deformities and orbital dystopia in Crouzon syndrome can be managed in patients as young as 5 to 7 years of age.[47] By this age, the cranial vault and orbits normally attain approximately 85 to 90% of their adult size.[43] When the upper midface and final cranial vault procedure is carried out at or after this age, the reconstructive objectives are to approximate adult dimensions in the cranio-orbitozygomatic region, with the expectation of a stable result (no longer influenced by growth) once healing has occurred (see Figure 46-4). Psychosocial considerations also support the upper midface and final cranial vault procedure taking place in patients 5 to 7 years of age. When the procedure is carried out at this age, the child may enter the first grade with an opportunity for satisfactory self-esteem. Routine orthognathic surgery will be necessary at the time of skeletal maturity to achieve an ideal occlusion, facial profile, and smile.

Orthognathic Procedures for Definitive Occlusal and Lower Facial Esthetic Reconstruction

Although the mandible has a normal basic growth potential in Crouzon syndrome, the maxilla does not. An Angle Class III

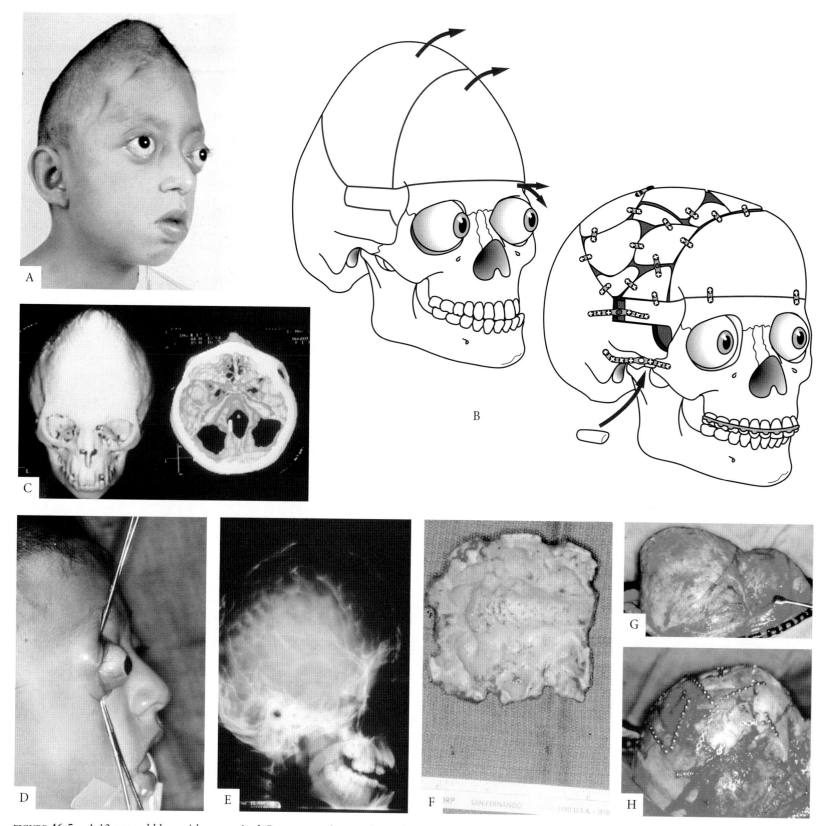

FIGURE 46-5 *A 12-year-old boy with unrepaired Crouzon syndrome who underwent total cranial vault and monobloc osteotomies with reshaping and advancement. A, Oblique view prior to surgery. B, The patient's craniofacial morphology before surgery. Osteotomy locations indicated. A second illustration after osteotomies completed with advancement, reshaping, and fixation. C, Three-dimensional CT scan views of cranial vault and cranial base prior to surgery. D, Intraoperative view with forceps placed at orbital rims indicating extent of proptosis. E, Lateral skull radiograph with "fingerprinting" indicating long-standing increased ICP. F, Inner table internal side of frontal bone indicating compression of brain against inner table of skull. G, Intraoperative lateral view of cranial vault and orbits through coronal incision before osteotomies. H, Same view after osteotomies, reshaping and stabilization of bone segments with miniplates and screws.*

(CONTINUED ON NEXT PAGE)

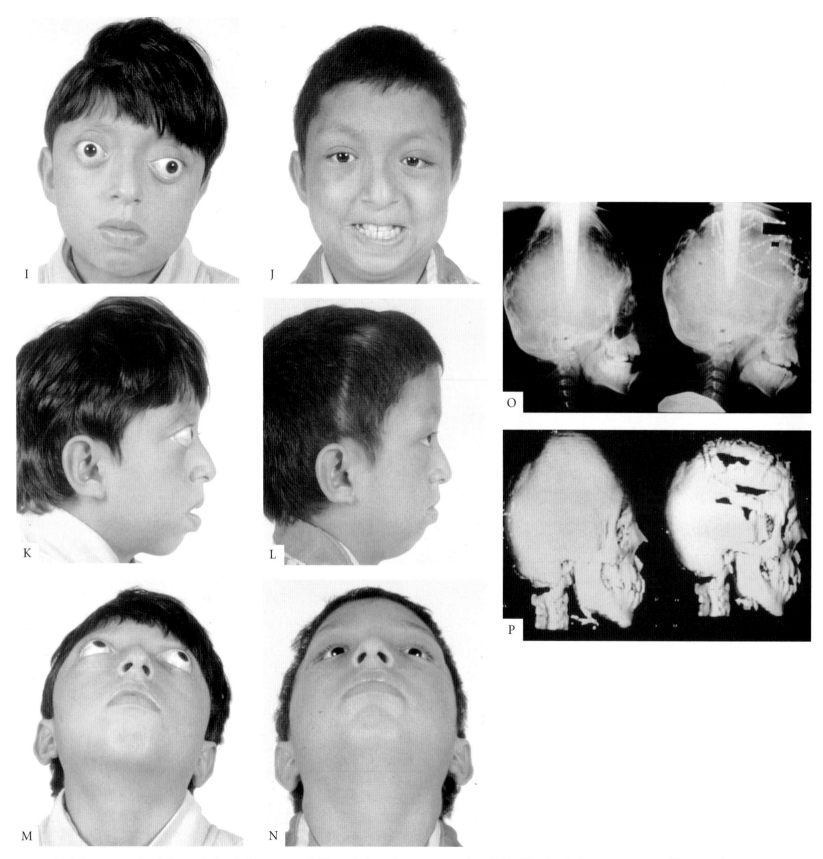

FIGURE 46-5 (CONTINUED)   I, *Frontal view before surgery.* J, *Frontal view after reconstruction.* K, *Profile view before surgery.* L, *Profile view after reconstruction.* M, *Worm's-eye view before surgery.* N, *Worm's-eye view after reconstruction.* O, *Comparison of lateral cephalometric radiographs before and after reconstruction.* P, *Comparison of three-dimensional CT scan views before and after reconstruction.* A, C–P reproduced with permission and B adapted from Posnick JC.[98]

malocclusion, resulting from maxillary retrusion, with anterior open bite often results. A Le Fort I osteotomy to allow for horizontal advancement, transverse widening, and vertical adjustment is generally required in combination with an osteoplastic genioplasty (vertical reduction and horizontal advancement) to further correct the lower face deformity. Secondary deformities of the mandible should be simultaneously corrected through sagittal split osteotomies. The elective orthognathic surgery is carried out in conjunction with orthodontic treatment planned for completion at the time of early skeletal maturity (approximately 13 to 15 years in girls and 15 to 17 years in boys) (Figure 46-6).

Apert Syndrome

Apert syndrome has previously been classified on the basis of its clinical findings.[85,86] Postmortem histologic and radiographic studies suggest that skeletal deficiencies in the patient with Apert syndrome result from a cartilage dysplasia at the cranial base, leading to premature fusion of the midline sutures from the occiput to the anterior nasal septum.[87–91] In addition, a component of the syndrome is four-limb symmetry complex syndactylies of the hands and feet (Figure 46-7). Fusion and malformation of other joints, including the elbows and shoulders, often occur. The soft tissue envelope also varies from that in Crouzon syndrome, with a greater downward slant to the canthi lateral and a distinctive, S-shaped upper eyelid ptosis. The quality of the skin often varies from normal, with acne and hyperhidrosis being prominent features. At the molecular level, one of two fibroblast growth factor receptor 2 (*FGFR2*) mutations involving amino acids (Ser252Trp and Pro253Arg) have been found to cause Apert syndrome in nearly all patients studied.[92–94]

Primary Cranio-orbital Decompression: Reshaping in Infancy

The initial craniofacial procedure for Apert syndrome generally requires bilater-al coronal suture release and anterior cranial vault and upper three-quarter orbital osteotomies to expand the anterior cranial vault and reshape the upper orbits and forehead (see Figure 46-1).[95,96] Our preference is to carry this out when the child is 9 to 11 months of age, unless signs of increased intracranial pressure are identified earlier in life. The main goals at this stage are to decompress the brain and provide increased space for it in the anterior cranial vault and to increase the orbital volume to decrease globe protrusion. The fronto-orbital surgical technique is similar to that described for Crouzon syndrome (Figure 46-8).

Further Craniotomy for Additional Cranial Vault Expansion and Reshaping in Young Children

As described for Crouzon syndrome, after the initial suture release, decompression, and reshaping carried out during infancy, the child is observed clinically at intervals by the craniofacial surgeon, pediatric neurosurgeon, pediatric ophthalmologist, and developmental pediatrician and undergoes interval CT scanning.[76,97,98] Should signs of increased ICP develop, further decompression with reshaping of the cranial vault to expand the intracranial volume is performed (Figure 46-9). In Apert syndrome the posterior cranial vault more commonly requires expansion. The technique is similar to that described for Crouzon syndrome.

Management of the "Total Midface" Deformity in Childhood

In Apert syndrome, for almost all patients, facial bipartition osteotomies combined with further cranial vault reshaping permit a more complete correction of the abnormal craniofacial skeleton than can be achieved through other midface procedure options (ie, monobloc or Le Fort III osteotomies). When using the facial bipartition approach, a more normal arc of rotation of the midface complex is achieved with the midline split. This further reduces the stigmata of the preoperative "flat, wide, and retrusive" facial appearance. The facial bipartition also allows the orbits and zygomatic buttresses as units to shift to the midline (correction of hypertelorism) while the maxillary arch is simultaneously widened. Horizontal advancement of the reassembled midface complex is then achieved to normalize the orbital depth and zygomatic length. The forehead is generally flat, tall, and retruded, with a constricting band just above the supraorbital ridge, giving the impression of bitemporal narrowing. Reshaping of the anterior cranial vault is simultaneously carried out (see Figures 46-8–46-10). See also Figure 46-9H for preoperative craniofacial morphology and planned and completed osteotomies and reshaping. Note that stabilization was achieved with cranial bone grafts and plate and screw fixation. A Le Fort III osteotomy is virtually never adequate for an ideal correction of the residual upper and midface deformity of Apert syndrome.

Orthognathic Procedures for Definitive Occlusal and Lower Facial Esthetic Reconstruction

The mandible has normal basic growth potential in Apert syndrome. The extent of maxillary hypoplasia will result in an Angle Class III malocclusion with severe anterior open-bite deformity. A Le Fort I osteotomy is required to allow for horizontal advancement, transverse widening, and vertical adjustment in combination with an osteoplastic genioplasty to vertically reduce and horizontally advance the chin, often combined with bilateral sagittal split osteotomies of the mandible. The elective orthognathic surgery is carried out in conjunction with detailed orthodontic treatment planned for completion at the time of early skeletal maturity (approximately 13 to 15 years in girls and 15 to 17 years in boys).

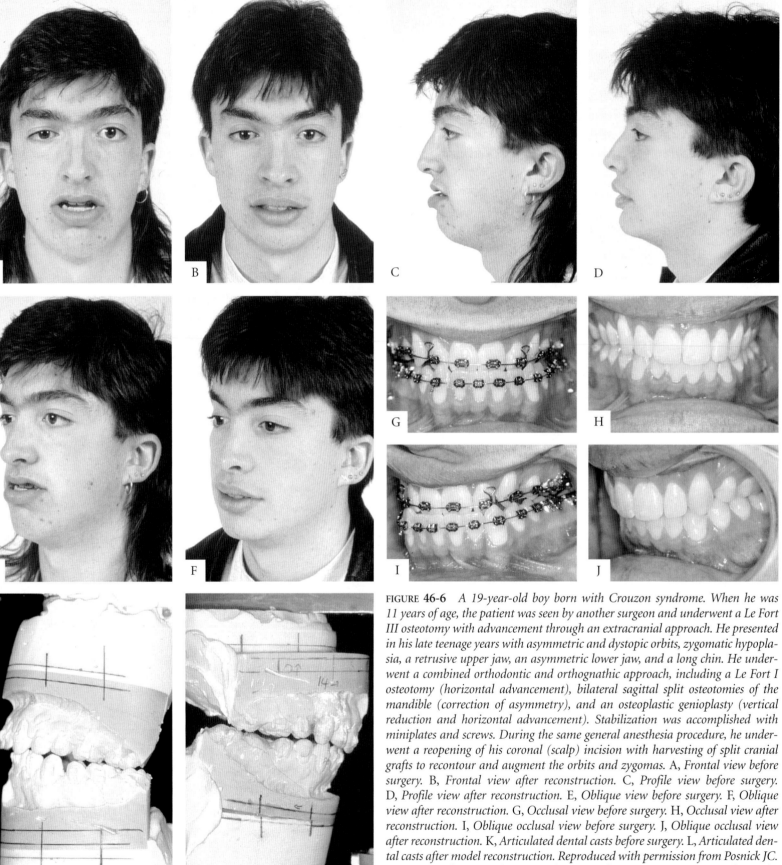

FIGURE 46-6 *A 19-year-old boy born with Crouzon syndrome. When he was 11 years of age, the patient was seen by another surgeon and underwent a Le Fort III osteotomy with advancement through an extracranial approach. He presented in his late teenage years with asymmetric and dystopic orbits, zygomatic hypoplasia, a retrusive upper jaw, an asymmetric lower jaw, and a long chin. He underwent a combined orthodontic and orthognathic approach, including a Le Fort I osteotomy (horizontal advancement), bilateral sagittal split osteotomies of the mandible (correction of asymmetry), and an osteoplastic genioplasty (vertical reduction and horizontal advancement). Stabilization was accomplished with miniplates and screws. During the same general anesthesia procedure, he underwent a reopening of his coronal (scalp) incision with harvesting of split cranial grafts to recontour and augment the orbits and zygomas. A, Frontal view before surgery. B, Frontal view after reconstruction. C, Profile view before surgery. D, Profile view after reconstruction. E, Oblique view before surgery. F, Oblique view after reconstruction. G, Occlusal view before surgery. H, Occlusal view after reconstruction. I, Oblique occlusal view before surgery. J, Oblique occlusal view after surgery. K, Articulated dental casts before surgery. L, Articulated dental casts after model reconstruction. Reproduced with permission from Posnick JC. Crouzon syndrome: evaluation and staging of reconstruction. In: Posnick JC, editor. Craniofacial and maxillofacial surgery in children and young adults. Philadelphia (PA): W.B. Saunders Co.; 2000. p. 299–300.*

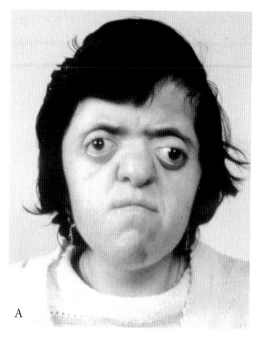

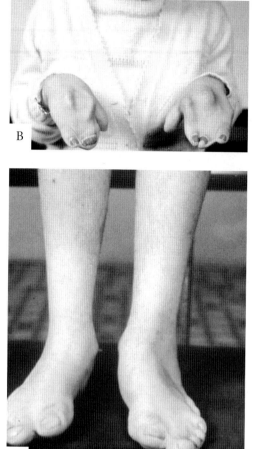

FIGURE 46-7 *A 28-year-old woman born with Apert syndrome. She was raised in Athens, Greece, and was unable to undergo craniofacial or extremity reconstruction. A, Frontal view. B, View of hands. C, View of feet. Reproduced with permission from Posnick JC. Apert syndrome: evaluation and staging of reconstruction. In: Posnick JC, editor. Craniofacial and maxillofacial surgery in children and young adults. Philadelphia (PA): W.B. Saunders Co.; 2000. p. 308.*

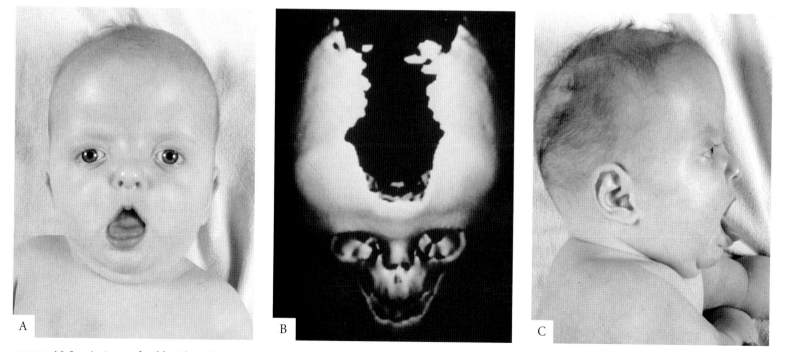

FIGURE 46-8 *A 6-month-old girl with Apert syndrome underwent anterior cranial vault and three-quarter orbital osteotomies with reshaping as described (see Figure 46-1). A, Frontal view before surgery. B, Three-dimensional CT scan view of cranial vault before surgery. C, Profile view before surgery.* (CONTINUED ON NEXT PAGE)

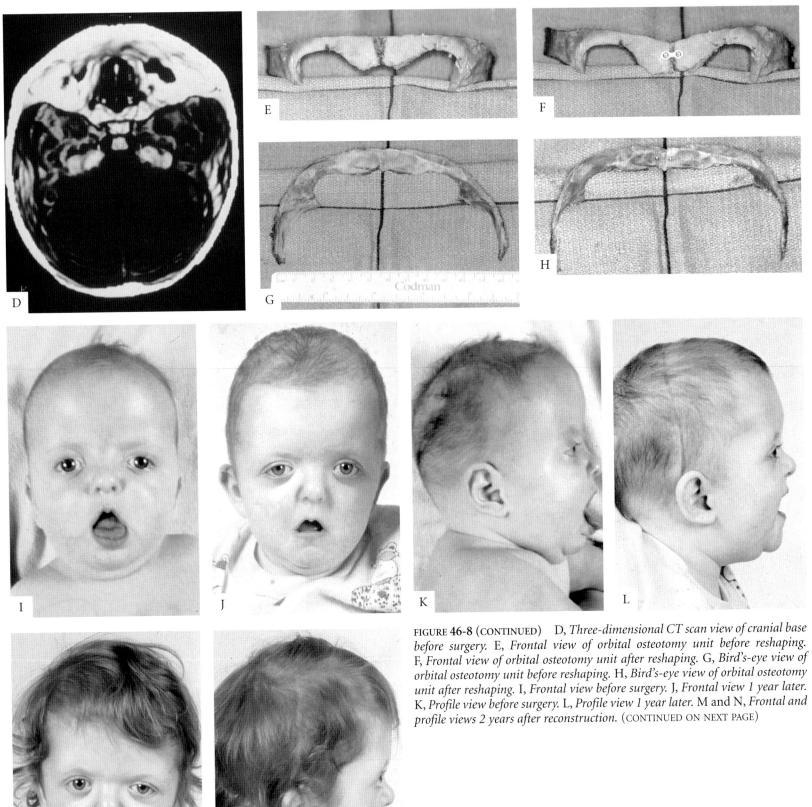

FIGURE 46-8 (CONTINUED) D, *Three-dimensional CT scan view of cranial base before surgery.* E, *Frontal view of orbital osteotomy unit before reshaping.* F, *Frontal view of orbital osteotomy unit after reshaping.* G, *Bird's-eye view of orbital osteotomy unit before reshaping.* H, *Bird's-eye view of orbital osteotomy unit after reshaping.* I, *Frontal view before surgery.* J, *Frontal view 1 year later.* K, *Profile view before surgery.* L, *Profile view 1 year later.* M and N, *Frontal and profile views 2 years after reconstruction.* (CONTINUED ON NEXT PAGE)

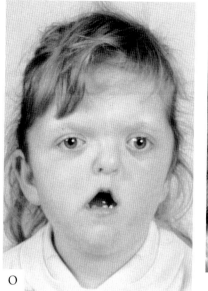
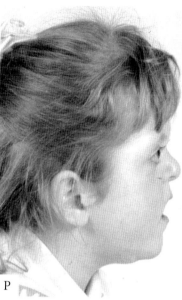
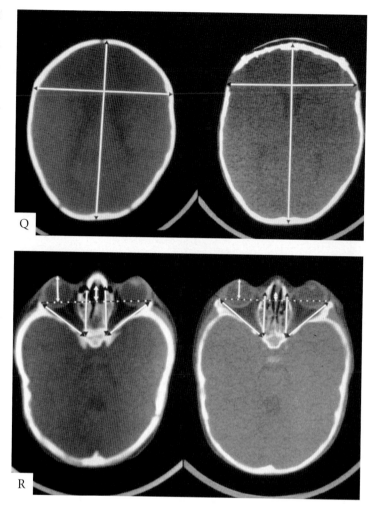

FIGURE 46-8 (CONTINUED)   *O and P, Frontal and profile views 3 years after first stage cranio-orbital reshaping; further staged reconstruction is required. Q, Comparison of standard axial CT slices through cranial vault before and 1 year after cranio-orbital reshaping. The cranial vault length (cephalic length) has increased from 115 to 158 mm. The anterior cranial vault width (intercoronal distance) has remained stable at 115 mm. R, Comparison of standard axial CT slices through midorbits before and 1 year after reconstruction. Marked globe protrusion of 16 mm has increased to 17 mm 1 year later. The anterior interorbital distance diminished from 29 to 25 mm, which still represented 137% of the age-matched control value. (Magnification of the individual CT scan images was not controlled for.) Reproduced with permission from Posnick JC et al.*[95]

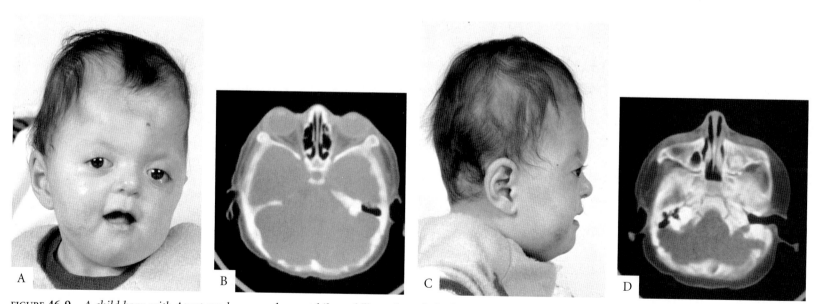

FIGURE 46-9   *A child born with Apert syndrome underwent bilateral "lateral canthal advancement" procedures when she was 6 weeks of age, carried out by the neurosurgeon working independently. At 18 months of age, she returned with turricephaly and a constricted anterior cranial vault requiring further cranio-orbital decompression and reshaping. At 5 years of age, she underwent anterior cranial vault and facial bipartition osteotomies with reshaping. As part of her staged reconstruction, she will require orthognathic surgery and orthodontic treatment planned for the teenage years. A, Frontal view at 8 months of age after lateral canthal advancement procedure with residual deformity. B, Axial-sliced CT scan through midorbits indicating dystopia, hypertelorism, and proptosis. C, Lateral view at 8 months of age. D, Axial-sliced CT scan through zygomatic arches indicating midface deficiency.* (CONTINUED ON NEXT PAGE)

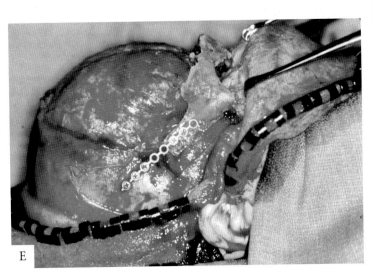

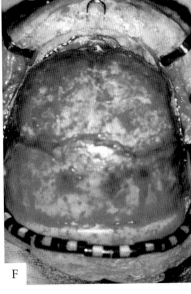

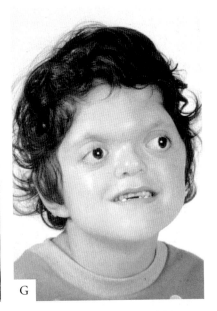

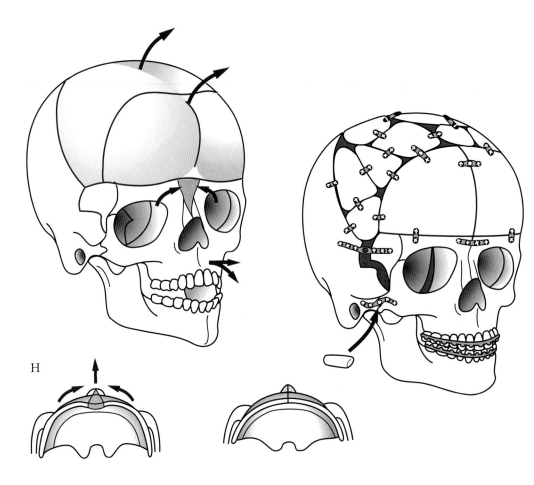

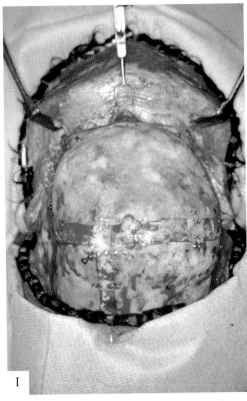

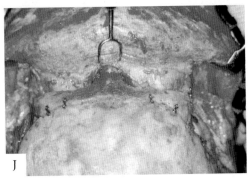

FIGURE 46-9 (CONTINUED)   E and F, *Lateral and bird's-eye view of cranio-orbital region after three-quarter orbital osteotomies and reshaping and anterior advancement.* G, *Frontal view at 5 years of age just prior to further anterior cranial vault and facial bipartition osteotomies.* H, *Craniofacial morphology with planned and completed osteotomies and reconstruction.* I and J, *Bird's-eye view of cranial vault and close-up view of upper orbits after osteotomies with reshaping.* (CONTINUED ON NEXT PAGE)

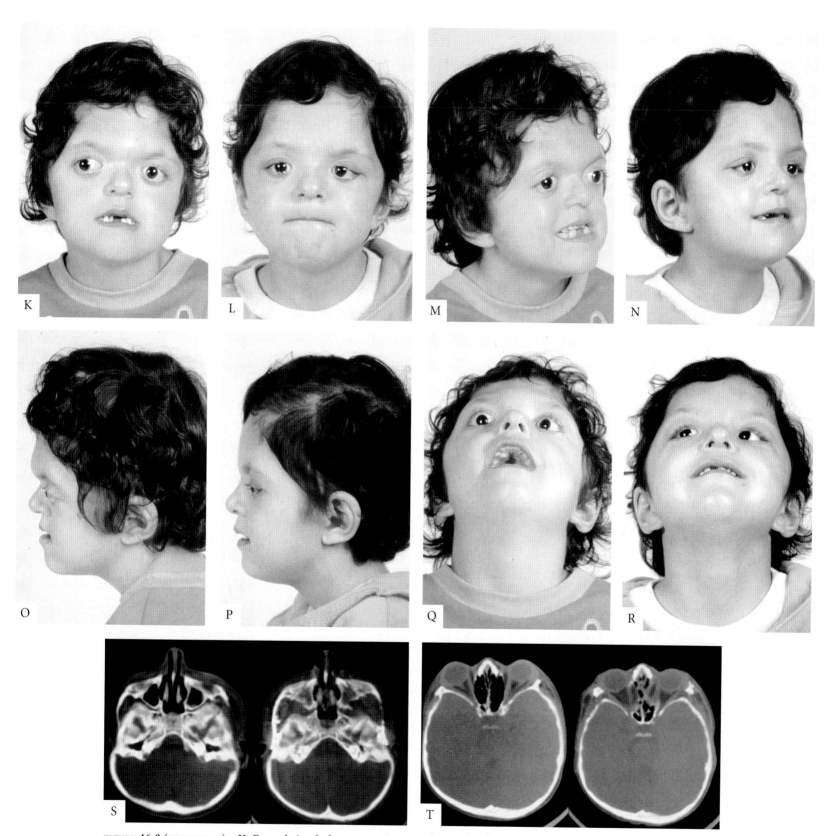

FIGURE 46-9 (CONTINUED)   K, *Frontal view before surgery.* L, *Frontal view after facial bipartition reconstruction.* M, *Oblique view before surgery.* N, *Oblique view after reconstruction.* O, *Profile view before surgery.* P, *Profile view after reconstruction.* Q, *Worm's-eye view before surgery.* R, *Worm's-eye view after reconstruction.* S, *Comparison of axial-sliced CT scans through zygomas before and after reconstruction, indicating a normalization of zygomatic arch length.* T, *Axial-sliced CT scan views through midorbits before and after reconstruction, indicating correction of orbital hyperteleorism and proptosis.* (CONTINUED ON NEXT PAGE)

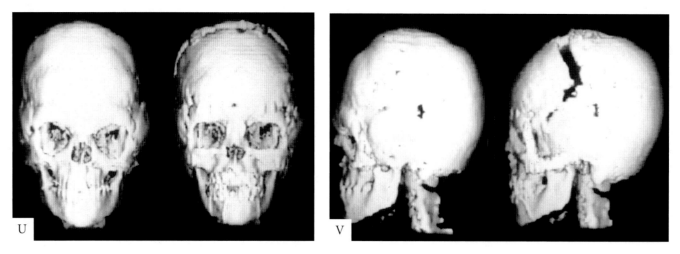

FIGURE **46-9** (CONTINUED) U and V, *Comparison of three-dimensional CT scan views of craniofacial region before and after reconstruction, including improved morphology of orbits. A–G, I–V reproduced with permission, and H adapted from Posnick JC. Apert syndrome: evaluation and staging of reconstruction. In: Posnick JC, editor. Craniofacial and maxillofacial surgery in children and young adults. Philadelphia (PA): W.B. Saunders Co.; 2000. p. 316.*

Pfeiffer Syndrome

In 1964, Pfeiffer described a syndrome consisting of craniosynostosis, broad thumbs, broad great toes, and occasionally partial soft tissue syndactyly of the hands.[99] This syndrome is known to have an autosomal dominant inheritance pattern with complete penetrance documented in all recorded two- and three-generation pedigrees.[100] Variable expressivity of the craniofacial and extremity findings is common (Figures 46-11 and 46-12). Although some authors have found clinical similarities in certain patients with Pfeiffer syndrome, Crouzon syndrome, and Jackson-Weiss syndrome, the three disorders are nosologically distinct.[47,101] According to Cohen, the phenotypes of the three conditions do not correlate well with the known molecular findings.[102] Patients with these three syndromes may have similar or even identical mutations in exon B of *FGFR2*, yet they breed true within families, an observation that is as yet unexplained by the molecular findings.[102,103]

Current thinking suggests that Pfeiffer syndrome is heterogeneous because it is caused by a single recurring mutation (Pro252Arg) of *FGFR1* and by several different mutations affecting *FGFR2*.[104,105]

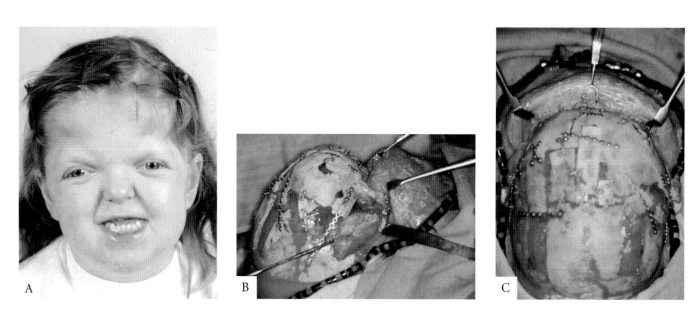

FIGURE **46-10** *A 5-year-old girl with Apert syndrome who underwent decompression and forehead and upper orbital reshaping at 6 months of age. She then presented to us with residual deformity requiring cranial vault and facial bipartition osteotomies with reshaping. She will require orthognathic surgery and orthodontic treatment later in the teenage years to complete her reconstruction. A, Frontal view before facial bipartition surgery. B, Intraoperative lateral view of cranial vault and orbits through coronal incision after reshaping. C, Bird's-eye view of cranial vault after osteotomies and reshaping and fixation of bone segments.* (CONTINUED ON NEXT PAGE)

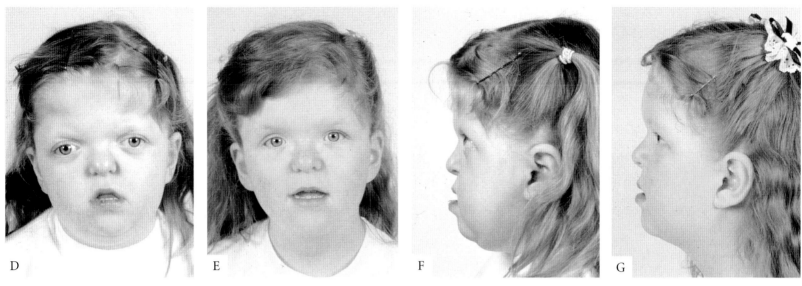

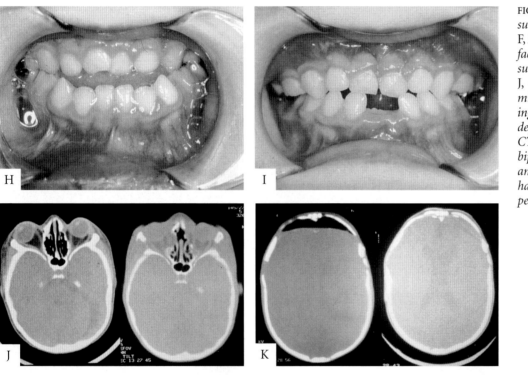

FIGURE **46-10** (CONTINUED)   D, *Frontal view before surgery. E, Frontal view 2 years after reconstruction. F, Profile view before surgery. G, Profile view 2 years after facial bipartition reconstruction. H, Occlusal view before surgery. I, Occlusal view 6 months after reconstruction. J, Comparison of axial-sliced CT scan views through midorbits before and after reconstruction, demonstrating improvement in orbital hypertelorism and orbital depth with diminished eye proptosis. K, Standard axial CT scan slices through cranial vault 1 week after facial bipartition (note dead space in the retrofrontal region), and at 1 year (notice that initial retrofrontal dead space has been resolved by brain expansion). Reproduced with permission from Posnick JC.[97]*

Cohen has reviewed the literature and further subgrouped Pfeiffer syndrome according to clinical features, associated low-frequency anomalies, and outcome. According to Cohen, Type I corresponds to the classic Pfeiffer syndrome and is associated with satisfactory prognosis. The Type II subgroup is associated with the cloverleaf skull anomaly while Type III is not. Both Types II and III have a less favorable outcome, with frequent death in infancy. The Type I variant frequently presents with bicoronal craniosynostosis and midface involvement. The longitudinal evaluation and staging of reconstruction depend on individual variations but is similar to that described for Crouzon syndrome.

Carpenter Syndrome

Carpenter syndrome is characterized by craniosynostosis often associated with preaxial polysyndactyly of the feet, short fingers with clinodactyly, and variable soft tissue syndactyly, sometimes postaxial ply- dactyly, and other anomalies such as congenital heart defects, short stature, obesity, and mental deficiency.[24] It was first described by Carpenter in 1901 and was later recognized to be an autosomal recessive syndrome. In general, the reconstructive algorithm described for Crouzon syndrome can be followed.

Saethre-Chotzen Syndrome

Saethre-Chotzen syndrome has an autosomal dominant inheritance pattern with

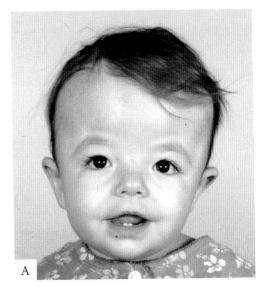

A

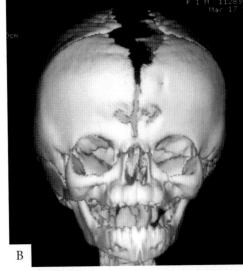

B

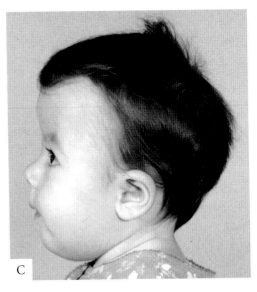

C

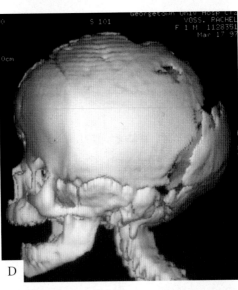

D

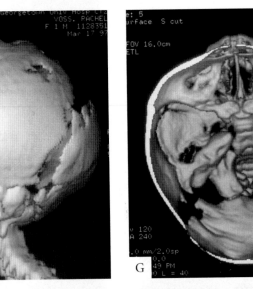

G

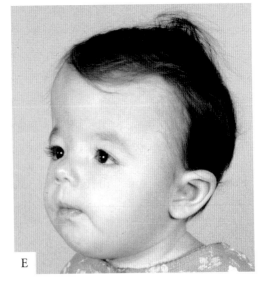

E

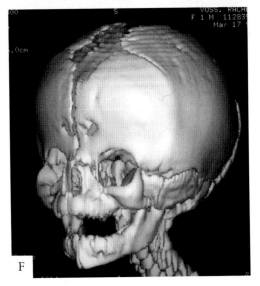

F

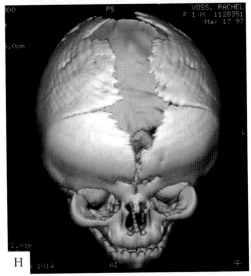

H

FIGURE 46-11   *A 2-month-old child born with Pfeiffer syndrome (Type I). She has bilateral coronal synostosis resulting in brachycephaly without suggestion of midface deficiency. A, Frontal view. B, Frontal view of CT scan. C, Profile view. D, Profile view of CT scan. E, Oblique view. F, Oblique view of CT scan. G, Cranial base view of CT scan. H, Craniofacial view of CT scan. Reproduced with permission from Posnick JC. Pfeiffer syndrome: evaluation and staging of reconstruction. In: Posnick JC, editor. Craniofacial and maxillofacial surgery in children and young adults. Philadelphia (PA): W.B. Saunders Co.; 2000. p. 344.*

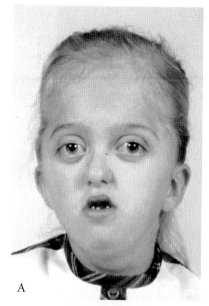
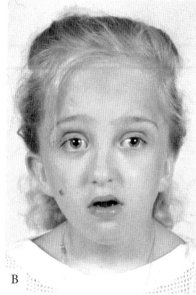
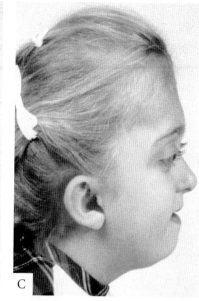
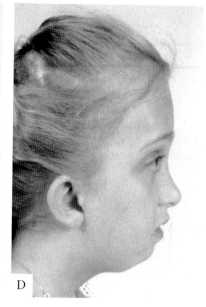

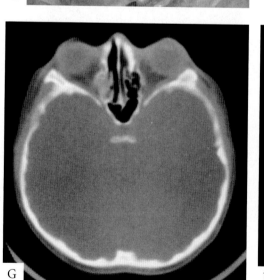
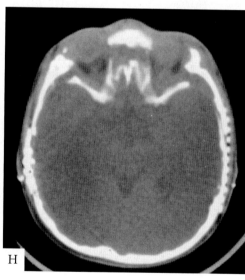

FIGURE **46-12** *A 6-year-old girl born with Pfeiffer syndrome (initially thought to have Crouzon syndrome). She underwent cranio-orbital decompression early in childhood. She presented to us with a constricted anterior cranial vault, orbital dystopia, and midface deficiency. She underwent anterior cranial vault and monobloc osteotomies with reshaping (see Figure 46-4). A, Frontal view before surgery. B, Frontal view after monobloc reconstruction. C, Profile view before surgery. D, Profile view after monobloc reconstruction. E, Occlusal view before surgery. F, Occlusal view after reconstruction. She still requires orthodontic treatment and orthognathic surgery, which is planned for the early teenage years. G and H, Comparison of axial CT slices through midorbits before and after reconstruction indicating decreased proptosis. Reproduced with permission from Posnick JC. Pfeiffer syndrome: evaluation and staging of reconstruction. In: Posnick JC, editor. Craniofacial and maxillofacial surgery in children and young adults. Philadelphia (PA): W.B. Saunders Co.; 2000. p. 349.*

a high degree of penetrance and expressivity.[106] Its pattern of malformations may include craniosynostosis, low-set frontal hairline, ptosis of the upper eyelids, facial asymmetry, brachydactyly, partial cutaneous syndactyly, and other skeletal anomalies. As part of the reconstruction, cranio-orbital reshaping will almost certainly be required and is similar to that described for Crouzon syndrome. Evaluation and management of the total midface deficiency and orthognathic deformities as decribed for Crouzon syndrome should be followed.

Cloverleaf Skull Anomaly

Kleeblattschädel anomaly (cloverleaf skull) is a trilobular-shaped skull secondary to craniosynostosis (Figure 46-13).[107,108] The cloverleaf skull anomaly is known to be both etiologically and pathogenetically heterogeneous. This anomaly is also non-specific: it may occur as an isolated anomaly or together with other anomalies, making up various syndromes (namely, Apert, Crouzon, Carpenter, Pfeiffer, and Saethre-Chotzen). The extent and timing of anterior cranial vault or upper orbital, posterior cranial vault, and midface reconstruction will be dependent on individual variation in the presenting deformity. In general, the protocol described for Crouzon syndrome can be followed.

Summary

Details of the timing and techniques for correction of the varied forms of craniofacial dysostosis syndromes differ from center to center. However, an essential element of successful rehabilitation is the delivery of care by committed, experienced, and technically skilled clinicians. The combined expertise of an experienced craniofacial surgeon and pediatric neurosurgeon working together to manage the cranio-orbital malformation and the experienced maxillofacial surgeon and orthodontist working together to manage the orthognathic deformity are essential to achieve maximum function and facial esthetics for each patient.

Our preferred approach for management of the craniofacial dysostosis syndromes is to stage the reconstruction to coincide with facial growth patterns, visceral (brain and eye) function, and psychosocial development. Recognition of the need for a staged reconstruction serves to clarify the objectives of each phase of treatment for the craniofacial surgeon, team, and most importantly the patient and patient's family.

By continuing to define our rationale for the timing and extent of surgical intervention and then evaluating both function and esthetic outcomes, we will further

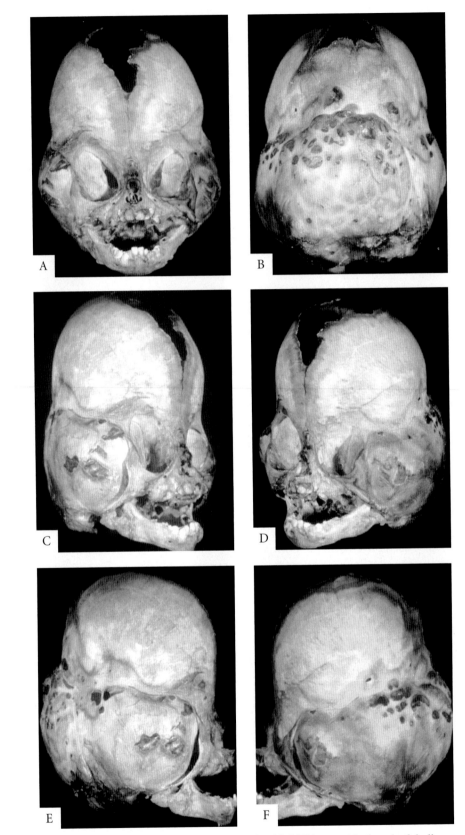

FIGURE 46-13 *The craniofacial skeleton of a 6-month-old child born with cloverleaf skull anomaly. He underwent tracheostomy and gastrostomy shortly after birth and died of pneumonia before craniofacial reconstruction could be undertaken. A, Frontal view. B, Posterior view. C, Right oblique view. D, Left oblique view. E, Left profile view. F, Right profile view. Reproduced with permission from Cloverleaf skull anomalies: evaluation and staging of reconstruction. In: Posnick JC, editor. Craniofacial and maxillofacial surgery in children and young adults. Philadelphia (PA): W.B. Saunders Co.; 2000. p. 364.*

improve the quality of life for the many hundreds of children born with syndromal forms of craniosynostosis. Our objective is to see each individual achieve personal success in life without special regard for the original malformation.

References

1. Cohen MM Jr. Sutural biology and the correlates of craniosynostosis. Am J Med Genet 1993;47:581–616.

2. Renier D. Intracranial pressure in craniosynostosis: Pre- and postoperative recordings. Correlation with functional results. In: Persing JA, Jane JA, Edgerton MT, editors. Scientific foundations and surgical treatment of craniosynostosis. Baltimore (MD): Williams & Wilkins; 1989. p. 263–9.

3. Gault DT, Renier D, Marchac D, Jones BM. Intracranial pressure and intracranial volume in children with craniosynostosis. Plast Reconstr Surg 1992;90:230–71.

4. Walia HK, Sodhi JS, Gupta BB, et al. Roentgenologic determination of the cranial capacity in the first four years of life. Ind J Radiol 1972;26:250.

5. Virchow R. Uber den cretinismus, nametlich in Franken, under uber pathologische: Schadelformen Verk Phys Med Gessellsch Wurszburg 1851;2:230–71.

6. Turvey TA, Gudeman SK. Nonsyndromic craniosynostosis. In: Turvey TA, Vig KWL, Fonseca RJ, editors. Facial clefts and craniosynostosis: principles and management. Philadelphia: W.B. Saunders Co.; 1996. p. 596–629.

7. Moss ML. The pathogenesis of premature cranial synostosis in man. Acta Anat (Basal) 1959;37:351–70.

8. Stewart RE, Dixon G, Cohen A. The pathogenesis of premature craniosynostosis in acrocephalosyndactyly (Apert syndrome): a reconsideration. Plast Reconstr Surg 1977; 59:699–703.

9. Pugeaut R. Le Probleme neuro chirurgical des craniostenoses. Cahier Med Lyon 1968; 44:3343.

10. Renier D, Sainte-Rose C, Marchac D, et al. Intracranial pressure in craniosynostosis. J Neurosurg 1982;57:370.

11. Siddiqi SN, Posnick JC, Buncic R, et al. The detection and management of intracranial hypertension after initial suture release and decompression for craniofacial dysostosis syndromes. Neurosurgery 1995; 36:703.

12. Turvey TA, Ruiz RL. Craniosynostosis and craniofacial dysostosis. In: Fonseca RJ, Baker SB, Wolford LM, editors. Oral and maxillofacial surgery. Philadelphia: W.B. Saunders Co.; 2000. p. 195–220.

13. Posnick JC. Craniofacial dysostosis syndromes: a staged reconstructive approach. In: Turvey TA, Vig KWL, Fonseca RJ, editors. facial clefts and craniosynostosis: principles and management. Philadelphia: W.B. Saunders Co.; 1996. p. 630–85.

14. Posnick JC. Quantitative computer tomographic scan analysis: normal values and growth patterns. In: Posnick JC, editor. Craniofacial and maxillofacial surgery in children and young adults. Philadelphia: W.B. Saunders Co.; 2000. p. 36–54.

15. Gault DT, Renier D, Marchac D, et al. Intracranial volume in children with craniosynostosis. J Craniofac Surg 1990;1:1.

16. Golabi M, Edwards MSB, and Ousterhout DK. Craniosynostosis and hydrocephalus. Neurosurgery 1987;21:63.

17. Hogan GR, Bauman ML. Hydrocephalus in Apert syndrome. J Pediatr 1971;79:782.

18. Fishman MA, Hogan GR, Dodge PR. The concurrence of hydrocephalus and craniosynostosis. J Neurosurg 1971;34:621.

19. Murovic JA, Posnick JC, Drake JM, et al. Hydrocephalus in Apert syndrome: a retrospective review. Pediatr Neurosurg 1993; 19:151–5.

20. Lauritzen C, Lilja J, Jarlstedt J. Airway obstruction and sleep apnea in children with craniofacial anomalies. Plast Reconstr Surg 1986;77:1–6.

21. Guilleminault C. Obstructive sleep apnea syndrome and its treatment in children: areas of agreement and controversy. Pediatr Pulmonol 1987;3:429–36.

22. Moore MH. Upper airway obstruction in the syndromal craniosynostoses. Br J Plast Surg 1993;46:355–62.

23. Drake AF, Sidman JD. Airway management. In: Turvey TA, Vig KWL, Fonseca RJ, editors. Facial clefts and craniosynostosis: principles and management. Philadelphia: W.B. Saunders Co.; 1996. p 174–82.

24. Gorlin RJ, Cohen MM Jr, Levin LS. Syndromes of the head and neck. 3rd ed. New York: Oxford University Press; 1990. p. 524–5.

25. Enlow DH, McNamara JA Jr. The neurocranial basis for facial form and pattern. Angle Orthod 1973;43:256–70.

26. Kreiborg S. Description of a dry skull with Crouzon syndrome. Scand J Plast Reconstr Surg 1982;16:245–53.

27. Marsh JL, Gado M. Surgical anatomy of the craniofacial dysostoses: insights from CT scans. Cleft Palate J 1982;19:212–21.

28. Freide H, Lilja J, Andersson H, Johanson B. Growth of the anterior cranial base after craniotomy in infants with premature synostosis of the coronal suture. Scand J Plast Reconstr Surg 1983;17:99–108.

29. Marsh JL, Vannier MW. The "third" dimension in craniofacial surgery. Plast Reconstr Surg 1983;71:759–67.

30. Kreiborg S. Apert and Crouzon syndromes contrasted. Qualitative craniofacial x-ray findings. J Dent Res 1985;64:203.

31. Marchac D. Radical forehead remodeling for craniosynostosis. Plast Reconstr Surg 1978;62:335–8.

32. Marchac D, Renier D, Jones BM. Experience with the "floating forehead." Br J Plast Surg 1988;41:1–15.

33. Posnick JC. The craniofacial dysostosis syndrome: current reconstructive strategies. Clin Plast Surg 1994;21:585–98.

34. Carr M, Posnick JC, Pron G, Armstrong D. Cranio-orbito-zygomatic measurements from standard CT scans in unoperated Crouzon and Apert infants: comparison with normal controls. Cleft Palate Craniofac J 1992;29:129–36.

35. Posnick JC, Al-Qattan MM, Armstrong D. Monobloc and facial bipartition osteotomies: quantitative assessment of presenting deformity and surgical results based on computed tomography scans. J Oral Maxillofac Surg 1995;53:358–67.

36. Kreiborg S. Crouzon syndrome. A clinical and roentgencephalometric study [thesis (disputats)]. Scand J Plast Reconstr Surg 1981;18 Suppl:198.

37. Posnick JC, Farkas LG. Anthropometric surface measurements in the analysis of craniomaxillofacial deformities: normal values and growth trends. In: Posnick JC, editor. Craniofacial and maxillofacial surgery in children and young adults. Philadelphia: W.B. Saunders Co.; 2000. p. 55–79.

38. Farkas LG, Posnick JC. Growth and development of regional units in the head and face based on anthropometric measurements. Cleft Palate Craniofac J 1992; 29:301–2.

39. Farkas LG, Posnick JC, Hreczko T. Anthropometric growth study of the head. Cleft Palate Craniofac J 1992;29:303–7.

40. Farkas LG, Posnick JC, Hreczko T. Growth patterns in the orbital region: a morphometric study. Cleft Palate Craniofac J 1992;29:315–7.

41. Farkas LG, Posnick JC, Hreczko T. Growth patterns of the face: a morphometric study. Cleft Palate Craniofac J 1992;29:308–14.

42. Waitzman AA, Posnick JC, Armstrong D, Pron GE. Craniofacial skeletal measurements based on computed tomography: part I.

Accuracy and reproducibility. Cleft Palate Craniofac J 1992;29:112–7.

43. Waitzman AA, Posnick JC, Armstrong D, Pron GE. Craniofacial skeletal measurements based on computed tomography. Part II. Normal values and growth trends. Cleft Palate Craniofac J 1992;29:118–28.

44. Vannier MW, Gado M, Marsh JL. Three-dimensional computer graphics for craniofacial surgical planning and evaluation. Comput Graph 1983;17:263.

45. Vannier MW, Pilgram TK, Marsh JL, et al. Craniosynostosis: diagnostic imaging with three-dimensional CT presentation. AJNR Am J Neuroradiol 1994;15:1861–9.

46. Kolar JC, Munro IR, Farkas LG. Patterns of dysmorphology in Crouzon syndrome: an anthropometric study. Cleft Palate J 1988;25:235–44.

47. Posnick JC, Ruiz RL. The craniofacial dysostosis syndromes: current surgical thinking and future directions. Cleft Palate Craniofac J 2000;37:433.

48. Kreiborg S, Pruzansky S. Roentgencephalometric and metallic implant studies in Apert syndrome. Abstract. Presented at the 50th General Session I.A.D.R. 1972. Las Vegas. 298:120[21].

49. Kreiborg S, Aduss H. Pre and post surgical facial growth in patients with Crouzon and Apert syndromes. Cleft Palate J 1986;23(suppl): 78–90.

50. Lannelongue M. De la craniectomie dans la microcephalie. Compte Rendu Acad Sci 1890;110:1382.

51. Lane LC. Pioneer craniectomy for relief of mental imbecility due to premature sutural closure and microcephalus. J Am Med Assoc 1892;18:49.

52. McCarthy JG, Epstein FJ, Wood-Smith D. Craniosynostosis. In: McCarthy JG, editor. Plastic Surgery. Volume 4. Philadelphia: W.B. Saunders Co.; 1990. p. 3013–53.

53. Gillies H, Harrison SH. Operative correction by osteotomy of recessed malar maxillary compound in case of oxycephaly. Br J Plast Surg 1950;3:123.

54. Tessier P. Osteotomies totales de la face: Syndrome de Crouzon, syndrome D'Apert: Oxycephalies, scaphocephalies, turricephalies. Ann Chir Plast 1967;12:273.

55. Tessier P. The definitive plastic surgical treatment of the severe facial deformities of craniofacial dysostosis: Crouzon and Apert diseases. Plast Reconstr Surg 1971;48:419.

56. Tessier P. Dysostoses cranio-faciales (syndromes de Crouzon et d'Apert): Osteotomies totales de la face. In: Transactions of the Fourth International Congress of Plas-

tic and Reconstructive Surgery. Amsterdam: Mosby; 1969. p. 774.

57. Tessier P. Relationship of craniosynostosis to craniofacial dysostosis and to faciosynostosis: A study with therapeutic implications. Clin Plast Surg 1982;9:531.

58. Tessier P. Autogenous bone grafts taken from the calvarium for facial and cranial applications. Plast Reconstr Surg 1971;48:224.

59. Tessier P. Total osteotomy of the middle third of the face for faciostenosis or for sequelae of the Le Fort III fractures. Plast Reconstr Surg 1971;48:533.

60. Tessier P. Traitement des dysmorphies faciales propres aux dysostoses craniofaciales (DGF), maladies de Crouzon et d'Apert. Neurochirurgie 1971;17:295.

61. Tessier P. Craniofacial surgery in syndromic craniosynostosis: craniosynostosis, diagnosis, evaluation and management. New York: Raven Press; 1986. p 321.

62. Tessier P. Recent improvement in the treatment of facial and cranial deformities in Crouzon disease and Apert syndrome. In: Symposium of Plastic Surgery of the Orbital Region. St. Louis (MO): C.V. Mosby Co.; 1976. p 271.

63. Tessier P. The monobloc frontofacial advancement: Do the pluses outweigh the minuses? [discussion] Plast Reconstr Surg 1993;91:988.

64. Rougerie J, Derome P, Anquez L. Craniostenosis et dysmorphies-cranio-faciales: Principes d'une nouvelle technique de traitement et ses resultats. Neurochirurgie 1972;18:429.

65. Hoffman HJ, Mohr G. Lateral canthal advancement of the supraorbital margin: a new corrective technique in the treatment of coronal synostosis. J Neurosurg 1976;45:376.

66. Whitaker LA, Bartlett SP, Schut L, et al. Craniosynostosis: an analysis of the timing, treatment and complications in 164 consecutive patients. Plast Reconstr Surg 1987;80:195.

67. Luhr HG. Zur Stabilen osteosynthese bei unterkieferfrakturen. Dtsch Zahnaerztl Z 1968;23:754.

68. Kaban LB, Conover M, Mulliken J. Midface position after LeFort III advancement: a long-term follow-up study. Cleft Palate J 1986;23(suppl):75–7.

69. Wolford LM, Cooper RL. Orthognathic surgery in the growing cleft patient and its effect on growth. Abstract. Presented at the American Association of Oral and Maxillofacial Surgeons Annual Scientific Sessions; 1987 Sep; Anaheim (CA): WB Saunders.

70. Wolford LM, Cooper RL, El Deeb M. Orthognathic surgery in the young cleft patient and the effect on growth. Abstract. Presented at the American Cleft Palate–Craniofa-

cial Association Annual Meeting; 1990 May; St. Louis (MO).

71. Posnick JC, Al-Qattan MM, Armstrong D. Monobloc and facial bipartition osteotomies reconstruction of craniofacial malformations: a study of extradural dead space. Plast Reconstr Surg 1996;97:1118.

72. Whitaker LA, Munro IR, Sayler KE, et al. Combined report of problems and complications in 793 craniofacial operations. Plast Reconstr Surg 1979;64:198.

73. David DJ, Cooter RD. Craniofacial infections in 10 years of transcranial surgery. Plast Reconstr Surg 1987;80:213.

74. Marsh JL, Galic M, Vannier MW. Surgical correction of craniofacial dysmorphology of Apert syndrome. Clin Plast Surg 1991;18:251.

75. Saltz R, Sierra D, Feldman D, et al. Experimental and clinical applications of fibrin glue. Plast Reconstr Surg 1991;88:1005.

76. Posnick JC. Craniosynostosis: surgical management in infancy. In: Bell WH, editor. Orthognathic and reconstructive surgery. Philadelphia: W.B. Saunders Co.; 1992. p. 1839.

77. Posnick JC. Brachycephaly: bilateral coronal synostosis without midface deficiency. In: Posnick JC, editor. Craniofacial and maxillofacial surgery in children and young adults. Philadelphia: W.B. Saunders Co.; 2000. p. 249–68.

78. Posnick JC. Crouzon syndrome: evaluation and staging of reconstruction. In: Posnick JC, editor. Craniofacial and maxillofacial surgery in children and young adults. Philadelphia: W.B. Saunders Co.; 2000. p. 271–307.

79. Posnick JC, Goldstein JA, Clokie C. Refinements in pterygomaxillary dissociation for total midface osteotomies: instrumentation, technique and CT scan analysis. Plast Reconstr Surg 1993;91:167–72.

80. Murray JE, Swanson LT. Midface osteotomy and advancement for craniosynostosis. Plast Reconstr Surg 1968;41:299–306.

81. Ortiz-Monasterio F, Fuente del Campo A, Carillo A. Advancement of the orbits and the midface in one piece, combined with frontal repositioning for the correction of Crouzon syndrome. Plast Reconstr Surg 1978;61:507–16.

82. Ortiz-Monasterio F, Fuente del Campo A. Refinements on the monobloc orbitofacial advancement. In: Caronni EP, editor. Craniofacial surgery. Boston: Little, Brown; 1985. p. 263.

83. Hogeman KE, Willmar K. On Le Fort III osteotomy for Crouzon disease in children: report of

a four year follow-up in one patient. Scand J Plast Reconstr Surg 1974;8:169–72.

84. Van der Meulen JC. Medial faciotomy. Br J Plast Surg 1979;32:339–42.

85. Cohen MM Jr. An etiologic and nosologic overview of craniosynostosis syndromes. Birth Defects Orig Artic Ser 1975;11:137–89.

86. Cohen MM Jr, Kreiborg S. The central nervous system in the Apert syndrome. Am J Med Genet 1990;35:36–45.

87. Kreiborg S, Prydsoe U, Dahl E, Fogh-Anderson. Calvarium and cranial base in Apert syndrome: an autopsy report. Cleft Palate J 1976;13:296–303.

88. Ousterhout DK, Melsen B. Cranial base deformity in Apert syndrome. Plast Reconstr Surg 1982;69:254–63.

89. Kreiborg S, Cohen MM Jr. The infant Apert skull. Neurosurg Clin North Am 1991; 2:551–4.

90. Cohen MM Jr, Kreiborg S. Skeletal abnormalities in the Apert syndrome. Am J Med Genet 1993;47:624–32.

91. Cohen MM Jr, Kreiborg S. The growth pattern in the Apert syndrome. Clin Genet 1993;47:617–23.

92. Park WJ, Theda C, Maestri NE, et al. Analysis of phenotypic features and FGFR2 mutations in Apert syndrome. Am J Hum Genet 1995;57:321–8.

93. Slaney SF, Oldridge M, Hurst JA, et al. Differential effects of FGFR2 mutations on syndactyly and cleft plate in Apert syndrome. Am J Med Genet 1996;58:923–32.

94. Cohen MM Jr. Transforming growth factor βs and fibroblast growth factors and their receptors: role in sutural biology and craniosynostosis. J Bone Miner Res 1997;12:322–31.

95. Posnick JC, Lin KY, Jhawar BJ, Armstrong D. Apert syndrome: quantitative assessment in presenting deformity and surgical results after first-stage reconstruction by CT scan. Plast Reconstr Surg 1994;93:489–97.

96. Posnick JC. Apert syndrome: evaluation and staging of reconstruction. In: Posnick JC, editor. Craniofacial and maxillofacial surgery in children and young adults. Philadelphia: W.B. Saunders Co.; 2000. p. 308–42.

97. Posnick JC. Craniofacial dysostosis: staging of reconstruction and management of the midface deformity. Neurosurg Clin N Am 1991;2:683–702.

98. Posnick JC. Craniofacial dysostosis: management of the midface deformity. In: Bell WH, editor. Orthognathic and reconstructive surgery. Philadelphia: W.B. Saunders Co.; 1992. p. 1888.

99. Pfeiffer RA. Dominant Erbliche Akrocephalosyndaktylie. *Z Kinderheilkd* 1964; 90:301–20.

100. Cohen MM Jr, editor. Craniosynostosis: diagnosis, evaluation, and management. New York: Raven Press; 1986.

101. Jabs EW, Li X, Scott AF, et al. Jackson-Weiss and Crouzon syndromes are allelic with mutations in fibroblast growth factor receptor 2. Nat Genet 1994;8:275–9.

102. Cohen MM Jr. Pfeiffer syndrome update, clinical subtypes, and guidelines for differential diagnosis. Am J Med Genet 1993;45:300–7.

103. Lajeunie E, Ma HW, Bonaventure J, et al. FGFR2 mutations in Pfeiffer syndrome. Nat Genet 1995;9:108.

104. Park WJ, Theda C, Maestri NE, et al. Analysis of phenotypic features and FGFR2 mutations in Apert syndrome. Am J Hum Genet 1995;57:321–8.

105. Rutland P, Pulley LJ, Reardon W. Identical mutations in the FGFR2 gene cause both Pfeiffer and Crouzon syndrome phenotypes. Nat Genet 1995;9:173–6.

106. Paznekas WA, Cunningham ML, Howard TD, et al. Genetic heterogeneity of Saethre-Chotzen syndrome, due to TWIST and FGFR mutations. Am J Hum Genet 1998;62:1370–80.

107. Cohen MM Jr. Cloverleaf syndrome update. Proc Greenwood Gene Center 1987;6: 186–7.

108. Cohen MM Jr. The cloverleaf anomaly: managing extreme cranio-orbito-facio-stenosis [discussion]. Plast Reconstr Surg 1993; 91:10–4.

Part 7

TEMPOROMANDIBULAR JOINT DISEASE

CHAPTER 47

Anatomy and Pathophysiology of the Temporomandibular Joint

Mark C. Fletcher, DMD, MD
Joseph F. Piecuch, DMD, MD
Stuart E. Lieblich, DMD

Classification

The temporomandibular joint (TMJ) is composed of the temporal bone and the mandible, as well as a specialized dense fibrous structure, the articular disk, several ligaments, and numerous associated muscles. The TMJ is a compound joint that can be classified by anatomic type as well as by function.

Anatomically the TMJ is a diarthrodial joint, which is a discontinuous articulation of two bones permitting freedom of movement that is dictated by associated muscles and limited by ligaments.[1] Its fibrous connective tissue capsule is well innervated and well vascularized and tightly attached to the bones at the edges of their articulating surfaces. It is also a synovial joint, lined on its inner aspect by a synovial membrane, which secretes synovial fluid. The fluid acts as a joint lubricant and supplies the metabolic and nutritional needs of the nonvascularized internal joint structures.

Functionally the TMJ is a compound joint, composed of four articulating surfaces: the articular facets of the temporal bone and of the mandibular condyle and the superior and inferior surfaces of the articular disk. The articular disk divides the joint into two compartments. The lower compartment permits hinge motion or rotation and hence is termed *ginglymoid*. The superior compartment permits sliding (or translatory) movements and is therefore called *arthrodial*. Hence the temporomandibular joint as a whole can be termed *ginglymoarthrodial*.

Bony Structures

The articular portion of the temporal bone (Figure 47-1) is composed of three parts. The largest is the articular or mandibular fossa, a concave structure extending from the posterior slope of the articular emi-

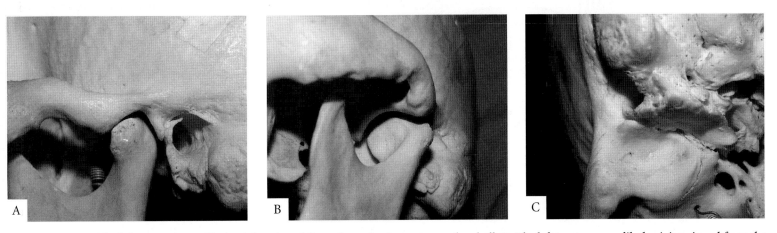

FIGURE 47-1 A, *The left temporomandibular joint viewed from the sagittal aspect on a dry skull.* B, *The left temporomandibular joint viewed from the oblique/coronal aspect on a dry skull.* C, *The left glenoid fossa and articular eminence.*

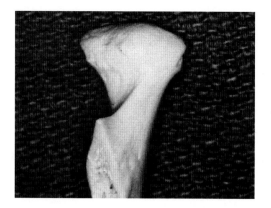

FIGURE 47-2   *The mandibular condyle. Reproduced with permission from Piecuch JF, Lieblich SE. Anatomy and pathology of the temporomandibular joint. In: Peterson LF, Indresano AT, Marciani RD, Roser SM. Principles of oral and maxillofacial surgery. Vol. 3. Philadelphia (PA): J.B. Lippincott Company; 1992. p. 1858.*

nence to the postglenoid process, which is a ridge between the fossa and the external acoustic meatus. The surface of the articular fossa is thin and may be translucent on a dry skull. This is not a major stress-bearing area. The second portion, the articular eminence, is a transverse bony prominence that is continuous across the articular surface

mediolaterally. The articular eminence is usually thick and serves as a major functional component of the TMJ. The articular eminence is distinguished from the articular tubercle, a nonarticulating process on the lateral aspect of the zygomatic root of the temporal bone, which serves as a point of attachment of collateral ligaments. The third portion of the articular surface of the temporal bone is the preglenoid plane, a flattened area anterior to the eminence.

The mandible is a U-shaped bone that articulates with the temporal bone by means of the articular surface of its condyles, paired structures forming an approximately 145° to 160° angle to each other. The mandibular condyle (Figure 47-2) is approximately 15 to 20 mm in width and 8 to 10 mm in anteroposterior dimension. The condyle tends to be rounded mediolaterally and convex anteroposteriorly. On its medial aspect just below its articular surface is a prominent depression, the pterygoid fovea, which is the site of attachments of the lateral pterygoid muscle.

Cartilage and Synovium

Lining the inner aspect of all synovial joints, including the TMJ, are two types of tissue: articular cartilage and synovium (Figure 47-3). The space bound by these two structures is termed the *synovial cavity*, which is filled with synovial fluid. The articular surfaces of both the temporal bone and the condyle are covered with dense articular fibrocartilage, a fibrous connective tissue. This fibrocartilage covering has the capacity to regenerate and to remodel under functional stresses. Deep to the fibrocartilage, particularly on the condyle, is a proliferative zone of cells that may develop into either cartilaginous or osseous tissue. Most change resulting from function is seen in this layer.

Articular cartilage is composed of chondrocytes and an intercellular matrix of collagen fibers, water, and a nonfibrous filler material, termed *ground substance*. Chondrocytes are enclosed in otherwise hollow spaces, called lacunae, and are arranged in three layers characterized by different cell shapes (Figure. 47-4A). The superficial zone contains small flattened cells with their long axes parallel to the surface.[2] In the middle zone the cells are larger and rounded and appear in columnar fashion perpendicular to the surface. The deep zone contains the largest cells and is divided by the "tide mark" below which some degree of calcification has occurred. There are few blood vessels in any of these areas, with cartilage being nourished primarily by diffusion from the synovial fluid.

Collagen fibers are arranged in arcades with an interlocking meshwork of fibrils parallel to the articular surface joining together as bundles and descending to their attachment in the calcified cartilage between the tide mark (Figure 47-4B). Functionally these arcades provide a framework for interstitial water and ground substance to resist compressive forces encountered in joint loading. Formed by intramembranous processes the TMJ's

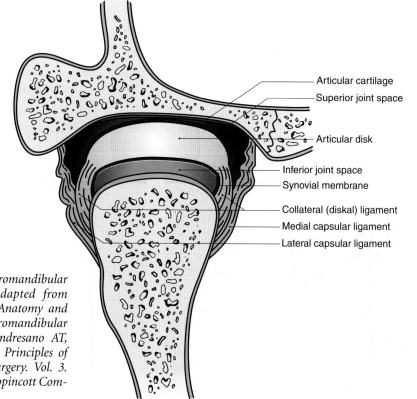

Articular cartilage
Superior joint space

Articular disk

Inferior joint space
Synovial membrane

Collateral (diskal) ligament
Medial capsular ligament
Lateral capsular ligament

FIGURE 47-3   *The temporomandibular joint (coronal view). Adapted from Piecuch JF, Lieblich SE. Anatomy and pathology of the temporomandibular joint. In: Peterson LF, Indresano AT, Marciani RD, Roser SM. Principles of oral and maxillofacial surgery. Vol. 3. Philadelphia (PA): J.B. Lippincott Company; 1992. p. 1859.*

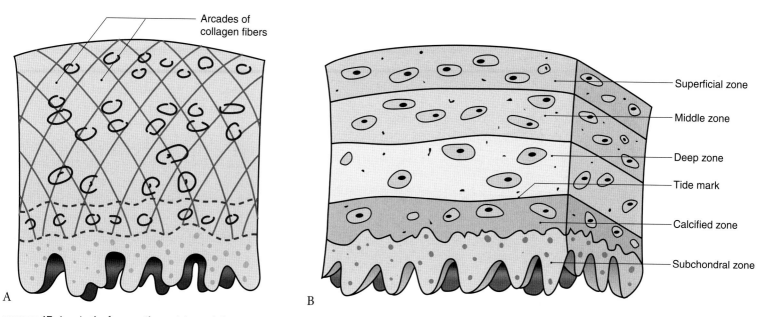

FIGURE 47-4   *Articular cartilage. Adapted from Albright JA and Brand RA.[2]*

articular cartilage contains a greater proportion of collagen fibers (fibrocartilage) than other synovial joints, which are covered instead by hyaline cartilage.

The ground substance contains a variety of plasma proteins, glucose, urea, and salts, as well as proteoglycans, which are synthesized by the Golgi apparatus of the chondrocytes. Proteoglycans are macromolecules consisting of a protein core attached to many glycosaminoglycan chains of chondroitin sulfate and keratan sulfate. Proteoglycans play a role in the diffusion of nutrients and metabolic breakdown products. Ground substance permits the entry and release of large quantities of water, an attribute thought to be significant in giving cartilage its characteristic functional elasticity in response to deformation and loading.

Lining the capsular ligament is the synovial membrane, a thin, smooth, richly innervated vascular tissue without an epithelium. Synovial cells, somewhat undifferentiated in appearance, serve both a phagocytic and a secretory function and are thought to be the site of production of hyaluronic acid, a glycosaminoglycan found in synovial fluid. Some synovial cells, particularly those in close approxi-

mation to articular cartilage, are thought to have the capacity to differentiate into chondrocytes. The synovium is capable of rapid and complete regeneration following injury. Recently, synovial cells (as well as chondrocytes and leukocytes) have been the focus of extensive research regarding the production of anabolic and catabolic cytokines within the TMJ.[3]

Synovial fluid is considered an ultrafiltrate of plasma.[2] It contains a high concentration of hyaluronic acid, which is thought to be responsible for the fluid's high viscosity. The proteins found in synovial fluid are identical to plasma proteins; however, synovial fluid has a lower total protein content, with a higher percentage of albumin and a lower percentage of α-2-globulin. Alkaline phosphatase, which may also be present in synovial fluid, is thought to be produced by chondrocytes. Leukocytes are also found in synovial fluid, with the cell count being less than 200 per cubic millimeter and with less than 25% of these cells being polymorphonuclear. Only a small amount of synovial fluid, usually less than 2 mL, is present within the healthy TMJ.

Functions of the synovial fluid include lubrication of the joint, phagocytosis of particulate debris, and nourishment of the

articular cartilage. Joint lubrication is a complex function related to the viscosity of synovial fluid and to the ability of articular cartilage to allow the free passage of water within the pores of its glycosaminoglycan matrix. Application of a loading force to articular cartilage causes a deformation at the location. It has been theorized that water is extruded from the loaded area into the synovial fluid adjacent to the point of contact. The concentration of hyaluronic acid and hence the viscosity of the synovial fluid is greater at the point of load, thus protecting the articular surfaces. As the load passes to adjacent areas the deformation passes on as well, while the original point of contact regains its shape and thickness through the reabsorption of water. Exact mechanisms of flow between articular cartilage and synovial fluid are as yet unclear. Nevertheless the net result is a coefficient of friction for the normally functioning joint—approximately 14 times less than that of a dry joint.

The Articular Disk

The articular disk (Figure 47-5) is composed of dense fibrous connective tissue and is nonvascularized and noninnervated, an adaptation that allows it to resist

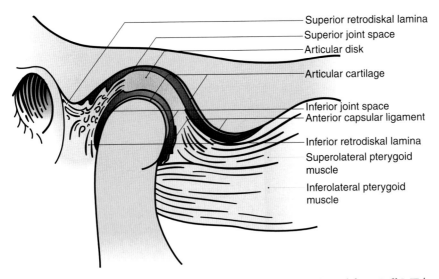

Superior retrodiskal lamina
Superior joint space
Articular disk

Articular cartilage

Inferior joint space
Anterior capsular ligament

Inferior retrodiskal lamina
Superolateral pterygoid muscle

Inferolateral pterygoid muscle

FIGURE 47-5   *The temporomandibular joint (lateral view). Adapted from Bell WE.[4]*

pressure.[4] Anatomically the disk can be divided into three general regions as viewed from the lateral perspective: the anterior band, the central intermediate zone, and the posterior band. The thickness of the disk appears to be correlated with the prominence of the eminence. The intermediate zone is thinnest and is generally the area of function between the mandibular condyle and the temporal bone. Despite the designation of separate portions of the articular disk, it is in fact a homogeneous tissue and the bands do not consist of specific anatomic structures. The disk is flexible and adapts to functional demands of the articular surfaces.[5] The articular disk is attached to the capsular ligament anteriorly, posteriorly, medially, and laterally.[6] Some fibers of the superior head of the lateral pterygoid muscle insert on the disk at its medial aspect, apparently serving to stabilize the disk to the mandibular condyle during function.

Retrodiskal Tissue

Posteriorly the articular disk blends with a highly vascular, highly innervated structure—the bilaminar zone, which is involved in the production of synovial fluid. The superior aspect of the retrodiskal tissue contains elastic fibers and is termed the *superior retrodiskal lamina*, which attaches to the

tympanic plate and functions as a restraint to disk movement in extreme translatory movements.[5] The inferior aspect of the retrodiskal tissue, termed the *inferior retrodiskal lamina*, consists of collagen fibers without elastic tissue and functions to connect the articular disk to the posterior margin of the articular surfaces of the condyle. It is thought to serve as a check ligament to prevent extreme rotation of the disk on the condyle in rotational movements.

Ligaments

Ligaments associated with the TMJ are composed of collagen and act predominantly as restraints to motion of the condyle and the disk. Three ligaments—collateral, capsular, and temporomandibular ligaments—are considered functional ligaments because they serve as major anatomic components of the joints. Two other ligaments—sphenomandibular and stylomandibular—are considered accessory ligaments because, although they are attached to osseous structures at some distance from the joints, they serve to some degree as passive restraints on mandibular motion.

The collateral (or diskal) ligaments (see Figure 47-3) are short paired structures attaching the disk to the lateral and medial poles of each condyle. Their function is to restrict movement of the disk away from

the condyle, thus allowing smooth synchronous motion of the disk-condyle complex. Although the collateral ligaments permit rotation of the condyle with relation to the disk, their tight attachment forces the disk to accompany the condyle through its translatory range of motion.[6]

The capsular ligament (see Figures 47-3, 47-5, 47-6, and 47-7) encompasses each joint, attaching superiorly to the temporal bone along the border of the mandibular fossa and eminence and inferiorly to the neck of the condyle along the edge of the articular facet. It surrounds the joint spaces and the disk, attaching anteriorly and posteriorly as well as medially and laterally, where it blends with the collateral ligaments. The function of the capsular ligament is to resist medial, lateral, and inferior forces, thereby holding the joint together. It offers resistance to movement of the joint only in the extreme range of motion. A secondary function of the capsular ligament is to contain the synovial fluid within the superior and inferior joint spaces.

The temporomandibular (lateral) ligaments (see Figure 47-7) are located on the lateral aspect of each TMJ.[5] Unlike the capsular and collateral ligaments, which have medial and lateral components within each

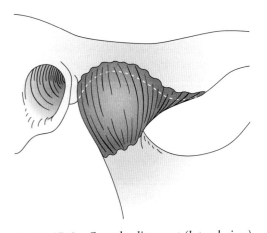

FIGURE 47-6   *Capsular ligament (lateral view). Adapted from Piecuch JF, Lieblich SE. Anatomy and pathology of the temporomandibular joint. In: Peterson LF, Indresano AT, Marciani RD, Roser SM. Principles of oral and maxillofacial surgery. Vol. 3. Philadelphia (PA): J.B. Lippincott Company; 1992. p. 1861.*

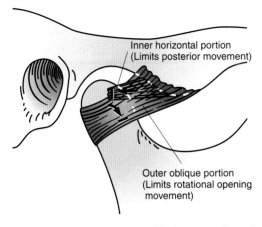

FIGURE 47-7 *Temporomandibular joint (lateral aspect). Adapted from Okeson JP.*

joint, the temporomandibular ligaments are single structures that function in paired fashion with the corresponding ligament on the opposite TMJ. Each temporomandibular ligament can be separated into two distinct portions, that have different functions.[6] The outer oblique portion descends from the outer aspect of the articular tubercle of the zygomatic process posteriorly and inferiorly to the outer posterior surface of the condylar neck. It limits the amount of inferior distraction that the condyle may achieve in translatory and rotational movements. The inner horizontal portion also arises from the outer surface of the articular tubercle, just medial to the origin of the outer oblique portion of the ligament, and runs horizontally backward to attach to the lateral pole of the condyle and the posterior aspect of the disk. The function of the inner horizontal portion of the temporomandibular ligament is to limit posterior movement of the condyle, particularly during pivoting movements, such as when the mandible moves laterally in chewing function. This restriction of posterior movement serves to protect the retrodiskal tissue.

The sphenomandibular ligament (Figure 47-8) arises from the spine of the sphenoid bone and descends into the fan-like insertion on the mandibular lingula, as well as on the lower portion of the medial side of the condylar neck.[1] The sphenomandibular ligament serves to some degree

as a point of rotation during activation of the lateral pterygoid muscle, thereby contributing to translation of the mandible.

The stylomandibular ligament (see Figure 47-8) descends from the styloid process to the posterior border of the angle of the mandible and also blends with the fascia of the medial pterygoid muscle. It functions similarly to the sphenomandibular ligament as a point of rotation and also limits excessive protrusion of the mandible.

Vascular Supply and Innervation

The vascular supply of the TMJ arises primarily from branches of the superficial temporal and maxillary arteries posteriorly and the masseteric artery anteriorly. There is a rich plexus of veins in the posterior aspect of the joint associated with the retrodiskal tissues, which alternately fill and empty with protrusive and retrusive movements, respectively, of the condyle-disk complex and which also function in the production of synovial fluid. The nerve supply to the TMJ is predominantly from branches of the auriculotemporal nerve with anterior contributions from the masseteric nerve and the posterior deep temporal nerve.[1] Many of the nerves

to the joint appear to be vasomotor and vasosensory, and they may have a role in the production of synovial fluid.

Musculature

All muscles attached to the mandible influence its movement to some degree. Only the four large muscles that attach to the ramus of the mandible are considered the muscles of mastication; however, a total of 12 muscles actually influence mandibular motion, all of which are bilateral.[1] Muscle pairs may function together for symmetric movements or unilaterally for asymmetric movement. For example, contraction of both lateral pterygoid muscles results in protrusion and depression of the mandible without deviation, whereas contraction of one of the lateral pterygoid muscles results in protrusion and opening with deviation to the opposite side.

Muscles influencing mandibular motion may be divided into two groups by anatomic position. Attaching primarily to the ramus and condylar neck of the mandible is the supramandibular muscle group, consisting of the temporalis, masseter, medial pterygoid, and lateral pterygoid muscles. This group functions predominantly as the elevators of the

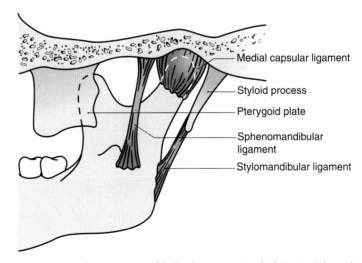

FIGURE 47-8 *Temporomandibular ligament (medial view). Adapted from Piecuch JF, Lieblich SE. Anatomy and pathology of the temporomandibular joint. In: Peterson LF, Indresano AT, Marciani RD, Roser SM. Principles of oral and maxillofacial surgery. Vol. 3. Philadelphia (PA): J.B. Lippincott Company; 1992. p. 1863.*

mandible. The lateral pterygoid does have a depressor function as well.[7] Attaching to the body and symphyseal area of the mandible and to the hyoid bone is the inframandibular group, which functions as the depressors of the mandible. The inframandibular group includes the four suprahyoid muscles (digastric, geniohyoid, mylohyoid, and stylohyoid) and the four infrahyoid muscles (sternohyoid, omohyoid, sternothyroid, and thyrohyoid). The suprahyoid muscles attach to both the hyoid bone and the mandible and serve to depress the mandible when the hyoid bone is fixed in place. They also elevate the hyoid bone when the mandible is fixed in place. The infrahyoid muscles serve to fix the hyoid bone during depressive movements of the mandible.

Supramandibular Muscle Group

The temporalis muscle (Figure 47-9) is a large fan-shaped muscle taking its origin from the temporal fossa and lateral aspect of the skull, including portions of the parietal, temporal, frontal, and sphenoid bones. Its fibers pass between the zygomatic arch and the skull and insert on the mandible at the coronoid process and anterior border of the ascending ramus down to the occlusal surface of the mandible, posterior to the third molar tooth.[1] Viewed coronally the temporalis muscle has a bipennate character in that fibers arising from the skull insert on the medial aspect of the coronoid process, whereas fibers arising laterally from the temporalis fascia insert on the lateral aspect of the coronoid process. In an anteroposterior dimension the temporalis muscle consists of three portions: the anterior, whose fibers are vertical; the middle, with oblique fibers; and the posterior portion, with semihorizontal fibers passing forward to bend under the zygomatic arch. The function of the temporalis muscle is to elevate the mandible for closure. It is not a power muscle. In addition contraction of the middle and posterior portions of the temporalis muscle can contribute to retrusive movements of the mandible. To a small degree unilateral contraction of the temporalis assists in deviation of the mandible to the ipsilateral side.

The masseter muscle (Figure 47-10), a short rectangular muscle taking its origin from the zygomatic arch and inserting on the lateral surface of the mandible, is the most powerful elevator of the mandible and functions to create pressure on the teeth, particularly the molars, in chewing motions. The masseter muscle is composed of two portions, superficial and deep, which are incompletely divided, yet have somewhat different functions. The superficial portion originates from the lower border of the zygomatic bone and the anterior two-thirds of the zygomatic arch and passes inferiorly and posteriorly to insert on the angle of the mandible. The deep head originates from the inner surface of the entire zygomatic arch and on the posterior one-third of the arch from its lower border. The deep fibers pass vertically to insert on the mandible on its lateral aspect above the insertion of the superficial head. The superficial portion in particular has a multipennate appearance with alternating tendinous plates and fleshy bundles of muscle fibers, which serve to increase the power of the muscle. Both the superficial and deep portions of the masseter muscle are powerful elevators of the mandible, but they function independently and reciprocally in other movements. Electromyographic studies show that the deep layer of the masseter is always silent during protrusive movements and always active during forced retrusion, whereas the superficial portion is active during protrusion and silent during retrusion.[8] Similarly the deep masseter is active in ipsilateral movements but does not function in contralateral movements, whereas the superficial masseter is active during contralateral movements but not in ipsilateral movements.

The medial pterygoid muscle (Figure 47-11) is rectangular and takes its origin from the pterygoid fossa and the internal surface of the lateral plate of the pterygoid process, with some fibers arising from the tuberosity of the maxilla and the palatine bone. Its fibers pass inferiorly and insert on the medial surface of the mandible,

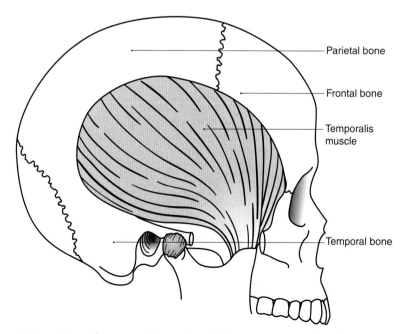

FIGURE 47-9   *The temporalis muscle with the zygomatic arch and masseter muscle removed. Adapted from Clemente CD.[51]*

Parietal bone

Frontal bone

Temporalis muscle

Temporal bone

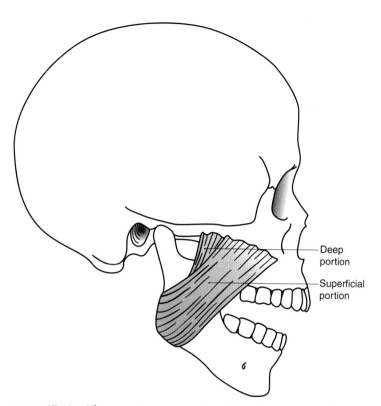

FIGURE **47-10**   *The masseter muscle. Adapted from Piecuch JF, Lieblich SE. Anatomy and pathology of the temporomandibular joint. In: Peterson LF, Indresano AT, Marciani RD, Roser SM. Principles of oral and maxillofacial surgery. Vol. 3. Philadelphia (PA): J.B. Lippincott Company; 1992. p. 1865.*

medial pole of the condyle. Anatomic studies have shown that the majority of the superior head fibers insert into the condyle rather than the disk.

The inferior and superior heads of the lateral pterygoid muscle function independently and reciprocally.[8,10] The primary function of the inferior head is protrusive and contralateral movement. When the bilateral inferior heads function together, the condyle is pulled forward down the articular eminence, with the disk moving passively with the condylar head. This forward movement of the condyle down the inclined plane of the articular eminence also contributes to opening of the oral cavity. When the inferior head functions unilaterally the resulting medial and protrusive movement of the condyle results in contralateral motion of the mandible. The function of the superior head of the lateral pterygoid muscle is predominantly involved with closing movements of the jaw and with retrusion and ipsilateral movement. A summary of the movements of the lateral pterygoid muscle and the other supramandibular muscles is given in Table 47-1.

inferiorly and posteriorly to the lingual. Like the masseter muscle the medial pterygoid fibers have alternating layers of fleshy and tendinous parts, thereby increasing the power of the muscle. The main function of the medial pterygoid is elevation of the mandible, but it also functions somewhat in unilateral protrusion in a synergism with the lateral pterygoid to promote rotation to the opposite side.

The lateral pterygoid muscle (see Figure 47-11) has two portions that can be considered two functionally distinct muscles. The larger inferior head originates from the lateral surface of the lateral pterygoid plate.[9] Its fibers pass superiorly and outward to fuse with the fibers of the superior head at the neck of the mandibular condyle, inserting into the pterygoid fovea. The superior head originates from the infratemporal surface of the greater sphenoid wing, and its fibers pass inferiorly, posteriorly, and outward to insert in the superior aspect of the pterygoid

fovea, the articular capsule, and the articular disk at its medial aspect, as well as to the

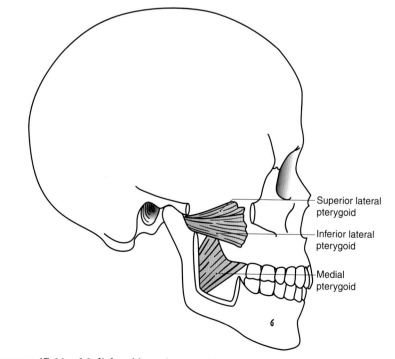

FIGURE **47-11**   *Medial and lateral pterygoid muscles. Adapted from Clemente CD.[51]*

Table 47-1   Contributions of the Supramandibular Muscles of Mastication to Movements of the Jaw as Confirmed by Electromyography

Muscles	Movement
Medial pterygoid	Closure, protrusion
Lateral pterygoid (inferior head)	Protrusion, opening contralateral
Lateral pterygoid (superior head)	Retrusion, closure, ipsilateral
Masseter, superficial layer	Protrusion, closure contralateral
Masseter, deep layer	Retrusion, closure ipsilateral
Temporalis, anterior portion	Closure
Temporalis, posterior portion	Retrusion, closure ipsilateral

Adapted from Gay T and Piecuch J.[8]

Inframandibular Muscle Group

The inframandibular muscles can be subdivided into two groups: the suprahyoids and the infrahyoids. The suprahyoid group consists of the digastric, geniohyoid, mylohyoid, and stylohyoid muscles; lies between the mandible and the hyoid bone; and serves to either raise the hyoid bone, if the mandible is fixed in position by the supramandibular group, or depress the mandible, if the hyoid bone is fixed in position by the infrahyoids. The infrahyoid group, consisting of the sternohyoid, omohyoid, sternothyroid, and thyrohyoid muscles, attaches to the hyoid bone superiorly and to the sternum, clavicle, and scapula inferiorly. This group of muscles can either depress the hyoid bone or hold the hyoid bone in position, relative to the trunk, during opening movements of the mandible.

Biomechanics of Temporomandibular Joint Movement

Complex free movements of the mandible are made possible by the relation of four distinct joints that are involved in mandibular movement: the inferior and superior joints—bilaterally. Two types of movement are possible: rotation and translation.

The inferior joints, consisting of the condyle and disk, are responsible for rotation, a hinge-like motion. The center of rotation is considered to be along a horizontal axis passing through both condyles.[4,5] In theory pure hinge motion of approximately 2.5 cm measured at the incisal edges of the anterior teeth is possible. Nevertheless most mandibular movements are translatory as well, involving a gliding motion between the disk and the temporal fossa, which are the components of the superior joints. The mandible and disk glide together as a unit because they are held together by the collateral ligaments. The maximum forward and lateral movement of the upper joint in translation is approximately 1.5 cm.

All movements of the mandible, whether symmetric or asymmetric, involve close contact of the condyle, disk, and articular eminence. Pure opening, closing, protrusive, and retrusive movements are possible as a result of bilaterally symmetric action of the musculature. Asymmetric movements, such as those seen in chewing, are made possible by unilateral movements of the musculature with different amounts of translation and rotation occurring within the joints on either side.

The positioning of the condyle and disk within the fossa, as well as the constant contact between the condyle, disk, and eminence, is maintained by continuous activity of the muscles of mastication, particularly the supramandibular group. The ligaments associated with the TMJ do not move the joint. Although they can be lengthened by movements of muscles, they do not stretch (ie, do not have an elastic recoil that returns them to a resting position automatically).

Instead the role of the ligaments is that of a passive restriction of movement at the extreme ranges of motion. During normal function rotational and translational movements occur simultaneously, permitting the free range of motion necessary in speaking and chewing.

Pathology of the Temporomandibular Joint

The demand for treatment of temporomandibular joint dysfunction (TMJD) is well known. Most studies estimate the prevalence of clinically significant TMJ-related jaw pain to be at least 5% of the general population. Approximately 2% of the general population seeks treatment for a TMJ-related symptom.[11,12] TMJD may be the result of muscular hyperfunction or parafunction, and/or underlying primary or secondary degenerative changes within the joint. It is important to note however that no single causative factor leading to TMJD has been unequivocally demonstrated in scientifically based studies.[13] Classification of TMJD is separated into nonarticular and articular categories and has been eloquently described by de Bont and colleagues.[13]

Nonarticular disorders include muscle disorders such as myofascial dysfunction, muscle spasm (with splinting, pain, and muscle guarding), and myositis. Articular disorders, often accompanied by internal derangement, include noninflammatory and inflammatory arthropathies, growth disorders, and connective tissue disorders. In diagnosing and treating TMJD it is helpful to assess patients with the above classification as a frame of reference Table 47-2. Treatment modalities can vary significantly depending on this classification.

Nonarticular Temporomandibular Disorders

Nonarticular TMJ disorders most commonly manifest as masticatory muscle dysfunction. Approximately one-half or more of all TMJDs are forms of masticatory

Table 47-2 General Classification of Synovial Disorders
Articular Disorders
Noninflammatory arthropathies
Primary osteoarthrosis (no clear
predisposing factor)
Secondary osteoarthrosis (trauma,
previous surgery, avascular necrosis)
Mechanical derangements
Bone and cartilage disorders with
articular manifestations
Inflammatory arthropathies
Synovitis
Capsulitis
Rheumatoid arthritis
Juvenile rheumatoid arthritis
Seronegative polyarthritis
Ankylosing spondylitis
Psoriatic arthritis
Reactive arthritis (bacterial, viral, fungal)
Growth disorders
Non-neoplastic: developmental
(hyperplasia, hypoplasia, dysplasia)
Non-neoplastic: acquired
(ie, condylolysis)
Neoplasm
Pseudotumors (synovial chondromatosis)
Benign (chondroma, osteotoma)
Malignant (primary, metastatic)
Diffuse connective tissue disorders
Miscellaneous articular disorders
Nonarticular Disorders
Muscle disorders
Muscle spasm (strain)
Myofascial pain and dysfunction (MPD)
Fibromyalgia
Myotonic dystrophies
Myositis ossificans progressiva
Growth disorders
Adapted from de Bont L et al.[13]

the supramandibular and inframandibular muscle groups on mandibular movement and function is evident in these conditions. Other nonarticular disorders include growth disorders affecting TMJ function and miscellaneous factors such as heterotopic bone formation leading to TMJD.

MPD is most commonly related to masseter or temporalis muscle spasm.[16] Additionally it can involve the pterygoids or any combination of the supramandibular or inframandibular muscle groups. Parafunctional habits such as bruxism and jaw clenching are thought to be the main contributors to MPD and have also been found to be causative in acute closed-lock conditions. The literature is replete with various treatment modalities for MPD. Such treatments include occlusal adjustments (for gross discrepancies), night-guard appliances (for joint unloading, jaw repositioning, and occlusal protection), nonsteroidal anti-inflammatory medications, muscle relaxants, and physical therapy. These treatment modalities, alone or in combination, remain the standard of care for the treatment of nonarticular TMJD, particularly MPD.

Fibromyalgia is a systemic condition marked by poor sleep, generalized pain with absence of localization to joints, and a history of somatization in other organ systems such as irritable bowel syndrome and headaches.[17] It is typically observed in an older population than MPD and has a female predilection. Fibromyalgia is often difficult to differentiate from MPD and is treated in similar fashion; that is, nonsurgically, with anti-inflammatory medications, dietary modifications, home-care techniques, bite appliances, and physical therapy. There appears to be a poorer overall response to the treatment of fibromyalgia when compared with MPD.

Rarely other nonarticular conditions such as myotonic dystrophy and myositis ossificans progressiva can lead to signifi-

cant loss of function and pain in the TMJ region. Myotonic dystrophy is a dominantly inherited multisystem disorder that may affect facial muscles in fully developed disease states.[18] This condition may contribute to atrophy and fibrosis of the supramandibular and inframandibular musculature. Clinically there are a variety of types of myotonic dystrophies. They tend to exert their pathologic effects in similar fashion, sometimes resulting in trismus, loss of function, and pain. Myositis ossificans progressiva is a rare condition resulting in fibrosis of soft tissues after apparent minor trauma. This condition has been reported to affect TMJ function after local trauma, including surgery, and can result in significant loss of mandibular range of motion, trismus, and pain.[19] Soft tissue ossification can sometimes occur after head trauma, severe burns, or neurogenic stimulus. In these cases heterotopic bone formation is observed and can lead to ankylosis in multiple joints throughout the body including the TMJ.[20]

Articular Temporomandibular Disorders

Noninflammatory articular disorders of the TMJ, the most common of which is osteoarthrosis, are often idiopathic. Osteoarthrosis can manifest as chondromalacia (softening of the cartilage), temporary or permanent disk displacement, degenerative changes within bone and cartilage often with osteophyte formation and remodeling, fibrosis, or any combination of the above. Noninflammatory articular disorders may also be secondary to trauma, infection, previous surgery, crystal deposition disorders (gout and pseudogout), avascular necrosis, or structural damage to joint cartilage resulting in disk displacement and/or perforation (Figure 47-12). TMJ disk displacement has been categorized through a widely accepted staging system by Wilkes, using such criteria as severity of displacement and chronicity (Table 47-3).[21]

myalgia.[14,15] They include such conditions such as acute muscle strain and spasm, myofascial pain and dysfunction (MPD), chronic conditions such as fibromyalgia, and less commonly, myotonic dystrophies and myositis ossificans. They invariably contribute to decreased mandibular range of motion and pain. The important role of

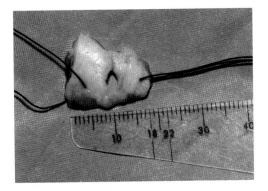

FIGURE 47-12   *Perforated disk (Wilkes stage V patient).*

Noninflammatory arthropathies are distinctly limited in their amount of overt inflammation and may be clinically silent or focal in nature. Alternatively if the condition becomes more severe, symptoms will ensue. If degenerative changes progress to synovitis, joint effusion (secondary to increased vascular permeability), or capsulitis, it is then considered to have transformed into an inflammatory arthropathy.

Inflammatory arthropathies are primarily due to such conditions as rheumatoid arthritis, juvenile rheumatoid arthritis, ankylosing spondylitis, psoriatic arthritis, or arthritis resulting from infectious causes (see Table 47-2). Secondary causes of inflammatory arthropathies include synovitis, capsulitis, traumatic arthritis, or acute inflamed crystal-induced arthritis, such as gout. As discussed previously noninflammatory arthropathies can progress to the inflammatory types through increasing concentrations of degradation products within the joint. Degenerative changes resulting in the release of inflammatory mediators have been demonstrated to worsen the degree of tissue destruction and dysfunction within the TMJ. This pathologic inflammatory cascade has been the primary focus of current TMJ research.

The past decade has shed new light on the cause and treatment of articular disorders (mainly, internal derangement) of the TMJ. Gross evaluation of disk position and disk integrity has traditionally been the mainstay of diagnosis and surgical treatment. More recently the physiologic activity of synovial cells, chondrocytes, and inflammatory cells in symptomatic joints have been associated with pathogenesis. This fundamental shift in focus has changed the primary treatment approach from openjoint surgery aimed at restoring the functional anatomy of the TMJ, to less invasive techniques directed toward lysis of adhesions and intracapsular lavage.[22] TMJ arthrocentesis and arthroscopy are thought to achieve an alteration in the joint milieu favoring a reduction in symptoms and improved joint function. Open-joint surgery nonetheless may still have a role in severe degenerative disease when preoperative criteria are met and surgery is indicated.

Milam and Schmitz have proposed a variety of molecular biologic mechanisms for TMJD.[23] Synovoid cells, chondrocytes, and inflammatory cells in the TMJ produce a physiologic balance between anabolic and catabolic cytokines.[23] Anabolic cytokines such as insulin-like growth factor-I and transforming growth factor beta are instrumental in the formation of extracellular joint matrix molecules. Collagen, proteoglycans, and glycoproteins are essential in load-bearing joints like the TMJ. Alternatively catabolic cytokines such as interleukin-1 (IL-1), IL-6, and tumor necrosis factor alpha (TNF-α) have been identified with the formation of proteases within the TMJ. These proteases (aspartic, cysteine, serine, and metalloproteases, among others) operate at low and neutral pH to exert their pathologic effects leading to degenerative changes.

Oxidative stress, often found associated with pathologic joints, is thought to contribute to free radical formation in the TMJ. The presence of free radicals has been postulated as an amplifying factor in the activation of cytokines, enzymes, neuropeptides, and arachidonic acid metabolites leading to degenerative joint disease.[24] Nitric oxide, a free radical involved in regulating vascular tone, has been observed at higher concentrations in arthritic joints. Nitric oxide has direct effects on prostaglandin synthesis and cyclooxygenase-2 enzymes leading to synovial inflammation and tissue destruction.[25] In a normal functioning joint a delicate balance is maintained between anabolic and catabolic mechanisms. In symptomatic joints catabolic processes have been found to exert greater overall effects thus disrupting the balance between anabolic physiologic maintenance and the negative effects of catabolic cytokines.

TMJ synovial fluid analysis has proven to be an excellent vehicle for evaluating the proposed contribution of cytokines, proteinases, and other catabolites to TMJD. Multiple independent studies support the hypothesis of catabolic imbalance within the joint. Kubota and colleagues demonstrated increased levels of IL-1β, IL-6, and active matrix metalloproteinases in TMJs with internal derangement and osteoarthritis when compared with control samples.[26] This study suggests the presence of elevated concentrations of these cytokines and proteinases serving as potential catabolic markers for cartilage degradation in the human TMJ. Murakami and colleagues reported high concentrations of chondroitin-4 and chondroitin-6 sulfates compared with hyaluronic acid in the TMJ synovial fluid of patients with internal derangement suggesting glycosaminoglycan components as markers of joint pathology.[27] Israel and colleagues demonstrated the prevalence of synovitis and osteoarthritis through arthroscopic evaluation in symptomatic TMJs.[28] These findings correlated with increased levels of keratan sulfate in the synovial fluid

Table 47-3 Wilkes Classification	
Stage I	Early reducing disk displacement
Stage II	Late reducing disk displacement
Stage III	Nonreducing disk displacement: acute/subacute
Stage IV	Nonreducing disk displacement: chronic
Stage V	Nonreducing disk displacement: chronic with osteoarthritis

of these joints suggesting its role as a potential biochemical marker for articular cartilage degradation.[28] Recently osteoclastogenesis inhibitory factor/osteoprotegerin (OCIF/OPG), a member of the TNF receptor family, has been studied in synovial fluid samples of TMJD patients.[29] Increased osteoclastic activity has been seen histologically in diseased mandibular condyles. Osteoclast differentiation requires cell-to-cell contact between osteoclast progenitors and bone marrow stromal cells. The presence of OCIF/OPG is thought to inhibit osteoclast differentiation by preventing the cell-to-cell contact needed for such activity. Synovial fluid samples in this study demonstrated decreased amounts of OCIF/OPG in osteoarthritic and internally deranged joints suggesting its physiologically important function in healthy joints. Although further investigation of synovial fluid components in TMJD is necessary to formulate definitive conclusions, it continues to shed new light on the pathogenesis and treatment of such disorders.

Treatment of patients with internal derangement of the TMJ typically begins with nonsurgical treatment modalities. Bite appliance therapy, diet modifications, nonsteroidal anti-inflammatory medications, muscle relaxants, moist heat or ice, and physical therapy have been found to be efficacious.[30] Surgical intervention is typically employed only after failure of nonsurgical treatment objectives.

A variety of surgical treatment modalities have been used in the treatment of articular TMJD. Arthrocentesis and TMJ arthroscopy have been found to be minimally invasive effective treatments for articular TMJD by decreasing pain and increasing mandibular range of motion. (Surgical techniques for arthroscopy are addressed in Chapter 49, "Temporomandibular Joint Arthrocentesis and Arthroscopy: Rationale and Technique.") Indications for these modalities include, but are not limited to, acute closed-lock degenerative joint disease accompanied by pain and limited range of

motion and joint effusion. Arthrocentesis and arthroscopy have also been reported to be useful in severe, often sudden onset, closed-lock disease due to an anchored or "stuck disk" phenomemon. This proposed phenomenon involves the disk becoming adherent to the glenoid fossa through increased intra-articular friction, with or without the formation of adhesions within the joint. Lysis of adhesions with joint lavage has been reported efficacious in restoring mandibular range of motion and decreasing pain in these clinical scenarios.[31,32] TMJ arthrocentesis and arthroscopy show promising results using the above criteria of pain symptoms and mandibular range of motion.[33] Based on the pathophysiology discussed in this chapter, a hypothesis explaining the efficacy of joint lavage relates to a proposed alteration in the biochemical constituents of the joint fluid, thus shifting the balance toward anabolic processes while reducing the amount of active catabolites contained within the joint.[34]

Indications for open arthrotomy include but are not limited to joint ankylosis, the need for reconstruction due to condylar resorption or growth disturbance, history of previous surgery, removal of foreign bodies, neoplasia, trauma, or severe degenerative disease precluding less invasive interventions. (Indications and techniques for open TMJ surgery are addressed more thoroughly in Chapter 50, "Surgery for Internal Derangements of the Temporomandibular Joint," and Chapter 51, "Management of the Patient with End-Stage Temporomandibular Joint Disease.") Open-joint surgery is primarily based on restoration of the functional anatomy of the TMJ when less invasive techniques are not feasible or unsuccessful. Recent data suggest comparable outcomes between open and closed surgery in the TMJ with lower morbidity associated with the latter.[35] Open TMJ surgery remains a viable treatment option at the end of the surgical treatment algorithm. New insight into the pathogenesis of TMJD has opened the

door to less invasive (albeit equally effective) treatment options for a large number of TMJD patients.

Infections of the Temporomandibular Joint

Infections of the TMJ are not common. Prompt diagnostic and therapeutic intervention is required when an infection of the TMJ is suspected because joint distention is usually painful and permanent changes in joint function can occur. On examination patients usually exhibit a posterior open bite on the ipsilateral side as a result of the increased joint fluid. The patient will also maintain a posture toward the contralateral side.[36] The surface overlying an infected joint is often warm, and fluctuance is occasionally felt.

The bacteria causing an infected joint are usually spread through a hematogenous route. The synovium is vascular and lacks a basement membrane, which permits bloodborne bacteria to gain access to the joint space.[37] Joints with underlying arthritic disease tend to be more susceptible to distant infection. Although the source of the bacteria is usually at a distant site, spread from dental infections of maxillary teeth has been reported in which the bacteria are thought to spread through the pterygoid plexus of veins to the joint.[38] Direct innoculation of a joint area following a traumatic injury is also possible. Complications of infections of the TMJ include fistula formation, fibrosis or bony ankylosis, temporal bone osteomyelitis, and intracranial abscess formation.

A thorough history and review of systems aids in the diagnosis of acute infectious arthritis of the TMJ. Active infection in adjacent sites, especially the ipsilateral maxillary molars, should be searched for. Other joints must be assessed to determine if they are involved. Initially aspiration of the joint should be considered to both relieve the pain from the joint capsular distention and to help in the identification of the infecting organism(s). The aspiration is performed by using a 20-gauge or larger needle under sterile conditions. The synovial fluid should be Gram stained and cultured for both aerobic and anaerobic bacteria. Sedation or general anesthesia may be required for the arthrocentesis.

In sexually active adults 60% of general acute infectious arthritis is due to *Neisseria gonorrhoeae*.[39] The majority of these patients have a prodrome of malaise, anorexia, headaches, fever, and chills. A few days of migratory arthritis usually precedes the localization of infection in one or two joints. Markowitz and Gerry reported a TMJ involvement rate of 3% in patients with disseminated gonococcal arthritis.[40] In children under 2 years of age almost 50% of acute infectious arthritis is due to *Haemophilus influenzae*. No reports of TMJ involvement are available. Other gram-positive cocci have been isolated from TMJ infections in all age groups, including staphylococci (particularly in the elderly) and β-hemolytic streptococci. The adherence characteristics of *Staphylococcus aureus* and *Neisseria gonorrhoeae* to synovium account for their prevalence.[41] Thus, the best choice for initial empiric antibiotic therapy for an acute infectious TMJ arthritis is an agent that combines a penicillin with a β-lactamase inhibitor. The combination of ampicillin and sulbactam will cover infections from the staphylococcal and streptococcal groups. Sulbactam, a derivative of penicillin, inactivates bacteria-produced β-lactamase and also has direct bactericidal activity against the *Neisseria* organisms. Therefore, this combination may have an advantage over the combination of a penicillin and clavulanic acid. It should be noted that bacterial resistance has become increasingly more problematic. Reference to up-to-date antibiotic regimens is recommended.

Effective treatment of septic arthritis by oral antibiotics has not been well studied, therefore the parenteral administration of antibiotics should be used initially.[37] Choices include ampicillin and sulbactam (Unasyn) 3 g intravenous (IV) every 6 hours, or clindamycin 600 mg IV every 6 hours in penicillin-allergic patients. A third generation cephalosporin, cefotaxime 6 to 12 g IV per day, could be used for a gram-negative infection in a nonhospitalized patient.[37] Tobramycin 3 mg/kg/day in four doses should be considered to treat a possible presence of *Pseudomonas aeruginosa* in infections that develop in hospitalized or immunocompromised patients.

The duration of treatment depends on the clinical response and the organism isolated. Based on information available for treatment of septic arthritis involving *Neisseria gonorrhoeae*, the patient with a septic TMJ could be placed on oral ampicillin or tetracycline after a 2-week course of IV therapy. Reportedly infections involving *Staphylococcus aureus* and gram-negative bacilli require 4 weeks of total therapy, and 2 to 3 weeks of therapy is adequate for streptococci and *Haemophilus* species.[42] Thus, it appears that a 30-day total course of antibiotic therapy for acute TMJ infection is appropriate.

In addition to culture and sensitivity testing, the aspirate from the infected joint should be submitted for white blood cell (WBC) count and differential, and examined for the presence of crystals and fibrinogen. Fibrinogen is usually present in the synovial fluid of acutely infected joints. Therefore, some of the synovial fluid collected should be placed into a heparinized tube to prevent clotting. It is important to note that ethylenediaminetetraacetic acid (EDTA) interferes with crystal analysis, therefore synovial fluid should not be placed in tubes containing it. The synovial fluid of an inflamed joint commonly contains greater than 2,000 WBC/mm^3 (normal < 200 WBC/mm^3). Septic joints normally have WBC counts greater than 50,000/mm^3. The cells are primarily mononuclear, as opposed to a predominance of polymorphonuclear cells in infected joint fluid. An exception to this occurs in fungal or mycobacterial joint infections in which the synovial fluid usually contains less than 20,000 WBC/mm^3 and shows a greater proportion of mononuclear cells.[43]

Following the institution of antibiotic therapy, lavage of the joint may be useful. Removing the joint fluid containing the products of the inflammation, reducing the bacterial load within the joint, and relieving the joint distention will usually markedly relieve the patient's symptoms and may also decrease the likelihood of spread to the temporal bone. Murakami and colleagues have reported on the use of the arthroscope for monitoring and treating an acutely infected TMJ.[38]

Following the resolution of an acute TMJ infection, a program must be started to minimize joint disability and to monitor for recurrence of infection. The acute inflammatory process that accompanies an infection can result in the deposition of fibrinogen and other products, which can predispose the joint toward a fibrous or bony ankylosis. Active range of motion exercises are started as soon as possible to prevent intra-articular adhesions. The patient's range of motion should be documented at weekly intervals. If the range of motion is still limited 1 month following the resolution of the infection, a brisement procedure or an arthroscopic procedure to lyse intra-articular adhesions should be considered. However, before this, extracapsular causes of limited opening, such as masseter muscle trismus, need to be differentiated from intracapsular disorders. Intracapsular restrictions are usually accompanied by restriction of lateral excursions to the contralateral side and deviation on opening. Recurrence of joint infection (of all joints) has been reported to occur at a rate of 10.5%.[44] Newman noted that infection recurred as long as 1 year following the initial episode.[44] The patient should be advised of this possibility.

Neoplastic Diseases

Tumors affecting the TMJ area are exceedingly rare. The tissues from which a neoplasm may arise include the synovium, bone, cartilage, and associated musculature. Neoplasms of this region can present with signs and symptoms similar to those occurring with internal derangement (preauricular pain and dysfunction) and thus can result in a delay in the diagnosis. The clinician should be aware of this when treating temporomandibular disorders, especially if the patient fails to respond to traditional therapy.

Benign Tumors

The most common benign bone tumors of the TMJ include the osteoma and condylar enlargement or condylar hypertrophy. Both present signs related to the increase in size of the condyle, a shift in the mandible to the contralateral side, and an ipsilateral open bite. Often the range of motion is decreased as the increased size of the condylar head prevents normal translation. Radiographs, including tomograms and computed tomography scans, should be obtained to delineate the extent of the condylar growth and to determine involvement of the glenoid fossa and associated structures. Radionuclide scans should be performed to determine if the process is still active and bone is being produced. Treatment includes a condylar head resection (partial or complete) for active lesions or a condyloplasty to reduce condylar size and restore the occlusion for nongrowing lesions. Condylar reconstruction is usually not necessary. The disk should be preserved or replaced (if it has been damaged) with a temporalis muscle flap or cartilage graft. Physical therapy is usually required to reduce dysfunction. Postoperative maxillomandibular fixation is not usually necessary, but guiding elastics may be helpful with muscle retraining. An active physical therapy program to reduce joint adhesions prevents permanent restriction of the joint.

Virtually all other benign bone tumors have been reported to occur in the TMJ. These bone tumors behave as they would in other areas of the mandible and therefore should be treated in a similar fashion.

Synovial Tumors

Synovial chondromatosis is the most commonly reported neoplasm of the TMJ synovium. Lustman and Zelster reported a series of 50 cases in which the mean age was 47 years.[45] This is in contrast to synovial chondromatosis involving other joints, which is more commonly found in the 20- to 30-year-old age group.[46] Pain and swelling of the preauricular area are the most common initial signs. Depending on the degree of calcification present, radiographs may reveal the presence of loose radiodense bodies within the joint. These loose bodies are formed by metaplastic synovial tissues. Foci of metaplastic synovium detach from the synovial lining and remain viable while suspended in the synovial fluid. While suspended they form a perichondrium and continue to grow and enlarge. Although the reason is unknown this process most frequently occurs in the superior joint space. The loose bodies are composed of cartilage containing multinucleated cells. The presence of cellular atypia and hyperchromatism is common and a careful review of all histologic material removed is necessary to rule out the possibility of chondrosarcoma.

Treatment of synovial chondromatosis involves extirpation of the loose bodies and removal of the synovial lining. Lustman and Zelster reported that a condylectomy was necessary in 13 of 47 cases to gain access to the anteromedial portion of the joint.[45] The condyle itself is not involved and therefore should only be removed for access. Recurrence of synovial chondromatosis is quite rare and is thought to be caused by an incomplete excision of the original lesions. No cases of TMJ synovial chondromatosis transforming into chondrosarcoma have been reported, although this has been reported in the knee.[47]

Ganglion Cysts

Ganglion cysts have also been reported to occur in association with the TMJ. These are cystic structures that arise subcutaneously in association with the joint capsule or tendon sheaths. Histologic examination of a ganglion reveals a true cyst, containing a mucinous fluid and hyaluronic acid. These lesions present as a preauricular mass and may produce classic "TMJ symptoms," such as pain and limitation of function. The swelling produced by the ganglion in the preauricular region can be confused with a parotid mass. Surgery is indicated to remove the cyst and reoccurrences have not been reported.[48]

Malignant Tumors

Malignancies of the TMJ are very rare and are usually the result of direct extensions of primary lesions of adjacent structures. Metastatic disease has been reported to involve the TMJ, but is more commonly found in the mandibular angle region. This may be due to the relative paucity of cancellous bone in the condylar head region.[49] The most common lesions to metastasize to the condyle are adenocarcinomas of the breast, kidney, and lungs. As with benign tumors the early signs of malignant disease of the TMJ are pain and dysfunction. Primary malignancies of the TMJ have been reported as intrinsic tumors of the condylar bone, disk, synovium, and cartilaginous linking. Typically patients with malignancies of the TMJ are older than the usual internal derangement patient. Patients with a history of preexisting malignant disease must undergo a thorough search for metastasis if TMJ symptoms develop. Radionuclide scans may be useful, although the inflammation from chronic synovitis can result in activity localizing in the condyle.[50] Patients presenting with a fracture of the condyle without a history of trauma should be suspect for the presence of a malignant lesion in the condyle.

Primary TMJ malignancies require aggressive therapy to prevent intracranial extension of the disease. Radiation, surgery, and chemotherapy are all appropriate means of treatment of diseases in this region. Radiation therapy can also be used for palliation in disseminated disease to control pain from the TMJ region and to prevent pathologic fractures.

References

1. DuBrul, EL. Sicher's oral anatomy. 7th ed. St. Louis (MO): C.V. Mosby; 1980. p. 146–61, 174–209.

2. Albright JA, Brand RA. The scientific basis of orthopedics. 2nd ed. Norwalk (CT): Appleton and Lange; 1987. p. 373–86.

3. Dijkgraaf LC, Milam SB. Osteoarthritis: histopathology and biochemistry of the TMJ. In: Piecuch JF, editor. Oral maxillofacial surgery knowledge update. Vol 3. Rosemont (IL): American Association of Oral and Maxillofacial Surgeons; 2001. p. 5–28.

4. Bell WE. Temporomandibular disorders: classification, diagnosis and management. 2nd ed. Chicago (IL): Yearbook Medical Publishers; 1986. p. 16–62.

5. Okeson JP. Management of temporomandibular disorders and occlusions. 2nd ed. St. Louis (MO): C.V. Mosby; 1989. p. 3–26.

6. Rayne J. Functional anatomy of the temporomandibular joint. Br J Oral Maxillofac Surg 1987;25:92–9.

7. Blackwood HJJ. Pathology of the temporomandibular joint. J Am Dent Assoc 1969;79:118.

8. Gay T, Piecuch J. An electromyographic analysis of jaw movements in man. Electromyogr Clin Neurophysiol 1986;26:365–84.

9. Carpentier P, Yung JP, Marguelles-Bonnet R, Meunissier M. Insertions of the lateral pterygoid muscle. J Oral Maxillofac Surg 1988;46:477–82.

10. McNamara JA. The independent functions of the two heads of the lateral pterygoid muscle. Am J Anat 1973;138:197–205.

11. Goulet JP, Lavigne GJ, Lund JP. Jaw pain prevalence among French speaking Canadians in Quebec and related symptoms of temporomandibular disorders. J Dent Res 1995; 74:1738–44.

12. DeKanter R, Kayser A, Battistuzzi P, et al. Demand and need for treatment of craniomandibular dysfunction in the Dutch adult population. J Dent Res 1992; 71:1607–12.

13. deBont L, Dijkgraaf L, Stegenga B. Epidemiology and natural progression of articular temporomandibular disorders. Oral Surg Oral Med Oral Pathol Oral Radiol Endod 1997;83:72–6.

14. Marbach JJ, Lipton JA. Treatment of patients with temporomandibular joint and other facial pain by otolaryngologists. Arch Otolaryngol 1982;108:102–7.

15. List T, Dworkin SF, Harrison R, Huggins K. Research diagnostic criteria/temporomandibular disorders: comparing Swedish and U.S. clinics [abstract]. J Dent Res 1996;75(special issue):352.

16. Laskin DM. Diagnosis and etiology of myofascial pain and dysfunction. Oral Maxillofac Surg Clin North Am 1995;7:73–8.

17. Demitrack M. Chronic fatigue syndrome and fibromyalgia dilemmas in diagnosis and clinical management. Psychiatr Clin North Am 1998;21:671–92.

18. Kiliardis S, Katsaros C. The effects of myotonic dystrophy and Duchenne muscular dystrophy on the orofacial muscles and dentofacial morphology. Acta Odontol Scand 1998;56:369–74.

19. Steiner M, Gould AR, Kushner GM, et al. Myositis ossificans traumatica of the masseter muscle: review of the literature and report of two additional cases. Oral Surg Oral Med Oral Pathol Oral Radiol Endod 1997;84:703–7.

20. Rubin M, Cozzi G. Heterotopic ossification of the temporomandibular joint in a burn patient. J Oral Maxillofac Surg 1986;44:897–9.

21. Wilkes CH. Internal derangement of the temporomandibular joint pathological variations. Arch Otolaryngol Head Neck Surg 1989;115:469–77.

22. Dolwick MF. Intra-articular disc displacement Part I: its questionable role in temporomandibular joint pathology. J Oral Maxillofac Surg 1995;53:1069–72.

23. Milam SB, Schmitz JP. Molecular biology of temporomandibular joint disorders: proposed mechanisms of disease. J Oral Maxillofac Surg 1995;53:1448–54.

24. Milam SB, Zardeneta G, Schmitz JP. Oxidative stress and degenerative temporomandibular joint disease: a proposed hypothesis. J Oral Maxillofac Surg 1998;56:214–23.

25. Takahashi T, Kondoh T, Ohtani M, et al. Association between arthroscopic diagnosis of osteoarthritis and synovial fluid nitric oxide levels. Oral Surg Oral Med Oral Pathol Oral Radiol Endod 1999;88:129–36.

26. Kubota E, Kubota T, Matsumoto J, et al. Synovial fluid cytokines and proteases as markers of temporomandibular joint disease. J Oral Maxillofac Surg 1998;56:192–8.

27. Murakami KI, Shibata T, Kubota E, Maeda H. Intra-articular levels of prostaglandin E2, hyaluronic acid, and chondroitin-4 and -6 sulfates in the temporomandibular joint synovial fluid of patients with internal derangement. J Oral Maxillofac Surg 1998;56:199–203.

28. Israel HA, Diamond BE, Said-Nejad F, Ratcliffe A. Correlation between arthroscopic diagnosis of osteoarthritis and synovitis of the human temporomandibular joint and keratin sulfate levels in the synovial fluid. J Oral Maxillofac Surg 1997;55:210–7.

29. Kaneyama K, Segami N, Nishimura M, et al. Osteoclastogenesis inhibitory factor/osteoprotegerin in synovial fluid from patients with temporomandibular disorders. Int J Oral Maxillofac Surg. 2003;32:404–7.

30. Okeson J. Nonsurgical treatment of internal derangements. Oral Maxillofac Surg Clin North Am 1995;7:63–71.

31. Nitzan D. The process of lubrication impairment and its involvement in temporomandibular joint disc displacement: a theoretical concept. J Oral Maxillofac Surg 2001;59:36–45.

32. Rao VM, Liem MD, Farole A, Razik A. Elusive "stuck" disk in the temporomandibular joint: diagnosis with MR imaging. Radiology 1993;189:823–7.

33. Goudot P, Jaquinet AR, Hugonnet S, et al. Improvement of pain and function after arthroscopy and arthrocentesis of the temporomandibular joint: a comparative study. J Craniomaxillofac Surg 2000;28:39–43.

34. Zardeneta G, Milam SB, Schmitz JP. Elution of proteins by continuous temporomandibular joint arthrocentesis. J Oral Maxillofac Surg 1997;55:709–16.

35. Holmlund AB, Axelsson S, Gynther G. A comparison of diskectomy and arthroscopic lysis and lavage for the treatment of chronic closed-lock of the temporomandibular joint: a randomized outcome study. J Oral Maxillofac Surg 2001; 59:972–7.

36. Bounds GA, Hopkins R, Sugar A. Septic arthritis of the temporomandibular joint: a problematic diagnosis. Br J Oral Maxillofac Surg 1987;25:61–7.

37. Simpson ML. Septic arthritis in adults. In: Gustilo RB, Grumminger RP, Tsukayama DT, editors. Orthopedic infection. Philadelphia (PA): WB Saunders; 1900. p. 286.

38. Murakami K, Matsumoto K, Iizuka T. Suppurative arthritis of the temporomandibular joint: report of a case with special reference to arthroscopic observations. J Maxillofac Surg 1984;12(1):41–5.

39. Parker RH. Acute infectious arthritis. In: Schlossberg D, editor. Orthopedic infection. New York (NY): Springer-Verlag; 1988. p. 69–75.

40. Markowitz HA, Gerry RG. Temporomandibular joint disease. Oral Surg Oral Med Oral Pathol 1950;3:75–9.

41. Eisenstein BI, Masi AT. Disseminated gonococcal infection and gonococcal arthritis. Semin Arthritis Rheum 1988;10:155–9.

42. Smith JW. Infectious arthritis. In: Mandell GL, Douglas RG, Bennett JE, editors. Principles and practice of infectious diseases. New York (NY): John Wiley & Sons; 1985. p. 697.

43. Mahowald ML, Messner RP. Chronic infective arthritis. In: Schlossberg D, editor. Orthopedic infection. New York (NY): Springer-Verlag; 1988. p. 76–95.

44. Newman JH. Review of septic arthritis throughout the antibiotic era. Ann Rheum Dis 1976;35:198–204.

45. Lustman J, Zelster R. Synovial chondromatosis of the temporomandibular joint. Int J Oral Maxillofac Surg 1989;18:90–4.

46. Orden A, Laskin DM, Leu D. Chronic preauricular swelling. J Oral Maxillofac Surg 1989;47:390–7.

47. King JW, Splut HJ, Fechner RE, Vanderpool DW. Synovial chondrosarcoma of the knee joint. J Bone Joint Surg 1967;49:1389–96.

48. Copeland M, Douglas B. Ganglions of the temporomandibular joint. Plast Reconstr Surg 1988;69:775–6.

49. Hartman GL, Robertson GR, Sugg WE, et al. Metastatic carcinoma of the mandibular condyle. J Oral Surg 1973;31:716–9.

50. Mizukawa JH, Dolwick MF, Johnson RP, et al. Metastatic breast adenocarcinoma of the mandibular condyle. J Oral Surg 1980;38:448–9.

51. Clemente CD, editor. Gray's anatomy of the human body. 30th ed. Philadelphia (PA): Lea & Febiger; 1985. p. 451.

CHAPTER 48

Nonsurgical Management of Temporomandibular Disorders

Vasiliki Karlis, DMD, MD
Robert Glickman, DMD

Temporomandibular disorder (TMD) is the general term used to describe the manifestation of pain and/or dysfunction of the temporomandibular joint (TMJ) and its associated structures. Up to 5% of the population are affected by TMD, with significantly more frequent and more severe signs and symptoms appearing in women and older adults.[1,2] The etiology of TMD is presumed to include trauma, parafunctional habits, malocclusion, joint overloading, arthritides, psychological factors, and ergonomic positioning of the head. The impact of psychological factors is difficult to calculate, but approximately 10 to 20% of patients with TMD also manifest some form of psychiatric illness.[3] As symptoms of TMD are quite variable and remain exceedingly difficult to attribute exclusively to one or more events (such as the true contribution or extent of involvement of muscles of mastication), the joint itself or psychological factors is best understood in terms of interdependence. When a diagnosis of TMD is suspected or confirmed, therapy should be directed to improve function and reduce pain and discomfort. There is ample literature to suggest that nonsurgical treatment modalities may account for as much as a 74 to 85% favorable response rate in patients with TMD.[4,5] In one study, Suvinen and colleagues reported that 81% of their

patients showed 50% or greater improvement after conservative physical therapy with a 6-month follow-up, attributing the improvement to a possible placebo-type effect.[6] Other sources report significant relief in 30 to 60% of patients when under some form of treatment.[7] Additionally, long-term follow-up studies have suggested that almost all patients with TMD will improve with time, regardless of the type of treatment they may receive.[4,8–12] Thus, it appears well established in the literature that the majority of patients with TMD achieve some relief of symptoms with nonsurgical therapy. The dilemma for the surgeon is exacerbated by the broad spectrum of results and claims that use a seemingly endless variety of surgical and nonsurgical strategies. Since the extent or severity of symptomatology is apparently unrelated to etiology, and the overwhelming number of symptoms respond to conservative management, the question of whether and how to incorporate surgical and nonsurgical treatment into the care of these patients becomes challenging for the attending physician. There are absolute indications where surgical intervention would be of primary benefit, and the questions would be whether there is still a role for nonsurgical therapy in these patients, and if so, when it should be instituted and for how long.

One approach is to consider the concept of nonsurgical versus surgical therapy misleading and incomplete. There are many times when it is inappropriate to consider surgery. At other times nonsurgical therapy precedes and almost always follows surgical intervention. Therefore, it is essential for the surgeon to have a deep appreciation of the available techniques and their limitations in order to know when and how to properly manage TMDs. The purpose of this chapter will be to delineate those techniques that are adjunctive or discriminating to surgical considerations.

Treatment Considerations

The primary goal in treatment of TMD is to alleviate pain and/or mandibular dysfunction. Pain and alterations in function (ie, mastication and speech) can become quite debilitating, greatly affecting oral health care and diminishing the quality of life for these individuals. Another critical objective relates to patient counseling and education on the predisposing factors for TMD. Depending on the degree of impairment, patients can often be assured that TMD is a benign condition and clinical improvement can be expected with appropriate therapy. However, it is prudent if not incumbent upon the surgeon to inform patients that complete elimination of symptoms is at times unattainable. Nonsurgical techniques that can decrease unintentional overloading of the masticatory system, eliminate pain, reduce dysfunction, decrease chronicity, and promote healing are essential in all phases of therapy. A patient home care program may prevent further injury and allow for a period of healing. In general patients can be instructed to limit mandibular function, modify habits, avoid stress, and start a home exercise program.[8]

Clicking and popping of the TMJ is quite common in TMD and normal joints. It is difficult to eliminate, usually reoccurs, and there is inconclusive evidence to suggest whether this poses a problem for the patient. There is considerable support that joint sounds without pain or dysfunction should not be treated (Table 48-1).

Once a diagnosis of TMD has been established, frequent follow-up appointments are necessary once therapy is instituted, to determine whether there is any improvement. Initial impressions may require modification after several weeks of therapy, and further diagnostic procedures may be warranted to rule out vascular, neurologic, neoplastic, psychological, or otolaryngologic abnormalities. TMD is a complex disorder that is molded by many interacting factors, and strong consideration should be given to a multidisciplinary approach. The role of the dentist, physical therapist, neurologist, psychologist/psychiatrist, anesthesiologist, and oral and maxillofacial surgeon cannot be understated, and should be key constituents of any facial pain/TMD center. We cannot precisely dictate timing or length of therapy. This must still be determined by the surgeon and based on severity of symptoms and supporting diagnostic parameters. As with other joints consideration must be given to rule out pathology, decrease inflammation, allow unimpeded joint motion, and restore range of motion. To accomplish this in a ginglymoarthrodial joint that is permanently attached to the opposite side and is intimately involved in oral health is indeed a challenge.

The remainder of this chapter provides basic guidelines for nonsurgical therapeutics. It is not intended to eliminate or preselect adjunctive dental or surgical treatment.

Nonsurgical Therapy

Diet

A soft diet is often overlooked in the management of TMD. A soft diet prevents overloading of the TMJ and decreases muscle activity that may be hyperactive. The extent of time that a patient should be placed on a soft food diet is dependent on the severity of symptoms. Patients should be instructed to cut their food into small pieces and abstain from eating chewy, hard, or crunchy foods. Uncooked vegetables and meats represent examples of foods that should not be eaten by these patients. A strict liquid diet is reserved for those patients experiencing severe TMD symptoms (Table 48-2).

Pharmacotherapy

Medications are often prescribed for managing the symptoms associated with TMD. Patients should understand that these medications may not offer the cure to their problem but can be a valuable adjunctive aid when prescribed as part of a comprehensive program. With pharmacotherapy there is always a danger of drug dependency and abuse, particularly with narcotics and tranquilizers. Since many TMD symptoms are periodic, there is a tendency to prescribe medications on a "take as needed" philosophy. This can provide brief periods of pain relief, but more frequent pain cycles can result in less effectiveness of the drugs and ultimate overuse or abuse of the medications.[12–15] The general recommendation is that when pharmacotherapy is employed, the medications should be prescribed at regular intervals for a specific period of time (eg, four times daily for 2 wk). The clinician must always be cognizant of potential personality traits that may contribute to drug dependence or abuse. Other obvious factors are concurrent medical ailments or medications, patient age, occupation, and each patient's attitude toward pharmacotherapy.

The most common pharmacologic agents used for the management of TMD are analgesics, anti-inflammatory agents, anxiolytic agents, antidepressants, muscle relaxants, antihistamines, and local anesthetics. Analgesics, corticosteroids, and anxiolytics are useful for acute TMD pain. Anti-inflammatory medications and antidepressants are primarily indicated for chronic pain management. Muscle relaxants, nonsteroidal anti-inflammatory drugs (NSAIDs), and local anesthetics can be used for both acute and chronic pain.

Analgesics   Analgesic medications are either opiate or nonopiate preparations. Nonopiate analgesics (salicylates and acetaminophen) can be added to the anti-inflammatory regimen to assist in pain relief. The salicylates (ASA) are commonly used in TMD and are the benchmark medications to which other analgesics are usually compared. Salicylates are antipyretic, analgesic, and anti-inflammatory. For

Table 48-1   Goals of Nonsurgical Therapy for Temporomandibular Disorders
Alleviate pain
Decrease or eliminate jaw dysfunction
Educate and counsel patients

Table 48-2   Soft Diet
Decreases muscle activity and loading forces on temporomandibular joints
Controls range of motion—hinge and sliding
Ranges from liquid diet to elimination of hard chewy food; involves cutting food into small pieces
Eliminates gum chewing

those patients who cannot take aspirin, a nonacetylated aspirin such as choline magnesium trisalicylate or salsalate may be effective. As with all salicylates, however, choline magnesium trisalicylate and salsalate should not be prescribed for children or teenagers with chickenpox, influenza, or flu symptoms or exposure.

Opioid analgesics (oxycodone, propoxyphene, and hydrocodone) should be prescribed only for moderate to severe pain of limited duration, due to the high potential for addiction. These drugs are often administered in conjunction with NSAIDs or acetaminophen (Vicodin, Lortab, Percocet, Darvocet, etc). They act on opioid receptors in the central nervous system, producing analgesia and sedation. Because patients can quickly become dependant on the narcotic analgesics, it is recommended that these drugs not be prescribed for longer than 2 to 3 weeks. Other side effects include constipation secondary to decreased gastric motility.

Anti-inflammatory Medications There are two types of anti-inflammatory medications useful in treating TMD: NSAIDs and corticosteroids (Figure 48-1). Glucocorticosteroids prevent the release of arachidonic acid, a key component of the inflammation cascade. NSAIDs inhibit cyclooxygenase, which inhibits prostaglandin synthesis from arachidonic acid.[16–18]

NSAIDs The advantages of NSAIDs in TMD patients are analgesia and their anti-inflammatory properties (Tables 48-3 and 48-4). NSAIDs may offer relief for patients with synovitis, myositis, capsulitis, symptomatic disk displacement, and osteoarthritis.[19] This type of therapy helps alleviate the inflammation, which thereby causes a decrease in pain perception. Side effects include gastric irritation, allergies, and liver dysfunction. An ideal NSAID would be one that has minimal gastric irritation, a quick onset with long-lasting effects, low dosage requirements, is tolerated at high levels,

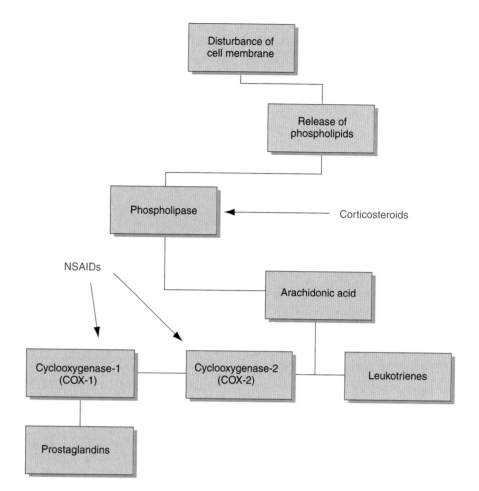

FIGURE 48-1 *Inflammation cascade. The corticosteriods prevent the release of arachidonic acid and thereby interrupt most of the inflammation cascade. The NSAIDs inhibit cyclooxygenase, which inhibits prostaglandin synthesis from arachidonic acid. NSAID = nonsteroidal anti-inflammatory drugs.*

and is low in cost. NSAIDs are divided into seven groups based on their chemical structure: salicylates (ASA), propionic acids (ibuprofen, naproxen), acetic acids (indomethacin, ketorolac), fenamic acids (meclofenamate), oxicams (piroxicam), and the cyclooxygenase (COX)-2 inhibitors (celecoxib, rofecoxib). The most common NSAIDs used are ibuprofen, diclofenac, and naproxen, but because of purported fewer gastrointestinal (GI) side effects and minimal effect on platelets, COX-2 inhibitors are becoming more popular. Recent studies have found that COX-2, an important inflammatory mediator, is present in the TMJ synovial tissue and fluid of patients with internal derangements. This offers the possibility that the COX-2 inhibitors might be more effective for TMJ

pain and arthralgias than other analgesics.[20,21] Enteric coating, prodrugs (nabumetone), taking agents after meals or in conjunction with antacids, and taking gastric protective agents (ranitidine and sucralfate) have been reported to reduce the gastric irritation from NSAIDs.[22]

Corticosteroids By completely blocking the arachidonic acid cascade, corticosteroids produce a greater anti-inflammatory response than do NSAIDs. Systemic steroids are indicated only for short-term therapy (5 to 7 d) due to their long-term possible complications. Osteoporosis, diabetes, hypertension, electrolyte changes, and clinical Cushing's disease are sequelae of long-term systemic corticosteroid treatment.[23] Steroids have also been directly injected into the TMJ

Table 48-3   Commonly Used Nonsteroidal Anti-inflammatory Agents

Category	Generic	Brand	Half-Life (hours)
Salicylates	Acetylsalicylic acid (aspirin)	Bayer	2.5
	Enteric coated	Ecotrin	2.5
	Aspirin with buffering agent	Bufferin	2.5
	Aspirin with caffeine	Anacin	2.5
	Diflunisal	Dolobid	8–12
	Choline magnesium trisalicylate	Trilisate	9–17
	Salsalate	Disalcid	16
Propionic acid	Ibuprofen	Motrin, Advil, Nuprin, Rufen	1.8–2.5
	Fenoprofen	Nalfon	2–3
	Suprofen	Suprol	2–4
	Naproxen	Naprosyn	12–15
	Naproxen sodium	Anaprox	12–15
Acetic acid	Indomethacin	Indocin	4.5–6
	Sulindac	Clinoril	7.8 (16.4)*
	Tolmetin	Tolectin	1–1.5
Fenamic acid	Meclofenamate	Meclomen	2 (3.3)*
	Mefenamic acid	Ponstel	2
Pyrazolones	Phenylbutazone	Butazolidin	84
Oxicam	Piroxicam olamine	Feldene	30–86
COX-2 inhibitors	Celecoxib	Celebrex	11–12
	Rofecoxib	Vioxx	17

*Active metabolite.
Adapted from Syrop SB.[25]

muscle, and cause sedation and may be selected according to their more favorable characteristics (ie, less sedation). The muscle relaxant properties may be used to decrease the effects of bruxism secondary to hyperactivity of muscles of mastication. It is recommended that the benzodiazepines not be used for more than a 2-week period because of the high potential for dependency, although this can be increased up to 3 weeks only at bedtime to control bruxism.[19] Buspar (azaspirodecanedione) is an anxiolytic; however, it does not produce either sedation or muscle relaxation. It may be used to control anxiety in TMD patients without producing drowsiness.

Antihistamines (promethazine and hydroxyzine) antagonize central and peripheral H_1 receptors, and have a sedative effect as well as anxiolytic properties. Antihistamines, unlike the benzodiazepines, do not have the potential for abuse. They can be used more safely in children and the elderly and for the treatment of vertigo and nausea that may accompany TMD.[25]

in an attempt to decrease inflammation or mediate the inflammatory response (ie, following arthroscopy), but long-term or excessive use is associated with condylar hypoplasia by inhibiting osteoblastic activity and increasing loss of calcium in the urine and GI tract.[24]

Anxiolytics Anxiolytic medications reduce the anxiety, insomnia, and muscle hyperactivity associated with TMD (Tables 48-5 and 48-6). These drugs often help the patient reduce the perception of, or reaction to, stress. Benzodiazepines (diazepam) decrease anxiety, relax skeletal

Antidepressants Antidepressants include monoamine oxidase inhibitors (MAOIs), tricyclic antidepressants, and selective serotonin reuptake inhibitors (Tables 48-7 and 48-8). They are pre-

Table 48-4   Nonsteroidal Anti-inflammatory Drugs: Ideal Properties

Minimal gastric irritation
Quick onset with long-lasting effects
Lower dosage
Tolerated at high levels
Low cost

Table 48-5   Commonly Used Benzodiazepines

Generic	Brand	Usual Dosage (mg/d)	Elimination (half-life [h])
Alprazolam	Xanax	0.5–1.5 (ddd)	12–15
Chlordiazepoxide	Librium	15–60 (ddd)	5–30
Diazepam	Valium	2–40 (ddd)	20–50
Flurazepam	Dalmane	30 (at bedtime)	47–100
Lorazepam	Ativan	2–6 (ddd)	10–18
Oxazepam	Serax	30–60 (ddd)	5–15
Prazepam	Verstran	20–40 (ddd)	30–100
Temazepam	Restoril	15–30 (at bedtime)	10–20
Triazolam	Halcion	0.25–0.5 (at bedtime)	1.5–5

ddd = divided daily doses
Adapted from Syrop SB.[25]

Table 48-6 Antianxiety Medications: Benzodiazepines

Bind GABA receptors

Serotonergic (5-HT) in the amygdala

Beneficial for treatment of anxiety, insomnia, muscle hypertonicity

Potential abuse

Avoid short-acting or high-potency drugs (ie, triazolam, alprazolam, lorazepam)

Taper gradually to avoid withdrawal, rebound anxiety

GABA = γ-aminobutyric acid; 5-HT = 5-hydroxy-tryptamine (serotonin).

Table 48-8 Antidepressant Medications

Tricyclics are most used and studied for chronic pain and depression

Monoamine oxidase inhibitors (MAOIs) not first choice due to adverse reactions

Selective serotonin reuptake inhibitors (SSRIs) such as fluoxetine can increase anxiety and bruxism

scribed for chronic pain, headaches, sleep disorders, obsessive-compulsive disorders, and central-mediated pain disorders. The relationship between pain and depression is a challenge and often necessitates treating both simultaneously. Depression in the TMD or chronic pain population is greater than in the general population. Studies report that up to 30% of TMD patients have major depression at the time of presentation for treatment, and up to 74% of patients with chronic TMD have had an episode of major depression.[26,27]

MAOIs are not routinely prescribed for TMD due to their numerous side effects and dietary restrictions. Benefits of tricyclic antidepressants have been well documented in chronic pain or depression populations and are probably due to analgesic and antidepressant actions. The analgesic properties are independent of the antidepressant effect, which requires higher doses. It has been shown that low doses of amitriptyline (10 mg) before sleep can have an analgesic effect on chronic pain but have no relationship to the antidepressant actions that require doses up to 20 times greater.[28] Tricyclic antidepressants may also help treat nocturnal bruxism and any sleep disturbance associated with TMD.[29] Side effects are related to anticholinergic activity causing xerostomia, constipation, blurred vision, and urinary retention. Selective serotonin reuptake inhibitors can also be used for treating the depressed TMD patient. These medications often need to be taken for several months and patients must be counseled appropriately. Fluoxetine (Prozac) may increase bruxism and anxiety and should be carefully monitored.

Muscle Relaxants Centrally acting muscle relaxants (cyclobenzaprine, methocarbamol, and carisoprodol) may be used to relax hyperactive musculature associated with TMD (Tables 48-9–48-11). These relaxants may also act as sedatives, and they are commonly combined with NSAID use. Cyclobenzaprine (Flexeril) has a similar chemical structure to the tricyclic antidepressants and if given over an extended period of time will produce antidepressant and sedative actions as well as the anticholinergic side effects of the tricyclics. Central muscle relaxants can be very effective for acute myofascial pain (ie, trauma).

One peripheral muscle relaxant, baclofen, has been used in myofascial pain but is best reserved for severe muscle spasm or neurogenic pain. Recently botu-linum toxin has been used to treat severe bruxism. By providing muscle relaxation, inflammation of the masseter muscle and TMJ capsule can be reduced.[30,31]

Local Anesthetics Local anesthetics act on the nerve cell membrane to prevent generation and conduction of impulses (Table 48-12). Local anesthetics can be used as diagnostic blocks intra-articularly and/or intramuscularly to alleviate pain and increase range of motion. For example, injection behind the maxillary tuberosity will permit the lateral ptery-goids to be anesthetized, thereby allowing maximal protrusion and retrusion of the mandible. There should be no vasoconstrictor used in conjunction with the anesthesia, as the decrease in blood flow may increase muscular pain. The intrinsic vasodilation effect of the anesthesia may improve perfusion and thereby further alleviate pain. It has been shown that an intra-articular injection of mepivacaine along with physiotherapy in patients with anteriorly displaced disks has yielded favorable results in pain relief and masticatory efficiency.[32]

Physical Therapy

There are many factors contributing to limited range of motion. They include muscular pain, anterior disk displacement (closed lock), and fibrotic scar tissue preventing rotation or translational movements. It is well accepted that immobilization has deleterious effects on both joints and muscles.

Table 48-7 Commonly Used Antidepressants

Generic	Brand	Dosage (mg/d)	Side Effects
Amitriptyline	Elavil	10–300	High
Desipramine	Norpramin	50–300	Moderate
Doxepin	Sinequan	25–300	High
Imipramine	Tofranil	20–300	Moderate
Nortriptyline	Pamelor,	25–150	Moderate
	Aventyl	25–150	
Fluoxetine	Prozac	5–20	Moderate

Table 48-9	Commonly Used Muscle Relaxants	
Generic	*Brand*	*Usual Dosage (mg/d; divided doses)*
Carisoprodol	Rela, Soma	1,000–1,400
Chlorzoxazone	Paraflex, Parafon Forte D.S.C.	750–3,000
Meprobamate	Miltown, Equanil	1,200–1,600
Methocarbamol	Robaxin	1,500–4,500
Cyclobenzaprine	Flexeril	5–30
Orphenadrine	Norflex, Disipal	150–300
Diazepam	Valium	2–40
Combination Fixed Dosage		
Meprobamate Aspirin	Equagesic	1–2 tablets 3 or 4 times daily
Orphenadrine Aspirin Caffeine	Norgesic	1–2 tablets 3 or 4 times daily

Adapted from Syrop SB.[25]

Immobilization may cause degenerative changes to the joint surfaces, synovial fluid, and surrounding tissues. Reduced motion also results in rapid muscle fatigue, muscle weakness, and contractures. Synovial fluid generation is reduced or halted when joints are immobile. Additionally it has been observed that the synovial fluid of patients with pain and limited motion often contains inflammatory byproducts. Kaneyama and colleagues listed a variety of cytokines such as interleukin (IL)-1β, tumor necrosis factor (TNF)-α, IL-6, and IL-8 in symptomatic joints, not observed in asymptomatic joints.[33] This high level of cytokine activity is believed to be related to the underlying pathogenesis of TMD. Cytokines such as IL-6 and IL-1β may induce the "inflammatory cascade." As a result of the release of proteinases, there may be destruction of articular cartilage and bone resorption. Each cytokine has its unique properties, not only affecting the surrounding tissues but also aiding in the release of other cytokines.[33] Thus, the role of functional motion and the synovium may be an indeterminate factor in the health of the TMJ (Table 48-13).

Exercise Therapy   Physical therapy and exercise are an important part of any TMD program. Mild or acute symptoms can be initially managed with soft diet, jaw rest, heat/ice packs, jaw/tongue posture opening exercises, lateral jaw movements, and passive stretching exercises. Once again the exact sequence of therapy is unknown but is usually based on degree of pain and limitation of function. Further reduction of pain and inflammation may require an office-based physical therapy program. From our experience, ultrasonography,

Table 48-10	Central Muscle Relaxants and Their Effects
Central Muscle Relaxants	
Carisoprodol (Rela, Soma) Chlorzoxazone (Paraflex) Methocarbamol (Robaxin) Cyclobenzaprine (Flexeril)	
Effects	
Tranquilizing effects General sedative effect on central nervous system No specific neurotransmitter No effect on skeletal muscle, motor end plate, or nerve fiber	

Table 48-11	Peripheral Muscle Relaxants
Peripheral Muscle Relaxants	
Baclofen (Lioresal) derivative of GABA that blocks spinal cord contraction reserved for severe muscle spasm, or neurogenic pain	
Botulinum toxin (Botox) is useful for management of oromandibular dystonia	
Effects	
Block synaptic transmission at neuromuscular junction Block muscle contraction	

GABA = γ-aminobutyric acid.

Table 48-12	Local Anesthetics
Act on nerve cell membrane to prevent generation and conduction of impulses	
Diagnostic blocks	
Muscle injection treatment to increase range of movement	

Table 48-13	Physical Therapy
Home Treatment Program (good for mild acute symptoms)	
Soft diet Decrease function Heat/ice packs Jaw/tongue posture opening exercise Lateral jaw movement Control passive motion (ie, Therabite)	
Office Treatment (reduction of pain and inflammation)	
Ultrasonography Transcutaneous electrical nerve stimulation Range of motion Soft tissue manipulation Trigger point injections Acupuncture (reestablishing proper energy flow by adding electric current or heat to the placed acupuncture needle)	

transcutaneous electrical nerve stimulation (TENS), soft tissue manipulation, trigger point injections, and acupuncture have also been advocated as effective in the management of the TMD patient.

Jaw exercise therapy can be described as passive, active, or isometric. Passive jaw exercise allows the patient to manually (or with a device such as Therabite Jaw Motion Rehabilitation System, Atos Medical, Milwaukee, WI, USA) increase interincisal opening (Figure 48-2). Passive jaw exercise has received a great deal of attention recently. Many authors report significant improvement in pain and mobility in the nonsurgical phase of treatment for TMD as well as for the postoperative TMD patients.[34–37] Passive jaw exercise is also very effective for patients experiencing muscular trismus and myofascial pain dysfunction (MPD). It may be contraindicated in patients with severely displaced disks, due to the possibility of damage to the disk or retrodiskal tissues.

Active exercise using the patient's jaw musculature may be incorporated into a home therapy program. One regimen allows the patient to activate, for example, their suprahyoid muscles (geniohyoid, mylohyoid, digastric, and stylohyoid), thereby inactivating the elevators of the jaw (medial pterygoid, masseter, temporalis). This may allow for relaxation of hyperactive muscles of mastication and may assist in increasing maximal incisal opening. In the active stretch phase patients are advised to keep their mouth open for several seconds and relax. They are instructed to open until they perceive pain and then advised to hold for several seconds and repeat this exercise several times a day. An active lateral stretch permitting the contralateral lateral pterygoid to be stretched may be accomplished by visualizing themselves in a mirror. In the active protrusion, also performed in front of the mirror, the mandible is protruded forward stretching the lateral pterygoids bilaterally. All active excursions are maintained for several seconds and slowly released.

Isometric exercises have been recommended for patients with severe pain and trismus. There is no movement during this exercise while the depressor muscles are activated, allowing for relaxation of the opposing elevator musculature (medial pterygoids, masseter, temporalis). These exercises are performed by holding the mandible stationary as the muscles are activated isometrically. The lateral pterygoids may also be exercised in a similar isometric fashion.

Mongini describes a three-stage office technique of mandibular manipulation for patients with pain, decreased mobility, and disk displacement without reduction.[38] Right and left lateral movements are initiated by the patient. The patient continues the movement while the clinician applies light pressure in the same direction, and in the last stage the mandible is moved to the opposite side with patient assistance.[38] Kurita and colleagues described a technique of placing one thumb on the last molar on the affected side while the other hand supports the head in the temporal region.[39] The mandible is then moved downward and forward. The patient is instructed to protrude and move their jaw laterally, and open their mouth while the clinician manipulates the jaw. Following this movement the mandible is pushed back so that the condyle is positioned posterosuperiorly in the glenoid fossa. Only 18% of the patients received significant benefit from the manipulation, and the more advanced the displacement, the less the success of the treatment.[39] Yuasa and Kurita suggested that physical therapy along with administration of NSAIDs (for a 4-week period) is a more effective way to treat TMJ disk displacement without osseous changes.[40] Nonetheless, there is no shortage of recommended exercises, and care must be taken to do no harm (Table 48-14).

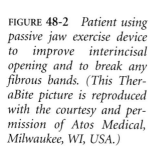

FIGURE **48-2** *Patient using passive jaw exercise device to improve interincisal opening and to break any fibrous bands. (This TheraBite picture is reproduced with the courtesy and permission of Atos Medical, Milwaukee, WI, USA.)*

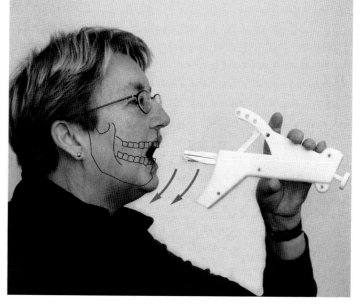

Table 48-14   Manual Therapy
Soft tissue technique
Massage, relaxation, stimulation, breaking scars, decreasing swelling, stretching
Manipulative therapy—spine realignment
Passive, quick, high-velocity, short-amplitude, thrust that forces the joint beyond its normal end range
Patient has no control; pain relief immediate but short lived

Thermal Agents Thermal agents are often incorporated in the management of TMD. The use of cold and heat can alleviate muscle pain and play an equal role during stretching and strengthening exercises.[41–43] Heat therapy has been reported to reduce muscle pain by increasing nerve conduction velocity and local vasodilatation.[43] Superficial heat therapy can be implemented with conductive (hot packs, paraffin, whirlpool) or radiant (infrared) agents. The most common types used are a moist hot washcloth, heating pad, or hydrocollator, a pad filled with clay and heated in a water bath to 70° to 88°C. It is wrapped in a towel and placed on the site for 15 to 20 minutes, causing a transient rise in skin temperature to about 42°C. The use of moist heating pads is an effective modality of treatment for myofascial pain associated with TMD.[44]

Cryotherapy is often used as an aid in stretching muscles in an attempt to increase maximal incisor opening limited by pain.[41] The pain perception model described by Melzack and Wall explains why cold therapy stimulates the large A delta fibers (temperature) inhibiting pain, which is stimulated by the small C fibers.[43] A physical therapist would place refrigerants on the skin in a sweeping motion followed by stretching of the musculature. Cold therapy should be used with caution because of the potential for increased joint stiffness, contracture, and immobility. Cold can also have analgesic effects after a therapeutic exercise regimen. Ice wrapped in a towel, fluoromethane spray, and reusable ice packs can all be used to deliver cryotherapy to the temporomandibular joint and related muscles. The stretch and spray technique, initially described by Modell and Simons and later modified by Travell and colleagues, is still a mainstay of office physiotherapy.[41,42] The therapist holds the fluoromethane spray about 30 to 45 cm from the patient and sprays in a sweeping motion multiple times, and this is then followed by stretching exercises.

Possible side effects include frostbite and the potential for joint stiffness. Many therapists follow cryotherapy with moist heat to prevent the muscles from contracting.

Ultrasonograpy and Phonophoresis Deep heat can be delivered by ultrasonography or phonophoresis. The ultrasound machine operates above audible frequency sound waves (0.75 to 1.0 MHz), which convert to heat while traveling through soft tissue. The ultrasound machine is applied to the skin along with an acoustic conductive gel, then moved slowly over the affected area in small circular movements. The operator must be careful not to keep the machine in one place for too long as it may cause overheating of the connective tissue, causing structural damage. The deep heat is intended to increase perfusion to the area, decreasing pain and increasing mobility.[45] Reported effects of ultrasound therapy include altered cell membrane permeability, intracellular fluid absorption, decreased collagen viscosity, vasodilatation, and analgesia. The beneficial effects to joints are reduced capsular contracture, break up of calcium deposits, and decreasing hyaluronic acid viscosity.[46] Because ultrasonography delivers heat to the deeper structures, it may have some advantage in treating tendonitis, capsulitis, muscle spasm, and tight ligaments.

Phonophoresis is an application of ultrasound heat therapy that incorporates a pad filled with a steroid or anesthetic cream placed over the affected area. As the ultrasound waves are applied, the medications perfuse into the tissues. The most common indication for phonophoresis is synovitis associated with painful jaw hypomobility. Contraindications for the use of ultrasonography and phonophoresis include areas that may have a reduced circulation, fluid-filled organs, eyes, radiation therapy sites, and malignant tissue. Ultrasound therapy should be used with extreme caution over active bone growth centers.[47]

Electrical Stimulation *Transcutaneous Electrical Nerve Stimulation* TENS has become a viable home therapy in treating TMD. The precise mechanism of action is unknown, but it has been suggested that the gate control theory, counter-irritation, neurohumoral substance release, and peripheral blockade are all involved.[48] TENS uses a low-voltage electrical current that is designed for sensory counterstimulation in painful disorders. It is used to decrease muscle pain and hyperactivity and for neuromuscular re-education.[49,50] TENS units are small and portable. Electrodes are placed along dermatomes or over acupuncture and trigger points. The patient can control the settings with variable frequency, amplitude, waveform, width, and pulse mode. Treatment can last several hours. TENS emits an asymmetric biphasic wave of 100 to 500 ms pulse. The efficacy of TENS for analgesia and muscle relaxation in myofascial pain has been documented.[51] Electrode placement is contraindicated over the carotid sinus, transcranially, directly on the spine, on a pregnant womb, or on patients with demand-type pacemakers.[52]

High-Voltage Stimulation High-voltage stimulation units deliver currents of positive and negative polarity with voltages greater than 100 V, which are delivered in a constant or intermittent pattern. The positive polarity produces vasoconstriction, whereas the negative polarity produces vasodilatation. The positive polarity reduces nerve irritability, and negative polarity enhances it. Negative polarity softens the affected tissue thus decreasing muscle tension. Treatment with high-voltage stimulation has improved jaw mobility and relieved pain intensity in TMD patients.[53] It can be used for pain relief, reduction of edema, and neuro muscular stimulation.[53]

Iontophoresis Iontophoresis transfers ions from a solution through intact skin by passing a direct current between two electrodes.[54] Positive ions are transmitted at the cathode, and negative ions are transmitted at the anode. Examples of negatively ionizing drugs are dexamethasone and methylprednisolone. Other drugs used in iontophoresis include lidocaine and salicylates. Iontophoresis was introduced in treating TMD and postherpetic neuralgia in 1982.[55] It appears to be most effective against inflammation, muscle spasm, and calcium deposits. The deep penetration of the medication aids in the treatment of severe joint inflammation and pain (Table 48-15).

Trigger Points and Muscle Injections A trigger point is an area of hyperirritability in a tissue that, when compressed, is locally tender, hypersensitive, and gives rise to referred pain and tenderness.[56] Trigger point development may be due to trauma, sustained contraction, or acute strain. When a needle penetrates this area it may cause a twitch response and referred pain.[56] Injection of local anesthetic agents without epinephrine may cause a temporary anesthesia, which enables the clinician to stretch the muscles in the affected area. A vasodilator effect of the local anesthetic may improve perfusion to the area, thus allowing harmful metabolites which may induce pain to be more readily removed by the vasculature.

Stress-Reduction Techniques

Relaxation and Biofeedback Relaxation and stress-reduction techniques for patients with TMD can be very effective treatment modalities. Various techniques

exist, an example being contracting and releasing skeletal muscles, starting from the feet and moving toward the head and neck region. Patients can also use audiotapes that teach breathing and specific relaxation techniques. Biofeedback techniques incorporate the use of electromyography (EMG) and skin temperature to measure the patient's physiologic function. The information is then conveyed back to the patient by a meter or sound. The patient can gauge their level of relaxation and measure progress accordingly.[57] The aim is to achieve pschycological self-regulation and to monitor the relationship between muscular tension and pain. In a review of the literature Crider and Glaros reported 69% of subjects rated as improved or symptom free following biofeedback and relaxation treatments, whereas only 35% of patients receiving placebo intervention showed any improvement.[58] Furthermore, on follow-up examination the patients showed no decline from post-treatment levels.[58] Scott and Gregg advocate that relaxation techniques and EMG feedback can yield good results, especially in patients who are not depressed and have temporomandibular pain for a short period of time.[59] The chief hurdle is the difficulty to motivate patients in pain (Table 48-16).

Acupressure and Acupuncture Acupressure and acupuncture may be implemented along with other modalities during nonsurgical treatment. Acupuncture uses the relationship between energy flow through meridians, natural elements, and positive and negative life forces. Fine nee-

Table 48-16 Behavioral Therapy
Components of Behavioral Therapy
Training the patient to recognize stress, anxiety, and depression

Relaxation training programs
    Biofeedback
    Self-hypnosis
    Meditation
    Cognitive therapy

Types of Behavioral Therapy
Psychiatric therapy
Pain clinic treatment (last resort)

dles are used to reestablish proper energy flow. There are several theories on the mechanism of action of acupuncture and acupressure. The first is the gate control theory, which states that the needle produces a painless stimulation, causing gates to close and preventing signal propagation to the spinal cord.[60] Other explanations include release of endorphins from the pituitary gland which block pain sensation, promotion of alpha waves (associated with stress reduction and relaxation), and rebalancing the electric ion flow pattern (when disrupted, it may elicit pain).[60] There are several different acupressure techniques including Jin Shin (two acupressure points held for 30 s to 5 m), Shiatsu (more rapid, held 3 to 10 s), reflexology (acupressure on feet, hands, and ears corresponding to areas of the body), Do-In (self-acupressure and breathing exercises), and G-Jo (acupressure for first aid purposes). Some studies have reported favorable results when these techniques are combined with other modalities (splint therapy), but overall data are limited.[61,62] These pain therapies can be offered as an alternative to conventional therapy.

Psychotherapy In some cases TMD may be the somatic expression of an underlying psychiatric or psychological disorder such as depression or conversion.[63,64] The

Table 48-15 Electrical Stimulation
Transcutaneous electrical nerve stimulation
Iontophoresis—direct current to drive drugs into tissue (hydrocortisone, lidocaine, salicylates); good for muscle spasm or inflammation
High-volume stimulation (100 V) (pumping effects of muscle contraction can increase circulation)

clinician should screen for personal or familial history of psychiatric disease, physical or sexual abuse, and substance abuse. Anxiety disorders occur at greater rates in patients with chronic pain.[65] Once identified these patients should be referred to a psychiatrist and/or psychologist for adjunctive treatment. Psychological treatments include behavioral therapy, cognitive-behavioral therapy, and self-management/support groups. Psychiatric treatments include medications with behavioral therapy. Often as a last resort TMD patients are referred to pain clinics for treatment, whether a psychological component exists or not, often out of frustration.

Occlusal Appliance Therapy

An occlusal appliance is a removable device, usually made of hard acrylic, which is custom fit over the occlusal surfaces of the mandibular or maxillary teeth. The splint is constructed so that there is even occlusal contact with the teeth of the opposing arch in centric and anterior contact only, in lateral and protrusive excursions of the mandible. The physiologic basis of treatment is not well understood but the effectiveness of the occlusal splint has been attributed to a decreased loading on the TMJs and reduction of the neuromuscular reflex activity. Alleviation of bruxism and MPD may be due to the change in vertical dimension, altering the proprioception in the postural position of the mandible.[66–68] There are generally two types of appliances: stabilization (flat plane) and anterior repositioning.

Table 48-17 Stabilization Appliance
Stabilizes temporomandibular joints
Redistribution of forces
Relaxation of masticatory muscle
Hard acrylic
Maxillary arch
Wear 24 h (except during meals)

Stabilization (Flat Plane) Appliance A stabilization appliance covers all the teeth in one arch and is indicated to relax the muscles of mastication, aid in joint stability, and protect teeth from bruxism (Table 48-17, Figures 48-3 and 48-4).[68,69] Additional indications for stabilization appliances may include myalgia, inflammation, and retrodiscitis secondary to trauma. With a stabilization appliance the condyles are placed in the most muscularly stable position while the teeth are contacting evenly and simultaneously.[70] There must be bilateral equal posterior contacts so that an environment of stable physiologic posture is possible. Canine guidance is created for protrusive and lateral excursions. As the patient's symptoms improve, the splint should be adjusted to maintain even contacts bilaterally. The splint is usually fabricated on the maxillary arch because it covers more tissue, especially with Class II or Class III patients where fabrication of a mandibular appliance can be difficult. On the other hand major advantages of the mandibular stabilization appliance include better speech and less visibility, which may contribute to better patient compliance.[70] The appliance should be worn 24 hours a day and taken out at mealtimes. Stabilization appliances can be weaned post-TMJ arthroscopy and/or as the patient's symptoms subside.

Major and Nebbe reported effective reduction in headaches and muscle pain using stabilization appliances, but occlusal stabilization appliances have limited value in reducing joint pain.[71] Lundh and colleagues concurred with the fact that the stabilization splints have little value in painful disk displacement without reduction.[72] Kai and colleagues reported that after treatment with a stabilization occlusal splint of the maxillary arch, clinical signs and symptoms of nonreducing anteriorly displaced disks decreased but osteoarthritic findings increased.[73]

Anterior Repositioning Appliance The anterior repositioning splint is an interoc-

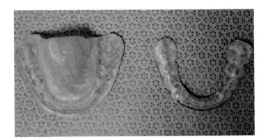

FIGURE **48-3** *Stabilization appliance. Hard acrylic full-coverage occlusal splints used for nonsurgical phase of treatment.*

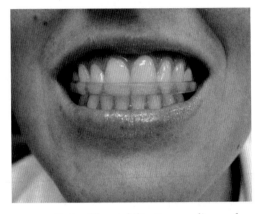

FIGURE **48-4** *The stabilization appliance does not change the anterior/posterior jaw position.*

clusal appliance that permits the mandible to assume a position more anterior than normal (Table 48-18, Figures 48-5 and 48-6). The purpose of these appliances is to alter the structural condyle-disk-fossa relationship in an effort to decrease joint loading.[74] Indications for this device are primarily disk derangement disorders. The maxillary appliance is preferred and it is fabricated with a guide ramp that permits the anterior repositioning of the mandible.[73] Anterior repositioning appliances are used less frequently because repositioning of the mandible over a period of time can result in irreversible occlusal changes such as posterior open

Table 48-18 Repositioning Appliance
In therapy it attempts to recapture the anterior displaced disk
Need for possible occlusal equilibration and constant adjustment

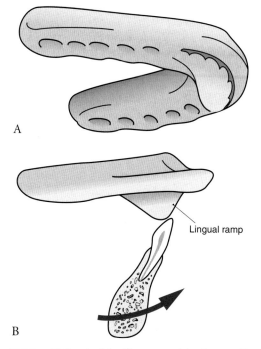

FIGURE **48-5** *A, Maxillary repositioning appliance. B, The lingual ramp engages the mandibular incisors and guides the lower jaw forward. A forward repositioner may carry a commitment to restore the patient to a new jaw position. Adapted from Syrop SB. Nonsurgical management of temporomandibular disorders. In: Peterson LJ, Indresano AT, Marciani RD, Roser SM. Principles of oral and maxillofacial surgery. Vol. 3. Philadelphia: J.B. Lippincott Company; 1992. p. 1917.*

bites, which could require extensive prosthetic rehabilitation.

Occlusal Adjustment There is a limited role for occlusal adjustment or selective grinding in the treatment of TMD.[75] The purpose of selectively grinding the teeth is

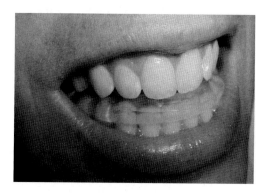

FIGURE **48-6** *Repositioning appliance. Hard acrylic repositioning appliance that changes the anterior/posterior jaw position and may require further dental rehabilitation.*

to permanently position the dentition into a better occlusion. It is an irreversible process and is best suited for the acute TMD symptoms arising from overcontoured restorations or postorthognathic surgery. In these select cases the occlusal equilibration allows for proper condylar positioning and prevents muscular problems associated with improper interferences.

Causes of Failure

As a singular modality it is very difficult to assess the clinical success or failures of nonsurgical treatments over time. DeLeeuw and colleagues reported long-lasting satisfactory results for patients treated with nonsurgical therapy for internal derangements and osteoarthrosis with a 30-year follow-up.[76] Symptoms such as joint noises persisted, whereas pain and discomfort generally subsided.

There are several possibilities that could explain the cause of failure of nonsurgical therapy for TMDs: incorrect history taking, improper diagnosis and treatment, lack of patient compliance, emotionally debilitated patient, or coexisting morbidities.[77] When significant symptoms persist after 3 to 6 months of nonsurgical therapy, alternative therapies and/or diagnoses should be considered, including surgery.

Summary

TMD is a complex disorder with common presenting signs and symptoms. In this chapter we have presented nonsurgical strategies used to alleviate the pain and dysfunction associated with the TMJ. Since an exact correlation between diagnosis and treatment is not always possible, success or failure with nonsurgical modalities is not a reliable outcome, even though this therapy may aid in diagnosis and be the first step for most patients. When surgery is indicated or evidence-based, nonsurgical techniques are a crucial adjunct perioperatively, if not forever.

References

1. deBont LGM, Kijkgraaf LC, Stegenga B. Epidemiology and natural progression of articular temporomandibular disorders. Oral Surg Oral Med Oral Path Oral Radiol Endod 1997;83:72–6.
2. Carlsson GE. Epidemiology and treatment needed for temporomandibular disorders. J Orofac Pain 1999;13:232–7.
3. Green CS. Orthodontics and temporomandibular disorders. Dent Clin North Am 1988;32(3):529–38.
4. Green CS, Laskin DM. Long term evaluation of treatment for myofascial pain dysfunction syndrome: a comparative analysis. J Am Dent Assoc 1983; 7:235–8.
5. Okeson JP, Hayes DK. Long term results of treatment for temporomandibular disorder: an evaluation by patients. J Am Dent Assoc 1986;12:473–8.
6. Suvinen TI, Hanes KR, Reade PC. Outcome of therapy in the conservative management of temporamandibular pain dysfunction disorder. J Oral Rehabil 1997;24:718–24.
7. Gaupp LA, Flinn DE, Weddige RL. Adjunctive treatment techniques. In: Tollinson CD, editor. Handbook of chronic pain management. Baltimore (MD): Williams & Wilkins; 1989. p. 174.
8. McNeill C, editor. Temporomandibular disorders: guidelines for classification, assessment and management. 2nd ed. Chicago (IL): Quintessence Publishing Co.; 1993.
9. Mejersjo C, Carlsson GE. Long-term results of treatment for temporomandibular pain-dysfunction. J Prosthet Dent 1983;49:805–15.
10. Nickerson JW, Boering G. Natural course of osteoarthrosis as it relates to internal derangement of the temporomandibular joint. Oral Maxillofac Surg Clin North Am 1989;1:27–46.
11. Greene CS, Marbach JJ. Epidemiologic studies of mandibular dysfunction: a critical review. J Prosthet Dent 1982;48:184–90.
12. Okeson JP. Management of temporomandibular disorders and occlusion. 2nd ed. St. Louis (MO): C.V. Mosby; 1989.
13. Fordyce WE. Behavior methods for chronic pain and illness. St Louis (MO): C.V. Mosby; 1976.
14. Black RG. The chronic pain syndrome. Surg Clin North Am 1975;55(4):999–1011.
15. Fordyce WE. On opioids and treatment targets. Am Pain Soc Bull 1991;1:1–13.
16. Samuelson B. An elucidation of arachadonic acid cascade. Drugs 1987;33 Suppl 1:2–9.
17. Simon LS, Mills JA. Non steroidal anti inflammatory drugs and their mechanism of action. Drugs 1987;33 Suppl 1:18–27.

18. Insel PA. Analgesic-antipyretics and antiinflammatory agents: drugs employed in the treatment of rheumatoid arthritis and gout. In: Gilman AG, Rall TW, Nies AS, et al., editors. Goodman and Gillman's the pharmacological basis of therapeutics. 8th ed. New York (NY): Pergamon Press; 1990. p. 485–521.

19. Syrop S. Pharmacologic management of myofascial pain and dysfunction. Oral Maxillofac Surg Clin North Am 1995;7:87–97.

20. Dimitroulis G, Gremillion HA, Dolwick FM, Walter JH. Temporomandibular disorders. 2. Nonsurgical treatment. Aust Dent J 1995;40(6):372–6.

21. Yoshida H, Fukumura S, Fujita M, et al. The expression of cyclo oxygenase-2 in human temporomandibular joint samples: an immunohistochemical study. J Oral Rehabil 2002; 29:1146–52.

22. Quinn J, Kent J, Moisc A, Lukiw W. Cyclooxygenase-2 in synovial tissue and fluid of dysfunctional temporomandibular joints with internal derangements. J Oral Maxillofac Surg 2000;58:1229–32.

23. Streeten DHP. Corticosteroid therapy, complication and therapeutic indication. JAMA 1975;232:1046–59.

24. Cowan J, Moenning JE, Bussard DA. Glucocorticoid therapy for myasthenia gravis resulting in resorption of the mandibular condyles. J Oral Maxillofac Surg 1995;53:1091–6.

25. Syrop SB. Pharmacological therapy. In: Kaplan AS, Assael LA, editors. Temporomandibular disorders—diagnosis and treatment. Philadelphia (PA): W.B. Saunders; 1991. p. 501–14.

26. Kinney RK, Gatchel RJ, Ellis E, et al. Major psychological disorders in TMD patients: impactions for successful management. J Am Dent Assoc 1992;123:49–54.

27. Magni G. On the relationship between chronic pain and depression when there is no organic lesion. Pain 1987;31:1–21.

28. Kerrick JM, Fine PG, Lipman AG, Love G. Low dose amitriptyline as an adjunct to opioids for postoperative orthopedic pain: a placebo controlled trial. Pain 1993;52:325–30.

29. Brown RS, Bottomley WK. The utilization and mechanism of action of tricyclic antidepressants in the treatment of chronic facial pain: a review of the literature. Anesth Prog 1990;37:223–9.

30. Tan E, Janovic J. Treating severe bruxism with botulism toxin. J Am Dent Assoc 2000; 131:211–6.

31. Freund B, Schwartz M, Symington JM. Botulism toxin: new treatment for temporomandibular disorders. Br J Oral Maxillofac Surg 2000;38:466–71.

32. Guarda NL, Tito R, Beltrame A. Treatment of temporomandibular joint closed lock using intra-articular injection of mepivacaine with immediate resolution durable in time (six month follow-up) [Italian]. Minerva Stomatol 2002;51(1–2):21–8.

33. Kaneyama K, Segami N, Nishimura M, et al. Importance of proinflammatory cytokines in synovial fluid from 121 joints with temporomandibular disorders. Br J Oral Maxillofac Surg 2002;418–23.

34. Israel H, Syrop S. The important role of motion in the rehabilitation of patients with mandibular hypomobility: a review of the literature. J Craniomandib Pract 1993;II(4):298–307.

35. Karlis V, Andreopoulos N, Kinney L, Glickman R. Effectiveness of supervised calibrated exercise therapy on jaw mobility and temporomandibular dysfunction. J Oral Maxillofac Surg 1994;52(8 Suppl 2):147.

36. Sebastian MH, Moffet BC. The effect of continuous passive motion on the temporomandibular joint after surgery. Oral Surg Oral Med Oral Pathol 1989;67:644–53.

37. Maloney G. Effect of a passive jaw motion device on pain and range of motion in TMD patients not responding to flat plane intraoral appliances. J Craniomandib Pract 2002;20(1):55–6.

38. Mongini F. A modified extraoral technique of mandibular manipulation in disk displacement without reduction. J Craniomandib Pract 1995;13(1):22–5.

39. Kurita H, Kurashina K, Ohtsuka A. Efficacy of a mandibular manipulation technique in reducing the permanently displaced temporomandibular joint disc. J Oral Maxillofac Surg 1999;57:784–7.

40. Yuasa H, Kurita K. Randomized clinical trial of primary treatment for temporomandibular joint disk displacement without reduction and without osseous changes: a combination of NSAIDs and mouth opening exercise versus no treatment. Oral Surg Oral Med Oral Pathol 2001;91(6):671–5.

41. Travell JG, Simons DG. Myofascial pain and dysfunction: the trigger point manual. Baltimore (MD): Williams & Wilkins; 1983.

42. Modell W, Travell J, Kraus H. Relief of pain by ethyl chloride spray. NY State J Med 1952;52:1550–8.

43. Melzack R, Wall P. Pain mechanisms: a new theory. Science 1965;150:971–9.

44. Nelson SJ, Ash MM. An evaluation of a moist heating pad for the treatment of TMJ / muscle pain dysfunction. Cranio 1988;6(4):355–9.

45. Vanderwindt D, Vanderheijden G, et al. Ultrasound therapy for musculoskeletal disorder: a systemic review. Pain 1999;81(3):257–71.

46. Ziskin MC, Michlovitz SL. Therapeutic ultrasound. In: Michlovitz SL, editor. Thermal agent in rehabilitation. Philadelphia (PA): F.A. Davis Co.; 1990. p. 141–69.

47. Adler RC, Adachi NY. Physical medicine in the management of myofascial pain and dysfunction: medical management of temporomandibular disorders. Oral Maxillofac Surg Clin North Am 1995;7(1):99–106.

48. Wolf SL. Neurophysiologic mechanisms in pain modulation: relevance to TENS. In: Manheimer JS, Lampe GN, editors. Clinical transcutaneous electrical nerve stimulation. Philadelphia (PA): F.A. Davis Co.; 1984. p. 41.

49. Clark GT, Adachi NY, Dornan MR. Physical medicine procedures affect temporomandibular disorders: a review. J Am Dent Assoc 1990;121:151–61.

50. Mohl ND, Ohrbach RK, Crowe HC, Gross AJ. Devices for the diagnosis and treatement of temporomandibular disorders. Part III. Thermography ultrasound, electrical stimulation and EMG biofeedback. J Prosthet Dent 1990;63:472–7.

51. Gold N, Greene CS, Laskin DM. Transcutaneous electrical nerve stimulation therapy for treatment of myofascial pain dysfunction syndrome. J Dent Res 1983;62:244.

52. Ersek RA. Transcutaneous electrical neurostimulation. Clin Orthop 1977;128:314–24.

53. Eisen AG, Kaufman A, Green CS. Evaluation of physical therapy for MPD syndrome. J Dent Res 1984;63(special issue):344, abstract 1561.

54. Lark MR, Gangarosa LP. Iontophoresis: an effective modality for the treatment of inflammatory disorders of the temporomandibular joint and myofascial pain. J Craniomandib Pract 1990;8:108–19.

55. Gangarosa LP, Mahan PE. Pharmacologic management of TMJ-MPDS. Ear Nose Throat J 1982;61:670.

56. Gerald MJ. Physical medicine modalities and trigger point injections in the management of temporomandibular disorders and assessing treatment outcome. Oral Surg Oral Med Oral Pathol Oral Radiol Endod 1997;83(1):118–22.

57. Kaplan AS, Assael LA. Temporomandibular disorders: diagnosis and treatment. Philadelphia (PA): W.B. Saunders Company; 1991. p. 522–5.

58. Crider AB, Glaros AG. A meta-analysis of EMG biofeedback treatment of temporomandibular disorders. J Orofac Pain 1999; 13(1):29–37.

59. Scott DS, Gregg JM. Myofacial pain of the temporomandibular joint: a review of the behavioral-relaxation therapies [review]. Pain 1980;9(2):231–41.

60. Matsumura WM. Use of acupressure techniques and concepts for nonsurgical management of TMJ disorders. J Gen Orthod 1993;4:5–16.

61. Matsumura TM, Ali NM. Evaluation of acupuncture and occlusal splint therapy in the treatment of temporomandibular joint disorders. Egypt Dent J 1995;41:1227–32.

62. Berry H, Fernandez L, Bloom B, et al. Clinical study comparing acupuncture, physiotherapy, injection, and oral anti-inflammatory therapy in shoulder cuff lesions. Curr Med Res Opin 1980;7:121–6.

63. Rugh JD. Psychological components of pain. Dent Clin North Am 1987;31:579–94.

64. Moss RA, Adams HE. The assessment of personality, anxiety and depression in mandibular pain dysfunction subjects. J Oral Rehabil 1984;11:233–7.

65. Katon W, Egan K, Miller D. Chronic pain: lifetime psychiatric diagnoses and family history. Am J Psychiatry 1985;142:1156–60.

66. Okeson JP, Kemper JT, Moody PM. A study of the use of occlusion splints in the treatment of acute and chronic patients with craniomandibular disorders. J Prosthet Dent 1982;48:708–12.

67. Okeson JP, Moody PM, Kemper JT, Haley J. Evaluation of occlusal splint therapy and relaxation procedures in patients with TMJ disorders. J Am Dent Assoc 1983;107:420–4.

68. Clark GT. A critical evaluation of orthopedic interocclusal appliance therapy: design, theory and overall effectiveness. J Am Dent Assoc 1984;108:359–64.

69. Rugh JD, Harlan J. Nocturnal bruxism and temporomandibular disorders. Adv Neurol 1988;49:329–41.

70. Okeson JP. Occlusal appliance therapy. In: Duncan LL, editor. Management of temporomandibular disorders and occlusion. 4th ed. Philadelphia (PA): Mosby Publishing; 1998. p. 474–502.

71. Major PW, Nebbe B. Use and effectiveness of splint appliance therapy: review of literature. J Craniomandib Pract 1997;15(2):159–66.

72. Lundh H, Per-Lenmart W, Eriksson L, et al. Temporomandibular disk displacement without reduction: treatment with flat occlusal splint versus no treatment. Oral Surg Oral Med Oral Pathol 1992; 73:655–8.

73. Kai S, Kai H, Tabata O, et al. Long-term outcomes of nonsurgical treatment in nonreducing anteriorly displaced disk of the temporomandibular joint. Oral Surg Oral Med Oral Pathol 1998;85:258–67.

74. Moloney F, Howard JA. Internal derangements of the temporomandibular joint. III. Anterior repositioning splint therapy. Aust Dent J 1986;31:30–9.

75. Clark GT, Adler RC. A critical evaluation of occlusal therapy. Occlusal adjustment procedures. J Am Dent Assoc 1985;110:743–50.

76. DeLeeuw R, Boering G, Stegenga B, et al. Symptoms of temporomandibular joint osteoarthrosis and internal derangement 30 years after nonsurgical treament. J Craniomandib Pract 1995;13(2):81–8.

77. Abdel-Fattah RA. Considerations before surgical intervention in management of temporomandibular joint disorders. J Craniomandib Pract 1997;15(1):94–5.

CHAPTER 49

Temporomandibular Joint Arthrocentesis and Arthroscopy: Rationale and Technique

Jeffrey J. Moses, DDS

Since the seventh century BC, papyrus images have revealed attempts at temporomandibular disorder (TMD) management through relocation of dislocations. Over a long and arduous route clinicians have sought to relieve the painful dysfunction of this structure through various mechanical, anatomic, and biochemical evaluations and correctional means. Through the relatively recent advances of technology, and partly because of the equivocal successes of historic management outcomes, modern maxillofacial surgeons now have the access to micronized minimally invasive techniques to assist in TMD management. From the diagnostic evidence produced by the thin intra-articular arthroscope and the evaluation of the fluid effudate comes new information turning this era into a valuable epoch of discovery. Successful long-term outcomes from relatively simplified therapeutics have led many surgeons to decrease the incidence of open-joint arthroplasties and their potential negative complication sequelae. While this chapter focuses on the techniques of arthroscopy and arthrocentesis, the current stage of the evolution of treatment philosophies and understanding of these techniques as applied to the pathophysiology of the discussed temporomandibular joint (TMJ) for successful outcome in patient management are emphasized.

History of Orthopedic Development

The development of biomechanical and optical accesses for the examination of intra-articular structures in the early twentieth century was accomplished by Kenji Tagaki in 1918 by his use of a 7.3 mm diameter pediatric cystoscope allowing him to examine a knee joint.[1] His later development of a 3.5 mm diameter scope made this procedure practical. Of historic significance, in 1921, Bircher published an independent report of the results of his arthroscopic studies of the knee joint using a laparoscope with gaseous distention of the joint space using oxygen or carbon dioxide.[2] Another report using arthroscopy was published by Kreyscher in 1925, predicting that it would become the definitive diagnostic modality for derangements of the knee.[3]

Following Tagaki's modification of the cystoscope and diameter reduction to 3.5 mm in the early 1930s and the use of saline for joint distention, several other pioneers went on to improve arthroscope design and used these in a patient series, publishing their clinical experiences.[4] Unfortunately, due to the technologic restraints at the time of lack of illumination and having only direct eyepiece visualization with electronic assistance, there was limited acceptance of this method as a valuable diagnostic modality.

A major turning point in the field came in the early 1950s with the recognition that the technologic advances in electronics and optical design could assist in endoscopic equipment development. This was appreciated and used by one of Tagaki's students, Masaki Watanabe. Watanabe and colleagues' design of the no. 21 arthroscope with 100° field of vision and a 6.5 mm diameter using tungsten light illumination and camera attachments turned the direction of this field of interest around.[5] The work done by Casscells as well as Jackson and Abe built on this foundation clinically, which was credited to Watanabe's performance of the first surgical procedure on the human knee joint in 1955.[6,7]

Enthused with the potential, Richard O'Conner returned home from a trip to Japan in 1970 and subsequently developed an operative arthroscope in 1974. He used this to perform a meniscal resection, the results of which he published in 1977.[8] A generalized instrumentation explosion, coupled with the development of motorized equipment by Lanny Johnson then ensued, which led to further technique developments in arthroscopic managements of intra-articular pathology.[9] Realizing that these techniques would be best learned in specifically designed courses with hands-on experience, in 1973, John Joyce III and Michael Hardy, an anatomist, organized the first of many courses that developed. This greatly enhanced the spread of this treatment modality throughout the orthopedic community. Many of these early courses were personally overseen by the pioneering experts, including Dr. Watanabe himself.

Development of Temporomandibular Joint Arthroscopy

A major breakthrough for small joint endoscopic access occurred in 1970 with the development of the Watanabe no. 24 Selfoc arthroscope with a 1.7 mm diameter.[10] This was introduced into the TMJ by Masatoshi Ohnishi using a fiberoptic light source and arthroscopic device manufactured by Olympus in the early 1970s. Ohnishi published both the puncture technique and the anatomic findings and later went on to describe the usefulness of this technique for clinical applications in the treatment of TMJ disease in 1980, including photographic documentation of normal anatomy as well as providing early information on traumatic pathology and joint fibrosis.[11–14]

In 1978 an animal study on rabbits by Hilsabech and Laskin demonstrated that TMJ arthroscopy was a safe technique that revealed the appearance of intra-articular structures.[15] In 1980 Williams tend Laskin went on to introduce pathologic conditions in the rabbit joint and concluded that these could be diagnosed by the arthroscope.[16] Holmlund and colleagues published similar results in 1986.[17] In 1982 Ken-Ischiro Murakami and Kazumasa Hoshino reported their procedural terminology and arthroscopic anatomy, excellently illustrating the human TMJ with color photography.[18] During a visit to the United States in 1984 Dr. Murakami introduced this concept to Bruce Sanders who, along with Joseph McCain but on separate US coastlines, began to perform the procedures clinically for patients with TMD. Drs. Ronald Kaminishi, Jeffrey Moses, Christopher Davis, as well as others were introduced to the puncture and arthroscopic visualization of the TMJ during this time. Wanting again to develop the training of this technique along the same lines as their orthopedic counterparts, the maxillofacial surgeons sought to develop educational symposia and hands-on training. The first international hands-on course using fresh cadaveric specimens for technique development was initiated by J.J. Moses in late 1985 and continued on through the sponsorship of The Pacific Clinical Research Foundation. Many of the initial surgeons exposed to the modality independently went on to develop a variety of techniques and courses using the communal efforts of the international pioneers at these sessions.

In 1985, with references to the arthroscopic observations, Murakami and Hoshino described histologic cellular characteristics of the inner surfaces of the TMJ.[19] Also in 1985 Holmlund and Hellsing published their landmark paper on the concept of reproducible puncture sites correlating measurements along the tragal-canthal line.[20] These are recommended for surgeons' early learning stages in technique development.[21]

Continued efforts by Murakami and Ono to improve surgical techniques were published in 1986, and McCain presented an abstract at the 1985 Annual Meeting of the American Association of Oral and Maxillofacial Surgeons (AAOMS) on his investigations.[22,23] A pivotal work was published in 1987 by Sanders in the treatment of closed lock condition with the surgical application of arthroscopic lysis and lavage over a 2-year period.[24]

In 1986 the first major didactic symposium on arthroscopy of the TMJ was guided by Drs. Kaminishi and Davis and sponsored by the Southern California Society of Oral and Maxillofacial Surgeons. This started the movement toward academic research and clinical investigations. Notably Dr. Ohnishi provided a demonstration of his puncture technique at this symposium, where many of the pioneers of this group began to prepare themselves for the 1986 meeting of the First Annual Symposium on Arthroscopy of the Temporomandibular Joint led by Dr. McCain, hosted in New York, and sponsored by the Hospital for Joint Diseases. It was at this subsequent meeting that the International Study Group (ISG) for the Advancement of Temporomandibular Joint Arthroscopy was formed. This pioneering group provided many of the national and international liaisons for future collaborations and collective dissemination of information, as well as expertise at the didactic and hands-on cadaveric symposium to follow.

An explosion of papers and presentations on multiple techniques, equipment development, and clinical studies ensued. Partly in an effort to curtail the potential for similar untoward sequelae as has been experienced in the field of open TMJ surgery in the past, the ISG worked together for the development of standards in credentialing, technique workshops, and recording of clinical results and provided clarification criteria for insurance coverage. As a result of much of this work the AAOMS formed an ad hoc committee and issued an official statement regarding TMJ arthroscopy, going on in 1988 to form an adjunctive insurance task force.

Important research over the early years contributed to knowledge showing that although disk position may be indicative of pathologic history, its lack of mobility more closely correlated to pathologic presence.[25] Also, the chronicity of the patient's TMD history seemed to lend itself to the development of articular remodeling in the absence of pain and limitation of motion in the postoperative phases.[26] Studies aimed at the identification of chemicophysiologic markers and mediators were done through joint fluid analysis. It was found that arthroscopic surgery was successful even in Wilkes stage III and stage IV diseases. Recently more work has been done on diskal reshaping procedures as well as arthroscopic functional diskectomy through superior-anterior capsular release combined with physical therapy for joint space enlargement.

Technique enhancements still on the horizon include early intervention with injectable joint lubricants like sodium hyaluronate (HA) following initial arthrocentesis or even the use of modified HA as an operating medium or for use as an intra-articular bandage.

Even though arthroscopic surgery is not the panacea for TMJ surgical care, it has proven itself as one of the basic techniques to be mastered by modern oral and maxillofacial surgeons in their complete management armamentarium.

Patient Selection and Evaluation

Although many patients present with pain in and around the TMJ, relatively few are selected for surgery. At the centers working with the Pacific Clinical Research Foundation, manned by teams of dentists, psychologists, physical therapists, and ancillary medical managers, only 10 patients in 400 evaluated actually have intracapsular joint derangements or pathology amenable to invasive procedures.

I have found arthroscopic management to be successful in 8 out of those 10 patients, with only 2 out of the original 400 requiring open surgery. A key to successful outcomes in any surgical care is careful patient selection and perioperative team management.

While patients certainly present with pain originating outside of the joint itself (such as atypical facial pain and neuralgias and some pains related to systemic diseases such as rheumatoid arthritis), for the purposes of this chapter we will limit our discussions to those with intracapsular etiology.

In general one has to screen the patient for the basic premise of pain origin. Is it from within the joint or from the muscles? As always there are etiologic factors affecting both possibilities that need to be identified. The most valuable screening technique comes through a valid history and physical examination that can be fairly succinct.

History

First it is comforting to the patient to address their primary chief complaint. This is done even though it is often secondary to the interest of the surgeon who wants to discover how it originated and what secondary damage has occurred so that corrections can be planned for the patient's condition and to prevent recurrence. This is done by asking the patient to identify the location, onset, and frequency of the pain, in addition to asking what the aggravating factors are and the maneuvers used to relieve the pain. Notice how the patient responds when answering the location question, whether they use a finger pointed to the joint as opposed to a flat hand palm placed on the face. The pointed location tends to lend credibility to capsular-intracapsular joint problems. The character and history of the progression of the joint noise is also helpful, paying close attention to how clicks proceeded to catching and locking, or crepitus. Also ask about the nonsymptomatic side since frequently there may be a history of the same sequence indicating the possibility of more advanced degenerative disease on that side, which will be evidenced on the radiograph and through the range of mandibular motion examination.

Patients often report pain in the shoulders and neck, headaches, earaches, and feelings of fullness in the ears or dulled hearing. It is important to inquire as to the patient's generalized physical or emotional status regarding recent pregnancy, childbirth, or menopause as well as their condition socially with jobs or family. This frequently adds significant overlay and insight to associated etiology and treatment management.

Positive answers to pointed questions regarding the history of recent or childhood trauma, habits of bruxism or clenching, and medications used, such as those initiating dyskinesia, should be explored. Also, one should inquire into past gnathologic treatments such as prior orthodontic care for closure of open bites, retrognathic treatment with class II elastics or positioners, extensive crown-and-bridge prosthetics, and equilibration for balancing contact occlusal interferences.

Physical Examination

The examination can likewise be fairly concise and takes a close second to the history in importance. The generalized physical examination can follow the focused joint and facial structure examination in order to let the patient know that their chief complaint has been heard, thus giving them more confidence and trust. Clinicians examine the location of pain, skeletofacial form, and the TMJ first followed by the nerve function, muscles, and dentition/occlusion. Initially noting the form of the skeletofacial structures, look for open bites, retrognathism (with or without deep bites), asymmetries of the jaw and facial bones, and pseudobites where the habitual position of the mandible is off of the skeletal position. Careful checking of capsular tenderness as well as palpating and auscultating for joint sounds, such as reciprocal clicks, pops, catching, and crepitus, all lend valuable information. Be certain to load the affected and nonaffected sides in occlusion to ascertain the effect on the pain as well.

Next generally check sensory nerve function and muscle response to cognitive motor stimulus. The muscle examination naturally follows with observations being made for hypertrophy, asymmetry, and tenderness to palpation. Frequently with longstanding symptoms a cascading of protective muscle splinting will lead to neck and shoulder symptoms. The ears and eyes are checked with notations for later specialist referrals if abnormalities are found or complaints are elicited.

Finally the teeth and occlusion are examined, looking for masked asymmetric skeletal characteristics secondary to orthodontic treatments applied during growth, pseudobite secondary to class II elastics, wear facets and balancing interferences, supraerupted teeth, or loss of posterior support. It is at this point that the mandibular range of motion is measured and observed, and deviations, limitations, or hypermobilities are noted.

Presurgical Diagnostics and Therapeutics

Following the history and physical examination and screening panoramic examination, clinicians usually initiate presurgical conservative therapy. The use of a presurgical orthotic appliance designed to deprogram the habitual occlusion and skeletal positions, as well as provide relief to the muscular splinting and resultant myositis, cannot be overemphasized. This not only assists physical therapists in their assessment and therapeutic care but also provides the surgeon with valuable information as to whether true skeletal asymmetries or open bites are preexisting, which may have been masked by neuromuscular programming through prior clinical care. Usually this is accomplished

with a maxillary splint built with cuspid guidance in order to prevent the dental movement and opening of the interdental spaces produced with clenching or bruxism. If an open bite exists, which would require a mandibular splint due to the undesirable excessive bulk of acrylic on a maxillary splint, the splint should also be designed for lateral disclusion using the bicuspid instead of the cuspid teeth.

The use of the orthotic splint appliance, combined with physical therapy and nonsteroidal anti-inflammatory drugs (NSAIDs), should allow most experienced physical therapists and surgeons to determine whether an intracapsular pathology will be responsive to nonsurgical therapy within a matter of 6 to 8 weeks.

Occasionally the decision is made for therapeutic muscular trigger-point injections or intracapsular superior joint compartment diagnostic blocks of diluted local anesthetic solution in order to segregate pain etiologic foci before proceeding to either arthrocentesis or combined arthroscopic surgery.

Imaging

Traditionally the panographic view is the first revealing image of the TMJ. Current concepts of management have been expanded through visualization of axially corrected sagittal tomography based on the submental vertex view with the alignment of the x-ray beam along the medial-lateral pole axis of each of the condyles, taken in the open mouth and closed occlusion positions. This is augmented by the coronal views in the protruded occlusion position with the incisors placed edge to edge in order to visualize the medial, lateral, and superior condylar anatomy in relation to the superior condyle's proximity along the functional area of the eminentia. These views can reveal osteophytes, erosions, and remodeling impingements that would otherwise be undetected from other bone imaging techniques.

For the shape, position, mobility, and intrinsic structural integrity of the disk itself, magnetic resonance imaging (MRI) has proven to be extremely reliable.[27] Whereas studies have shown that history and clinical examination are reliable for predicting similar MRI diagnosis for anterior disk displacements without reduction, and arthroscopic examinations have been shown to be statistically reliable for disk displacements as well, additional information of disk immobility with normal disk position and diskal structure and integrity loss with myxomatous changes can be ascertained by MRI, proving its overall value and reliability for additional soft tissue information compared with other techniques such as arthrography.[28,29]

For patients with conditions that are suspect for partial bony ankylosis, which occurs with the advanced disease process associated with repetitive surgery or with a fibrous ankylosis, a computerized axial tomography scan will sometimes provide the best possible information. Whether one chooses to proceed with arthroscopy on basic imaging techniques and the history and physical examination alone or to add more sophisticated imaging to the presurgical diagnostic package is a decision to be made by each clinician who is involved with the individual patient.

Indications and Contraindications

Indications

Early meetings of the International Study Group for the Advancement of TMJ Arthroscopy were convened to formulate international consensus on the various indications and contraindications for TMJ arthroscopy. Resolutions were forwarded for acceptance to the AAOMS, which finalized the position paper on TMJ arthroscopy in 1988.[30] This paper separated indications for diagnostic and operative arthroscopy with generalized examples given of patients in whom disorders were found that were not explained by other means and for which a diagnostic confirmation would affect the patient's care and outcome. It also included indications for diagnostic arthroscopy in order to enhance treatment decisions. Examples include the following:

- Biopsy of suspected lesions or disease
- Confirmation of other diagnostic findings that could warrant surgical intervention
- Unexplained persistent TMJ pain that is nonresponsive to medical therapy

The indications for surgical arthroscopy are matched carefully with the diagnosis before application. Helpful criteria of disease staging should be applied through the combined use of the Wilkes staging classification for internal joint derangement (Table 49-1), which was based on clinical, radiologic, and anatomic divisions, and the Bronstein and Merrill arthroscopic staging of internal joint derangements (Table 49-2) correlated at the time of arthroscopic surgery. Intraoperatively, internal joint surface procedures are applied individually to the significant finding.

Internal joint derangement (IJD) is known to be a preoperative indication for surgical arthroscopy. The AAOMS position paper defines IJD as a disruption of the internal aspects of the TMJ with either diskal displacements or alterations in the normal dynamic motions of the intracapsular elements. This would include adhesions or impingements in the face of even normal disk position. The paper goes on to describe surgical arthroscopy as indicated for joint conditions that constitute a disability for the patient and which are refractory to medical treatments and require structural modification.[30]

Whereas internal derangements associated with hypomobility due to adhesions, disk immobility, and disk displace-

ments with blockade are likely candidates for structural modifications, those joints with recent trauma, degenerative disease, synovial disease, and even hypermobility are included in the conditions indicated for arthroscopic surgical intervention.

Table 49-1   Wilkes Staging Classification for Internal Derangement of the Temporomandibular Joint

I. Early Stage
   A. Clinical: no significant mechanical symptoms other than early opening reciprocal clicking; no pain or limitation of motion
   B. Radiologic: slight forward displacement; good anatomic contour of the disk; negative tomograms
   C. Anatomic/pathologic: excellent anatomic form; slight anterior displacement; passive incoordination demonstrable

II. Early/Intermediate Stage
   A. Clinical: one or more episodes of pain; beginning major mechanical problems consisting of mid- to late-opening loud clicking, transient catching, and locking
   B. Radiologic: slight forward displacement; beginning disk deformity of slight thickening of posterior edge; negative tomograms
   C. Anatomic/pathologic: anterior disk displacement; early anatomic disk deformity; good central articulating area

III. Intermediate Stage
   A. Clinical: multiple episodes of pain; major mechanical symptoms consisting of locking (intermittent or fully closed), restriction of motion, and difficulty with function
   B. Radiologic: anterior disk displacement with significant deformity/prolapse of disk (increased thickening of posterior edge); negative tomograms
   C. Anatomic/pathologic: marked anatomic disk deformity with anterior displacement; no hard tissue changes

IV. Intermediate/Late Stage
   A. Clinical: slight increase in severity over intermediate stage
   B. Radiologic: increase in severity over intermediate stage; positive tomograms showing early to moderate degenerative changes—flattening of eminence; deformed condylar head; sclerosis
   C. Anatomic/pathologic: increase in severity over intermediate stage; hard tissue degenerative remodeling of both bearing surfaces (osteophytosis); multiple adhesions in anterior and posterior recesses; no perforation of disk or attachments

V. Late Stage
   A. Clinical: crepitus; scraping, grating, grinding symptoms; episodic or continuous pain; chronic restriction of motion; difficulty with function
   B. Radiologic: disk or attachment perforation; filling defects; gross anatomic deformity of disk and hard tissues; positive tomograms with essentially degenerative arthritic changes
   C. Anatomic/pathologic: gross degenerative changes of disk and hard tissues; perforation of posterior attachment; multiple adhesions; osteophytosis; flattening of condyle and eminence; subcortical cystic formation

Adapted from Bronstein SL and Thomas M.[79]

Contraindications

Even though there are relatively few absolute contraindications to joint arthroscopy, it is generally recognized that underlying medical instabilities, overlying skin infections, and risks associated with

Table 49-2   Bronstein and Merrill Arthroscopic Staging of Internal Joint Derangements Correlated with the Wilkes Staging

I. Early Stage

Roofing, 80% (closed position) to 100% (open or protrusive positions); incipient bilaminar zone elongation; normal disk flexure at junction of diskal eminence and superior lamina; normal synovium; incipient loss of articular surface smoothness; normal superior compartment recesses and vascularity

II. Early/Intermediate

Roofing, 50% (closed) to 100% (open or protrusive); bilaminar elongation with decreased flexure; early adhesive synovitis with beginning adhesion formation; slight lateroanterior capsular prolapse

III. Intermediate

Advanced bilaminar elongation with accordion-shaped redundancy and loss of flexure; prominent synovitis; diminished lateral recess; advanced adhesion formation; anterior pseudowall formation in substage B

Substage A: Roofing, 5% (closed) to < 15% (open or protrusive); chondromalacia grades I–II (softening, blistering, or furrowing)

Substage B: No roofing, more severe anterior recess changes; chondromalacia grades II–III (blistering, furrowing, ulceration, fraying, fibrillation, surface rupture)

IV. Intermediate/Late

Increase over intermediate stage disease; hyalinization of posterior attachment; chondromalacia grades III–IV (ulceration, fraying, furrowing, fibrillation, surface rupture, cratering, bone exposure)

V. Late Stage

Prominent fibrillations on articular surfaces; perforation; retrodiskal hyalinization; false-capsule formation anteriorly; generalized adhesions; advanced synovitis; chondromalacia grade IV (cratering, bone exposure)

Adapted from Bronstein SL and Thomas M.[79]

malignant tumor seeding represent relative contraindications.[31]

Arthroscopic Instrumentation and Anesthesia Consideration

Surgeons performing arthroscopic surgery should be familiar with not only the surgical technique but the supportive electronics and operating room set-up as well. As a guide for the surgeon a recommended schematic of room set-up is shown in Figure 49-1.

Video Monitoring Equipment

Even though the interior surfaces of the joint can be visualized directly via the eyepiece, most arthroscopists prefer to use video electronic enhancement and documentation equipment. A video monitor and recording device are placed at the head of the patient, easily orienting everyone in attendance to the 12:00 (twelve o'clock) position of the joint with the video camera attached to the arthroscopic eyepiece. A video monitoring cart (Figure 49-2) contains the monitor, light source, and recording units with the cumbersome cords draped on the contralateral side of the patient's head to the surgeon's position. The clear imaging of the joint allows all people involved with the case to clearly participate with interest. This has the additional benefit of allowing them to better anticipate the progress and needs of the surgeon.

Irrigation System

A constant flow of irrigation fluid is essential to providing a clear view of the joint surfaces through the distention of the potential joint space, as well as for washing blood and debris away from the lens objective. The inflow is attached to the arthroscopic cannula, and an outflow needle is placed elsewhere in the joint space. The diameter of the outflow portal should be of a lesser size than the inflow portal, which allows a slight pressure differential in order to maintain sufficient joint distention.

For routine arthroscopic procedures a 1½ inch 18-gauge short-beveled needle is ideal. If laser débridement is anticipated a second arthroscopic cannula with a stopcock and rubber obturator should be placed so that the outflow volume can be adjusted to the higher flows of irrigation fluid required for the prevention of excessive thermal synovial damage that is possible from the heat generated by the laser photovaporization. Additional benefits of the irrigation include those associated with the therapeutic effects of lavage and arthrocentesis.[32]

The components of a simplified approach to an irrigation system include several units of extension tubing with Luer-loc attachments, a 30 mL or 60 mL syringe, a three-way stopcock, the arthroscopic cannula, and a 1½ inch 18-gauge short-beveled needle. For most cases the drainage may be collected in a small basin with the end of the exit tubing taped to the basin's edge, allowing the surgical technician visible evidence that the fluid pushed into the point is equal to that coming back out to prevent extravasation into the periarticular tissues.

Alternatively for the higher volumes necessary in cases requiring laser-assisted techniques, a pneumatic-assisted compression unit may be used instead of the syringes to provide constant pressure on a 500 mL bag of irrigation solution. This provides a consistent joint distention as well as a cooling flow of solution across the joint surfaces. The outflow in these cases is usually voluminous and is collected in an

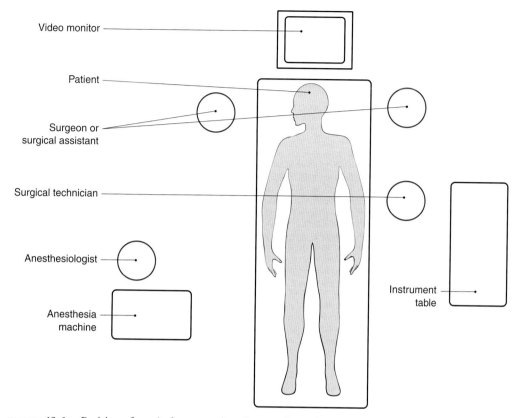

- Video monitor
- Patient
- Surgeon or surgical assistant
- Surgical technician
- Anesthesiologist
- Anesthesia machine
- Instrument table

FIGURE **49-1** *Position of surgical team and equipment for arthroscopic surgery. The surgeon and surgical assistant may change positions freely without disturbing the positions of the equipment or other persons helping.*

orthopedic shoulder arthroscopy bag, which has a drainage portal at the apex.

Arthroscope

The manufacturers use four basic techniques for arthroscope construction. The early design, in 1966, of the rod-lens endoscope by H.H. Hopkins improved the traditional achromatic lens system, which made arthroscopic examination

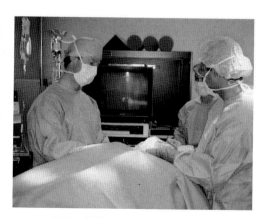

FIGURE **49-2** *Video monitoring cart.*

practical by reducing the diameter of the instrument. By placing at least two different types of glass into the system, secondary advancements made color correction possible. This led to brighter images due to a reduced separation of spaces between the rod lenses when compared with the achromatic focusing lens system, and lessened the likelihood of breakage.[5]

A third advance came with the development of a unique type of glass with a nonuniform refractive index called the Selfoc lens. The characteristic of this gradient-index system is that curved surfaces are not required, and the spacing between the lenses could be eliminated using optional cements which allowed a thinner diameter with brighter images and an equivalent breakage resistance.[33] The glass structure itself provides the focusing power of the system (Figure 49-3).

In the fourth alternative, optical lenses are placed at either end of a fiberoptic relay, focusing the image along the fiber relay, which transmits the image from the objective to the output ocular lens or eyepiece. These are primarily used in work requiring extreme flexibility such as vascular exploration. However, there are new disposable fiberscopes now available for needle access to the small joint.

No matter whether a rod lens or Selfoc lens is used in arthroscopic surgery, any bending of the lens sheath will produce a dark halo crescent and heralds possible lens damage or fracture.

Visual Fields and Angles

The angle of vision consists of the angle formed extending from the outermost margin of the objective lens to the subject viewed.

The field of vision consists of the three-dimensional circular area within those angles of the angle of vision.

The angle of inclination is commonly termed the direction of view, which can be altered by the lens construct itself. Usual angles of inclination are 10°, 30°, and 70°. Through the careful use of rotation of the angled arthroscope in an arc-like fashion, a wider field of vision can be produced (Figure 49-4).

Another valuable insight into the optical characteristics of the arthroscope is the fact that the field of view will be dimmed by magnification without providing increased resolution. Light transmission is critical in order to keep the image definition clear and is reduced by increasing the angle of inclination from 0° to 70° incrementally.

A good general rule to remember is that as the diameter of the scope decreases and the angle of the scope increases, the apparent field of view and brightness of the image decreases.

There are two ways to overcome these obstacles: (1) through the use of an integrated video arthroscopic system with zoom camera couplers, and (2) through the enhancement of light. Even though a quartz-halogen light may be sufficient for

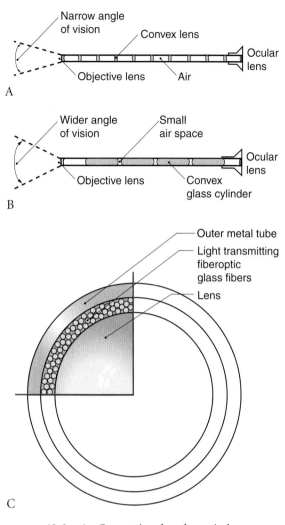

A, *Conventional endoscopic lens system showing the narrow angle of vision.* B, *Rod-lens system showing the wider angle of vision.* C, *Cross-sectional representation of endoscope.*

FIGURE **49-3**

direct visualization in small joints, video work is greatly improved through the use of a xenon or mercury-xenon arc lamp light source.

The light transmission through the arthroscope is accomplished by the light fibers surrounding the lens system (see Figure 49-3) and is connected at the side of the arthroscope to a fiber light-cord coupler, which, in turn, attaches it to the light source. This light source is usually fitted with an automatic light level adjustment system connected to the camera's console for a feedback loop (Figure 49-5).

Instruments: Cannula, Trocars, Obturators, Elevators

The cannula is a sheath through which either the arthroscope or the instruments may be passed into the joint space repeatedly. A Luer-loc attachment together with stopcock valve is used for inflow where the cannula is housing the arthroscope and used for outflow when on a second cannula that is used for instrumentation access.

Excess outflow can be restricted by partly closing the valve and adding a rubber stopper with a small hole through which the instruments are passed during a triangulation procedure. These cannulae are passed into the joint space after intro-

ducing the sharp trocar into the cannula, which is used to puncture through the skin and joint capsule. The joint capsule is distended with irrigation solution during this maneuver from a needle injection (see section in this chapter "Functional Anatomy and Joint Entry Techniques"). The blunt obturator then replaces the sharp trocar within the cannula as further entry into the joint is accomplished, in order to avoid scuffing of the articular cartilage.

In the superior joint space, after visual confirmation of joint space access has been achieved, the blunt trocar can sometimes be incorrectly used as a release elevator. This can often lead to bending of the cannula and, with repetition, can lead to eventual breakage. It is recommended to use a hardened metal release elevator if further procedures are anticipated (Figure 49-6).

A series of dilation cannulae are also available for enlarging the diameter of the access tube in order to facilitate the use of graspers to remove debris or broken instruments.

Specialized Instruments

A variety of hand and motorized instrumentation is available to the arthroscopic surgeon. The most commonly used are the hooked probe, grasping and biopsy or cutting forceps, scissors, and retrograde (pull) knives. Again, sufficient cannulae diameters to incorporate the grasping forceps after it holds the object are critical in providing a safe and smooth retrieval of the object without having to remove the cannula along with the grasper. This avoids the risk of subcutaneous loss of the object on the way out of the joint space.

Lasers

The use of laser energy in arthroscopic surgery has fought a long battle for acceptance. The carbon dioxide laser proved ineffective for practical reasons relating to the joint insufflation with gasses.[33,34] The neodymium:yttrium-aluminum-garnet (Nd:YAG) laser was abandoned because it was shown to result in

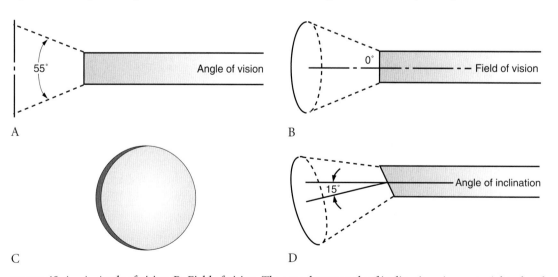

FIGURE **49-4** A, *Angle of vision.* B, *Field of vision. The zero degree angle of inclination gives a straight-ahead view.* C, *Dark crescent at the edge of the field of vision caused by bending of the arthroscope.* D, *Angle of inclination (direction of view). Rotation of an arthroscope with an oblique angle of inclination around its axis increases the field of vision.*

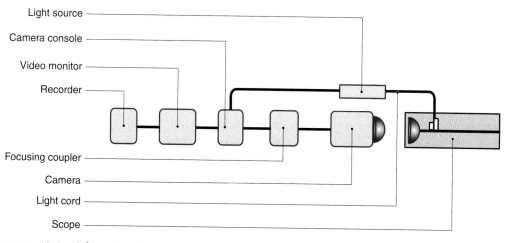

FIGURE **49-5** *Schematic of equipment hook-up sequence.*

excessive depth of tissue damage.[35] However-er, the holmium:YAG (HO:YAG) laser seems to have won approval within the orthopedic community and has been shown to be effective for the TMJ reduction of synovial and vascular hyperplasias, as well as débridement of fibrous tissues.[36] It can be used for the release of the anterior capsule and, in the defocused mode, used for reduction of chondromalacia. Once again generalized synovial damage must be avoided through the use of copious irrigation during the use of laser energy within the joint compartment.

Anesthesia and Medication Considerations

TMJ arthroscopy can be performed in the outpatient or inpatient setting. When local anesthesia alone is used auriculotemporal and intracapsular anesthetic blocks are placed. This technique is usually reserved

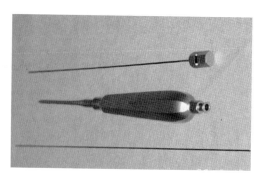

FIGURE **49-6** *Moses' release elevator, trocar, and switching stick.*

for fine-needle diagnostic arthroscopy. Alternatively it can be performed combined with intravenous sedation for lysis of adhesions as well as eminentia release capsular stretch procedures.

Whereas most surgeons tend to segregate the general anesthesia requirements from the surgical, modern oral and maxillofacial surgeons naturally integrate the two for enhanced outcome. Initially led by requests for controlled hypotension required for beneficial effects during orthognathic surgery, considerations followed that were specific to the arthroscopic surgical arena.

Requests are made for the anesthesiologist to administer certain drugs at the onset of the intravenous (IV) access, as well as muscle relaxants, and even to perform deep extubations at the conclusion of surgery. Injection of methylprednisolone at 125 mg for adults and 40 mg for children is given in order to help stabilize the mast cell membranes to help to inhibit the release of histamines due to tissue injury and to reduce the postoperative edema. Even though postoperative infections are rare, a cephalosporin antibiotic is usually given as well for prophylaxis.

With the anesthesiologist located at the position indicated on Figure 49-1, clear access is given to the surgeons while still affording the anesthesiologist the patient's arm or hand for IV access as needed. Mus-

cle relaxants are given with sufficient length of duration for the entire case in order to allow the surgical assistant better ease of joint mobilization, yielding the surgeon sufficient space for instrumentation.

Even in cases of anticipated short duration it is helpful to explain the requirement for absolute muscular relaxation to the anesthesiologist ahead of time and to allow sufficient postsurgical time for the chemical reversal agents to work adequately for extubation. The surgeon can use this time to organize progress notes or findings and procedural dictation. Also for the more involved cases, a preemergence extubation can help to prevent the Valsalva response to the endotracheal tube and thus limit intra-articular bleeding and hematoma formation.[37]

Biomechanics of Articular Pathology and Arthroscopic Management

The etiology of pain in the TMJ diagnosed with IJD is unclear. Certain surgical anatomy of the TMJ is important to understand as it relates to the biomechanics of the functioning joint in order to effectively treat the dysfunctional state of the patient.

Clinical observations and findings of the synovial lining of the TMJ and correlation of findings of disk perforations, mobility, and blockade also significantly guide the arthroscopic surgeons in their management decisions.

There are many theories regarding TMJ dysfunction. However, the following question arises in almost every discussion: What are the causes of the pain, and why can one joint with disk displacement not hurt whereas another, perhaps with a less serious problem, severely tender?

Part of the answer involves the histochemical characteristics of pain mediators within the joint fluid, but the direct and indirect results of inflammation and resulting fibrosis on the capsule, associated tissues, and musculature also play a role in pain symptoms.[38]

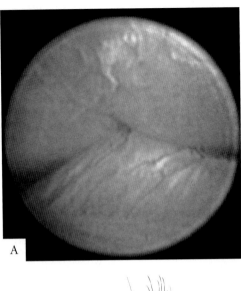

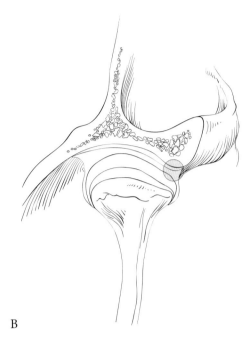

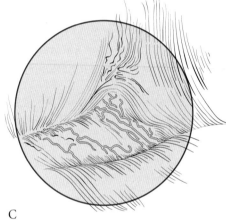

FIGURE 49-7 A, *Arthroscopic photograph of endaural view of disk impingement under articular tubercle. Reproduced with permission from Moses JJ.[47] B, Drawing of location of the endaural view seen in A. C, Drawing of endaural photograph seen in A. B and C adapted from Moses JJ.[47]*

tioning simultaneously (Figure 49-8).[46] An understanding of the force on the load-bearing surfaces with the structural inherent rotational and translational forces and their combined effects on rotational force, moments, torque, and shear, are essential in helping to understand the reasons that lateral condylar pole, eminential, and capsular pathologies are present in higher frequency than at the medial joint location.

This has led to the investigation of the lateral TMJ articulation by coronal MRI and by axial-corrected tomographic laminograms, both taken in the anteroposterior (AP) protruded jaw position performed on patients who had failed nonsurgical efforts to correct TMJ dysfunction and yet did not exhibit classic disk displacement.[47] These cases were further investigated by direct arthroscopic examinations from the AP view via endaural puncture access. It has become apparent that there is a process of pathology occurring which ranges from seemingly minor capsulitis with proliferative synovial changes to frank degenerative disease with disk/capsular impingements (see Figure 49-7).

Disk displacement actually may occur late in the pathophysiology of internal joint derangement (Table 49-3). Early inflammatory changes, initiated by macrotrauma or microtrauma, may lead to a loss of the lubricating nature of the HA and chondroitin sulfate within the synovial fluid. Capsulitis itself, with the synovium proliferating in an attempt to repair or regenerate damaged intracapsular structures, combines with inflammation and leads to the production of hyaluronidase, which breaks down the HA within the TMJ. A loss of lubrication ensues, leading to increased surface "stickiness," resulting in capsular fibrosis and relative immobility of the TMJ, especially within the superior joint compartment, on attempted translatory movements of the mandible.

A review of studies of similar joint pain and restricted mobility in the shoulder with acromial impingement syndrome shows striking resemblances to observations made on the TMJ (Figure 49-7).[39–45] Additional studies performed on the basic biomechanics of the TMJ have shown that with jaw rotational mechanics, the linear velocity of rotation (V) will differ between the medial and lateral poles as a consequence of an orthopedic system with two joints func-

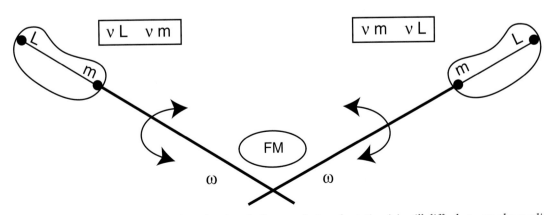

FIGURE 49-8 *With jaw rotational mechanics, the linear velocity of rotation (v) will differ between the medial and lateral poles. Given a fixed measurable angular velocity of rotation (r), the velocity of point m (medial pole) will differ from point L (lateral pole). FM = rotational force movement.*

Table 49-3 Progressive Stages of Impingement Lesions

Stage	Diagnosis	Clinical Course	Treatment
I. Inflammation	Acute capsulitis and synovitis	Reversible	NSAIDs, rest, physical therapy, OSA, intracapsular irrigations, and lavage
II. Fibrosis	Chronic adhesive capsulitis, proliferative synovitis, diskal displacement or immobility, synovial plicae	Recurrent pain with activity	Arthroscopic lysis of adhesions, lateral eminencia release and capsular stretch, lavage, physical therapy, OSA
III. Bony remodeling and attachment migration	Diskal displacement or immobility, hyperplastic eminencia tubercle, degenerative joint disease	Progressive disability	Lateral eminencia release, capsular stretch, lateral eminencia osteoplasty, physical therapy, OSA

NSAIDs = nonsteroidal anti-inflammatory drugs; OSA = orthotic splint appliance.

If allowed to mature the adhesions may vascularize and become part of the restrictions (Figure 49-9). On attempted opening, lateral adhesive components can cause incoordination of disk/condyle/eminence dynamics. Strain is placed on the lateral disk attachments as the condyle is forced to begin translation from within the inferior joint compartment. The disk, while relatively immobile in its relationship to the articular eminence, may or may not be displaced at this time (Figure 49-10).

Over a period of time, translation, solely in the inferior joint compartment, may cause a gradually increasing laxity of the lateral disk attachment, allowing the anatomic migration of the disk anteromedially. The patient may also experience a "closed lock," depending on the morphologic changes within the disk and its ability to form a mechanical obstruction (Figure 49-11).

As the disk slowly migrates forward and medially, movement within the superior joint compartment generally remains minimal. The inferior joint compartment begins to act as the translatory compartment for the "wide-open" mouth position.

Anterior disk displacement traditionally has been diagnosed via arthrographic studies and now with MRI. A sagittal view may reveal a well-placed disk; however, the MRI coronal view allows diagnosis of medial or lateral disk displacement, as MRI correlative studies on more than 100 arthroscopic confirmations of disk displacement have shown that disks that appeared in normal anatomic position on sagittal views were actually rotated on their condyles with medial displacement (Figure 49-12).

Diagnosis of disk pathologies based on two-dimensional studies can be misleading. In some cases the posterior band almost becomes longitudinally placed anteroposteriorly along the lateral rim of the condyle. This may lead to a "bulging" out of the capsule on coronal MRI (Figure 49-13). In other cases images of a disk more medially displaced may have a "sucked-in" appearance of the lateral capsule on coronal MRI, which is termed lateral capsular prolapse (Figure 49-14). Lateral capsular prolapse may play a role in the development of the lateral impingement phenomenon.

As disk displacement progresses anteromedially the lateral attachment

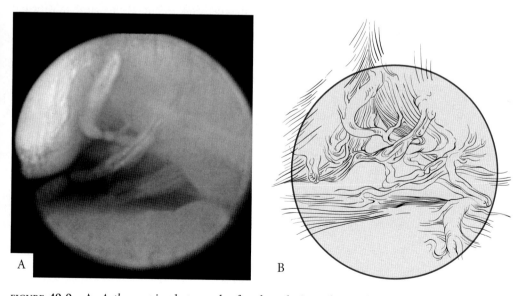

FIGURE **49-9** A, *Arthroscopic photograph of endaural view of articular eminence, demonstrating inflamed synovial proliferative tissue and early adhesions. Reproduced with permission from Moses JJ.*[47] *B, Drawing of the endaural view seen in A. Location of this tissue is the same as that seen in A. Adapted from Moses JJ.*[47]

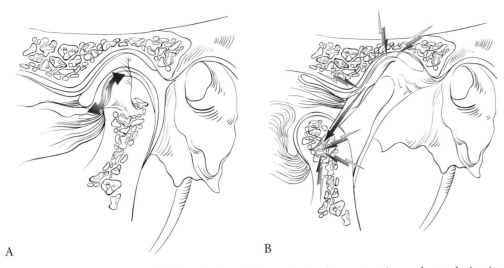

A   B

FIGURE **49-10** A, *Drawing depicting relative disk immobility after maturation and vascularization of adhesions: translation is forced to occur in the lower compartment.* Arrows *indicate the movement of the condyle under the immobile disk.* B, *Eventually there is laxity of the lateral disk attachments and increased translatory movements in the lower joint compartment.* Arrow *indicates the location of the lateral diskal attachment, which is strained and possibly painful. Adapted from Moses JJ.*[47]

migrates forward as a result of the gradual and progressive pull of the condyle, which stretches it during attempted translation in the inferior joint space.[46–48] The attachment carries with it the bone of the condylar lateral pole, developing the anterior beaking or "lipping" commonly seen in sagittal tomography (Figure 49-15). "Beaking" represents an adaptation of condylar remodeling to forces placed on it rather than a true osteophyte.

If the load is not redistributed, areas of perforation can occur, and further degenerative changes may develop along with adaptive remodeling of both hard and soft tissues (Figure 49-16).[49] The concept of load distribution is a fundamental biomechanical principle that is crucial to the understanding of joint structure and function. The entire physiologic function of the joint and its associated structures is load distribution, and damage occurs when factors inhibit this function. Dysfunction occurs when metaplasia and adaptive remodeling cannot repair this damage by restructuring load distribution.

A review of arthroscopic cases reveals that the majority of pathologic adhesions

and restricted motion lie within the lateral third of the joint. The soft tissues of the capsule become fibrotic and constricted, with inactivity and/or inflammation restricting mandibular movement. From the endaural arthroscopic approach, viewing anteriorly along the lateral trough of the superior compartment, inflamed synovial proliferation and projection are seen, as well as adhesions binding the disk to the eminence and capsule, leading to restricted mobility and possible pain (see Figure 49-9).

In the advanced stage, areas of lateral condylar resorption, best seen in AP tomograms (Figure 49-17), correlate with the hypertrophic articular tubercles that impinge on the lateral third of the disk (Figure 49-18A–C). If the joint space has diminished with degenerative changes, this becomes especially important as the condyle will articulate more heavily in the lateral area on protrusive and opening movements (Figure 18D and E). In my experience disk perforation occurs most frequently in the lateral posterior bilaminar zone/disk junction correlating with this lateral impingement.

Pain itself is not a disease. "Pain merely halts the function to allow healing. The gradual increase in function allows the programming of mesenchymal cell differentiation."[50] The goals of treatment should include decreasing functional load and increasing the capacity of cells to accomplish articular remodeling.

Clinical studies using the lateral eminence release and capsular stretch procedures, combined with routine arthroscopic lysis of adhesions and lavage, have relieved both pain and restricted mandibular mobility in over 92% of patients (see Table 49-3).[27] Patients with lateral tubercle impingements on the disk seem to require additional eminoplasty, which gains joint space and

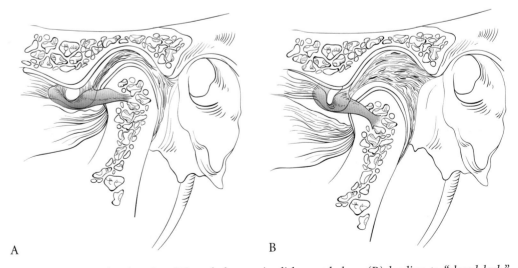

A   B

FIGURE **49-11** *Disk migration (A) and changes in disk morphology (B) leading to "closed lock." Superior compartment adhesions restrict translatory movements. Adapted from Moses JJ.*[47]

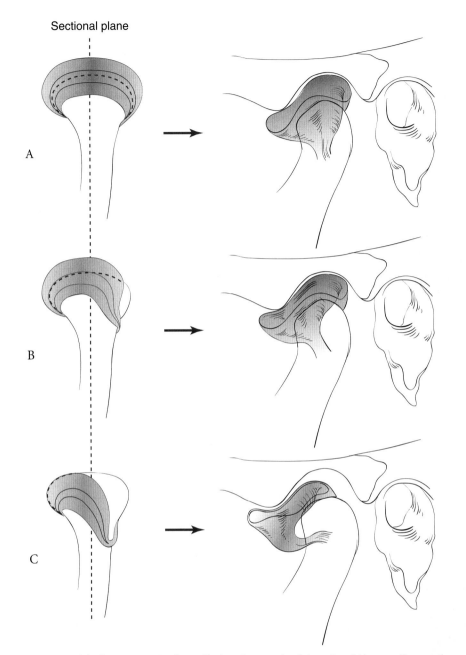

FIGURE **49-12** *Disk that appears to be well placed on sagittal imaging (A) actually may be rotated on the condyle with medial displacement (B) and in time may suffer increased laxity of the lateral collateral disk attachments (C). Adapted from Moses JJ.*[47]

ing occurs long-term following arthroscopic procedures (Figure 49-20).

In a study using standardized tomography, Moses in 1994 showed that disk and capsule mobilizations have effectively restored function with pain reduction, while correlation to chronicity seems to dictate whether or not articular remodeling occurs.[26]

In certain cases, when the chronicity of the displacement has led to anterior disk displacement, the morphology of the disk can "ball" up and effect a blockade to condylar anterior movements. This phenomenon is termed *obstructive disk blockade*. The traditional approach to this condition's management is either through open or closed surgical attempts to reshape and reposition the disk or complete disk extirpation.[53–55]

An arthroscopic surgical alternative is that consisting of an anterior capsular release performed with either the HO:YAG laser or pull-knife assistance under arthroscopic guidance via triangulation portal access. Care is taken not to violate the pterygoid muscle during this procedure, keeping the dissection on top of this structure. This procedure, termed *anterior capsular release*, allows the opening of the anterior joint compartment for functional remodeling to occur during the postoperative rehabilitation enlarging the space for the disk to move.[56]

Functional Anatomy and Joint Entry Techniques

Over the past 15 years arthroscopy of the TMJ region has gained popularity as both a diagnostic tool and as a therapeutic mode for procedures involving IJD and intracapsular dysfunctional pathology. Although this popularity gave rise to many proposed procedures and techniques, which give the surgeon many choices on which to base their treatments, the fundamentals all remain the same. As the skill of surgeons advances, desired access for visibility and instrumentation has led to the increased use of angled view and alternate entry portals combined with triangulation techniques.

relieves load concentration from that area (Figure 49-19).[51]

MRI analysis study revealed a consistent result of no change in disk position in the closed-mouth status, both before and after arthroscopic surgery in 92 patients.[52] The study revealed an increase in mobility of the disk following arthroscopic release that was directly correlated with the clinical success of

pain reduction and restoration of normal mandibular function.

The mobilization of tissues within and around the joint, combined with reduction of load concentrations, enhances mesenchymal cell reprogramming, allowing potential formation of pseudodisk articulations and condylar remodeling. Studies are in progress at the present time to investigate whether condylar remodel-

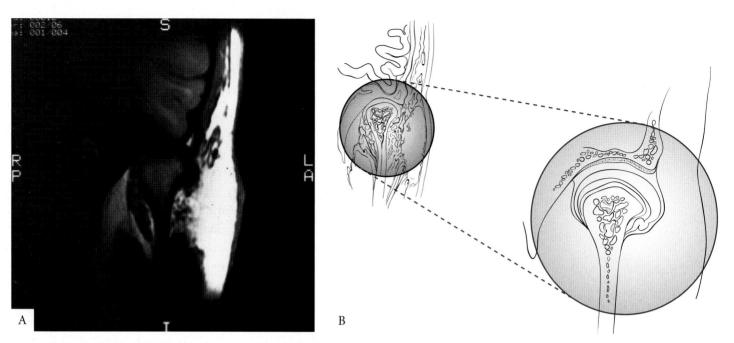

FIGURE **49-13**   A, *Magnetic resonance image, coronal view, of the temporomandibular joint, demonstrating lateral capsular bulge. Reproduced with permission from Moses JJ.[47] B, Drawing of the image shown in A. Adapted from Moses JJ.[47]*

General Principles

In any arthroscopic surgical procedure involving small joints it is important to adhere to some basic technical points:

1. The joint should remain fully distended, allowing easier trocar puncture and minimizing the risk of iatrogenic intracapsular damage.
2. The skin should be punctured with a sharp trocar.
3. All intra-articular procedures should be done with care to prevent articular surface damage.
4. Attention should be given to preserve as much healthy synovium as possible in order to enhance its physiologic effects on the joint.
5. The joint space should be kept expanded during instrumentation by a slow infusion irrigation system.

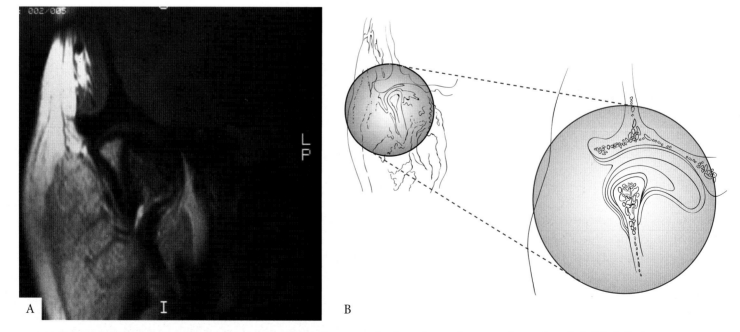

FIGURE **49-14**   A, *Magnetic resonance image, coronal view, demonstrating lateral capsular concavity and medial diskal displacement. Reproduced with permission from Moses JJ.[47] B, Drawing of the image shown in A. Adapted from Moses JJ.[47]*

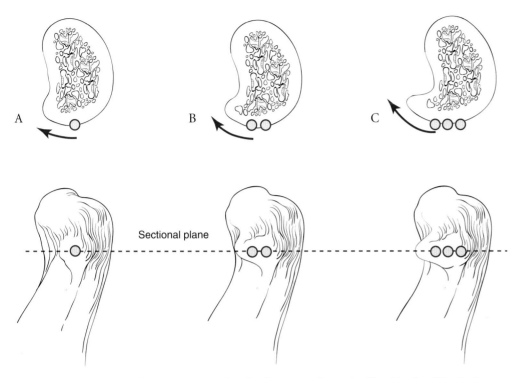

FIGURE **49-15** *Drawing depicting progressive development of anterior "beaking" or "lipping" commonly seen on sagittal tomograms. Adapted from Moses JJ.*[47]

Puncture Anatomy and Landmarks

The anatomic landmarks relevant for open joint surgery also apply for arthroscopic surgery.

The frontal branch of the facial nerve appears to be the most likely nerve structure to be involved. Whereas Greene and colleagues reported a mean distance of 22.5 mm from this branch as it crossed the zygomatic arch to the posterior aspect of the tragus with a range of 16 to 29 mm, Al Kayat and Bramley reported the mean distance of 20 mm from its crossing measured to the anterior margin of the bony auditory meatus with a range of 8 to 35 mm.[57,58]

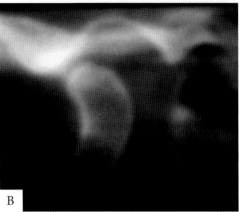

FIGURE **49-17** A, *Coronal tomogram taken in slightly protruded position showing bony lateral impingement and prominent articular remodeling of lateral one-third of the condyle. B, Sagittal tomogram of the same temporomandibular joint. Reproduced with permission from Moses JJ.*[47]

The tympanic plate was found by Greene and colleagues to be 7 mm anterior to the posterior tragus (range 6 to 9 mm) and perpendicular to the skin at a mean depth of 25.4 mm (range 19 to 32 mm).[57]

Finally, even though the mean distance of the superficial temporal vessels from the posterior aspect of the tragus has been measured at 12.8 mm, there is some variance and this structure occasionally can be vulnerable to puncture lacerations.[57]

There have been reports of cases of arteriovenous fistulas developing as a result of puncture through these structures, requiring subsequent vessel ligations.[59]

An important point to remember during the puncture procedure is the visualization of the directional axis of the trocar angle, which should be anterior

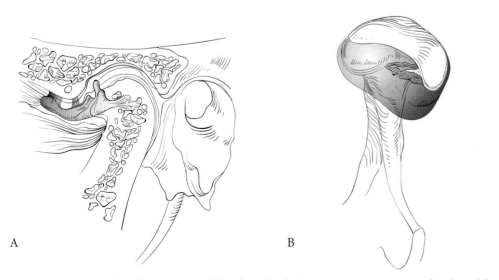

FIGURE **49-16** *Further degeneration of hard and soft tissues in response to undistributed load.* A, *Diskal lateral ligamental and bony changes. B, Disk perforation. Adapted from Moses JJ.*[47]

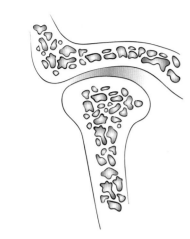

A

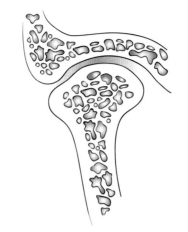

B

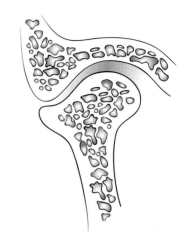

C

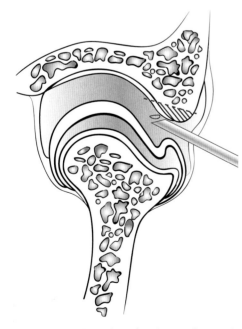

D

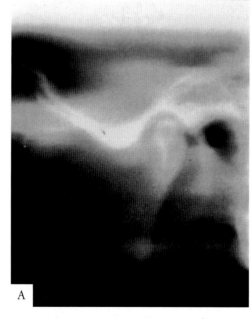

E

FIGURE **49-18** *Drawings showing advanced stages of condylar remodeling and/or resorption. Areas of lateral condylar resorption correlate with hypertrophic articular tubercles (A–C) in response to disk displacement and loss of joint space. D, Sagittal view of degenerative joint closed mouth view. E, Sagittal view of degenerative joint—protruded jaw position. The dashed line sectional plane correlates with the coronal view in C. Degenerative joint with bony changes evident. Adapted from Moses JJ.[47]*

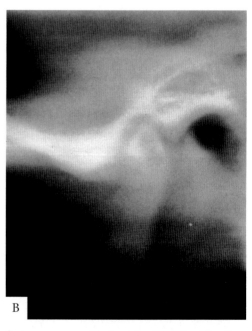

FIGURE **49-19** *Drawing showing arthroscopic osteoplasty of hypertrophic articular tubercle. Adapted from Moses JJ.[47]*

FIGURE **49-20** A, *Preoperative sagittal tomogram of a temporomandibular joint (TMJ) with adhesions. B, One-year postoperative sagittal tomogram of same TMJ showing adaptive remodeling following lysis of adhesions and joint lavage. Reproduced with permission from Moses JJ[47]*

and superior just above the "finger-palpated" lip of the glenoid fossa and not perpendicular or posteriorly directed in order to avoid middle ear or vessel damage. A frequently overlooked situation leading to a loss of perceived direction is improper head positioning. The head should be turned away from the operator and as flat to the operating table as possible.

Several authors have advocated marking the skin with points measured at 10 mm, 15 mm, and 20 mm along the line drawn from the posterior aspect of the midtragus to the lateral canthus. These positions can be helpful for orientation early in the learning curve for the arthroscopist. After time, however, the size and weight of the patient as well as their age can lead to variations of this.[60] Experience has shown the initial palpation with the mandibular mobilization by the surgical assistant to be more relevant and valuable than measurements alone.

The surgeon can often palpate the pulse of the superficial temporal vessels and the posterior aspect of the condyle while putting the fingernail side of the surgeon's digit along the inferior lip of the glenoid fossa with the mandible distracted downward and forward by the assistant.

Arthroscopic Approaches

The initial puncture of the TMJ is done with a needle and irrigation solution and is administered for joint distention of the potential space of the superior joint compartment. A detailed description of the initial joint puncture and the superior posterolateral and endaural approaches will follow this overview of the various approaches to the joint compartments (Figure 49-21).

Because many of our radiology imaging procedures cannot accurately visualize early lateral capsular synovial proliferation (see Figure 49-9), capsular herniations (Figure 49-22), or diskal impingements (see Figure 49-7), various approaches to capsular access become important to the arthroscopic surgeon in correctly diagnos-

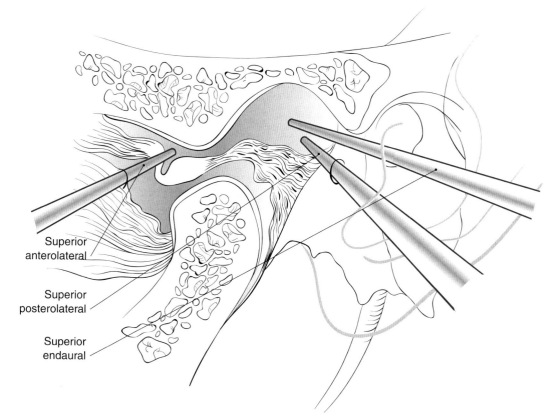

Superior anterolateral

Superior posterolateral

Superior endaural

FIGURE **49-21**   *Arthroscopic approaches to the temporomandibular joint. Adapted from Moses JJ.*[47]

ing intra-articular pathologies for the application of treatment modalities.

Superior Posterolateral Approach

In this technique the mandible is distracted downward and forward, producing a triangular depression in the front of the tragus.[61] This depression represents an area bordered superiorly by the glenoid fossa, anteroinferiorly by the dorsal aspect of the condylar head, and posteriorly by the external auditory canal. It is at the roof of this depression, above the gloved fingernail of the surgeon's digit outlining the inferior aspect of the glenoid fossa, that the trocar is inserted. The trocar is directed anterosuperiorly toward the posterior slope of the eminentia. This provides access to the posterosuperior joint space and allows visualization of the superior joint space. The areas that are difficult to visualize are the superoanterior synovial pouch and the medial paradiskal synovial groove.

Inferior Posterolateral Approach

This is a variation of the inferolateral approach, in that the trocar is directed against the lateral posterior surface of the mandibular head.[62] The inferoposterior synovial pouch and posterior condylar surface can then be examined.

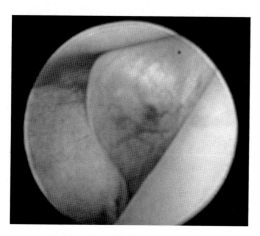

FIGURE **49-22**   *Capsular herniations noted in the medial wall of a right temporomandibular joint. Reproduced with permission from Moses JJ.*[47]

Superior Anterolateral Approach

In this technique the trocar is directed superiorly, posteriorly, and medially along the inferior slope of the articular eminence after first locating the prominence of the lateral articular tubercle as a landmark. The mandibular condyle is distracted inferiorly and positioned posteriorly by the surgical assistant. This approach allows anterosuperior joint compartment instrumentation or visualization.

Inferior Anterolateral Approach

This is a technically more difficult approach than those described above and allows observation of the lower anterior synovial pouch. In this technique the condylar head and articular tubercle are palpated.[62] The trocar is then inserted at a point anterior to the lateral pole of the condylar head and immediately below the articular tubercle. This places the trocar in the lower anterior synovial pouch, adjacent to the anterior aspect of the condylar head. The technique allows observation of the lower anterior synovial pouch.

Endaural Approach

This access is initiated by a trocar entering the posterosuperior joint space from a point 1 to 1.5 cm medial to the lateral edge of the tragus through the anterior wall of the external auditory meatus. The trocar is directed in an anterosuperior and slightly medial direction toward the posterior slope of the eminentia. This approach provides access and visualization of the posterior superior joint space as well as the medial and lateral paradiskal troughs. Its detailed technique will be covered in this chapter under "Endaural Arthroscopic Approach: Rationale/Technique."

Joint Distention and Trocar Puncture Technique

The arthroscopic surgical procedures are typically carried out with the patient under general anesthesia via nasal endo-tracheal intubation and complete neuromuscular relaxation throughout the procedure (Figure 49-23). A 1½ inch 20-gauge short-beveled needle is introduced into the posterior aspect of the superior joint compartment, testing the depth and direction for subsequent trocar/cannula placement. Iced heparinized lactated Ringer's solution (2000 IU of heparin/L Ringer's lactate) is administered via a syringe as a joint distension medium (Figure 49-24). To facilitate this maneuver the mandible is distracted downward and forward by the surgical assistant.

The mandibular condyle is then repositioned downward and backward, and a short-beveled 18-gauge outflow needle is attached to the catheter tubing and directed from an anterior lateral approach into the anterior aspect of the superior joint compartment (see Figure 49-24). By slow injection of iced heparinized Ringer's lactate solution, irrigation of the superior joint compartment should be noted as fluid emerges from the outflow extension tubing. The 20-gauge needle is then removed.

Distention of the capsule is maintained by the slow infusion of the Ringer's solution temporarily applied to the outflow portal 18-gauge needle prior to trocar puncture. This procedure allows a more distinct feel of the puncture into the joint, which should be done with a sharp trocar. Skin incisions are not required.

Superoposterior Lateral Approach

The sharp trocar is placed into the cannula and, with a fingerstop applied to the cannula grip to prevent inadvertent excessive puncture depth, the trocar is directed into the point above the palpating digit's fingernail location at the inferior aspect of the glenoid fossa. It is aimed anterosuperiorly toward the posterior slope of the eminence.

The sharp trocar is then replaced with the blunt obturator and further entry into the joint is executed. The syringe of Ringer's solution is then removed from the outflow tubing and connected to the irrigation tubing attached to the arthroscopic cannula stopcock. Bubbles are displaced from the cannula by flushing with irrigation fluid as the arthroscope is placed in the sheath. Examination of the superior joint compartment is then initiated, and systematic examination of the joint is performed prior to further instrumentation.

Lateral Eminentia Release and Capsular Stretch Procedures

Even though these procedures should technically be listed under surgical instrumentation, their importance is assigned not only to therapeutic management but also to the creation of soft tissue mobilization necessary for further joint exploration into the anterosuperior compartment by the endoscope.

Errors in Entry

Occasionally the arthroscopist will encounter difficulty in entry to the superior joint compartment. Most commonly this is due to insufficient joint distention by the irrigation solution. If severe fibrous strands are encountered in a joint not suspected of fibrous ankylosis, the inadvertent positioning of the scope cannula into the retrodiskal tissue is likely to be the cause. In this case removal of the scope from the cannula is recommended, and a repeat process of standardized puncture for superior posterolateral approach with the blunt

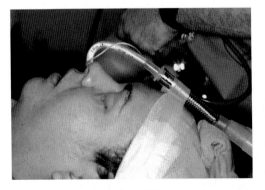

FIGURE **49-23** *Example of hair taped on head-wrap and endotracheal tube stabilizer pad. Reproduced with permission from Moses JJ.*[47]

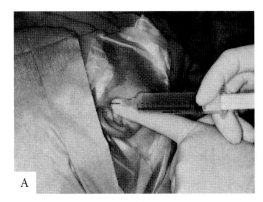

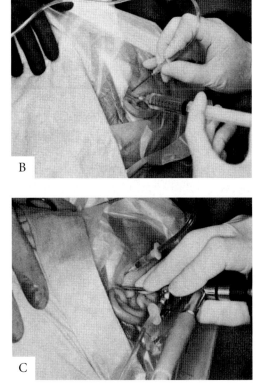

FIGURE 49-24 *Initial steps in endaural approach. A, Injection of heparinized Ringer's lactate to distend joint. B, Placement of outflow needle in anterolateral aspect of joint. C, Arthroscopic examination of joint via inferolateral approach. Reproduced with permission from Moses JJ.[47]*

probe is done. Only after confirmation of actual joint space access is visually achieved through the camera image can further instrumentation be initiated.

Endaural Arthroscopic Approach: Rationale/Technique

Certain limitations have become evident using the traditional posterolateral and anterolateral arthroscopic approaches to the TMJ. This is especially true for visualization of the lateral trough and anterolateral joint space or where access for instrumentation to the medial and lateral paradiskal grooves is required. Clear visualization of those areas is impeded using the currently available 15° angled scopes and lateral portals.[63]

To solve these visualization and access problems the endaural entry portal provides clear visualization and enhances instrumentation to the medial and, especially, the lateral spaces (Figure 49-25). This new approach also provides better access for the retrieval of loose bodies and broken instruments. Working with the arthroscope in the endaural portals permits access to other portals for instrumentation.

In order to perform this technique a 30° angled arthroscope is recommended, which increases the panoramic visualization of the joint. The off-axis viewing angulation changes as the scope is rotated and permits a more comprehensive examination of the TMJ in areas difficult to examine with conventional 15° arthroscopes. In order to visualize the lateral capsule and attachment areas it is important to obtain

an arthroscope that has the visual axis oriented toward the light cord, preventing the impediment of having the light cord forced against the patient's temporal area. Because this is a deviation from the usual manufacturer's product it must be specifically requested during the ordering process.

For the surgeon inexperienced in this technique it is best initially to penetrate the superior joint space from the standard superior posterolateral approach. Once this has been accomplished the arthroscope is then rotated and angled superiorly, posteriorly, and laterally so that the light shines through the anterior wall of the external auditory canal (Figure 49-26). This spot is usually located approximately 1 to 1.5 cm medial to the lateral edge of the tragus in the external auditory canal (Figure 49-27). While the mandible is distracted downward and forward, the anterior wall of the external auditory canal is perforated with the sharp trocar and 30° arthroscopic cannula. The cannula and trocar are angled anterosuperiorly and slightly medially, perpendicular to the posterior slope of the articular eminence. Most important, these instruments enter into the joint above the level of the arthroscope in order to ensure superior compartment puncture (Figure 49-28). Penetration should be carried to a depth of no greater than 1.5 cm using the cannula

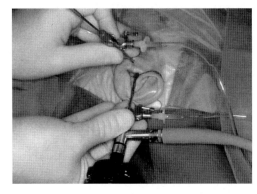

FIGURE 49-25 *Clinical view of an arthroscope in the temporomandibular joint that has been placed through the endaural portal. The working portal is now located in the superior posterolateral location. Reproduced with permission from Moses JJ.[47]*

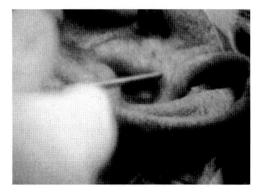

FIGURE 49-26 *The arthroscope via the inferolateral portal is angled so that the light from the scope is transilluminated through the tragal cartilage, identifying the site for endaural puncture into the joint. Reproduced with permission from Moses JJ.[47]*

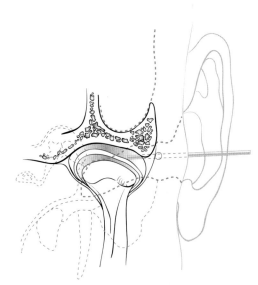

FIGURE **49-27** *Diagram indicating approximate site of puncture for the endaural approach. Coronal section is positioned just anterior to the cartilaginous meatus and tragus. Adapted from Moses JJ.*[47]

markings as a guide. Visual confirmation of the penetration into the joint space can then be made using the arthroscope, which has been placed in the inferolateral portal. Additional confirmation that the endaural cannula tip lies within the superior joint space can be ascertained when removal of the trocar results in an outflow of irrigation fluid from the endaural cannula. The arthroscope, with the attached fiberoptic cable and inflow tubing, can then be removed from the inferolateral cannula and connected to the endaural cannula. The inferolateral cannula can then be sealed off with a rubber cap to prevent excessive outflow when the TMJ is being irrigated, and the cannula can be used as a working portal while visualization is accomplished via the endaural portal.

By rotating the arthroscope, the medial, lateral, and superior aspects of the TMJ can be examined. This approach is especially helpful in visualizing the anterolateral synovial space, which is difficult to do from either the superior posterolateral or anterolateral portal (Figure 49-29). This technique also allows the superior posterolateral or anterolateral portal to be

used for the instrumentation if necessary (see Figures 49-28 and 49-30).

As skill is acquired, direct puncture through the anterior wall of the external auditory canal into the TMJ can be performed after initial joint distention, without the need for superior posterolateral cannulation. Following the arthroscopic surgical procedure the lateral puncture site receives pressure and round bandage dressings. No sutures are necessary. The endaural puncture is difficult to dress and is left as is. Usually if there is minimal manipulation through this portal, the cartilaginous elastic memory of the canal serves to close the puncture site. A routine otoscopic examination is always made following arthroscopy to visualize the external acoustic meatus and tympanic membrane in order to confirm that no iatrogenic damage has been caused by the procedure.

Perioperative

Preoperative Management

In the preanesthesia holding room several preparatory functions usually help in man-

agement. First, the anesthesiologist assesses the interincisal opening of the patient to determine the extent of the physical blockage versus that of painful restriction. Then, the intravenous line for early administration of the corticosteroid, methylprednisolone, is initiated in order to prepare the patient's mast cell membrane stability which assists in prevention of excessive histamine release on surgical tissue insult. This steroid is followed by an intramuscular injection of 80 mg methylprednisolone acetate at the termination of the case.

Finally, the patient's hair is bundled into a pillowcase and the case is taped to the forehead and nape of the neck with the excess rolled into a "bun" on top of the forehead. This is used to help support the nasoendotracheal tube after intubation (see Figure 49–23). Paper tape is placed along the sideburn hair, holding it up and out of the field. Paper tape with benzoin is used in order to help prevent the "lifting" off of the tape when the surgical prep is applied.

Postoperative Management

Cloth adhesive strips or the ends of cloth bandages are applied to the skin punctures,

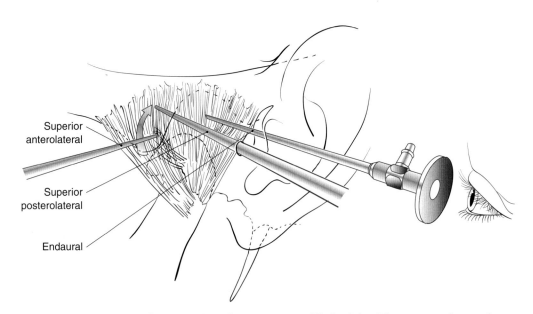

FIGURE **49-28** *Diagram of puncture into the temporomandibular joint. The trocar and cannula are directed anterosuperiorly and medially, perpendicular to the posterior slope of the articular eminence and above the inferolateral cannula. The probes, located in either of the working portals, may now be used for the lateral eminence release and the capsular stretch (see arrow). Adapted from Moses JJ.*[47]

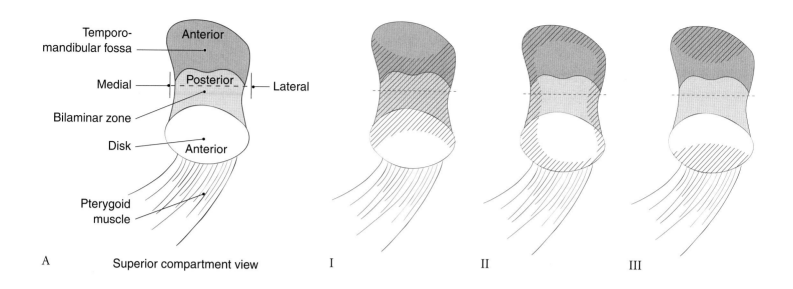

A, Superior compartment view   I   II   III

B

C, Inferior compartment view   I   II

FIGURE 49-29 *Visible fields with the various arthroscopic approaches: oriented to the left temporo-mandibular joint (TMJ) with the roof of the TMJ folded upward. Areas depicted with diagonal lines are difficult to observe arthroscopically. A, Superior compartment, orientation of the sectional planes: I is superior anterolateral area, II is superior posterolateral view, III is inferior anterolateral view. B, Superior and inferior compartment views. C, Inferior compartment, orientation of the sectional planes: I is inferior anterolateral view, II is inferior posterolateral view. Adapted from Moses JJ.*[47]

and an injection of diluted 10 mg triamcinolone acetate is made into the superior joint compartment and another portion directed into the tendon of the deep belly of the masseter muscle as it inserts under the root of the zygomatic arch anterior to the eminentia.

Otoscopic examination of the external auditory meatus is done, confirming the removal of the protective cottonoid pack and the absence of any tympanic membrane damage. The orthotic splint is applied to the patient's teeth, while still sedated if possible, in order for the neurologic reprogramming to assist in the patient's adjustment to its fit as the joint edema resolves. The patient should keep the head slightly elevated for the first 12 to 24 hours postoperatively and avoid any increased abdominal pressure or Valsalva's maneuvers.

Jaw closure compression pressure is used over the TMJ puncture sites on extubation unless the patient is extubated "deep" while still anesthetized in order to help prevent bleeding and hematoma intra-articularly.

The dressing is removed the next morning and the adhesive strips are removed. The skin punctures may be washed gently with soapy water and rinsed. They are then coated with a light coat of antibiotic ointment.

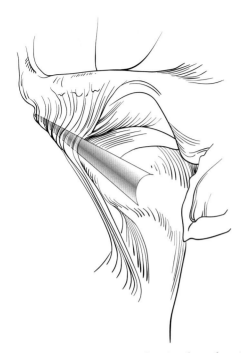

FIGURE **49-30** *Diagram showing lateral eminence release. Adapted from Moses JJ.*[47]

Postoperative Medications

Routine NSAIDs are given for the postoperative month and muscle relaxants for the first week. Oral cephalosporin following the intraoperative IV bolus of 1 g cephalosporin antibiotics are routinely given for the first week as well. Cortisporin otic suspension eardrops are prescribed for the first 7 to 10 days with 2 drops in the ear canal of the affected side. Narcotic pain medications are rarely, if ever, indicated.

Physical Therapy

Preparatory physical therapy evaluation and management are imperative for a predictable outcome. The patterns for exercise and postoperative mobilization will be well understood and compliance established. Active exercises for the patient consist of opening the jaw, moving it to each side, and protruding the jaw, with each movement performed to the fullest extent ten times and repeated ten times daily for 10 days minimum (Rule of 10's). More important, however, is the passive joint mobilization applied to the patient by the physical therapist. The joint distraction

and mobilization, along with adjunctive therapies, will increase success rates dramatically. This therapy usually can be prescribed with visits three times a week for the first 3 weeks postoperatively, twice a week for the next 2 weeks, and once a week for the next month (Rule of 3-2-1).

Appliance Therapy

An occlusal splint should have been applied postoperatively to deprogram the muscles from periodontal membrane neuromuscular feedback. Occasional skeletofacial deformities of asymmetry or mandibular hypoplasia may be thus revealed, especially in cases where orthodontic elastics have been used during growth and pseudobites have developed.

Sometimes the splint used preoperatively for myositis reduction and other dental attempts for TMJ management may not be applicable for postoperative use following the release of intra-articular pathology. This is explained to the referring clinician as well as the patient, and the new orthotic splint appliance is placed on the patient's teeth on emergence from anesthesia.

The routine use of the splint is dictated by the presence or absence of skeletofacial deformity, muscular symptoms, and the inability to wean off of the device without symptoms. At first the splint is worn full-time (day and night), noting that is is especially needed during meals, explaining its similarity to a crutch after knee surgery. If the patient requires orthodontics in preparation for orthognathic surgery, it is usually recommended to maintain the splint on the maxilla while the opposing arch is aligned and leveled and then switch over if necessary to the other arch.

If there is no further concern for either myositis/bruxism control or skeletofacial deformity stabilization, then weaning of the splint from full-time use is indicated. One splint usage routine (Rule of 4's) proven effective is for the patient to wear the splint full-time, including during meals, for 1 month postoperatively until symptoms

and range of motion are normalized. Then weaning takes place over the next 5 months, allowing the patient to reduce wear each month by any selected 4 hours of their choosing, with the exception being the times worn during sleep. This routine yields the final fifth month of wear for nocturnal use only. Many patients wish to maintain the use of the splint at night and a decision can be made at the 6-month postoperative visit, whether this is indicated.

Complications

One might expect there to be a large increase in the complication rate for TMJ arthroscopy when compared with the orthopedic experiences due to the close proximity of many anatomic structures in the head and neck region and their relative complexity of function. At first glance the multicenter retrospective study in 1987 of 2,225 cases showed a global complication rate significantly larger than that reported in a prospective study from orthopedic literature for knees.[64–66] The differences in these studies, however, must be measured by the severe limitations of a retrospective design and reliance on surgeon's recall.

One significant conclusion to the multicenter study was that the majority of the complications were perioperative in nature and resolved relatively quickly postoperatively without long-term sequelae. With the learning curve of arthroscopic advancements behind us in this area, the various individual reports of usual and unusual complications have led to a better understanding of prophylactic measures that assist the current surgeon.[67]

Extravasation

Whether or not a mechanical pump or hand-operated syringe is used, extravasation is a continual risk for arthroscopic procedures. Complications include pharyngeal embarrassment of airway requiring overnight hospitalization, periorbital and temporal edema, and transient cranial nerve V and VII effects.[68] Techniques of constant inflow-outflow volume monitoring during the procedure with the outflow tubing lifted by taping the end to the edge of a basin help reduce the likelihood of extravasation. Limiting the number of punctures laterally and preventing unnecessary medial capsular wall punctures will keep extravasation down as well.

Procedures should be kept to a minimum duration, and if anterior release procedures are required, they should be done at the end of all the other procedures performed within the joint to help keep the hydraulic distention present and avoid early extravasation limiting operating time.

Neurologic Injury

Nerve injury comprises one of the largest categories of complication reported in the longer retrospective studies.[64,65] By far the most common are those to the peripheral source of the sensory nerve V and its various branches. While the auriculotemporal branch is most frequently affected, it is commonly transient in its hypoesthesia and usually resolves within 6 months.[69] The other nerve that is at risk for damage is the inferior alveolar branch which, while usually only transiently affected by extravasation, can be iatrogenically damaged by mandibular angle clamps placed for jaw manipulation.[70,71] Safer methods of manipulation have been described that use the assistant's hands and thumbs on the teeth for joint positioning or mobilization.[72] The motor cranial nerve VII (temporozygomatic and masseteric branches) has been reported damaged in arthroscopic procedures, with reporting rates ranging from 0.56% to 4%. The damage typically resolved within 6 months according to reports reviewed.[64,65,73,74] Management of injury to these motor branches is done postoperatively in a similar fashion to that occurring after open surgery, with artificial tears, eye patching, physical therapy, electrostimulation, and oculoplastic consultation if needed.

Finally one must constantly be aware of the variation of anatomy present with-

in the TMJ. Rare cases of glenoid fossa defects can result in middle cranial fossae perforation, and more commonly giant cell erosion of bone from previous implant surgery can lead to increased risks of cerebrospinal fluid leakage as well.[75] Management includes identification, neurosurgical consultations, hospitalization, observation with elevated head and rest, and rarely application of subarachnoid drain placement. Fortunately in most cases the dura seals and the leak resolves.

Vascular

Intraoperative intra-articular hemorrhage as well as retrodiskal hemorrhages can occur with inadvertent medial wall puncture and anterior capsular release. This can sometimes be stopped by the mild hydraulic pressure produced by blocking the outflow portal and allowing inflow pressure to build. If this fails, removal of the instruments and firm compression of the joint, both by shutting the teeth together and lateral compression with gauze overlying the joint capsule, is warranted for a few minutes. Vasoconstrictors may be introduced into the joint space to assist this maneuver.

Another hemorrhagic complication of arthroscopy involves inadvertent puncture or laceration of the overlying vessels on entry. These may include, but are not limited to, superficial temporal artery/vein (A/V), transverse facial A/V, or even the masseteric artery. Very rarely will this event cause such vigorous bleeding as to require intraoperative ligation or subsequent management of an arteriovenous fistula, evidenced by later "whooshing" sounds overlying the joint preauricularly.[59,65,76] Usually this event can be managed by the application of pressure with gauze overlying the vessel, with the patient's head turned to the opposite side and supported by the operating table headrest, thus allowing continuance of the surgery after homeostasis is achieved.

Intra-articular

The small size of the TMJ and the fact that any joint space is in fact only a potential joint space requires constant hydraulic and mechanical distention in order to negotiate instrumentation safely and without causing unnecessary joint surface scuffing and damage. Entry into the joint space through the capsule may be made with a sharp trocar initially, with the irrigation fluid distending the space, but a blunt trocar should then be used to explore the entry success in order to minimize the possibility of scuffing and damage. Additionally a lateral eminence release and a capsular stretch should be employed early in the procedure to allow easy movements of instruments from the posterior to the anterior recess in order to minimize surface damage and potential instrument breakage.

Instrument Breakage

Due to the minimally invasive nature of arthroscopy and size restraints on the mechanical instruments, metallurgic strengths are sometimes exceeded even with the most careful of techniques. Instrument manufacturers have been encouraged to produce "shear points" within their instruments which, on breakage, keep all of the metallic pieces together. These act as a "fuse" breaker, failing just before the functioning edge of their instrument breaks off into the joint space. Not all manufacturers use this principle, however, and the surgeon must be prepared to retrieve broken instrumentation parts from the joint space, either arthroscopically or via open arthrotomy, thus making it imperative to include this possibility on the operation consent form.

Arthroscopic retrieval can be performed through the use of dilation cannulas, which gradually enlarge the access portal to a size sufficient for the grasper or magnetic retriever to hold the broken fragment and come back through the sheath intact without becoming trapped. If restriction occurs and the sheath has to be removed with the fragment, then there is a strong possibility that the fragment may be lost into the soft tissue between the capsule and the skin. As in standard practice, instrument breakage should require incident reporting.

Otologic

One of the earlier complications of arthroscopic surgery reported was that of injury to the tympanic membrane and the middle ear ossicles and permanent hearing loss.[73,77] In retrospect it is seen that the anatomic course of the auditory meatus is anterior and medial. This fact, combined with a patient's head position, in anything other than a near-horizontal ear-flat-to-the-table position portends an increased risk of trocar puncture from the posterolateral approach. One must keep constant vigilance to the direction of the entry trocar anteriorly and superiomedially *combined* with an awareness of the positioned direction of the patient's head at the onset of surgery.

Other rare otologic events include laceration of the external auditory canal.[64,65] Treatment usually involves observation, antibiotic drops, or occasional hemostatic control.

More minor events otologically include otitis externa and otitis media, as well as tympanic membrane perforation resulting from too vigorous canal preparation.[78] Otitis can occur spontaneously postsurgically or from an inadvertent contaminant such as cotton pieces left in the canal.[72] It is therefore prudent for the surgeon to use an otoscope postoperatively to visualize and dry the canal prior to case conclusion, as well as to prescribe medication such as an antibiotic hydrocortisone suspension for eardrops postoperatively. Patients with nonresolving otologic issues or tympanic membrane damage are referred to an otolaryngology specialist for consultation.

Infection

The low overall infection rate of 1% following arthroscopic surgery of the TMJ follows that of the orthopedic literature.[64,66] Even the relative contraindication of puncturing through overlying skin infection has had modifications to allow entry into suppurative arthritis with therapeutic benefit and no adverse postoperative dissemination of infection or cellulitis.[65,75] Although infections are rare, the standard regimen at present for prophylaxis remains at a 1 g bolus of cephalosporin plus oral coverage of cephalosporin 500 mg every 6 hours for 5 days.[27,68,70] Prophylactic antibiotic corticosteroid eardrops are used for 5 days as well.[27,68]

Burns

Various procedures using electrocautery and laser have led to concerns regarding adequate protection of tissues to prevent adverse affects. The use of electrocautery within the joint for reduction of inflammatory or granulation tissue can rarely lead to inadvertent contact of the active electrode's end with the metal of the cannula. This can lead to accidental thermal injury.[79]

Additionally, without copious amounts of irrigating solution to flush and cool the synovial lining of the joint, HO:YAG laser débridements can cause thermal damage to these important cells, inhibiting their natural physiologic function of phagocytosis and production of joint lubricants. Not only should the modern arthroscopist have mechanical hand-eye coordination but an awareness of physiologic colateral effects of surgery as well.

Subcutaneous Fat Atrophy

Subcutaneous fat atrophy has been reported both in the literature and in the community anecdotally.[32] Triamcinolone is frequently used within the superior joint space postoperatively at the case conclusion and in subsequent visits for management of recurrent fibrosis or ankylosis. Its use in both the reduction of deep masseter tendonitis by injection and in reduction of capsulitis by iontophoresis is also common. Even though subcutaneous fat atrophy is rare in occurrence, low concentrations and limiting administrations of triamcinolone can be helpful in limiting risk.

Anesthetic Complication

Manipulation of the jaw has been shown to have occasional effects on the carotid body and thus to result in unexpected bradycardia. If such an event is not reversed by relaxing the jaw position, atropine may be administered. Conversely occasionally epinephrine (1:200,000) is administered to assist in hemostasis during arthroscopic surgery *after* the initial examination is complete, so as not to mask the grading of the synovitis. This hemostatic vasoconstrictor may occasionally cause cardiac arrhythmias. Any persistent premature ventricular contractions or ventricular irritabilities may be treated with intravenous lidocaine if indicated.

Outcomes and Discussion

Over the past decade numerous researchers have shown the effectiveness of TMJ arthroscopy, both in the diagnosis and the surgical management of TMJ articulopathies.[71,80–85]

Although numerous techniques have been developed for both open and arthroscopic surgical management, it would appear that the more complex the procedure applied, the more difficult the postoperative management is, with resulting diminishment of success rates. The overriding factors of similarity for all procedures seem to include the following:

1. Preoperative splint and physical therapy management
2. Release of capsular restrictions, either through incision or blunt obturator release and stretch
3. Release of intra-articular fibrosis and restrictions

4. Application of postoperative physical therapy joint mobilization

The disk position, with the exception of the severely shredded or morphologically obstructed disk, does not appear to affect the patient's outcome of comfort with jaw movements and clinical success.[25,86] While techniques designed to alter the position of the disk, restrict hypermobility, and the like are certainly sometimes indicated, caution must be taken to rein in the enthusiasm for adding yet more complexity to a system that responds very well to simplicity and is adaptive in its articular remodeling and functional response. Even disks that are perforated and joints with Grades III and IV degeneration respond well to the arthroscopic approach.[75]

Further advancements in arthroscopic techniques and treatment modalities are certainly arising and each advance is weighed with these risk-benefit ratios.

References

1. Tagaki K. Practical experience using Tagaki's arthroscope. J Jpn Orthop Assoc 1933;8:132.
2. Bircher E. Die Arthro endoskopie. Zentralbl Chir 1921;48:1460.
3. Kreyscher P. Semilunar cartilage disease: a plea for early recognition by means of the arthroscope and early treatment of this condition. IMG 1925;47:290.
4. Burmann MS, Finkelstein H, Mayer L. Arthroscopy of the knee joint. J Bone Joint Surg 1934;16A:225.
5. Watanabe M, Bechtol R, Nottage W. History of arthroscopic surgery. In: Shahriaree H, editor. O'Connor's textbook of arthroscopic surgery. Philadelphia (PA): Lippincott; 1984. p. 1–6.
6. Casscells SW. Arthroscopy of the knee joint. J Bone Joint Surg 1971;53A:287.
7. Jackson RW, Abe I. The role of arthroscopy in the management of disorders of the knee: an analysis of 200 consecutive examinations. J Bone Joint Surg 1972;54B:310.
8. O'Conner RL. Arthroscopy. Philadelphia (PA): Lippencott; 1977.
9. Johnson LI. Arthroscopic surgery: principles and practice. St. Louis (MO): Mosby; 1986.
10. Watanabe M. Arthroscopy of small joints. Tokyo and New York: Igaku-Shoin; 1985.
11. Ohnishi M. Clinical studies on the intra-articular puncture of the temporomandibular joint. J Jpn Stomat 1970;37:14.
12. Ohnishi M. Arthroscopy of the temporomandibular joint. J Jpn Stomat 1975;42:207.
13. Ohnishi M. Diagnostic application of arthroscope to ankylosis of the temporomandibular joint. Jpn J Oral Surg 1976;22:436.
14. Ohnishi M. Clinical application of arthroscopy in temporomandibular joint diseases. Bull Tokyo Med Dent Univ 1980;27:141.
15. Hilsabech RB, Laskin DM. Arthroscopy of the temporomandibular joint of the rabbit. J Oral Surg 1978;36:938.
16. Williams RA, Laskin DM. Arthroscopic examination of experimentally induced pathologic conditions of the rabbit temporomandibular joint. J Oral Surg 1980;38:652.
17. Holmlund A, Hellsing G, Bang G. Arthroscopy of the rabbit temporomandibular joint. Int J Oral Maxillofac Surg 1986;15:170.
18. Murakami K-I, Hoshino K. Regional anatomical nomenclature and arthroscopic terminology in human temporomandibular joints. Okajimas Folia Anat Jpn 1982;58:4–6.
19. Murakami K-I, Hoshino K. Histological studies on the inner surfaces of the articular cavities of human temporomandibular joints with special references to arthroscopic observations. Anat Anz 1985;160:167.
20. Holmlund A, Hellsing G. Arthroscopy of the temporomandibular joint. Int J Oral Surg 1985;14:169.
21. McCain JP. An illustrated guide to temporomandibular joint arthroscopy. Andover (MA): Dyonics, Inc.; 1987.
22. Murakami KI, Ono T. Temporomandibular joint arthroscopy by inferolateral approach. Int J Oral Maxillofac Surg 1986;15:410.
23. McCain JP. Proceedings of the American Association of Oral and Maxillofacial Surgery TMJ Arthroscopy Symposium Session, Annual Meeting Sept 1985. J Oral Maxillofac Surg.
24. Sanders B. Diagnostic and surgical arthroscopy of the temporomandibular joint: clinical experience with 137 procedures over a 2-year period. J Craniomandib Disord Facial Oral Pain 1987;1(3):202.
25. Moses JJ, Sartoris D, Glass R, et al. The effect of arthroscopic surgical lysis and lavage of the superior joint space on TMJ disc position and mobility. J Oral Maxillofac Surg 1989;47:674–8.
26. Moses JJ, Lo HH. Tomographic changes of the TMJ following arthroscopic surgery with lysis and lavage and eminentia release. J Orofac Pain 1994;8:407–12.
27. Moses JJ, Poker ID. TMJ arthroscopic surgery: an analysis of 237 patients. J Oral Maxillofac Surg 1989; 47:790–4.
28. Emshoff R, Brandimaier I, Schmid C, et al. Bone marrow edema of the mandibular condyle related to internal derangement, osteoarthrosis, and joint effusion. J Oral Maxillofac Surg 2003;61(1):35–40.
29. Moses JJ, Salinas E. MRI or arthrographic diagnosis of TMJ internal derangement: correlation comparison study with arthroscopic surgical confirmation. Oral Surg Oral Med Oral Pathol 1993;75:268–72.
30. Bronstein SL, Thomas M. Arthroscopy of the temporomandibular joint. Philadelphia (PA): W.B. Saunders Co.; 1991. p. 347–50.
31. Shahriaree H. O'Connor's textbook of arthroscopic surgery. Philadelphia (PA): J.B. Lippencott; 1984. p. xi, 1, 237.
32. Nitzan DW, Price A. The use of arthrocentesis for the treatment of osteoarthritic temporomandibular joints. J Oral Maxillofac Surg 2001;59(10):1154–9.
33. Hopkins H. Optical principles of the endoscope. In: Berci G, editor. Endoscopy. New York (NY): Appleton-Century-Crofts; 1976. p. 3–26.
34. Bradrick JP, Eckhauser ML, Indresano AT. Morphologic and histologic changes in canine temporomandibular joint tissues following arthroscopic guided neodymium:YAG laser exposure. J Oral Maxillofac Surg 1989;47(11):1177–81.
35. Bradrick JP, Eckhauser ML, Indresano JP. Early response of canine temporomandibular joint tissues to arthroscopically guided neodymium:YAG laser wounds. J Oral Maxillofac Surg 1992;50(8):835–42.
36. Hendler BH, Gateno J, Mooar P, Sherk HHL. Holmium:YAG laser arthroscopy of the temporomandibular joint. J Oral Maxillofac Surg 1992;50(9):931–4.
37. Jones BR, Moses JJ. Anesthesia for temporomandibular joint arthroscopy. Anesthes Clin North Am 1989;7(3):693–705.
38. Alstergren P, Kopp S. Prostaglandin E$_2$ in temporomandibular joint synovial fluid and its relation to pain and inflammatory disorders. J Oral Maxillofac Surg 2000;58(2):180–6.
39. Neer CS II. Anterior acromioplasty for the chronic impingement syndrome in the shoulder: a preliminary report. J Bone Joint Surg 1972;54A:41.
40. Hawkins RF, Kennedy JC. Impingement syndrome in athletes. Am J Sports Med 1980;8:151.
41. Neer CS II. Impingement lesions. Clin Orthop 1983;173:70.
42. Pujadas GM. Coracoacromial ligament syndrome. J Bone Joint Surg 1979;52A:136.
43. Post M, Cohen J. Impingement syndrome: a review of late state II and early state III lesions. Orthop Trans 1985;9:48.

44. Raggio CL, Warren RF, Sculco T. Surgical treatment of impingement syndrome: 4-year follow-up. Orthop Trans 1985;9:48.

45. Backwood HJJ. Arthritis of the mandibular joint. Br Dental J 1963;115:317.

46. Kirk WS, Kirk BS. Basic biomechanics for temporomandibular surgeons. Presented at the American Society of TMJ Surgeons' Annual Conference; March 2003; Laguna Beach (CA).

47. Moses JJ. Articular pathology: disc displacement and lateral impingement syndrome. In: Bronstein SC, Thomas M, editors. Arthroscopy of the temporomandibular joint. Philadelphia (PA): W.B. Saunders Co.; 1991. p. 249–57.

48. Juniper RP. The pathogenesis and investigation of TMJ dysfunction. Br J Oral Maxillofac Surg 1987;25:105–12.

49. Tay David KL. The pathogenesis of disc displacement in the temporomandibular joint: a reassessment of the role of closed-lock positions. J Gnathol 1987;6(1).

50. Moffett BC, Johnson LC, McCabe JB, Askew HC. Articular remodeling in the adult human temporomandibular joint. Am J Anat 1964;115:119–42.

51. Moses JJ, Topper DC. Use of new arthroscopic joint spreader/stabilizer. Oral Surg Oral Med Oral Rad J 1991;71:535–7.

52. Moses JJ, Poker I. Correlation studies of effects of TMJ arthroscopic surgical lysis of superior joint compartment adhesions and lavage. J Oral Maxillofac Surg 1989;47:674–8.

53. Kondoh T, Hamada Y, Kamei K, Seto K. Simple disc reshaping surgery for internal derangement of the temporomandibular joint: 5-year follow-up results. J Oral Maxillofac Surg 2003;61:41–8.

54. Mazzonetto R, Spagnoli DB. Long-term evaluation of arthroscopic discectomy of the temporomandibular joint using the holmium YAG laser. J Oral Maxillofac Surg 2001;59(9):1018–23.

55. Eriksson L, Westesson PL. Discectomy as an effective treatment of temporomandibular joint internal derangement: a 5-year clinical and radiographic follow-up. J Oral Maxillofac Surg 2001;59(7):750–8.

56. Moses JJ. TMJ arthroscopic surgery: rationale and technique. Proceeding of the American Association of Oral and Maxillofacial Surgeons 82nd Annual Meeting. J Oral Maxillofac Surg 2000;58(8).

57. Greene MW, Hacknewy FL, Van Sickles JE. Arthroscopy of the temporomandibular joint: an anatomic perspective. J Oral Maxillofac Surg 1989;47:386.

58. Al-Kayat A, Bramley P. A modified preauricular approach to the temporomandibular joint and malar arch. Br J Oral Surg 1979;17:91.

59. Moses JJ, Topper DC. Arteriovenous fistula: an unusual complication associated with arthroscopic TMJ surgery. J Oral Maxillofac Surg 1990;18:1220–2.

60. Moses JJ, Hosaka H. Pediatric arthroscopic surgery: a case report with special surgical considerations. J Oral Maxillofac Surg 1992;7:81–99.

61. Murakami K, Takatoki O. Temporomandibular joint arthroscopy by inferolateral approach. Int J Oral Surg 1986;15:410–7.

62. Watanabe M. Arthroscopy of the temporomandibular joint. In: Arthroscopy of small joints. New York (NY): Igaku Shoin; 1985.

63. Moses JJ, Poker ID. Temporomandibular joint arthroscopy: the endaural approach. Int J Oral Maxillofac Surg 1989;18:347–51.

64. Carter JB, Testa L. Complications of TMJ arthroscopy: a review of 2,225 cases. Review of the 1988 Annual Scientific Sessions abstracts. J Oral Maxillofac Surg 1988;46:M14–5.

65. Greene MW, Van Sickels JE. Survey of TMJ arthroscopy in oral and maxillofacial surgery residency programs. J Oral Maxillofac Surg 1989;47:574–6.

66. Small NC. Complications in arthroscopic surgery performed by experienced arthroscopists. J Arthrosc Rel Surg 1988;4:215–21.

67. Tsuyama M, Kondoh T, Seto K, Fukuda J. Complications of temporomandibular joint arthroscopy: a retrospective analysis of 301 lysis and lavage procedures performed using the triangulation technique. J Oral Maxillofac Surg 2000;58(5):500–5.

68. White RD. Retrospective analysis of 100 consecutive surgical arthroscopies of the temporomandibular joint. J Oral Maxillofac Surg 1989;47:1014–21.

69. Carter JB, Schwaber MK. Temporomandibular joint arthroscopy: complications and their management. Oral Maxillofac Surg Clin North Am 1989;1(1): 185–99.

70. Tarro AW. Arthroscopic diagnosis and surgery of the temporomandibular joint. J Oral Maxillofac Surg 1988;46:282–9.

71. Heffez L, Blaustein D. Diagnostic arthroscopy of the temporomandibular joint. I: normal arthroscopic findings. Oral Surg 1987; 64:653–70.

72. Sanders B. Arthroscopic surgery of the temporomandibular joint: treatment of internal derangement with persistent closed lock. Oral Surg 1986;62:361–72.

73. Applebaum EL, Berg LF, Kumar A, et al. Otologic complications following temporo-

mandibular joint arthroscopy. Ann Otol Rhinol Laryngol 1988; 97:675–9.

74. Indreasano AT. Arthroscopic surgery of the temporomandibular joint: report of 64 patients with long-term follow-up. J Oral Maxillofac Surg 1989; 47:439–41.

75. Murakami K, Matsumoto K, Iizuka T. Suppurative arthritis of the temporomandibular joint: report of a case with special reference to arthroscopic observations. J Maxillofac Surg 1984;12:41–5.

76. Preisler SA, Koorbusch GF, Olson RAJ. An acquired arteriovenous fistula secondary to temporomandibular joint arthroscopy: report of a case. J Oral Maxillofac Surg 1991;49:187–90.

77. Van Sickels JE, Nishioka GJ, Hegewald MD, et al. Middle ear injury resulting from temporomandibular joint arthroscopy. J Oral Maxillofac Surg 1987;45:962–5.

78. Tarro AW. Arthroscopic treatment of anterior disc displacement: a preliminary report. J Oral Maxillofac Surg 1989;47:353–8.

79. Bronstein SL, Thomas M. Arthroscopy of the temporomandibular joint. Philadelphia (PA): W.B. Saunders Co.; 1991. p. 320.

80. Goss AN, Bosanquet AG. Temporomandibular joint arthroscopy. J Oral Maxillofac Surg 1986;44:614.

81. Murakami K, Matsuki M, Iizulea T, et al. Diagnostic arthroscopy of the TMJ: differential diagnosis in patients with limited jaw opening. J Craniomandib Pract 1986;4:118.

82. Blaustein D, Heffez L. Diagnostic arthroscopy of the temporomandibular joint. II Arthroscopic findings of arthrographically diagnosed disk displacements. Oral Surg Oral Med Oral Pathol 1988;65:135.

83. Holmlund A, Hellsing G. Arthroscopy of the temporomandibular joint: occurrence and location of osteoarthrosis and synovitis in a patient material. Int J Oral Maxillofac Surg 1988;17:36.

84. Goss AN, Bosanquet A, Tideman H. The accuracy of temporomandibular joint arthroscopy. J Craniomaxillofac Surg 1987;15:99.

85. Uriell P, Bertolucci L, Swaffer C. Physical therapy in the postoperative management of temporomandibular joint surgery. J Craniomandib Pract 1989;7:27.

86. Montgomery MT, Van Sickels JE, Thrash WJ, et al. Signs and symptoms, patient satisfaction and meniscal position following arthroscopic TMJ surgery. Paper presented at the 70th Annual Meeting and Scientific Sessions of the American Association of Oral and Maxillofacial Surgeons; 1989 Sep 30; Boston (MA). J Oral Maxillofac Surg.

CHAPTER 50

Surgery for Internal Derangements of the Temporomandibular Joint

Leslie B. Heffez, DMD, MS

The chapter on surgery for internal derangements of the temporomandibular joint (TMJ) written for the first edition, published in 1992, has stood the test of time. The surgical procedures described are still being performed today, which is indicative of their acceptance within the surgical community and perhaps of their success. The history of TMJ surgery has paralleled the rise and subsequent all but disappearance of the western cowboy. New surgical techniques that neglected to pay attention to the fundamental underlying symptoms and etiology have been heralded as panaceas, only to rapidly fade into obscurity, leaving a trail of iatrogenia. The new TMJ surgeon must be wary of this past. However, prudence should not lead to avoidance of surgery as a treatment modality.

According to Annandale, Sir Astley Cooper was the first to suspect the existence of altered condyle disk-fossa relations.[1] Later the term *internal derangement* was adopted to describe any pathologic entity that interfered with the smooth function of the TMJ. The term is currently used exclusively to describe alterations in disk-fossa relations. Historically, clinicians have recognized that surgery for internal derangements should be reserved for patients with

pain or dysfunction that is severe and disabling and is refractory to nonsurgical management. These conditions still form the basic indications for surgery. Open surgery of the TMJ for primary disease has undergone a complete metamorphosis as a result of the research and clinical results of surgical arthroscopy. At one time only a handful of surgeons professed the viability of function with a displaced disk and argued against surgical repositioning. Today the tables are reversed, and the majority of surgeons recognize that an internal derangement does not imply an ipso facto need for surgery. Furthermore, the presence of persistent symptoms in light of an internal derangement does not imply that surgical correction is necessary or imminent. Only if the mechanical obstruction is felt to be the primary etiology behind the symptoms is surgery indicated. This philosophy has resulted in a dramatic reduction in the number of open surgical procedures performed. This reduction has, in turn, resulted in dramatically fewer cases deemed to have an iatrogenic pathology; we continue to grapple with the 1980 to 1990 vestiges of such cases.

The chapter begins with sections on criteria for diagnosis and goals for surgical

intervention. A brief discussion of surgical anatomic considerations is followed by a description of the classic surgical approaches to the joint capsule and capsular incisions. A critical review of the history, indications, rationale for performance, and techniques of primary operations of the TMJ is then presented. Numerous references are made to those authors who have fueled the development of surgery for internal derangements. In my discussions I have used the term *posterior attachment* to describe tissue that is an extension of the retrodiskal tissue and inserts onto the posterior aspect of the disk. When the adjective *remodeled* is used to qualify an intraarticular structure, as in *remodeled posterior attachment,* the structure is considered pathologic.

Criteria for Diagnosis

Internal derangements are classically divided into two groups: reducing disk displacements and nonreducing disk displacements. Qualifying descriptors are sometimes included, such as the direction of displacement, degree of displacement, and presence of a perforation. Unfortunately, these large diagnostic rubrics fail to identify the finer stages of the disease process. Disk morphology and severity of displacement are only gross indicators of the disease process. Although more complicated classifications such as the Wilkes classification exist, the treatments applied to the diagnostic categories have been diverse, rendering specific recommendations ill advised. It suffices to say that an astute clinician must be armed with that rare commodity of common sense rather than a rigid algorithm of treatment modalities. The research and clinical work emanating from arthroscopic trials will, in the future, establish more specific diagnostic criteria for establishing treatment protocols.

In the surgical decision-making process the specific diagnosis is only one piece of information necessary to make the decision to perform surgery. Surgery should be considered when the dysfunction or pain cannot be corrected to a level of patient satisfaction by nonsurgical modalities. Cookbook approaches to the diagnosis and surgical management of internal derangements should not be used. It is important to consider that no dysfunction is identical to another when the surgeon factors into the treatment equation the patient's perception of his or her problem, the effect on daily routine, and the patient psyche. The diagnosis of an internal derangement is achieved predominantly through clinical skills. Imaging of the joint usually is most useful only in the later planning stages of surgery, rather than during the establishment of a working diagnosis. There is the occasional instance in which a diagnostic dilemma exists and magnetic resonance imaging (MRI) is required to elucidate the case.

For the sake of discussion, the condition internal derangement can be identified in three different clinical settings. The first is the occurrence of a primarily functional disturbance. In this condition the chief complaint is functional. The patients may describe a need to perform a special maneuver with the mandible to achieve a wide opening, or they may describe an annoying terminal jolting associated with closing. Joint pain is typically not chronic and appears to be related to the instability of the condyle-disk relations. Pain occurs with the sudden separation of joint surfaces during disk reduction or displacement. However, pain may not be a feature. Most of these cases demonstrate a reducing disk displacement, in which the disk represents a mobile mechanical obstacle and the condyle is not permanently restricted in its range of motion. Reduction refers to the ability of the condyle to negotiate around the disk. The disk's recoil potential is minimal in the pathologic condition. The inferior surface of the disk is typically bulged and histologically is the site of increased proteoglycan deposition. If pain and dysfunction persist despite treatment of a coexistent parafunctional habit, surgery should be considered. These patients are best managed with open surgery and reduction of the obstructing portions of the articular disk. Diskoplasty, partial diskectomy, or full diskectomy may be performed, depending on the degree of disk atrophy and deformation. Disk repositioning should be considered only when the disk is minimally deformed and of near-normal length. Clinical indicators for surgical intervention of this condition are rare. Some clinicians prefer to perform arthroscopic disk-stabilizing procedures using suturing or sclerosing techniques.

The second clinical setting in which internal derangements are identified is the condition of closed lock. *Closed lock* refers to an acute or chronic limitation of movement of the condyle owing to an intra-articular disturbance. Patients experiencing closed lock often complain of muscle dysfunction secondary to efforts to reach a baseline mouth opening.

The coexistence of muscle dysfunction and an internal derangement does not imply a relationship. A large segment of the general population have minimal signs and symptoms associated with internal derangements. Careful recording of the chief and ancillary complaints is imperative, with attention being paid to the details of onset and duration of facial pain and joint noise, timing of symptoms of facial tightness, inability to open or close the mouth, and distribution of headaches. Concomitant sources of pain need to be identified and consultations with neurology, otolaryngology, psychology, or general dentistry, as required, obtained. The history of previous treatment is equally important.

There are usually a number of factors that are considered in the etiology of closed lock, including intracapsular and extracapsular inflammation and adhesions, muscle tension or spasm, disk displacement, synovial fluid viscosity, and reduction in synovial lubrication.

The closed lock phenomenon may resolve spontaneously or gradually over a period of weeks to months. Hence, it is important to evaluate the patient on several visits to effectively note a response to nonsteroidal anti-inflammatory agents and muscle relaxants. In the absence of pain, many patients are able to tolerate the restriction in mouth opening, which gradually improves over several months to years.

MRI of the closed lock condition usually demonstrates a displaced disk, with various degrees of deformation. In some patients the disk appears in a normal position but is unable to be displaced down the slope of the eminence. Although not the subject of this chapter, it suffices to say that T1 and T2 (or gradient echo imaging) in sagittal planes is required to delineate intra-articular fluid, interstitial inflammation, and disk morphology. Magnetic resonance images demonstrate that the condyle is unable to displace the disk anterior enough to reach the apex of the eminence or beyond. On fast magnetic resonance or T2 images, inflammatory fluid or increased vascularity appears as a high signal intensity (Figure 50-1).

Adhesions associated with closed lock cannot be definitively identified on an MRI scan. They are suspected when there

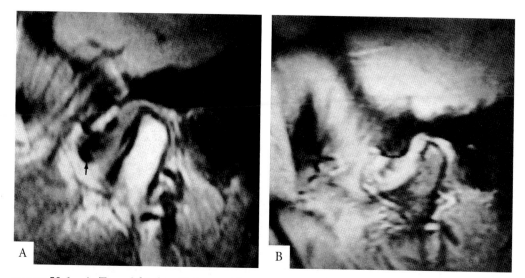

FIGURE 50-1 A, *T1-weighted sagittal magnetic resonance image demonstrating a dislocated disk. Note the low signal intensity, which represents a portion of the deformed disk* (arrow). B, *Fast imaging (GRASS [gradient recalled acquisition in steady state]) of the same section demonstrates the presence of extra-articular and intra-articular fluid or an increase in vascularity in the anterior regions of the joint. These changes may be partly responsible for the closed lock phenomenon.*

is a confluence of the low signal intensities of the condyle and glenoid fossa without intervening intermediate signal intensity. Arthrocentesis followed by arthroscopic lysis of superior joint space adhesions, lavage, and manipulation are the treatments of choice for this condition. Open surgical procedures are indicated when arthroscopy has failed to resolve the restriction in opening. The choice of open procedure largely depends on disk anatomy and position.

The third clinical setting is the internal derangement condition of disk displacement that reduces on opening and is associated with persistent preauricular pain refractory to nonsurgical therapy. This is the most difficult of the three conditions to treat and requires long-term therapy with control of parafunctional habits. The clinician must ask whether the pain is occurring from hypermobility caused by contralateral hypomobility, acute or chronic separation of disk surfaces during displacement and reduction, noncompliance with diet restrictions, or persistent parafunctional or work-related habits. There are indications for surgical intervention; however, it is this condition that

carries the greatest peril of being rendered into the painful operated ankylosed joint after several fruitless surgeries.

Arthrocentesis has supplanted arthroscopic surgery as the most successful treatment modality. It should be attempted before performing any open surgical procedure. The type of open procedure is governed by the degree of disk morphology. The key to arthroscopy is to remove the source of the persistent inflammation including the vascular retrodiskal tissue and hyperplastic inflamed synovium.

Goals of Surgery

The general goals of any surgical intervention are to return the patient to a regular diet, with some limitations, and to establish an adequate functional range of motion. Each patient's complaints must be individually analyzed, and specific outcomes set for the operation. Postoperatively the surgeon should evaluate the patient's response to therapy according to whether the patient feels there has been a total eradication, significant reduction, or minimal reduction of his or her complaints, or no change or worsening of the condition. It is unreasonable for the surgeon to evaluate the results

of an operation on the basis of attainment of a finite mouth opening. Many patients are quite satisfied with reductions in their mouth opening as long as their facial pain is relieved. The goals for all surgical procedures should include preservation of articular tissue to permit normalization and regeneration of synovium, and a restoration of the articular relations to permit the joint structures to adapt and function through an adequate range of motion. The remodeled disk is only one element of the degenerative process. Joint function may be asymptomatic and satisfactory in the presence of various types of internal derangement. Thus, surgically returning a displaced disk to the ideal position found in a healthy joint may not be appropriate for an individual patient. To illustrate this point, one would not reposition a disk in a joint in which the articular tissue is so severely damaged that it is incapable of healing. In this situation removing the disk is recommended. Repositioning the disk is recommended in the patient with minimal changes in the joint structures, in whom symptoms have persisted despite nonsurgical and arthroscopic intervention. As indicated above, this condition is indeed rare.

Additional magnetic resonance and arthroscopic information about the structure and function of the joint in health and disease is needed to establish reliable indicators and predictors of surgical outcome.

Surgical Approaches

The classic surgical approaches to the TMJ may be classified as preauricular, endaural, and postauricular. The choice of approach is usually a matter of surgeon's preference and is based on his or her ability and experience. Cosmetic considerations may also influence the choice of approach.

Surgical Anatomic Considerations

Anterior to the auricle, the auricularis anterior and superior muscles overlie the superficial temporalis fascia and the temporalis fascia. These muscles are incised in the classic preauricular and endaural approaches. The fascia superficial to the muscles is thin and a dull white. This layer is confluent with the galea aponeurotica above and the parotideomasseteric fascia below. The temporalis fascia is a tough fibrous connective tissue structure, substantially thicker than the overlying superficial fascia. It is stark white and extends from the superior temporal line of the temporal bone to the zygomatic arch. The deep surface furnishes one of the origins of the temporalis muscle. Inferiorly, at a variable distance, the fascia splits into two well-defined layers (Figure 50-2). The outer layer attaches to the lateral margin of the superior border of the zygomatic arch, and the inner layer to the medial margin. A small quantity of fat, the zygomatico-orbital branch of the temporal artery, and zygomaticotemporal branch of the maxillary nerve are located between the fascial layers. The splitting of the fascial layers is most noticeable at the level of the zygomatic arch. Posteriorly, superior to the glenoid fossa, the separation is not as well-defined (Figure 50-3).

The superficial temporal vessels are typically located in the superficial fascia below the auricularis anterior muscle. The vessels are often visible, invested in the superficial fascia without incising the muscle. The superficial temporal vein lies posterior to the artery and the auriculotemporal nerve immediately behind the vessels. The superficial temporal vessels and auriculotemporal nerve appear to take on a horizontal course once the flap is fully developed and reflected anteroinferiorly.[2]

Numerous authors have studied the facial nerve's anatomic relations to determine clinically applicable landmarks for its main trunk, temporofacial division, and temporal branches. Al-Kayat and Bramley noted that the facial nerve bifurcated into temporofacial and cervicofacial components within 2.3 cm (range 1.5–2.8 cm) inferior to the lowest concavity of the bony external auditory canal and within 3.0 cm (range 2.4–3.5 cm) in an inferoposterior direction from the postglenoid tubercle.[3] The temporal nerve branches lie closest to the joint and are the most commonly injured branches during surgery. These nerves are located in a condensation of superficial fascia, temporalis fascia, and periosteum as they cross the zygomatic arch. The most posterior temporal branches lie anteriorly to the postglenoid tubercle. Their location was measured by Al-Kayat and Bramley as 3.5 ± 0.8 cm from the anterior margin of the bony external auditory canal (Figure 50-4).[3]

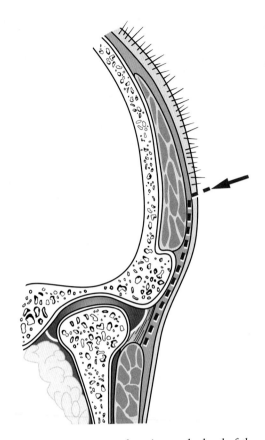

FIGURE 50-3 *Coronal section at the level of the glenoid fossa. The splitting of the temporalis fascia is not as well-defined* (broken line).

Thus, the two potential sources of facial nerve injury are dissection anterior to the posterior glenoid tubercle where the temporal branches cross the arch, and aggressive retraction at the inferior margin of the flap where the main trunk and temporofacial division are located.

Preauricular Approach

Historically, a myriad of preauricular incisions have been proposed. Many of the earlier designs afforded good access but increased the risk of facial nerve injury and compromised esthetics. The preauricular incisions used today are essentially modifications of the Blair curvilinear or inverted-L incision.[4] This approach has become the favorite chosen by oral and maxillofacial surgeons. The technique is an incision commencing from within the temporal hairline and extending inferiorly

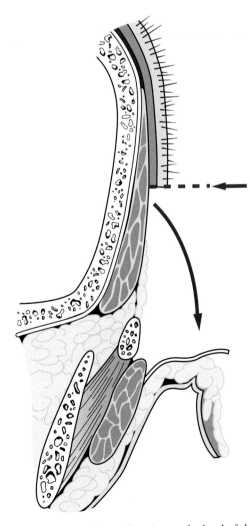

FIGURE 50-2 *Coronal section at the level of the zygomatic arch. Two well-defined layers of temporalis fascia are noted* (arrows).

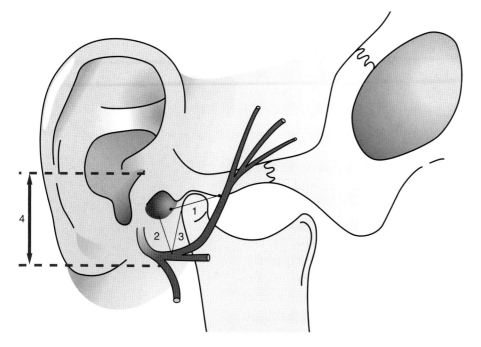

FIGURE 50-4 *Landmarks for the location of the temporal branches and main trunk of the facial nerve: (1) the distance between the anterior margin concavity of the meatus to the zygomatic arch (3.5 ± 0.8 cm); (2) the distance between the inferior margin of the meatus to the trunk (2.3 ± 0.28 cm); (3) the distance between the postglenoid tubercle to the main trunk (3.0 ± 0. 31 cm); (4) the distance from the tragus to the facial nerve trunk is variable.*

into a preauricular crease immediately anterior to the auricle. The exact length and decision to incorporate an anterior temporal extension are governed largely by the nature of the surgical procedure. For some surgeons, the approach for diskectomy requires a smaller incision than that for diskoplasty.

The incision is approximately 3 to 4 cm in length and consists of two limbs: a small superior curved limb (1–2 cm) and an inferior vertical limb anterior to the tragus (variable distance approximately 1–2 cm) (Figure 50-5). The junction of these limbs is the site of attachment of the superior aspect of the helix to the temporal tissue. The extent of the superior limb of the preauricular incision is dictated by the amount of access required, which may not be determined until the dissection has reached the lateral TMJ ligament and capsule. The incision is usually not extended as inferiorly as the lobule of the ear.

The incision should be placed posteriorly to the superficial temporal vessels

and auriculotemporal nerve and within a preauricular crease. The skin and subcutaneous tissues are incised the length of the entire incision. The deeper dissection is begun in the temporal region by sharply dissecting progressively through the auricularis anterior and superficial

fascial layers to the stark white temporalis fascia (Figure 50-6). A retractor is placed on the anterior flap, and tension is applied in a forward direction. The dissection over the zygomatic arch is addressed. The anatomic layers in this region are usually not clearly defined. There is a condensation of tissues consisting variably of the auricularis interior, superficial fascia, temporalis fascia, periosteum, and occasionally cartilage. This tissue is incised to the level of fibrous connective tissue. A retractor is placed in the incision opposite the tragus, and forward traction is applied to the flap. This results in the definition of a cleft between the perichondrium and cartilage of the external auditory canal and the parotideomasseteric fascia. The perichondrium is followed medially with sharp dissection (Figure 50-7). Care should be exercised not to proceed perpendicularly to the skin surface, as the external auditory canal inclines anteromedially at approximately 45° to the surface. The dissection is continued along the outer surface of the external auditory

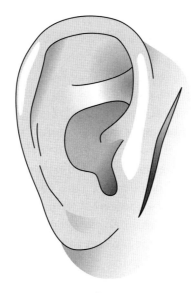

FIGURE 50-5 *Preauricular incision.*

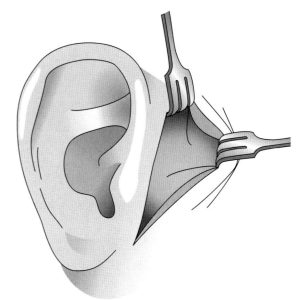

FIGURE 50-6 *The preauricular incision has been carried sharply through the skin, subcutaneous tissue, superficial temporal fascia, auricularis anterior and superior, and outer layers of the temporal fascia. The flap is reflected anteroinferiorly, revealing the inner layer of the temporal fascia.*

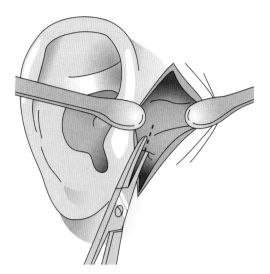

FIGURE 50-7   *The parotideomasseteric fascia is sharply dissected from the perichondrium of the external auditory canal* (broken line).

canal until the lateral TMJ ligament is reached.

When the condyle and its overlying temporomandibular ligament are palpated, the flap is reflected inferiorly and anteriorly forward with a combination of sharp

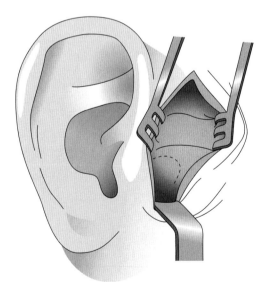

FIGURE 50-8   *Retraction is accomplished by using a self-retaining retractor positioned between the external auditory canal and flap and a right-angle retractor at the interior portion of the flap. The condyle* (dotted line) *is noted under the lateral TMJ ligament and/or simply the lateral capsule depending on the depth of the reflection.*

and blunt dissections. Scissors may be used to cut some fascial attachments to the lateral TMJ ligament. The blades of the scissors are held parallel to the ligament to ensure that the joint is not violated. The flap is reflected as far forward as the midportion of the anterior tubercle. The surgeon can now see the bulging of the lateral pole of the condyle under cover of the lateral ligament and capsule. Gentle manipulation of the jaw to cause movement of the condyle helps to orient the surgeon. The deep surface of the flap and the tissues overlying the zygomatic arch may be touched with a nerve stimulator to ascertain the location of the facial nerve. Retraction is accomplished using a self-retaining retractor (eg, cerebellar Weitlaner or a Dolwick-Reich) placed between the flap and the perichondrium. A small right-angled retractor may be placed at the inferior portion of the flap (Figure 50-8).

Endaural Approach

Rongetti described a modification of Lempert's endaural approach to the mastoid process for surgical improvement of otosclerosis, for approaching the TMJ.[5,6] The endaural incisions employed today either incorporate the anterior wall of the external auditory canal, or the tragus, or simply the skin overlying the mental aspect of the tragus (Figure 50-9).

The incision begins well within the external auditory meatus at the superior mental wall. At this level the incision is made down to the bone and extended in a curvilinear fashion upward hugging the anterior helix (see Figure 50-9). It becomes less penetrating as it approaches the superior surface, ending at about the level of the inferior tragus. The incision is deepened to the level of the temporalis fascia. The incision is now continued inferiorly, with the knife in continuous contact with the tympanic plate, to make a semicircular incision to the inferior point of the meatus. The incision is then continued

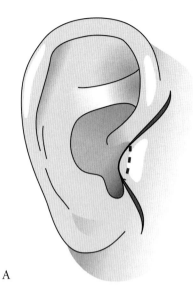

A

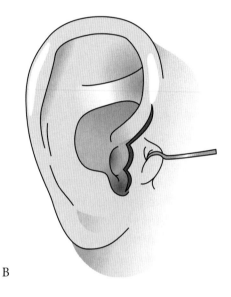

B

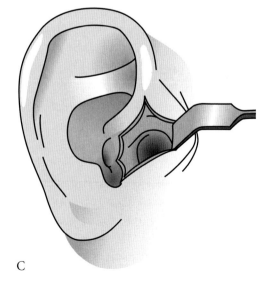

C

FIGURE 50-9   A–C, *Endaural approach according to J. R. Rongetti. Adapted from Rongetti JR.*[5]

anteroinferiorly to fall into the incisura intertragica, ending just before it approaches the surface. The application of forward traction on the inner aspect of the tragus assists the surgeon in completing the incision. Sharp dissection is carried deeply for some distance along the perichondrium. The flap is then reflected en masse anteroinferiorly off the lateral capsule and ligament.

The advantages of this incision lie in its excellent access to the lateral and posterior aspects of the joint, good exposure of the anterior aspect, and its esthetic value. The access afforded through this approach is equal to that obtained through the preauricular approach. Disadvantages lie in the potential for perichondritis and an esthetic compromise if tragal projection is lost.

Postauricular Approach

In the postauricular approach the incision is made posterior to the ear and involves the sectioning of the external auditory meatus.[7] Excellent posterolateral exposure is afforded with this technique. The flap, once reflected, contains the entire auricle and superficial lobe of the parotid gland. A perimeatal approach combining the preauricular and postauricular incisions has also been described.[8,9]

The incision in the postauricular approach begins near the superior aspect of the external pinna and is extended to the tip of the mastoid process. The superior portion may be extended obliquely into the hairline for additional exposure. The incision is made 3 to 5 mm parallel and posterior to the postauricular flexure (Figure 50-10). The dissection is performed through the posterior auricular muscle to the level of the mastoid fascia, which is contiguous with the temporalis fascia. A combination of blunt and sharp dissections is used to isolate the cartilaginous portion of the external auditory canal. A blunt instrument is placed in the external auditory canal to assist in the

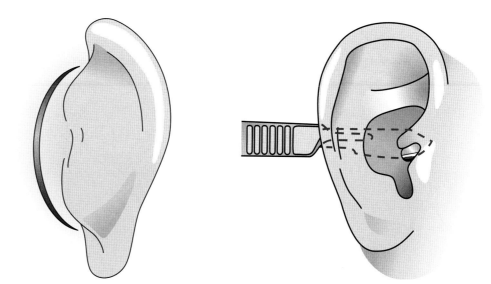

FIGURE 50-10 *Postauricular approach. The incision is placed 3 to 5 mm parallel and posterior to the postauricular flexure.*

transsection of the external auditory canal. The transsection may be partial or complete, depending on the need for exposure. The incision should leave 3 to 4 mm of cartilage on the medial aspect to permit adequate reapproximation of the canal (Figure 50-11). This technique helps to prevent meatal stenosis. The incision is carried through the outer layer of the temporalis fascia, continuing inferiorly, reflecting the parotideomasseteric fascia off the zygomatic arch and lateral TMJ ligament (Figure 50-12). A self-retaining retractor is used to maintain exposure. The advantages of the postauricular approach lie in the predictability of the anatomic exposure. Dissection to the joint is rapid with minimal bleeding. The approach offers an alternative for a patient who has had previous procedures in this region. This approach may not be desirable in the patient susceptible to keloid formation, owing to the potential for a keloid to develop in the meatus. Meatal atresia has been reported with this technique.[10] The risk of facial nerve injury is not eliminated. Paresthesia in the area of the posterior aspect of the auricle usually occurs and lasts 3 to 4 months.

FIGURE 50-11 *The external auditory canal is sectioned, leaving 3 to 4 mm of cartilage on the medial aspect to assist reapproximation of the canal.*

Capsular Incisions

Hori\zontal Incision Over the Lateral Rim of the Glenoid Fossa The lateral ligament, capsule, and periosteum are reflected inferiorly en masse. Diskal or posterior attachment connections, or both, to the lateral capsule are dissected sharply with scissors to the level of the condylar neck (Figure 50-13A). Posterior dissection is performed diligently to avoid severing the retrodiskal tissue. This portion of the dissection exposes the superior joint space (Figure 50-13B). A Freer septum elevator

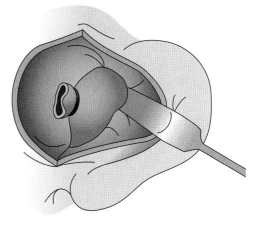

FIGURE 50-12 *The external auditory canal has been sectioned and the flap retracted forward.*

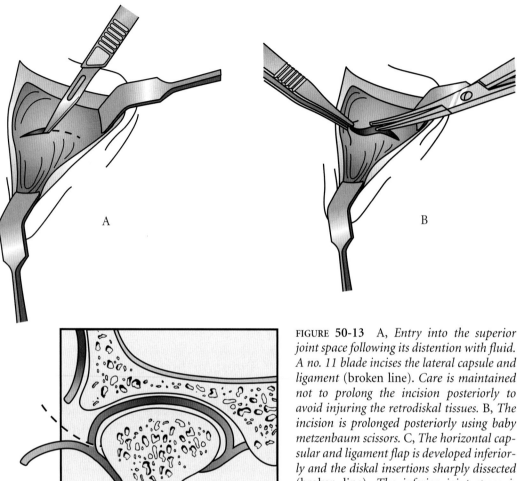

FIGURE **50-13** A, *Entry into the superior joint space following its distention with fluid. A no. 11 blade incises the lateral capsule and ligament (broken line). Care is maintained not to prolong the incision posteriorly to avoid injuring the retrodiskal tissues. B, The incision is prolonged posteriorly using baby metzenbaum scissors. C, The horizontal capsular and ligament flap is developed inferiorly and the diskal insertions sharply dissected (broken line). The inferior joint space is defined by incising along the superolateral aspect of the condyle. A Freer septum elevator is used to define the joint spaces.*

may be used to define and explore the space. The posterior attachment and disk attachments are then severed sharply at the lateral pole of the condyle from within the developed flap. The Freer septum elevator is used to reflect the posterior attachment and disk superiorly off the head of the condyle to expose the inferior joint space. A periosteal elevator may be used to stretch the capsule and lateral ligament flap outward to form a pocket (Figure 50-13C).

There is a risk of reflecting the fibrous connective tissue that lines the glenoid fossa when this approach is used (Figure 50-14A). The surgeon may form the incorrect assumption that he or she is stripping adhesions from the temporal bone while defining the space. The result may be a

partial or total synovectomy of the superior joint space. Prearthrotomy arthroscopic examinations have alerted clinicians to this error. The ability of the pathologic joint to regenerate this synovium and fibrous connective tissue layer has not been determined.

Horizontal Incision Below the Lateral Rim of the Glenoid Fossa   A no. 11 blade may be used to puncture into the superior joint space at the level of the lateral disko-capsular sulcus (Figure 50-14B). The opening is then lengthened anteriorly and posteriorly using sharp-pointed scissors. A dissection technique, similar to that described in the foregoing approach, is used to define the superior joint space. A

dissection is then carried inferiorly removing the attachment of the capsule to the disk and exposing the inferior joint space. There is less risk of injury to the retrodiskal tissue with this approach; the risk to the fibrocartilage is also reduced. This is the approach I favor.

Horizontal Incisions Above and Below the Disk   The horizontal approach above and below the disk (Figure 50-14C) leaves some of the capsule and ligament attached to the disk or remodeled retrodiskal tissue.

L-Shaped Incision   A horizontal incision is made at or below the lateral rim of the glenoid fossa. The horizontal incision is then joined by either an anterior (Figure 50-14D) or posterior (Figure 50-14E) vertical extension. The posterior vertical incision carries the risk of severing the retrodiskal tissue. The anterior vertical incision should not be placed farther anteriorly than the tubercle to avoid injury to the facial nerve. The capsule and ligament are then reflected either anteroinferiorly or posteroinferiorly.

T-Shaped Incision   A horizontal incision is joined by a vertical incision to create a T-shaped incision over the midportion of the glenoid fossa (Figure 50-14F).

Cross-Hair Incision   Dissection of the posterior attachment of the lateral ligament and capsule may be tedious with the cross-hair incision (Figure 50-14G).

Open-Sky Incision   In the open-sky incision two horizontal incisions are joined by a central vertical incision (Figure 50-14H).

Vertical Incision   After a vertical incision is made, the capsular flaps are reflected anteriorly and posteriorly to expose the posterior attachment and disk (Figure 50-14I). Closure of the capsule is often difficult to attain following open surgical procedures. When diagnostic arthroscopy precedes the

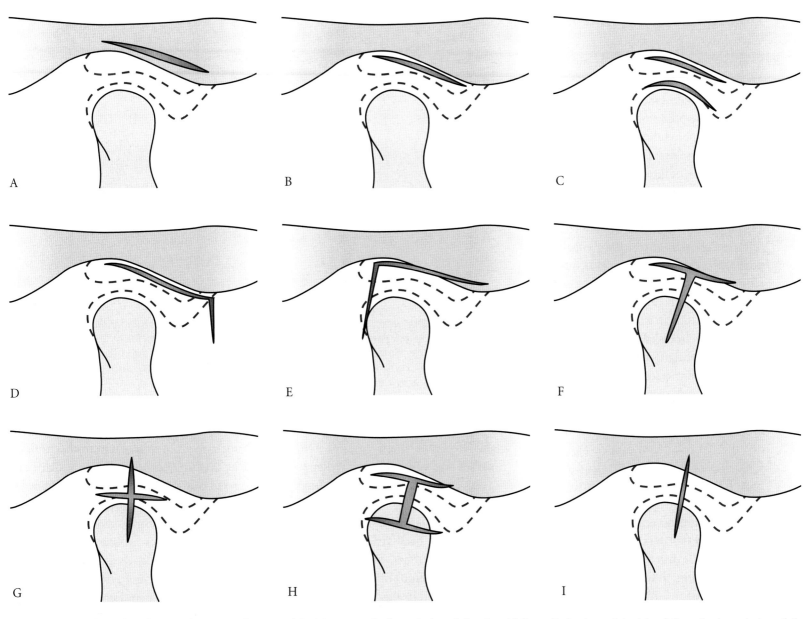

FIGURE **50-14** *Capsular incision designs: A, horizontal incision over the lateral rim of the glenoid fossa; B, horizontal incision below the lateral rim of the glenoid fossa; C, horizontal incisions above and below the disk; D and E, L-shaped incision; F, T-shaped incision; G, cross-hair incision; H, open-sky incision; I, vertical incision. The lateral pole of the condyle and lateral aspect of the remodeled posterior attachment* (broken lines) *are illustrated.*

arthrotomy, the inflow and outflow ports violate the capsule, making watertight closure extremely difficult. Support for the lateral ligament can be obtained by raising a temporalis muscle and fascia flap, about 2 cm in length, pedicled inferiorly, and rotated inferiorly over the lateral rim of the glenoid fossa and sutured to the lateral capsular tissue. The pedicle stabilizes the flap but has not been shown to contain nutrient vessels. Closure of the capsule may not be critical to the success of the

diskectomy procedure, and in some cases the closure may restrict mandibular motion.[11,12] However, closure of the capsule and ligament after disk repositioning lends stability to the diskorrhaphy.

Operative Procedures

A concerted comparative evaluation of different surgical techniques is difficult because for many years there was no uniform set of criteria for selection of patients or compilation and evaluation of results.

Criteria and guidelines for disk surgery were initially developed in 1984 by the American Association of Oral and Maxillofacial Surgeons (AAOMS).[13] The criteria were established through a literature review and consensus. In 1990 a standards and criteria document was published by the AAOMS.[14] The document established indications for surgery, identified markers for favorable and unfavorable results, and outlined risk factors. These publications have laid the groundwork for peer review.

Disk-Repositioning Procedures

The goal of disk-repositioning procedures is to relocate the disk so that its posterior band can be returned to the normal condyle-disk-fossa relationship. Essentially, the repositioning places the posterior band over the superior or superoanterior surface of the condyle. This retropositioning is accomplished by one of three procedures: plication in which the remodeled posterior attachment is folded on itself and the lateral tissues are approximated (Figure 50-15); full-thickness excision in which a wedge-shaped portion of the posterior attachment is removed and the lateroposterior tissues are approximated (Figure 50-16); or partial-thickness excision in which the superior lamina of the retrodiskal tissue and posterior attachment are removed, without violation of the inferior joint space, and the lateroposterior tissues are approximated (Figure 50-17).

When the disk displaces, the pathologic changes are not seen uniformly throughout the entire lateromedial extent of the joint. Typically, the medially displaced disk must be rotated posterolaterally to achieve a correct condyle-disk-fossa relation; therefore, a greater amount of tissue is plicated or excised laterally rather than medially. Rarely, the disk may be displaced in the lateral direction, in which event the reverse would be true.

The technical improvements in TMJ arthrography in the 1970s stimulated interest in correcting disturbances in the condyle-disk-fossa relations,[15] and the

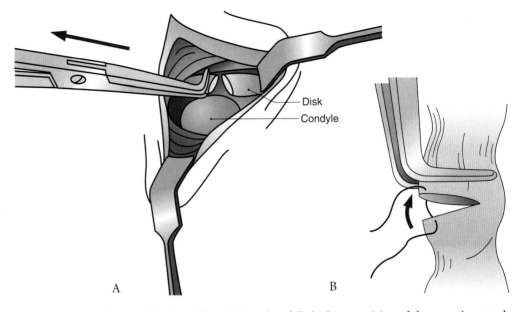

FIGURE 50-16 *Disk repositioning achieved through a full-thickness excision of the posterior attachment. Retention of disk position is through sutures placed on posterior and lateral margins. A, A clamp has been placed over the posterior attachment. The* arrow *represents the direction of pull of the clamp to complete the incision and reveal the condylar surface. B, View from above demonstrating the wedge-shaped resection (*arrow *indicates the direction of closure).*

concept that disk repair procedures were a viable answer to many cases of TMJ dysfunction was re-introduced.[16] Reports on the outcome of disk repair procedures have indicated an 80% or greater success rate.[17–19] The latter assumes an accurate diagnosis has been made. Surgeon diagnostic acumen has evolved with time. Although the results of the procedures may have been good in the 1980s, readers must be cautious as the indications for performing the procedure have changed and hence the outcomes may be misleading given the new subset of surgical candidates.

The histologic basis for performing surgery within vascular retrodiskal tissue was described in animals by Wallace and Laskin and by Zeitler and colleagues.[20,21] Synoviocytes play an important role in the healing process. Stimulated by inflammation, synoviocytes proliferate and migrate to fill the surgically created gap in the tissues.[22–24] The synoviocytes produce ground substance and collagen fibers and phagocytose the debris. The degree of tissue vascularity and the distance from capsular and synovial vasculature have also been described as important factors in the healing process. [25,26]

Extrapolations to the clinical situation must be made from these results as an animal model for TMJ pathology is lacking. In the human, variable decreases in the vascularity of the remodeled posterior attachment are believed to occur with an increasing duration of displacement and load. The disk-repositioning techniques thus involve a repair in the pathologic remodeled retrodiskal tissue with a variable degree of vascularity. The primary source of nourishment to the repositioned

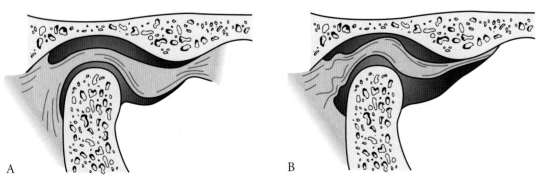

FIGURE 50-15 *Disk repositioning achieved through plication of the posterior attachment. Retention of disk position is through sutures to the lateral capsule ligament. A, Preoperative location. B, Postoperative location.*

disk appears to be through the synovium on the medial aspect of the disk and posterior recesses of the joint spaces. Thus, a critical aspect of the successful surgical repair in the retrodiskal tissue appears to be the rapid migration of synoviocytes to the area of the surgical repair. Smith and Walters followed up 12 patients for 1 year and reported success suturing tears in the avascular portion of the disk.[27] Others, however, have reported that suturing anything but vascularized tissue results in failure of the repair.[20,28]

With an increasing displacement of the disk, the retrodiskal tissue comes into contact with the condole and sustains increasing loading. The loading results in decreased vascularity of the retrodiskal tissue. With the reduction in retrodiskal tissue vascularity, this tissue becomes transformed into a pseudodisk. MRI of chronically displaced retrodiskal tissues demonstrates a signal intensity of the tis-

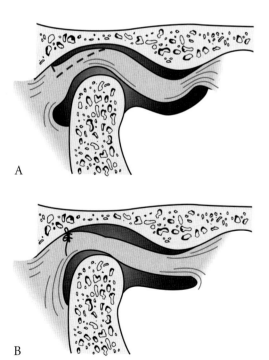

FIGURE 50-17 *Disk repositioning achieved through a partial-thickness excision of the superior lamina of the retrodiskal tissue. The inferior joint space is not violated. A, Outline of a partial-thickness excision of the superior lamina. B, Excision is closed, resulting in posterior repositioning of the disk.*

sue that resembles the disk. In fact, radiologists may inaccurately describe a disk fragmentation because only a portion of the displaced disk may display its original signal intensity. The remainder, owing to alterations in the glycoprotein distribution and hence the attraction of water, demonstrate a moderate signal intensity. With increasing displacement of the disk, the superior joint space does not accommodate for the increase in length of the retrodiskal tissue. Rather, the disk undergoes atrophy, deformation (buckling), and absorption into the anterior capsule. These changes can make anatomic repositioning of the disk impossible.

Disk repositioning without diskoplasty is indicated in the following instances:

- There is minimal disk displacement
- The disk is of near-normal length
- The disk structure is near normal (bow-tie)

The rationale behind repositioning is founded on the belief that the disease process is reversible or can be halted by normalizing the position of the disk. In addition, removal of the posterior attachment overlying the condyle is intended to remove a source of localized inflammation. The repositioned disk facilitates movement of the condyle previously blocked by the displaced disk, provides joint stabilization, and improves articular cartilage nutrition and lubrication. Moreover, the rationale is that the workload of the masticatory muscles is reduced when the obstructing disk is repositioned.

Before performing disk-repositioning procedures in patients with satisfactory disk morphology, adequate trials of nonsurgical therapy should be undertaken to determine whether the patient can be made symptom free despite disk displacement. In 1989, reports were published demonstrating, by postarthroscopic MRI, persistent disk displacement despite the resolution of pain and increase in mandibular mobility.[29,30] These reports,

and the appearance of anterior disk displacement in patients without any history of TMJ symptoms, support the execution of nonsurgical therapy prior to deciding whether it is necessary to perform disk-repositioning surgery.

Deformation of the disk in all planes is an important feature to recognize when planning a repositioning procedure. When a bulge-shaped disk is of appropriate length and can be repositioned, a diskoplasty may be performed to minimize the change in the occlusion.[31] It has been reported that during function, the fiber arrangement and proteoglycan distribution of the repositioned disk change to those of a normal disk and that diskoplasty therefore would be unnecessary.[32] More evidence is still required to substantiate these changes.

In general, the limiting factor to disk repositioning is the degree of lateral disk atrophy or resorption. Despite severe lateral atrophy, the most medial aspect of the disk may have a normal length and shape (Figure 50-18). Disk shortening may preclude disk repositioning without an extensive release of the anterolateral disk attachments, calling into question the procedure of repositioning.

Disk Repositioning and Diskoplasty A rosette-shaped disposable orthopedic meniscus knife, typically used for orthopedic arthroscopic procedures, is used to effect a release of the disk from its most anterior and lateral attachments (Figure 50-19). This is accomplished by gently prodding the knife along the inside perimeter of the capsule (Figure 50-20). As the dissection is performed under cover of the capsule, there is no danger of injuring the facial nerve. Disk mobility is evaluated by applying posterolateral traction with a forceps (Figure 50-21). A DeBakey bulldog vascular clamp is inserted to the medial limit of the posterior attachment and guided posteriorly as far as possible in the glenoid fossa (see Figure 50-20B). The

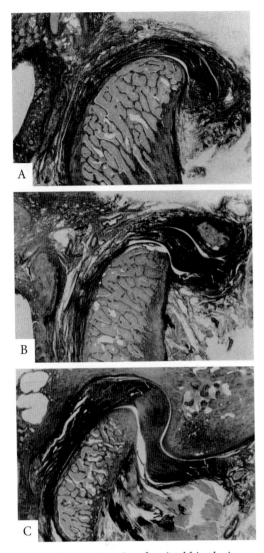

FIGURE **50-18** *A series of sagittal histologic sections through a joint, demonstrating partial disk displacement. Note the change in disk length and morphology as one moves from lateral (A) to medial (C)(hematoxylin eosin stain; macroscopic section).*

clamp greatly assists in the control of hemorrhage from the retrodiskal tissue, stabilization of the posterior attachment during tissue excision, and stabilization of the posterior attachment during suturing.[33] The design of the instrument minimizes tissue damage. A wedge of remodeled posterior attachment is excised, leaving a 1 mm margin anterior to the beaks of the clamp. This permits suturing of the disk to the retrodiskal tissue without removal of the clamp. Range of motion is then verified. Tissue forceps are used to stabilize and slightly evert the disk so that the infe-

rior surface may be sculpted with meniscus knives (Figure 50-22). The tissue is closed with nonresorbable suture on an S-2 spatula needle (Figure 50-23). Once the disk has been sutured into its new position, its lateral rim is sutured to the lateral capsule ligament.

Operative difficulties with the repositioning techniques include control of hemorrhage from the retrodiskal tissue and access to the medial aspect of the fossa. Bleeding may be controlled by using the DeBakey clamp before sectioning the posterior attachment. Access to the medial aspect of the joint is greatly improved when the anterior attachment is released, permitting the surgeon to draw the disk outward posterolaterally while it remains pedicled to the medial attachment. Interestingly, the problem of access was one of the impetuses for combining disk repositioning with a condylar and/or eminential arthroplasty.

Disk Repositioning and Arthroplasty

Several operators have advocated combining an arthroplasty of the condyle or eminence with disk repositioning.[16,32,34–36] Arthroplasty reduces the amount of posterolateral repositioning required and therefore permits repositioning of an atrophic disk (Figure 50-24). The current trend, however, is to avoid removal of any normal articular bone since the postoperative healing phase already involves some loss of bone substance, which may be additive and result in occlusal disturbances. In addition, postoperative bleeding from cut bone surfaces into the joint can result in fibrous adhesions of the disk or fibrous/bony ankylosis of the joint.

A 2 to 4 mm condylar-eminence arthroplasty procedure can be performed with rotary or hand instruments. Hand instruments such as fine chisels are preferable to avoid heat generation (Figure 50-25). Bone files should be used judiciously because, once the compact bony layer is interrupted, the trabeculae of bone can be

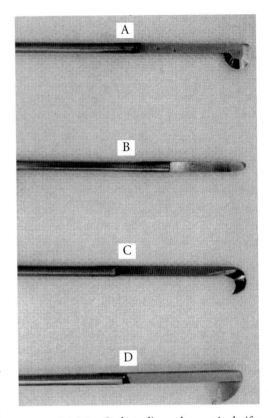

FIGURE **50-19** *Orthopedic arthroscopic knifes (blade handles are not illustrated):* A, *rosette minimeniscus curved;* B, *curved (right or left available);* C, *sickle;* D, *retrograde.*

easily and rapidly removed. A periosteal elevator may be used to burnish sharp edges. Care should be exercised not to exaggerate the arthroplasty in the lateral condylar regions while accessing the medial condylar region. In some cases an arthroplasty of the eminence is essentially a lateral tuberculectomy for access and decompression of the anterior recess of the superior joint space (Figure 50-26).[36,37] Disk repositioning is then performed through the plication or excision technique. The capsule is closed in the customary fashion. Intermaxillary fixation or training elastics are used for 1 to 3 weeks to allow muscular adaptation and dental compensations to occur.

Repair of Perforated Posterior Attachment

Perforations rarely occur within the disk proper but rather within the lateral third of the remodeled posterior attachment.[38,39]

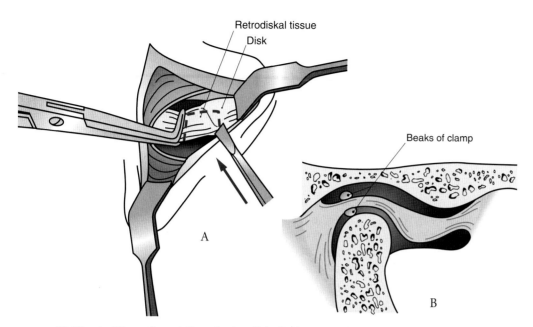

FIGURE 50-20 A, *View of partially reducing disk displacement from above and slightly posterior. Note that when the medial portion of the disk is in the normal position, that portion of the disk may be preserved. Note the path of incision of the crescent-shaped mini-meniscus knife* (broken line). *B, Positioning of the beaks of the DeBakey clamp on retrodiskal tissue.*

condylar movement. This procedure is performed rarely and only in those patients refractory to intra-articular steroid injection, arthrocentesis, or arthroscopy.

Management of Small Perforations When primary closure of a small perforation (1–3 mm) is planned, the atrophic displaced disk is repositioned posteriorly to only a minor degree. If the disk is to be fully repositioned, the margins of the perforation should be excised and the posterior attachment on the posterior edge of the disk approximated to the tympanic portion of the retrodiskal tissue. Anterolateral release of the diskal attachments is usually necessary to mobilize the disk posteriorly. The margins of the perforation are oversewn in a straight-line fashion with a nonresorbable material. The repair procedure is often performed in conjunction with an arthroplasty to reduce sharp bony spurs that may be present.

When the disk is perforated, it may be secondary to a developmental rather than a pathologic process. Condylar overgrowth often occurs in the areas of the perforations; therefore, an arthroplasty is frequently performed in conjunction with the procedure. The repaired remodeled retrodiskal tissue is intended to maintain the shape of the articular surface and to prevent ankylosis. Repair of a perforation without repositioning the disk is successful only if the disk is atrophied and is not an obstruction to

Management of Large Perforations Large perforations are usually grafted after excision of the edges. The disk is not repositioned. In many cases this procedure is a partial diskectomy (Figures 50-27 and 50-

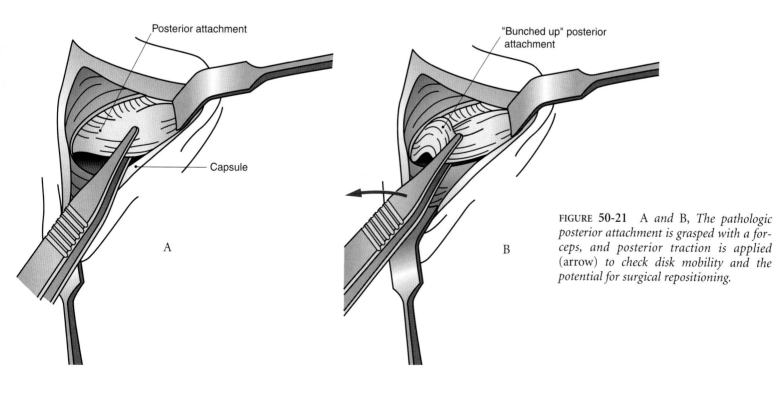

FIGURE 50-21 A *and* B, *The pathologic posterior attachment is grasped with a forceps, and posterior traction is applied* (arrow) *to check disk mobility and the potential for surgical repositioning.*

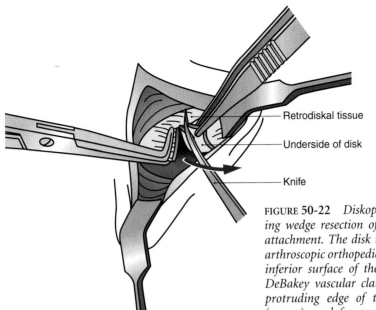

Retrodiskal tissue

Underside of disk

Knife

FIGURE 50-22   *Diskoplasty is performed following wedge resection of the pathologic posterior attachment. The disk is slightly evened, and an arthroscopic orthopedic knife is used to sculpt the inferior surface of the bulge-shaped disk. The DeBakey vascular clamp is in place. Note the protruding edge of the posterior attachment (arrow) used for reapproximation to the disk and lateral capsule.*

postoperative import of ankylosis largely depends on the efficacy of physical therapy, the surface area affected, and ability of synovium to regenerate.

The rationale for electing to perform a partial diskectomy rather than a disk repositioning is based on the belief that those factors responsible for the initial disk displacement are often not adequately controlled or identified and thus eventually cause redisplacement of the disk. Usually osseous remodeling changes have occurred to accommodate the change in disk position. Sprinz described the histologic basis for the partial diskectomy procedure.[42] Surgically created defects within the rabbit meniscus healed uneventfully if the defects

28). The graft material is laid over the perforation and posterior attachment. Autografts (dermal) and homografts have been used (Figure 50-29). The free edges of the graft are sutured to the underlying posterior attachment and disk. Typically, medial sutures are difficult to place. A suturing technique using an S-2 spatula or RD-1 needle is recommended.

Disk-Removal Procedures

Partial Diskectomy   The partial diskectomy procedure is used to correct partial reducing disk displacement.[12,40] The goal of the procedure is to excise the pathologic posterior attachment and that portion of the displaced atrophic/resorbed disk that represents an obstruction or is presumed to be responsible for terminal jolting. The portion of the disk that is properly positioned, usually the medial aspect of the disk, is left in place. This procedure was recently re-described under the term *disk reshaping*.[41] Kondoh and colleagues reported a favorable 5-year outcome in their patients.[41] The absence of portions of the TMJ disk may predispose the joint to areas of fibrous or bony ankylosis. The

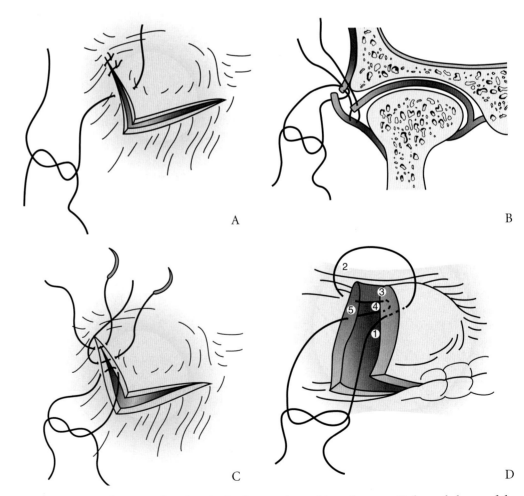

A

B

C

D

FIGURE 50-23   *Disk reapproximation: A, simple posterior and lateral sutures; B, layered closure of the superior and inferior lamina; C, figure-of-8 closure; D, the order of passage of the figure-of-8 suture labeled 1 to 5.*

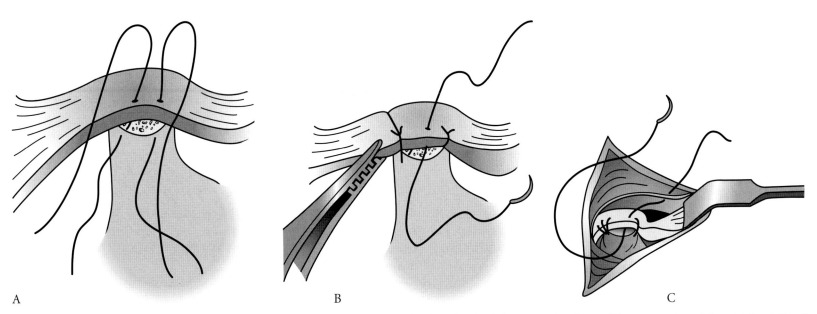

A   B   C

FIGURE **50-24**   *A–C, Disk repositioning with arthroplasty according to Walker and Kalamchi. The disk is sutured to the condyle stump. Adapted from Walker RV and Kalamchi S.[32]*

were close to the vascular periphery. In the rabbit knee meniscus subjected to partial meniscectomy, the replacement tissue appeared to be derived from the synovium of the articular capsule.[43]

Preoperative confirmation of a partial reducing disk using MRI or arthrotomographic images is imperative in deciding whether to perform this procedure. After exposure of the joint spaces, the DeBakey

clamp is inserted to the medial limit of the posterior glenoid fossa. Retrodiskal tissue and displaced portions of the disk are then

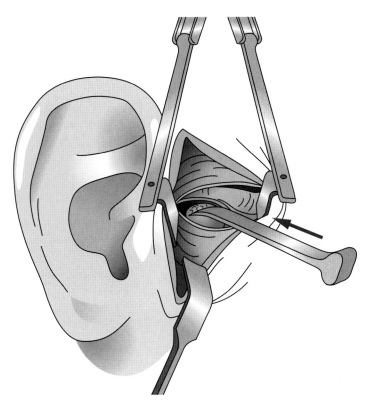

FIGURE **50-25**   *Condylar arthroplasty using an osteotome. An osteophyte has already been excised. The direction of the osteotome (arrow) is indicated in order to skim the condylar surface. Self-retaining and right-angle retractors are in place.*

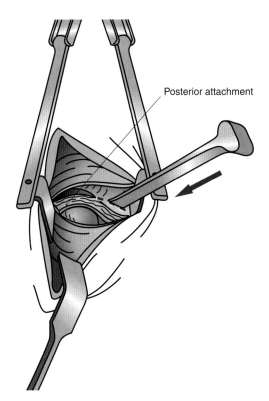

Posterior attachment

FIGURE **50-26**   *Lateral tuberculectomy may be performed to acquire access to the anterior glenoid and eminence regions (broken line indicates bone to be excised and arrow indicates direction of osteotome).*

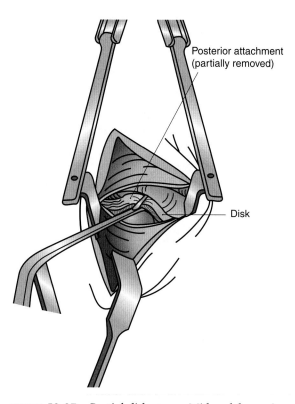

FIGURE **50-27** *Partial diskectomy. Midcondylar region is illustrated. Bulge portions of the disk are excised in a piecemeal fashion using otologic basket forceps. Portions of the excised disk partially excised are hatched exposing the remodeled disk in cross-section.*

removed in a piecemeal fashion using otologic basket forceps (see Figure 50-27). The tissues are removed until the properly positioned disk is noted. The surgeon may then graft the surgical site with an autologous dermal graft. The graft is sutured to a cuff of tissue left at the circumference of the surgically created perforation (see Figures 50-28 and 50-29). In some cases the surgeon may elect not to graft the artificially created perforation. Capsular and skin closures are accomplished in the customary fashion. Following extirpation of the disk portion in question, joint movement is simulated to ensure that there is smooth condylar movement in lateral and anterior planes. The procedure can produce excellent immediate gratification to the patient and improve joint function. However, complete smooth excision of the inferior aspect of the disk is required to prevent reoccurrence. A perforation is sometimes intentionally created to

remove the obstacle. The displaced disk is essentially changed to a displaced meniscus. The perforation is rarely problematic for the patient as it is created anterior to the condyle. The perforation repair described earlier is performed over the head of the condyle; such perforations can lead to chronic pain refractory to steroid injection.

Total Diskectomy Total diskectomy is the procedure in which the remodeled posterior attachment and entire disk are excised. It is the most extensively used and reported surgical procedure, having been applied from as early as the 1900s. Total diskectomy has been used to treat the full gamut of internal derangements, without consideration for the degree of displacement of disk morphology, with generally good to excellent results.[44–50]

Despite the reported successes with diskectomy,[51–53] the more sophisticated diskoplasty techniques supplanted the diskectomy during the 1970s to mid-1980s.[51–53] In the 1980s diskectomy became popular once again following the introduction of implantable biomaterials that were used as disk replacements.

Diskectomy is indicated in those situations for which disk repositioning is not feasible because of disk atrophy, deformation, or severe degeneration. A joint with an atrophied, deformed, or degenerated disk cannot be rejuvenated because some of the associated pathologic changes—collagen fiber reorientation, increased ground substance, presence of elastic fibers in all disk zones, cartilaginous deposits, and increased vascularity—are irreversible. The goal of surgery is to assist the host to adapt to the pathology at hand by removing the physical impediment to movement and the pathologic posterior attachment.

Bowman studied the results of total diskectomy in 52 patients followed over 3 months to 22 years.[12] Thirty of his patients were studied for 4 years or more. Subsequently, in 1986, Eriksson and West-

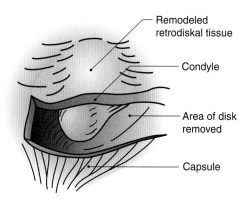

FIGURE **50-28** *For repair of a large perforation, a partial diskectomy is performed first. A portion of the disk and the retrodiskal tissue may be retained.*

esson reported a follow-up (mean 29 yr) on 15 of Bowman's patients.[40] Bowman's observations, which have been corroborated by others,[10,54,55] form the basis of much of the discussion that follows.

Total diskectomy deprives the joint of the posterior attachment and posterior aspect of the remodeled disk. In the diseased state these tissues serve as the shock absorbers for the bony surfaces. The residual "normal" synovium is responsible for the lubrication and nutrition of the articular surfaces. The absence of retrodiskal tissue may interfere with the normal flow and diffusion of synovial fluid.[56] With diskectomy, the surgeon probably transforms a joint into what more appropriately would be described as two bones in close apposition. As a result, several adaptive changes

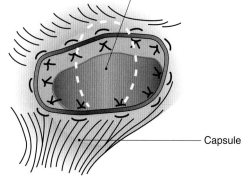

FIGURE **50-29** *A dermal graft covers the surgically created perforation. The edges of the graft overlay the disk, retrodiskal tissue, and lateral capsule to assist in suturing.*

rapidly occur. These changes are reflected in the manner in which the joint functions and how it appears radiographically. Many clinical examples of such a bony arrangement providing the patient with adequate pain-free function may be drawn from the reconstructive literature.

Clinicians often observe the loss or reduction of gliding motion in the joint with nonreducing disk displacement. In this situation the joint behaves principally as a ginglymoid joint. Initially there is limited translational capability. As healing progresses and osseous remodeling occurs, the rotational (hinge) movement becomes minimal and the gliding motion predominates. The patient must rapidly regain mobility through prescribed physical therapy to prevent the development of ankylosis.

Adult cartilage derives its nutrients solely from synovial fluid. The prolonged contact of bony surfaces following meniscectomy may interfere with diffusion of nutrients from the synovial fluid. The decreased diffusion of nutrients to cartilage may result in the eventual resorption of noncalcified cartilage.

After a diskectomy some masticatory muscle and joint tenderness can be expected for a variable period, extending from several weeks to months. The patient at first favors mastication on the operated side. Later, when healing is advanced, mastication is performed on the nonoperated side. An opening deviation of as much as 8 to 9 mm may occur toward the operated side. The deviation appears to be a normal compensatory function secondary to the loss of posterior attachment and synovium, the change in the joint architecture, and areas of fibrous ankylosis. Counteracting the lateral deviation actively or passively causes pain in the operated joint.

Hypermobility of the nonoperated joint may develop or increase after diskectomy. Limitation of mandibular movement on the operated side appears to be responsible for the hypermobility. The

hypermobility may be responsible for awakening symptoms of a quiescent internal derangement. Capsular tightening procedures have been performed in conjunction with diskectomy to reduce condylar hypermobility (Figure 50-30).[57–59] Physical therapy greatly assists the control of the ipsilateral deviation and hence contralateral hypermobility.

Joint crepitations or "snappings" often occur postoperatively. The snappings have been attributed to the condyle rubbing on residual nonextirpated portions of the disk and usually cease after several months. Patients often report an alteration in their bite, although rarely as a major complaint. The thicker the retrodiskal tissue removed, the greater is the anticipated change in occlusion. The sensation of an altered bite usually resolves within a week to several months, with resolution of intra-articular edema, clot retraction, and dental compensations. Occlusal equilibration is rarely indicated.

There is considerable variation in the ability of each patient and joint to adapt to the postdiskectomy state. Individual factors, such as inclination of the eminence, state of preoperative symptoms, loss of molar support, and amount of postoperative remodeling, do not seem to play a substantial role.

Clinicians are often alarmed by the degree of osseous remodeling observed

after a diskectomy. The morphologic and radiologic changes observed in the TMJ concur with those observed in experimental diskectomy.[41,60] After approximately 1 year the morphologic appearance of the condyle and temporal bone appear similar to those observed in a typical arthrodial joint, that is, there are planar (flat) articular surfaces. This is reflected by the manner in which the joint is observed to function. Agerberg and Lundberg described erosion of the articular surfaces and interruptions of the cortical outline on transcranial radiographs.[61] The osseous changes appeared primarily in the lateral and anterior aspects of the joint. The posterior aspects were least affected. Remodeling changes have even been identified in the lateral third of the contralateral (nonoperated) joint.[62,63] However, this was not confirmed by Bowman.[12] Agerberg and Lundberg concluded that the remodeling process stabilized after 2 years.[61] They used the term *remodeling* and not osteoarthrosis to describe the radiographic changes because the osseous changes occurred in the absence of symptoms. The bony changes appear similar to those that are observed longitudinally with chronic disk displacement, suggestive of the same mechanism. The rate of remodeling, however, is accelerated in the postdiskectomy state. A similar observation has been made in the postmeniscectomy human knee joint.[64]

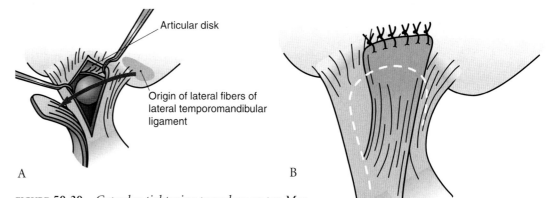

FIGURE 50-30 *Capsular tightening procedure as per Martin and colleagues. The lateral ligament is reflected from the zygomatic arch* (arrow) *(A) and then sutured posterior to its anatomic origin (B). Adapted from Martin BC et al.*[59]

Diskectomy without Replacement Disk extirpation is facilitated when the atrophic disk is severed from its anterior and lateral attachments and then retracted laterally and posteriorly to complete the incisions. This approach permits the surgeon to verify the ability of the disk to be repositioned posteriorly before excision. With severe atrophy of the disk, substantial resistance to posterolateral traction is noted. A hemostatic clamp is positioned across the anterior attachment to serve as a guide plane for the knife, which is used to sever the attachment lateromedially (Figure 50-31). As the posterior attachment demonstrates a variable degree of vascularity changes, the DeBakey bulldog vascular clamp or straight mosquito clamp may be applied here before severing the posterior attachment. Next, a hemostat is used to apply outward traction to the tissue to be extir-

pated (Figure 50-32). A meniscus knife is used to sever the medial attachments. When the remodeled posterior attachment and disk are extirpated, the retrodiskal tissue is electrocauterized to control bleeding. Care is taken not to disrupt the fibrous connective tissue lining of the fossa and condyle. The morphology of the condyle and glenoid fossa often prevent excision in one piece. Incomplete excision of the posterior attachment over the lateral pole of the condyle may account for some cases of failure with diskectomy. After the disk and posterior attachment are excised, the surgeon should verify that there is not a significant diaphragm of irregular posterior attachment tissue that remains laterally around the head of the condyle.

With the disk and posterior attachment removed, mandibular range of motion is simulated by manipulating the mandible in lateral and protrusive excursions. Joint noises, characterized as snappings, may indicate a disk remnant. Disk remnants are usually located on the medial aspect of the joint cavity. The surgeon should remove all disk remnants that appear to impede movement.

Disk Replacements

Autogenous, homologous, and alloplastic replacements for the disk have been used following diskectomy to prevent or reduce intra-articular adhesions, osseous remodeling, and recurrent pain. In addition, the interpositional material was believed to decrease joint noises by dissipating loading forces on the osseous surfaces. The effectiveness of interpositional grafts in reducing adhesions, protecting the articular surfaces, and diminishing pain and postdiskectomy joint noise has not been substantiated. The use of these materials is sporadic and according to operator preference.

The dermal graft may be harvested from the buttock, upper lateral thigh, groin, or the inner aspect of the upper extremity. When the thigh is selected as the donor site, a dermatome may be used to

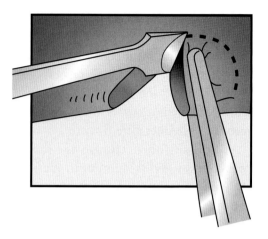

FIGURE 50-32 *An arthroscopic knife severs the posterior attachment* (broken line), *guided by the clamp. The clamp retracts the disk anterolaterally for visibility.*

raise the skin (0.30–0.38 mm) and then the dermis (0.46–0.51 mm). The dermatome width should be set to take the dermal graft 20 to 30% larger than is required to compensate for immediate contraction of the graft. Bleeding in the donor site should then be thoroughly controlled to prevent hematoma formation under the skin, which is replaced over the donor site. Adhesive strips may be applied, or the skin edges may be sutured with 5-0 nylon. The surgical site is then dressed with an occlusive dressing. Postoperatively the donor site should be checked for seroma formation during the first 48 hours.

Alternatively, when size requirements are minimal, the graft may be harvested freehand. An elliptic wedge of epidermis and underlying dermis is harvested. The underlying surface of the dermis must be defatted before being implanted. The defatted graft is trimmed and sutured to the retrodiskal tissue and the anterior and lateral capsular attachments.

The dermal graft is believed to function as a framework for the new disk. Vascularization of the graft is probably derived from the joint periphery.[20,21,28,42] The vascular retrodiskal tissue provides pluripotential cells and synoviocytes to participate in the healing process. Dermal grafts implanted in the primate TMJ were

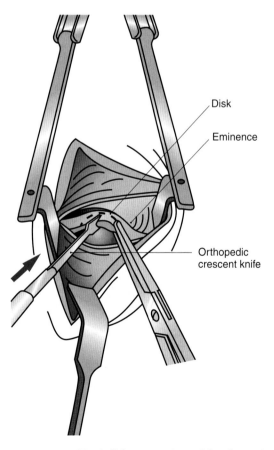

FIGURE 50-31 *Total diskectomy. A straight clamp is inserted onto the anterior attachment. A meniscus knife separates the anterior attachment guided by the clamp. The* arrow *represents the direction of the incision.*

Disk

Eminence

Orthopedic
crescent knife

reported to be viable at postoperative week 36.[65] The collagen and elastic elements of the dermal graft were reported to persist, whereas the dermal appendages atrophied.[66,67] Chao and colleagues reported, however, that the dermal grafts were completely repaired by fibrous tissue.[68]

The temporalis muscle has been used as an interpositional material. The flap may be pedicled in a variety of ways, some of which risk the blood supply owing to torsion of the pedicle. Advantages of this technique over a free graft include its stability, owing to its connection at the base (Figure 50-33), its availability at the same surgical site, and its lack of morbidity.

Feinberg and Larsen described a technique that pedicled the posterior temporalis

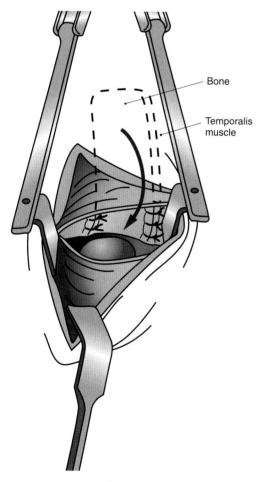

FIGURE **50-33** *Disk replacement using temporalis mucle/fascial graft* (broken line) *pedicled from above the glenoid fossa and rotated inward* (arrow). *Lateral, anterior, and posterior sutures hold the graft in place.*

muscle fibers anteriorly.[69] A 1 cm–wide paddle is developed above the posterior root of the zygomatic arch. The paddle is elevated and rotated anteriorly and inferiorly around the posterior root of the zygomatic arch. The muscle is then sutured to the retrodiskal tissues (Figure 50-34).

Sanders and Buoncristiani described a technique for using the temporalis myofascial flap for interpositional tissue in TMJ reconstruction.[70] The shape and size of the flap is outlined by incising posteriorly near the postglenoid spine of the joint through temporalis fascia muscle and periosteum. This incision is extended superiorly near the temporal line. Subperiosteal dissection elevates the amount of flap needed from the temporal bone. A transverse incision is made at the superior portion anteriorly to create a 3 cm–wide flap. The width should be greater than the anteroposterior coverage desired in the joint to allow flap contraction. An anterior incision is made parallel to the posterior incision. The superior aspect of the anterior incision is carried to bone in this thin area of the temporalis. Inferiorly, as the arch is approached, the muscle thickens; therefore, the dissections are not carried completely through muscle to bone. Blunt dissection is carried inferiorly to a point just medial to the arch to permit adequate mobility of the flap. Branches of the temporal artery found in this area are preserved if possible. The length of the flap is usually 5 cm.

The flap is fully reflected off the bone, and resorbable interrupted sutures are placed in several areas on the edge of the flap through fascia, muscle, and the periosteum to keep the layers from separating. Holes are drilled in the bone of the lateral lip of the glenoid fossa posteriorly and anteriorly before placement of the flap into the joint. One suture is placed through bone anteriorly near the eminence, and a second posterior suture is placed near the postglenoid spine. Two additional sutures hold the medial edge to

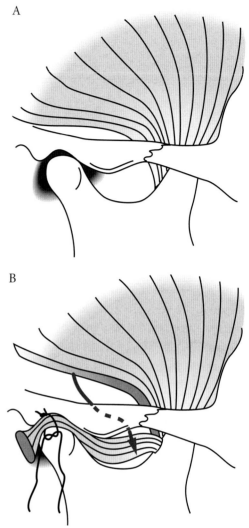

FIGURE **50-34** A *and* B, *Disk replacement using temporalis muscle/fascial graft pedicled anteriorly and rotated anteriorly and inferiorly around (beneath) the posterior root of the zygomatic arch* (arrow). *The graft is sutured to the retrodiskal tissues.*

anterior and posterior medial tissues. These medial sutures are sometimes difficult or impossible to secure, and the sutures through lateral bone are usually adequate to hold the flap in place. A cosmetic temporal defect may result depending on the thickness of tissue harvested.

Autogenous fascia interpositional grafts were described in 1911 for use as interpositional material in gap arthroplasties for ankylosis.[71,72] The attractiveness of this material lies in its resistance to resorption, response to mechanical stress, and biocompatibility.[73–75]

Autogenous conchal cartilage was first used as a disk replacement by Perko, according to Witsenburg and Freihofer.[76] Cartilage harvested from the cavum conchae results in minimal esthetic compromise. The graft can be tailored to fit the condyle or glenoid fossa. Notably, the quality and thickness of the aural cartilage is variable. In some cases an iatrogenic tear in the cartilage may occur during the harvesting process.

The procedure to obtain chondral cartilage as interpositional material for TMJ reconstruction has been described by Hall and Link.[77] A 3 to 4 cm postauricular incision is made on the ear a few millimeters lateral to the auriculocephalic sulcus and is carried through to the perichondrium. The middle division of the posterior auricular artery may be encountered and ligated or cauterized. A careful supraperichondral dissection with a fine dissecting scissors exposes the surface of the cartilage. A scalpel is used to cut through the cartilage in the shape of the desired amount of graft, usually 1.5 by 2.5 cm. It is important not to extend to the rim of the antihelix to avoid permanent deformity of the ear. Subperichondral dissection between the skin of the bowl and cartilage permits the cartilage to be removed without tearing it or perforating the skin. The ear is packed with gauze or other material to maintain the shape of the bowl and to apply pressure to the skin. The pressure pack is maintained for 48 hours.

Timmel and Grundschober and Boyne and Stringer reported the use of lyophilized dura in both the porcine and human TMJ.[78,79] Foreign body reactions were always associated with the material. There was gradual replacement of the material with fibrous connective tissue, although they noted this was not complete by 120 to 130 days. There is increasing resistance among surgeons toward using fresh homologous materials owing to the possibility of transmitting communicable diseases. Relatively recently Creutzfeldt-Jakob disease has been transmitted to a patient who received lyophilized dura.[80]

In the future surgeons may be able to use tissue explants or biocompatible allogeneic collagen sheets as disk replacements.[81]

Alloplastic Materials The requirements for an ideal alloplastic implant are that it be biocompatible, easily secured, adaptable to the variable morphology of the recipient site, and resistant to the compressive and shear forces of the joint. Currently there is no alloplastic material or technique that fulfills all of these requirements. Computeraided design using three-dimensional computed tomography images of the TMJ may bring us closer to defining the ideal characteristics and design of the various components of the TMJ.

Silicone elastomer is a rarely used implantable material. It is exclusively and rarely used in the TMJ for temporary use, but even in this application it is not free of problems. Its sole reputed advantage is that the material does not incorporate into the surrounding tissues. In the past when it was used as a permanent implant, the material's properties were responsible for its migration through stabilizing wires. Gallagher and Wolford suggested that this lack of stability resulted in the loss of as many as one-third of all implants placed following condylectomy.[82] Continued loading of silicone elastomer interpositional implants by the condyle has led to fragmentation and foreign body reactions because of its high coefficient of friction and poor wear characteristics under direct function.[83] Recognition of the limitation of this material led to the abandonment of the permanent silicone implant elastomer and its subsequent rare use as only a temporary implant replacement.

Implants laminated with a composite of polytetrafluoroethylene (PTFE) and aluminum oxide were used extensively in the early and mid-1980s.[84,85] The PTFE material's ultraporosity and wetability permitted rapid ingrowth of fibrous connective tissue to facilitate anchorage of the prosthesis. The polytef surface on which the condyle interfaced was chosen to provide a smooth surface resistant to shear and compressive forces.

In the mid-1980s reports of problems with the PTFE implant began to surface.[84] Patients reported pain, swelling, joint crepitus, and limitation of range of motion resistant to conservative management. In such TMJ reconstructions the PTFE implants that were removed demonstrated perforations, shredding, and displacement. Severe osseous remodeling changes, particularly of the condyle, were reported.[86] Previous reports indicated that the PTFE-carbon implants elicited a severe histiocytic foreign body reaction,[87] similar to what was being reported as happening in the human TMJ. Because of the growing number of failures with PTFE, in 1990 the Food and Drug Administration formally withdrew the PTFE implant from the market and cautioned that patients should be closely followed up for progressive bony changes using radiographic studies at 6-month intervals.

Temporary Implant Insertion To date only the high-performance polymeric silicone implant has been considered for temporary (retrievable) implant insertion. The paddle-shaped implant is inserted with the neck of the paddle rolled over the zygomatic arch (Figure 50-35). Several tacking sutures are placed to the temporalis fascia. Retrieval is planned for 2 to 6 months postoperatively. As the polymeric silicone material is never incorporated into the host, the implant is easily removed at a second operation under local anesthesia. The fibrous connective tissue that encapsulates the implant is left in place to act theoretically as the permanent layer between the condyle and the fossa. However, at the time of retrieval of the temporary implant, the fibrous connective tissue encapsulation may be incomplete. As a result, this procedure has dropped out of favor.

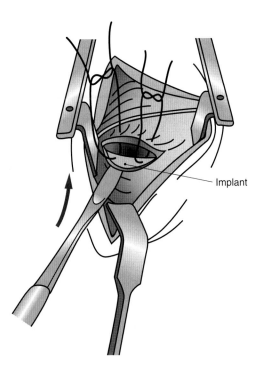

— Implant

FIGURE **50-35** *Temporary (retrievable) polymeric silicone implant inserted. The paddle extension is sutured to the temporalis fascia. A Freer elevator holds the implant in place (arrow) while the sutures are secured.*

Condylectomy

Low condylectomy or simply condylectomy is the procedure that is defined as the removal of the entire condylar process. The procedure used to be performed to increase the joint space to alleviate pressure on nerve endings,[48] but it has largely been abandoned in the surgical repertoire for treatment of internal derangements because of problems of reduced condylar mobility, mandibular deviations, and open bite.

High condylectomy is the removal of only the articular surface of the condyle. The disk is left intact to prevent ankylosis and to promote healing. This contrasted with the radical condylectomy in which the tendon of the lateral pterygoid muscle was released. Only slight mandibular deviation was reported in patients after high condylectomy.[88–94]

When the condylar or eminence articular surfaces appear intact, most clinicians are reluctant to shave the osseous surfaces. Arthroplasty is performed when the rate

and distribution of bone remodeling have resulted in mechanical interferences.

Condylotomy

The condylotomy procedure is an osteotomy performed through the condylar neck. Campbell, one of the originators of the technique, made the observation that symptoms of TM dysfunction disappeared after condylar fractures.[95] This led to his application of the closed condylotomy to patients with TMJ symptoms refractory to nonsurgical therapy. The rationale behind its use in treatment of internal derangements was to produce anteromedial displacement of the condyle to change the condyle-disk-fossa relation, increase joint space, shorten the lateral pterygoid muscle, and alter load forces.[88,96–100]

Originators of the technique performed a closed osteotomy with a Gigli wire saw with the intent of creating an anteromedial fracture dislocation. Intermaxillary fixation was sometimes applied in the immediate postoperative period. Today, when the procedure is performed, the intraoral route used for the vertical mandibular ramus osteotomy is employed.

Postoperative Management

Surgery should reduce painful symptoms to a level that represents little or no concern to the patient. It is important to weigh the contribution of masticatory muscle myalgia to the patient's chief complaint. Although joint surgery can relieve the joint pain, in many cases it may be ineffectual in controlling muscle discomfort. Nonsurgical management of the muscle disorders must continue in many patients after surgery for internal derangements. Joint surgery does not restore the joint to its prepathologic state. The patient should understand that biting force may be reduced and jaw fatigue may become apparent with heavy meals or long conversations. After primary surgery (ie, no previous TMJ surgery), one should strive for the following passive range-of-motion

parameters: maximum interincisal opening of 35 to 40 mm, lateral excursive movements of 4 to 6 mm, and protrusive excursive movements of 4 to 6 mm. However, success should not be measured by the attainment of a finite measurement. A patient's overall success should be measured by the eradication or diminution of the preoperative complaints. Surgery is rarely performed to correct purely functional complaints. Elimination of pain during function is usually the predominant concern for the patient, who is willing to accept some compromise in degree of opening and lateral excursions.

Bite appliances should be used to maintain a stable occlusal relation in the immediate postoperative phase. This is particularly important after disk repositioning. The appliance is frequently adjusted as the edema resolves and disk tissues heal. The patient should be able to return to a normal mechanical diet with minimal dietary restrictions. Restricted foods include such items as French bread, toffee apples, and popcorn. A stable acceptable occlusion should be maintained. Joint sounds may develop or persist, but the asymptomatic sounds should be of minimal concern to the patient.

Postoperative outcomes may be influenced by several factors, including concomitant facial pain from other sources, degenerative bony changes, advanced morphologic changes in the disk, perforation of the posterior attachment, poorly controlled parafunctional habits, malocclusion, psychological overlay, previous TMJ surgery, history of facial nerve paralysis or orofacial numbness, history of infection, or systemic diseases affecting the muscles, ligaments, or bone.[14]

Historically, clinicians emphasized restricted joint function after joint surgery. The clinician must balance his desire to rapidly and actively restore a normal range of motion with the capacity of the joint and facial muscles to adapt. Some latitude must be maintained on the part of the clinician in dealing with a patient's rehabilitation schedule. Care should be exercised in the rehabilitative process of the patient with bilateral joint disease whose operation was unilateral. Diet restrictions are important. Excessive lateral excursive movements to the ipsilateral side may contribute to the exacerbation of contralateral symptoms. There is no cookbook recipe to postoperative management of these patients. Some patients, regardless of the procedure, achieve an acceptable range of motion within 7 to 14 days, with minimal effort on their part. Others need to follow a strict physical therapy regimen. The help of a physical therapist may sometimes be enlisted to regain joint mobility, especially when patient cooperation with a home exercise program is questionable. In general, some light passive opening and protrusion stretching exercises are prescribed four times a day beginning 5 days postoperatively. With disk repair procedures the physical therapy exercises should be more gradual.

Patients should be maintained on a full-liquid to soft diet for the first 2 postoperative weeks. Heat may be applied before and after exercises to improve comfort. Splint therapy is routinely used when a large parafunctional component is present. Some authors advocate using anterior repositioning devices to permit healing of suture sites following disk repositioning. Patients should be encouraged to chew gum after 4 weeks to improve lateral excursive movements.

Complications

Complications may arise immediately (intraoperatively or within 24 hr) or be delayed (> 24 hr).

Transient neuropraxia of the temporal branches of the facial nerve occurs in as many as 20 to 30% of cases. Typically, the injury is of little significance to the patient and resolves within 3 to 6 months. The incidence increases when a separate skin flap is raised.[101] Rarely, the zygomatic

branches and, even more rarely, the entire temporofacial division may be injured. Injury to the chorda tympani from aggressive condylar retraction in the medial aspect of the fossa may occur rarely as well. Neuropraxia of the inferior alveolar and, less commonly, the lingual nerves may result from clamp placement for joint manipulation. Auriculotemporal syndrome (gustatory sweating, Frey's syndrome) has been reported as a result of the dissection of the joint.

Hemorrhage from the retrodiskal tissue may interfere with performance of the disk repair. Temporary control may be obtained with seating of the condyle in the glenoid fossa. Electrocautery, injection of epinephrine, or application of hemostatic agents while maintaining the mandible in the closed position may be necessary.

Infections rarely occur. Microorganisms cultured may originate from the skin or external auditory meatus flora. Auriculitis and external otitis are more likely to occur with the postauricular and endaural approaches. To avoid contamination an ear packing is avoided as it frequently becomes dislodged during surgery. In addition, the ear is not suctioned during surgery. When the wound is closed the external auditory canal is irrigated gently with saline via an 18-gauge angiocatheter.

Postoperatively, joint sounds are a frequent occurrence, regardless of the surgery. The sounds following diskectomy may be the loudest. In some patients the sounds may be obtrusive enough to disturb them. The surgeon should delay reintervention until the patient is reevaluated at 6 to 12 months, as some sounds may become inconsequential to the patient.

Summary

Remarkably good success has been reported with several surgical procedures, which differ in their fundamental approach to the problem and their aggressiveness. Most of these techniques share common denominators: first, a lateral approach to the capsule

and ligament; second, a severing of the posterior attachment-disk attachments to the capsule once the superior joint space is accessed; and, third, a blunt delineation of the joint spaces. Although the capsule and ligament tissues are approximated at the conclusion of the procedure, the patient is encouraged to function on the operated joint. Long before arthroscopic surgery, Toller recognized the importance of mobilizing the condyle-disk-fossa relations to achieve a successful result.[102] He devised the lateral capsular arrangement procedure. It remains to be determined whether disk repositioning, posterior attachment repair, diskectomy, high condylectomy, and even condylotomy derive some or all of their therapeutic benefits through a lateral capsule and ligament release and mobilization of the disk complex. Arthrocentesis and arthroscopic surgical procedures for treatment of the closed lock condition appear to be therapeutic through the same mechanism.[103]

Open surgical approaches to TMJ internal derangements are now relegated to a tertiary line of care following nonsurgical therapy and arthrocentesis/arthroscopy for most conditions. They do, however, have a clear indication for certain mechanical conditions directly attributed to a disk obstruction.

Much of what was written in the previous edition of this chapter has stood the test of time. As we increase our understanding of the pathology, open surgical procedures are being performed for specific well-defined conditions. However, the new TMJ surgeon will never quite appreciate the experience that comes with performance of arthrotomy procedures. Arthroscopy developed as a consequence of this experience. Now, as we regress with progress, arthrocentesis with and without steroid injection, a procedure performed by many surgeons years before the pathology of the joint was even elucidated, has become a mainstay for treatment. This treatment alone has significantly reduced the need to intervene via arthrotomy.

References

1. Annandale T. On displacement of the interarticular cartilage of the lower jaw and its treatment by operation. Lancet 1887;1:411.

2. Warwick R, Williams P, editors. Gray's anatomy. 35th ed. Philadelphia: WB Saunders; 1973. p. 1011–5.

3. Al-Kayat A, Bramley P. A modified pre-auricular approach to the temporomandibular joint and malar arch. Br J Oral Surg 1979–80; 17:91.

4. Blair VP. Operative treatment of ankylosis of the mandible. South Surg Gynecol 1913;26:436.

5. Rongetti JR. Meniscectomy—a new approach to the temporomandibular joint. Arch Otolaryngol 1954; 60:566–72.

6. Lempert J. Improvement of hearing in cases of otosclerosis. Arch Otolaryngol 1938; 28:818–23.

7. Alexander RW, James RB. Postauricular approach for surgery of the temporomandibular articulation. J Oral Surg 1985; 33:346–500.

8. Dolwick MF, Kretzschmar DP. Morbidity associated with the preauricular and perimeatal approaches to the temporo-mandibular joint. J Oral Maxillofac Surg 1982; 40:699–700.

9. Eggleston DJ. The perimeatal exposure of the condyle. J Oral Surg 1978;36:369–71.

10. Husted E. Surgical diseases of the temporomandibular joint. Acta Odontol Scand 1956;14:119.

11. Bowman K. A new operation for luxation in the temporomandibular joint. Acta Chir Scand 1970;136:391.

12. Bowman K. Temporomandibular joint arthrosis and its treatment by extirpation of the disc. Acta Chir Scand 1947;95 Suppl 118:156.

13. American Association of Oral and Maxillofacial Surgeons. 1984 criteria for TMJ meniscus surgery. Chicago: AAOMS; 1984.

14. American Association of Oral and Maxillofacial Surgeons. 1990 standards and criteria of surgical procedures. Chicago: AAOMS; 1990.

15. Wilkes CH. Structural and functional alterations of the temporomandibular joint. Northwest Dent 1978;57:287–94.

16. McCarty WL, Farrar WB. Surgery for internal derangements of temporomandibular joint. J Prosthet Dent 1979;42:191–6.

17. Bronstein SL, Tomasetti BJ, Ryan DE. Internal derangements of the temporomandibular joint: correlation of arthrography with surgical findings. J Oral Surg 1981;39:572–84.

18. Dolwick MF, Riggs RR. Diagnosis and treatment of internal derangements of the temporomandibular joint. Dent Clin North Am 1983;27:561–72.

19. Merrill HG. Historical perspectives and comparisons of TMJ surgery for internal derangements and arthropathy. J Craniomandib Pract 1986;4:74–85.

20. Wallace DW, Laskin DM. Heating of surgical incisions in the disc and retrodiscal tissue of the rabbit temporomandibular joint. J Oral Maxillofac Surg 1986;44:965–71.

21. Zeitler DL, Olson R, Krizan K, Fonseca R. Healing of meniscus surgery in cynomolgus monkey temporomandibular joints. In: Case reports and outlines of scientific sessions. Proceedings of the 66th Annual Meeting of the AAOMS; New York. September 1984. p. 49.

22. Kim JM, Moon MS. The effect of synovectomy upon regeneration of the meniscus in rabbits. Clin Orthop 1979;141:287–94.

23. Heatley FW. The meniscus—can it be repaired? An experimental investigation in rabbits. J Bone Joint Surg 1980;62B:397–402.

24. Arnoczky SP, Warren RF. The microvasculature of the meniscus and its response to injury. An experimental study in the dog. Am J Sports Med 1983;11:131–41.

25. Stingl J. Blood supply of the temporomandibular joint in man. Folia Morphol 1965; 13:20–6.

26. Satko CR, Blaustein DI. Revascularisation of the rabbit temporomandibular joint after surgical intervention: a histologic and microangiographic study. J Oral Maxillofac Surg 1986;44:871–6.

27. Smith D, Walters PJ. An alternative to meniscectomy in repair of tears in the temporomandibular meniscus. In: Case reports and outlines of scientific sessions. Proceedings of the 65th Annual Meeting of the AAOMS; 1983 Sept; Las Vegas. 1983.

28. Marciani RD, White DK, Traurig H, Roth GI. Healing following condylar shave in the monkey temporomandibular joint. J Oral Maxillofac Surg 1988;46: 1071–6.

29. Gabler M, Perry H, Schwartz C, et al. Effect of arthroscopic TMJ surgery on articular disk position. Proceedings of the 18th Annual Session of the AADR [special issue]. J Dent Res 1989;68:310.

30. Montgomery M, Van Sickels J, Harms S, Thrash W. Arthroscopic TMJ surgery. Effects on signs, symptoms and disc position. J Oral Maxillofac Surg 1989; 47:1263.

31. Heffez L, Jordan S. A classification of temporomandibular joint disk morphology. Oral Surg 1988;67:11–9.

32. Walker RV, Kalamchi S. A surgical technique for management of internal derangements of the temporomandibular joint. J Oral Maxillofac Surg 1987; 45:299–305.

33. Saunderson SR, Dolwick MR. Increased hemostasis in temporomandibular joint surgery with the DeBakey clamp. J Oral Maxillofac Surg 1983;91:271–2.

34. Mercuri LG, Campbell HL, Shanaskin RC. Intraarticular meniscus dysfunction surgery—a preliminary report. Oral Surg 1982;54:6.

35. Hall MB. Meniscoplasty of the displaced temporomandibular joint meniscus without violating the inferior joint space. J Oral Maxillofac Surg 1984;42:788–92.

36. Weinberg S, Cousens C. Meniscocondylar plication: a modified operation for surgical repositioning of the ectopic temporomandibular joint meniscus. Oral Surg 1987;63:393–402.

37. Weinberg S. Eminectomy and meniscorrhaphy for internal derangements of the temporomandibular joint. Oral Surg 1984;57:241–9.

38. Blackwood HJJ. Pathology of the temporomandibular joint. J Am Dent Assoc 1969; 79:118–24.

39. Isaacson A, Isberg A, Johansson AS, Larson O. Internal derangement of the temporomandibular joint: radiographic and histologic changes associated with severe pain. J Oral Maxillofac Surg 1986;44:771–8.

40. Eriksson L, Westesson P-L. Diskectomy in the treatment of anterior disk displacement of the temporomandibular joint. A clinical and radiological one-year follow-up study. J Prosthet Dent 1986;55:106–16.

41. Kondoh T, Hamada Y, Kamei K, Seto K. Simple disc reshaping surgery for internal derangement of the temporomandibular joint: 5-year follow-up results. J Oral Maxillofac Surg 2003;61:41–8.

42. Sprinz R. Further observations on the effect of surgery on the meniscus of the mandibular joint in rabbits. Arch Oral Biol 1961; 5:195–201.

43. Walmsley R, Bruce J. The early stages of replacement of the semilunar cartilages of the knee in rabbits after operative excision. J Anat Lond 1937;72:260.

44. Pringle J. Displacement of the mandibular meniscus and its treatment. Br J Surg 1918;6:385–9.

45. Ashhurst A. Recurrent unilateral subluxation of the mandible excision of the interarticular cartilage in cases of snapping jaw. Ann Surg 1921;73:712.

46. von Stapelmohr S. Stir les craquements de l'articulation temporo-maxillaire et les luxations habituelles de la machoire. Acta Chir Scand 1929;65:1.

47. Bellinger DH. Internal derangements of the temporomandibular joint. J Oral Surg 1952;10:47.

48. Agerberg C, Carlsson CE. Behandlingresultat after oprativa ingrepp i kakleder. Sver Tandlak Tidskr 1969;61:1204.

49. Silver CM. Long-term results of meniscectomy of the temporomandibular joint. J Craniomandib Pract 1984;3:46–57.

50. Hall HD. Meniscectomy for damaged discs of the temporomandibular joint. South Med J 1985;78:569–72.

51. Poswillo D. The late effects of mandibular condylectomy. Oral Surg 1972;33:500–12.

52. Hiltebrandt C. Das artikulationgleichgewicht, ein wort ohne inhalt! Zahnarztl Rundschau 1940;43:1592.

53. Staz J. The treatment of disturbances of the temporomandibular joint. J Dent Assoc S Afr 1951;6:314.

54. Kiehn CL, Des Prez JD. Meniscectomy for internal derangement of temporomandibular joint. Br J Plast Surg 1962;15:199–204.

55. Dingman HO, Moorman WC. Meniscectomy in the treatment of lesions of the temporomandibular joint. J Oral Surg 1951;9:214–24.

56. Salter RB, Field P. The effects of continuous compression on living articular cartilage. J Bone Joint Surg 1960;42A:31.

57. Morris J. Chronic incurring temporomaxillary subluxation: surgical consideration of snapping jaws with report of successful operative result. Surg Gynecol Obstet 1930; 50:983.

58. Gordon SD. Surgery of the temporomandibular joint. Am J Surg 1958;95:263–6.

59. Martin BC, Trabue JC, Leech TR. The surgical treatment of chronic derangements of the temporomandibular joint. Plast Reconstr Surg 1957;19:131–6.

60. Dubecq XJ. Recherches morphologiques, physiologiques et cliniques sur le menisque mandibulaire: luxation habituelle et craquements temporomaxillaires. J Med Bordeaux 1937;114:125.

61. Agerberg C, Lundberg M. Changes in the temporomandibular joint after surgical treatment. A radiologic follow-up study. Oral Surg 1971;32:865–75.

62. Prentiss HJ. A preliminary report upon the temporomandibular articulation in the human type. Dent Cosmos 1918;6:505.

63. Vaughan HC. A study of the temporomandibular articulation. J Am Dent Assoc 1943;19:1501.

64. Collins DH, McElligott TF. Sulphate ($^{35}SO_4$) uptake by chondrocytes in relation to histological changes in osteoarthritic human articular cartilage. Ann Rheum Dis 1960; 19:318–30.

65. Tucker MR, Jacoway JR, White RP Jr. Autogenous dermal grafts for repair of temporomandibular joint disc perforations. J Oral Maxillofac Surg 1986;94:781–90.

66. Georgiade N, Altany F, Pickrell K. An experimental and clinical evaluation of autogenous dermal grafts used in the treatment of temporomandibular joint ankylosis. Plast Reconstr Surg 1957;19:321–90.

67. Stewart HM, Hann JR, Detomas DC, et al. Histologic fate of dermal grafts following implantation for temporomandibular joint meniscal perforation: a preliminary study. Oral Surg 1986;62:481–5.

68. Chao LS, Hinton RJ, Babler WJ, et al. Autogenous dermal graft as a TMJ disc replacement in rabbits. Proceedings of the 18th Annual Session of the AADR [special issue]. J Dent Res 1989;68:309.

69. Feinberg SE, Larsen PE. The use of a pedicled temporalis muscle-pericranial flap for replacement of the TMJ disc: preliminary report. J Oral Maxillofac Surg 1989; 47:142–6.

70. Sanders B, Buoncristiani RO. Temporomandibular joint arthrotomy; management of failed cases. Oral Maxillofac Surg Clin North Am 1989;1:944.

71. Lewis D, Davis C. Experimental direct transplantation of tendon and fascia. JAMA 1911;57:540.

72. Narang R, Dixon RA. Temporomandibular joint arthroplasty with fascia lata. Oral Surg 1975;39:45–50.

73. Miller TA. Temporalis fascia grafts for facial and nasal augmentation. Plast Reconstr Surg 1988;81:524–33.

74. Kiqppachne WW, Hunt TK, Jackson DS, et al. Effects of function on grafts of autologous and homologous connective tissue. Surg Forum 1961;12:97–9.

75. Kirppachne WV, Hunt TK, Jackson DS, et al. Studies on the effect of stress on transplants of autologous and homologous connective tissue. Am J Surg 1962; 104:267–72.

76. Witsenburg B, Freihofer HP. Replacement of the pathological temporomandibular disc using autogenous cartilage of the external ear. Int J Oral Surg 1984;13:401–5.

77. Hall HD, Link JJ. Diskectomy alone with ear cartilage in joint reconstruction. Oral Maxillofac Surg Clin North Am 1989;2.

78. Timmel R, Grundschober F. The interposition of Lyodura in operations of ankylosis of the temporomandibular joint. An experimental study using pigs. J Maxillofac Surg 1982; 10:193–9.

79. Boyne PJ, Stringer DE. Allogeneic freeze-dried dura as meniscus replacement in temporomandibular joint surgery [IADR/AADR abstracts]. J Dent Res 1981;64:286.

80. Centers for Disease Control. Possible association between dura mater graft and Creutzfeldt-Jakob disease. MMWR Morb Mortal Wkly Rep 1987;Feb:6.

81. Feinberg SE, McDonell EJ. The use of a collagen sheet as a disc replacement in the rabbit temporomandibular joint. J Oral Maxillofac Surg 1995;53:535–42.

82. Gallagher DM, Wolford LM. Comparison of Silastic and Proplast implants in the temporomandibular joint after condylectomy for osteoarthritis. J Oral Maxillofac Surg 1985;40:627–30.

83. Dolwick M, Aufdemorte Cornelius TB. Histopathologic findings in internal temporomandibular joint derangements. IADR Abstr 1984;265.

84. Turlington EC, Welch SR. Foreign body reaction to Teflon-Proplast fossa implants in TMJ arthroplasty (poster session). In: Annual Scientific Meeting of the AAOMS; New Orleans. Sept 1986.

85. Bronstein SL. Retained alloplastic temporomandibular joint disk implants: a retrospective study. Oral Surg 1987;64:135–45.

86. Wade M, Catto D, Florine B. Assessment of Proplast implants and meniscoplasties as TMJ surgical procedures. In: Case reports and outlines of scientific sessions. In: Proceedings of the 68th Annual Meeting of the AAOMS; New Orleans. 1981 Sept. p. 28.

87. Homsy CA, Kent JN, Hinds EC. Materials for oral implantation—biology and functional criteria. J Am Dent Assoc 1973; 86:817–32.

88. Christensen RW. Chronic unilateral dislocation of the temporomandibular joint treated surgically by a high condylectomy. Oral Surg 1960;13:12–22.

89. James B. The surgical treatment of mandibular joint disorders. Ann R Coll Surg Engl 1911;99:310.

90. Cherry CQ, Frew A. High condylectomy for treatment of arthritis of the temporomandibular joint. J Oral Surg 1971; 35:285–8.

91. Guralnick W, Kaban LB, Merrill RG. TMJ afflictions. N Engl J Med 1975;299:123–9.

92. Dunn MJ, Benza R, Moran D, Sanders J. Temporomandibular joint condylectomy: a technique and postoperative follow-up. Oral Surg 1981;51:363–74.

93. Marciani RD, Ziegler RC. Temporomandibular joint surgery: a review of 51 operations. Oral Surg 1983;56:472–6.

94. Nespeca JA, Griffin JM Temporomandibular

joint surgery—a three year study. J Hawaiian Dent Assoc 1983;14(2):9–10.

95. Campbell W. Clinical and radiological investigations of the mandibular joints. Br J Radiol 1961;38:401–21.

96. Ward TC. Surgery of the mandibular joint. Ann R Coll Surg Engl 1961;18:139.

97. Sada V. Experience in surgical treatment of temporomandibular joint arthrosis by the Ward technique. Trans Cong 1st Int Assoc Oral Surg 1967;265–7.

98. Tasamen A, Lamberg M. Closed condylotomy in the treatment of osteoarthrosis of the temporomandibular joint. Int J Oral Surg 1978;7:1–6.

99. Poswillo D. Surgery of the temporomandibular joint. Oral Rev 1974;6:87–118.

100. Buckerfleld JP. The applied anatomy of closed condylotomy. Br J Oral Surg 1978;15:245–52.

101. Brown RW, Hall AB, Lebowitz MS. Facial nerve injury during TMJ surgery: a comparison of two dissection techniques. In: Case reports and outlines of scientific sessions. J Oral Maxillofac Surg 1985;43:20–3.

102. Toller PA. Temporomandibular capsular rearrangement. Br J Oral Surg 1074;11:207–12.

103. Nitzan DW, Dolwick MF, Heft MW. Arthroscopic lavage and lysis of the temporomandibular joint: a change in perspective. J Oral Maxillofac Surg 1990;48:798–801.

CHAPTER 51

Management of the Patient with End-Stage Temporomandibular Joint Disease

Stephen B. Milam, DDS, PhD

The patient with end-stage temporomandibular joint (TMJ) disease is typically characterized by a protracted history of multiple therapeutic interventions, often including multiple TMJ surgeries. The patient with end-stage TMJ disease commonly suffers from unrelenting pain and severe limitation of jaw movement. In addition, some patients with end-stage TMJ disease may also endure facial deformities, sensory or motor abnormalities, dysfunctional malocclusions, and upper airway compromise. The suffering of these unfortunate individuals is often compounded by their compromised position in managed health care systems and mounting personal debt. Understandably, virtually all patients with end-stage TMJ disease exhibit signs and symptoms of depression, often straining relationships with significant others.

Several factors likely contribute to the evolution of end-stage TMJ disease. The progression of some TMJ disorders may be influenced by variables such as sex (ie, mediated by sex hormones such as estrogen and prolactin), genetic backdrop (eg, predisposition to rheumatoid arthritis is associated with some estrogen receptor polymorphisms), nutritional status, age, and psychological stress (eg, plasma levels of nerve growth factor, an endogenous

peptide implicated in the genesis of some muscular and neurogenic pains, are elevated in humans following psychological stress). In addition, it is clear that many patients with end-stage TMJ disease also suffer from iatrogenic injury.

Currently the prognosis for recovery of the patient with end-stage TMJ disease is extremely poor. Clearly, the best strategy is prevention. How can risks for developing end-stage TMJ disease be reduced?

Basic Elements of Care

Effective management of any TMJ disorder is primarily dependent on three elements of care: an accurate diagnosis, careful patient selection, and effective perioperative patient management (Table 51-1).

An accurate assessment of a patient's condition(s) is an absolute requirement for the selection of an effective treatment. The experienced clinician recognizes that many painful conditions of the head and neck region can mimic a TMJ disorder. For example, it is well known that some masticatory myalgias can produce pain of various qualities (ie, ranging from aching sensations to "stabbing" or "throbbing" pains) that may be felt in the area of one or both TMJs.[1] Furthermore, some of these painful conditions, such as the masticatory myalgias, may also be associated with

restricted jaw movement and may be exacerbated by such movement. Similarities between many painful head and neck disorders with respect to clinical presentation can pose a significant challenge for the clinician to derive an accurate diagnosis. Failure to do so can lead to the initiation of an ineffective and perhaps damaging treatment that may ultimately contribute to clinical anomalies that characterize end-stage TMJ disease.

Proper patient selection is important since, although appropriate surgical objectives and proper technique are obviously significant determinants of treatment outcome, a patient's commitment and ability to perform critical perioperative tasks (eg, regular exercises, nutritional maintenance, abstinence from unhealthy habits) may be the single most important determinant of the outcome of surgical treatment of a TMJ disorder. Therefore, the clinician must accurately assess the patient's willingness

Table 51-1 Basic Elements of Surgical Care
Accurate diagnosis
Careful patient selection
Effective perioperative management
Pain management
Restoration of jaw movement

and ability to comply with an often-difficult perioperative regimen. Depending on the condition, patients who are unwilling or unable to comply with a demanding but essential perioperative regimen may not be viable candidates for the indicated surgery. Failure to recognize this limitation preoperatively often leads to a significantly compromised surgical outcome.

It is also important to delineate realistic objectives of therapy, including surgery, and to recognize the limitations of each approach. Experienced surgeons often reliably achieve TMJ surgical objectives, including excision of neoplastic or diseased tissues, relief of physical obstructions to joint movement, and restoration of important anatomic relationships. However, even the most experienced surgeon may not reliably achieve some treatment objectives such as relief of pain. Clinicians may sometimes recommend treatment by default (eg, other approaches have failed to provide adequate pain relief) without clearly delineated and reliably achieved treatment objectives. Such an approach has significant potential for worsening the patient's overall condition by iatrogenic injury. All recommended treatments should be based on an accurate diagnosis, and a plan based on well-delineated achievable treatment objectives.

Perioperative Management

Patients with end-stage TMJ disease suffer primarily from persistent pain and restricted jaw function. Recent evidence suggests that some persistent pain may result from neuroplastic changes evoked in nociceptive pathways of the central nervous system (CNS) by intense stimulation or nerve injury. There is also strong evidence that these changes may be prevented or significantly obtunded by preemptive techniques that reduce or block CNS responses to surgical stimulation (ie, preemptive analgesia). Two primary goals of perioperative management of the operated TMJ patient are pain control (ie, using

preemptive analgesia techniques) and establishment and maintenance of acceptable joint movements (ie, mandibular range of motion). These goals are not exclusive. Patients who suffer from temporomandibular pain are often noncompliant with recommended jaw exercises that must be performed to achieve and maintain physiologic joint movements.

Pain-Control Strategies

With few exceptions, pain is the primary chief complaint of patients with TMJ disease and is often the principal limiting factor in the patient's willingness to comply with physical therapy designed to restore jaw movements. In addition, patients suffering from persistent pain often exhibit clinical signs of depression. They are often socially withdrawn, and interpersonal relationships with significant others may become compromised. Therefore, effective pain control strategies must be identified, preferably in the preoperative period, and implemented aggressively to ensure an optimum surgical outcome and to sustain an acceptable quality of life for the patient (Table 51-2).

Preemptive Analgesia

Effective postsurgical pain control begins in the operating room. It is now recognized that methods that limit CNS neuronal activation by surgical stimulation may significantly reduce pain in the postsurgical period and may also reduce the liability for the development of some persistent pains. The term *preemptive analgesia* is used to describe methods that apparently reduce postsurgical pain by protecting the CNS from surgical stimulation. The concept is based on recent observations that collectively indicate that nociceptive processing is highly dynamic. Nociception and subsequent pathway sensitization likely involves de novo protein synthesis and even establishment of novel connections by neurons in the affected pathway.[2–4] The old view that nociceptive

pathways are merely static conductors of neural signals generated by noxious stimuli appears to be invalid. We now know that gene transcription is induced in stimulated neuronal populations.[5,6] Some neuropeptides that are translated from these genes may facilitate future neural activities by receptive field expansion or by facilitation of specific interneuronal interactions. The term *neuroplasticity* is often used to refer to the dynamic state of stimulated neural pathways. These, and perhaps other more ominous changes (ie, neuronal death from excessive stimulation), may be fundamental to the development of some chronic pain states. Fortunately, these CNS responses may be significantly attenuated by preemptive analgesic techniques.[3,7]

Table 51-2   Pain Management
Perioperative
Preemptive analgesic techniques
• Regional anesthesia
• Opioid-based general anesthesia
• Ketamine
• Ketorolac
Immediate postsurgical period
• Regional anesthesia
• Opioids (patient controlled analgesia or scheduled regimens)
• Ketorolac
Long term
Pharmacologic
• Tricyclic antidepressant (eg, amitripty-line)
• Opioids (scheduled dosing)
• GABAergics (eg, baclofen, gabapentin)
• Nonopioid analgesics (for pain associated with inflammation)
Nonpharmacologic
• Regular exercise
• Acupuncture
• Biofeedback
• Transcutaneous electrical nerve stimulation
• Heat/cold packs
GABA = γ-aminobutyric acid.

Techniques From animal and clinical studies there is evidence that protracted neural responses to painful stimuli can be modified or prevented by the following: (1) neural blockade with local anesthetics,[8–10] (2) administration of opioids,[11–15] (3) administration of N-methyl-D-aspartate receptor antagonists (eg, MK801, ketamine, dextrophan),[16–18] or (4) administration of ketorolac, a peripherally and centrally acting nonopioid analgesic.[19–21] These agents must be administered *prior* to noxious stimulation to prevent CNS changes that may be related to the development of postsurgical pain, and perhaps persistent pain. It is interesting to note that a general anesthetic state does not prevent neuroplastic changes induced by surgical stimulation, unless the general anesthetic technique employs high-dose opioids or ketamine. Neural impulses from surgical stimulation apparently reach the CNS evoking sensitization despite the fact that overt signs of surgical stimulation (ie, patient movement, heart rate, systemic blood pressure) are blocked by general anesthesia. This stimulus-dependent neural sensitization, characterized by receptive field expansion and the "wind-up" phenomenon,[2,3] has been attributed to postsurgical hyperesthesia and pain.

When regional anesthesia is employed as an adjunct to general anesthesia, there is strong evidence that postoperative pain is significantly reduced, consistent with current models of central sensitization and neuroplasticity. However, to ensure that neural activities induced by surgical stimulation are fully blocked, the surgeon must administer regional anesthesia *prior* to surgical stimulation. If necessary during long procedures, the surgeon should reanesthetize the operative field and not rely solely on a general anesthetic state for CNS protection.

Jebeles and colleagues studied the effects of preemptive regional anesthesia on postsurgical discomfort associated with tonsillectomy and adenoidectomy performed under general anesthesia.[22] Twenty-two children were given either bupivacaine or saline infiltrations in the peritonsillar regions prior to surgical stimulation. For this study postsurgical analgesics were standardized for all subjects and postsurgical pain was assessed over a 10-day period by three dependent measures (ie, constant pain, pain evoked by swallowing a standard volume of water, and the time required to drink 100 mL of water based on the assumption that the rate-limiting factor for this activity is throat pain). All three dependent measures confirmed that subjects given bupivacaine regional anesthesia with general anesthesia experienced significantly less pain over a 10-day postsurgical period compared with the saline-injected group.[22] Other studies have provided similar evidence that regional anesthesia, provided prior to surgical stimulation, can significantly reduce pain following craniotomy and bone harvesting from the iliac crest.[23,24] To date no published papers have documented the efficacy of preemptive regional anesthesia on postoperative pain, or on the subsequent development of chronic pain, in the operated patient with TMJ disease. Nevertheless, existing evidence strongly suggests that the use of regional anesthesia as an adjunct to general anesthesia will significantly reduce postsurgical pain in such a patient.

Opioids administered *prior* to surgical stimulation may also reduce postsurgical hyperesthesia believed to be due to central sensitization. For example, isoflurane or isoflurane and nitrous oxide, administered in a concentration sufficient to suppress cardiovascular responses to surgical stimuli (ie, minimum alveolar concentration that blocks adrenergic responses [MACBAR]), do not inhibit formalin-induced hyperesthesia.[25] Formalin injected intradermally provides a potent noxious stimulus that results initially in a volley of neural activity that sensitizes central nociceptive neurons in the pathway. This observation reinforces previous studies indicating that general anesthesia alone does not offer protection against central sensitization. However, morphine administered *prior* to formalin injection significantly reduces postinjection hyperesthesia in this model.[25] In fact, a significant reduction in formalin-induced hyperesthesia was also observed even if morphine was reversed by naloxone shortly after the formalin injection was administered, indicating that even a brief exposure to an opioid prior to noxious stimulation is sufficient to prevent or significantly reduce stimulation-induced hyperesthesia.[25] Likewise, alfentanil reduces capsaicin-induced hyperalgesia in human subjects, but only if this agent is administered prior to capsaicin administration.[26] Capsaicin is a vanilloid extracted from peppers that is known to selectively stimulate C-fiber neurons expressing the vanilloid receptor (VR-1). Stimulation of C-fiber neurons by capsaicin administration produces receptive field expansion and hyperesthesia by mechanisms that involve central sensitization.[3] Notably, alfentanil did not effectively reduce pain scores, flare response, or secondary hyperalgesia when administered *after* an intradermal injection of capsaicin in these human studies.[26] These studies highlight the fact that, as is apparent for regional anesthesia, opioids are only optimally effective as modulators of central sensitization and subsequent hyperalgesia if they are administered prior to surgical stimulation.

Ketorolac is a peripherally and centrally acting nonopioid analgesic that is also an effective preemptive analgesic.[19–21] In a randomized double-blind trial involving 48 patients undergoing ankle fracture surgery, ketorolac 30 mg administered prior to surgical stimulation significantly reduced postsurgical pain relative to the same amount of ketorolac administered after stimulation.[20]

Preemptive Analgesia and Persistent Pain
Some preemptive analgesia techniques significantly reduce postsurgical pain. There is also evidence that preemptive analgesia may provide some protection against the development of some chronic pain states. Bach and colleagues reported one of the few investigations designed to assess the impact of preemptive analgesia on the evolution of a chronic pain state.[27] In this clinical study 25 elderly patients scheduled for a below-the-knee amputation received either treatment with epidural bupivacaine and/or morphine to produce a pain-free state for 3 days prior to surgery, or no pretreatment (control group). All patients subsequently underwent amputation under spinal anesthesia. After 6 months, none of the patients assigned to the presurgery analgesia group experienced phantom limb pain.[27] However, 38% of the subjects who did not receive the presurgical pain treatment had phantom limb pain at the 6-month postamputation period. Furthermore, 27% of these subjects experienced persistent phantom limb pain at the 1-year follow-up period.[27]

Recommendations   It is recommended that, when feasible, an opioid-based or opioid-supplemented general anesthetic technique be employed for TMJ surgery. Also, regional anesthetic should be administered to cover the entire surgical field *prior* to surgical stimulation. During long procedures, the surgical field should be reanesthetized periodically. If there are no contraindications (eg, bleeding concerns), some consideration can also be given to ketorolac administration (ie, 0.5 mg/kg or 30 mg IV) *prior* to surgical stimulation. Finally, postoperative pain should also be well controlled with a combination of regional anesthesia and opioid or ketorolac analgesia. These regimens may significantly reduce postsurgical pain facilitating a shortened convalescence, and may also protect the patient from

CNS responses to surgical stimulation that may be involved in the genesis of some chronic pain states.

Postsurgical Pain Management and Pharmacologic Approaches

Effective pain management permits immediate postsurgery physical therapy by improving patient compliance, which is crucial to the establishment and maintenance of an acceptable mandibular range of motion. Based on the studies cited above, it is reasonable to assume that a continuation of effective pain control beyond the intraoperative period may offer some additional benefits in the prevention of some protracted (ie, chronic) pain states, although this remains a subject for future studies. The most common methods of postsurgical pain management incorporate a combination of opioid and nonopioid analgesics. In some instances other medications (eg, tricyclic antidepressants [TCAs], γ-aminobutyric acid [GABA]-ergics) may also offer significant pain relief for the patient with end-stage TMJ disease. Finally, some patients may benefit from nonpharmacologic approaches (eg, walking 30 min/d for 6d/wk, acupuncture, cold or hot pack applications, hypnosis, meditation, progressive relaxation, biofeedback).that can be used as a substitute for (eg, the medication-intolerant patient) or in tandem with pharmacologic approaches.

Nonopioid Analgesics   Nonopioid analgesics, including salicylates (eg, acetylsalicylic acid), *p*-aminophenols (eg, acetaminophen), arylacetic acids (eg, indomethacin), arylpropionic acids (eg, ibuprofen), and keto-enolic acids (eg, piroxicam), are commonly used to manage pain that is associated with inflammation. Nonopioid analgesics block the synthesis of prostaglandins (PGs) from arachidonic acid by the action of cyclooxygenases (COXs) (Figure 51-1). Some PGs (eg, PGE$_2$) are known to sensitize peripheral nociceptors contributing to the development of hyperalgesia.

Two isoforms of COX are known (COX-1 and COX-2). COX-1 is constantly expressed in most tissues to provide a steady production of PGs that are required for many normal cellular functions.[28–30] On the other hand, COX-2 is an inducible COX. It is not typically expressed under normal conditions, but, rather, it is synthesized in response to injury accounting for the increased production of PGs associated with inflammation.[28,31,32] Studies indicate that some PGs (eg, PGE$_2$) sensitize sensory neurons to stimulation by other biochemicals, including bradykinin and histamine.[33] It is generally felt that PGs play an important role in the genesis of inflammatory pain via this mechanism. PGs, specifically PGE$_2$, have been detected in lavage fluid or synovial fluid samples obtained from symptomatic human TMJs in concentrations ranging from 0.1 to 3.5 ng/mL.[34,35] These concentrations are above the dissociation constants for prostanoid receptors (ie, the concentration required for receptor binding) and are therefore physiologic. Nonopioid analgesics are believed to exert their primary effects by inhibiting the synthesis of PGs in peripheral tissues, including the TMJ.

Some nonopioid analgesics may produce analgesia by central mechanisms, perhaps by suppressing COX activity in CNS neurons or adjacent glial cells. An intrathecal administration of acetylsalicylate produced analgesia in humans suffering from late-stage cancer pain.[36] Furthermore, central injections of nonopioid analgesics produce antinociception in several animal models of pain.[37,38] Therefore, it appears that some nonopioid analgesics may relieve some types of pain by both central and peripheral mechanisms.

Side Effects   As noted above, it is currently believed that basal levels of PGs are generated under normal circumstances in tissues by the action of COX-1.[30] PGs regulate important physiologic processes in several tissues, including gastric

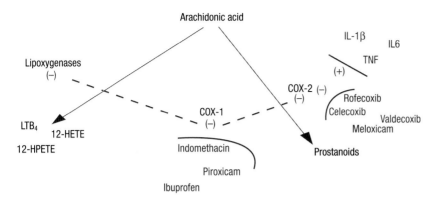

FIGURE 51-1 *Proinflammatory molecules derived from arachidonic acid. Proinflammatory prostanoids and leukotrienes (LTs) are derived from arachidonic acid liberated from cell membrane phospholipids by phospholipases. Prostanoids are generated by the actions of cyclooxygenases (COX-1 and COX-2). COX-2 is an inducible form that is synthesized by cells stimulated by molecules produced after injury (eg, interleukin-1β [IL-1β], tumor necrosis factor [TNF], IL-6). Leukotrienes are generated by the actions of lipoxygenases. 12-hydroxyeicosatetraenoic acid (12-HETE) and 12-hydroperoxyeicosatetraenoic acid (12-HPETE) may be capable of stimulating nociceptors by direct action (ie, by binding vanilloid receptor 1; see text). Selective COX-2 inhibitors (eg, rofecoxib, celecoxib, meloxicam, and valdecoxib) block the activity of COX-2, thereby reducing prostanoid synthesis under inflammatory conditions. Nonselective COX inhibitors (eg, indomethacin, piroxicam, and ibuprofen) inhibit both COX-1 and COX-2 activities. At higher doses these drugs may also inhibit lipoxygenases.*

mucosa, kidney, bone, and cartilage.[39–44] For example, in the stomach nonopioid analgesic suppression of PG synthesis results in an increase in gastric acid secretion since PGs inhibit this process.[39] Also, the secretion of gastric mucus that provides a protective coating of the stomach lining is inhibited by some nonopioid analgesics. These combined effects, in susceptible individuals, can produce gastrointestinal irritation and bleeding. In fact, chronic users of nonopioid analgesics have a threefold greater risk of serious gastrointestinal complications compared with the risk in nonusers.[45]

Selective COX-2 Inhibitors

Relatively selective COX-2 inhibitors have been introduced for clinical use in an attempt to reduce systemic side effects associated with chronic nonopioid analgesic consumption. Four relatively selective COX-2 inhibitors are available in the United States at the present time: celecoxib, meloxicam, rofecoxib, and valdecoxib. There has been a general misperception that these agents provide superior analgesia relative to the traditional nonselective COX inhibitors. However, clinical trials have generally not supported this notion. For example, ibuprofen provides superior analgesia to celecoxib following third molar extraction with a similar side-effect profile.[46] Therefore, the primary indication for the use of relatively selective COX-2 inhibitors appears to be the control of inflammatory pain in patients with gastrointestinal or renal disorders. However, it should be noted that these agents do not prevent serious gastrointestinal or renal side effects, although the incidence of their occurrence may be relatively low.

Leukotrienes: a Target for Future Therapies

Leukotrienes are generated from arachidonic acid by the action of lipoxygenases. Leukotrienes (LTs), particularly LTB₄, are proinflammatory molecules that promote leukocyte chemotaxis, sensitize nociceptors, stimulate free radical production, and promote bone and cartilage destruction. LTB₄ has been detected in lavage fluids obtained from symptomatic human TMJs.[34]

In addition to well-documented effects on bone and cartilage catabolism, some lipoxygenase products may also play an important role in nociception; they appear to be endogenous analogs of capsaicin.[47,48] As noted above, the pepper extract capsaicin selectively stimulates nociceptors. The tertiary structures of 12-hydroxyeicosatetraenoic acid and 12-hydroperoxyeicosatetraenoic acid are very similar to that of capsaicin.[47] Furthermore, these lipoxygenase products are capable of stimulating nociceptors in a concentration-dependent fashion. This evoked activity can be inhibited by antagonists for the primary capsaicin receptor VR-1.[47] These findings indicate that some lipoxygenase products are capable of directly stimulating nociceptors. By this mechanism, these arachidonic acid products could contribute to inflammatory pain. Therefore, lipoxygenase inhibitors may have significant analgesic properties, in addition to potential inhibitory effects on LT-mediated bone and cartilage catabolism.

Recommendations

At the present time the efficacies of nonopioid analgesics employed to manage pain in the patient with end-stage TMJ disease have not been determined. Some nonopioid analgesics to treat arthritic pain are effective. Therefore, one may expect to see beneficial responses to nonopioid analgesics when a significant inflammatory component underlying reported TMJ pain is suspected.

Nonopioid analgesics vary considerably in relative potency. All clinically available nonopioid analgesics suppress PG synthesis to a variable extent (ie, they differ in relative potencies for COX-1 and COX-2 inhibition) in either peripheral or CNS tissues. Some nonopioid analgesics also block LT synthesis in the recommended dose range. LTs, as noted in the previous discussion, can promote potentially detrimental effects in inflamed tissues, and some lipoxygenase products may be endogenous algesics. At the present time specific LT inhibitors are not available for clinical use, although compounds have been identified that hold future promise.[49] Therefore, nonopioid analgesics that inhibit both PG and LT pathways may be preferred.

All nonopioid analgesics achieve synovial fluid concentrations that are above their median effective dose (ED_{50}) following the administration of their recommended oral dose. Therefore, it is difficult to favor one nonopioid analgesic over another in this respect.

Nonopioid analgesics may be indicated when an inflammatory component of the patient's condition is suspected (ie, joint effusion, acute localized pain, local swelling, or acute posterior open bite). Clearly, nonopioid analgesics may offer significant benefits in the postsurgical period, perhaps used in combination with opioids. Given well-documented potentially serious side effects, nonopioid analgesics should be discontinued if a brief trial fails to provide significant clinical benefit or if the patient experiences side effects. If benefits are not apparent after a reasonable trial period (ie, 7–10 d) or if side effects are observed, the drug should be withdrawn. If the nonopioid is found to be effective, it can be continued. However, patients receiving nonopioid analgesics should be monitored on a regular basis for drug side effects. Furthermore, periodic tapered withdrawal trials should be performed to reassess the need for the drug.

Opioids   Opioids elicit their physiologic effects via interactions with one or more subclasses of opioid receptors located in the CNS and in peripheral tissues. Three classes of opioid receptor are known to exist, designated μ-opioid receptor (MOR), δ-opioid receptor (DOR), and κ-opioid receptor (KOR). In addition, at least two subclasses of MOR and DOR receptors and four subclasses of the KOR receptor have been identified.[50,51] Opioids

affect neurons and some non-neural cells such as leukocytes by several mechanisms, including inhibition of cyclic adenosine monophosphate (cAMP) formation, activation of G_o or $G_{i/o}$ proteins, or altered Ca^{++} or K^+ translocation.[52–54] Increasing evidence suggests that analgesia may be produced by opioid effects in the CNS, spinal cord, or peripheral tissues. Some types of pain may be refractory to opioid effects. For example, it is generally believed that opioids are ineffective for the relief of neurogenic pain, although there is recent evidence to the contrary.[55]

In animal models of TMJ injury, activation of neurons in multiple areas of trigeminal nuclei can be demonstrated by expression of Fos.[56] Fos is a transcription factor that regulates the expression of specific genes in all cells including neurons. In neurons Fos expression is used as a measurement of activation and is typically determined using standard immunohistochemical approaches employing monospecific antibodies directed against Fos. Systemically administered morphine significantly reduces Fos expression in the trigeminal nucleus following acute TMJ stimulation in the rat.[56]

Peripheral Mechanisms of Opioid Analgesia
For many years clinicians have been aware of the analgesic effects of peripherally administered opioids. Chase reported that local application of small amounts of morphine was effective in relieving toothache.[57] Hargreaves and colleagues have recently validated this early observation.[58] In this latter study endodontic patients diagnosed with acute dental infection were administered morphine (0.4 mg), lidocaine, or saline by intraligamentous injection in a randomized double-blinded fashion. These investigators found that at one-tenth the systemic dose required to relieve dental pain, morphine administered locally (ie, by intraligamentous injection) produced significant pain relief. This supports the belief that opioids can produce

relief of some types of pain by actions in peripheral tissues.

There is additional support for the concept that opioids may provide relief of TMJ pain by peripheral action. In the rat TMJ MOR has been detected at nerve terminals supplying both anterior and posterior synovial tissues, as well as other cell types, presumed to be resident macrophages, mast cells, and endothelial cells.[59] In other articular joints local injections of opioids can suppress the release of neuropeptides from peripheral nerve terminals supplying the injected joint.[60] Some neuropeptides, such as substance P and calcitonin gene–related peptide, are proinflammatory and have been detected in nerve terminals supplying the TMJ and in synovial fluid samples recovered from symptomatic TMJs.[61–64] Released of these neuropeptides into articular tissues can generate a variety of inflammatory responses that may underlie joint pain and disease. The term *neurogenic inflammation* is used to describe this phenomenon. It is speculated that the intra-articular administration of an opioid into the TMJ could inhibit neurogenic inflammation by blocking the release of proinflammatory neuropeptides from stimulated nerve terminals located in the TMJ. Opioids employed in this fashion could be effective "anti-inflammatory" agents if this model is correct.

Despite clinical and animal studies that suggest that peripherally administered opioids produce analgesic responses, studies examining the effects of intra-articular morphine on TMJ pain remain equivocal.[65–67] In the largest of the three published studies to date, 53 patients diagnosed with unilateral TMJ arthralgia or osteoarthritis were assigned to one of three groups receiving a single intra-articular injection of 1 mg morphine sulfate, 0.1 mg morphine sulfate, or saline.[67] The dependent measures employed in this study included pain at rest, assessed by a standard visual analog scale, pain at maximum opening, pressure pain threshold, and mandibular range of motion measurements (ie, maximum vertical opening, lateral and protrusive movements). Significant group differences in pain at maximum opening were not observed until 4 days after the injection in subjects given the 0.1 mg morphine dose. Subjects reported less pain at maximum opening indicating that intraarticular morphine lessened mechanical allodynia (ie, pain with non-noxious mechanical stimulation or movement). However, no dose response was observed (ie, the higher dose of morphine did not produce a similar or greater effect), and pain at rest was not affected by intraarticular morphine. The pressure pain threshold was significantly elevated (ie, more pressure required to produce pain) at the 1-week follow-up period in patients given the 0.1 mg dose of morphine.

Several factors may govern responses to locally administered opioids. Opioids do not produce measurable effects when administered into normal peripheral tissues.[68–70] However, when injected into inflamed peripheral tissues, opioids may reduce pain,[58,71] inhibit plasma extravasation and edema,[72,73] and alter leukocyte function.[74,75] Animal studies have demonstrated potent effects of opioids injected into inflamed tissues.[76] For example, PG-induced hyperalgesia is suppressed by nanomolar concentrations of opioids.[76] The primary mechanism(s) by which opioids exert their influence in inflamed peripheral tissues is unknown. From previous studies of opioid receptor distribution in the TMJ, it appears that a variety of cells, including neurons, leukocytes, synoviocytes, and endothelial cells, can respond to peripherally administered opioids.[59] Therefore, it is likely that opioids exert their effects on both neural and non-neural cell populations in inflamed tissue. It is also possible that some inflammatory molecules (eg, bradykinin, PGs) may "sensitize" opioid receptors to opioid stimulation.

Factors Affecting Response to Peripheral and Central Opioids Responses to peripherally administered opioids may be sex dependent. Cai and colleagues examined jaw muscle electromyographic activity in the rat following an injection of glutamate, an algesic amino acid, into the TMJ.[77] Peripherally applied morphine significantly reduced glutamate-evoked muscle activity in male Sprague-Dawley rats but not when administered to female animals. This observation is consistent with sex-based differences in neural responses following systemically administered opioids. Brainstem neural responses to intense noxious stimulation of the TMJ are obtunded by a prestimulation systemic administration of morphine in male rats to a much greater extent than is observed in female animals.[5] Morphine is predominantly a MOR agonist. Interestingly, a KOR agonist was found to attenuate brainstem responses to TMJ stimulation in the female to a greater extent than in the male.[5] These observations indicate that sex hormones may differentially regulate the expression of different opioid receptor types, and that males and females may therefore differ significantly in responses to different opioids (eg, MOR agonists vs KOR agonists). Further research is clearly needed in this area to confirm sex-based differences in opioid receptor expression in the CNS and in peripheral tissues such as the TMJ.

Another factor that may govern responsiveness to opioids is the genetic backdrop of the patient. Polymorphisms of opioid receptor genes could account for some of the variability observed in response to opioids. Polymorphisms are subtle gene mutations that result in the production of a protein, in this case an opioid receptor that differs from native protein with respect to structure and function. Some gene polymorphisms may perturb function of the protein, whereas others may enhance function. Studies are needed to determine whether polymor-

phisms of opioid receptors explain apparent individual differences in clinical response to either peripherally or systemically administered opioids.

Chronic Opioid Therapy Drug dependency or addiction, reinforcing drug-seeking behavior, drug-induced depression, drug tolerance, and fear of government prosecution are frequently cited reasons for avoiding opioids in management protocols for chronic pain patients. Until recently each of these concerns was considered a valid reason for avoiding opioid therapy. However, recent evidence suggests that the risk of addiction may be extremely low in chronic pain patients with no prior history of substance abuse.[78] Drug use alone does not appear to be the major determinant of addiction. Rather, other factors such as social, psychological, and economic conditions appear to contribute more to addictive behavior.[79] Psychiatric consultation may be valuable in the identification of individuals with true addictive behavior.

Despite clinical impressions to the contrary, studies have not validated concerns regarding development of opioid tolerance. These data indicate that the analgesic potency of opioids seldom declines over time, unless there is a worsening of the patient's physical condition.[80–82] Furthermore, cross-tolerance is often incomplete in patients who do exhibit signs of opioid tolerance.[83,84] In these instances switching to another narcotic can produce an analgesic response. Future studies are required to determine the true benefits and risks of protracted opioid therapy to manage persistent pain experienced by the patient with end-stage TMJ disease.

Indications for Opioid Therapy Opioids do not appear to be effective for all types of pain. It is often difficult to determine whether the apparent lack of efficacy observed in some patients is due to this fact or if the dose administered is simply inadequate. However, a rational approach that can be employed to confirm the analgesic efficacy of opioid therapy for a specific patient is suggested in a study conducted by Dellemijn and Vanneste.[55] These investigators used an active placebo (diazepam) and an inactive placebo (saline) to demonstrate the analgesic efficacy of an opioid (fentanyl) in patients suffering from neuropathic pain. In this particular study diazepam was no more effective than saline as an analgesic. However, diazepam did produce a sedative effect similar to that produced by fentanyl and was therefore suitable for use as an active placebo. Using this experimental design, the investigators demonstrated the analgesic efficacy of fentanyl for control of neuropathic pain. A similar approach could be employed to determine whether opioid therapy would provide effective analgesia for a particular patient with end-stage TMJ disease. In this way, the clinician could provide a better estimate of the benefit-to-risk ratio of opioid therapy.

As-needed dosing schedules for opioids are avoided. It is preferable to dose opioids on a scheduled basis for optimum control of pain. For example, if the patient indicates that pain is worse in the late morning and afternoon hours, then an adequate loading dose of the opioid should be administered 1 to 2 hours prior to the morning peak pain period with supplemental dosings at 3- to 6-hour intervals depending on the drug. During the titration period patients may be asked to log their pain using a 0 to 10 intensity scale at hourly intervals. Dose adjustments can then be made based on patient reports of pain. Some consideration should be given to the use of long-acting opioids or alternate delivery systems (eg, transdermal, implanted infusion pumps) in those instances when severe protracted pain is controlled by opioid therapy. This approach may be more cost effective and can provide better long-term pain relief.

TCAs Imipramine was the first TCA found to possess analgesic properties.[85,86] Since that time numerous well-controlled trials have documented pain relieving effects of TCAs.[87–90]

Mechanism of Antinociception TCAs produce significant analgesia independent of their antidepressant effects. For example, analgesic effects of TCAs are observed in pain patients with normal mood.[91,92] Furthermore, TCA-induced analgesia is typically observed prior to antidepressant effects and at doses that are generally believed to be too low for any significant antidepressant effect.[93–95]

Amitriptyline and imipramine, antidepressants with antinociceptive actions, are potent inhibitors of serotonin reuptake.[96] Though these agents have no direct effect on norepinephrine reuptake, their metabolites are also potent norepinephrine reuptake inhibitors.[96] In vivo, these TCAs can be viewed as mixed monoamine reuptake inhibitors (ie, they inhibit the reuptake of both serotonin and norepinephrine).

TCAs enhance the biologic activities of serotonin and norepinephrine by reuptake blockade. Monoamine receptor occupancy is increased by reuptake inhibitors (ie, TCAs) resulting in an antinociceptive effect. There is recent evidence that monoamines may be important modulators of temporomandibular pain.[97] This is strongly suggested in studies investigating the relative sensitivities of patients who express different versions of the catechol *O*-methyltransferase (COMT) gene (ie, polymorphisms) to painful masseter muscle stimulation. COMT is an enzyme that regulates noradrenergic neurotransmission by catecholamine metabolism. The gene for COMT exists in a variety of forms created by subtle mutations (ie, polymorphisms). A COMT gene polymorphism exists at codon 158 (a codon is a three-nucleotide deoxyribonucleic acid sequence that encodes a specific amino acid of the encoded protein, in this instance COMT), where a valine code is substituted by a methionine code. This substitution results in a COMT variant that is three to four times less active than the native COMT. Individuals who are homozygous for this COMT variant report significantly more pain following a hypertonic saline injection of the masseter muscle relative to those individuals who express the normal variant.[97] Interestingly, these individuals also show a reduction in endogenous opioid responses to this stimulation in discreet regions of the thalamus as assessed by functional magnetic resonance imaging studies.

Efficacy for Relief of Muscular Pain Amitriptyline significantly reduces the duration and frequency but not the intensity of chronic tension-type headaches.[89,98] However, selective serotonin reuptake inhibitors do not appear to affect chronic tension-type headaches.[89] Appropriately controlled clinical studies have also provided evidence that amitriptyline is effective in relieving pain associated with fibromyalgia.[99–103] However, sustained clinical improvement occurs in a relatively small percentage of fibromyalgia patients given this agent.

Efficacy for Relief of Neuropathic Pain As appears to be the case for relief of muscular pain, antidepressants with mixed serotonin and norepinephrine reuptake inhibition (eg, amitriptyline) are more efficacious than relatively selective reuptake blockers (eg, predominant norepinephrine reuptake inhibition by desipramine; predominant serotonin reuptake inhibition by paroxetine or citalopram) with respect to relief of neuropathic pain.[92,104–108] The efficacy of mixed serotonin and norepinephrine reuptake inhibitors has been demonstrated for various types of neuropathic pain. For example, 53% of patients with neuropathic pain following treatment of breast cancer had a > 50% reduction in pain at a median daily dose of 50 mg of amitriptyline.[105] Amitriptyline has also been shown to be more effective than placebo for relief of pain associated with diabetic neuropathy, postherpetic neuropathy, and central lesions.[92,104–108] Some multiply operated patients with end-stage TMJ disease may suffer from neuropathic pains, typically described as "sharp" or "burning," that likely result from traumatic injury to peripheral neurons during surgery. When this is suspected, it may be appropriate to consider a mixed serotonin and norepinephrine reuptake inhibitor (eg, amitriptyline).

Dosing Recommendations There is a tremendous intersubject variability in the pharmacokinetics of some TCAs. This is believed to be due, in part, to expressed polymorphisms of the sparteine/debrisoquin oxygenase system that governs metabolism of the TCAs.[109] Given the wide intersubject variability in TCA pharmacokinetics, standard-dose regimens may be poorly tolerated or ineffective for a particular individual. Therefore, these drugs should be titrated to effect. It should be also remembered that only 50 to 70% of patients are responders (ie, individuals who experience a desired effect), and often the response to the drug is modest. Although there is a general perception that the analgesic response to TCAs is delayed, studies have actually documented a relatively rapid analgesic response to these agents. In fact, as previously mentioned, measurable antinociceptive effects have been observed after a single dose.[95] Therefore, an analgesic response should be expected within 1 week of the administration of an effective TCA dose, but a maximum response may not be observed for 4 to 6 weeks.

For most patients amitriptyline is the TCA of choice for pain management in the patient with end-stage TMJ disease. Other TCAs (eg, desipramine) may be less effective for relief of pain owing to their relative

selectivities for monoamine reuptake inhibition. In most instances amitriptyline may be administered as a single dose given at bedtime. An initial dose of 10 to 25 mg is typical for this application. The dose may be increased at 2-week intervals to a range of 10 to 75 mg/d based on subjective pain reports by the patient and drug tolerance. It should be recognized that a therapeutic window has been observed for some TCAs, with maximum analgesic responses typically observed at lower doses.[110,111] For this reason a ceiling dose of 75 mg (1 mg/kg) amitriptyline for an adult is recommended. If significant pain relief is not observed after trial dosing up to this recommended ceiling, then the agent should be withdrawn by a tapering regimen. If significant pain relief is observed, then the agent should be continued at the effective dose. Periodic tapered withdrawals of the agent are recommended to ascertain the need for continued dosing.

TCAs can usually be administered with few side effects observed at recommended doses. However, side effects including morning sluggishness, urinary retention, weight gain from enhanced appetite, sleep disturbances, and constipation are reported by some patients. Serious side effects, such as cardiac dysrhythmias/myocardial infarction, seizures, stroke, agranulocytosis, and thrombocytopenia, are very rare with low-dose regimens in patients who are not otherwise medically compromised. TCAs should be administered cautiously in patients with a history of cardiovascular disease, seizure disorders, or urinary retention or who concurrently take medications that can influence monoamine activities (eg, antidepressants/antipsychotics, tramadol).

Drug-Induced Bruxism and Jaw Clenching Patients with end-stage TMJ disease may be subjected to drugs that can exacerbate their condition by induction of focal dystonias leading to increased bruxism or jaw clenching. For example, bilateral masticatory myalgia with TMJ symptoms was ob-

served shortly after the administration of sustained-release bupropion in a 44-year-old man for relief of depression secondary to chronic lower back pain and tension headaches.[112] These temporomandibular symptoms developed within 48 hours of a dose adjustment from 150 mg/d of sustained-release bupropion to 300 mg/d. Furthermore, these symptoms resolved completely with withdrawal of the medication. Dystonic reactions to some antipsychotic and antidepressant medications may result from an acute reduction in dopaminergic activity in the brain.[113,114] Ninety percent of these reactions occur within 3 to 5 days of drug initiation or dose adjustment.[112] Selective serotonin reuptake inhibitors (eg, fluoxetine, citalopram, paroxetine, and sertraline) may evoke this response. Ironically, some patients with end-stage TMJ disease are placed on these agents to manage the inevitable depression that occurs in this group of patients. In some of these patients, it is conceivable that the antidepressant could worsen their condition by evoking focal dystonic reactions or bruxism affecting the masticatory and cervical musculature. Such a response could provoke additional muscle pain and may even aggravate a TMJ condition by increasing mechanical loads.

Opioid addiction may be associated with exaggerated oromotor behavior and signs and symptoms of temporomandibular dysfunction. Winocur and colleagues studied 55 individuals who were addicted to opioids and were receiving treatment at a methadone clinic.[115] A sex-, age-, and socioeconomic class–matched nonaddict group served as the control in this study. The addicted group exhibited a higher frequency of bruxism and jaw clenching, as well as morning headache, TMJ noises, and masticatory muscle tenderness. It is unclear from this study whether the apparent effects on the stomatognathic system were a direct manifestation of chronic opioid use or a mere reflection of a personality disorder that led to an opioid addiction.

Nevertheless, many patients with end-stage TMJ disease undergo chronic opioid therapy for pain management. In some instances it is possible that induction of focal dystonias in patients with end-stage TMJ disease by opioids could exacerbate their condition, resulting in an escalation in pain that could be confused with opioid tolerance. If this phenomenon is suspected, then a tapered withdrawal of the opioid should be initiated. Contrary to the reaction expected with an opioid-tolerant patient, opioid withdrawal in this instance may provide paradoxic pain relief.

GABAergics   GABA is an inhibitory neurotransmitter that has been implicated in nociception modulation.[116–118] GABA effects are mediated via at least two different types of GABA receptors: $GABA_A$ and $GABA_B$.[119,120] A third GABA receptor, $GABA_C$, may also exist, but its distribution appears to be exclusively restricted to the retina of the eye.[121]

$GABA_B$ receptors are inhibitory G-protein coupled receptors that attenuate neural activities.[120,122] The classic agonist for the $GABA_B$ receptor is baclofen. Baclofen administered either systemically or intrathecally suppresses allodynia and hyperalgesia in animal models of pain.[123,124] In a clinical study of lower back pain, 30 to 80 mg/d baclofen was found to be superior to placebo as an analgesic.[125]

Gabapentin has been used to reduce pain associated with some neuropathic states including pain that is sympathetically maintained.[126] Gabapentin appears to elicit this effect by increasing the endogenous synthesis of GABA. Gabapentin's analgesic effects appear to be pain-type specific. In acute pain animal models, gabapentin does not produce analgesia.

Based on available data, it may be reasonable to consider a trial of baclofen (30–80 mg/d) or gabapentin (300–1800 mg/d) for patients with end-stage TMJ disease who may be suffering from a neuropathic component of pain. As previously mentioned, this might result from previous injury to neurons innervating tissues of the TMJ region. However, given the limited data demonstrating efficacy for temporomandibular pain, particularly in the patient with end-stage TMJ disease, these agents should be reserved for use after other approaches have been tried.

Sympathetically Maintained Pain

Sympathetically maintained pain (SMP), reflex sympathetic dystrophy, causalgia, and most recently complex regional pain syndrome (CRPS) are terms often used by clinicians in reference to a syndrome(s) characterized by continuous burning pain believed to be associated with abnormal nociception affected by activity in the sympathetic nervous system. CRPS typically follows traumatic injury to the affected region. Some multiply operated patients with end-stage TMJ disease with localized tactile or mechanical allodynia and burning pain complaints may be suffering from sympathetically driven pain. However, the incidence of CRPS in patients with end-stage TMJ disease is unknown.

Clinical Presentation   Signs or symptoms of CRPS occurring with an incidence of 75% or greater include weakness (95%), pain (93%), altered skin temperature (92%), skin color change (92%), limited range of motion (88%), and hyperesthesia (75%).[127] Less common findings include edema, altered hair growth, tremor, hyperhidrosis, muscle/skin atrophy, and bone resorption.[127]

The mechanism(s) underlying the development of CRPS is unknown. However, there is emerging evidence that suggests that this condition may result from neuroplastic changes induced by peripheral sensory nerve injury. In animals the sprouting of sympathetic neurons into sensory ganglia (ie, dorsal root ganglia) has been observed after injury to peripheral sensory nerves. This sprouting may be induced by a neurotrophic substance, known as nerve growth factor (NGF), that is released into injured tissues.[128–132] A similar response is observed in animals in which NGF is administered intrathecally.[132] These data are consistent with the belief that CRPS results from an abnormal sympathetic input to sensory ganglia following peripheral sensory nerve injury. This abnormal sympathetic input may be made possible by the development of physical connections between sympathetic neurons and primary afferent sensory neurons. Injury may elicit this abnormal response via molecular intermediates, specifically NGF. Clearly this phenomenon does not occur in all individuals who sustain injuries to sensory peripheral nerves. Future research is needed to confirm this model and to determine risk factors that govern an individual's susceptibility to the development of CRPS.

Treatment   Over 25 treatments for CRPS have been reported in the literature.[133] The most common therapeutic approach has involved the interruption of sympathetic activity via a stellate ganglion block. An effective stellate ganglion block may produce protracted pain relief (ie, lasting longer than the duration of anesthetic blockade), although this effect is usually transient. Other pharmacologic interventions (eg, phentolamine, prazosin, bretylium, guanethidine, calcitonin, nifedipine, gabapentin) and surgical sympathectomy have also been employed with inconsistent results.[133] With new information concerning the molecular events that may underlie the development of CRPS, it is hoped that more effective therapies will be developed in the near future.

Physical Therapy

A primary goal of all therapies directed to the management of the patient with end-stage TMJ disease is to restore normal joint function (ie, joint movement). Patients with end-stage TMJ disease typically exhibit severely restricted jaw movements. Pain and intra-articular fibrosis or fibro-osseous ankylosis often coexist to restrict jaw movement. For this reason, pain management must be effective for optimum patient compliance with prescribed physical therapy.

Passive jaw exercises are effective at improving joint function if they are performed regularly over an extended period of time. Two devices are currently commercially available that facilitate passive motion of the TMJ. Alternatively, passive motion exercises can be performed with simple finger crossover maneuvers or with tongue depressor blades.

A simple but effective protocol incorporating passive motion exercises to increase mandibular movements in the patient with end-stage TMJ disease involves repetitive (10–12 times daily) vertical opening exercises. For these exercises the patient is given a number of tongue depressor blades that, when inserted between the maxillary and mandibular teeth, produce an opening of the jaws that is barely tolerated by the patient. The patient is instructed to apply these tongue depressor blades hourly (8–10 times daily) for 2 to 3 minutes. On the first day of each week, the patient is instructed to increase the total number of tongue depressor blades used by addition of one blade. This approach permits tissues to gradually adapt to advancing jaw movements and is generally well tolerated by the majority of patients with end-stage TMJ disease.

Therapy for Periarticular Ectopic Bone Formation

Periarticular ectopic bone formation is viewed as a significant postsurgical complication with a negative impact on functional outcomes in some patients with end-stage TMJ disease. Ectopic bone may form in adjacent native periarticular tissues or proximate to alloplastic materials used to reconstruct the TMJ. In either instance, periarticular ectopic bone formation is viewed as pathologic since it typically restricts normal joint movement and may contribute to ongoing pain.

The pathogenesis of periarticular ectopic bone formation is poorly understood. It has been suggested that displaced osteogenic precursor cells are stimulated to form ectopic bone by inflammatory mediators formed in response to surgical insult.[134] Alternatively, osteoinductive molecules (eg, bone morphogenetic proteins) may be dispersed into periarticular tissues during surgery, resulting in the stimulation of resident pluripotent cells and subsequent ectopic bone synthesis. In addition, there may be other factors, such as genetics, sex hormones, systemic disease (eg, ankylosing spondylitis, Paget's disease), or other local conditions, that could also contribute to the formation of ectopic bone in periarticular tissues of the TMJ.

Two strategies have been employed in an attempt to prevent or minimize periarticular ectopic bone formation in either orthopedic surgery patients or those with TMJ disease. These are low-dose radiation therapy, and nonsteroidal anti-inflammatory drug (NSAID) therapy.

Low-Dose Radiation Therapy Some clinicians have advocated the use of low-dose radiation to prevent or minimize postsurgical fibro-osseous ankylosis of the TMJ.[135–138] This approach is based on an earlier report indicating that low-dose radiation may be effective at preventing the formation of ectopic bone following hip arthroplasty.[139] For prevention of periarticular ectopic bone formation of the TMJ, fractionated total doses of 10 to 20 Gy have been used. One study reported that 10 Gy dosing was as effective as higher-dose regimens.[136]

Timing appears to be critical for optimum results from low-dose radiation therapy. It is believed that low-dose radiation therapy elicits its effect on ectopic bone formation by prohibiting the proliferation of pluripotent cells that are precursors to osteoblasts. Therefore, it is rec-ommended that low-dose radiation therapy be initiated within 4 days of surgery to provide optimum suppression of ectopic bone formation. Although there is some concern that early postsurgical radiation may have a detrimental impact on wound healing, in a recent study of the efficacy of a single dose of 600 cGy administered between postsurgical days 2 and 4 (mean 3.2 d), radiation did not appear to significantly impact wound healing after hip arthroplasty.[140]

Radiation therapy was used to prevent ectopic bone formation in the periarticular region of the TMJ in a 53-year-old man.[137] This individual sustained mandible fractures in an automobile accident and subsequently underwent five operations to correct a TMJ ankylosis suffered as a complication of his injury. Over an 18-year period, the patient suffered from a significant limitation of jaw movement, with reported maximum interincisal movements as low as 6 mm. Following his final TMJ arthroplasty, the patient underwent fractionated cobalt radiation therapy consisting of ten sessions beginning on the first postoperative day. The patient received a total radiation dose of 20 Gy in equal fractions. He apparently tolerated the procedure well without significant complications. At the 3-year follow-up, the patient had sustained a maximum interincisal distance of 25.5 mm.[137]

Schwartz and Kagan provided a report describing a similar beneficial effect of fractionated radiation (ie, 20 Gy in 10 fractions) in a 51-year old man who experienced a zygomatico-coronoid ankylosis following a depressed fracture of the zygomatic arch.[138] This condition was surgically treated with a 5 mm gap arthroplasty with placement of an intervening sheet of silicone rubber. Postsurgical radiation was initiated 1 week after the operation. At a 19-month follow-up, the patient exhibited a 40 mm maximum interincisal distance. Although the patient initially complained of xerostomia and had some loss of facial hair, there were no reported lasting ill effects from this treatment.

Experiences with 10 patients suffering from bony ankylosis of the TMJ were reported by Durr and colleagues.[136] Four men and six women (median age 32.5 yr, range 14–59 yr) with a previous history of TMJ ankylosis underwent TMJ arthroplasties and immediate postsurgical (ie, 1–3 d) radiation therapy consisting of 10 to 11.2 Gy in five fractions over a 5-day period. The median follow-up for this reported case series was 19 months (range 7–31 mo). Only three patients (ie, 30%) were followed up for > 2 years postoperatively. Forty percent of the patients in this series experienced some recurrence of ectopic bone formation as assessed radiographically. A parotitis was identified in 30% of the patients in this series. However, the radiation therapy did not appear to interfere with healing, and there were no other reported complications.

Reid and Cooke have reported the largest case series to date involving postoperative radiation therapy to manage ectopic bone formation of the TMJ in 14 patients with histories of multiple TMJ surgeries.[135] Each patient underwent TMJ arthroplasty with total joint reconstruction using an alloplastic prosthesis. The majority of these patients received a fractionated 10 Gy radiation dose beginning on the first postoperative day. However, some patients treated early in the series received a fractionated 20 Gy radiation dose. Patients in this series were followed up postoperatively with a mean follow-up of 4.2 years (range 1–9.6 yr). The recurrence rate for ectopic bone formation at the 1-year follow-up was 21%. However, long-term follow-up revealed ectopic bone formation in 75% of the patients seen at 5 years and 100% (*n* = 2) of patients examined at the 9-year follow-up (Figure 51-2). Consistent with earlier reports, no significant persistent side effects of radiation therapy were noted.

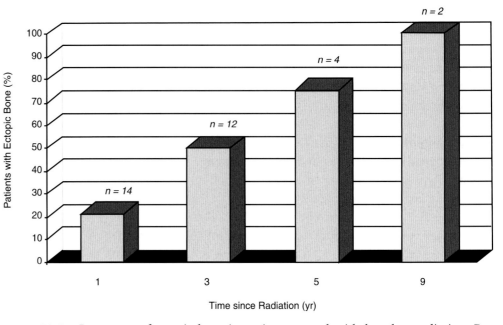

FIGURE 51-2   *Recurrence of ectopic bone in patients treated with low-dose radiation. Data adapted from Reid R and Cooke H.[135]*

A major concern with the use of low-dose radiation for the treatment of ectopic bone formation in the TMJ area is the potential for induction of neoplasias. Despite the fact that there have been no reported cases of malignant transformation associated with low-dose radiation therapy used to manage periarticular ectopic bone formation in the TMJ area, this concern seems justified based on a report by Ron and colleagues.[141] These investigators examined 10,834 patients who had undergone low-dose radiation therapy for the treatment of ringworm infection of the scalp (ie, tinea capitis). All irradiated subjects received treatment (mean radiation dose 1.5 Gy) before the age of 16 years. Controls included 10,834 nonirradiated age- and sex-matched individuals not related to the radiated subjects, serving as a general population control, and 5,392 nonirradiated siblings of the subjects. The subjects were monitored for up to 33 years for the development of benign and malignant neural tumors. Tumors developed in 73 individuals, 60 among irradiated subjects, 8 in the general population control group, and 5 among siblings of irradiated subjects. Overall, there was a sevenfold increase in neoplasms of the nervous system in individuals who had undergone low-dose radiation therapy. Twenty-four malignant neoplasias were identified in this study, with 18 occurring in irradiated patients, 4 in the general population control group, and 2 in siblings of irradiated subjects. There was a 4.5-fold increase in the incidence of malignant neoplasias in patients who underwent low-dose radiation therapy relative to the control groups. The cumulative risk of developing a neural tumor over a 33-year period was significantly higher in the irradiated group (0.84 ± 0.16%) than in the controls (0.09 ± 0.03%). It should be noted that there was a prolonged latency of tumor occurrence (mean 17.6 yr after radiation exposure). From this study it appears that the risk of radiation-associated tumors was highest between 15 and 24 years postradiation. This has significance in light of the fact that the longest published follow-up for any case series reporting the effects low-dose radiation therapy for management of ectopic bone formation in the TMJ area is 9 years (only two patients).[135] It should be noted that patients receiving radiation therapy for tinea capitis in this study were significantly younger (< 16 yr old) than the TMJ patients reported in the series cited above. It is possible that the risk of radiation-associated neoplasia may be age dependent. However, this assumption has not yet been validated in appropriately designed studies.

In summary, the evidence supporting the use of low-dose radiation therapy to prevent or minimize ectopic bone formation in periarticular regions of the TMJ is supplied by case summaries that report beneficial effects with 10 to 20 Gy exposures in fractionated doses initiated within 4 days of surgery. However, it should be recognized that definitive studies (ie, appropriately blinded and controlled) have not been reported to date. In the absence of these studies, the true efficacy of this therapy remains obscure. Furthermore, there is evidence that such therapy may pose significant long-term health risks.[141]

NSAID Therapy Several studies have provided evidence that NSAIDs may be effective retardants of ectopic bone formation.[140,142–145] The mechanism(s) by which these drugs elicit this effect is currently unknown. However, the effect is believed to be secondary to the ability of these drugs to inhibit prostanoid, and perhaps LT, synthesis associated with normal inflammatory responses to injury.

Kienapfel and colleagues compared the effects of indomethacin, a nonselective COX inhibitor (also capable of inhibiting lipoxygenase), with those of low-dose radiation therapy employed to prevent ectopic bone formation after hip arthroplasty.[140] For this study 154 patients scheduled for hip arthroplasty to treat various degenerative arthritides were randomly assigned to one of three groups: (1) low-dose radiation treatment (600 cGy administered as a single dose between postoperative days 2 and 4); (2) indomethacin treatment (50 mg administered orally twice a day beginning

on postoperative day 1 and continuing until postoperative day 42); or (3) control (no postoperative radiation or NSAID). Patients assigned to the indomethacin treatment group who were either at risk for NSAID-induced gastrointestinal disease or who developed dyspepsia with the therapy were given cimetidine 200 mg (H$_2$ receptor antagonist) concomitantly.

All subjects enrolled in the study were assessed clinically and radiographically 18 months after surgery.[140] Ectopic bone formation was significantly inhibited by both treatment conditions relative to the control. Furthermore, both treatments were found to be equally effective. Surgical wound secretions were more persistent in the radiated subjects postoperatively, but neither treatment group subsequently exhibited signs of poor wound healing that were significantly different from the control. The incidence of dyspepsia was higher in the indomethacin-treated group, but gastrointestinal bleeding was not detected in this group.

Other NSAIDs have been used to prevent or minimize ectopic bone formation following hip arthroplasty, including ibuprofen, ketorolac, and diclofenac.[142,143,145] All of these agents are nonselective COX inhibitors (ie, they block by COX-1 and COX-2). At the present time it is not known whether the selective COX-2 inhibitors are effective retardants of ectopic bone formation.

To date there have been no reported studies of NSAID use for the management of ectopic bone formation of the TMJ. Therefore, the efficacy of these agents for this specific application remains to be demonstrated. However, based on the orthopedic surgery literature, it may be prudent to consider NSAID therapy for patients who are at risk for ectopic bone formation following TMJ surgery. The potential gastrointestinal and renal complications associated with this approach should not be underestimated. Patients undergoing NSAID therapy to prevent or

minimize ectopic bone formation should be properly monitored. If indicated, misoprostol or an H$_2$ receptor antagonist should be administered concomitantly to reduce the potential for serious gastrointestinal complications.

Conclusions

The patient with end-stage TMJ disease is typically afflicted by severe unrelenting pain, restricted jaw function, facial deformity, depression, compromised interpersonal relationships, and financial hardships. Given the complexities involved, these patients pose a significant challenge for the most experienced clinicians. A coordinated team of specialists best provides optimum care. However, in most communities this level of care is not available. The local oral and maxillofacial surgeon is often looked on as the specialist who will manage these complicated cases. For the multiply operated patient with end-stage TMJ disease, few surgical options are viable. In these instances medical management is advised with primary treatment objectives typically being pain management and improvement in jaw movements. When surgery is contemplated, it is imperative that the surgeon complete an accurate assessment of the patient's condition. The surgeon must establish realistic surgical objectives based on this assessment. Finally, the surgeon must exercise good judgment in the selection of patients for surgery. Patients who are incapable or unwilling to comply with demanding but essential postsurgery rehabilitation programs may not be viable candidates for surgery, even when feasible surgical objectives are identified.

References

1. Travell JG, Simons DG. Myofascial pain and dysfunction: the trigger point manual. 1. Baltimore: Williams and Wilkins; 1983.
2. Mendell LM, Wall PD. Response of single dorsal cord cells to peripheral cutaneous unmyelinated fibres. Nature 1965;206:97–9.
3. Woolf CJ, King AE. Dynamic alterations in the

cutaneous mechanoreceptive fields of dorsal horn neurons in the rat spinal cord. J Neurosci 1990;10:2717–26.

4. Owens CM, Zhang D, Willis WD. Changes in the response states of primate spinothalamic tract cells caused by mechanical damage of the skin or activation of descending controls. J Neurophysiol 1992;67:1509–27.

5. Bereiter DA. Sex differences in brainstem neural activation after injury to the TMJ region. Cells Tissues Organs 2001;169:226–37.

6. Bereiter DA, Bereiter DF. Morphine and NMDA receptor antagonism reduce c-fos expression in spinal trigeminal nucleus produced by acute injury to the TMJ region. Pain 2000;85:65–77.

7. Woolf CJ, Chong MS. Preemptive analgesia—treating postoperative pain by preventing the establishment of central sensitization. Anesth Analg 1993;77:362–79.

8. Giannoni C, White S, Enneking FK, et al. Ropivacaine with or without clonidine improves pediatric tonsillectomy pain. Arch Otolaryngol Head Neck Surg 2001;127:1265–70.

9. Goodwin SA. A review of preemptive analgesia. J Perianesth Nurs 1998;13:109–14.

10. Goldstein FJ. Preemptive analgesia: a research review. Medsurg Nursing 1995;4:305–8.

11. Gilron I, Quirion R, Coderre TJ. Pre- versus post-formalin effects of ketamine or large-dose alfentanil in the rat: discordance between pain behavior and spinal Fos-like immunoreactivity. Anesth Analg 1999;89:128–35.

12. Kelly DJ, Ahmad M, Brull SJ. Preemptive analgesia I: physiological pathways and pharmacological modalities. Can J Anaesth 2001;48:1000–10.

13. Kilickan L, Toker K. The effect of preemptive intravenous morphine on postoperative analgesia and surgical stress response. Panminerva Med 2001;43:171–5.

14. Subramaniam B, Pawar DK, Kashyap L. Preemptive analgesia with epidural morphine or morphine and bupivacaine. Anaesth Intensive Care 2000;28:392–8.

15. Chiaretti A, Viola L, Pietrini D, et al. Preemptive analgesia with tramadol and fentanyl in pediatric neurosurgery [discussion]. Childs Nerv Sys 2000;16:93–9

16. Dickenson AH, Sullivan AF. Evidence for a role of the NMDA receptor in the frequency dependent potentiation of deep rat dorsal horn nociceptive neurones following C fibre stimulation. Neuropharmacol 1987; 26:1235–8.

17. Haley JE, Sullivan AF, Dickenson AH. Evidence for spinal N-methyl-D-aspartate receptor involvement in prolonged chemical noci-

cpetion in the rat. Brain Res 1990; 518:218–26.

18. Torrebjork HE, Lundberg LE, LaMotte RH. Centeral changes in processing of mechanoreceptive input in capsaicin-induced secondary hyperalgesia in humans. J Physiol 1992; 448:765–80.

19. Mixter CGR, Hackett TR. Preemptive analgesia in the laparoscopic patient. Surg Endosc 1997;11:351–3.

20. Norman PH, Daley MD, Lindsey RW. Preemptive analgesic effects of ketorolac in ankle fracture surgery [comment]. Anesthesiology 2001;94:599–603.

21. Wittels B, Faure EA, Chavez R, et al. Effective analgesia after bilateral tubal ligation. Anesth Analg 1998;87:619–23.

22. Jebeles JA, Reilly JS, Gutierrez JF, et al. Tonsillectomy and adenoidectomy pain reduction by local bupivacaine infiltration in children. Int J Pediatr Otorhinolaryngol 1993;25:149–54.

23. Honnma T, Imaizumi T, Chiba M, et al. Preemptive analgesia for postoperative pain after frontotemporal craniotomy. No Shinkei Geka 2002;30:171–4.

24. Hoard MA, Bill TJ, Campbell RL. Reduction in morbidity after iliac crest bone harvesting: the concept of preemptive analgesia. J Craniomaxillofac Surg 1998;9:448–51.

25. Abram SE, Yaksh TL. Morphine, but not inhalation anesthesia, blocks post-injury facilitation: the role of preemptive suppression of afferent transmission. Anesthesiology 1993;78:713–21.

26. Wallace MS, Braun J, Schulteis G. Postdelivery of alfentanil and ketamine has no effect on intradermal capsaicin-induced pain and hyperalgesia. Clin J Pain 2002;18:373–9.

27. Bach S, Noreng MF, Tjellden NU. Phantom limb pain in amputees during the first 12 months following limb amputation, after preoperative lumbar epidural blockade. Pain 1988;33:297–301.

28. Hla T, Ristimaki A, Appleby S, et al. Cyclooxygenase gene expression in inflammation and angiogenesis [review]. Ann N Y Acad Sci 1993;696:197–204.

29. Crofford LJ, Wilder RL, Ristimaki AP, et al. Cyclooxygenase-1 and -2 expression in rheumatoid synovial tissues. Effects of interleukin-1 beta, phorbol ester, and corticosteroids. J Clin Investig 1994;93:1095–101.

30. O'Neill GP, Ford HA. Expression of mRNA for cyclooxygenase-1 and cyclooxygenase-2 in human tissues. FEBS Lett 1993;330:156–60.

31. Hla T, Neilson K. Human cyclooxygenase-2 cDNA. Proc Natl Acad Sci U S A 1992; 89:7384–8.

32. Ristimaki A, Garfinkel S, Wessendorf J, et al. Induction of cyclooxygenase-2 by interleukin-1 alpha. Evidence for post-transcriptional regulation. J Biol Chem 1994; 269:11769–75.

33. Hua XY, Jinno S, Back SM, et al. Multiple mechanisms for the effects of capsaicin, bradykinin, and nicotine on CGRP release from tracheal afferent nerves: role of prostaglandins, sympathetic nerves, and mast cells. Neuropharmacol 1994;33:1147–54.

34. Quinn JH, Bazan NG. Identification of prostaglandin E2 and leukotriene B4 in the synovial fluid of painful, dysfunctional temporomandibular joints. J Oral Maxillofac Surg 1990;48:968–71.

35. Murakami K-I, Shibata T, Kubota E, et al. Intra-articular levels of prostaglandin E2, hyaluronic acid, and chondroitin-4 and -6 sulfates in the temporomandibular joint synovial fluid of patients with internal derangement. J Oral Maxillofac Surg 1998; 56:199–203.

36. Devoghel JC. Small intrathecal doses of lysine-acetylsalicylate relieve intractable pain in man. J Int Med Res 1983;11:90–1.

37. Malmberg AB, Yaksh TL. Antinociceptive actions of spinal nonsteroidal anti-inflammatory agents on the formalin test in the rat. J Pharmacol Exp Ther 1992;263:136–46.

38. Malmberg AB, Yaksh TL. Antinociception produced by spinal delivery of the S and R enantiomers of flurbiprofen in the formalin test. Eur J Pharmacol 1994;256:205–9.

39. Wallace JL. Prostaglandins, NSAIDs, and cytoprotection. Gastroentrol Clin North Am 1992;21:631–41.

40. Clive DM, Stoff JS. Renal syndromes associated with nonsteroidal antiinflammatory drugs. N Engl J Med 1984;310:563–72.

41. Morita I, Suzuki Y, Toriyama K, et al. Induction of cyclooxygenase in osteoblasts and bone metabolism. Adv Prostaglandin Thromboxane Leukot Res 1991;21B:839–42, .

42. Bell NH, Hollis BW, Shary JR, et al. Diclofenac sodium inhibits bone resorption in postmenopausal women. Am J Med 1994; 96:349–53.

43. Kemick ML, Chin JE, Wuthier RE. Role of prostaglandins in differentiation of growth plate chondrocytes. Adv Prostaglandin Thromboxane Leukot Res 1989;19:423–6.

44. Goldring MB, Sohbat E, Elwell JM, et al. Etodolac preserves cartilage-specific phenotype in human chondrocytes: effects on type II collagen synthesis and associated mRNA levels. Eur J Rheumatol Inflamm 1990;10:10–21.

45. Gabriel SE, Jaakkimainen L, Bombardier C.

Risk of serious gastrointestinal complications related to use of nonsteroidal anti-inflammatory drugs. Ann Intern Med 1991;115:787–96.

46. Doyle G, Jayawardena S, Ashraf E, et al. Efficacy and tolerability of nonprescription ibuprofen versus celecoxib for dental pain. J Clin Pharmacol 2002;42:912–9.

47. Hwang SW, Cho H, Kwak J, et al. Direct activation of capsaicin receptors by products of lipoxygenases: endogenous capsaicin-like substances. Proc Natl Acad Sci U S A 2000;97:6155–60.

48. Shin J, Cho H, Hwang SW, et al. Bradykinin-12-lipoxygenase-VR1 signaling pathway for inflammatory hyperalgesia. Proc Natl Acad Sci U S A 2002;99:10150–5.

49. Flynn DL, Belliotti TR, Boctor AM, et al. Styrylpyrazoles, styrylisoxazoles, and styrylisothiazoles. Novel 5-lipoxygenase and cyclooxygenase inhibitors. J Med Chem 1991;34:518–25.

50. Jiang Q, Takemori AE, Sultana M, et al. Differential antagonism of opioid delta antinociception by [D-ala2,Leu5,Cys6]-enkephalin and naltrindole 5'-isothiocyanate: evidence for delta receptor subtypes. J Pharmacol Exp Ther 1991;257:1069–75.

51. Pasternak GW. Pharmacological mechanisms of opioid. Clin Neuropharmacol 1993;16:1–18.

52. Yoshimura M, North RA. Substantia gelatinosa neurones in vitro hyperpolarized by enkephalin. Nature 1983;305:529–30.

53. Carter BD, Medzihradsky F. G$_o$ mediates the coupling of the mu opioid receptor to adenyl cyclase in cloned neural cells and brain. Proc Natl Acad Sci U S A 1993;90:4062–6.

54. Grudt TJ, Williams JT. Kappa-opioid receptors increase potassium conductance. Proc Natl Acad Sci U S A 1993;90:11429–32.

55. Dellemijn PLI, Vanneste JAL. Randomized double-blind active-placebo-controlled crossover trial of intravenous fentanyl in neuropathic pain. Lancet 1997;349:753–8.

56. Bereiter DA, Bereiter DF, Ramos M. Vagotomy prevents morphine-induced reduction in Fos-like immunoreactivity in trigeminal spinal nucleus produced after TMJ injury in a sex-dependent manner. Pain 2002;96:205–13.

57. Chase H. Sensitive dentine. Dent Cosmos 1867;8:635–7.

58. Hargreaves KM, Keatin K, Cathers S, et al. Analgesic effects of morphine after PDL injection in endodontic patients. [abstract]. J Dent Res 1991;70:445.

59. Hayashi K, Sugisaiki M, Ota S, et al. mu-Opioid receptor mRNA expression and immunohistochemical localization in the rat temporomandibular joint. Peptides 2002;23:889–93.

60. Yaksh TL. Substance P release from knee joint afferent terminals: modulation by opioids. Brain Res 1988;458:319–24.

61. Ichikawa H, Matsuo S, Wakisaka S, et al. Fine structure of calcitonin gene-related peptide-immunoreactive nerve fibres in the rat temporomandibular joint. Arch Oral Biol 1990;35:727–30.

62. Appelgren A, Appelgren B, Eriksson S, et al. Neuropeptides in temporomandibular joints with rheumatoid arthritis: a clinical study. Scand J Dent Res 1991;99:519–21.

63. Holmlund A, Ekblom A, Hansson P, et al. Concentrations of neuropeptides substance P, neurokinin A, calcitonin gene–related peptide, neuropeptide Y and vasoactive intestinal polypeptide in synovial fluid of the human temporomandibular joint. A correlation with symptoms, signs and arthroscopic findings. Int J Oral Maxillofac Surg 1991;20:228–31.

64. Kido MA, Kiyoshima T, Kondo T, et al. Distribution of substance P and calcitonin gene–related peptide-like immunoreactive nerve fibers in the rat temporomandibular joint. J Dent Res 1993;72:592–8.

65. Bryant CJ, Harrison SD, Hopper C, et al. Use of intra-articular morphine for postoperative analgesia following TMJ arthroscopy. Br J Oral Maxillofac Surg 1999;37:391–6.

66. Furst IM, Kryshtalskyj B, Weinberg S. The use of intra-articular opioids and bupivacaine for analgesia following temporomandibular joint arthroscopy: a prospective, randomized trial. J Oral Maxillofac Surg 2001;59:979–84.

67. List T, Tegelberg A, Haraldson T, et al. Intra-articular morphine as analgesic in temporomandibular joint arthralgia/osteoarthritis. Pain 2001;94:275–82.

68. Yuge O, Matsumoto M, Kitahaa L, et al. Direct opioid application to peripheral nerve does not alter compound action potentials. Anesth Analg 1985;64: 667–71.

69. Senami M, Aoki M, Kitahata L, et al. Lack of opiate effects on cat C polymodal nociceptive fibers. Pain 1986;27:81–90.

70. Stein C, Millan M, Shippenberg T, et al. Peripheral effects of fentanyl upon nociception in inflamed tissue of the rat. Neurosci Lett 1988;84:225–8.

71. Stein C, Comisel K, Haimerl E, et al. Analgesic effect of intraarticular morphine after arthroscopic knee surgery. N Engl J Med 1991;325:1123–6.

72. Bartho L, Szolscanyi J. Opiate agonists inhibit neurogenic plasma extravasation in the rat. Eur J Pharmacol 1981;73:101–4.

73. Barber A. Mu- and kappa-opioid receptor agonists produce peripheral inhibition of neu-rogenic plasma extravasation in rat skin. Eur J Pharmacol 1993;236:113–20.

74. Ruff M, Wahl S, Mergenhagen S, et al. Opiate receptor-mediated chemotaxis for human monocytes. Neuropeptides 1985;5:363–366.

75. Sibinga NES, Goldstein A. Opioid peptides and opioid receptors in cells of the immune system. Ann Rev Immunol 1988;6:219–49.

76. Ferriera S, Nakamura M. Prostaglandin hyperalgesia II: the peripheral analgesic activity of morphine, enkephalins and opioid antagonists. Prostaglandins 1979;23:53–60.

77. Cai BB, Cairns BE, Sessle BJ, et al. Sex-related suppression of reflex jaw muscle activity by peripheral morphine but not GABA. Neuroreport 2001;12:3457–60.

78. Portenoy RK. Chronic opioid therapy for nonmalignant pain: from models to practice. APS J 1992;1:285–8.

79. Robins LN, David DH, Nurco DN. How permanent was Vietnam drug addiction? Am J Public Health 1974;64:38–43.

80. Kanner RM, Foley KM. Patterns of narcotic drug use in cancer pain clinic. Ann N Y Acad Sci 1981;362:161–72.

81. Foley KM. Clinical tolerance to opioids. In: Basbaum AI, Bessons JM, editors. Towards a new pharmacology of pain. Philadelphia: John Wiley and Sons; 1991. p. 181–197.

82. Brescia FJ, Portenoy RK, Ryan M. Pain, opioid use and survival in hospitalized patients with advanced cancer. J Clin Oncol 1992;10:149–55.

83. Houde RW. Systemic analgesics and related drugs: narcotic analgesics. In: Bonica JJ, Ventafriddas V, editors. Advances in pain research and therapy. Vol. 2. New York: Raven; 1979. p. 263–73.

84. Inturrisi CE, Foley KM. Narcotic analgesics in the management of pain. In: Kuhar M, Pasternaks GW, editors. Analgesics: neurochemical, behavioral, and clinical perspectives. New York: Raven; 1984. p. 257–88.

85. Kuhn R. Treatment of depressive states with imipramine hydrochloride. Am J Psychiatry 1958;115:459–64.

86. Paoli F, Darcourt G, Corsa P. Note preliminaire sur l'action de l'imipramine dans les etats douloureux. Rev Neurol 1960;2:503–4.

87. Acton J, McKenna JE, Melzack R. Amitriptyline produces analgesia in the formalin pain test. Exp Neurol 1992;117:94–6.

88. Bendtsen L, Jensen R, Olesen J. Amitriptyline, a combined serotonin and noradrenaline re-uptake inhibitor, reduces exteroceptive suppression of temporal muscle activity in patients with chronic tension-type headache. Electroencephalogr Clin Neurophysiol 1996;101:418–22.

89. Bendtsen L, Jensen R, Olesen J. A non-selective (amitriptyline), but not a selective (citalopram), serotonin reuptake inhibitor is effective in the prophylactic treatment of chronic tension-type headache. J Neurol Neurosurg Psychiatry 1996;61:285–90.

90. Brown RS, Bottomley WK. Utilization and mechanism of action of tricyclic antidepressants in the treatment of chronic facial pain: a review of the literature. Anesth Prog 1990;37:223–9.

91. Max MB, Zeigler D, Shoaf SE, et al. Effects of a single oral dose of desipramine on postoperative morphine analgesia. J Pain Symptom Manage 1992;7:454–62.

92. Max MB, Lynch SA, Muir J, et al. Effects of desipramine, amitriptyline, and fluoxetine on pain in diabetic neuropathy. N Engl J Med 1992;326:1250–6.

93. Leijon G, Boivie J. Central post-stroke pain—a controlled trial of amitriptyline and carbamazepine. Pain 1989;36:27–36.

94. Kvinesdal B, Molin J, Froland A, et al. Imipramine treatment of painful diabetic neuropathy. JAMA 1984;251:1727–30.

95. Coquoz D, Porchet HC, Dayer P. Central analgesic effects of desipramine, fluvoxamine, and moclobemide after single oral dosing: a study in healthy volunteers. Clin Pharmacol Ther 1993;54:339–44.

96. Hall H, Ogren SO. Effects of antidepressant drugs on different receptors in the brain. Eur J Pharmacol 1981;70:393–407.

97. Zubieta J-K, Heitzeg MM, Smith YR, et al. COMT $val^{158}met$ genotype affects m-opioid neurotransmitter responses to a pain stressor. Science 2003;299:1240–3.

98. Gobel H, Hamouz V, Hansen C, et al. Chronic tension-type headache: amitriptyline reduces clinical headache duration and experimental pain sensitivity but does not alter pericranial muscle activity readings. Pain 1994;59:241–9.

99. Bryson HM, Wilde MI. Amitriptyline. A review of its pharmacological properties and therapeutic use in chronic pain states. Drugs Aging 1996;8:459–76.

100. Godfrey RG. A guide to the understanding and use of tricyclic antidepressants in the overall management of fibromyalgia and other chronic pain syndromes. Arch Intern Med 1996;156:1047–52.

101. Goldenberg DL. A review of the role of tricyclic medications in the treatment of fibromyalgia syndrome. J Rheumatol Suppl 1989; 19:137–9.

102. Goldenberg D, Mayskiy M, Mossey C, et al. A randomized, double-blind crossover trial of fluoxetine and amitriptyline in the treatment of fibromyalgia. Arthritis Rheum 1996;39:1852–9.

103. Scudds RA, McCain GA, Rollman GB, et al. Improvements in pain responsiveness in patients with fibrositis after successful treatment with amitriptyline. J Rheumatol Suppl 1989;19:98–103.

104. Bowsher D. The effects of pre-emptive treatment of postherpetic neuralgia with amitriptyline: a randomized, double-blind, placebo-controlled trial. J Pain Symptom Manage 1997;13:327–31.

105. Eija K, Tiina T, Pertti NJ. Amitriptyline effectively relieves neuropathic pain following treatment of breast cancer. Pain 1996;64:293–302.

106. Eisenberg E, Yaari A, Har-Shai Y. Chronic, burning facial pain following cosmetic facial surgery. Ann Plast Surg 1996;36:76–9.

107. Jett MF, McGuirk J, Waligora D, et al. The effects of mexiletine, desipramine and fluoxetine in rat models involving central sensitization. Pain 1997;69:161–9.

108. McQuay HJ, Tramer M, Nye BA, et al. A systematic review of antidepressants in neuropathic pain. Pain 1996;68:217–27.

109. Brosen K, Gram LF. Clinical significance of the sparteine/debrisoquin oxidation polymorphism. Eur J Clin Pharmacol 1989;36:537–47.

110. Diamond S, Balters BJ. Chronic tension headache-treated with amitriptyline—a double-blind study. Headache 1971;1:110–6.

111. Watson C. Therapeutic window for amitriptyline analgesia. Can Med Assoc J 1984;130:105–6.

112. Detweiler MB, Harpold GJ. Bupropion-induced acute dystonia. Ann Pharmacother 2002;36:251–4.

113. Miller LG, Jankovic J. Persistent dystonia possibly induced by flecainide. Mov Disord 1992;7:62–3.

114. Gerber PE, Lynd LD. Selective serotonin-reuptake inhibitor-induced movement disorders. Ann Pharmacother 1998;32:692–8.

115. Winocur E, Gavish A, Volfin G, et al. Oral motor parafunctions among heavy drug addicts and their effects on signs and symptoms of temporomandibular disorders. J Orofac Pain 2001;15:56–63.

116. Burt DR, Kamatchi GL. GABA$_A$ receptor subtypes: from pharmacology to molecular biology. FASEB J 1991;5:2916–23.

117. Goodchild CS, Serrao JM. Intrathecal midazolam in the rat: evidence for spinally mediated analgesia. Br J Anaesth 1987;59:1563–70.

118. Crawford ME, Jensen FM, Toftdahl DB, et al. Direct spinal effect of intrathecal and extradural midazolam on visceral noxious stimulation in the rabbit. Br J Anaesth 1993;70:642–6.

119. Dunn SMJ, Bateson AN, Martin IL. Molecular neurobiology of the GABA$_A$ receptor. Int Rev Neurobiol 1994;36:51–96.

120. Bowery NG. GABA$_B$ receptor pharmacology. Annu Rev Pharmacol Toxicol 1993; 33:109–47.

121. Djamgoz MBA. Diversity of GABA receptors in the vertebrate outer retina. Trends Neurosci 1995;18:118–20.

122. Mott DD, Lewis DV. Bridging the cleft at GABA synapses in the brain. Int Rev Neurobiol 1994;36:97–223.

123. Hao JX, Xu XJ, Wiesenfeld-Hallin Z. Allodynia-like effect in rat after ischemic spinal cord injury photochemically induced by laser irradiation. Pain 1991;45:175–85.

124. Hao JX, Xu XJ, Yu YX, et al. Baclofen reverses the hypersensitivity of dorsal horn wide dynamic range neurons to mechanical stimulation after transient spinal cord ischemia: implications for a tonic GABAergic inhibitory control of myelinated fiber input. J Neurophysiol 1992;68:392–6.

125. Dapas F, Hartman SF, Martinez L, et al. Baclofen for the treatment of acute low-back syndrome: a double-blind comparison with placebo. Spine 1985;10:345–9.

126. Mellick LB, Mellick GA. Successful treatment of reflex sympathetic dystrophy with gabapentin. Am J Emerg Med 1995;13:96.

127. Veldman PH, Reynen HM, Arntz IE, et al. Signs and symptoms of reflex sympathetic dystrophy: prospective study of 829 patients. Lancet 1993;342:1012–6.

128. Jones MG, Munson JB, Thompson SW. A role for nerve growth factor in sympathetic sprouting in rat dorsal root ganglia. Pain 1999;79:21–9.

129. McLachlan EM, Hu P. Axonal sprouts containing calcitonin gene–related peptide and substance P form pericellular baskets around large diameter neurons after sciatic nerve transection in the rat. Neuroscience 1998;84:961–5.

130. Ramer MS, French GD, Bisby MA. Wallerian degeneration is required for both neuropathic pain and sympathetic sprouting into the DRG. Pain 1997;72:71–8.

131. Ramer M, Bisby M. Reduced sympathetic sprouting occurs in dorsal root ganglia after axotomy in mice lacking low-affinity neurotrophin receptor. Neurosci Lett 1997;228:9–12.

132. Woolf CJ. Phenotypic modification of primary sensory neurons: the role of nerve growth factor in the production of persistent pain. Philos Trans R Soc Lond B Biol Sci 1996;351:441–8.

133. Tanelian DL. Reflex sympathetic dystrophy. A reevaluation of the literature. Pain Forum 1996;5:247–56.

134. Puzas JE, Miller MD, Rosier RN. Pathologic bone formation. Clin Orthop 1989;245:269–81.

135. Reid R, Cooke H. Postoperative ionizing radiation in the management of heterotopic bone formation in the temporomandibular joint. J Oral Maxillofac Surg 1999;57:900–6.

136. Durr ED, Turlington EG, Foote RL. Radiation treatment of heterotopic bone formation in the temporomandibular joint articulation. Int J Radiat Oncol Biol Phys 1993;27:863–9.

137. Robinson M, Arnet G. Cobalt radiation to prevent reankylosis after repeated surgical failures: report of case. J Oral Surg 1977;35:850–4.

138. Schwartz HC, Kagan AR. Zygomatico-coronoid ankylosis secondary to heterotopic bone formation: combined treatment by surgery and radiation therapy—a case report. J Maxillofac Surg 1979;7: 158–61.

139. Coventry MB, Scanlon PW. The use of radiation to discourage ectopic bone. A nine-year study about the hip. J Bone Joint Surg 1981;63:201–8.

140. Kienapfel H, Koller M, Wust A, et al. Prevention of heterotopic bone formation after total hip arthroplasty: a prospective randomised study comparing postoperative radiation therapy with indomethacin. Arch Orthop Trauma Surg 1999;119:296–302.

141. Ron E, Modan B, Boice JD, et al. Tumors of the brain and nervous system after radiotherapy in childhood. N Engl J Med 1988; 319:1033–9.

142. Elmstedt E, Lindholm TS, Nilsson OS, et al. Effect of ibuprofen on heterotopic ossification after hip replacement. Acta Orthop Scand 1985;56:25–7.

143. Pritchett JW. Ketorolac prophylaxis against heterotopic ossification after hip replacement. Clin Orthop 1995;314:162–5.

144. Sodemann B, Persson PE, Nilsson OS. Prevention of heterotopic ossification by nonsteroid antiinflammatory drugs after total hip arthroplasty. Clin Orthop 1988;237:158–63.

145. Wahlstrom O, Risto O, Djerk K, et al. Heterotopic bone formation prevented by diclofenac. Prospective study of 100 hip arthroplasties. Acta Orthop Scand 1991; 62:419–21.

CHAPTER 52

Hypomobility and Hypermobility Disorders of the Temporomandibular Joint

Meredith August, DMD, MD
Maria J. Troulis, DDS, MSc
Leonard B. Kaban, DMD, MD

Hypomobility

Etiology

The etiology of mandibular hypomobility is varied, and successful treatment requires an understanding of the underlying disorder. Trauma is the most commonly identified cause, followed by infection (odontogenic, otitis media, and mastoiditis). Various systemic disease states have been associated with hypomobility, including ankylosing spondylitis, rheumatoid arthritis, and other collagen vascular diseases such as scleroderma. Iatrogenic causes have also been identified and include the sequelae of high-dose radiation involving the muscles of mastication, craniotomy procedures, and, uncommonly, orthognathic surgery. Internal temporomandibular joint (TMJ) derangements may also lead to chronic hypomobility problems. Traumatic perinatal events and neuromuscular conditions can result in hypomobility in infancy. In general terms, congenital ankylosis is defined as limited interincisal opening noted at birth with no

known causative factor. Table 52-1 lists the etiologic factors associated with mandibular hypomobility.

Classification

Various classification schemes have been proposed to describe hypomobility.[1–3]

Trismus is most commonly found in conjunction with spasm of the muscles of mastication. It can be secondary to myofascial pain dysfunction, infection, trauma, tumors, and various medications as well as psychiatric and neurologic factors. Ankylosis may be classified according to location (intra-articular vs extra-articular), type of tissue involved (bony, fibrous, or mixed), and the extent of fusion (complete vs incomplete). True ankylosis is caused by either fibrous or bony fusion of the structures contained within the TMJ capsule and, in its most severe state, is characterized by a bony union of the condyle to the glenoid fossa. True ankylosis has been further classified into subtypes depending on the anatomic positioning of the condyle and the extent of bridging bone. Topazian proposed a

three-stage classification to grade complete ankylosis as follows: stage I, ankylotic bone limited to the condylar process; stage II, ankylotic bone extending to the sigmoid notch; and stage III, ankylotic bone extending to the coronoid process.[4] Other classification schemes have also been proposed.[5] However, the utility of these designations in terms of treatment planning is questionable. So-called false ankylosis (pseudoankylosis), in contrast, describes limited mobility based on extra-articular factors such as fibrosis, mechanical obstruction (eg, zygomatic arch fracture), muscle spasm, or other pathologies.

Clinical Presentation

Patients with fibrous or bony ankylosis present with restricted mandibular motion and, depending on the patient's age and the condition's etiology, may have an abnormality in mandibular size and shape. Unilateral pathology in children may result in significant problems with lower facial symmetry. A shortened ramus on the affected side is usually accompanied by a prominent antegonial notch

Table 52-1   Etiologic Factors Associated with Hypomobility of the Mandible
Trismus
Odontogenic: myofascial pain, malocclusion, erupting teeth
Infection: pterygomandibular, lateral pharyngeal, temporal
Trauma: fracture of the mandible, muscle contusion
Tumors: nasopharyngeal tumors, tumors that invade jaw muscles
Psychologic: hysteric trismus
Pharmacologic: phenothiazines
Neurologic: tetanus
Pseudoankylosis
Depressed zygomatic arch fracture
Fracture dislocation of the condyle
Adhesions of the coronoid process
Hypertrophy of the coronoid process
Fibrosis of the temporalis muscle
Myositis ossificans
Scar contracture following thermal injury
Tumor of the condyle or coronoid process
True ankylosis
Trauma: intracapsular fracture (child), medial displaced condylar fracture (adult),
obstetric trauma, intracapsular fibrosis
Infection: otitis media, suppurative arthritis
Inflammation: rheumatoid arthritis, Still's disease, ankylosing spondylitis,
Marie-Strümpell disease, psoriatic arthritis
Surgical: postoperative complications of temporomandibular joint or orthognathic surgery

noted on radiographs. Such unilateral mandibular growth disturbances have secondary effects on the maxillary occlusal plane and midfacial structures (pyriform rims and bony orbits).

Ankylosis in adults is characterized by limited jaw opening and decreased translation, but the morphologic characteristics found in the growing patient are frequently absent. Loss of condylar structure and mandibular angle prominence is seen in cases caused by rheumatologic disease, specifically scleroderma. An associated anterior open bite is frequently noted with the loss of ramus/condyle height (Figure 52-1). Unilateral cases with a traumatic etiology may result in malocclusion and ipsilateral dental prematurities. A physical examination is helpful in identifying whether the process is bilateral or unilateral and may be suggestive of the etiology.

Imaging Assessment

In addition to the clinical examination, radiographic assessment is critical in evaluating and treating patients with hypomobility disorders. Plain radiographs are limited in delineating the true extent of the deformity. What can be identified with these studies are the presence or absence of a TMJ space, obvious bony abnormalities in the region of the joint, and coronoid hyperplasia. Sanders and colleagues have reported that conventional radiographs underestimate the extent of bony ankylosis and give little information about the anatomy medial to the condyle.[6] The use of computed tomography (CT) scans (including axial, coronal, and sagittal views with three-dimensional reconstruction) is helpful in fully defining the extent of ankylosis as well as the relationship of the ankylotic mass to important anatomic

structures, especially at the skull base (pterygoid plates, carotid canal, jugular foramen, and foramen spinosum) (Figure 52-2).[7,8] Often in post-traumatic cases the distance between the maxillary artery and the medial pole of the condyle is reduced—a contrast CT helps to determine this distance. Fusion of the ankylotic mass to the base of the skull can also be appreciated on CT scans. Since adequate treatment requires the removal of the mass in toto, knowledge of this anatomy preoperatively is critical to surgical planning and long-term success.

Magnetic resonance imaging (MRI) has had a great impact on TMJ evaluation, especially regarding the delineation of meniscal position. Diagnosis of fibrous ankylosis is possible with the use of MRI, but the CT scan is superior in demonstrating bony pathology.[9]

Post-traumatic Hypomobility

Trauma is the most common cause of bony and fibrous ankylosis as reported by multiple authors.[10–12] It is hypothesized that the formation of an intra-articular hematoma with subsequent scarring and new bone formation is the common precipitant. Most often, a medially displaced fracture dislocation of the condyle is found. Subsequent hypomobility is of particular concern in growing children in whom the development of hypomobility can have significant impact on facial

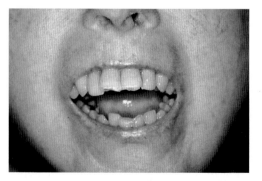

FIGURE **52-1**   *Patient with systemic sclerosis (scleroderma) demonstrating a limitation in jaw opening and skin changes characterized by perioral furrows and telangiectasia.*

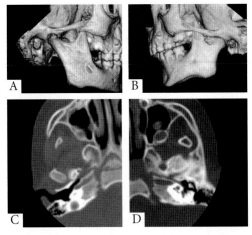

FIGURE 52-2 *Three-dimensional (A, B) and axial (C, D) computed tomography scans of a patient with extensive bony ankylosis of the left temporomandibular joint. Note the comparison with the unaffected right side (A, C). Coronoid hyperplasia is also seen on the affected left side (B, D).*

growth (Figure 52-3). In addition, resultant hypomobility can lead to speech impairment, difficulty with chewing, poor oral hygiene, limited access to dental care, and possible airway compromise. In large reviews of pediatric facial fractures, the condylar and subcondylar regions were

involved in > 40% of cases.[13,14] In many cases a direct blow to the chin with transmission of the impact force to the condyles resulted in the fracture. Prolonged immobilization, secondary to treatment with maxillomandibular fixation, splinting, or mechanical obstruction can lead to subsequent ankylosis.

Extra-articular ankylosis can also occur with coronoid fractures and fractures of the zygomatic arch. In both cases the resultant hematoma may calcify, resulting in a fusion of the coronoid process to the zygomatic arch.

Myositis ossificans traumatica (MOT), or fibrodysplasia ossificans circumscripta, is generally associated with a traumatic event or repeated episodes of minor trauma and can result in mandibular hypomobility.[15,16] The precise mechanism remains to be elucidated but appears to involve fibrous metaplasia and subsequent ossification of both soft tissues and muscle after bleeding and myonecrosis. Histologically, both mature and woven bone can be noted (sometimes in distinct zones), and both

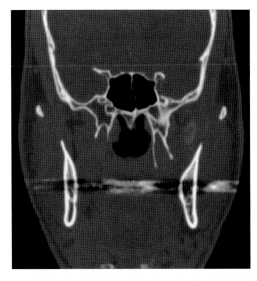

FIGURE 52-4 *Computed tomography scan of patient with myositis ossificans traumatica demonstrating a focus of calcification within the medial pterygoid muscle on the left side.*

osteoblasts and osteocytes are abundant. MOT is characterized by soft tissue ectopic ossifications and is relatively uncommon in the head and neck regions. Of all reported cases involving the muscles of mastication, the masseter is most commonly affected. MOT involving the medial pterygoid muscle and secondary to local anesthesia injections has also been reported.[17] Diagnosis is confirmed by identification of calcifications within the muscles of mastication on CT scans (Figure 52-4). Minimal response is found with physical therapy and stretching exercises; consequently, surgical treatment is often undertaken to remove the ectopic bone. Other treatment modalities include acetic acid iontophoresis, magnesium therapy, and the use of etidronate sodium.[18,19] Since repeated relapses and refractory cases are common, the use of multiple treatment modalities may be associated with the best outcome.

Postinfectious Hypomobility

A TMJ infection resulting in hypomobility is most commonly the result of contiguous spread from an odontogenic infection, otitis media, or mastoiditis.[20, 21] In the era of aggressive antibiotic treatment of infection,

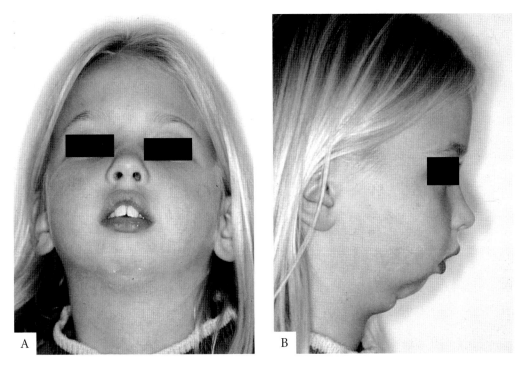

FIGURE 52-3 *A and B, Evident mandibular growth disturbance is noted in this child who has had bilateral condylar fractures. Note the submental scar secondary to a laceration sustained at the time of the bony injury.*

such reported cases are now relatively uncommon. Hematogenous spread of infection has also been reported in association with disease states such as tuberculosis, gonorrhea, and scarlet fever.

Various case series describe deep fascial space infections manifesting themselves as hypomobility and often being misdiagnosed at initial presentation.[22,23] Odontogenic infection is commonly associated with trismus. In such cases associated symptoms (fever, dysphagia) are likely present, and CT scanning is invaluable in determining a diagnosis and in treatment planning. Medial pterygoid abscess formation or fibrosis secondary to hematoma organization can be precipitated by an inferior alveolar nerve block or posterior superior alveolar block. A history of recent dental treatment should suggest this possibility; the use of CT imaging can help delineate the anatomy of the masticator and pharyngeal spaces.

Mass lesions (both benign and malignant) can also result in mandibular hypomobility. Squamous cell carcinoma of the tongue base or tonsillar pillar is often accompanied by trismus. Masses involving the mandibular condyle invariably affect range of motion and need to be included in the differential diagnosis of hypomobility.

Hypomobility following Radiation Therapy

Mandibular hypomobility is a common sequela of the treatment of head and neck malignancies (Figure 52-5). The resultant fibromyositis caused by radiation therapy may exacerbate the postsurgical problems caused by large ablative procedures.[24] Goldstein and colleagues reviewed the effects of tumoricidal radiation therapy on restricted mandibular opening and found a linear dose-related effect.[25] Mandibular dysfunction increased as the dose to the pterygoid muscles increased. The authors reported diminution in opening with doses as low as 15 Gy. Pow and colleagues reported that 30% of patients treated for

nasopharyngeal carcinoma with high-dose radiation therapy had significant trismus compared with age-matched nonradiated control subjects.[26] Radiation therapy for primary tumors of the retromolar trigone was associated with a 12% incidence of long-term trismus. This association, compounded by resultant xerostomia, severely compromises the ability of these patients to maintain oral health.

The efficacy of early interventional physical therapy has been described. Buchbinder and colleagues compared the outcome of unassisted exercise, mechanically assisted exercise with the use of tongue blades, and use of the Therabite System in radiated patients.[27] All patients presented with an interincisal opening of < 30 mm. The response to each therapy was recorded every 2 weeks over a 10-week period. All groups showed improvement over the first 4 weeks, but the group using a mechanical exercising device (ie, Therabite System) continued to demonstrate an improvement of maximal interincisal opening (MIO) over the full 10-week period that was significantly greater than that of the other two groups.

Postcraniotomy Hypomobility

Mandibular hypomobility after intracranial surgical procedures is an uncommon yet reported phenomenon.[28,29] Mechanistically, this problem is secondary to neurosurgical procedures performed through the temporal bone requiring an incision of the temporalis muscle. Subsequent fibrosis of the muscle may then result in limited opening, which is best treated with coronoid resection followed by vigorous physical therapy. The incidence of this problem is not known, but a review by Kawaguchi and colleagues reported limited mouth opening in as many as 33% of patients undergoing frontotemporal craniotomy procedures.[30] Although most are self-limiting, persistent hypomobility can severely compromise subsequent airway and anesthesia management in these

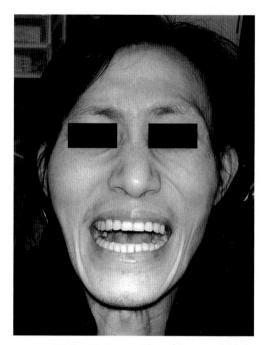

FIGURE **52-5** *Patient with a history of high-dose radiation therapy and subsequent reirradiation for recurrence of nasopharyngeal carcinoma. Note the severe temporal atrophy and the limitation in opening.*

patients and needs to be recognized. The maximal opening is not improved with the use of muscle relaxants or local or general anesthesia. Patients who have undergone skull base surgery may also manifest severe hypomobility postoperatively. If such surgery requires the dissection of the temporalis muscle inferior to the zygoma, pseudoankylosis of the mandible may be encountered.

Inflammatory and Rheumatologic Causes

Ankylosing spondylitis (Bekhterev's disease) is a chronic and progressive inflammatory condition most commonly affecting the sacroiliac joints and the spine. The male-to-female ratio of incidence is reported to be 2.4:1, and the severity and extension of the disease in male patients is found to be more severe. TMJ involvement in ankylosing spondylitis has been reported in between 1 and 22% of affected individuals and can include severe bony deformation and ankylosis.[31,32] The most commonly reported radiographic findings in the condyle and glenoid fossa region include flattening, erosions, sclerosis, osteophytes, subcortical cysts, and bony erosion at the insertion of the masseter (angle of the jaw) and temporalis muscles (coronoid process). One large prospective study evaluating 50 patients with ankylosing spondylitis did not show any correlation between the bony severity noted in the cervical spine and TMJ abnormalities.[33] These authors reported a 22% incidence of TMJ involvement, either clinical or radiographic. Because the majority of patients reported no pain or limitation in function, the radiographic findings included in this study may well have represented early changes in the disease process.

TMJ involvement in rheumatoid arthritis follows the same destructive path as do other joints. Generally, the severity of joint dysfunction is correlated with the stage of rheumatoid arthritis. Radiographically, the most common findings in the condylar region are the following: sclerosis (75%), erosion (50%), and flattening (30%).[34] These bony changes commonly result in progressive malocclusion secondary to the loss of ramus/condyle height and subsequent apertognathia. Juvenile rheumatoid arthritis is chronic arthritis diagnosed in childhood before the age of 16 years. It is estimated that > 60% of patients with juvenile rheumatoid arthritis manifest TMJ involvement.[35] However, multiple authors point out that despite radiographic and morphologic changes in the joint, a minority of affected children (generally < 25%) report pain with function.[36,37] Svensson and colleagues report that restricted mouth opening was a more common finding.[38] The duration of active disease and a history of pain with function correlate positively with progressive TMJ dysfunction. With active disease in growing children, abnormalities in facial growth, mandibular hypoplasia, and hypomobility are common problems (Figure 52-6).

Scleroderma (progressive systemic sclerosis) is a disorder of unknown etiology affecting multiple organ systems and char-acterized by abundant fibrosis of the skin, blood vessels, and visceral organs. It is believed that abnormalities in small blood vessels result in the progressive thickening and fibrotic changes noted in affected tissues, particularly those of the gastrointestinal tract, heart, lung, and kidney as well as diffuse skin involvement. Mandibular movement can become severely limited in affected individuals secondary to facial skin fibrosis and atrophy of the muscles of mastication (particularly the masseter and medial pterygoid muscles).[39] Bony changes in the mandible are also reported and include severe resorption of the angles, condyles, and coronoid processes (osteolysis).[40] The bony lesions are believed to be of ischemic origin but may be exacerbated by the tightness of the tissue in the region of the mandibular angles causing pressure resorption as well. In addition to the severe limitation in jaw movement, the small mouth orifice and progressive malocclusion make oral function and access to dental care problematic for these patients.

Hypomobility following Orthognathic Surgery

Hypomobility following orthognathic surgery has been reported by multiple authors and appears to be most commonly associated with the bilateral sagittal split osteotomy.[41,42] This postoperative limited opening has been commonly attributed to muscle atrophy and soft tissue scar formation. Atrophic muscular changes seem to be exacerbated by prolonged use of maxillomandibular fixation, and the advent of rigid internal fixation appears to have limited this problem. Intra-articular pathology (edema, hemorrhage) as well as condylar torque may also result in hypomobility. In such cases rigid internal fixation may predispose to this problem. Van Sickels and colleagues have hypothesized that condylar torque at the time of the bilateral sagittal split osteotomy may cause impingement of the condyle against the disk, causing a mechanical impediment to opening.[43]

Management of hypomobility after orthognathic surgery depends on the underlying cause. Trauma to the muscles of mastication is best managed postoperatively by vigorous physical therapy protocols. Those patients who fail to improve within the first 3 months need to be carefully evaluated for an intra-articular source of the problem. Edema, bleeding, and fibrosis within the joint space can frequently be managed by arthrocentesis procedures, especially when recognized early. If a mechanical obstruction to opening is suspected, CT is a helpful diagnostic aid. Condylar torque is best treated by reoperation with appropriate positioning of the proximal segment.[44]

General Treatment Considerations

The treatment goal for all hypomobility states is the restoration of normal and comfortable jaw motion and prevention of disease progression. Reversible causes such as muscular hyperactivity or spasm, infectious and inflammatory causes, and medication-induced limitations must be identified and treated. Restoration of function in cases of

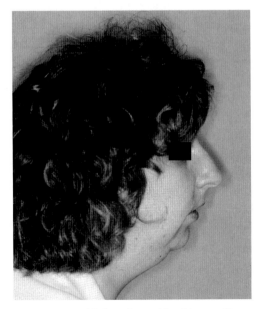

FIGURE 52-6 *Adult patient with a history of juvenile rheumatoid arthritis affecting the temporomandibular joints and resulting in a mandibular growth disturbance and hypomobility.*

ankylosis can be difficult. Proper treatment requires excision of the involved structures and immediate reconstruction. Many operative techniques have been described in the literature, with varying and often less than satisfactory results. As mentioned above, understanding the etiology and anatomy of the problem is critical and can be greatly aided with CT.

The gap arthroplasty is a procedure that creates a new area of articulation distal to the fused TMJ and ankylotic segment.[45,46] Advocates of this procedure describe its simplicity. However, the creation of a pseudoarticulation significantly shortens the ramus height, and the procedure is associated with a high degree of reported reankylosis. Development of postoperative malocclusion and a decreased range of motion are the most common problems associated with this procedure as reported by Rajgopal and colleagues.[47] Because of these limitations, the use of the gap arthroplasty to treat ankylosis has been largely abandoned.

Temporomandibular ankylosis is more commonly treated with complete excision of the ankylotic mass and, if required, by subsequent joint reconstruction. Our protocol for the treatment of ankylosis follows that documented by Kaban and colleagues, a sequential protocol for the treatment of TMJ ankylosis that is based on aggressive resection of the ankylotic mass.[48] Wide intraoperative exposure is required, and special attention is directed to the medial aspect of the joint to ensure that bony, fibrous, and granulation tissue are completely removed. In addition to this aggressive resection of the bony and fibrous mass, dissection and stripping of the temporalis, masseter, and medial pterygoid muscles followed by ipsilateral coronoidectomy are performed in all cases through the same incision. Longstanding ankylosis frequently results in muscle fibrosis and coronoid hyperplasia. After this resection is completed, the MIO is measured. If it is found to be < 35 mm,

a contralateral coronoidectomy is performed via an intraoral approach to attain the desired level of opening. Because complete resection of the ankylotic mass frequently results in substantial loss of ramus height, subsequent reconstruction must address this fact and attempt to restore occlusion as well as function. Commonly, a temporalis fascia flap and costochondral graft are employed to both line the glenoid fossa and create ramus height. The patient is placed into maxillomandibular fixation following the reconstruction, and the teeth are placed into a prefabricated occlusal splint. Fixation is maintained for approximately 10 days and after release a strict protocol of physiotherapy is employed. Overall results have been excellent with this approach. After 1 year MIO was maintained at > 35 mm in all 18 patients included in the report. Furthermore, absence of pain with function was reported in all but two patients (Figure 52-7).[48]

Recently, the Kaban protocol has been modified to substitute ramus/condyle reconstruction using distraction osteogenesis, when possible, instead of costochondral grafting.[49] This protocol has the major advantage of eliminating the donor site operation and allowing for immediate vigorous TMJ mobilization. The surgical procedure for the release of the ankylosis is identical to that described above. After the release the jaw is mobilized and the glenoid fossa lined with a temporalis myofascial flap if the native disk is unavailable. The remaining mandibular stump is reshaped to create a narrow and rounded top. A corticotomy is created distally, leaving sufficient bone to serve as a transport disk. The distraction device is secured, the corticotomy completed, and the mobility of the segments tested. Distraction then proceeds at 1 mm/d until the desired length is achieved. The patient begins a program of active jaw motion exercises immediately postoperatively (Figure 52-8).

The use of total joint prostheses has an interesting history in the TMJ. Advocates

describe two major advantages over autogenous reconstruction: (1) the absence of a donor site and (2) the ability of the patient to return to function more quickly. However, multiple complications have been reported—some with devastating consequences for patients.[50–52] Foreign body reaction to any alloplast may occur. In its most severe form, extensive bony erosion in the area of the glenoid fossa has been found. Fragmentation of alloplastic material secondary to function with a migration of particles into contiguous tissue and regional lymph nodes has also been reported. Progressive wear may result in a loosening and fracture of the prosthesis. In addition, the lack of growth potential precludes the use of these joint-replacement systems in young children. Recurrent ankylosis after prosthesis placement has also been reported, with periprosthetic calcifications most commonly seen in younger patients.

TMJ reconstruction with a variety of autogenous tissues has been described. When the extent of bony resection does not severely shorten ramus height, autogenous interpositional grafts may be employed. These include skin, temporal muscle, cartilage, and fascia. A recent review by Chossegros and colleagues has demonstrated superior results (defined by the authors as an interincisal opening of 30 mm or greater over a follow-up period of 3 yr) using full-thickness skin grafts and temporalis muscle.[53] Various bone grafts (costochondral, sternoclavicular, iliac crest, and metatarsal head) have been used to reconstruct ramus height after the resection of ankylosis. First described in the 1920s, the costochondral graft for TMJ reconstruction was popularized in later years by Poswillo, and MacIntosh and Henny.[54,55] Autogenous tissue (particularly the costochondral graft) has the advantage of being biologically acceptable and possessing growth and remodeling potentials that make it a particularly attractive reconstructive choice in the growing child. Potential problems with its use include fracture, resorption, donor site

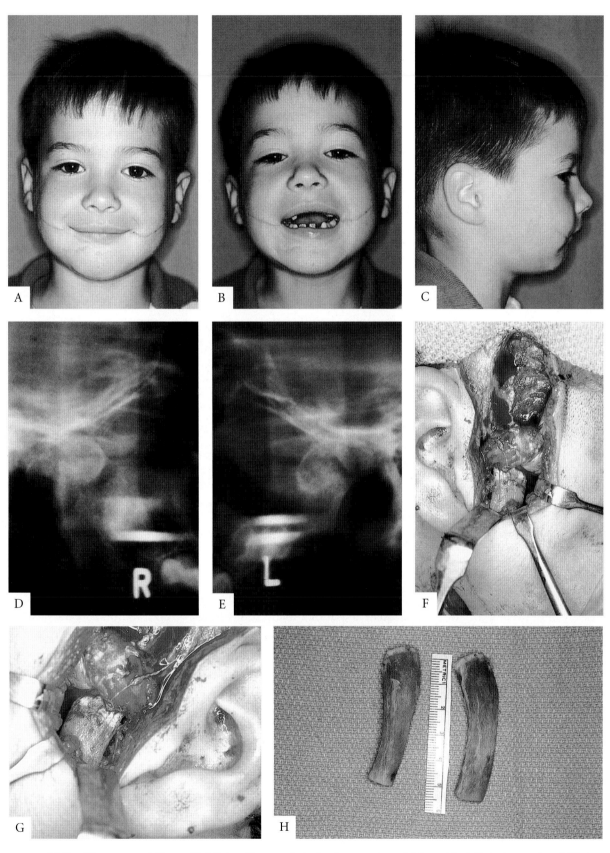

FIGURE 52-7   *Three-year-old boy with bilateral bony ankylosis after a motor vehicle accident that also produced bilateral lacerations of the commissures. Frontal photograph (A), frontal maximal incisal opening (B), and lateral photograph (C). Note the limited opening. Right (D) and left (E) panoramic views of the ankylotic masses of the temporomandibular joints (TMJs). Right (F) and left (G) TMJs exposed after the dissection was completed. H, Harvested costochondral grafts with 1–2 mm cartilaginous caps.* (CONTINUED ON NEXT PAGE)

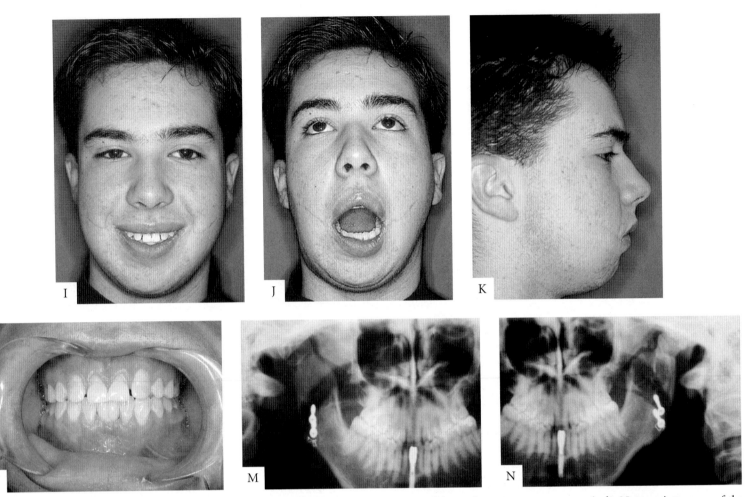

FIGURE **52-7** (CONTINUED)   *Frontal (I), frontal opening (J), and lateral (K) facial views of the patient 11 years postoperatively. Note maintenance of the normal MIO. L, Intraoral views. Right (M) and left (N) panoramic radiographs show remodeling of the costochondral grafts. Reproduced with permission from Kaban LB. Acquired temporomandibular deformities. In: Kaban LB, Troulis MJ, editors. Pediatric oral and maxillofacial surgery. St. Louis (MO): Elsevier; 2004. p. 361–5.*

morbidity, recurrence of ankylosis, and a variable growth behavior of the graft in situ.

Complications Associated with Treatment

Various complications have been reported secondary to the treatment of ankylosis. Dolwick and Armstrong caution that a severe limitation of opening can make the palpation of landmarks difficult and increases the surgical risks.[56] The aggressive bony removal and recontouring that is often required can increase the risk of development of an aural-TMJ fistula if the tympanic plate is displaced posteriorly. In addition, stenosis of the external auditory meatus and subsequent hearing impairment may follow tympanic plate displacement.

Recurrent ankylosis may result from inadequate initial treatment. It most commonly occurs on the medial aspect of the condyle where surgical access is most difficult. Such maneuvers as the postoperative use of nonsteroidal anti-inflammatory drugs and vigorous physical therapy limit problems with recurrent hypomobility.[57,58]

In pediatric patients treated for ankylosis, the expected outcome may be less sanguine.[59] The improvement in interincisal opening, despite strict adherence to the above treatment protocol and compliance with physical therapy regimens, is often significantly less than 35 mm. Posnik and Goldstein reviewed the outcome of nine children and demonstrated a mean MIO of 24.8 mm in unilateral cases and

17.5 mm in bilateral cases measured an average of 2 years postoperatively.[60] The authors caution that improvement in bilateral congenital cases is particularly problematic and may be confounded by the associated neuromuscular and atrophic changes found in these patients.

Peripheral nerve injuries are possible sequelae of all TMJ operations, with the upper branches of the facial nerve being the most vulnerable. Parotid gland injury with subsequent sialocele and fistula formation has also been reported.

As previously described, the costochondral graft is the most commonly used autogenous material for TMJ reconstruction. However, its growth pattern can be unpredictable. Linear overgrowth

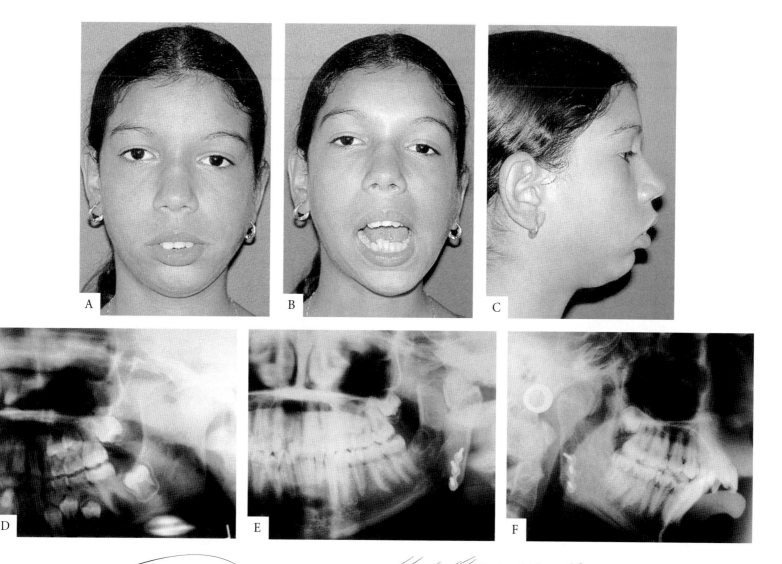

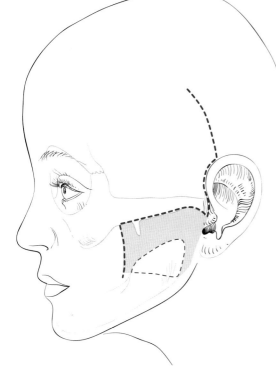

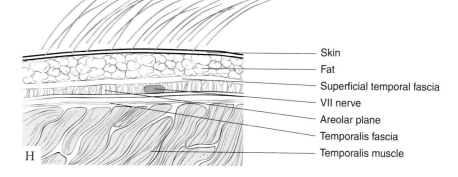

FIGURE 52-8 *Thirteen-year-old female with recurrent ankylosis of the left temporomandibular joint (TMJ) secondary to trauma sustained in a motor vehicle accident. Frontal (A), frontal at maximum incisal opening (MIO) (B), and lateral facial photos (C) of a teenage female with recurrent ankylosis of the left TMJ. D, Panoramic radiograph prior to the first operation demonstrates bony ankylosis of the left TMJ. E, Panoramic radiograph after the patient developed re-ankylosis. She had had a condylectomy and coronoidotomy at another institution. The TMJ was reconstructed with a costochondral graft. There was no soft tissue lining in the joint. F, Lateral cephalogram documenting the mandibular retrognathism. G, Diagram of operative plan, the ankylosis release is carried out via a preauricular incision (outlined in dashed blue line). Excision of the ankylotic mass and coronoidectomy is shown by the shaded area. H, Diagram of the layers of the scalp.* (CONTINUED ON NEXT PAGE)

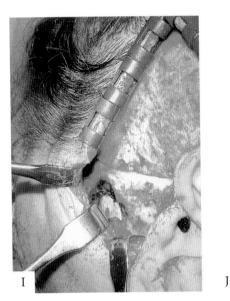

I

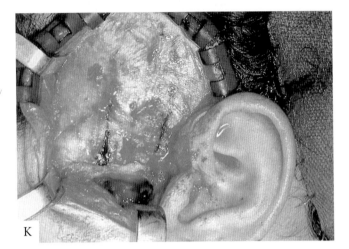

J

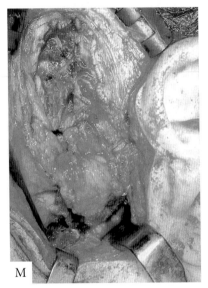

K

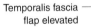

Temporalis fascia
flap elevated

L

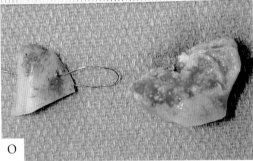

M

Temporalis fascia
wrapped around
zygomatic arch

N

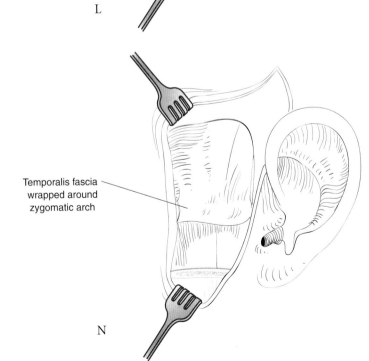

O

FIGURE 52-8 (CONTINUED)   I, *Intraoperative view after dissection was completed. Note the bony ankylotic mass and the coronoid process with obliteration of the sigmoid notch. J, Diagram of the bone removed (shaded area) and the proposed reconstruction using a distraction device (Synthes Maxillofacial, Paoli, PA) instead of a costochondral graft.* K, *Temporalis flap is outlined with* malachite green. *The flap is dissected and rotated over the arch (L) and sutured in place (M, N).* O, *Specimen: ankylotic mass and coronoid process.* (CONTINUED ON NEXT PAGE)

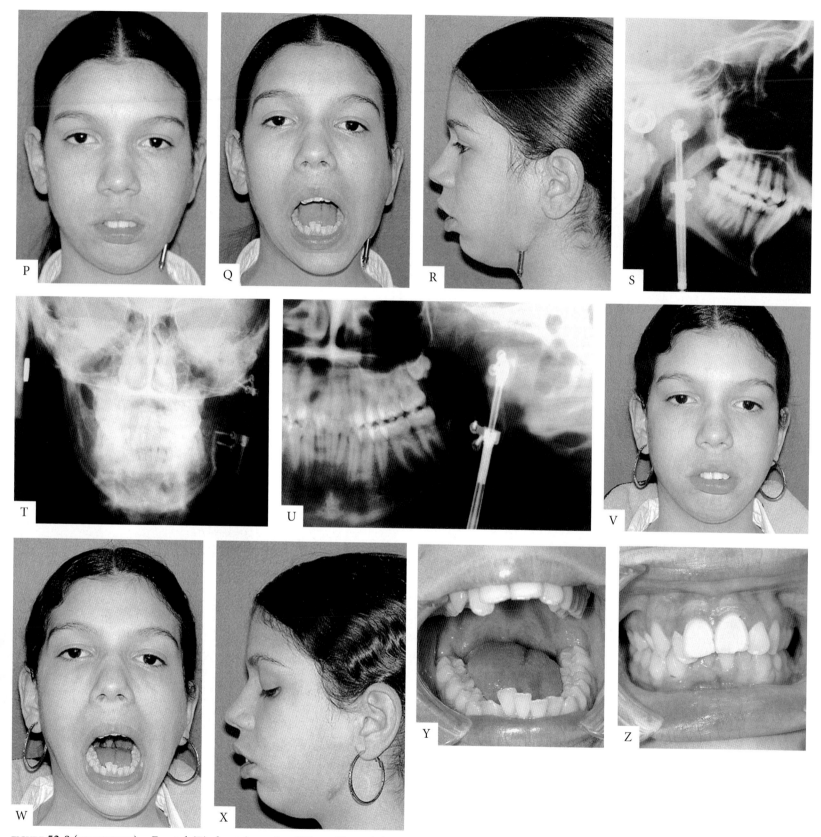

FIGURE 52-8 (CONTINUED) *Frontal (P), frontal opening (Q), and lateral (R) photographs at end distraction. The patient was mobilized and started on physical therapy immediately postoperatively. She was comfortable because there was no donor site operation and no period of maxillomandibular fixation. Lateral (S) and anterior-posterior (A-P) (T) designated as cephalogram and panoramic radiograph (U) at the end of distraction osteogenesis demonstrating the lengthened mandibular ramus. Frontal (V), frontal opening (W), and lateral (X) photographs 1 year after completion of treatment. The patient maintained her TMJ motion and will be beginning presurgical orthodontic treatment to correct her preexisting malocclusion. Open (Y) and closed (Z) intraoral views with the patient opening 39 mm at 1 year.* (CONTINUED ON NEXT PAGE)

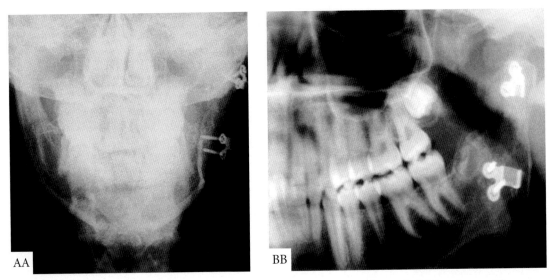

FIGURE **52-8** (CONTINUED)   *A-P cephalogram (AA) and panoramic radiograph (BB) at 1 year. The ramus lengthening is demonstrated by the space between the retained footplates. A–F, I, K, M and O–BB reproduced with permission and G, H, J, L, N adapted from Kaban LB. Acquired temporomandibular deformities. In: Kaban LB, Troulis MJ, editors. Pediatric oral and maxillofacial surgery. St. Louis (MO): Elsevier; 2004. p. 354–7.*

with the subsequent development of asymmetry and malocclusion has been reported by multiple authors.[61,62] The frequency is more common in the growing patient. Munro and colleagues reported 2 of 22 cases of considerable linear overgrowth with resultant chin deviation and development of a Class III malocclusion.[61] Perrott and colleagues reported 3 of 26 cases of lateral bony overgrowth (tumor-like overgrowth), with an evident preauricular fullness and subsequent limitation of opening. However, no cases of linear overgrowth were found in that series of patients.[62]

Postoperative Physical Therapy

Patients with hypomobility disorders require aggressive physical therapy programs, often in conjunction with surgical treatment, to maintain a functional MIO. Various rehabilitation programs have been described in the literature, and approaches include unassisted exercise, tongue-blade and finger-stretch exercises, manual exercisers, and mechanically assisted mandibular motion devices (Figure 52-9). Manipulation under general anesthesia may also be required in refractory or recurrent cases.

Most authors agree that the duration of physical therapy should be prolonged well after a desired MIO is achieved to prevent subsequent relapse.[63]

Hypermobility

Classification

Mandibular subluxation occurs when there is a momentary inability to close the mouth from a maximally open position. It is defined as a self-reducing partial dislocation of the TMJ, during which the condyle passes anterior to the articular eminence. In distinction, dislocation may be considered a long-lasting inability to close the mouth. Subluxation of the condyle may be an early feature of TMJ pathology in a subset of patients. It is often associated with an abnormally wide opening while eating or yawning. Extended periods of mouth opening (eg, during dental treatment or endotracheal anesthesia) may also precipitate subluxation. Subluxation may occur secondary to acute trauma or following a seizure and is also associated with systemic diseases such as Ehlers-Danlos syndrome and Parkinson's disease.

Etiology

TMJ dislocation is defined as an internal derangement characterized by a condylar position anterior and superior to the articular eminence that is not self-reducing. Recurrent dislocation is a relatively unusual problem. Much like subluxation, the etiology is varied. It is observed most frequently in patients with neurologic and connective tissue disorders, those with TMJ dysfunction, and those being treated with phenothiazines and other neuroleptic agents (Table 52-2).

Extrinsic trauma, especially that sustained while the mouth is open, may result in dislocation. Wide opening of any type as well as capsular laxity may be etiologic. Muscular problems secondary to medication use or neurologic disorders may be associated. The problem may be unilateral or bilateral, and patients generally present with associated muscle spasm and pain.

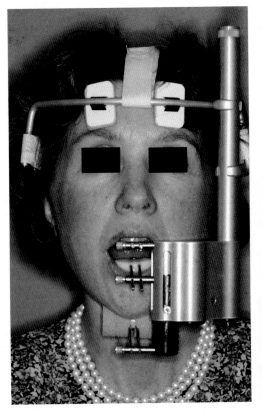

FIGURE **52-9**   *Photograph demonstrating a continuous passive motion device used in the postoperative management of hypomobility.*

Table 52-2 Causes of Hypermobility

Intrinsic trauma: overextension injury
    Yawning
    Vomiting
    Wide biting
    Seizure disorder

Extrinsic trauma
    Trauma: flexion-extension injury to the
        mandible, intubation with general
        anesthesia, endoscopy, dental
        extractions, forceful hyperextension
    Connective tissue disorders:
        hypermobility syndromes,
        Ehlers-Danlos syndrome, Marfan
        syndrome
    Miscellaneous causes: internal
        derangement, dyssynchronous
        muscle function, contralateral
        intra-articular obstruction,
        lost vertical dimension,
        occlusal discrepancies
    Psychogenic: habitual dislocation,
        tardive dyskinesia
    Drug induced: phenothiazines

Treatment Considerations

In the absence of pain, subluxation requires no specific treatment since it is self-reduced by the patient. When associated with wide mouth opening, conscious efforts to avoid this are usually successful at preventing recurrent subluxation. Patients are advised to modify their diets, and dental treatment is done over multiple shorter appointments. The use of bite-blocks during procedures can also be helpful. In cases in which extreme laxity in the joint results in continued problems, surgical intervention may be warranted.

Reduction of mandibular dislocation should be done precipitously before muscle spasm becomes severe and makes the procedure more difficult. Reduction is accomplished by pressing the mandible downward and then backward to relocate the condyle within the glenoid fossa (Figure 52-10). In acute cases this can generally be accomplished without the use of

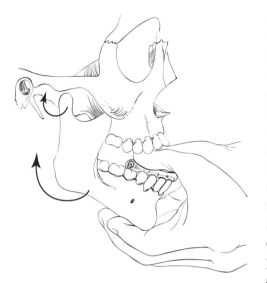

FIGURE 52-10 *Bimanual mandibular manipulation in a downward-posterior direction to disengage the condyle from its open-locked position posterior to the articular eminence. Adapted from Rotskoff KS. Management of hypomobility and hypermobility disorders of the temporomandibular joint. In: Peterson LJ, Indresano AT, Marciani RD, Roser SM. Principles of oral and maxillofacial surgery. Vol. 3. Philadelphia: J.B. Lippincott Company; 1992: p. 2009*

anesthesia. In cases of prolonged or chronic dislocation, the use of muscle relaxants and analgesics may be required. If reduction cannot be thus achieved, general anesthesia may be required. After reduction the mandible should be immobilized for several days to allow for capsular repair, muscle rest, and prevention of recurrence.[64,65]

Chronic dislocation usually requires a more interventional approach. The use of various sclerosing agents has been described in the past. However, caustic agents can result in progressive damage to other joint structures, and multiple reports of misapplications and complications have resulted in the abandonment of this technique. Surgical treatments of various types are reported. Identification of etiology is important when considering surgical correction. In cases of extreme joint laxity, mechanical tightening may be indicated. Plication procedures involve fastening the condyle to a fixed structure to maintain its position within the glenoid fossa. Certain authors advocate the creation of a mechanical impediment to translation by altering the conformation of the articular eminence. Procedures targeting a decrease in muscle pull can also be effective.

Plication procedures are aimed at limiting mandibular motion and may be accomplished in various ways. Removal of redundant capsular tissue (Figure 52-11) is a relatively simple method for addressing laxity, and a review by MacFarlane reported excellent long-term results.[66] Plication of the condyle to the temporal bone and of the coronoid process to the zygomatic arch have also been described. Multiple materials have been used for plication procedures, including both resorbable and nonresorbable sutures and wire. Miniplates and surgical anchors have also been used in both the lateral

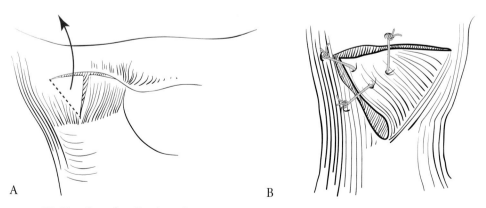

A   B

FIGURE 52-11 *Capsular plication. The exposed lateral capsule is incised (A) and sutured back on itself (B) to tighten and limit capsular laxity. Adapted from Rotskoff KS. Management of hypomobility and hypermobility disorders of the temporomandibular joint. In: Peterson LJ, Indresano AT, Marciani RD, Roser SM. Principles of oral and maxillofacial surgery. Vol. 3. Philadelphia: J.B. Lippincott Company; 1992: p. 2010*

pole of the condyle and the posterior roof of the zygomatic arch. Wolford and colleagues have described the threading of heavy suture material between the eyelets of the surgical anchors, thereby preventing condylar dislocation.[67]

Mechanical impediments to condylar translation effectively deepen the glenoid fossa. Bone and cartilage grafts (cranial, iliac crest, rib, tibial) have been used for this purpose. Nonautogenous material has also been onlayed to the articular eminence. In 1943 LeClerc and Girald described a procedure for inferior displacement of the zygomatic arch to prevent translation (Figure 52-12).[68] Access was gained through an extended preauricular incision, and dissection of the zygomatic arch was performed. An oblique osteotomy downward and forward then allowed the arch to be moved inferiorly. Chossegros and colleagues reported excellent success using this technique in 36 patients with chronic and recurrent dislocation.[53]

The eminectomy procedure was first introduced by Myrhaug in 1951 as a treatment for chronic and habitual dislocation of the condyle.[69] In addition to the standard open eminectomy, reports describing the use of the arthroscope for this purpose have recently appeared in the literature.[70] Both procedures involve the removal of a portion of the articular tubercle and eminence to allow the condyle to move freely.

Concerns regarding the use of the eminectomy procedure include the following: hypermobility of the joint with further damage to contiguous tissues; significant and often bothersome TMJ noise (clicking and crepitation) with function; the potential for facial nerve injury; recurrent dislocation; and inadvertent temporal lobe exposure (anatomic variant).[71]

Reported success rates of surgery to treat dislocation vary considerably. Recurrent dislocation following standard eminectomy procedures ranges from 7 to 33%.[72–74] Patients with significant ligamentous laxity or predisposing conditions (eg, seizure disorders) are prone to recurrent problems. Arthroscopic eminectomy, owing to technical limitations, prevents the complete removal of the medial aspect of the eminence. The consequence of this in terms of recurrence remains to be elucidated.[72,73]

If muscular hyperactivity is associated with chronic recurrent dislocation, removal of the insertion of the lateral pterygoid muscle (lateral pterygoid myotomy) may be an effective treatment. Bowman has reported good success with this procedure,[74] but subsequent animal studies have shown lateral pterygoid electromyographic activity returning to baseline several months after the procedure.[75] However, the long-term efficacy often attributed to this procedure may be sec-

ondary to scarring anterior to the joint capsule, thereby limiting condylar excursion.[76]

The injection of botulinum toxin type A into the lateral pterygoid muscles has also been proposed as a treatment for chronic and recurrent dislocation of the mandible. Ziegler and colleagues reviewed 21 patients treated in this fashion. Injections were given on a 3-month basis with only 2 of 21 patients suffering further dislocations. No adverse side effects were reported in this series.[77] Botulinum toxin type A has an associated latency of 1 week, and its duration of action is between 2 and 3 months. Injections should not be done more often than every 12 weeks to avoid the development of antibodies. An injection dose of between 10 and 50 U into the targeted muscle is usually sufficient.

Clark reviewed the use of botulinum toxin for the treatment of mandibular motor disorders, as well as for the treatment of facial spasm, and expanded on the potential side effects of such treatment.[78] Although local side effects are unusual, the two most common problems encountered were alterations in salivary consistency and an inadvertent weakness of swallowing, speech, and facial muscles. These complications were more commonly reported with lateral pterygoid, soft palate, and tongue injections and were found to be dose dependent.

Summary

This chapter summarizes the spectrum of mobility problems that can affect the TMJ and contiguous structures. The varied etiologic factors associated with hypo- and hypermobility have been reviewed; an understanding of the etiology in each particular case is imperative for appropriate treatment to be rendered. Fortunately, improved imaging techniques, including three-dimensional CT, can be invaluable adjuncts to the history and physical examination. In cases of ankylosis, the extent and nature of the problem is best appreciated with these CT images. Altered anatomy and

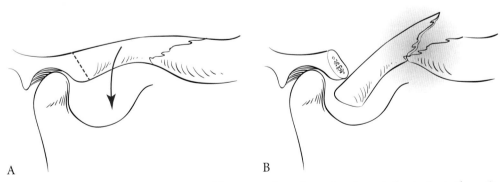

A   B

FIGURE 52-12 *LeClerc procedure. A, An oblique cut using a fissure bur is created anterior to the articular eminence to decrease the frequency of condylar dislocation by obstructing the path of condylar movement. B, The osteotomized segments of the articular eminence are made to overlap one another. Adapted from Rotskoff KS. Management of hypomobility and hypermobility disorders of the temporomandibular joint. In: Peterson LJ, Indresano AT, Marciani RD, Roser SM. Principles of oral and maxillofacial surgery. Vol. 3. Philadelphia: J.B. Lippincott Company; 1992: p. 2010*

the extent of bony bridging can be assessed preoperatively. In addition to operative intervention, long-term success in the management of ankylosis requires aggressive physical therapy programs and longitudinal follow-up.

Hypermobility (both subluxation and dislocation) is similarly reviewed. Again, understanding the causative factors (ligamentous laxity, shallow eminentia, muscular hyperactivity) helps one to focus the treatment planning and to minimize problems with recurrence.

References

1. Aggarwal S, Mukhopakhyay S, Berry M, Bhargava S. Bony ankylosis of the temporomandibular joint: a computed tomographic study. Oral Surg Oral Med Oral Pathol 1990;69:128–32.

2. Chandra P, Dave PK. Temporomandibular joint ankylosis. Prog Clin Biol Res 1985; 187:449–58.

3. El-Mofty S. Ankylosis of the temporomandibular joint. Oral Surg Oral Med Oral Pathol 1972;33:650–60.

4. Topazian RG. Etiology of ankylosis of the temporomandibular joint: analysis of 44 cases. J Oral Surg 1964;22:227–33.

5. Adekeye EO. Ankylosis of the mandible; analysis of 76 cases. J Oral Maxillofac Surg 1983;41:442–9.

6. Sanders R, MacEwan CJ, McCulloch AS. The value of skull radiography in ophthalmology. Acta Radiol 1994;35:429–33.

7. El-Hakim IE, Metwalli SA. Imaging of temporomandibular joint ankylosis. A new radiographic classification. Dentomaxillofac Radiol 2002;31:19–23.

8. de Bont LG, van der Kuijl B, Stegenga B, et al. Computed tomography in the differential diagnosis of temporomandibular joint disorders. Int J Oral Maxillofac Surg 1993; 22:200–9.

9. Roberts D, Schenck J, Joseph P. Temporomandibular joint: magnetic resonance imaging. Radiology 1985;154:829–30.

10. Chidzonga MM. Temporomandibular joint ankylosis: review of thirty-two cases. Br J Oral Maxillofac Surg 1999;37:123–6.

11. de Burgh JE. Post-traumatic disorders of the jaw joint. Ann R Coll Surg Engl 1982; 64:29–36.

12. Guralnick WC, Kaban LB. Surgical treatment of mandibular hypomobility. J Oral Surg 1976;34:343–8.

13. Marianowski R, Martins CC, Potard G, et al. Mandibular fractures in children—long term results. Int J Pediatr Otorhinolaryngol 2003;67:25–30.

14. Zachariades N, Papavassiliou D, Koumoura F. Fractures of the facial skeleton in children. J Craniomaxillofac Surg 1990;18:151–3.

15. Aoki T, Naito H, Ota Y, Shiiki K. Myositis ossificans tramatica of the masticatory muscles: review of the literature and report of a case. J Oral Maxillofac Surg 2002;60:1083–8.

16. Parkash H, Goyal M. Myositis ossificans of the medial pterygoid muscle. A cause for temporomandibular joint ankylosis. Oral Surg Oral Med Oral Pathol 1992;73:27–8.

17. Luchetti W, Cohen RB, Hahr GV, et al. Severe restriction in jaw movement after routine injection of local anesthetic in patients who have fibrodysplasia ossificans progressiva. Oral Surg Oral Med Oral Pathol Oral Radiol Endod 1996;81:21–5.

18. Wieder DL. Treatment of myositis ossificans with acetic acid iontophoresis. Phys Ther 1992;72:133–7.

19. Steidl L, Ditmar R. Treatment of soft tissue calcifications with magnesium. Acta Univ Palacki Olomuc Fac Med 1991;130:273–87.

20. Faerber TH, Ennis RL, Allen GA. Temporomandibular joint ankylosis following mastoiditis; report of a case. J Oral Maxillofac Surg 1990;48:866–70.

21. Hadlock TA, Ferraro NF, Rahbar R. Acute mastoiditis with temporomandibular joint effusion. Otolaryngol Head Neck Surg 2001;125:111–2.

22. Cohen SG, Quinn PD. Facial trismus and myofascial pain associated with infectious and malignant disease. Oral Surg Oral Med Oral Pathol 1988;65:538–44.

23. Leighty SM, Spach DH, Myall RW, Burns JL. Septic arthritis of the temporomandibular joint: review of the literature and report of two cases in children. Int J Oral Maxillofac Surg 1993;22:292–7.

24. Huang CJ, Chao KS, Tsai J, et al. Cancer of the retromolar trigone: long-term radiation therapy outcome. Head Neck 2001;23:758–63.

25. Goldstein M, Maxymiw WG, Cummings BJ, Wood RE. The effects of antitumor irradiation on mandibular opening and mobility: a prospective study of 58 patients. Oral Surg Oral Med Oral Pathol Oral Radiol Endod 1999;88:365–73.

26. Pow EH, McMillan AS, Leung WK, et al. Oral health condition in southern Chinese after radiotherapy for nasopharyngeal carcinoma: extent and nature of the problem. Oral Dis 2003;9:196–202.

27. Buchbinder D, Currivan RB, Kaplan AJ, Urken ML. Mobilization regimens for the prevention of jaw hypomobility in the radiated patient: a comparison of three techniques. J Oral Maxillofac Surg 1993;51:863–7.

28. Hollins RR, Moyer DJ, Tu HK. Pseudoankylosis of the mandible after temporal bone attached craniotomy. Neurosurgery 1988; 22:137–9.

29. Nitzan DW, Azaz B, Constantini S. Severe limitation in mouth opening following transtemporal neurosurgical procedures: diagnosis, treatment, and prevention. J Neurosurg 1992;76:623–5.

30. Kawaguchi M, Sakamoto T, Furuya H, et al. Pseudoankylosis of the mandible after supratentorial craniotomy. Anesth Analg 1996;83:731–4.

31. Resnick D. Temporomandibular joint involvement in ankylosing spondylitis. Radiology 1974;112:587–91.

32. Ramos-Remus C, Major P, Gomez-Vargas A, et al. Temporomandibular joint osseous morphology in a consecutive sample of ankylosing spondylitis patients. Ann Rheum Dis 1997;56:103–7.

33. Locher MC, Felder M, Sailer HF. Involvement of the temporomandibular joints in ankylosing spondylitis (Bechterew's disease). J Craniomaxillofac Surg 1996;24:205–13.

34. Voog U, Alstergren P, Eliasson S, et al. Inflammatory mediators and radiographic changes in temporomandibular joints of patients with rheumatoid arthritis. Acta Odontol Scand 2003;61:57–64.

35. Bakke M, Zak M, Jensen BL, et al. Orofacial pain, jaw function and temporomandibular disorders in women with a history of juvenile chronic arthritis or persistent juvenile chronic arthritis. Oral Surg Oral Med Oral Pathol Oral Radiol Endod 2001;92:406–14.

36. Larheim TA, Hoyeraal HM, Stabrun AE, Haanaes HR. The temporomandibular joint in juvenile rheumatoid arthritis. Radiographic changes related to clinical and laboratory parameters in 100 children. Scand J Rhuematol 1982;11:5–12.

37. Olson L, Eckerdal O, Hallonsten AL, et al. Craniomandibular function in juvenile chronic arthritis. A clinical and radiographic study. Swed Dent J 1991;15:71–83.

38. Svensson B, Larsson A, Adell R. The mandibular condyle in the juvenile chronic arthritis patients with mandibular hypoplasia. Int J Oral Maxillofac Surg 2001;30:300–5.

39. Seifert MH, Steigerwald JC, Cliff MM. Bone resorption of the mandible in progressive systemic sclerosis. Arthritis Rheum 1975;18:507–12.

40. Haers PE, Sailer HF. Mandibular resorption due to systemic sclerosis. Case report of

surgical correction of a secondary open bite deformity. Int J Oral Maxillofac Surg 1995;24:261–7.

41. Hori M, Okaue M, Hasegawa M, et al. Worsening of pre-existing TMJ dyfunction following sagittal split osteotomy: a study of three cases. J Oral Sci 1999;41:133–9.

42. Feinerman DM, Piecuch JF. Long term effects of orthognathic surgery on the temporomandibular joint. Comparison of rigid and nonrigid methods. Int J Oral Maxillofac Surg 1995;24:268–72.

43. Van Sickels JE, Tiner BD, Alder ME. Condylar torque as a possible cause of hypomobility after sagittal split osteotomy: report of three cases. J Oral Maxillofac Surg 1997; 55:398–402.

44. Sanders B, Kaminishi R, Buoncristiani R, Davis C. Arthroscopic surgery for treatment of temporomandibular joint hypomobility after mandibular sagittal osteotomy. Oral Surg Oral Med Oral Pathol 1990;69:539–41.

45. Roychoudhury A, Parkash H, Trikha A. Functional restoration by gap arthroplasty in temporomandibular joint ankylosis: a report of 50 cases. Oral Surg Oral Med Oral Pathol Oral Radiol Endod 1999;87:166–9.

46. Sawhney CP. Bony ankylosis of the temporomandibular joint: follow-up of 70 patients treated with arthroplasty and acrylic spacer interposition. Plast Reconstr Surg 1986; 77:29–40.

47. Rajgopal A, Banerji PK, Batura V, Sural A. Temporomandibular ankylosis. A report of 15 cases. J Oral Maxillofac Surg 1983;11:37–41.

48. Kaban LB, Perrott DH, Fisher K. A protocol for management of temporomandibular joint ankylosis. J Oral Maxillofac Surg 1990; 48:1145–51.

49. Kaban LB. Acquired temporomandibular deformities. In: Kaban LB, Troulis MJ, editors. Pediatric oral and maxillofacial surgery. St. Louis: Elsevier; 2004. p. 353–5.

50. Mercuri LG. The use of alloplastic protheses for temporomandibular joint reconstruction. J Oral Maxillofac Surg 2000;58:70–5.

51. Kent JN, Misiek DJ. Controversies in disc and condyle replacement for partial and total temporomandibular joint reconstruction. In: Worthington P, Evans JR, editors. Controversies in oral and maxillofacial surgery. Philadelphia: WB Saunders; 1994. p. 397–435.

52. Henry CH, Wolford LM. Treatment outcomes for temporomandibular joint reconstruction after Proplast-Teflon implant failure. J Oral Maxillofac Surg 1993;51:352–8.

53. Chossegros C, Guyot L, Cheynet F, et al. Comparison of different materials for interpositon arthroplasty in treatment of temporomandibular joint ankylosis surgery: long-term follow-up in 25 cases. Br J Oral Maxillofac Surg 1997;35:157–60.

54. Poswillo DE. Biological temporomandibular joint reconstruction. Annu Meet Am Inst Oral Biol 1975;3(7):72–82.

55. MacIntosh RB, Henny FA. A spectrum of applications of autogenous costochondral grafts. J Maxillofac Surg 1977;5:257–67.

56. Dolwick MF, Armstrong JW. Complications of temporomandibular joint surgery. In: Kaban LB, Pogrel MA, Perrott DH, editors. Complications in oral and maxillofacial surgery. Philadelphia: WB Saunders; 1997. p. 89–103.

57. Topazian RG. Comparison of gap and interpositional arthroplasty in the treatment of TMJ ankylosis. J Oral Surg 1966;24:405–9.

58. Padgett GC, Robinson DW, Stephenson KL. Ankylosis of the temporomandibular joint. Surgery 1948;24:426–32.

59. Oji C. Fractures of the facial skeleton in children: a survey of patients under the age of 11 years. J Craniomaxillofac Surg 1998;26:322–5.

60. Posnick JC, Goldstein JA. Surgical management of temporomandibular joint ankylosis in the pediatric population. Plast Reconstr Surg 1993;91:791–8.

61. Munro IR, Phillips JH, Griffin G. Growth after construction of the temporomandibular joint in children with hemifacial microsomia. Cleft Palate J 1989;26:303–11.

62. Perrott DH, Umeda H, Kaban LB. Costochondral graft construction/reconstruction of the ramus/condyle unit: long-term follow-up. Int J Oral Maxillofac Surg 1994;23:321–8.

63. Friedman MH, Weisberg J, Weber FL. Postsurgical temporomandibular joint hypomobility. Rehabilitation technique. Oral Surg Oral Med Oral Pathol 1993;75:24–8.

64. Caminiti MF, Weinberg S. Chronic mandibular dislocation: the role of non-surgical and surgical treatment. J Can Dent Assoc 1998;64:484–91.

65. Hoard MA, Tadje JP, Gampper TJ, Edlich RF. Traumatic chronic TMJ dislocation: report of an unusual case and discussion of management. J Craniomaxillofac Trauma 1998;4:44–7.

66. MacFarlane WI. Recurrent dislocation of the mandible: treatment of seven cases by a simple surgical method. Br J Oral Surg 1977;14:227–9.

67. Wolford LM, Pitta MC, Mehra P. Mitek anchors for treatment of chronic mandibular dislocation. Oral Surg Oral Med Oral Pathol Oral Radiol Endod 2001;92:495–8.

68. LeClerc G, Girald G. Un nouveau procede de butee dans le traitment chirurgical de la luxation recidivante de la manchoire inferieure. Mem Acad Chir (Paris) 1943;69:457–9.

69. Myrhaug H. A new method of operation for habitual dislocation of the mandible—review of former methods of treatment. Acta Odontol Scand 1951;9:247–61.

70. Sato J, Segami N, Nishimura M, et al. Clinical evaluation of arthroscopic eminoplasty for habitual dislocation of the temporomandibular joint: comparative study with conventional open eminectomy. Oral Surg Oral Med Oral Pathol Oral Radiol Endod 2003;95:390–5.

71. Undt G, Kermer C, Rasse M. Treatment of recurrent mandibular dislocation, part II: eminectomy. Int J Oral Maxillofac Surg 1997;26:98–102.

72. Westwood RM, Fox GL, Tilson HB. Eminectomy for the treatment of recurrent temporomandibular joint dislocation. J Oral Surg 1975;33:774–9.

73. Courtemanche AD, Son-Hing QR. Eminectomy for chronic recurring subluxation of the temporomandibular joint. Ann Plast Surg 1979;3:22–5.

74. Miller GA, Murphy EJ. External pterygoid myotomy for recurrent mandibular dislocation. Review of the literature and report of a case. Oral Surg Oral Med Oral Pathol 1976;42:705–16.

75. Burke RH, McNamara JA Jr. Electromyography after lateral pterygoid myotomy in monkeys. J Oral Surg 1979;37:630–6.

76. Sindet-Pedersen S. Intraoral myotomy of the lateral pterygoid muscle for treatment of recurrent dislocation of the mandibular condyle. J Oral Maxillofac Surg 1988;46:445–9.

77. Ziegler CM, Haag C, Muhling J. Treatment of recurrent temporomandibular joint dislocation with intramuscular botulinum toxin injection. Clin Oral Investig 2003;7:52–5.

78. Clark GT. The management of oromandibular motor disorders and facial spasms with injections of botulinum toxin. Phys Med Rehabil Clin N Am 2003;14:727–48.

Part 8

ORTHOGNATHIC SURGERY

Craniofacial Growth and Development: Current Understanding and Clinical Considerations

Peter M. Spalding, DDS, MS, MS

This chapter will provide a summary of the current understanding of prenatal and postnatal craniofacial growth and its relevance for clinical treatment. Although there clearly is awareness of the importance of genetic and environmental influences on craniofacial growth and development, the control and precise biologic mechanisms are not well understood and continue to be fertile areas of investigation. The chapter will review human morphogenesis, prenatal and postnatal growth and development, the factors that influence these phases of growth and development, and the orthopedic and orthodontic clinical considerations that will determine whether surgical intervention will be necessary to achieve optimum cosmetic and functional craniofacial treatment outcomes.

Prenatal Craniofacial Development

Human prenatal development can be conveniently divided into the embryonic period, from fertilization through the eighth week of development, and the fetal period, continuing from the ninth to the fortieth week at birth. The embryonic period is characterized by new tissue differentiation and organogenesis, whereas the fetal period is distinguished by growth and expansion of the basic structures already formed.

During the first few days following the formation of the single-cell zygote at conception, four mitotic divisions occur to form the 16-cell morula. After entering the uterus the morula develops into a 100-cell blastocyst consisting of an outer (trophoblast) and inner (embryoblast) cell mass. The trophoblast further differentiates to form the placenta and other peripheral embryonic structures, whereas the embryoblast differentiates into the future embryo. At the end of the first week the blastocyst adheres to the uterine endometrium to begin implantation. During the second week the embryoblast forms a bilaminar disk composed of two germ layers: the ectoderm, forming the amniotic cavity floor; and the endoderm, lying beneath and forming the yolk sac floor. Later the ectoderm will form a variety of epidermal structures including dental enamel, oral mucosa and nasal epithelia. The endoderm will later form the pharyngeal epithelium. By the end of the second week the endoderm develops a thickened area called the prechordal plate, located at the cranial end of the bilaminar disk, that prefaces the development of the head (Figure 53-1).

Embryonic Period

Germ Layer Formation Craniofacial embryogenesis begins during the third week of gestation, when gastrulation and neurulation occur. Gastrulation is the process whereby the bilaminar disk is converted into a trilaminar one with the appearance of the third germ layer, the mesoderm, forming between the other two from ectodermal cell proliferation and differentiation in the caudal area of the disk. The prominence created from this proliferation forms a craniocaudal midline furrow termed the primitive streak. Cell proliferation and differentiation of the cranial end of the primitive streak forms the notochord around which the axial skeleton will form.

Neural Tube Formation Neurulation, occurring at the same time as gastrulation during the third week and continuing through the fourth week, is a process that results in the formation of the neural tube,

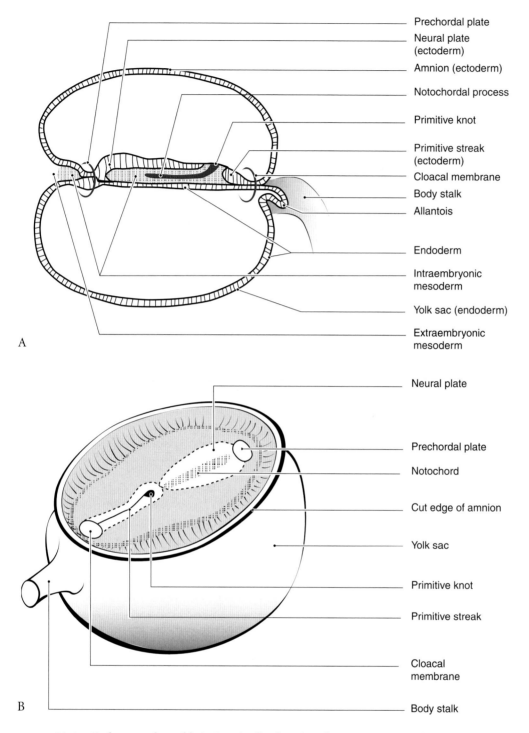

Prechordal plate
Neural plate (ectoderm)
Amnion (ectoderm)
Notochordal process
Primitive knot
Primitive streak (ectoderm)
Cloacal membrane
Body stalk
Allantois
Endoderm
Intraembryonic mesoderm
Yolk sac (endoderm)
Extraembryonic mesoderm

A

Neural plate
Prechordal plate
Notochord
Cut edge of amnion
Yolk sac
Primitive knot
Primitive streak
Cloacal membrane
Body stalk

B

FIGURE 53-1 *Embryo 14 days old. A, Longitudinal section showing amnion (above) and yolk sac (below). Adapted from Sperber G. Craniofacial development. Hamilton (ON): BC Decker Inc; 2001. p.19. B, Dorsal surface view with the amnion cover removed, showing the embryonic disk. Adapted from Sperber G. Craniofacial development. Hamilton (ON): BC Decker Inc; 2001. p.20.*

the primordium of the central nervous system. Neurulation is characterized by development of the neural plate from the ectoderm overlying the notochord. As the neural plate grows caudally toward the primitive streak, the lateral edges of the neural plate rise up to create neural folds, forming the neural groove between them. Mesoderm on either side of the groove develops into paired blocks of tissue called somites (ultimately 48 somite pairs will develop). In the fourth week the neural folds begin to fuse at the midline in the central part of the embryo, at the level of the fourth to fifth somite, to form the neural tube (Figure 53-2). The neural tube continues to form toward the cranial and caudal ends, completing caudal formation by the time about 20 somite pairs are present. The anterior portion of the neural tube develops into the forebrain, midbrain, and hindbrain. After neural tube closure is complete on day 28, the two hemispheres of the brain begin development, increasing in size to eventually cover the roof of the brain stem. The otic, optic, and olfactory placodes develop in association with the forebrain neuroectoderm.

Cell Population Origin, Migration, and Interaction By the end of the fourth week multipotential neural crest cells arising from the neural folds must translocate or migrate from the dorsal margins of the closing neural tube to specific locations along hyaluronate-rich fibronectin-lined extracellular pathways.[1] The migration of neural crest cells follows a proper sequence and distinct pathways over extensive distances, but there is evidence that the cells have an ability to differentiate into a variety of derivatives (Figure 53-3).[2] There is growing evidence that neural crest cell differentiation is not predetermined but dependent on their epithelial-mesenchymal cellular interactions with tissues along the route to their final destinations.[3] Multiple genes, in particular a class of homeobox-containing transcription factors, affect subpopulations of neural crest cells that help regulate their migration and determine the pattern and position of structures within the pharyngeal arches.[4] All of the skeletal and connective tissue of the face, with the exception of dental enamel, is derived from neural crest cells, whereas skeletal and connective tissue of the trunk is mesodermal in origin. Many craniofacial malformations are produced from faulty neural crest formation or

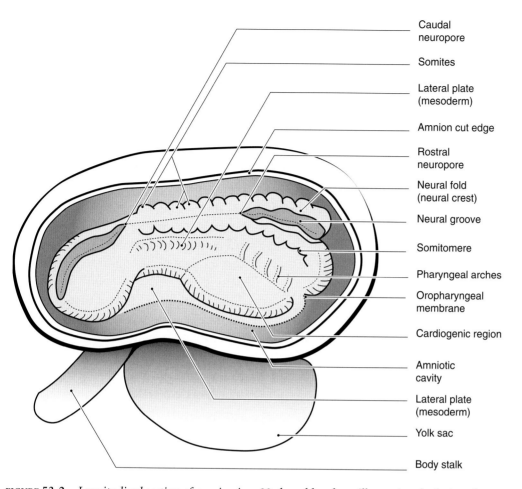

Caudal neuropore

Somites

Lateral plate (mesoderm)

Amnion cut edge

Rostral neuropore

Neural fold (neural crest)

Neural groove

Somitomere

Pharyngeal arches

Oropharyngeal membrane

Cardiogenic region

Amniotic cavity

Lateral plate (mesoderm)

Yolk sac

Body stalk

FIGURE 53-2 *Longitudinal section of amnion in a 23-day-old embryo illustrating the fusion of neural folds and the initial formation of somites. Adapted from Sperber G. Craniofacial development. Hamilton (ON): BC Decker Inc; 2001. p.21.*

migration, loss of neural crest cells, or flawed epithelial-mesenchymal interaction during this fourth week of gestation.

Development of Facial Primordia The pharyngeal arches, which give rise to most of the head and neck structures, develop during the fourth week as a result of neural crest migration (Figures 53-3 and 53-4). They consist of four bilaterally paired arches on the ventral external surface of the human embryo. Facial development occurs between the fourth and eighth weeks of gestation. Development of the face begins with five prominences or primordia surrounding the stomatodeum or primitive mouth cavity. The primordia form from the first pair of pharyngeal arches arising from neural crest ectomesenchyme and include the single median frontonasal primordium, the paired maxillary primordia, and the paired mandibular primordia. Recent studies indicate that these facial primordia may be initiated through different morphogenetic mechanisms. They are composed of different neural crest cells, have their outgrowth regulated by different

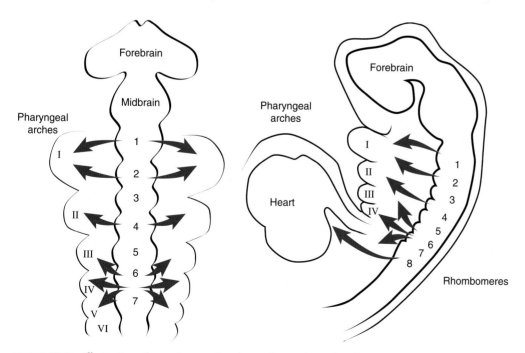

FIGURE 53-3 *Illustration of neural crest migration pathways from rhombomeres 1 to 7 to pharyngeal arches I to VI, from dorsal (left) and lateral (right) views. Adapted from Sperber GH. Pathogenesis and morphogenesis of craniofacial developmental anomalies. Ann Acad Med Singapore 1999;28:708–13.*

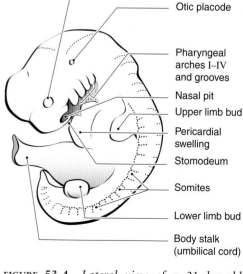

Optic placode

Otic placode

Pharyngeal arches I–IV and grooves

Nasal pit

Upper limb bud

Pericardial swelling

Stomodeum

Somites

Lower limb bud

Body stalk (umbilical cord)

FIGURE 53-4 *Lateral view of a 31-day-old embryo showing somites along the back and development of the pharyngeal arches and limb buds. Adapted from Sperber G. Craniofacial development. Hamilton (ON): BC Decker Inc; 2001. p. 24.*

genes, and have different responses to teratogenic agents.[5] The facial primordia merge when the epithelium between them breaks down, followed by invasion of the mesenchyme and coalescence of the adjoining prominences (Figure 53-5). Initially the mandibular primordia merge in the midline to form the chin and lower lip. At the same time nasal placodes form in the inferior and lateral portion of the frontonasal primordium. On either side of

these nasal placodes, medial and lateral nasal primordia develop. The medial nasal primordia move toward each other and merge in the midline early in the sixth week, forming the central part of the upper lip and the primary palate, including the maxillary incisors and their surrounding alveolar bone. There still is some controversy regarding the origin of the central part of the upper lip, which some believe is of frontonasal primordial origin.[6] The

maxillary primordia move medially as well, merging with the lateral and medial nasal primordia during the sixth week, to complete formation of the upper lip. At this same time the maxillary and mandibular primordia merge laterally, determining the width of the mouth. Merging of facial primordia requires disintegration of surface epithelia in order to permit the underlying mesenchymal cells to unite (Figure 53-6). The groove between the primordia is gradually filled out by proliferation of the mesenchyme so that the primordia appear to merge. Facial clefting is a result of failure of epithelial disintegration and lack of merging. Facial primordial growth and merging is dependent on ectodermal-mesenchymal interactions that appear to be regulated by the secreted protein sonic hedgehog (SHH).[5] Mutations in SHH that prevent its signaling during early neural plate patterning cause midline defects that range from hypotelorism and cleft lip/palate to holoprosencephaly and cyclopia.[7] There is also evidence that adequate epidermal growth factor receptor signaling is necessary for sufficient secretion of matrix metalloproteinases for normal facial development.[8] From 5 weeks' gestation to the early part of the fetal period at 9 weeks, there is medial migration of the eyes, assisted by frontal and temporal lobe expansion and greater proliferation of the lateral facial regions relative to the central face, resulting in facial expansion and interocular reduction.

The nasal placodes that formed at about 5 weeks each are separated inferiorly by a nasal groove. With continued proliferation of mesenchyme, the placodes submerge to form the nasal pits, the precursors to the anterior nares. As the nasal pits continue to submerge with the proliferating mesenchyme, they are eventually separated from the stomatodeum by only a thin oronasal membrane. This membrane will rupture at the beginning of the seventh week, forming a continuous nasal and oral cavity.

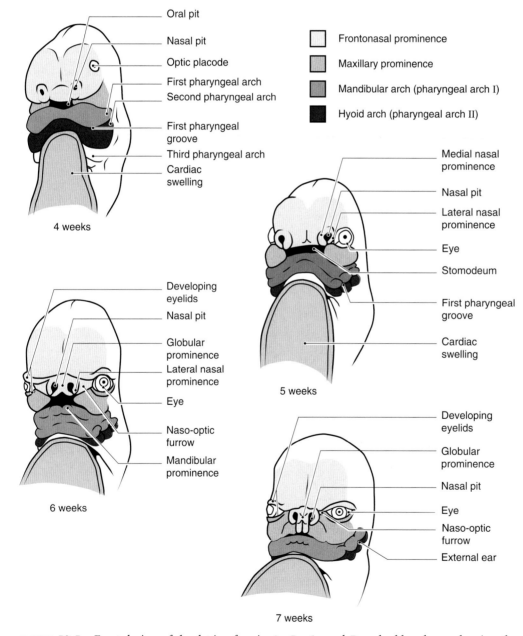

FIGURE 53-5 *Frontal view of developing face in 4-, 5-, 6-, and 7-week-old embryos showing the merging of facial primordia (prominences). Adapted from Sperber G. Craniofacial development. Hamilton (ON): BC Decker Inc; 2001. p. 32.*

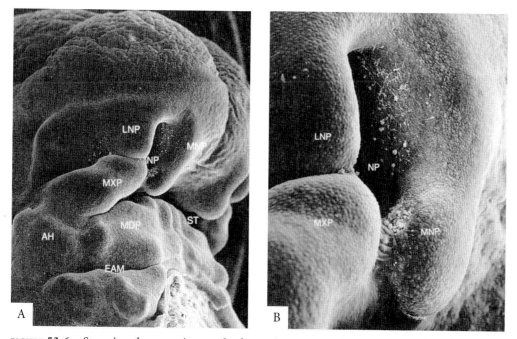

FIGURE 53-6 *Scanning electron micrograph of a 41-day-old human embryo. A, Craniofacial region. LNP = right lateral nasal primordium; MNP = right medial nasal primordium; NP = right nasal pit; MXP = right maxillary primordium; AH = right auricular hillock; EAM = right external acoustic meatus; MDP = mandibular prominence; ST = left side of stomodeum. B, Enlarged view, showing the epithelial bridges between the merging right maxillary primordium (MXP) and the right medial nasal primordium (MNP). Failure of these primordia to merge together with the lateral nasal primordium (LNP) results in cleft of the lip. Reproduced with permission from Hinrichsen K. The early development of morphology and patterns of the face in the human embryo. In: Advances in anatomy, embryology and cell biology. Vol. 98. New York: Springer-Verlag; 1985.*

Formation of Neurocranium and Viscerocranium Formation of the craniofacial bones begins with development of the cartilaginous and membranous precursors to the neurocranium and viscerocranium during the latter part of the fifth week of gestation (Figure 53-7). The membranous neurocranium (desmocranium) that will give rise to the flat bones of the calvaria is connective tissue derived from the paraxial mesoderm and neural crest. The cartilaginous neurocranium (chondrocranium) that will form the cranial base is cartilage from neural crest origin. Cartilage maturation occurs in a caudal-rostral sequence. The membranous viscerocranium that will give rise to the maxilla, zygomatic bone, squamous temporal bone, and mandible is derived from the neural crest. The cartilaginous viscerocranium that will form the middle ear ossicles, styloid process of the temporal bone, hyoid bone, and laryngeal cartilages is from neural crest ectoderm.

Endochondral ossification centers occur in the cartilaginous components and intramembranous ossification centers form in the membranous components of the neurocranium and viscerocranium. Osteoblast differentiation with the onset of mineralization results from a rapid angiogenic process with vascular ingrowth closely surrounding the center of ossification. The earliest ossification of the craniofacial bones begins in the seventh and eighth weeks of gestation. There are eventually 110 ossification centers, nearly all of which appear between 6 and 12 weeks' gestation, that develop in the embryo to form 45 bones at birth, which ultimately form 22 bones in the adult.

Ossification The onset of ossification generally follows the chronologic sequence of mandible, maxilla, palatine, cranial base, and cranium, with intermembranous centers usually preceding endochondral

centers.[9] Ossification of the mandible begins in the mental foramen region. Endochondral ossification of Meckel's cartilage occurs anteriorly to this area and intramembranous ossification occurs posteriorly. The condylar cartilage forms at the posterior end of this intramembranous portion, independently of Meckel's cartilage. Maxillary ossification begins in the area of the infraorbital foramen. Intramembranous ossification occurs anteriorly and posteriorly to this region. The vertical portion of the palatine bone then begins intramembranous ossification in the region of the palatine nerve, followed by ossification of the anterior, then posterior borders of the incisive foramen, spreading through the hard palate from the canine area. Following ossification of the main portion of the mandible and maxilla, during the sixth week of gestation, endochondral ossification of the cranial base occurs in the midline from the foramen magnum to the nasal bone, and intramembranous ossification occurs laterally. Finally intramembranous ossification of the cranial bones follows.

Final Tissue Differentiation Interaction between pharyngeal endoderm and neural crest tissue, followed by oral ectoderm proliferation, produces identifiable odontogenic tissue by the end of 4 weeks' gestation. There are four origin sites of odontogenic epithelium for both the maxillary and mandibular arches, appearing at the end of 5 weeks' gestation. The primary anterior and first molar tooth germs appear at 6 weeks' gestation, followed by development of the primary second molar germs at 7 weeks. Apposition of bone on the alveolar margins of the maxilla and mandible in the presence of developing tooth germs form the initial alveolar processes.

The latest orofacial structure to reach completion at the end of the embryonic period is the secondary palate, developing from the paired lateral palatine shelves of

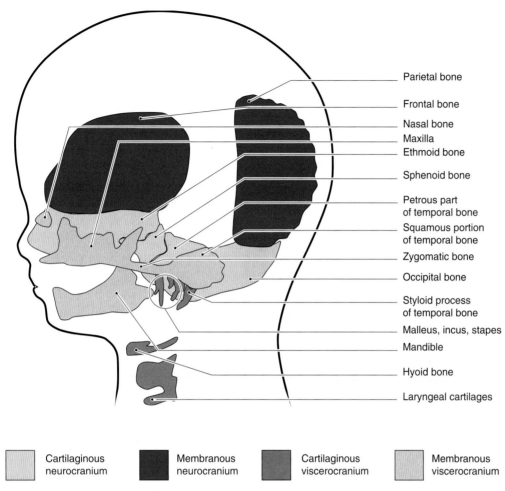

Parietal bone

Frontal bone

Nasal bone

Maxilla

Ethmoid bone

Sphenoid bone

Petrous part
of temporal bone

Squamous portion
of temporal bone

Zygomatic bone

Occipital bone

Styloid process
of temporal bone

Malleus, incus, stapes

Mandible

Hyoid bone

Laryngeal cartilages

Cartilaginous
neurocranium

Membranous
neurocranium

Cartilaginous
viscerocranium

Membranous
viscerocranium

FIGURE 53-7   *Lateral view of 20-week-old embryo illustrating initial development of the cartilaginous and membranous neurocranium and viscerocranium. Adapted from Moore KL, Persaud TVN. The developing human: clinically oriented embryology. 5th ed. Philadelphia (PA): W.B. Saunders; 1993. p. 361.*

the maxilla. These shelves are oriented vertically with the tongue interposed, but the tongue and floor of the oral cavity descend as the nasal chambers expand laterally and inferiorly (Figure 53-8). As this occurs the palatal shelves become elongated and elevate medially toward each other, beginning fusion at the end of the eighth week and completing in the ninth week of gestation. There is evidence that transforming growth factor (TGF)-β3 is intimately involved in regulating secondary palatal fusion by mediating the breakdown of the midline epithelial seam prior to fusion.[10]

Fetal Period

The fetal period begins during the eighth week, at 60 days' gestation, lasting until birth at 40 weeks, and overall somatic growth follows a cephalocaudal growth gradient (Figure 53-9). There is a prenatal growth spurt between 20 and 30 weeks' gestation with the peak growth velocity at 27 to 28 weeks being approximately 2.5 cm per week. The prenatal spurt in weight is slightly later at 30 to 40 weeks' gestation with a peak at 34 to 36 weeks.[11] The rate steadily decreases during the last trimester and continues to decline after birth until adulthood, with two exceptions. The first is a small "midgrowth" spurt that occurs in many children at 6 to 8 years old that has been attributed to increased adrenal secretion of androgenic hormones. The second is a dramatic endocrine mediated "pubertal growth" spurt during adolescence. Growth of the craniofacial complex during the fetal period is characterized by a

constant rate during the second trimester. The craniofacial skeletal components increase more in the anteroposterior dimension than in the vertical or transverse, with the exception of the mandible which increases more in the transverse dimension in order to maintain appropriate articulation.[12]

During the fetal period the neurocranium undergoes precocious development relative to the viscerocranium with earlier brain and neurocranial bone vault growth than facial and masticatory portions of the skull. This results in an early proportional predominance of the neurocranium over the face that only reduces to an 8:1 proportion by birth. The brain nearly doubles in size from 4 months to birth, achieving about 25% of its adult dimension. The formation and maintenance of cranial sutures are regulated by tissue interactions with the underlying dura mater as the brain develops.[13] A number of growth factors have been identified that regulate cranial bone growth and suture fusion, including TGF-β1, TGF-β2, and TGF-β3, bone morphogenetic protein (BMP)-2, BMP-7, fibroblast growth factor (FGF)-4, insulin-like growth factor (IGF)-I, and SHH.[14,15] Transcription factors MSX2 and TWIST also play a role in suture development, binding to target effector genes to determine their expression.[16] The eyeballs grow concurrently with the early brain growth, increasing facial expansion and separating the neural and facial skeletons to increase skull height.

The cranial base growth parallels the rapid growth of the cranial vault during the fetal period. The anterior cranial base grows sevenfold while the posterior cranial base increases fivefold. The intraethmoidal and intrasphenoidal synchondroses close before birth.

The ossification centers that begin the formation of the facial bones late in the embryonic period enlarge during the early fetal period until most of the bones have developed into a definitive shape by

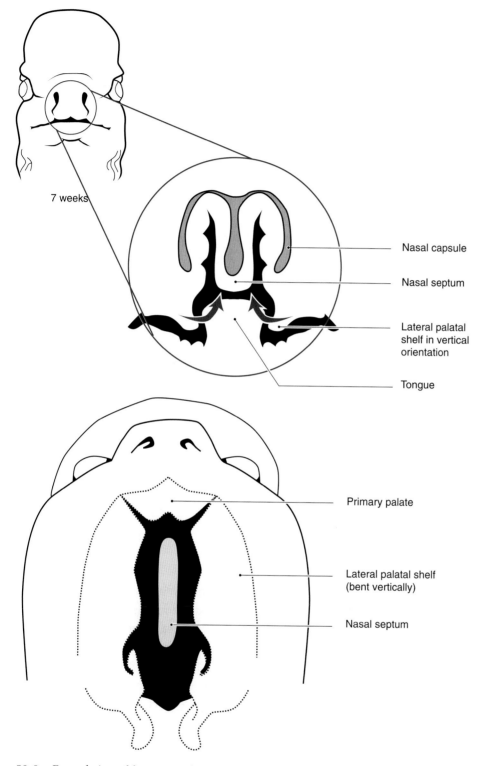

the developing tooth buds of the primary and permanent dentitions. Although the tooth germs start to develop as early as 6 weeks' gestation, the onset of dental mineralization does not begin until ossification has occurred. The maxilla demonstrates a rapid height increase associated with dental development.[17] Once the primary teeth have erupted, these same anterior areas undergo resorption rather than deposition to produce the descent of the maxilla with continued growth. Meanwhile the posterior, infraorbital, and lingual surfaces of the maxilla are depository in both fetal and postnatal development. The fetal temporal bone grows faster in height than width while the lateral and inferior margins of the zygomatic bone grow faster than its orbital margin.[17]

The paranasal sinuses, including the maxillary, sphenoidal, frontal, and ethmoidal, begin developing at the beginning of the fetal period. Pneumatization begins first with the maxillary sinus, starting at 5 months' gestation. It is proposed that a septomaxillary ligament, attached to the sides and anteroinferior border of the nasal septum and inserted in the nasal spine, transmits septal growth, pulling the maxilla downward. Between the tenth week of gestation and birth, the nasal septum increases its vertical height sevenfold. The nasal septum growth, together with neural growth and facial sutural growth, transposes the maxilla inferiorly and anteriorly. The frontomaxillary, frontonasal, frontozygomatic, frontoethmoidal, and ethmoidolmaxillary sutures grow predominantly in a vertical direction. The temporozygomatic and nasomaxillary sutures contribute most of the anteroposterior change. The intermaxillary and zygomaticomaxillary sutures provide most of the transverse expansion of the face. Overall the middle and lower thirds of the face develop primarily in a downward and slightly forward direction away from the cranial base due to brain development, maxillary and palatine sutural growth, and possibly nasal septum growth.

Nasal capsule

Nasal septum

Lateral palatal shelf in vertical orientation

Tongue

Primary palate

Lateral palatal shelf (bent vertically)

Nasal septum

A

FIGURE 53-8 *Frontal view of face, coronal section of the stomodeum, and inferior view of the palate in 7- and 12-week-old embryos. A, Embryo at 7 weeks showing palatal shelves vertically oriented. Adapted from Sperber G. Craniofacial development. Hamilton (ON): BC Decker Inc; 2001. p. 41, 114.* (CONTINUED ON NEXT PAGE)

14 weeks. At this time they begin to remodel as they continue to grow by intramembranous and/or endochondral ossification. The anterior aspects of the maxilla, mandible, and zygoma of the fetal and early postnatal face undergo deposition. This early anterior deposition is necessary to permit adequate osseous mass for

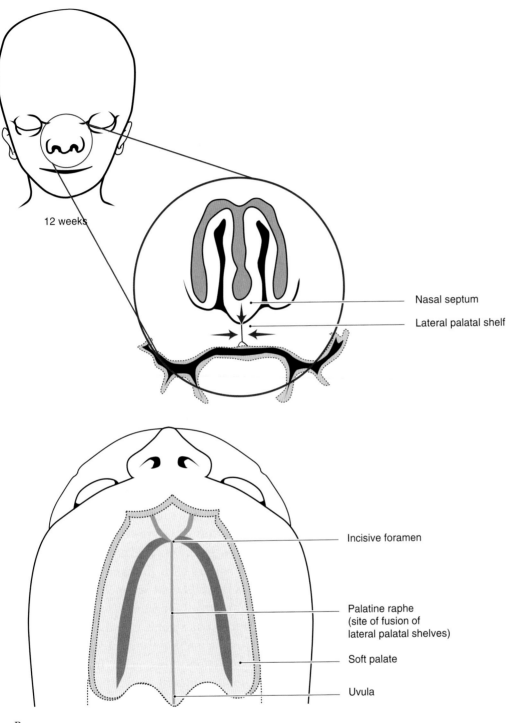

12 weeks

Nasal septum

Lateral palatal shelf

Incisive foramen

Palatine raphe
(site of fusion of
lateral palatal shelves)

Soft palate

Uvula

B

FIGURE 53-8 (CONTINUED)   B, *Embryo at 12 weeks showing fusion following elevation of palatal shelves. Adapted from Sperber G. Craniofacial development. Hamilton (ON): BC Decker Inc; 2001. p. 41, 116.*

Although the mandible is larger than the maxilla during the embryonic period, the mandible approximates the size of the maxilla within the first month of the fetal period. The three secondary cartilages of the mandible do not appear until the tenth and fourteenth weeks of gestation, forming on the lateral and superior aspects of the condylar processes. This secondary type of cartilage differs morphologically from epiphyseal and synchondrosal cartilage.[18] Two of these secondary cartilages forming at the mental protuberance and the coronoid process ossify before birth, leaving only the cartilage on the condylar head as a site of postnatal mandibular endochondral growth. This cartilage never undergoes complete ossification, providing a means for absorbing functional forces and retaining growth potential throughout life. Between the thirteenth and twentieth weeks of gestation, the mandible lags behind the maxilla again while there is a transition from Meckel's cartilage to condylar cartilage as the primary growth site. During the third trimester there is a significant deepening of the corpus in association with the developing dentition. The mandibular ramus growth rate is greater than the growth rate of the mandibular body during this time.[19] At the time of birth the mandible usually is equal in size again to the maxilla, although it is often in a retrognathic position relative to the maxilla.

Development of the permanent tooth germs begins at 16 weeks' gestation, with the first permanent molar germs developing posteriorly from the dental lamina followed by the permanent anterior tooth germs emerging from the lingual side of the primary enamel organs. At birth the primary tooth crowns are still not completely calcified, as the first permanent molars begin to calcify.

Postnatal Craniofacial Development

Skeletal Development

Development and completion of craniofacial growth follow the overall somatic

Although the midsagittal part of the middle face entirely consists of nasal septal cartilage during the fetal period, ossification leaves only a small anterior part of this cartilage remaining postnatally. Currently there is controversy regarding the role of the nasal septum in postnatal facial growth. Some believe it is limited to a compensatory and biomechanical role, and others believe it serves a more extensive role, particularly in promoting vertical maxillary growth.

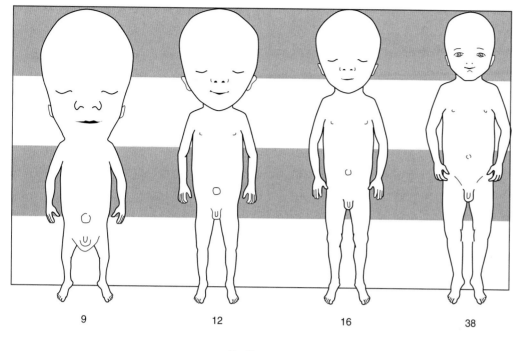

controls. Our understanding of postnatal craniofacial growth has developed in part from cross-sectional anatomic and histologic studies of human cadavers and skeletal material. What has been particularly helpful in supplementing this material is a number of North American longitudinal craniofacial growth records and longitudinal implant (used for stable reference points) studies that were gathered from the 1940s to the mid-1960s before radiation hygiene and human subject research standards became more stringent.[21]

9   12   16   38

Fertilization age in weeks

FIGURE 53-9   *Changing fetal body proportions with all stages drawn to the same total height. At the start of the fetal period, the head is about half the length of the fetus, and by birth, it is one-quarter the length. Adapted from Moore KL, Persaud TVN. The developing human: clinically oriented embryology. 5th ed. Philadelphia (PA): W.B. Saunders; 1993. p. 97.*

Cranial Vault   At birth the cranial bones are separated by sutures with fontanelles where the corners of the bones meet, permitting compression of the skull during the birthing process (Figure 53-11). Postnatal bone growth results in narrowing of the sutures with all of the fontanelles closing within the first 2 years. The pressures exerted by the developing brain determine the size and shape of the cranium. As the brain expands, the pressure creates tension across the sutures and compression against the cranial bones, resulting in intramembranous bone growth by suture and surface apposition. Remodeling of the cranial bones to a flatter shape is necessary to adapt to the expanding surface of the brain. This occurs primarily from endocranial resorption and ectocranial apposition. Although suture apposition

cephalocaudal growth gradient throughout prenatal and postnatal growth, with cranial vault growth completing before the cranial base, followed by the nasomaxilla and finishing with the mandible. During postnatal growth the neurocranium continues to develop ahead of the viscerocranium (Figure 53-10). It increases from about 30% of its ultimate adult size at the time of birth to 50% by 6 months of age, and 75% by 2 years of age, and nearly 90% by 3 years of age. By 5 years of age, the orbits have reached nearly 80% of their adult size.[20] This is why a child of this age appears to have a disproportionately large cranium and eyes. After birth the neurocranium increases about five times in size, whereas the viscerocranium increases about ten times in size. There is also a difference in the amount of postnatal increase in the three dimensions, with the vertical increasing by about 200%, the anteroposterior by somewhat less, and the transverse by the least at approximately

75%. By 10 years of age the neurocranial growth is nearly 95% complete, while facial growth is only about 60% complete.

The craniofacial complex can be divided conveniently into four primary units: the cranial vault, the cranial base, the nasomaxilla, and the mandible. Each of these units has its growth regulated to some extent by both intrinsic and extrinsic

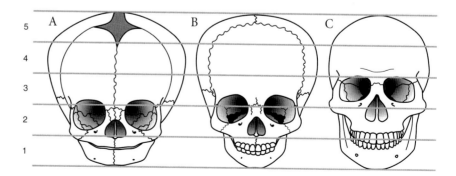

FIGURE 53-10   *Changing proportions of the postnatal skull with all stages enlarged to the same skull height and oriented in the Frankfurt horizontal plane with skull height divided into fifths. A, Neonate, showing the viscerocranium representing one-fifth of the total height; B, 3-year-old and C, adult showing the proportional increase in the height of the viscerocranium relative to the neurocranium. Adapted from from Sarnat BG. Normal and abnormal craniofacial growth. Some experimental and clinical considerations. Angle Orthod 1983;53:263.*

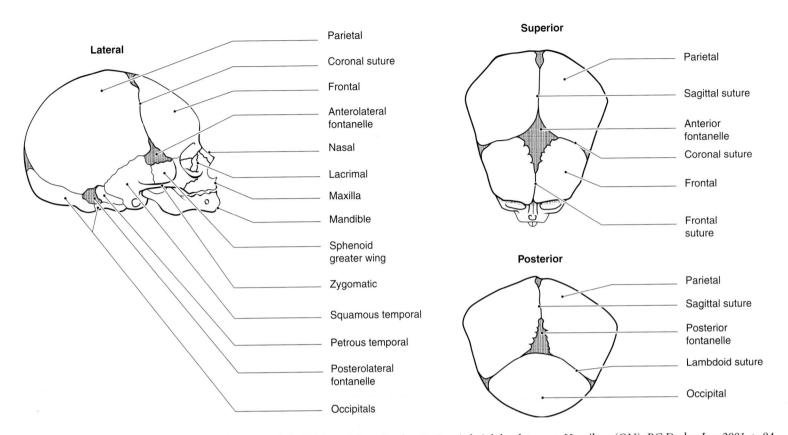

FIGURE 53-11 *Fontanelles and sutures of the neonatal skull. Adapted from Sperber G. Craniofacial development. Hamilton (ON): BC Decker Inc; 2001. p. 84.*

plays a larger role than surface apposition in overall cranial vault capacity, the postnatal shape primarily is determined by extrinsic factors.

By 6 to 7 years of age the inner table of the cranial bones becomes stable due to the cessation of cerebral growth. However, the outer table continues to remodel in response to extracranial muscular forces. The temporal muscles tend to laterally compress the cranium, forming temporal sulci and zygomatic arches. The lateral and posterior cervical muscles insert primarily on the squamous part of the temporal and occipital bones, influencing their shape. Even after attainment of the adult form, the cranial bones continue to thicken during adulthood.

Cranial Base Compared with the other craniofacial units the shape of the cranial base is relatively stable during growth, due likely to its greater intrinsic growth potential. Perhaps more than any other cranio-facial area, growth of the cranial base is genetically predetermined and influenced the least by functional matrices.[22,23] However, prenatal brain growth may provide a minor extrinsic influence, causing some flattening of the cranial base, since this does not occur with anencephaly. In addition there is recent evidence that chondral growth of the cranial base can be altered with mechanical forces.[24]

The anterior cranial base matures earlier than the posterior cranial base with the posterior intraoccipital synchondroses closing during the second and third years postnatally and the anterior intraoccipital synchondroses closing at 3 to 4 years of age (Figure 53-12). The sphenoethmoidal synchondrosis closes at about 6 years of age. Although the spheno-occipital synchondrosis is not a main growth site before birth, it provides the greatest contribution to cranial base growth postnatally, delaying fusion until adolescence. The prolonged postnatal growth period of the spheno-occipital synchondrosis permits posterior growth of the maxilla to provide adequate bone for the developing posterior permanent teeth and adequate space for the nasopharynx. In addition to endo-chondral bone growth, intramembranous remodeling of the cranial base occurs, including apposition on the basioccipital bone and anterior margin of the foramen magnum, resulting in continued lengthening of the posterior cranial base even after adolescence. Enlargement of the sella turcica continues postnatally, with the anterior wall stabilizing at about 6 years of age and the posterior wall continuing to resorb until late adolescence.

Nasomaxilla The prenatal precocity of neurocranial growth relative to the face becomes less predominant postnatally. Nevertheless considerable postnatal displacement of the nasomaxilla downward and forward occurs due to continued growth of the brain and cranial base. This

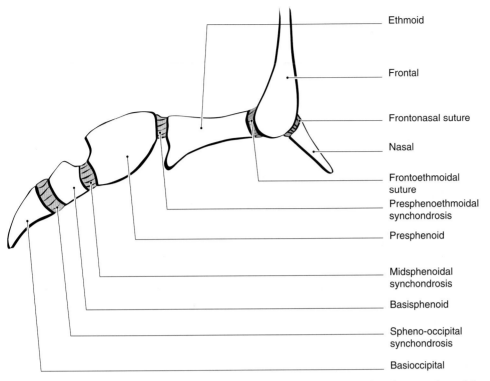

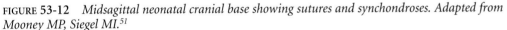

FIGURE 53-12 *Midsagittal neonatal cranial base showing sutures and synchondroses. Adapted from Mooney MP, Siegel MI.*[51]

inferior and anterior maxillary transposition is augmented by the sutural growth between the cranial base and maxilla and growth of the nasal septum. Following birth the vertical growth of the maxilla continues with contributions from the frontomaxillary, frontonasal, frontozygomatic, frontoethmoidal, and ethmoidal-maxillary sutures and possibly the nasal septum (Figure 53-13). The vertical descent of the maxilla is further increased by remodeling with resorption on the nasal surfaces and the simultaneous apposition on the oral surfaces. Anteroposterior growth continues with temporozygomatic and nasomaxillary sutural growth and transverse growth from intermaxillary and zygomaticomaxillary sutures. The resulting downward and forward translation displaces adjacent bones and permits adequate space for the developing nasopharynx and growth at the posterior aspect

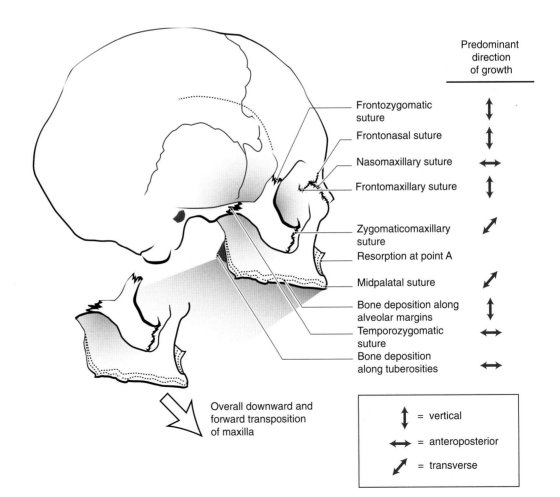

FIGURE 53-13 *Nasomaxillary intramembranous growth at various sites, resulting in an overall downward and forward transposition of the maxilla relative to the cranial base. Adapted from Sperber G. Craniofacial development. Hamilton (ON): BC Decker Inc; 2001. p. 107.*

of the maxilla and maxillary tuberosities to provide adequate space for the development and eruption of the maxillary molars. Following the postnatal growth of the facial sutures, they serve as sites of fibrous union where some remodeling still can take place. In fact a number of cranial and facial sutures are interdigitated but still not fused even beyond 50 years of age.

Growth determinants for postnatal nasomaxillary growth are not well understood and include a variety of intrinsic and extrinsic factors. Passive displacement secondary to brain and cranial base growth, and perhaps nasal septal growth guidance, are the most significant influences on the downward and forward movements of the maxilla after birth until about the seventh postnatal year. From that age through adolescence these influences dramatically decrease as sutural growth and surface intramembranous growth predominate. Maxillary growth also depends to some extent on various functional matrices. The orbits' early response to eyeball growth and their functional movement, the influence of respiration on the nasal cavity, the influence of oral function in determining tuberosity, palatal and alveolar development, and the surrounding facial soft tissues all contribute functional roles in determining growth and remodeling of the nasomaxilla.[25]

Significant remodeling must occur in order to maintain the general shape of the maxilla as it is displaced downward. As mentioned above, resorption of the nasal side of the maxilla, providing nasal cavity enlargement, occurs concomitantly with apposition on the oral side, resulting in descent of the maxilla. Although secondary pneumatization of the maxillary sinus begins prenatally, it does not occur for the other paranasal sinuses until after birth (first 2 years for ethmoidal and frontal sinuses and 6 to 7 years for sphenoidal sinuses). The vertical growth of the maxillary alveolar process is rapid during dental eruption, surpassing the vertical

descent of the palate threefold. The alveolar development contributes to the depth and width of the palate and vertical height of the face. Considerable resorption of the anterior surface of the maxilla minimizes the overall forward displacement of the maxilla and creates a deeper supra-alveolar concavity while increasing the relative prominence of the anterior nasal spine. Transverse growth occurs by lateral displacement of the maxillary bodies by means of the midpalatal suture and bone resorption on the lateral borders of the nasal cavity. Transverse development of the maxillary alveolar process continues with buccal eruption of the posterior teeth. Growth of the midpalatal suture ends after the first two postnatal years, but the suture remains patent until late adolescence, with fusion usually not being complete until the third decade.

Mandible   The mandible has the most delayed growth and the most postnatal growth of all the facial bones. Although usually in a retrognathic position relative to the maxilla at birth, there is rapid postnatal growth that corrects this discrepancy. The right and left bodies of the mandible are still separate at birth, uniting at the midline mental symphysis during the first year of life. The primary sites of mandibular postnatal growth are the endochondral apposition occurring at the condylar cartilages, and the intramembranous apposition on the posterior aspects of the rami and the alveolar ridges (Figure 53-14). Remodeling in the form of resorption of the anterior surface of the condyle, the anterior contours of the ramus, and the inner surface of the mandibular body are integrated with the posterior apposition. The growth of the condylar cartilages contributes most of the total ramus height, whereas growth of alveolar bone contributes about 60% to the mandibular body height.[26] Proliferation of condylar cartilage results in superior and posterior growth of the condylar heads, displacing

the mandible downward and forward in concert with the maxilla. Condylar growth appears to involve the sequential involvement of transcription factor SOX9, expressed by chondrocytes, which regulates the synthesis of Type II collagen, Type X collagen secreted as matrix, and vascular endothelial growth factor secreted to regulate the neovascularization of the cartilage.[27] At birth the inclination of the mandibular condyles is more horizontal, resulting in a greater increase in length than height. During childhood the inclination becomes more vertical so that condylar growth results in a greater increase in height than length. However, there is great variability in this inclination within the general population, influencing the degree to which the mandibular growth is expressed in a forward anteriorly rotating, as opposed to downward posteriorly rotating, direction. Simultaneous remodeling of the inferior mandibular border tends to reduce the effect of this rotation on facial morphology. Although minimal maxillary growth occurs after about 10 years of age, mandibular growth continues longer, to

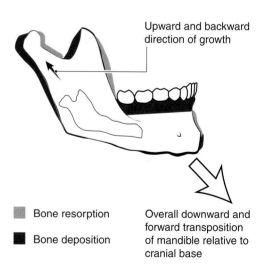

Upward and backward direction of growth

▨ Bone resorption

■ Bone deposition

Overall downward and forward transposition of mandible relative to cranial base

FIGURE **53-14** *Mandibular intramembranous and endochondral growth, resulting in an overall downward and forward transposition of the mandible relative to the cranial base. An outline of the fetal mandible is superimposed on the adult mandible for size and shape comparison. Adapted from Sperber G. Craniofacial development. Hamilton (ON): BC Decker Inc; 2001. p. 130.*

the end of adolescent growth. This differential growth, typically characterized by a peak in the rate of mandibular growth at puberty, usually results in the final correction of the mandibular position relative to the maxilla.

If the cranial base is the craniofacial skeletal unit whose growth is least determined by extrinsic factors, the mandible is the opposite extreme with its growth highly dependent on the postnatal functional demands placed on it. It has a great capacity to adapt to mandibular displacement and accommodate to lingual and labial soft tissue and muscular function. The condylar inclination, dictating the type of mandibular rotation, is determined by these secondary functional influences. The relevant functional matrices include the lateral pterygoid attached to the condylar neck, the growth and function of the tongue, the masticatory muscles attached to the buccal and lingual aspects and to the coronoid process, and the facial soft tissue and musculature, all influencing the ultimate size and shape of the mandible. For this reason the mandible, more than any other part of the craniofacial complex, may have a low intrinsic growth potential that is significantly increased and regulated in response to functional demand.

Dental Development

The alveolar processes contribute a great portion of the vertical height of the lower face. Their development is entirely dependent on the presence and eruption of the primary and permanent dentition. Just as vertical appositional alveolar growth accompanies vertical dental eruption, transverse apposition complements transverse dental eruption. This minor contribution to the transverse dimension of the alveolar processes continues until about 7 years of age, with eruption of the permanent incisors. Further transverse dentoalveolar growth is minimal, occurring with eruption of the premolars and canines. Facial growth and the concomitant

increase in the size of the jaws occur posteriorly, creating additional space for the dentition only in the molar region.

Eruption of the maxillary teeth enhances the vertical dimension of the maxilla with posterior development of the maxillary tuberosities to accommodate the development and eruption of the maxillary posterior teeth. In the mandible, resorption of the anterior ramal borders provides room for the development and eruption of the mandibular posterior teeth. Eruption of the mandibular teeth enhances the vertical growth of the mandible and also contributes to the height of the face. However, compensatory condylar growth must occur to prevent the mandible from rotating posteriorly as the maxilla grows downward and the dentition erupts. Dental emergence into the oral cavity begins at approximately the sixth postnatal month, and the primary dentition is established by 2.5 years of age. The primary incisors begin to exfoliate at 6 to 7 years of age, and the permanent dentition begins to emerge with eruption of the mandibular incisors and first molars. The permanent dentition is established by 12 to 14 years of age except for the eruption of the third molars, contributing to the vertical dimension of the lower face during adolescent growth.

Facial Development

The growth of the facial soft tissue follows the underlying facial bones but is not directly correlated with bone growth. Facial soft tissue is thicker relative to the underlying skeletal tissue in the young child due to subcutaneous fat. This is one of the reasons it is more challenging to assess potential underlying skeletal discrepancies in the young child based only on a clinical appraisal. The thicker soft tissue envelope, together with the relative retrognathic position of the mandible, creates a more convex profile in infancy and early childhood. Lip thickness increases until it reaches a maximum at the end of

the pubertal growth spurt, then decreasing in late teens and adulthood.[28,29] These later changes, combined with continued forward nasal growth as well as anterior mandibular and chin projection, leave the lips with a more retrusive appearance and the nose and chin with a more prominent appearance. These changes usually create a flatter facial profile in older adolescents and adults. This tendency is even greater on average in males than females, due to the less common presence of subcutaneous fat, combined with more nasal growth and anterior mandibular and chin projection in males.

The facial soft tissue also follows the cephalocaudal growth gradient, with the soft tissue of the lower face growing more in magnitude and duration than the upper face. The vertical length of the upper lip is a smaller proportion of lower face height in the preadolescent, often resulting in lack of resting lip apposition. During and following pubertal growth the upper lip proportion increases with greater vertical lip growth than the underlying vertical skeletal growth, creating a more likely chance of resting lip apposition in adults.[30]

There is significant growth in the length of the nose during adolescence, influencing the facial balance between the nose, lips, and chin.[31] In fact the vertical nasal growth is much greater than anteroposterior or transverse nasal growth. Nasal growth during adolescence is primarily limited to cartilage and soft tissue since the nasal bones usually have completed growth earlier. The nasal shape often changes prior to adolescence with the upper nasal dorsum developing superiorly and anteriorly, with the lower nasal dorsum more often following the lower facial growth pattern. In other words, individuals who have a more anterior and superior rotational pattern of lower face growth will exhibit a similar rotation of the lower nasal dorsum. There is some evidence that skeletal Class II jaw relationships usually demonstrate a more prominent nasal bridge and convex dorsum than balanced jaw relationships.[32]

The upper third of the face grows the most rapidly early in life due to brain growth and achieves its ultimate size earliest, finishing most growth by 12 years of age. Orbital height already reaches 55% of its adult height at birth and 94% by 7 years of age.[33] The middle and lower thirds of the face are less affected by brain growth, growing more slowly and for a longer time. Most of the middle third growth is completed later during puberty, with the lower third of the face continuing to grow beyond puberty into adulthood.

In addition to this vertical sequential growth gradient, craniofacial growth does not take place at an equal rate in the three planes of space. The completion of growth follows a sequence where transverse growth finishes first, followed by anteroposterior and finally vertical growth. The face reflects the early transverse neural expansion of the cranium, the early fusion of the mandibular symphysis, and the early growth cessation of the midpalatal suture during the first few years of life. This presents clinically as a disproportionately wide face relative to the height in the infant and young child. As the maxilla and mandible displace and grow downward and forward, the anteroposterior and vertical growth begin to take proportionately greater roles. The growth rate of the maxilla slows down after about 10 years of age, and together with anterior maxillary resorption, reduces the relative anterior projection of the midface. The maxillary length reaches maturity prior to the upper facial height, which is followed by mandibular length and finally ramus height.[34] The somewhat retrognathic position of the mandible at birth is usually corrected early in postnatal life. The mandible grows for a longer duration than the maxilla, typically undergoing a growth spurt at puberty. Anteroposterior growth is accompanied and then followed by vertical facial growth, often continuing well beyond puberty, even in to the third and fourth decades.

There are gender differences in facial growth, with males characteristically having volume changes of greater magnitude than females. Females have much less nasal growth on average, with many not even exhibiting a pubertal nasal growth spurt, in contrast to males who characteristically have a nasal growth spurt throughout puberty. Females have earlier soft tissue growth that follows their earlier puberty and they have greater lip thickness at all ages. The flattening of the facial profile during adolescence is less dramatic in females, due in part to their fuller lips, but also due to females having less forward mandibular growth projection and chin growth. Females have on average more late vertical maxillary growth than males. If mandibular growth is not matching these late maxillary changes, the mandible translates downward and backward, resulting in a more convex profile. Not only are male facial volume changes on average greater in magnitude, but the duration of the changes is longer, and there is more predominance of volume increase in the lower third of the face.[35] Males are on average more likely to have late mandibular growth that may be beneficial in improving a maxillary protrusion or mandibular retrusion, but is disadvantageous when a mandibular prognathism or maxillary retrusion is present prior to late growth.

Growth and Facial Changes during Adulthood

There has been awareness since the late nineteenth century that human growth continues beyond adolescence, at least until the fourth or fifth decade of life.[36] Nevertheless investigators in the mid-twentieth century were surprised to find that facial growth continues into the sixth decade of life.[37] More recently it was found that the craniofacial complex remodels throughout adulthood, with thickening of the frontal region of the cranium and a symmetric modest increase in the size of the cranium, cranial base, maxilla, and mandible.[38,39]

During the past two decades there have been a number of longitudinal craniofacial growth studies that have examined changes during adulthood.[40–44] Evaluation of the serial cephalometric radiographs revealed that craniofacial growth continues with increases in both anteroposterior and vertical dimensions at all age levels, similar to the changes seen during adolescence, but of a much lesser magnitude and rate. Females grow less and their craniofacial growth is expressed more vertically with posterior mandibular rotation, whereas males tend to grow with anterior mandibular rotation during adulthood, thereby straightening their profile (Figure 53-15).

Typical lip changes during adulthood include less prominence with decreased thickness and thinning of the vermilion, with male lips continuing to appear more retrusive with age. Female lips generally do not become more retrusive and their lower lip thickness tends to increase slightly. The lips become positioned more inferiorly, resulting in less vertical display of maxillary incisors and less lip separation.[45] The nose continues to increase in size in all dimensions, but more so in males, with the nasal tip dropping inferiorly.[46] There is deepening of the nasolabial folds and the oral commissures tend to sag inferiorly. There is more prominence of the pogonion due to continued soft tissue increase, but this is typically limited to males.

The biologic regulator mechanism for initiating and directing craniofacial growth and dental eruption timing, pattern, and rate remains a poorly understood phenomenon. It is clear that it is a complex mechanism, influenced by an intricate interaction of genetic, epigenetic, and local environmental factors.

Factors Influencing Craniofacial Growth

Craniofacial growth is a complex process influenced by both prenatal and postnatal genetic and environmental factors. The principal influence on craniofacial growth

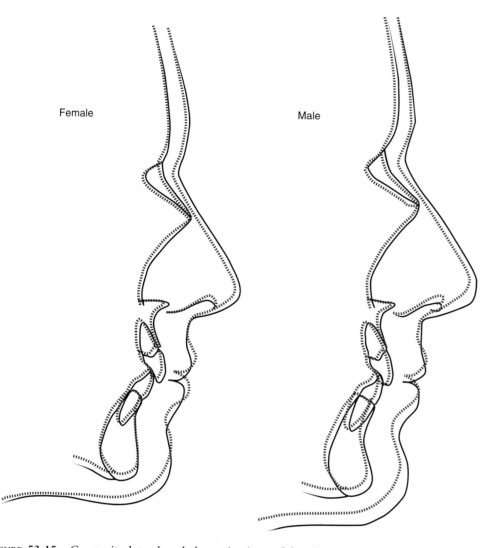

Female   Male

FIGURE **53-15** *Composite lateral cephalometric views of female and male showing longitudinal growth changes from young adult (broken line at mean age 17) to middle age adult (solid line at mean age 47 to 51). Note the continued downward and forward skeletal and soft tissue growth with relative flattening of the lips. Adapted from Behrents RG.*[40]

Genetic Craniofacial malformations arise from disturbance in morphogenesis as early as the germ layer formation to the final formation of organ systems at the end of the embryonic period. The fourth to eighth weeks' gestation is a particularly critical time because this is the period when neural crest migration is at its most active, the facial primordia and dental laminae are forming, and neurovascular bundles are being generated prior to facial bone ossification. Malformations are caused from chromosome abnormalities or single gene mutations, or are multifactorial (genetic and/or teratogenic) in origin. Growth retardation, premature death, and mental retardation seem to be more frequent in autosomal recessive or X-linked syndromes.[48] Craniofacial malformations range from acephaly to mild facial defects such as a microform cleft or notching of the lip. Cranial malformations include premature or delayed fusion of the cranial sutures, due to mutations in fibroblast growth factor receptors and the transcription factor MSX2, associated with syndromes such as trisomy 21 and cleidocraniodysostosis or with simply a deformation craniosynostosis.[49,50] Cranial base malformations usually are related to malformations that affect cartilage growth such as achondroplasia. Apert, Crouzon, and Pfeiffer syndromes involve premature fusion of multiple facial and cranial sutures as well as cranial base synchondroses.[51] Many facial malformations originate from a deficiency, incomplete migration, or failure in cytodifferentiation of neural crest tissue during embryogenesis.[52] The result is a failure in normal formation of the skeletal and connective tissue portions of the facial primordia. Nasomaxillary malformations include deficiencies and/or absence of facial bones that occur in ectodermal dysplasia or mandibulofacial dysostosis, as well as facial clefts that are associated with over 250 syndromes. The most common craniofacial malformation is unilateral cleft lip,

and morphogenesis is one of multifactorial genetic control. However, the interaction of this genetic control with environmental factors is a complex one, and it is usually impossible to accurately differentiate between these influences.

Prenatal Factors

Prenatal defects of craniofacial development can be classified conveniently into three categories: (1) malformation—a morphologic defect of an organ, part of an organ, or larger region of the body resulting from an intrinsically abnormal developmental process, which is intrinsically

determined due to the genome or a teratogen, and occurs during the embryonic period; (2) deformation—an abnormal form, shape, or position of a part of the body caused by mechanical forces, which is influenced directly by the fetal environment; and (3) disruption—a morphologic defect of an organ, part of an organ, or a larger region of the body resulting from the extrinsic breakdown of, or an interference with, an originally normal developmental process, which also occurs during the fetal period and may result from intrauterine pressure as well, but can be of metabolic, vascular, and/or teratogenic origin.[47]

affecting 1 in 700 to 800 births. Malformations that affect the mandible range from the rare absence (agnathia), to various forms of micrognathia, associated with a number of syndromes, such as mandibulofacial dysostosis (Treacher Collins syndrome) or Turner syndrome, to macrognathia, associated with hyperpituitarism or hemifacial hypertrophy.

Two more common chromosomal disorders that result in growth retardation are Down syndrome and Turner syndrome, both of which are characterized by short stature and brachycephaly. The protruding tongue typical of Down syndrome usually results in an anterior openbite, whereas a narrow high-arched palate often is seen with Turner syndrome. The Russell-Silver syndrome is a chromosomal disorder characterized by poor fetal and postnatal growth and small triangular facies. Other syndromes associated with prenatal growth retardation include Bloom syndrome, de Lange syndrome, leprechaunism (mutations of the insulin receptor gene), Ellis-van Creveld syndrome, Aarskog syndrome, Rubenstein-Taybi syndrome, Perheentupa syndrome, Dubowitz syndrome, and Johanson Blizzard syndrome.[53]

Single-gene disorders that result in fetal overgrowth include Sotos syndrome, Weaver syndrome, and Beckwith-Wiedemann syndrome. Sotos syndrome includes craniofacial features of macrocephaly, dolichocephaly, a prominent forehead, hypertelorism, prominent ears, high-arched palate, and mandibular prognathism. The Beckwith-Wiedemann syndrome, another example of uniparental disomy, is associated with excessive somatic and specific organ growth (eg, macroglossia) apparently caused by excess IGF-II. In spite of the overgrowth with these disorders that extends from the fetal period into early childhood, both lead to early epiphyseal fusion, resulting in adult short stature. Klinefelter syndrome (XXY) is a chromosomal disorder that leads to postnatal extended growth from pubertal failure, resulting in tall adult stature.

An example of a single-gene growth disorder is achondroplasia, the most common form of human dwarfism, which is autosomal dominant with complete penetrance, involving mutations in the *FGFR3* gene. Since the primary cartilage of the cranial base synchondroses is affected, and not the secondary cartilage of the mandibular condyles, midfacial hypoplasia resulting in a Class III skeletal discrepancy is the usual facial outcome. A single-gene disorder that leads to postnatal overgrowth resulting in tall adult stature is Marfan syndrome.

Environmental Prenatal environmental growth factors are those not directly determined by the genome, including cytoplasmic and extracellular contents in the embryo or fetus and the placenta, influenced by the mother and her interaction with the external environment. Some of these environmental factors may be internal (such as focal embryonic hemorrhages) or external (from maternal malnutrition, metabolic factors, and disease, or exposure to pollutants, chemicals, drugs, infectious agents, or radiation), and may impair normal growth or act as teratogens during either the embryonic or fetal period if the maternal exposure is large or frequent enough (Figure 53-16).

Cytomegalovirus and rubella are examples of pathogens that can cause microcephaly, hydrocephaly, and microphthalmia. Glucocorticoids, phenytoin, ethyl alcohol, tobacco smoke, aspirin, and retinoic acid (a vitamin A metabolite) are examples of an ever-increasing number of substances that are being identified as teratogens, causing cleft lip and palate as well as other craniofacial anomalies.[54] Teratogens have distinct mechanisms of action and are selective to certain target cells, but the severity of the resulting malformation is variable. It is speculated that the range of phenotypic effects caused by a teratogen is due to factors that include the concentration or method of delivery, the timing and

duration of exposure, variations in susceptibility, and synergistic interactions among teratogenic compounds.[55] Even in the absence of any detectable malformations, serious long-term physical and mental development can result from drug intake during pregnancy.

When the fetal period begins, environmental factors can still have a profound growth effect on the developing fetus. Maternal malnutrition adversely affects fetal growth.[56] Maternal diet composition is relevant, with a high-protein diet being associated with increased linear fetal growth and a high-fat diet linked to an increased birth weight. Maternal consumption of alcohol, recreational drugs, or tobacco all have an important negative influence on growth in utero as well as during the first year of life.[57–59] Even maternal exposure to passive tobacco smoke reduces fetal growth.[60] Frequent high maternal noise exposure has been shown to adversely affect prenatal growth, perhaps related to the stress imposed.[61] Maternal pathology such as rubella is particularly detrimental if it occurs in the first trimester, causing a growth deficit with no long-term recovery.[62]

Intrauterine pressures can result in deformations or disruptions. Intrauterine restrictions can result in mild to severe deformations that can present as mild facial or cranial asymmetry. Some isolated forms of craniosynostosis, causing cranial deformations such as plagiocephaly, may be caused from intrauterine mechanical factors.[63] These deformations may resolve after birth with catch-up growth but usually require orthopedic or surgical intervention during infancy. Another deformation is the Robin sequence whereby retrognathia from posterior restraint of the mandible forces the developing tongue into a posterior position, often acting as a mechanical obstruction that prevents elevation of the palatal shelves, resulting in an isolated cleft palate. A disruption is a typically more serious anomaly than a deformation, from the

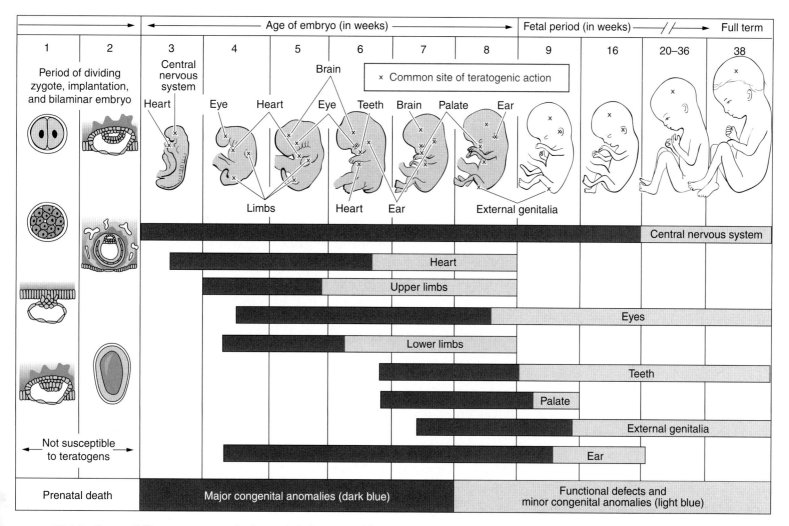

FIGURE **53-16** *Susceptibility to teratogens during periods in prenatal human development. During the first two weeks' gestation, damage from the teratogen results in death of the conceptus, or damages only a few cells, allowing recovery by the embryo to develop without birth defects. Dark blue indicates highly sensitive periods when major defects may be produced (eg, amelia, absence of limbs). Light blue indicates less sensitive periods when minor defects may be produced (eg, hypoplastic thumbs). Adapted from Moore KL, Persaud TVN. The developing human: clinically oriented embryology. 5th ed. Philadelphia (PA): W.B. Saunders Co.; 1973. p. 156.*

standpoint of both treatment and future growth, because it presents as a morphologic and functional defect that requires surgical repair. An example of a disruption is where a strand of torn amnion or amniotic band is swallowed by the fetus, resulting in a facial cleft that is not located at a site of embryonic fusion.

The hormonal regulation of fetal growth is not well understood. Fetal androgens appear to be growth promoters. At midgestation the level of gonadotropin is similar to pubertal levels.[64] Although there is some evidence that estrogen promotes fetal bone development, there are also data that suggest that it inhibits fetal

growth.[65,66] There is a marked and progressive increase in prolactin during late gestation. Before 12 weeks' gestation, maternal hypothyroidism can have long-term deleterious effects on hearing and intelligence, but neither maternal nor fetal hypothyroidism has an appreciable effect on fetal length or weight. However, when both conditions are present, linear growth is still unaffected but there is incomplete pulmonary, cardiovascular, and skeletal maturation.[67] Although poorly understood, insulin appears to have an important role in regulation and promotion of fetal growth. Maternal diabetes increases fetal length and weight, whereas fetal

insulin deficiency results in decreased length and weight at birth.[68]

Although growth hormone (GH) is essential for postnatal growth, growth in utero and probably in the first 2 years of life is largely GH independent.[69,70] Nevertheless IGF-I and -II play important roles in determining fetal growth, but the specific nature of these roles are not well understood. IGF-II is important in supporting fetal growth during early gestation whereas IGF-I has a greater role during later gestation and especially in postnatal life.[71] The fetal roles of growth factors such as nerve, epidermal, and platelet-derived growth factors also remain unclear. Other fetal growth factors include hematopoietic growth factors, fibroblast growth factors, vascular endothelial growth factor, and members of the TGF-β family.[72]

The placenta functions as an additional endocrine organ, providing a secondary source of hypothalamic, pituitary, adrenal, and gonadal hormones and growth factors.[73] Placental GH and lactogen can alter the production of maternal IGF-I.[71] Maternal IGF-I in turn affects placental nutrient transport, increasing fetal growth.[74] Lactogen regulates maternal glucose, amino acid, and lipid metabolism, facilitating nutrient transport to the fetus. Disruption of placental GH or lactogen production can occur from vascular disease, infection, or intrinsic placental abnormalities, impairing fetal growth.[75]

Postnatal Factors

The size of infants in the first months of life is more related to the prenatal environment than parental height. If prenatal factors caused only mild growth attenuation and it occurred during the last trimester, then postnatal catch-up growth is feasible.

An area of craniofacial growth can be differentiated as a growth center or growth site. A growth center is where there is primarily intrinsic genetic growth control with a minimal environmental or functional role. Although a growth site also is controlled to some extent by genetic programming, it is more vulnerable to extrinsic growth control, being dependent more on the functional influence of the surrounding tissues. Cranial base synchondroses, where endochondral ossification of primary cartilage occurs, represent growth centers. The role of the cartilaginous nasal septum as a growth center or site remains controversial. There is a clearer understanding that the endochondral growth of the secondary cartilage of the mandibular condyles acts as a growth site, being greatly influenced by mandibular and soft tissue function. Areas of membranous bone growth resulting from sutural or periosteal ossification are primarily growth sites and represent the bulk of the remaining craniofacial complex. There are exceptions, such as craniosynostosis, that can be due to an underlying genetic cause. Membranous ossification by sutural and periosteal remodeling is essentially the only type of craniofacial bone growth that occurs after adolescence throughout adulthood.

Genetic Heritability appears to have an effect on somatic growth, from a greater to lesser extent in the following order: skeletal length, skeletal breadth, weight, circumference, and skin folds. By the same token skeletal tissues respond less to changes in the nutritional environment than soft tissues.[76] The timing and pace of maturation is also genetically controlled to a large degree. The extent to which heredity is the cause of postnatal growth that results in jaw discrepancies is controversial. It appears that the genetic influence is particularly important for excessive mandibular growth and excessive vertical facial growth.[77,78] It is speculated that probably no more than 50% of facial skeletal variation is due to the genetic component with the remaining half or more due to environmental influence.[79] Functional forces have a crucial influence in modifying craniofacial bone growth. Although genetic influence is important, the membranous viscerocranium is determined to a great extent by functional influences, with these extrinsic factors having the greatest control over mandibular growth.

Environmental There is a multitude of postnatal environmental factors that interact with genetic control mechanisms, including functional, traumatic, endocrine, nutritional, pathologic, psychological, cultural, and climatic, or seasonal factors.

The functional environment is determined by neuromuscular behavior necessary for survival such as respiration, mastication, deglutition, speech, and posture. However, it is clear that functional influences at rest (ie, postural activity or the presence of a pathologic mass) are much more important than transient muscle contractions and mandibular movement in influencing craniofacial growth.[80] Chronic pressure alters regional skeletal growth and may be used to improve or correct some craniofacial deformities.[81] Habitual behavior such as non-nutritive sucking and other oral or postural habits also may have an impact on growth if it is present with great enough frequency and duration.[82,83] Mastication limited to one side for sufficient duration can cause asymmetric mandibular growth.[84] There is some evidence that diet consistency has an effect on mandibular morphology.[85,86]

The extent of masticatory muscular and dental development can modify the morphology of skeletal superstructures, including the temporal fossae and sagittal crests, the zygomatic arches, the lateral pterygoid plates, the angular and coronoid processes and rami of the mandible, and parts of the temporomandibular joints.[87] The size and function of masticatory muscles has been correlated with facial morphology.[88–90] Other studies have demonstrated an atrophic effect from muscle denervation.[91,92] However, it also is clear that external craniofacial bone growth nevertheless can occur in the absence of any muscle function.[93,94]

Growth deficiency due to neuromuscular deficits can occur in muscle weakness conditions such as muscular dystrophy. The difficulty in returning function to the area makes such conditions particularly resistant to treatment. However, if the muscle is normal, it appears that the normal force range of masticatory muscular function in the general population does not significantly affect facial growth.[95] Long-term impairment of nasal breathing historically has been viewed as a cause of long face deformity, but this assumption continues to be controversial.[96] There is less disagreement about a relationship between nasal obstruction and facial deformity than there is with the extent and duration of mouth breathing necessary to cause a deformity.

Postnatal surgery during infancy for congenital malformations such as cleft lip and palate introduces scarring that is responsible for some midfacial growth attenuation. Typical surgery to close palatal clefts requires that mucoperiosteal flaps be raised and moved medially and posteriorly. This results in denuded bony areas that will heal with the formation of scar tissue bands of variable size and elasticity. This scar tissue usually connects across the maxilla and includes the palatal bones and possibly the pterygoid plates. It is thought that the presence of this scar tissue during postnatal growth compromises midfacial growth.[97] The longer postnatal surgery can be delayed, the less growth is affected.

Perinatal or postnatal trauma to the craniofacial complex can modify growth if there is limitation of blood supply or mechanical constriction due to scarring. Extensive midfacial trauma can cause midface growth deficiency as a result of the loss of intrinsic nasal septal growth or from a structural collapse that prevents normal morphologic expression of growth.[98] Untreated burns of the head and neck can cause significant craniofacial dysmorphology.[99] Neurologic damage may lead to muscle paralysis that can alter craniofacial form due to decreased muscle function. There should be caution when considering early craniofacial reconstructive surgery, since the surgery itself may produce additional scarring that can exacerbate the growth attenuation. There is no evidence that the use of rigid plate fixation for trauma reconstruction causes restrictive growth effects in addition to the trauma alone.[100] With trauma involving the mandible, mandibular function must be maintained, often requiring physical therapy

and the use of a functional appliance. As long as mandibular ankylosis is prevented, surgery should be avoided when treating condylar fractures in children.[101]

Endocrine disturbances originating from pathology or the environment are among the most potent regulators of postnatal growth. The primary growth promoting hormone, GH, is secreted by the pituitary and regulated by somatostatin and GH-releasing hormone release from the hypothalamus. Studies have demonstrated increased GH secretion throughout the day and night in the newborn. However, IGF-I levels are lower at birth and gradually increase during childhood and into adolescence, indicating an early immaturity in the feedback loop. Although the growth process in utero and in the first months after birth is more nutritionally dependent than GH dependent, this changes during the first year of life, with full GH dependence attained during the second year.[70] GH has been shown to have a direct stimulatory effect on cartilage growth, whereas IGF-I acts as a secondary stimulatory effector.[102]

Most of our present understanding of the endocrine influence on craniofacial growth has developed from assessing children who have diagnosed endocrine disorders. GH-deficient children have excess subcutaneous fat and overall delayed facial and cranial base development, resulting in infantile, but proportional, facies. Dental development is delayed as well but to a much lesser degree than facial or somatic growth. In contrast the craniofacial growth is disproportionate in an autosomal recessive condition known as Laron syndrome where there is IGF-I deficiency in spite of increased serum GH levels.[103] There is a normal calvarium with small facial bones, resulting in the forehead appearing large and prominent relative to the small recessed face.[104] This suggests that some areas of the face are more directly affected by GH than IGF-I.

GH excess, usually a consequence of a pituitary adenoma, results in gigantism if it occurs prior to the end of adolescence and presents with overall larger craniofacial dimensions. Acromegaly is the outcome if the GH excess is produced following adolescence, characterized by increased periosteal bone that includes cranial thickening, increased size of the frontal sinuses, prominent supraorbital ridges, and nasal enlargement as well as renewed mandibular condylar cartilage growth, leading to mandibular prognathism.

Hypothyroidism will decrease GH release and results in delayed bone and dental development.[105] The craniofacial outcome of this deficiency differs from GH deficiency primarily by the smaller cranium. Anabolic steroids increase craniofacial growth but may lead to excessive anterior maxillary growth in high doses.[106] Testosterone, GH, and IGF-I accelerate endochondral and intramembranous craniofacial skeletal growth as well as statural height. Estrogen appears to decrease endochondral growth.[107,108]

Although glucocorticoid production is necessary for normal growth, glucocorticoid therapy in the prepubertal child must be carefully managed to avoid its inhibitory effect on GH and IGF-I production, resulting in short stature.[109] Though there are no clinical studies indicating the effect on craniofacial growth, animal model studies have suggested a retarding effect on mandibular condylar cartilage growth and acceleration in dental eruption.[110,111]

Poor nutrition, hygiene, and health adversely affect growth. Insufficient caloric and protein intake is the most common cause of growth failure worldwide.[112] Growth deficiency from malnutrition is proportional to the severity of the nutritional deficit. Malnutrition is associated with increased GH but decreased production of IGF-I, reallocating calories from anabolic to survival requirements.[113] It is estimated that 55% of the morphologic variation of the cranium is due to nutritional factors.[114]

Because of the early rapid growth of the brain, the cranium is affected more by infant malnutrition than the rest of the craniofacial complex. The size of the neurocranium decreases in rats subjected to malnutrition.[115] A diet deficient in calcium and vitamin D resulted in cranial dimensional changes in rats.[116] It is thought that maternal vitamin A deficiency alters endocrine function that causes a disturbance in chondrogenesis, reducing the cranial base.[117] Nasomaxillary hypoplasia in humans can be related to maternal vitamin K deficiency induced in rats, causing limited nasal septal cartilage growth.[118] Protein malnutrition in rats decreases the length of the skull relative to the width.[119,120] Voluntary undernutrition has become more common during adolescence, especially with females trying to decrease weight for athletics and those with anxiety about obesity. This may develop into extreme eating disorders such as anorexia or bulimia, which may result in impaired growth, delayed puberty, and osteopenia.[121]

Chronic disease such as congenital heart disease, malabsorption syndrome (eg, chronic inflammatory disease, cystic fibrosis, celiac disease), chronic renal or liver disease, chronic anemia, inborn errors of metabolism, chronic infections (eg, tuberculosis, acquired immunodeficiency syndrome), severe asthma, or other chronic pulmonary disease can adversely affect growth.[122] There are a variety of mechanisms causing the growth deficits from these conditions, including reduced nutritional intake, metabolic disbalance, hypoxia, chronic metabolic acidosis protein loss, and often the treatment for the pathology itself.[123] Medications that limit potential growth include chronic adrenal steroid therapy (used for asthma, nephritic syndrome, lupus, and other chronic diseases) and cytostatics (for cancer treatment). Irradiation of the head and face for childhood cancer can result in severe hypoplasia of soft and hard tissues.[124,125] If cranial irradiation is required in cases of leukemia and tumors of the central nervous system, hypothalamic function can be damaged, affecting the release of hypothalamic and pituitary hormones, notably GH.

Chronic psychological trauma, emotional deprivation, or psychosocial stress can have a profound effect on somatic growth, causing a functional and reversible GH deficiency, often mimicking growth disorders that are caused from endocrine or nutritional deficiencies.[126]

Additional less important factors have been shown to have a significant influence on postnatal growth and development. These include climate, altitude, exposure to environmental pollutants, and noise.[127–130] Future research will increase our understanding of the role that these and other yet unidentified environmental factors play in altering human genetic growth potential.

Orthopedic and Orthodontic Clinical Considerations

Orthopedic Treatment for Growth Modification

Just as our understanding of craniofacial growth is continually evolving, the application of this knowledge to clinical practice is also in a constant state of flux. This application is particularly important in order to determine the appropriate use of growth modification for treatment of craniofacial skeletal discrepancies.

A harmonious esthetic facial appearance and balanced dentoskeletal segments facilitating a functional occlusion are both goals that orthodontists and oral maxillofacial surgeons work to achieve by means of orthodontic treatment combined with orthognathic surgery. However, before a surgical correction is contemplated in a growing patient, a determination should be made if the patient is a candidate for orthopedic treatment that may modify craniofacial growth to improve the skeletal imbalance to a favorable esthetic and functional outcome without the need for orthognathic surgery. It is well known that craniofacial orthopedic devices can generate forces that cause stress in sutures capable of modifying suture growth.[131] As indicated earlier in the chapter, almost 50% of the total cumulative growth of the midface and mandible remains between the ages of 10 years and adulthood, making it possible to have an orthopedic treatment effect on the jaws during this time.

In spite of over a century of clinical experience with orthopedic facial appliances, it remains controversial as to what extent growth can be predictably and permanently modified by orthopedic treatment. Although there is consensus that there is an important genetic influence on the outcome of craniofacial growth, there is a wide range of views regarding the amount in which postnatal factors, particularly orthopedic treatment, influence this outcome. Views range from the belief that orthopedic alteration of jaw relationships is predictable and stable, to the contrasting opinion that facial growth is primarily determined genetically and cannot be significantly altered by orthopedic treatment. The reality is likely to be somewhere between these two extreme views. It has been proposed that the typical range of skeletal malocclusions include individuals with normal gene polymorphisms for signaling molecules and growth factors that attenuate the capacity of tissues and cells to reliably respond to orthopedic treatment.[132]

The efficacy of craniofacial growth modification has been a controversial subject for more than a century. At the onset of the twentieth century there was universal confidence by the orthodontic profession that forces applied through the dentition to the growing face could effectively treat craniofacial skeletal discrepancies. After the 1920s there was a decline in this conviction by North American orthodontists. With the invention of the cephalostat, more precise skeletal assessment of treatment outcomes became possible during the 1950s. This resulted in renewed faith in growth modification, with the demonstration of skeletal changes from the use of extraoral force applied with a cervical headgear.

In Europe there was less controversy regarding craniofacial growth modification efficacy throughout the first half of the twentieth century. European orthodontists relied primarily on removable "functional" appliances, designed to provide forces from facial muscles and soft tissue function, for facial orthopedic treatment. The separate philosophical paths taken by European and American orthodontists united in the 1960s, resulting in a more global acceptance of either extraoral (headgear) or intraoral (functional) appliances, or a combination of both to facilitate craniofacial orthopedic treatment. This acceptance gained support and enthusiasm from results of basic research conducted during the 1970s using animal models. Although this enthusiasm reached its peak in the 1980s, it was considerably moderated in the 1990s from clinical experiences and the results of retrospective clinical studies. There remains little argument that some craniofacial growth modification is feasible, but there continues to be controversy over the nature and extent of the skeletal change possible in individual patients as well as the optimal treatment timing and appliance type. In addition a reliable and accurate method of predicting the direction, timing, and magnitude of craniofacial growth for an individual has not been devised.

The aim of craniofacial growth modification is to alter the growth pattern by changing the relationships of the jaws. If the skeletal unit is too large, the aim of the orthopedic treatment is to attenuate or redirect its growth to improve its relationship relative to the opposing jaw. If the jaw is too small, the growth modification treatment is aimed at enhancing or redirecting its growth relative to the larger skeletal unit. Virtually all of the growth modification appliances to date have been "tooth-borne" to some extent, so that the orthopedic forces applied to the skeletal units also create stress to the teeth that results in some dental movement. Although the goal of craniofacial growth modification is to limit the changes to the skeletal units with minimal movement of the teeth, the reality is that the treatment is a combination of skeletal and dentoalveolar changes.

There is growing evidence that the long-term success of many forms of growth modification requires that the treatment be continued until facial growth is nearly complete, making early treatment a less efficient way to treat many jaw discrepancies. The following discussion will summarize the facial orthopedic options we have for clinical application of our present understanding of craniofacial growth in the three planes of space.

Transverse Orthopedic Treatment Since transverse growth reaches completion earlier than anteroposterior or vertical craniofacial growth, it follows that transverse skeletal problems should be addressed early. The most common transverse skeletal problem is maxillary constriction, which can be treated in the preadolescent child, even as early as during the primary dentition. The most recent federal epidemiologic study, the National Health and Nutrition Estimates Survey (NHANES-III) conducted from 1989 through 1994, indicates the prevalence of posterior crossbite is about 5% of the US population.[133] Significant facial or mandibular asymmetry represents about 0.1% of the total population.[134] Although maxillary orthopedic expansion devices have been used since 1860, they fell out of favor for a few decades prior to the 1940s due to unsubstantiated concerns regarding their safety and effectiveness.[135] Orthopedic expansion of the maxilla can be achieved with a variety of toothborne appliances (Figure 53-17). These appliances apply moderate to high forces to the teeth that are transmitted as stresses to the maxilla, primarily distracting the midpalatal sutures but also producing less pronounced stresses to the sphenoid and zygomatic bones and other adjacent structures.[136] Within days following initial expansion, new bone forms, eventually depositing both perpendicular and parallel to the edges of the expanded sutures.[137] Although a large amount of the skeletal

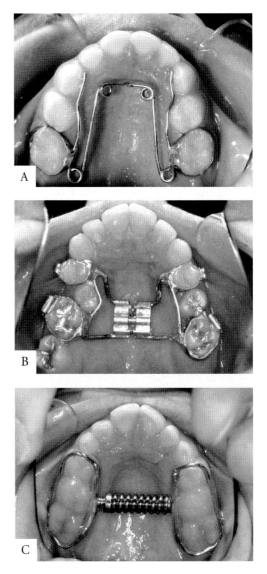

FIGURE **53-17** *Types of maxillary orthopedic expansion appliances. A, Quad-helix: An effective skeletal expansion appliance in the primary dentition. B, Banded Hyrax: This traditional jackscrew also can be used as an activation component for an appliance bonded to the maxillary posterior teeth. C, Bonded Minne-expander: This spring-loaded component also can be used as an activation component for an appliance banded to the maxillary posterior teeth.*

expansion relapses during retention, overall stability is good if the extent of sutural patency and magnitude of expansion are great enough. A potential additional benefit to improvement in interarch transverse compatibility is an increase in arch perimeter made possible by the maxillary orthopedic expansion.[138]

Although complete fusion of the midpalatal suture usually does not occur until the third postnatal decade, the process leading to fusion is a gradual one, characterized by progressive sutural interdigitation and ossification.[139] For this reason more effective sutural separation, requiring less force and concomitant dental expansion, is possible in the younger child, especially prior to puberty, during a "phase 1" treatment in the mixed or early permanent dentition. Treatment prior to the pubertal growth velocity peak may result in greater long-term skeletal craniofacial transverse width.[140] Treatment may even be indicated as early as the primary dentition in the presence of a transverse functional shift. This compensatory functional problem can result in asymmetric condylar positioning that may lead to asymmetric mandibular growth and uneven remodeling of the glenoid fossae, possibly resulting in permanent facial asymmetry, even if the constricted maxillary arch is corrected at a later date.[141] Maxillary constriction without a transverse functional shift does not carry the same urgency and is conveniently treated closer to the onset of puberty during the early permanent dentition.[142]

Maxillary orthopedic expansion in late adolescent or postadolescent patients should be attempted with caution. Even if skeletal expansion is possible in these older patients, the extent of circum-maxillary sutural patency is limited enough to compromise stability of the treatment outcome. It is appropriate to confirm intermaxillary expansion with an occlusal radiograph in these patients, since the development of a midline diastema may only indicate bending of maxillary bones.

If the expansion is limited to lateral tipping of maxillary posterior teeth, buccal alveolar bone height reduction and gingival recession may occur. It usually is more prudent to consider surgically assisted palatal expansion for late adolescent or postadolescent patients to avoid periodontal compromises and instability.

The expansion appliance can be banded or bonded to the maxillary posterior teeth with a spring-loaded or nonspring-loaded palatal jackscrew that usually is activated by the patient 0.5 mm per day, delivering from 2 to more than 10 pounds of force (this may increase to cumulative loads of 20 pounds or more with multiple activations in the absence of adequate sutural separation). The conventional description for the expansion induced with this appliance is "rapid palatal expansion." However, it is possible to affect slower expansion with less frequent activations, requiring more active treatment time, but less retention time to ensure stability.[143] It is possible to achieve skeletal expansion with simpler appliances such as a W-arch or Quad-helix, provided that the patient is in the primary or very early mixed dentition, when the maxillary sutures are more patent or when a cleft of the hard palate is present (Figure 53-18).

Since all of these expansion appliances are toothborne, unwanted dentoalveolar expansion is an inevitable consequence.[144,145] An additional undesirable outcome is the long-term loss of about 30% of the skeletal expansion achieved during active treatment due to the rebound of stretched palatal tissues.[146] To compensate for these effects, maxillary expansion should be continued until adequate overexpansion is achieved, usually to the extent that the lingual cusps of the maxillary molars are opposing the buccal cusps of the mandibular molars (Figure 53-19). Once adequate expansion has been accomplished, at least 3 to 6 months of retention is necessary to permit new bone

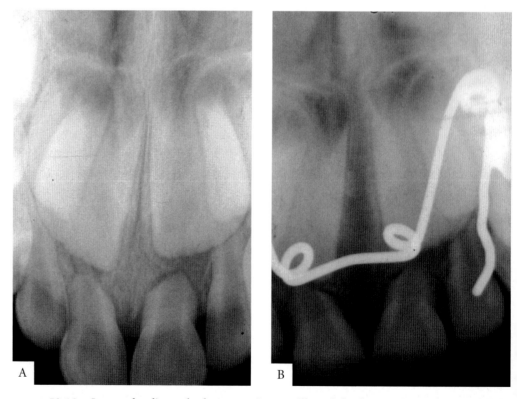

FIGURE 53-18 *Intraoral radiographs demonstrating maxillary skeletal expansion with a Quad-helix during the primary dentition. Note the distraction of the midpalatal suture.* A, *Before expansion.* B, *After initial expansion.*

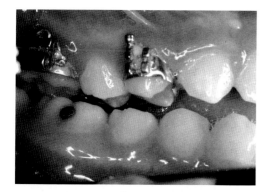

FIGURE 53-19　*Maxillary overexpansion to compensate for dentoalveolar expansion and skeletal rebound. Note that the lingual cusps of the maxillary posterior teeth are occluding with the buccal cusps of the mandibular posterior teeth.*

to fill in the spaces created by maxillary separation and to permit time for dissipation of reaction forces stored in the facial bones that promote relapse. The overexpansion permits the orthodontist to upright the posterior teeth in their alveolar housing without compromising the transverse occlusal correction following retention. Osseointegrated attachments may hold future promise for a means of expanding the maxilla without buccally tipping posterior teeth (Figure 53-20).[147]

A less common transverse skeletal problem than maxillary constriction is asymmetric mandibular deficiency, usually caused from a previous trauma associated

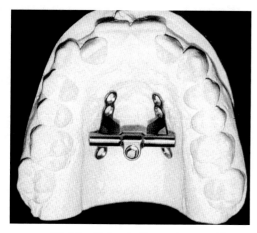

FIGURE 53-20　*Palatal distraction appliance. Reproduced with permission from Gerlach KL, Zahl C. Traversal palatal expansion using a palatal distractor. J Orofac Orthop 2003; 64:444.*

with unilateral mandibular condylar fracture or hemifacial microsomia, a congenital facial asymmetry. In both of these conditions the affected side exhibits growth deficiency relative to the unaffected or normal side, resulting in a mandibular deviation toward the affected side. If left untreated in a growing individual, the alveolar processes compensate with limited eruption of the maxillary posterior teeth on the affected side and excessive eruption of the maxillary posterior teeth on the unaffected side, resulting in an occlusal cant that is higher on the affected side. It is best to start orthopedic treatment with these individuals prior to the pubertal growth spurt, as early as patient compliance will permit. The goal is to maximize the growth expression on the deficient side and minimize dentoalveolar compensation. The orthopedic appliance of choice is an asymmetric "hybrid" functional appliance that is constructed to posture the mandible forward on the affected side, bringing the chin to the midline.[148] Posterior dental eruption is attenuated on the unaffected side with a bite block and eruption is facilitated on the affected side with a buccal shield and the absence of interocclusal acrylic (Figure 53-21). Since untreated mandibular asymmetries of this nature invariably worsen with growth, orthopedic treatment is considered successful if the asymmetry remains stable or improves. Treatment should not continue if progressive asymmetry is apparent in spite of reliable appliance use by the patient.

Anteroposterior Orthopedic Treatment: Class II　A Class II skeletal relationship can be the result of a retrusive and/or deficient mandible, a protrusive or vertically excessive maxilla, or a combination of these skeletal problems. The prevalence of this type of malocclusion is about 15 to 20% of the US population, with about 2% severe enough to be considered as handicapping.[133,134] Prospective clinical studies have supported that early growth modification therapy may lead to an improve-

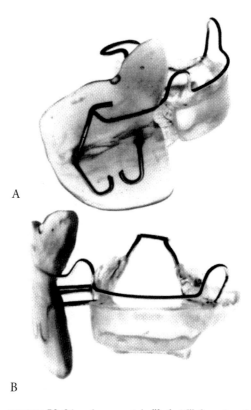

A

B

FIGURE 53-21　*Asymmetric "hybrid" functional appliance: A, right lateral view; B, frontal view. On the left, unaffected side, posterior dental eruption is restricted with an interocclusal acrylic block. On the right, affected side, the mandible is postured forward and posterior dental eruption is encouraged with a buccal shield and absence of an interocclusal acrylic block. Reproduced with permission from Proffit WR, Fields HW. Contemporary orthodontics. 3rd ed. St. Louis (MO): Mosby; 2000. p. 370.*

ment in the skeletal Class II malocclusion.[149–151] It should be kept in mind that regardless of whether orthopedic treatment is attempted during active facial growth, approximately 10% of patients ultimately require orthognathic surgery to fully correct the Class II malocclusion.[150]

The headgear has been used as a means of Class II orthopedic treatment in North America since the late nineteenth century (Figure 53-22). An orthopedic force ranging from 16 to more than 32 ounces is delivered using elastic traction from the headgear to a cervical or cranial attachment for 12 to 14 hours per day, usually for 9 to 12 months. Theoretically the force is transmitted in a posterior and

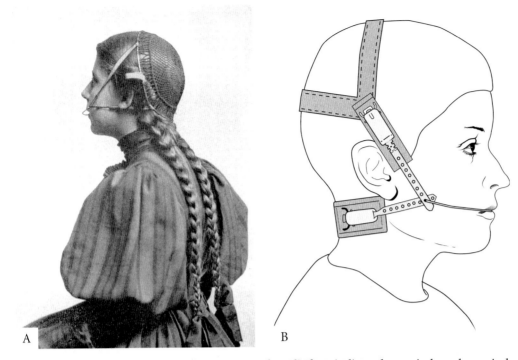

FIGURE **53-22** *Headgear, past and present. An orthopedic force is directed posteriorly and superiorly to the maxilla, attenuating circum-maxillary sutural growth. A, Headgear from the late nineteenth century. Reproduced from Angle EH. Treatment of malocclusion of the teeth. Philadelphia (PA): S.S. White Dental Manufacturing Co; 1907. p. 234. B, Contemporary headgear. The appliance is fabricated with more durable materials and has additional calibration and safety features but the overall design has changed little in over a century. Adapted from McNamara JA, Brudon WL. Orthodontics and dentofacial orthopedics. Ann Arbor (MI): Needham Press, Inc.; 2001. p. 365.*

superior direction via the teeth through the maxilla to compress the circum-maxillary sutures, limiting or redirecting maxillary growth. Since the introduction of standardized cephalometric radiographs, many clinical studies have demonstrated that maxillary growth can be altered with the use of the headgear.[152–170] These clinical data have been supported by primate studies demonstrating that extraoral orthopedic force directed against the maxilla attenuates forward growth and alters bone apposition at the maxillary sutures.[171–179] There are some studies that suggest that mandibular growth may be enhanced as well. Since the headgear is a toothborne appliance, there is some maxillary dental retraction that accompanies the skeletal change. Another dentoalveolar effect is the attenuation of maxillary molar eruption, resulting in anterior and superior mandibular rotation. There is some support for this being the only clinically rele-

vant skeletal effect.[180] A significant treatment effect usually requires that a headgear be worn 12 to 16 hours per day with a superior and posterior force of one pound or more per side. Human GH and other endocrine factors that promote growth and dental eruption are primarily released during the evening and night.[181–183] It is fortuitous that this is the only time of day that one can reliably expect an adolescent to wear a headgear. Since it is a removable appliance, few adolescents after the peak of the pubertal growth spurt will reliably wear the appliance.

The alternative orthopedic method for treating a Class II skeletal relationship is the Class II functional appliance, which has been used since the early twentieth century in Europe and since the 1960s in North America. These appliances include the removable toothborne activator, bionator, and twin block, the removable and primarily tissueborne Fränkel (functional

regulator) appliance, or the fixed toothborne Herbst appliance (Figure 53-23). All of these appliances position the mandibular condyles downward and forward away from the glenoid fossae. Theoretically the distracted condylar positions reduce the normal compressive joint pressure on the growing condylar cartilage and the forward mandibular posturing alters muscle tension on the condyles, stimulating or accelerating the endochondral condylar growth more than would normally occur.[184] There is some support from animal studies that a histologic increase in condylar growth can be achieved.[185–187] However, clinical studies have not confirmed that a greater absolute growth is the long-term treatment outcome.[149,150] Some retrospective clinical studies have supported the assertion that clinically significant lengthening of the mandible can be achieved with functional appliances.[188–198] Others have refuted this assertion.[158,199–217] Much of the skeletal change demonstrated with a functional appliance may result from forces against the maxilla, similar to those applied with a headgear, that are created from the stretched facial muscles and soft tissues attempting to return the postured mandible back to its posterior and superior position.[158,202,203,208,218–222] Because of the toothborne nature of this appliance, dentoalveolar changes accompany the skeletal changes, including maxillary dental retraction and mandibular dental protrusion.

Clinical studies have demonstrated few differences in treatment outcome when comparing the skeletal response between headgear and functional appliance treatment.[168,193,223] However, there appears to be more of a maxillary effect with headgears.[150,158,161,168] There is more of a mandibular effect with functional appliances.[149,150,168,192,205] Most functional appliances need to be worn for the same daily duration as the headgear (exceptions are the Fränkel and Herbst appliances which

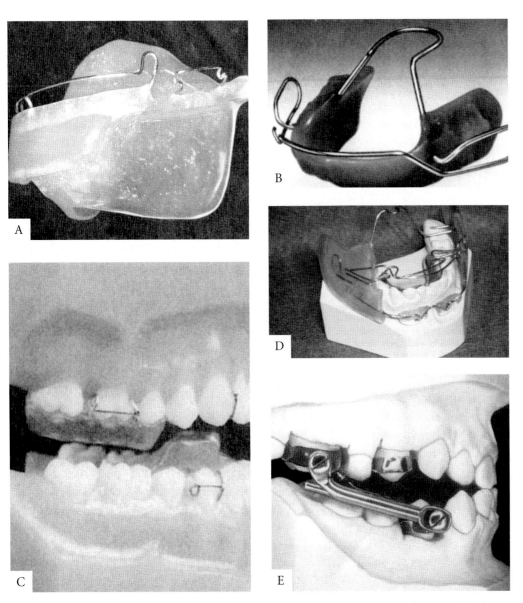

FIGURE **53-23**   *Class II functional appliances. All of these appliances position the mandible downward and forward, distracting the condyles from the glenoid fossae. This simultaneously creates posterior and superior forces to the maxilla from the facial muscles and soft tissues attempting to return the mandible to its normal position. A, Activator. B, Bionator. C, Twin block. D, Fränkel. E, Fixed Herbst. An alternative is to utilize occlusal acrylic and bond the maxillary portion of the appliance with a removable acrylic splint for the mandibular arch. A , C, and D reproduced with permission from Bishara SE. Textbook of orthodontics. Philadelphia (PA): W.B. Saunders; 2001. p. 345. B reproduced with permission from Graber TM, Vanarsdall RL. Orthodontics: current principles and techniques, 3rd ed. St. Louis (MO): Mosby; 2000. p. 488. E reproduced with permission from McNamara JA, Brudon WL. Orthodontics and dentofacial orthopedics. Ann Arbor (MI): Needham Press, Inc.; 2001. p. 287.*

al appliance (Figure 53-24).[204,224–227] This approach was intended to provide greater cumulative skeletal growth effects than use of either appliance alone, but this has yet to be demonstrated by clinical studies.

Although there is greater general acceptance that treatment with a headgear or functional appliance may achieve an improved long-term treatment outcome, there continues to be controversy over the optimum treatment time in the growing child. It has already been demonstrated that orthopedic Class II treatment in the very young child, in the primary or early mixed dentition, results in substantial relapse and recurrence of the original facial skeletal pattern by late adolescence.[228] However, there is great debate regarding the efficacy of orthopedic treatment during later mixed dentition as the first phase of a two-phase treatment versus delaying orthopedic treatment until definitive orthodontic treatment during puberty, after the eruption of the permanent dentition. Many orthodontists historically have preferred the earlier first phase since there is substantial potential growth remaining, compliance in wearing the orthopedic appliance often is greater, and the arch space for the remaining erupting dentition may be improved. The advocates for a delayed one-phase treatment have contended that comparable skeletal treatment effects can be achieved during definitive orthodontic treatment, without putting the patient through an unnecessary initial phase.[229,230] Recent prospective randomized clinical trials have supported this position, demonstrating that early skeletal improvement achieved from these appliances seems to represent accelerated growth and can be used just as effectively later during pubertal growth.[149–151] They also showed that there was substantial individual growth variability with no reliable predictors for a favorable growth response identified, and early treatment did not reduce the need for dental extraction or orthognathic

are worn full-time) for a significant treatment effect. Much like the headgear, dependable wear is more realistic during the evening and at night when the most active facial growth and dental eruption usually occur. However, like the headgear, its removable nature prevents it from being

reliably worn by most adolescents after the peak of their pubertal growth spurt.

In the late 1960s, when European and American facial orthopedic philosophies were becoming more fully integrated, a method was introduced in Europe using a headgear in combination with a function-

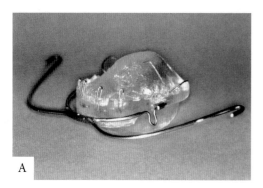

A

FIGURE **53-24** *Combination headgear and removable functional appliance. The interocclusal acrylic permits the orthopedic force to be transmitted further anteriorly and superiorly through the center of the maxilla. A, Intraoral part of appliance with headgear tubes embedded in the interocclusal acrylic. B, Extraoral part of appliance. Reproduced with permission from Bishara SE. Textbook of orthodontics. Philadelphia (PA): W.B. Saunders; 2001. p. 341.*

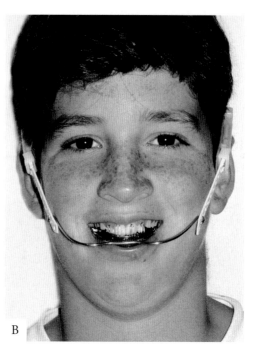

B

surgery during the definitive phase. These studies indicate that there is no adequate additional benefit in treatment outcome to justify the greater burden to the patient, their parents, and the orthodontist, as represented by an early phase that precedes the definitive phase of orthodontic treatment.

It can be concluded from past retrospective and more recent prospective clinical trials that headgear treatment tends to have more of a maxillary restrictive effect whereas functional appliances have more of a mandibular enhancing effect. Either approach can be satisfactory and should be selected on the basis of patient acceptance of the appliance and dentoalveolar side effects (there is more maxillary dental retrusion with headgear and more mandibular protrusion with a functional appliance). It appears that orthopedic treatment during the mixed dentition can only be justified where there is increased trauma risk (due to excessive overjet), sufficient esthetic concern by the patient, or a precocious adolescent growth spurt that substantially precedes dental development. Treatment at an earlier age has been further justified by the argument that there is lack of reliable means of

predicting mandibular growth and that improved cooperation usually is present with the younger patient.[231]

Although improvement in skeletal discrepancy is expected, the Class II correction usually is due to a combined response of both the dentoalveolar and skeletal segments. Both headgear and Class II functional appliance use can be effective in limiting downward and forward eruption of the maxillary molars. However, the functional appliance tends to promote upward and forward eruption of mandibular molars, which may complement the correction in deep overbite cases but is counterproductive in patients with a long face. Since Class II orthopedic appliances are toothborne, there may be some unwanted dentoalveolar change, including retraction of maxillary anterior teeth and protraction of mandibular anterior teeth. This compensatory change may be undesirable if the skeletal discrepancy ultimately requires orthognathic surgery for correction. With the advent of osseointegrated attachments there may be the future possibility of preventing unwanted dentoalveolar change by attaching a force system directly to these

attachments rather than using tooth-borne attachments.

Anteroposterior Orthopedic Treatment: Class III A Class III skeletal relationship can be the result of a retrusive and/or deficient maxilla, a large and/or prognathic mandible, or most often, a combination of these skeletal problems. The prevalence of this type of malocclusion is about 3 to 5% of the US population, with about 0.3% severe enough to be considered as handicapping.[133,134] Since the late nineteenth century, when headgear was being used for Class II skeletal problems, the chin cup was the appliance used for orthopedic treatment of skeletal Class III problems (Figure 53-25). Theoretically an orthopedic force is transmitted to the mandibular condyles, compressing the condylar cartilage and limiting endochondral growth in order to decrease the ultimate length of the mandible.[232] Primate studies suggest that mandibular growth can be limited with heavy full-time forces directed against the condyles.[233] Full-time wear is unrealistic with humans and most clinical studies have demonstrated that mandibular growth is not restrained, but rather vertically redirected from chin cup wear, resulting in decreased chin prominence at the expense of increased face height.[234–238] Studies also have suggested that the long-term stability of these changes is poor.[239,240] Treatment with a chin cup may be an acceptable option for an individual with mandibular excess associated with decreased facial height but is contraindicated where there is a normal or excessive facial height, since the treatment outcome simply would be trading one deformity for another.

Class III functional appliances also have been developed, limiting eruption of mandibular posterior teeth and promoting eruption of maxillary posterior teeth. These functional appliances have few advocates due to their effectiveness being limited to dentoalveolar changes and their inability to promote forward maxillary growth or attenuate mandibular growth.[241]

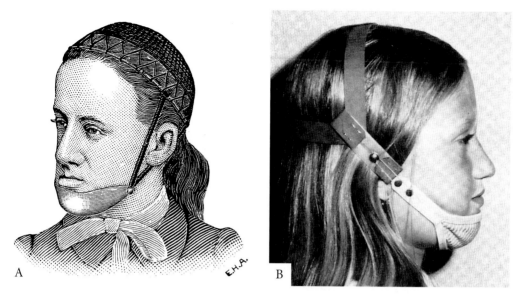

FIGURE 53-25 *Class III chin cup appliance. A retractive orthopedic force is directed against the chin posteriorly and superiorly toward the condylar heads. A, Chin cup from the late nineteenth century. Reproduced from Angle EH. Treatment of malocclusion of the teeth. Philadelphia (PA): S.S. White Dental Manufacturing Co; 1907. p. 194. B, Contemporary chin cup, with minimal change in design, but fabricated with more comfortable and durable materials. Reproduced with permission from Proffit WR, Fields HW. Contemporary orthodontics. 3rd ed. St. Louis (MO): Mosby; 2000. p. 271.*

Jean Delaire, a French dentist, was responsible for developing the protraction headgear or facemask, the most effective orthopedic appliance for skeletal Class III problems since its introduction in the early 1970s (Figure 53-26).[242] Delaire recognized that the offending jaw in many of the skeletal Class III problems was the maxilla, so he departed from the historic focus on the mandible and directed treatment at the retrusive or deficient maxilla. The appliance creates tension in the circum-maxillary sutures with elastics from the maxillary dental arch to a frame that uses the forehead and chin to dissipate the force anteriorly. Primate studies have demonstrated adaptive responses of the sutures to the stress from the distraction forces produced by this appliance.[137]

Depending on the developmental stage and size of the patient, a protractive force ranging from 2 to 4 pounds is applied to the facemask in an anterior and slightly inferior direction relative to the occlusal plane for 12 to 16 hours per day, usually for 6 to 9 months. Clinical studies have demonstrated clinically relevant

maxillary skeletal protraction downward and forward on average with this appliance, with some concomitant protraction of the maxillary teeth due to the tooth-borne nature of the intraoral part of the appliance.[243–246] However, as with other forms of craniofacial orthopedic treatment, there is substantial variability and an unpredictable patient response to the appliance, ranging from no appreciable skeletal change to about 5 mm anterior maxillary movement.[247] It is important to achieve overcorrection of the anterior crossbite and anterior overbite since there is some relapse following discontinuation of treatment.[248] Additional effects of maxillary orthopedic protraction often include rotation of the maxilla downward in the posterior and upward in the anterior, downward and backward rotation of the mandible, and retraction of the mandibular incisors due to the reactive posterior force dissipated on the chin. These additional orthopedic and dentoalveolar changes that accompany maxillary skeletal protraction would be contraindicated for a Class III pattern with excessive vertical

development or where mandibular excess is the underlying cause of the problem.[249]

The timing of facemask therapy usually is recommended for patients in the primary to early mixed dentition (ie, ages 4 to 8), due to the increased patency of the maxillary sutures and compliance with appliance wear at this age.[250,251] As the patient ages there is more interdigitation and ossification of the sutures, resulting in less skeletal and more dental response to the protraction forces. Nevertheless most clinical studies have found few differences between early and late treatment up until puberty.[251–254]

The stability of maxillary orthopedic protraction with a facemask is variable and dependent on favorable facial growth following active treatment. However, it is common for the original facial growth pattern to resume after treatment, often resulting in relapse of the skeletal discrepancy. The best overall success rate at the end of adolescent growth cannot be expected to be more than 50%.[255] One should expect that about 20% of these patients will ultimately require orthognathic surgery to fully correct the Class III malocclusion.[248] The patients who relapse usually have mandibular growth during late adolescence that overwhelms the earlier correction. Long-term efficacy of facemask treatment has not been fully studied.

Class III orthopedic appliances, as with Class II devices, result in dentoalveolar movements that accompany the skeletal changes. Treatment with the facemask causes protraction of maxillary anterior teeth and retraction of mandibular anterior teeth. The development of osseointegrated attachments may make it possible to transmit the orthopedic protraction force to intraoral skeletal attachments that prevent undesirable dentoalveolar changes.[256]

Vertical Orthopedic Treatment Vertical maxillary excess presents with a maxilla that is inferiorly positioned, resulting in excessive vertical display of maxillary

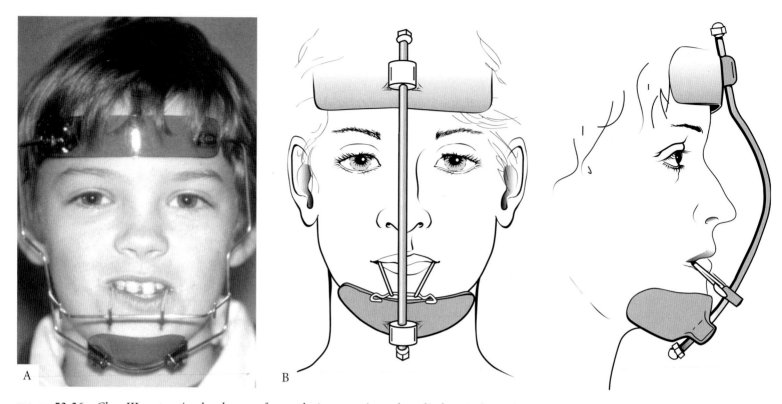

FIGURE **53-26**   *Class III protraction headgear or facemask. A protractive orthopedic force is directed downward and forward, with the force being dissipated on the forehead and chin, distracting the circum-maxillary sutures to augment anterior maxillary growth. A, Delaire design. Reproduced with permission from Proffit WR, Fields HW. Contemporary orthodontics. 3rd ed. St. Louis (MO): Mosby; 2000. p. 516. B, Petit design (frontal and lateral views). Adapted from McNamara JA, Brudon WL. Orthodontics and dentofacial orthopedics. Ann Arbor (MI): Needham Press, Inc.; 2001. p. 378.*

incisors relative to the upper lip, and downward and backward rotation of the mandible, resulting in an increased mandibular plane angle and lower face height. The prevalence of vertical facial problems is less than 5% of the US population with about 0.3% considered as handicapping.[133,134]

The orthodontist presently does not have very effective nonsurgical options to manage vertical skeletal problems. Orthopedic treatment strategy is directed at restraining vertical maxillary growth and posterior dental eruption in order to promote anterior and superior mandibular rotation. A high-pull headgear is used to apply a superior intrusive force of 2 to 4 pounds to inhibit eruption of maxillary posterior teeth and compress circum-maxillary sutures to limit the downward development of the maxilla. With exceptional daily (14 to 16 hours) and long-term (throughout adolescent growth)

wear, mandibular growth may be redirected in a more anterior than downward direction, improving a Class II skeletal discrepancy with vertical maxillary excess. However, this is counterproductive when treating vertical maxillary excess with a normal or prognathic mandible, since any decrease in vertical maxillary development would promote anterior mandibular rotation, thereby aggravating the Class III malocclusion. An alternative to the use of high-pull headgear is a removable orthopedic appliance that incorporates interocclusal acrylic bite blocks in order to stretch the facial musculature and soft tissue beyond the normal resting vertical dimension, creating a reactive intrusive force against the mandibular as well as maxillary teeth.[257,258] As with the high-pull headgear option, exceptional daily and long-term wear is necessary to obtain any appreciable benefit. Repelling magnets have been embedded in the opposing

acrylic bite blocks to accentuate the intrusive force.[259–261] Most of the treatment benefit from this method appears to be limitation of posterior vertical dentoalveolar development rather than any appreciable skeletal effect.[261–263]

A significant treatment effect by either the headgear or interocclusal bite block is rare since it is dependent on the patient wearing the appliance at least 14 to 16 hours per day over a number of years. In fact significant clinical benefit from the use of interocclusal acrylic alone may require closer to 16 to 24 hours per day. As with the Class II orthopedic methods these two methods have been combined into one appliance with the hope that this approach may provide greater cumulative skeletal growth effects than use of either appliance alone.[264] In combination with the interocclusal bite block the force transmitted by the headgear can be distributed over all of the teeth contacting the acrylic, and the force vector can be directed further forward and more vertically, closer to the maxillary center of resistance (see Figure 53-24).

Use of either or both of these orthopedic appliances to treat vertical maxillary excess is particularly challenging since it is impossible to direct the force in a straight vertical manner. Both methods include some posteriorly directed force to the maxilla that is not appropriate unless the maxilla is protrusive as well as inferiorly positioned. It also is counterproductive in a patient with maxillary vertical excess combined with a Class III skeletal relationship. Just as the protraction headgear should not be used with this individual to address the anteroposterior skeletal problem, the high-pull headgear and/or interocclusal bite block are contraindicated in this same clinical situation to address the vertical excess.

No studies to date have been able to demonstrate long-term stability with any nonsurgical orthopedic methods for correcting vertical maxillary excess, with or without an anterior open bite.[265] Achieving stability is particularly difficult due to the extended duration of vertical facial growth, often continuing well beyond adolescence.[40] For a successful outcome orthopedic treatment may have to be extended over a number of years, from the time of the mixed dentition through definitive orthodontic treatment in the permanent dentition, perhaps including a removable orthopedic appliance even during orthodontic retention. This extended treatment makes the vertical plane of space the most difficult to successfully manage by the orthodontist attempting facial growth modification. Osseointegrated attachments hold promise as a means of anchorage to potentially permit more effective treatment of skeletal vertical problems in the future.[266]

Conclusion Facial orthopedic treatment may be effective in resolving mild to mod-

erate skeletal discrepancies in some patients. An orthopedic phase should be attempted with a specific treatment time frame established in order to assess treatment progress toward successful correction. This time frame must be honored in order to prevent protracted treatment with excessive dental compensations that need to be reversed for surgical correction. The orthodontist attempting growth modification must be mindful of the duration and extent of treatment to prevent excessive length and morbidity of the orthodontic treatment. If significant skeletal improvement is not being achieved within 6 to 8 months of starting orthopedic treatment, the case needs to be reevaluated and the growth modification treatment likely abandoned as a treatment choice.

It has become clear that there is great variability in individual treatment response, even when factoring out wear compliance and duration of treatment. It has not been possible to identify the variables to explain why some patients respond well and some do not demonstrate any significant skeletal improvement with treatment regardless of their facial morphology or the severity of their skeletal discrepancy. It is anticipated that future research will reveal the variables that will enable the clinician to predict treatment response.

It also is expected that research will provide a greater understanding of the nature and extent of facial growth modification possible in individual patients as well as the type of appliance and timing of treatment to achieve the best outcome. The development of intraoral osseointegrated attachments holds promise for a future means of dissipating orthopedic forces to prevent unwanted dentoalveolar changes that presently occur with our toothborne appliances. Analogous attachments are presently undergoing clinical testing for surgically assisted orthopedic movements associated with distraction osteogenesis.[267,268] Recent and future advances in developmental biology and genomics hold

great promise in increasing our understanding of the molecular and genetic mediators of craniofacial growth.[132] This understanding will be crucial for us to make constructive modifications of our treatment methods to target these mediators in order to prevent or correct a craniofacial anomaly or developmental deformity.

Orthodontic Camouflage: Orthopedic Consequence versus Surgical Preparation

Orthodontic camouflage, rather than orthognathic surgery, may indeed be an appropriate treatment choice for some mild and moderate skeletal malocclusions in patients who are beyond the pubertal growth spurt. The treatment goal, however, must include a realistic outcome characterized by an acceptable dental and facial esthetic appearance with favorable dental function and occlusion. Since esthetic appearance is subjective in nature, it is essential to have the patient and parent perceptions dictate whether camouflage is a reasonable option.

Most mild and some moderate skeletal Class II malocclusions can be effectively camouflaged with extraction of two maxillary premolars and retraction of maxillary anterior teeth, leaving the posterior teeth in a Class II occlusion. However, these cases should mainly be limited to those that present without significant dental crowding, some protrusion of the maxillary incisors, and where there is not significant maxillary gingival display on smiling. If the maxillary incisors are normally or palatally inclined prior to treatment, orthodontic retraction of these teeth may result in an even poorer esthetic result than the original problem even if the occlusion is acceptable. The unesthetic appearance includes not just the incisor inclination but often an unattractive retrusive upper lip and increased gingival exposure during smiling as well. This is why the recent introduction of palatal implants as orthodontic anchorage, which provide the opportunity for the orthodontist to retract maxillary incisors even further than was previously possible, is a mixed blessing.

It is more challenging to camouflage Class III than Class II skeletal malocclusions since considerable natural dentoalveolar camouflage (proclined maxillary incisors, lingually inclined mandibular incisors) is often already present prior to treatment. Additional maxillary incisor proclination may be unesthetic, and further lingual inclination of mandibular incisors usually accentuates an already prominent chin. For this reason extraction of mandibular premolars to permit more retraction of mandibular incisors to obtain positive overjet often compromises the esthetic outcome. If interarch tooth size compatibility can be maintained, extraction of one mandibular incisor rather than two premolars may provide an acceptable compromise.

Camouflage of an anterior open bite that is due to maxillary vertical excess has been notoriously unsuccessful in the past. Recently an orthodontic technique for stably extruding anterior teeth has been introduced.[269] Unfortunately this only exacerbates the excessive vertical display of maxillary gingiva and anterior teeth.

Summary

The surgeon's understanding of craniofacial growth has an important impact on clinical treatment decisions to alter craniofacial morphology. This understanding is relevant to the appreciation of the role of orthopedic treatment in the prepubertal and pubertal patient to limit or preclude the need for corrective surgery at a later age. Clinically relevant modification of craniofacial growth is possible, but substantial advances will be necessary to elucidate how growth modification can be accomplished in a controlled and predictable manner to achieve an efficacious outcome. Optimal timing and stability of craniofacial surgery are dependent on a thorough appreciation of the sequence, timing, magnitude, and differential expression of craniofacial growth. The recent dramatic advances in developmental genetics and molecular biology, highlighted by complete mapping of the human genome, usher in a new millenium that promises to bring an explosive increase to our understanding of the complex interactions of the genetic and environmental influences that determine human craniofacial morphogenesis, prenatal development, and postnatal growth. A thorough understanding of these genomic and epigenetic factors will be necessary to determine the best timing and method of clinical intervention to achieve the optimum treatment outcome.

References

1. Kontges G, Lumsden A. Rhombencephalic neural crest segmentation is preserved throughout craniofacial ontogeny. Development 1996;122:3229–42.
2. Bronner-Fraser M, Fraser SE. Application of new technologies to studies of neural crest migration and differentiation. Am J Med Genet Suppl 1988;4:23–39.
3. Smith I, Thorogood P. Transfilter studies on the mechanism of epithelio-mesenchymal interaction leading to chondrogenic differentiation of neural crest cells. J Embryol Exp Morphol 1983;75:165.
4. Krumlauf R, Marshall H, Studer M, et al. Hox homeobox genes and regionalisation of the nervous system. J Neurobiol 1993;24:1328–40.
5. Young DL, Schneider RA, Hu D, Helms JA. Genetic and teratogenic approaches to craniofacial development. Crit Rev Oral Biol Med 2000;11:304–17.
6. Warbrick JG. The early development of the nasal cavity and upper lip in the human embryo. J Anat (Lond) 1960;94:351–62.
7. Hu D, Helms JA. The role of sonic hedgehog in normal and abnormal craniofacial morphogenesis. Development 1999;126:4873–84.
8. Fujino M, Osumi N, Ninomiya Y, et al. Disappearance of epidermal growth factor receptor is essential in the fusion of the nasal epithelium. Anat Sci Int 2003;78:25–35.
9. Kjaer I. Human prenatal craniofacial development related to brain development under normal and pathologic conditions. Acta Odontol Scand 1995;53:135–43.
10. Brunet CL, Sharpe PM, Ferguson MW. Inhibition of TGF-beta 3 (but not TGF-beta 1 of TGF-beta 2) activity prevents normal mouse embryonic palate fusion. Int J Dev Biol 1995;39:345–55.
11. Cameron N. Human growth and development. London: Academic Press, Elsevier Science; 2002. p. 6–7, 85.
12. Houpt MI. Growth of the craniofacial complex of the human fetus. Am J Orthod 1970;58:373–83.
13. Opperman LA, Passarelli RW, Morgan EP, et al. Cranial sutures require tissue interactions with dura mater to resist osseous obliteration in vitro. J Bone Miner Res 1995;10:1978–87.
14. Roth DA, Gold LI, Han VK, et al. Immunolocalization of transforming growth factor beta 1, beta 2, and beta 3 and insulin-like growth factor 1 in premature cranial suture fusion (see comments). Plast Reconstr Surg 1997;99:300–9; discussion 310–6.
15. Kim HJ, Rice DP, Kettunen PJ, Thesleff I. FGF-, BMP- and Shh-mediated signaling pathways in the regulation of cranial suture morphogenesis and calvarial bone development. Development 1998;125:1241–51.
16. Nah H. Suture biology: lessons from molecular genetics of craniosynostosis syndromes. Clin Orthod Res 2000;3:37–45.
17. Plavcan JM, German RZ. Quantitative evaluation of craniofacial growth in the third trimester human. Cleft Palate Craniofac J 1995;32:394–404.
18. Rönning O. Basicranial synchondroses and the mandibular condyle in craniofacial growth. Acta Odontol Scand 1995;53:162–6.
19. Bareggi R, Sandrucci MA, Baldini G, et al. Mandibular growth rates in human fetal development. Arch Oral Biol 1995;40:119–25.
20. Bentley RP, Sgouros S, Natarajan K, et al. Normal changes in orbital volume during childhood. J Neurosurg 2002;96:742–6.
21. Hunter WS, Baumrind S, Moyers RE. An inventory of United States and Canadian growth record sets: preliminary report. Am J Orthod Dentofac Orthop 1993;103:545–55.
22. Copray JC, Jansen HW, Duterloo HS. Growth and growth pressure of mandibular condylar and some primary cartilages of the rat in vitro. Am J Orthod Dentofac Orthop 1986;90:19–28.
23. Peltomaki T, Kylamarkula S, Vinkka-Puhakka H, et al. Tissue-separating capacity of growth cartilages. Eur J Orthod 1997;19:473–81.
24. Wang X, Mao JJ. Chondrocyte proliferation of the cranial base cartilage upon in vivo mechanical stresses. J Dent Res 2002;81:701–5.
25. Kiliaridis S. Masticatory muscle influence on craniofacial growth. Acta Odontol Scand 1995;53:196–202.

26. Sarnat BG. Normal and abnormal craniofacial growth. Angle Orthod 1983;53:263–89.

27. Rabie ABM, Hägg U. Factors regulating mandibular condylar growth. Am J Orthod Dentofac Orthop 2002;122:401–9.

28. Mamandras AH. Linear changes of the maxillary and mandibular lips. Am J Orthod 1988;94:405–10.

29. Nanda RS, Meng H, Kapila S, Goorhuis J. Growth changes of the soft tissue profile. Angle Orthod 1990;60:177–90.

30. Vig PS, Cohen AM. Vertical growth of the lips: a serial cephalometric study. Am J Orthod 1979;75:405–15.

31. Subtelny JD. A longitudinal study of soft tissue facial structures and their profile characteristics defined in relation to underlying skeletal structures. Am J Orthod 1959;45:481–507.

32. Chaconas SJ. A statistical evaluation of nasal growth. Am J Orthod 1969;56:403–14.

33. Scott JH. Growth of human face. Proc R Soc Med 1953;47:91–100.

34. Buschang PH, Baume RM, Nass GG. A craniofacial growth maturity gradient for males and females between 4 and 16 years of age. Am J Phys Anthropol 1983;61:373–81.

35. Ferrario VF, Sforza C, Poggio CE, Schmitz JH. Craniofacial growth: a three-dimensional soft-tissue study from 6 years to adulthood. J Craniofac Genet Dev Biol 1998;18:138–49.

36. Hrdlička A. Growth during adult life. Proc Am Phil Soc 1936;76:847–97.

37. Hooton EA, Dupertuis CW. Age changes and selective survival in Irish males. In: American Association of Physical Anthropology. Studies in physical anthropology. No. 2. New York (NY): Wenner-Gren Foundation; 1951. p. 1–130.

38. Israel H. Recent knowledge concerning craniofacial aging. Angle Orthod 1973;43:176–84.

39. Lewis AB, Roche AF. Late growth changes in the craniofacial skeleton. Angle Orthod 1988;58:127–35.

40. Behrents RG. Growth in the aging craniofacial skeleton. Craniofacial growth monograph series. Monograph 17. Ann Arbor: Center for Human Growth and Development, University of Michigan; 1985.

41. Bishara SE, Treder JE, Jakobsen JR. Facial and dental changes in adulthood. Am J Orthod Dentofac Orthop 1994;106:175–86.

42. Formby WA, Nanda RS, Currier GF. Longitudinal changes in the adult facial profile. Am J Orthod Dentofac Orthop 1994;105:464–76.

43. West KS, McNamara JA. Changes in the craniofacial complex from adolescence to midadulthood: a cephalometric study. Am J Orthod Dentofac Orthop 1999;115:521–32.

44. Akgül AA, Toygar TU. Natural craniofacial changes in the third decade of life: a longitudinal study. Am J Orthod Dentofac Orthop 2002;122:512–22.

45. Dickens ST, Sarver DM, Proffit WR. Changes in frontal soft tissue dimensions of the lower face by age and gender. World J Orthod 2003;3:313–20.

46. Fanouns N. Aging lips: esthetic analysis and correction. Facial Plast Surg 1987;4:179–83.

47. Spranger J, Benirschke K, Hall JG, et al. Errors of morphogenesis: concepts and terms. Recommendations of an international working group. J Pediatr 1982;100:160–5.

48. Wilson GN. Genomics of human dysmorphogenesis. Am J Med Genet 1992;42:187–96.

49. Jabs EW, Muller U, Li X, et al. A mutation in the homeodomain of the human MSX2 gene in a family affected with autosomal dominant craniosynostosis. 1993;75:443–50.

50. Bellus GA, Gaudenz K, Zackai EH, et al. Identical mutations in three different fibroblast growth factor receptor genes in autosomal dominant craniosynostosis syndromes. Nat Genet 1996;14:174–6.

51. Mooney MP, Siegel MI. Understanding craniofacial anomalies: the etiopathogenesis of craniosynostoses and facial clefting. New York (NY): Wiley-Liss, Inc.; 2002.

52. Johnston MC, Bronsky PT. Abnormal craniofacial development: an overview. Crit Rev Oral Biol Med 1995;6:368–422.

53. Jones KL. Smith's recognizable patterns of human malformation. Philadelphia (PA): W.B. Saunders; 1988.

54. Shepard TH. Catalog of teratogenic agents. Baltimore (MD): Johns Hopkins University Press; 1995.

55. Gorlin RJ, Cohen MM, Levin LS. Syndromes of the head and neck. New York (NY): Oxford University Press; 1990.

56. Edwards LE, Alton IR, Barrada MI, Hakansen EY. Pregnancy in the underweight woman: course, outcome, and growth patterns of the infant. Am J Obstet Gynecol 1979; 135:297–302.

57. Abel EL. Consumption of alcohol during pregnancy: a review of effects on growth and development of offspring. Hum Biol 1982;54:421–53.

58. Zuckerman B, Frank DA, Hingson R, et al. Effects of maternal marijuana and cocaine use on fetal growth. N Engl J Med 1989;320:762–8.

59. Haste FM, Anderson HR, Brooke O, et al. The effects of smoking and drinking on the anthropometric measurements of neonates. Paediatr Perinatal Epidemiol 1991;5:83–92.

60. Misra DP, Nguyen RH. Environmental tobacco smoke and low birth weight: a hazard in the workplace. Environ Health Perspect 1999; 107:897–904.

61. Ando Y, Hattori H. Statistical studies on the effects of intense noise during human fetal life. J Sound Vibr 1973;27:101–10.

62. Lejarraga H, Peckham C. Birth weight and subsequent growth of children exposed to congenital rubella in utero. Arch Dis Child 1974;49:50–8.

63. Higginbottom MC, Jones KL, James HE. Intrauterine constraint and craniosynostosis. Neurosurgery 1980;6:39–44.

64. Gluckman PD. Fetal hypothalamic-pituitary relationships: a review with particular reference to experimental studies of the somatotropic axis. In: Sizonenko PC, Aubert ML, editors. Developmental endocrinology. Serono Symposia Publications. Vol 67. New York (NY): Raven Press; 1990.

65. Abdul-Karim RW, Marshall CD. Influence of maternal oophorectomy on the collagen and calcium contents of fetal bone. Obstet Gynecol 1969;34:837–40.

66. Abdul-Karim RW, Nesbitt REL Jr, Drucker MH, Rizk PT. The regulatory effect of estrogens on fetal growth. I. Placental and fetal body weights. Am J Obstet Gynecol 1971; 109:656–61.

67. de Zegher F, Pernasetti F, Vanhole C, et al. The prenatal role of thyroid hormone evidenced by fetomaternal Pit-1 deficiency. J Clin Endocrinol Metab 1995;80:3127–30.

68. Warshaw JB. Intrauterine growth restriction revisited. Growth Genet Horm 1992;8:5–8.

69. D'Ercole AJ, Applewhite GT, Underwood LE. Evidence that somatomedins are synthesized by multiple tissues in the fetus. Dev Biol 1980;75:315–28.

70. Hindmarsh PC. Endocrinology of growth. In: Cameron N, editor. Human growth and development. London: Academic Press, Elsevier Science; 2002. p. 85–101.

71. Evain-Brion D. Hormonal regulation of fetal growth. Horm Res 1994;42:207–14.

72. Rotwein P. Peptide growth factors other than insulin-like growth factors or cytokines. In: Degroot LJ, Jameson JL, editors. Endocrinology. 4th ed. Philadelphia (PA): W.B. Saunders; 2001. p. 461–76.

73. Siler-Khodr TM. Endocrine and paracrine function of the human placenta. In: Polin RA, Fox WW, editors. Fetal and neonatal physiology. 2nd ed. Philadelphia (PA): W.B. Saunders; 1998. p. 89–102.

74. Hall K, Enberg G, Hellem E, et al. Somatomedin levels in pregnancy: longitudinal study in healthy subjects and patients with growth hormone deficiency. J Clin Endocrinol Metab 1984;59:587–94.

75. Li Y, Behringer RR. Esx1 is an X chromosome-imprinted regulator of placental development and fetal growth. Nature Genet 1998;20:309–11.

76. Towne B, Demerath EW, Czerwinski SA. The genetic epidemiology of growth and development. In: Cameron N, editor. Human growth and development. London: Academic Press, Elsevier Science; 2002. p. 103–37.

77. Litton SF, Ackermann LV, Isaacson RJ, Shapiro BL. A genetic study of class III malocclusion. Am J Orthod 1970;58:565–77.

78. El-Gheriani AA, Maher BS, El-Gheriani AS, et al. Segregation analysis of mandibular prognathism in Libya. J Dent Res 2003;82:523–7.

79. Proffit WR. The development of dentofacial deformity: influences and etiologic factors. In: Proffit WR, White RP, Sarver DM, editors. Contemporary treatment of dentofacial deformity. St. Louis (MO): Mosby; 2003. p. 58.

80. Proffit WR. Equilibrium theory revisited. Angle Orthod 1978;48:175–86.

81. Buchman SR, Bartlett SP, Wornom IL III, Whitaker LA. The role of pressure on regulation of craniofacial bone growth. J Craniofac Surg 1994;5:2–10.

82. Schumacher GH. Factors influencing craniofacial growth. In: Normal and abnormal bone growth: basic and clinical research. Alan R. Liss, Inc.; 1985. p. 3–22.

83. Kean MR, Houghton P. The role of function in the development of human craniofacial form: a perspective. Anat Rec 1987;218:107–10.

84. Poikela A, Kantomaa T, Pirttiniemi P. Craniofacial growth after a period of unilateral masticatory function in young rabbits. Eur J Oral Sci 1997;105:331–7.

85. Bouvier M, Hylander WL. The effect of dietary consistency on gross and histologic morphology in the craniofacial region of young rats. Am J Anat 1984;170:117–26.

86. Luca L, Roberto D, Francesca SM, Francesca P. Consistency of diet and its effects on mandibular morphogenesis in the young rat. Prog Orthod 2003;4:3–7.

87. Gionhaku N, Lowe AA. Relationship between jaw muscle volume and craniofacial form. J Dent Res 1989;68:805–9.

88. Ingervall B, Thilander B. Relation between facial morphology and activity of the masticatory muscles. J Oral Rehab 1974;1:131–47.

89. Weijs WA, Hillen B. Relationships between masticatory muscle cross-section and skull shape. J Dent Res 1984;63:1154–7.

90. van Spronsen PH, Weijs WA, Valk J, et al. A comparison of jaw muscle cross-sections of long-face and normal adults. J Dent Res 1992;71:1279–85.

91. Gardner DE, Luschei ES, Joondeph DR. Alterations in the facial skeleton of the guinea pig following a lesion of the trigeminal motor nucleus. Am J Orthod 1980;78:66–80.

92. Wolf G, Koskinen-Moffett L, Kokich V. Migration of craniofacial periosteum in guinea-pigs with unilateral masticatory muscle paralysis. J Anat 1985;140:259–68.

93. Hirabayashi S, Harii K, Sakuri A, et al. An experimental study of craniofacial growth in a heterotopic rat head transplant. Plast Reconstr Surg 1988;82:236–43.

94. Sakurai A, Hirabayashi S, Harii K, Fukuda O. Experimental studies on complete global brain ischemia using the isohistogenic infantile head transplant model in Lewis rats. J Reconst Microsurg 1989;5:145–50.

95. Proffit WR, Fields HW. Occlusal forces in normal and long face children. J Dent Res 1983;62:571–4.

96. Vig KW. Nasal obstruction and facial growth: the strength of evidence for clinical assumptions. Am J Orthod Dentofac Orthop 1998;113:603–11.

97. Ross RB. The clinical implications of facial growth in cleft lip and palate. Cleft Palate J 1970;7:37–47.

98. Moyers RA, McNamara JA. Factors affecting growth of the midface. In: McNamara JA Jr, editor. Craniofacial growth monograph series. Monograph 6. Ann Arbor: Center for Human Growth and Development, University of Michigan; 1976. p. 43–59; 169–204; 239–49.

99. Katsaros J, David DJ, Griffin PA, Moore MH. Facial dysmorphology in the neglected paediatric head and neck burn. Br J Plast Surg 1990;43:232–5.

100. Laurenzo JF, Canady JW, Zimmerman MB, Smith RJ. Craniofacial growth in rabbits. Effects of midfacial surgical trauma and rigid plate fixation. Arch Otolaryngol Head Neck Surg 1995;121:556–61.

101. Proffit WR, White RP, Sarver DM. Contemporary treatment of dentofacial deformity. St. Louis (MO): Mosby; 2003. p. 43–51, 587–96.

102. Ohlsson C, Isaksson O, Lindahl A. Clonal analysis of rat tibia growth plate chondroctes in suspension culture — differential effects of growth hormone and insulin-like growth factor I. Growth Regul 1994;4:1–7.

103. Berg MA, Argente J, Chernausek S, et al. Diverse growth hormone receptor gene mutations in Laron syndrome. Am J Hum Genet 1993;52:998–1005.

104. Schaefer GB, Rosenbloom AL, Guevara-Aguirre J, et al. Facial morphometry of Ecuadorian patients with growth hormone receptor deficiency. J Med Genet 1994;31:635–9.

105. Pirinen S. Endocrine regulation of craniofacial growth. Acta Odontol Scand 1995;53:179–85.

106. Barrett RL, Harris EF. Anabolic steroids and craniofacial growth in the rat. Angle Orthod 1993;63:289–98.

107. Petrovic A, Stutzmann J, Gasson N. La taille définitive de la mandibule est-elle, comme telle, prédéterminée génétiquement? Orthod Fr 1979;50:751–67.

108. Riesenfeld A. Endocrine and biomechanical control of craniofacial growth: an experimental study. Hum Biol 1974;46:531–72.

109. Rivkees SA, Danon M, Herrin J. Prednisone dose limitation of growth hormone treatment of steroid-induced growth failure. J Pediatr 1994;125:322–5.

110. Maor G, Silberman M. Studies of hormonal regulation of the growth of the craniofacial skeleton. IV. Specific binding sites for glucocorticoids in condylar cartilage and their involvement in the biological effects of glucocorticoids on cartilage cell growth. J Craniofac Gen Devel Biol 1986;6:189–202.

111. Teng C-M, Sobkowski J, Johnston L. The effect of cortisone on the eruption rate of root resected incisors in the rat. Am J Orthod Dentofac Orthop 1989;95:67–71.

112. Graham GC, Adrianzen T, Rabold J, Mellits ED. Later growth of malnourished children. Am J Dis Child 1982;136:348–52.

113. Soliman AT, Hassan AEHI, Aref MK, et al. Serum insulin-like growth factors I and II concentrations and growth hormone and insulin responses to arginine infusion in children with protein-energy malnutrition before and after nutritional rehabilitation. Pediatr Res 1986;20:1122–30.

114. Pucciarelli HM. The effects of race, sex, and nutrition on craniofacial differentiation in rats. A multivariate analysis. Am J Phys Anthropol 1980;53:359–68.

115. Pucciarelli HM. Growth of the functional components of the rat skull and its alteration by nutritional effects. A multivariate analysis. Am J Phys Anthropol 1981;56:33–41.

116. Engstrom C, Linde A, Thilander B. Craniofacial morphology and growth in the rat. Cephalometric analysis of the effects of a low calcium and vitamin D-deficient diet. J Anat 1982;134:299–314.

117. Baume LJ, Franquin J-C, Körner WW. The prenatal effect of maternal vitamin A deficiency on the cranial and dental development of the progeny. Am J Orthod 1972;62:447–60.

118. Howe AM, Webster WS. Vitamin K — its essential role in craniofacial development. A review of the literature regarding vitamin

K and craniofacial development. Aust Dent J 1994;39:88–92.

119. Li KW. Dietary protein deficiency reduces serum growth hormone and skeletal growth. J Dent Res 1995;74:254.

120. Miller JP, German RZ. Protein malnutrition affects the growth trajectories of the craniofacial skeleton in rats. J Nutr 1999;129:2061–9.

121. Russell GFM. Premenarchal anorexia nervosa and its sequelae. J Psychiatr Res 1985;19:363–9.

122. Salzer HR, Haschke F, Wimmer M, et al. Growth and nutritional intake of infants with congenital heart disease. Pediatr Cardiol 1989;10:17–23.

123. Cameron N. Human growth and development. London: Academic Press, Elsevier Science; 2002. p. 41.

124. Berkowitz RJ, Neuman P, Spalding PM, et al. Developmental orofacial deficits associated with multimodal cancer therapy: case report. Pediatr Dent 1989;11:227–31.

125. Cohen SR, Bartlett SP, Whitaker LA. Reconstruction of late craniofacial deformities after irradiation of the head and face during childhood. Plast Reconstr Surg 1990;86:229–37.

126. Powell GF, Brasel JA, Blizzard RM. Emotional deprivation and growth retardation simulating idiopathic hypopituitarism. N Engl J Med 1967;276:1271–83.

127. Bogin B. Patterns of human growth. Cambridge: Cambridge University Press; 1988.

128. Frisancho AR. Human adaptation and accommodation. Ann Arbor: University of Michigan Press; 1993.

129. Schell LM, Knutsen KL. Environmental effects on growth. In: Cameron N, editor. Human growth and development. London: Academic Press, Elsevier Science; 2002. p. 165–95.

130. Schell LM, Norelli RJ. Airport noise exposure and the postnatal growth of children. Am J Phys Anthropol 1983;61:473–82.

131. Mao JJ, Wang X, Kopher RA. Biomechanics of craniofacial sutures: orthopedic implications. Angle Orthod 2003;73:128–35.

132. Carlson DS. Biological rationale for early treatment of dentofacial deformities. Am J Orthod Dentofac Orthop 2002;121:554–8.

133. Brunelle JA, Bhat M, Lipton JA. Prevalence and distribution of selected occlusal characteristics in the US population, 1988–1991. J Dent Res 1996;75:706–13.

134. Proffit WR. The development of dentofacial deformity: influences and etiologic factors. In: Proffit WR, White RP, Sarver DM, editor. Contemporary treatment of dentofacial deformity. St. Louis (MO): Mosby; 2003. p. 23–4.

135. Haas AJ. Rapid expansion of the maxillary dental arch and nasal cavity by opening the mid-palatal suture. Angle Orthod 1961;31:73–90.

136. Jafari A, Shetty S, Kumar M. Study of stress distribution and displacement of various craniofacial structures following application of transverse orthopedic forces: a three-dimensional FEM study. Angle Orthod 2003;73:12–20.

137. Wagemans PAHM, van de Velde J-P, Kuijpers-Jagtman AM. Sutures and forces: a review. Am J Orthod Dentofac Orthop 1988;94:129–41.

138. McNamara JA. Early intervention in the transverse dimension: is it worth the effort? Am J Orthod Dentofac Orthop 2002;121:572–4.

139. Melsen B, Melsen F. The postnatal development of the palatomaxillary region studied on human autopsy material. Am J Orthod 1982;82:329–42.

140. Baccetti T, Franchi L, Cameron CG, McNamara JA Jr. Treatment timing for rapid maxillary expansion. Angle Orthod 2001;71:343–50.

141. Pirttiniemi P, Kantomaa T, Lahtela P. Relationship between craniofacial and condyle path asymmetry in unilateral cross-bite patients. Eur J Orthod 1990;12:408–13.

142. Revelo B, Fishman LS. Maturational evaluation of ossification of the mid-palatal suture. Am J Orthod Dentofac Orthop 1994;105:288–92.

143. Hicks EP. Slow maxillary expansion: a clinical study of the skeletal vs. dental response to low magnitude force. Am J Orthod 1978;73:121–41.

144. Krebs AA. Expansion of mid palatal suture studied by means of metallic implants. Acta Odontol Scand 1959;17:491–501.

145. Wertz RA. Skeletal and dental changes accompanying rapid midpalatal suture opening. Am J Orthod 1970;58:41–66.

146. Krebs AA. Rapid expansion of mid palatal suture studied by fixed appliance. An implant study over a 7 year period. Trans Eur Orthod Soc 1964;141–2.

147. Mommaerts MY. Transpalatal distraction as a method of maxillary expansion. Br J Oral Maxillofac Surg 1999;37:268–72.

148. Vig PS, Vig KW. Hybrid appliances: a component approach to dentofacial orthopedics. Am J Orthod 1986;90:273–85.

149. Keeling SD, Wheeler TT, King GJ, et al. Anteroposterior skeletal and dental changes after early class II treatment with bionators and headgear. Am J Orthod Dentofac Orthop 1998;113:40–50.

150. Tulloch JFC, Philips C, Proffit WR. Benefit of early class II treatment: progress report of a two-phase randomized clinical trial. Am J Orthod Dentofac Orthop 1998;113:62–72.

151. Ghafari J, Shofer FS, Jacobsson-Hunt U, et al. Headgear versus functional regulator in the early treatment of class II, division I malocclusion: a randomized clinical trial. Am J Orthod Dentofac Orthop 1998;113:51–61.

152. Kloehn S. Guiding alveolar growth and eruption of the teeth to reduce treatment time and produce a more balanced denture and face. Angle Orthod 1947;17:10–33.

153. Poulton DR. Change in class II malocclusions with and without occipital headgear therapy. Angle Orthod 1959;29;234–50.

154. Ricketts RM. The influence of orthodontic treatment in facial growth and development. Angle Orthod 1960;30:103–33.

155. Wieslander L. The effects of orthodontic treatment on the concurrent development of the craniofacial complex. Am J Orthod 1963;49:15–27.

156. Poulton DR. A three-year survey of class II malocclusions with and without headgear therapy. Angle Orthod 1964;34:181–93.

157. Creekmore TD. Inhibition or stimulation of the vertical growth of facial complex, its significance to treatment. Angle Orthod 1967;37:285–97.

158. Jakobsson SO. Cephalometric evaluation of treatment effect on class II, division 1, malocclusions. Am J Orthod 1967;53:446–56.

159. Ringenberg QM, Butts WC. A controlled cephalometric evaluation of single-arch cervical traction therapy. Am J Orthod 1970;57:179–85.

160. Barton JJ. High-pull headgear vs. cervical traction: a cephalometric comparison. Am J Orthod 1972;62:517–29.

161. Wieslander L. The effect of force on craniofacial development. Am J Orthod 1974;65:531–8.

162. Cross JJ. Facial growth: before, during and following orthodontic treatment. Am J Orthod 1977;71:68–78.

163. Melsen B. Effects of cervical anchorage during and after treatment: an implant study. Am J Orthod 1978;73:526–40.

164. Baumrind S, Molthen R, West EE, et al. Mandibular plane changes during maxillary retraction. Part 1 and 2. Am J Orthod 1978;74:32–40, 603–20.

165. Mills CM, Holman RG, Graber TM. Heavy intermittent cervical traction in class II treatment: a longitudinal cephalometric assessment. Am J Orthod 1978;74:361–79.

166. Brown P. A cephalometric evaluation of high-pull molar headgear and facebow neck strap therapy. Am J Orthod 1978;74:621–32.

167. Baumrind S, Molthen R, West EE, Miller DM. Distal displacement of the maxilla and upper first molar. Am J Orthod 1979;75:630–40.

168. Baumrind S, Korn EL, Molthen R, West EE.

Changes in facial dimensions associated with the use of forces to retract the maxilla. Am J Orthod 1981;80:17–30.

169. Howard RD. Skeletal changes with extraoral traction. Eur J Orthod 1982;4:197–202.

170. Firouz M, Zernik J, Nanda R. Dental and orthopedic effects of high-pull headgear in treatment of class II, division 1 malocclusion. Am J Orthod Dentofac Orthop 1992;102:197–205.

171. Sproule WR. Dentofacial changes produced by extraoral cervical traction to the maxilla of the Macaca mulatta: a histologic and serial cephalometric study. Am J Orthod 1969;56:532–3.

172. Fredrick DL. Dentofacial changes produced by extraoral cervical traction to the maxilla of the Macaca mulatta: a histologic and serial cephalometric study [dissertation]. University of Washington; 1969.

173. Droschl H. The effect of heavy orthopaedic forces on the maxilla of the growing Siamiri sciureus (squirrel monkey). Am J Orthod 1973;63:449–61.

174. Thompson RW. Extraoral high-pull forces with rigid palatal expansion in the macaca mulatta. Am J Orthod 1974;66:302–17.

175. Elder JR, Tuenge RH. Cephalometric and histologic changes produced by extra-oral high pull traction to the maxilla of Macaca mulatta. Am J Orthod 1974;66:599–617.

176. Meldrum RJ. Alterations in the upper facial growth of Macaca mulatta resulting from high-pull headgear. Am J Orthod 1975;67:393–411.

177. Yamamoto J. Effects of extraoral forces in the dentofacial complex of the Macaca irus. J Jpn Orthod 1975;34:173–97.

178. Triftshauser R, Walters RD. Cervical retraction of the maxilla in the Macaca mulatta monkey. Angle Orthod 1976;46:37–46.

179. Brandt HC, Shapiro PA, Kokich VG. Experimental and postexperimental effects of posteriorly directed extraoral traction in adult Macaca fascicularis. Am J Orthod 1979;75:301–17.

180. Dermaut LR, Aelbers CMF. Orthopedics in orthodontics: fiction or reality: a review of the literature, Part II. Am J Orthod Dentofac Orthop 1996;110:667–71.

181. Born J, Muth S, Fehm HL. The significance of sleep onset and slow wave sleep for nocturnal release of growth hormone (GH) and cortisol. Psychoneuroendocrinology 1988;13:233–43.

182. Stevenson S, Hunziker EB, Hermann W, et al. Is longitudinal bone growth influenced by diurnal variation in the mitotic activity of chondrocytes of the growth plates? J Orthop Res 1990;8:132–5.

183. Risinger RK, Proffit WR. Continuous overnight observation of human premolar eruption. Arch Oral Biol 1996;41:779–89.

184. Carlson DS. Growth of the temporomandibular joint. In: Zarb GA, Carlsson GE, Sessle B, Mohl ND, editors. Temporomandibular joint. 2nd ed. Copenhagen: Munksgaard; 1994. p.128–58.

185. Petrovic AG. Experimental and cybernetic approaches to the mechanism of action of functional appliances on mandibular growth. In: McNamara JA, Ribbens KA, editors. Malocclusion and the periodontium. Craniofacial growth monograph series. Monograph 15. Ann Arbor: Center for Human Growth and Development, University of Michigan; 1984. p. 213–68.

186. McNamara JA, Bryan FA. Long-term mandibular adaptations to protrusive function in the rhesus monkey (Macaca mulatta). Am J Orthod Dentofac Orthop 1987;92:98–108.

187. Rabie ABM, She TT, Hägg U. Functional appliance therapy accelerates and enhances condylar growth. Am J Orthod Dentofac Orthop 2003;123:40–8.

188. Marshchner JF, Harris JE. Mandibular growth and class II treatment. Angle Orthod 1966;36:89–93.

189. Parkhouse RC. A cephalometric appraisal of cases of Angle's class II, division 1, malocclusion treated by the Andresen appliance. Dent Pract Dent Rec 1969;19:425–33.

190. Woodside DG, Reed RT, Doucet JD, et al. Some effects of activator treatment on the growth rate of the mandible and position of the midface. In: Cook JT, editor. Transactions of the Third International Orthodontic Congress. St. Louis (MO): C.V. Mosby Co.; 1975. p. 459–80.

191. Pancherz H. The effect of continuous bite-jumping on the dentofacial complex: a follow-up study after Herbst appliance treatment of class II malocclusion. Eur J Orthod 1981;3:49–60.

192. Luder HU. Effects of activator treatment — evidence for the occurrence of two different types of reaction. Eur J Orthod 1981;3:205–22.

193. Righellis EG. Treatment effects of Fränkel, activator and extraoral traction appliances. Angle Orthod 1983;53:107–21.

194. Wieslander L. Intensive treatment of severe class II malocclusions with a headgear-Herbst appliance in the early mixed dentition. Am J Orthod 1984;86:1–13.

195. McNamara JA, Bookstein FL, Shaughnessy TG. Skeletal and dental relationships following functional regulator therapy on class II patients. Am J Orthod 1985;88:91–110.

196. Remmer KR, Mamandras AH, Hunter WS, et al. Cephalometric changes associated with treatment using the activator, the Fränkel appliance, and the fixed appliance. Am J Orthod 1985;88:363–72.

197. DeVincenzo JP, Huffer R, Winn MA. A study in human subjects using a new device designed to mimic the protrusive functional appliances used previously in monkeys. Am J Orthod Dentofac Orthop 1987;91:213–24.

198. Jakobsson SO, Paulin G. The influence of activator treatment on skeletal growth in Angle class II: 1 cases. A roentgenocephalometric study. Eur J Orthod 1990;12:174–84.

199. Björk A. The principle of the Andresen method of orthodontic treatment, a discussion based on cephalometric x-ray analysis of treated cases. Am J Orthod 1951;37:437–58.

200. Softley J. Cephalometric changes in seven "post normal" cases treated by the Andresen method. Dent Rec 1953;73:485–94.

201. Björk A. Variability and age changes in overjet and overbite: report from a follow-up study of individuals from 12 to 20 years of age. Am J Orthod 1953;39:779–801.

202. Meach CL. A cephalometric comparison of bony profile changes in class II, division 1 patients treated with extraoral force and functional jaw orthopedics. Am J Orthod 1966;52:353–70.

203. Trayfoot J, Richardson A. Angle class II, division 1, malocclusions treated by the Andresen method. Br Dent J 1968;124:516–9.

204. Hasund A. The use of activators in a system employing fixed appliances. Trans Eur Orthod Soc 1969;329–41.

205. Harvold EP, Vargervik K. Morphogenetic response to activator treatment. Am J Orthod 1971;60:478–90.

206. Stöckli PW, Dietrich UC. Experimental and clinical findings following functional forward displacement of the mandible. Trans Eur Orthod Soc 1973;435.

207. Woodside DG. Some effects of activator treatment on the mandible and the midface. Trans Eur Orthod Soc 1973;443–7.

208. Dietrich UC. Aktivator — mandibuläre Reaktion. Schweiz Monatsschr Zahnheilkd 1973;83:1093–104.

209. Wieslander L, Lagerström L. The effect of activator treatment on class II malocclusions. Am J Orthod 1979;75:20–6.

210. Forsberg CM, Odenrick L. Skeletal and soft tissue response to activator treatment. Eur J Orthod 1981;3:247–53.

211. Calvert FJ. An assessment of Andresen therapy on class II division 1 malocclusion. Br J Orthod 1982;9:149–53.

212. Creekmore TD, Radney LJ. Fränkel appliance

therapy: orthopedic or orthodontic? Am J Orthod 1983;83:89–108.

213. Gianelly AA, Brosnan P, Martignoni M, Bernstein L. Mandibular growth, condyle position, and Fränkel appliance therapy. Angle Orthod 1983;53:131–42.

214. Janson I. Skeletal and dentoalveolar changes in patients treated with a bionator during pre-pubertal and pubertal growth. In: McNamara JA, Ribbens KA, Howe RP, editors. Clinical alteration of the growing face. Craniofacial growth monograph series. Monograph 14. Ann Arbor: Center for Human Growth and Development, University of Michigan; 1983. p. 131–54.

215. Mills JRE. Clinical control of craniofacial growth: a skeptic viewpoint. In: McNamara JA, Ribbens KA, Howe RP, editors. Clinical alteration of the growing face. Craniofacial growth monograph series. Monograph 14. Ann Arbor: Center for Human Growth and Development, University of Michigan; 1983. p. 17–39.

216. Looi LK, Mills JR. The effect of two contrasting forms of orthodontic treatment on the facial profile. Am J Orthod 1986;89:507–17.

217. Nelson C, Harkness M, Herbisson P. Mandibular changes during functional appliance treatment. Am J Orthod Dentofac Orthop 1993;104:153–61.

218. Moss JP. Cephalometric changes during functional appliance therapy. Trans Eur Orthod Soc 1962;327–41.

219. Evald H, Harvold EP. The effect of activators on maxillary-mandibular growth and relationships. Am J Orthod 1967;37:18–25.

220. Freunthaller P. Cephalometric observations in class II, division 1 malocclusions treated with the activator. Angle Orthod 1967;37:18–25.

221. Hotz R. Application and appliance manipulation of functional forces. Am J Orthod 1970;58:459–78.

222. Ahlgren J, Laurin C. Late results of activator-treatment: a cephalometric study. Br J Orthod 1976;3:181–7.

223. Baumrind S, Korn EL, Isaacson JR, et al. Quantitative analysis of the orthodontic and orthopedic effects of maxillary retraction. Am J Orthod 1983;84:384–98.

224. Teuscher UM. A growth-related concept for skeletal class II treatment. Am J Orthod 1978;74:258–75.

225. Bass NM. Dento-facial orthopaedics in the correction of the class II malocclusion. Br J Orthod 1982;9:3–31.

226. Stöckli PW, Teuscher UM. Combined activator headgear orthopedics. In: Graber TM, Swain BF, editors. Orthodontics: current principles and techniques. St. Louis (MO): C.V. Mosby Co.; 1985. p. 405–83.

227. Lagerström LO, Nielsen IL, Lee R, Isaacson RJ. Dental and skeletal contributions to occlusal correction in patients treated with the high-pull headgear-activator combination. Am J Orthod Dentofac Orthop 1990;97:495–504.

228. Wieslander L. Long-term effect of treatment with the headgear-Herbst appliance in the early mixed dentition. Stability or relapse? Am J Orthod 1993;104:319–29.

229. Pancherz H. The effects, limitations, and long-term dentofacial adaptations to treatment with the Herbst appliance. Semin Orthod 1997;3:232–43.

230. von Bremen J, Pancherz H. Efficiency of early and late class II division 1 treatment. Am J Orthod Dentofac Orthop 2002;121:31–7.

231. Bishara SE. Facial and dental changes in adolescents and their clinical implications. Angle Orthod 2000;70:471–83.

232. Yamada S, Saeki S, Takahashi I, et al. Diurnal variation in the response of the mandible to orthopedic force. J Dent Res 2002;81:711–5.

233. Campbell PM. The dilemma of class III treatment: early or late? Angle Orthod 1983;53:175–91.

234. Thilander B. Chin-cap treatment for Angle. Class III malocclusion: a longitudinal study. Trans Eur Orthod Soc 1965;41:311–27.

235. Vego L. Early orthopedic treatment of cl. II skeletal patterns. Am J Orthod 1976;70:59–69.

236. Graber L. Chin cup therapy for mandibular prognathism. Am J Orthod 1977;72:23–41.

237. Allen RA, Connolly IH, Richardson A. Early treatment of incisor relationship using the chincap appliance. Eur J Orthod 1993;15:371–6.

238. Sugawara J, Mitani H. Facial growth of skeletal class III malocclusion and the effects, limitations, and long-term dentofacial adaptations to chincap therapy. Semin Orthod 1997;3:244–54.

239. Sakamoto T, Iwase I, Uka A, Nakamura S. A roentgenocephalometric study of skeletal changes during and after chin cap treatment. Am J Orthod 1984;85:341–50.

240. Sugawara J, Asano T, Endo N, Matani H. Long-term effects of chincup therapy on skeletal profile in mandibular prognathism. Am J Orthod 1990;98:127–33.

241. Robertson NRG. An examination of treatment changes in children treated with the functional regulator of Fränkel. Am J Orthod 1983;83:299–309.

242. Delaire J. Considérations sur la croissance faciale (en particulier du maxillaire supérieur). Déductions thérapeutiques. Rev Stomatol 1971;72:57–76.

243. Jackson GW, Kokich VG, Shapiro PA. Experimental and postexperimental response to anteriorly directed extraoral force in young Macaca nemestina. Am J Orthod 1979; 75:318–33.

244. Takada K, Petdachai S, Sakuda M. Changes in dentofacial morphology in skeletal class III children treated by a modified maxillary protraction headgear and a chin cup: a longitudinal cephalometric appraisal. Eur J Orthod 1993;15:211–21.

245. Ngan P, Hagg U, Yiu C, et al. Treatment response to maxillary expansion and protraction. Eur J Orthod 1996;18:151–68.

246. Nartallo-Turley PE, Turley PK. Cephalometric effects of combined palatal expansion and facemask therapy on class III malocclusion. Angle Orthod 1998;68:217–24.

247. Ngan PW, Hagg U, Yiu C, Wei SHY. Treatment response and long-term dentofacial adaptations to maxillary expansion and protraction. Semin Orthod 1997;3:255–64.

248. Williams MD, Sarver DM, Sadowsky PL, Bradley E. Combined rapid maxillary expansion and protraction facemask in the treatment of class III malocclusions in growing children: a prospective long-term study. Semin Orthod 1997;3:265–74.

249. da Silva Filho OG, Magro AC, Capelozza Filho L. Early treatment of the class III malocclusion with rapid maxillary expansion and maxillary protraction. Am J Orthod 1998;113:196–203.

250. Baccetti T, McGill JS, Franchi L. Skeletal effects of early treatment of Class III malocclusion with maxillary expansion and face-mask therapy. Am J Orthod 1998;113:333–43.

251. Kapust AJ, Sinclair PM, Turley PK. Cephalometric effects of face mask/expansion therapy in class III children: a comparison of three age groups. Am J Orthod Dentofac Orthop 1998;113:204–12.

252. Baik HS. Clinical results of the maxillary protraction in Korean children. Am J Orthod 1995;108:583–92.

253. Merwin D, Ngan P, Hagg U, et al. Timing for effective application of anteriorly directed orthopedic force to the maxilla. Am J Orthod 1997;112:292–9.

254. Gallagher RW, Miranda F, Buschang PH. Maxillary protraction: treatment and posttreatment effects. Am J Orthod 1998;113:612–9.

255. Ngan P. Biomechanics of maxillary expansion and protraction in class III patients. Am J Orthod Dentofac Orthop 2002;121:582–3.

256. Smalley WM, Shapiro PA, Hohl TH, et al. Osseointegrated titanium implants for maxillofacial protraction in monkeys. Am J Orthod Dentofac Orthop 1988;94:285–95.

257. Woodside DG, Altuna G, Harvold E, et al. Primate experiments in malocclusion and bone induction. Am J Orthod Dentofac Orthop 1983;83:460–8.

258. Lundstrom A, Woodside DG. Longitudinal changes in facial type in cases with vertical and horizontal mandibular growth directions. Eur J Orthod 1983;5:259–68.

259. Dellinger EL. A clinical assessment of the active vertical corrector — a nonsurgical alternative for skeletal open bite treatment. Am J Orthod Dentofac Orthop 1986;89:428–36.

260. Kalra V, Burstone CJ, Nanda R. Effects of a fixed magnetic appliance on the dentofacial complex. Am J Orthod Dentofac Orthop 1989;95:467–78.

261. Kuster R, Ingervall B. The effect of treatment of skeletal open bite with two types of bite-blocks. Eur J Orthod 1992;14:489–99.

262. Iscan HN, Sarisoy L. Comparison of the effects of passive posterior bite-blocks with different construction bites on the craniofacial and dentoalveolar structures. Am J Orthod Dentofac Orthop 1997;112:171–8.

263. Barbre RE, Sinclair PM. A cephalometric evaluation of anterior open bite correction with the magnetic active vertical corrector. Angle Orthod 1991;61:93–102.

264. Galleto L, Urbaniak J, Subtelny JD. Adult anterior open bite. Am J Orthod Dentofac Orthop 1990;97:522–6.

265. Shapiro PA. Stability of open bite treatment. Am J Orthod Dentofac Orthop 2002;121:566–8.

266. Umemori M, Sugawara J, Mitani H, et al. Skeletal anchorage system for open-bite correction. Am J Orthod Dentofac Orthop 1998;115:166–74.

267. Sawaki Y, Ohkubo H, Hibi H, Ueda M. Mandibular lengthening by distraction osteogenesis using osseointegrated implants and an intraoral device: a preliminary report. J Oral Maxillofac Surg 1996;54:594–600.

268. Cohen SR. Craniofacial distraction with a modular internal distraction system: evolution of design and surgical techniques. Plast Reconstr Surg 1999;103:1592–607.

269. Kim YH, Han UK, Lim DD, Serraon MLP. Stability of anterior open bite correction with multiloop edgewise therapy: a cephalometric follow-up study. Am J Orthod Dentofac Orthop 2000;118:43–54.

CHAPTER 54

Database Acquisition and Treatment Planning

Marc B. Ackerman, DMD
David M. Sarver, DMD, MS

Until the turn of the twenty-first century, treatment planning in orthognathic surgery was based primarily on a system of clinical observation, a static set of records (models, radiographs), with the major thrust of treatment being directed toward satisfying lateral cephalometric goals. These goals might include particular measurements (sella-nasion–A point and A point–nasion–B point differences) or analytical norms (Steiner, Ricketts), or even comparison of lateral head film tracings of persons with craniofacial skeletal dysplasia[1-3] to templates having average skeletal proportions derived from longitudinal growth studies.[4] The most significant shortcoming of this reliance on the lateral cephalogram as the primary determinant of treatment goal setting is that it did not take into account the resting and dynamic hard–soft tissue relationships, which are the most critical aspects in treatment planning in both orthodontics and orthognathic surgery. Furthermore, cephalometric analysis quantifies dentoskeletal relationships in angular and linear measures, which are not entirely representative of the multidimensional interrelationship of craniofacial parts. That is to say, the integumental soft tissue drape may sometimes be inconsistent with the underlying skeletal framework in a given patient.

Whereas the skeletal framework may be reasonably stable post-adolescence, the soft tissues are more subject to maturational and age-related changes. The cephalometric approach to treatment planning is now considered "Procrustean," after the story based on Greek mythology. As the story goes, Procrustes was an innkeeper with only one bed. If a traveler was too tall for the bed, Procrustes would cut off the traveler's feet so that he or she would fit the bed. A traveler who was too short would be stretched on a rack to likewise fit the bed in length. This charming story relates to this chapter in that by applying the same hard tissue cephalometric analysis to all patients, all of our patients end up being crammed into the same bed!

The contemporary approach to the surgical orthodontic treatment of dentofacial deformity will illustrate the use of dentofacial proportionality in the place of applying absolute linear or angular norms to the individual patient. Patient-specific treatment planning will be the focus of this chapter.

Contemporary Orthognathic Treatment Planning

The emphasis in this chapter on orthognathic diagnosis and treatment planning is intended to lead us into a new era and methodology of patient analysis and treatment goal setting. In modern orthognathic surgery, treatment goals are determined through systematic clinical examination and quantification of the patient's dentofacial characteristics. Therefore, the purpose of this chapter will be to introduce the reader to a method of systematic dentofacial analysis in all three dimensions with emphasis on both static and dynamic relationships, as well as both functional and esthetic objectives.

Problem-oriented treatment planning has served us very well in the past several decades, by focusing on the problems in need of correction, including the identification of solutions for each problem. The natural progression of problem-oriented treatment planning should now include the identification of favorable attributes as well as the problems. The reason for this next step is the realization that focusing solely on the problems and their solutions may result in a treatment plan which potentially has a negative effect on the positive attributes in that patient. A classic orthodontic example is where the extraction of maxillary premolars in the correction of a skeletal Class II malocclusion, while satisfying functional and occlusal issues, may result in profile flattening and an unfortunate effect on facial appearance. In the orthognathic arena, a good example is the widening of the alar base secondary to maxillary advancement and/or impaction. The goal of orthognathic treatment is the optimization of negative attributes, while at the same time preserving those attributes that are deemed favorable (Figure 54-1).

This systematic approach to clinical examination of the patient is essential for the development of an optimization-oriented database. All clinically detectable deviations from the optimal range fall into the two broad categories of function and esthetics.

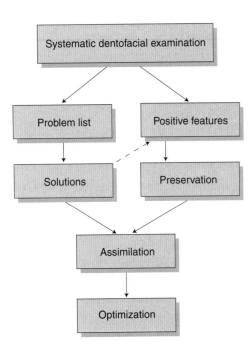

FIGURE 54-1 *Contemporary treatment planning flow chart. After the clinical examination and databasing of the quantitative measurements, both problems and positive attributes are identified. Solutions for the problems are identified and the* dotted arrow *indicates that each potential solution can negatively impact a positive feature. Therefore, the advantage of measuring both problems and positive features permits the clinician to recognize the potential negative impact that any given solution has on the positive attributes. This "decision tree" leads to correction of the problems but also preservation of the positive attributes. The clinician then assimilates all of this information for optimization of treatment.*

Function and Dentofacial Deformity

Patients with severe discrepancies in the size and position of their jaws and their teeth often have difficulty in oral function. Certain foods may be difficult to incise and chew. Speech may also be affected by jaw deformity. If the patient cannot bring the tongue and lips into the proper position, it may not be possible to produce a specific sound properly. Besides careful examination of the patient, it is doubtful that diagnostic tests of function that can be carried out in the dental or surgical office are useful. The relationship of temporomandibular (TM) joint problems to severe malocclusion and dentofacial deformities is complex but important. Although there is some evidence that patients with specific types of malocclusion are more susceptible to TM joint problems, the increased risk is relatively small.[5] In general terms, patients with dentofacial deformity are similar to patients with normal facial proportions in the prevalence of TM joint problems.[6]

Appearance and Dentofacial Deformity

Appearance and dentofacial esthetics can be divided into three subcategories: macroesthetics, miniesthetics, and microesthetics (Figure 54-2). The specific concerns of the patient can be elucidated through open-ended doctor-patient communication and then integrated into the diagnostic decision tree. The surgeon and orthodontist should be sensitive to the patient's esthetic desires, balancing them against cultural and familial standards. The physical burden of treatment is borne by the patient and must be weighed when determining the extent of surgical intervention. For example, when deciding whether treatment should involve orthodontics alone, orthodontics and orthognathic surgery, or acceptable orthodontic camouflage, the patient should understand the risk-benefit ratio of any given treatment sequence.

Data Collection

Primary data collection begins at the clinical examination and is supplemented with static and dynamic recordings of the patient in three spatial dimensions. Record taking should replicate the functional and esthetic presentation of the patient. Findings from the clinical examination should either be confirmed or challenged by data obtained from the records. The analysis of the clinical database will generate a diagnostic summary and optimized problem list. An emerging soft-tissue paradigm in surgical orthodontic treatment planning has refocused analysis on facial proportionality and balance versus reliance on normative data derived from cephalometrics.[7] The art of surgical orthodontics rests in the ability to envisage the patient's desired three-dimensional soft tissue outcome and then retroengineer the dental and skeletal hard tissues to produce such a change. The concept of retroengineering will be explained later in this chapter under technological applications to orthognathic treatment planning.

In today's clinical environment there are three methods of data collection. The first and most commonly used method includes still photography, study models, and cephalometric radiographs. The second is the use of databasing programs to document direct clinical measurement of the patient's resting and dynamic relationships. The third involves the use of digital video to record the dynamics of facial movement. This methodology as it currently exists does not dynamically quantify movement. Expect to see greater recognition of the value of this technology, which should lead to research into the quantification of dynamic facial movements.

Conventional Records

Standard orthodontic records have not changed significantly in many years, but contemporary records in surgical orthodontic treatment are changing rapidly.

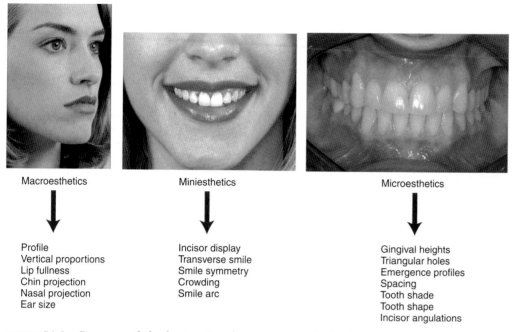

Macroesthetics	Miniesthetics	Microesthetics
Profile Vertical proportions Lip fullness Chin projection Nasal projection Ear size	Incisor display Transverse smile Smile symmetry Crowding Smile arc	Gingival heights Triangular holes Emergence profiles Spacing Tooth shade Tooth shape Incisor angulations

FIGURE 54-2   *Recommended subcategories of appearance and esthetics.*

Surgical orthodontics demands treating all dimensions of patients. In clinical practice, standard records include film or digital photographs, radiographs, and study models (whether plaster, mounted or unmounted, or electronic models). The facial images, which are universally considered standard records, include frontal at rest, frontal smile, and profile at rest images. Whereas these orientations do provide an adequate amount of diagnostic information, they do not contain all of the information needed for three-dimensional visualization and quantification. Orthognathic surgery requires expansion of the database compared to conventional orthodontic treatment.

The suggested records can be divided into two groups—static and dynamic. The accepted facial photographic recordings should include frontal smile close-up, oblique facial smile, oblique smile close-up, and profile smile.[8]

Direct Measurement as a Biometric Tool

The goal of the clinical examination is to quantitatively assess soft and hard tissue attributes of the dentofacial complex, and record what elements are satisfactory and which are in need of optimization. Clinical examination procedures vary greatly among practitioners. Measurement should be thorough, systematic, and consistent, thus minimizing the chance that something of importance will be overlooked. We want to avoid the situation where the clinician performs a cursory examination, jotting down brief notes as to abnormalities that are observed without recording any other descriptive data. This practice is often justified by the assumption that most diagnostic decisions can be made from the records after the patient leaves. This is a poor diagnostic technique for several reasons.

First, static records cannot reflect the dynamic relationships that are important in the overall functional assessment of the patient. For example, the simple idea of the relationship of the upper incisor at rest and on smile is not reflected on radiographs or models and is poorly evaluated in photographs. Second, information that may have not looked important enough to write down during a cursory examination may be important later, and thus would be unavailable because it was not recorded.

Third, a thorough and comprehensive examination record that includes normal observations is an accurate medicolegal document. It is hard for an unhappy patient to charge negligence when it is clear that the information was obtained and used. The more thorough and well documented the record is, the more valuable it is if problems arise.

Contemporary clinical examination uses a computer-databasing program to facilitate data entry, and these data are then merged into reports and treatment planning screens or forms.[9] Each clinical characteristic in the examination has a pop-up menu containing all of the possible descriptions for that particular trait (Figure 54-3). By using a computer interface, the surgeon or orthodontist saves valuable time in both the clinical examination and diagnostic and treatment planning work-up. The information is then stored for recall and analysis, and can even have predefined parameters that identify problematic measurements automatically.

As an example of how this interface facilitates the examination of dynamic hard–soft tissue relationships, we suggest that the following frontal measurements be performed systematically in evaluation of anterior dental display, both at rest and at smile:

- Philtrum height: The philtrum height is measured in millimeters from subnasale (the base of the nose at the midline) to the most inferior portion of the upper lip on the vermilion tip beneath the philtral columns. The absolute linear measurement is not particularly important, but what is significant is its relationship to the upper incisor, and the commissures of the mouth. In the adolescent, it is common to find the philtrum height to be shorter than the commissure height, and the difference can be explained in the differential in lip growth with maturation.

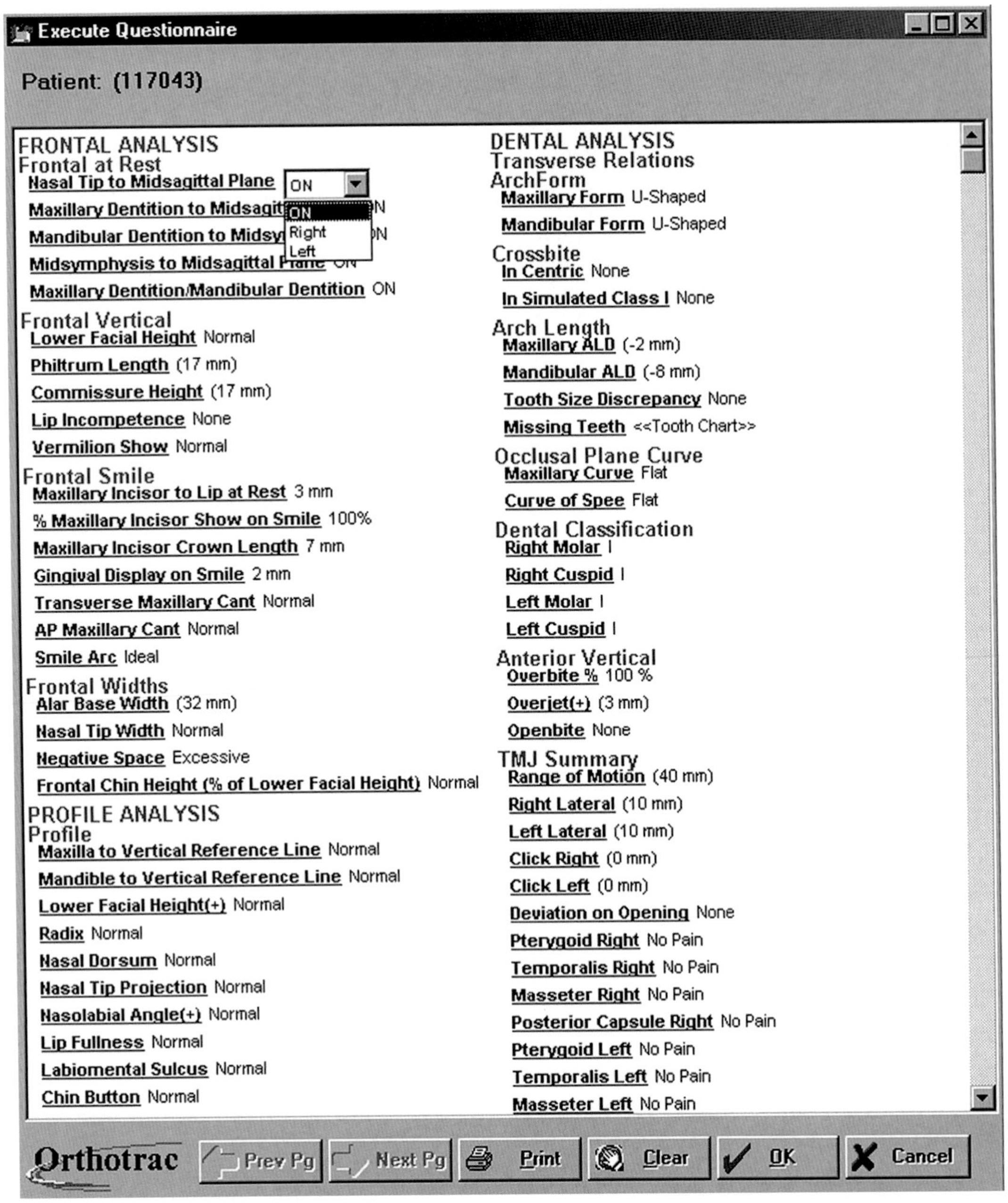

Execute Questionnaire

Patient: (117043)

FRONTAL ANALYSIS
Frontal at Rest
Nasal Tip to Midsagittal Plane   ON
Maxillary Dentition to Midsagit... ON
Mandibular Dentition to Midsy... ON
Midsymphysis to Midsagittal Plane ON
Maxillary Dentition/Mandibular Dentition ON
Frontal Vertical
Lower Facial Height Normal
Philtrum Length (17 mm)
Commissure Height (17 mm)
Lip Incompetence None
Vermilion Show Normal
Frontal Smile
Maxillary Incisor to Lip at Rest 3 mm
% Maxillary Incisor Show on Smile 100%
Maxillary Incisor Crown Length 7 mm
Gingival Display on Smile 2 mm
Transverse Maxillary Cant Normal
AP Maxillary Cant Normal
Smile Arc Ideal
Frontal Widths
Alar Base Width (32 mm)
Nasal Tip Width Normal
Negative Space Excessive
Frontal Chin Height (% of Lower Facial Height) Normal
PROFILE ANALYSIS
Profile
Maxilla to Vertical Reference Line Normal
Mandible to Vertical Reference Line Normal
Lower Facial Height(+) Normal
Radix Normal
Nasal Dorsum Normal
Nasal Tip Projection Normal
Nasolabial Angle(+) Normal
Lip Fullness Normal
Labiomental Sulcus Normal
Chin Button Normal

DENTAL ANALYSIS
Transverse Relations
ArchForm
Maxillary Form U-Shaped
Mandibular Form U-Shaped
Crossbite
In Centric None
In Simulated Class I None
Arch Length
Maxillary ALD (-2 mm)
Mandibular ALD (-8 mm)
Tooth Size Discrepancy None
Missing Teeth <<Tooth Chart>>
Occlusal Plane Curve
Maxillary Curve Flat
Curve of Spee Flat
Dental Classification
Right Molar I
Right Cuspid I
Left Molar I
Left Cuspid I
Anterior Vertical
Overbite % 100 %
Overjet(+) (3 mm)
Openbite None
TMJ Summary
Range of Motion (40 mm)
Right Lateral (10 mm)
Left Lateral (10 mm)
Click Right (0 mm)
Click Left (0 mm)
Deviation on Opening None
Pterygoid Right No Pain
Temporalis Right No Pain
Masseter Right No Pain
Posterior Capsule Right No Pain
Pterygoid Left No Pain
Temporalis Left No Pain
Masseter Left No Pain

Orthotrac Prev Pg Next Pg Print Clear OK Cancel

FIGURE 54-3 *A computer-databasing program facilitates data entry, and these data are then merged into reports and treatment planning screens or forms. Each clinical characteristic in the examination has a pop-up menu containing all of the possible descriptions for that particular trait.*

- Commissure height: The commissure height is measured from a line constructed from the alar bases through subspinale, then from the commissures perpendicular to this line.
- Interlabial gap: The interlabial gap is the distance in millimeters between the upper and lower lips, when lip incompetence is present.
- Amount of incisor show at rest: The amount of upper incisor show at rest is

a critical esthetic parameter because one of the inevitable characteristics of an aging tooth-lip relationship is diminished upper incisor show at rest and on smile. For example, an adult patient who displays 3 mm of gingival display on smile and 3 mm of upper incisor at rest should only carefully consider maxillary incisor intrusion or maxillary impaction to reduce gingival display, since reduction in gingival dis-

play also results in diminished incisor show at rest and during conversation (a characteristic of the aging face).

- Amount of incisor display on smile: On smile, patients will either show their entire upper incisor, or only a percentage of the incisor. Measurement of the percentage of incisor display, when combined with the crown height measured next, leads the clinician to decide how much tooth movement is required to attain the appropriate smile for that patient.
- Crown height: The vertical height of the maxillary central incisors in the adult is measured in millimeters and is normally between 9 and 12 mm, with an average of 10.6 mm in males and 9.6 mm in females. The age of the patient is a factor in crown height because of the rate of apical migration in the adolescent.
- Gingival display: There is variability in what is esthetically acceptable for the amount of gingival display on smile, but it is important to always remember the relationship between gingival display and the amount of incisor shown at rest. In broad terms, it is better for a patient to be treated less aggressively in reducing smile gumminess when considering that the aging process will result in a natural diminishment of this characteristic. A gummy smile is often more esthetic than a smile with diminished tooth display.
- Smile arc: The smile arc should be defined as the relationship of the curvature of the incisal edges of the maxillary incisors and canines to the curvature of the lower lip in the posed social smile.[10,11] The ideal smile arc has the maxillary incisal edge curvature parallel to the curvature of the lower lip upon smile, and the term *consonant* is used to describe this parallel relationship. A *nonconsonant* or flat smile arc is characterized by the

maxillary incisal curvature being flatter than the curvature of the lower lip on smile. The smile arc relationship is not as quantitatively measurable as the other attributes, so the qualitative observation of consonant, flat, or reverse smile arcs is generally cited.

Is it important to measure these above-described characteristics in orthognathic cases? The following case illustrates the significance of resting and dynamic soft tissue measurement, and how surgical or orthodontic treatment planning is determined by direct measurement as much as it is by cephalometric analysis. The role of cephalometrics will be discussed later in this chapter, and the emphasis will be less on static comparisons to norms and more on its coordination with the soft tissue overlay of the face and the use of predictive algorithms to arrive at final macrotreatment decisions.

The patient in Figure 54-4 was a 16-year-old male who presented for an opinion relative to his chief complaint of excessive gingival display on smile, or a "gummy smile" (see Figure 54–4A). He had finished orthodontic treatment about 1 year earlier, and when his mother asked the

orthodontist if something could be done, the orthodontist felt that the only way to improve that smile characteristic was to consider surgical maxillary superior repositioning via Le Fort I osteotomy. A referral to the oral and maxillofacial surgeon was recommended, and maxillary impaction was recommended, but the surgeon felt that he wanted to wait until the patient had reached full physical maturity. The patient's mother felt further investigation was warranted.

The examination revealed a well-treated orthodontic case with excellent occlusion, and the macrorelations were also quite normal in terms of profile and facial proportion. The anterior tooth-lip relationships were as follows:

- Resting relationships (see Figure 54-4B)
  Philtrum height: 25 mm
  Commissure height: 25 mm
  Maxillary incisor at rest: 2 mm

- Dynamic relationships (see Figure 54-4C)
  Percentage of maxillary incisor display on smile: 100%
  Maxillary incisor crown height: 8 mm
  Gingival display on smile: 4 mm
  Smile arc: consonant

It is instructive to outline the etiologies of excessive gingival display on smile and characteristics seen with each in order to demonstrate the decision-making process in problem-oriented treatment planning with optimization.

- Vertical maxillary excess: Characterized by a disproportionately long lower facial height, lip incompetence, excessive incisor display at rest, and excessive gingival display on smile
- Short philtrum: The philtrum height shorter than the commissure, excessive incisor display at rest, and a reverse resting upper lip line
- Excessive smile curtain: Excessive animation of the upper lip on smile, displaying more tooth and gingiva than desired
- Short crown height: If the anterior incisor height is short, excessive gingival display may result

In this case, vertical maxillary excess was ruled out because facial proportionality was normal, no lip incompetence was present, and only 2 mm of upper incisor showed at rest. The second possibility, a short philtrum, was ruled out since the philtrum and commissure heights were

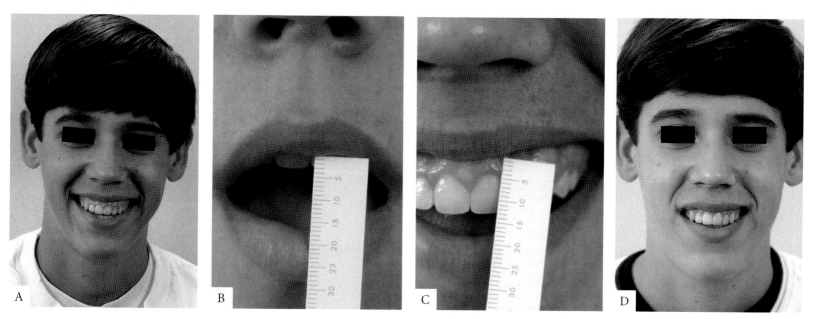

FIGURE **54-4**   A–D, *Case illustration of direct measurement of lip-tooth-gingival relationships.*

the same, and no reverse upper lip resting characteristics were noted. The third possibility, excessive curtain, was eliminated because the vermilion was adequate on smile and the margins of the commissure and philtrum even on posed smile. The fourth possibility, short crown height, was significant since the maxillary incisors measured to be only 8 mm in height.

Therapeutic options to decrease gingival display included maxillary impaction, orthodontic intrusion of maxillary incisors, or periodontal crown lengthening.

- Maxillary impaction: A 4 mm superior repositioning of the maxilla would decrease the gumminess of the smile, but would result in a −2 mm upper incisor show at rest, greatly hastening the aging characteristics of the face and smile.
- Orthodontic intrusion of the maxillary anterior teeth: This would likewise result in reduction of incisor display at rest but would also flatten the already consonant smile arc.
- Periodontal crown lengthening: The increase in anterior crown height decreases the gumminess of the smile (appropriate because the teeth are short), and optimizes treatment by *not* decreasing incisor display at rest and by maintaining the consonant smile arc.

After discussing all these options with the family, the family decided to proceed with the third and recommended option of crown lengthening, with an excellent outcome (see Figure 54-4D).

In summary, this case demonstrates the new direction in dentofacial treatment planning, even though the final result was not an orthognathic treatment plan. This case was selected to make the point that through careful observation and measurement, the appropriate treatment plan was delivered.

Digital Videography

Dynamic recording of patient's facial motion is accomplished with the use of digital videography.[12] This technology may be used to document and evaluate such characteristics as range of mandibular motion on opening and laterotrusive movements, deviations on opening, smile, and speech. Digital video and computer technology have primarily been used to record anterior tooth display during speech and smiling. Digital videos can be recorded in a standardized fashion with the camera at a fixed distance from the subject. We recommend that these images be taken in a standard format with emphasis on natural head position, so that future analysis and research possibilities may be maximized. We also recommend that video be taken in the frontal, oblique, and lateral dimensions. Clinically, an example of where this technology is most relevant is the patient with an asymmetric smile. The question that arises is whether or not the patient has a dental asymmetry, skeletal asymmetry, or asymmetric movement of the lip curtain during animation. The single smile photograph cannot corroborate the clinical impression gained during the data collection process. The video clip may be reviewed and evaluated during all planning phases of treatment as well as for comparison of the orthognathic treatment effects (Figure 54-5).

Systematic Clinical Examination of Dentofacial Deformity

We have previously discussed the importance of clinical observation and direct measurement of the interaction of hard and soft tissues in planning appropriate combined orthodontic and orthognathic treatments of dentofacial deformity. In this section, we will describe the components of the examination from the macro-, mini-, and microperspectives.

Macroesthetic Examination: Frontal View

The facial areas for macroesthetic examination, as investigated from the frontal view, can be summarized as follows:

- Vertical proportions
  Facial heights:
    Lower third
- Transverse proportions
  Rule of fifths
    Middle fifth
      Inner canthi
      Alar base
    Medial two-fifths
      Outer canthi
      Gonial angles of mandible
    Outer two-fifths
      Ear deformity
      Ear projection
  Nasal anatomy
    Alar base
    Columella
    Nasal tip
    Dorsum
- Transverse symmetry
  Nasal tip to midsagittal plane
  Maxillary dental midline to mid sagittal plane
  Mandibular dental midline to symphysis
  Mandibular asymmetry with or without functional shift
  Maxillomandibular asymmetry
  Chin asymmetry

The starting point for the macroesthetic examination is the frontal perspective. Transverse and vertical relationships comprise the major components of the frontal examination and analysis. As emphasized in our introduction, the *proportional* relationship of height and width is far more important than absolute values in establishing overall facial type. Faces can be broadly categorized as either mesocephalic, brachycephalic, or dolichocephalic (Figure 54-6).[13] The differentiation between these facial types has to do with the general proportionality of facial breadth to facial height, with brachycephalic faces being broader and shorter in comparison to the longer and more narrow dolichocephalic faces. Generally, the most attractive faces tend to have common

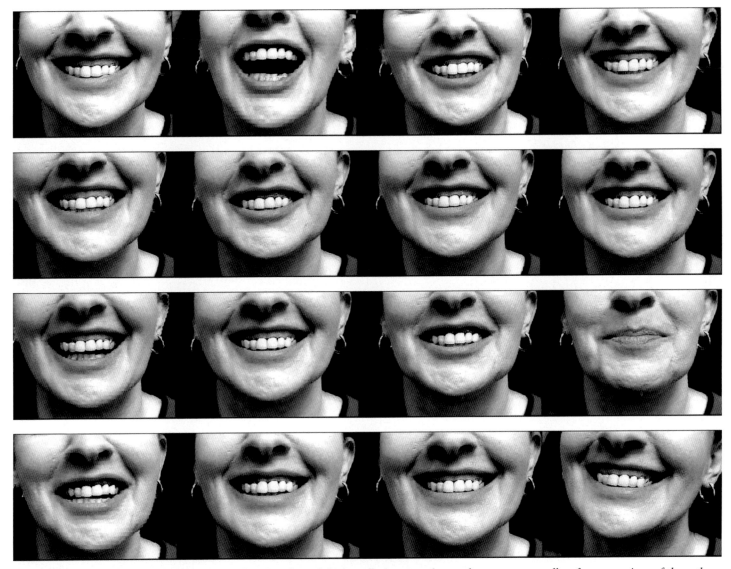

FIGURE 54-5 *The video clip may be reviewed and evaluated during all planning phases of treatment as well as for comparison of the orthognathic treatment effects.*

proportions and relationships that generally differ from normative values.[14]

Vertical Facial Proportions The ideal face is vertically divided into equal thirds by horizontal lines adjacent to the hairline, the nasal base, and menton (Figure 54-7A). Surgical orthodontic treatment is in a large part limited to the lower facial third. Measurement of the upper face is often hindered by the variability in identification of broad landmarks such as the location of the hairline and radix.

We will begin our clinical examination with the evaluation of lower facial height. In the ideal lower third of the face, the upper lip makes up the upper third, and the lower lip and chin compose the lower two-thirds (Figure 54-7B). Disproportion of the vertical facial thirds may be a result of many dental and skeletal factors, and these proportional relationships may help us define the contributing factors related to vertical dentofacial deformities.

In the following sections, we present case illustrations of orthognathic changes in vertical proportionality.

Short Vertical Proportions The patient in Figure 54-8 presented for correction of her Class II deep bite secondary to her mandibular deficiency. Her anterior vertical relationships were characterized by a short lower facial third relative to her upper thirds (see Figure 54-8A and B). In addition, the lower third was comprised of a 45:55 vertical relation of the upper lip to lower lip and chin height. Recalling that the ideal proportions of the lower face are one-third upper lip and two-thirds lower lip and chin, the treatment plan was clearly a result of the direct clinical examination rather than any cephalometric standard. Other important clinical measurements entered into the decision process. Differential diagnosis for a short lower facial height included the following:

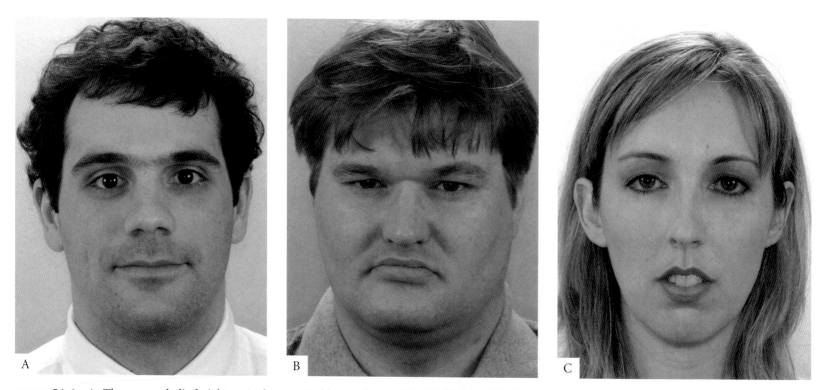

FIGURE 54-6   A, *The mesocephalic facial type is characterized by equal vertical facial thirds.* B, *The brachycephalic facial type appears square with a diminished lower third.* C, *The dolichocephalic facial type appears ovoid with an increased lower third.*

- Vertical maxillary deficiencies, which are then characterized by the following characteristics:

    Short lower facial third
    Diminished maxillary incisor display at rest
    Diminished incisor display on smile

- Diminished chin height, ascertained through the proportionality in the lower face rather than a linear cephalometric value
- Posterior dental collapse secondary to the loss of posterior dental support

The functional goal of mandibular advancement to correct the Class II dentoskeletal relationship was obvious, but an esthetic adjunctive consideration was a vertical genioplasty to optimize the macroesthetics of her vertical facial thirds. The final diagnosis depended not only on the vertical facial proportionality but on the measurement of the resting tooth-lip relationships as well in order to more clearly define the etiology of the lower facial height. In this case, our patient displayed 3 mm of maxillary incisor at rest, and all of her maxillary incisor on smile (see Figure 54-8C), which was inconsistent with vertical maxillary deficiency. Since the chin height was short, the final diagnosis was mandibular deficiency with short chin height. Therefore, the recommended treatment plan was

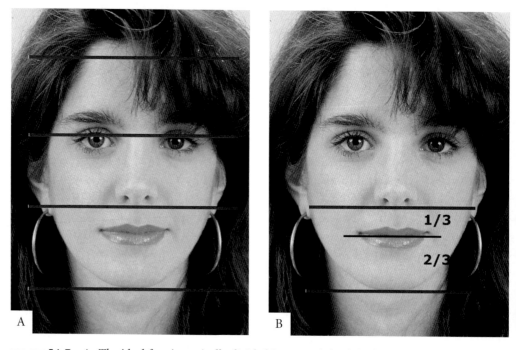

FIGURE 54-7   A, *The ideal face is vertically divided into equal thirds by horizontal lines adjacent to the hairline, the nasal base, and menton.* B, *In the ideal lower third of the face, the upper lip makes up the upper third, and the lower lip and chin compose the lower two-thirds.*

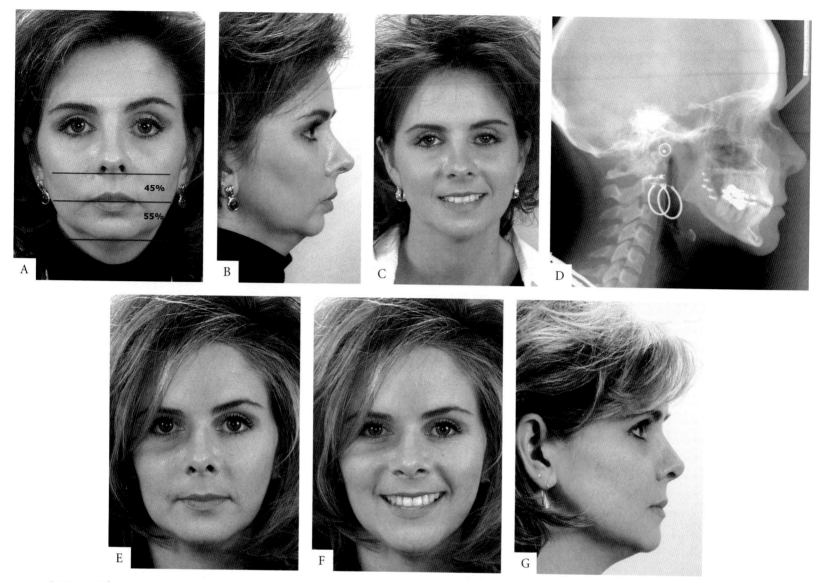

FIGURE 54-8 A, *This patient was referred for correction of her Class II deep bite secondary to her mandibular deficiency. B, Evaluation of her anterior vertical relationships was characterized by a short lower facial third relative to her upper thirds. The lower third was comprised of a 45:55 vertical relationship of the upper lip to lower lip and chin height. The ideal proportions of the lower face are one-third upper lip and two-thirds lower lip and chin; thus the treatment plan was derived from the direct clinical examination of this patient rather than any cephalometric standard. C, Our patient displayed 3 mm of maxillary incisor at rest, and all of her maxillary incisors on smile, inconsistent with vertical maxillary deficiency. D, The treatment plan was orthodontic preparation for mandibular advancement and vertical genioplasty. E, The post-treatment frontal view demonstrating balance of the vertical facial thirds. F, The vertical incisor position at smile was maintained, while the lower facial third was vertically augmented. G, The profile view shows improved mandibular projection relative to the upper face, improved chin-neck angle, and improved chin-neck length.*

orthodontic preparation for mandibular advancement and vertical genioplasty (see Figure 54-8D) to increase the lower facial height (see Figure 54-8E–G).

Long Vertical Proportions Long lower facial height is due to one of two possibilities: (1) vertical maxillary excess (VME) or (2) excessive chin height. The clinical keys that may be associated with VME are

gummy smile, open bite, lip incompetence, and steep mandibular plane as evidenced by gonial angle form. Excessive chin height is measured from the lower vermilion to the soft tissue menton. The clinical keys that may be associated with excessive chin height are lower facial third disproportionate from the one-third upper lip to two-thirds low lip and chin ratio, and the absence of VME characteristics.

The patient in Figure 54-9A was referred for correction of an anterior open bite and a gummy smile. Our systematic examination revealed the following problem list and characteristics:

- Frontal proportions at rest
  1. Long lower facial third
  2. Disproportion of chin height with the upper lip occupying 25% of the

lower facial third and the lower lip and chin occupying 75% of the lower third of the face
3. Lip incompetence of 5 mm
4. 8 mm of maxillary incisor display at rest
5. Midsymphysis to right 3 mm with no functional shift
6. Lip strain on closure (Figure 54-9B)

Clinical assessment of the frontal resting macroesthetic evaluation: This patient had most of the macrocharacteristics of vertical maxillary excess with a long lower facial height and excessive incisor display at rest. Excessive chin height was also a contributor to the lower facial height disproportion, as is evidenced by the upper lip and chin height clinical proportions.

- Frontal proportions on smile (Figure 54-9C)
  1. 100% of maxillary incisor displayed on smile
  2. Excessive gingival display on smile with 3 mm gingival display at the right cuspid and 5 mm at the left with a transverse cant to the palatal plane
  3. Transverse cant to the maxilla with the left side down 2 mm more than the left

Clinical assessment of the frontal dynamic (smiling) macroesthetic evaluation: A gummy smile was present but with normal incisor crown height. This would exclude cosmetic periodontal crown lengthening as the primary therapeutic choice for improvement of the gummy smile. The asymmetry of the maxilla is in compensation for the mandibular asymmetry, and results in a canted frontal occlusal plane and smile line.

- Oblique at-rest facial observation (Figure 54-9D)
  1. Excessive lower facial height
  2. Lip strain and excessive chin height

3. Flat labiomental sulcus
4. Nasal form judged to be quite adequate

Clinical assessment of the oblique macroesthetic evaluation: The flattened labiomental sulcus was secondary to the excessive lower facial height, lip incompetence, and chin deficiency.

- Oblique smiling facial observation (Figure 54-9E)
  1. No noticeable anteroposterior cant to the maxillary occlusal plane
  2. The smile arc was consonant
  3. The excessive gingival display was also evident on the oblique smile

Clinical assessment from the oblique smiling macroesthetic evaluation: Since the smile arc was consonant, alteration of the palatal plane would not have been indicated either through surgery or orthodontic incisor repositioning.

- Profile evaluation (Figure 54-9F)
  1. Long lower facial third
  2. Long chin height
  3. Flat labiomental sulcus
  4. Lip strain on closure

Clinical assessment of the profile macroesthetic evaluation: As would be expected from the frontal and oblique characteristics, the lateral profile reflected the overall skeletal and dental characteristics of vertical maxillary excess, but the chin deficiency that became evident on the oblique view was clearly demonstrated on the profile view.

The functional problem of the anterior open bite in this nongrowing patient necessitated superior repositioning of the maxilla to correct the functional complaint (Figure 54-9G–K). The exact surgical movements were directed by the clinical examination and measurements. Because the patient had the clinical diag-

nosis of vertical maxillary excess, maxillary impaction was indicated, but some discretionary decisions were needed for appropriate position of the maxilla from the esthetic standpoint. From the frontal dimension, the left side of the maxilla was impacted 2 mm more than the right in order to level the smile line. The differential degree of impaction reflected the degree of the maxillary compensation for the mandibular asymmetry.

Transverse Facial Proportions The assessment of the transverse components of facial width is best described by the rule of fifths.[9] This method describes the ideal transverse relationships of the face. The face is divided sagittally into five equal parts from helix to helix of the outer ears (Figure 54-10). Each of the segments should be one eye distance in width. Each transverse fifth should be individually examined and then assessed as a complete group.

The middle fifth of the face is delineated by the inner canthus of the eyes. A vertical line from the inner canthus should be coincident with the alar base of the nose. Variation in this facial fifth could be due to transverse deficiencies or excesses in either the inner canthi or alar base. For example, hypertelorism in craniofacial syndromes can create disproportionate transverse facial esthetics.

A vertical line from the outer canthus of the eyes frames the medial three-fifths of the face, which should be coincident with the gonial angles of the mandible. Although disproportion may be very subtle, it is worth noting since our treatments can positively change the shape or relative proportion of the gonial angles.

The outer two-fifths of the face is measured from the lateral canthus to lateral helix of the ear, which represents the width of the ears. Unless this abnormality is part of the chief complaint, prominent ears are often a difficult feature to discuss with the patient because laypeople only recognize its effect on the face in severe cases. However,

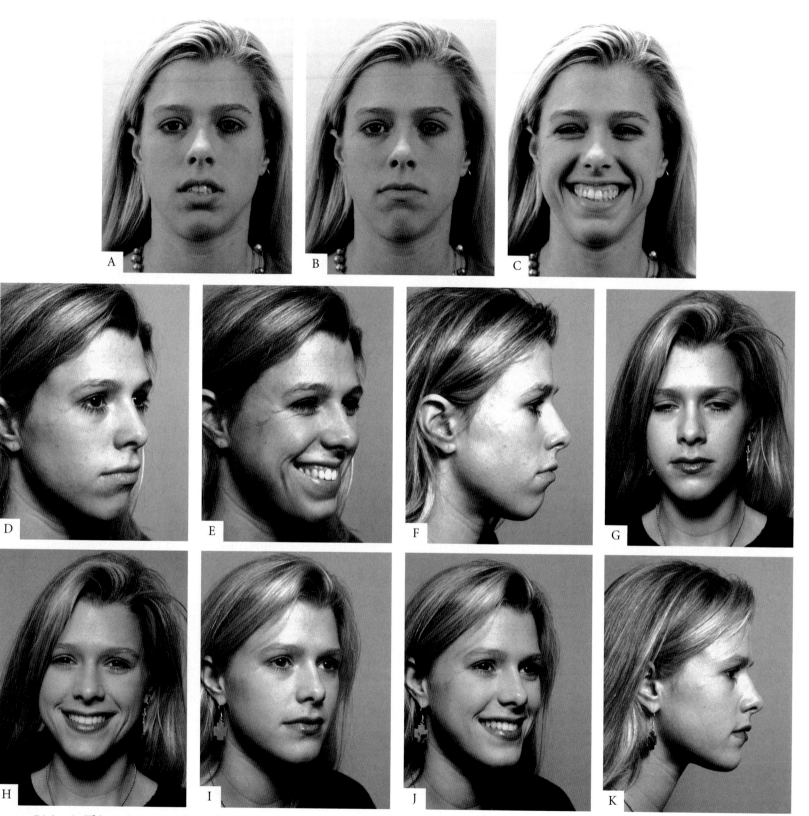

FIGURE 54-9 *A, This patient was referred for correction of an anterior open bite and a gummy smile. B, Lip strain on closure. C, Frontal proportions on smile with 100% of maxillary incisor displayed. There was excessive gingival display on smile with 3 mm gingival display at the right cuspid and 5 mm at the left with a transverse cant to the palatal plane. Transverse cant to the maxilla with the left side down 2 mm more than the left. D, Oblique at-rest facial observation with excessive lower facial height, lip strain and excessive chin height, and a flat labiomental sulcus. The nasal form was judged to be quite adequate. E, Oblique smiling facial observation with no noticeable anteroposterior cant to the maxillary occlusal plane. The smile arc was consonant. The excessive gingival display was also evident on the oblique smile. F, Profile evaluation with emphasis on a long lower facial third, long chin height, a flat labiomental sulcus, and lip strain on closure. G–K, The functional problem of the anterior open bite in this nongrowing patient necessitated superior repositioning of the maxilla to correct the functional complaint. The exact surgical movements were obtained from the clinical examination and measurements (see text).*

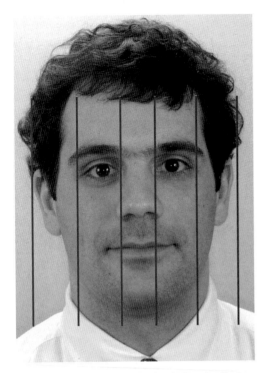

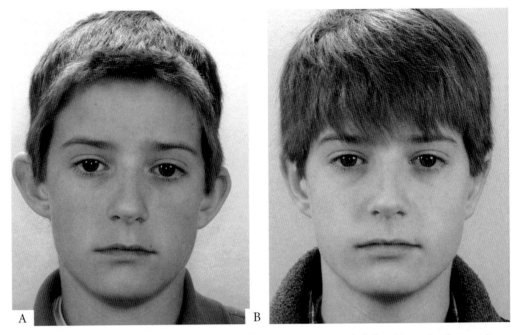

FIGURE **54-11**   A, *An otoplastic surgical procedure was recommended for this patient's prominent ears. B, The facial transverse fifths were improved, resulting in a dramatic facial improvement.*

FIGURE **54-10**   *The face is divided sagittally into five equal parts from helix to helix of the outer ears. The middle fifth of the face is delineated by the inner canthus of the eyes, the inner corner of the eye containing the lacrimal duct. A line from the inner canthus should be coincident with the ala of the base of the nose. A vertical line from the outer canthus of the eyes frames the medial two-fifths of the face, which should be coincident with the gonial angles of the mandible. The outer two-fifths of the face is measured from the lateral canthus to the lateral helix, which represents the width of the ears. Another significant frontal relationship is the mid-pupillary distance, which should be transversely aligned with the commissures of the mouth.*

studies clearly indicate that large ears are judged by laypeople to be one of the most unesthetic features, particularly in males. Otoplastic surgical procedures are relatively atraumatic and can dramatically improve facial appearance. In orthognathic cases in which this disproportion is noted by the clinician, we feel that failure to mention this feature violates informed consent. Therefore, otoplasty should be presented as a treatment option, whether received positively or not. These procedures can be performed on adolescents and adults as is illustrated in Figure 54-11A and B.

Another significant frontal relationship is the midpupillary distance, which should be transversely aligned with the commissures of the mouth.[15] Although this is considered the ideal transverse facial proportionality, there is little that can be done therapeutically to correct this disproportion, except in craniofacial synostosis such as Apert syndrome.

Nasal anatomy in the transverse plane should also be assessed through proportionality. The width of the alar base should be approximately the same as the intercanthal distance, which should be the same as the width of an eye. If the intercanthal distance is smaller than an eye width, it is better to keep the nose slightly wider than the intercanthal distance. The width of the alar base is heavily influenced by inherited ethnic characteristics.

Asymmetry of the face is a somewhat natural occurrence. Systematic examination of the patient's facial symmetry should be directly measured in the frontal plane. The following measures compose this portion of the clinical examination.

Nasal Tip to Midsagittal Plane   Having the patient elevate the head slightly and then visualizing the nasal tip in relation to the midsagittal plane provides the best view to evaluate the position of the nasal tip (Figure 54-12). Any deviation of the nasal tip should be noted in relation to the maxillary midline. The clinician should not make the mistake of treating the maxillary midline to a distorted nose. An attempt to obtain the etiology of nasal tip asymmetry is recommended. The

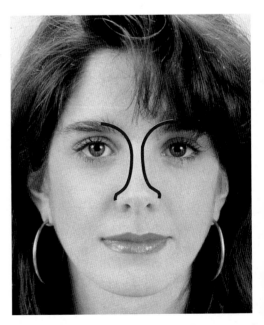

FIGURE **54-12**   *The "gull in flight" contour of the base of the nose.*

patient should be questioned as to any previous history of nasal trauma or nasal surgery for a deviated septum. Patients may then be advised appropriately as to whether this deviation is severe enough to consider correction.

Maxillary Dental Midline to Midsagittal Plane

The maxillary dental midline should be recorded relative to the midsagittal plane. A discrepancy could be due to either dental factors or skeletal maxillary rotation. Maxillary rotation is a rarely occurring clinical finding and is usually accompanied by posterior dental crossbite. The dental features of maxillary midline discrepancies will be discussed in both the miniesthetic and microesthetic perspectives.

Mandibular Dental Midline to Midsymphysis

The mandibular dental midline to midsymphysis relationship is best visualized by standing behind the patient and then viewing the lower arch from above (Figure 54-13). The patient should open his or her mouth in order for the clinician to view the lower arch and its relationship to the body of the mandible and symphysis. Lower dental midline discrepancies are usually due to tooth related issues such as dental crowding with shifted incisors, premature exfoliation of primary teeth and subsequent space closure in preadolescents, congenitally missing teeth, or

an extracted unilateral tooth. If the lower dental midline is not coincident with the midsymphysis, it usually indicates a dental shift. However, chin asymmetry should also be considered.

Mandibular Asymmetry with or without Functional Shift

Mandibular asymmetry is suspected when the midsymphysis is not coincident with the midsagittal plane. An important diagnostic factor is whether a lateral functional shift is present secondary to a functional shift of the mandible due to crossbite. When the patient is manipulated into centric relation, a bilateral, end-to-end crossbite usually is present, and as the patient moves the teeth into full occlusion, the patient must choose a side to move his or her mandible into maximum intercuspation. This lateral shift is indicative not of true mandibular asymmetry but of transverse maxillary deficiency and a resultant functional shift of the mandible.

True mandibular asymmetry is suspected when, in closure into centric relation, no lateral functional shift occurs. The truly asymmetric mandible may be due to an inherited asymmetric facial growth pattern or a result of localized or systemic factors. A thorough history of traumatic injuries and a review of systems of the patient will help ascertain potential etiologies of true mandibular asymmetry.

Chin Asymmetry

Facial asymmetry in some cases may be limited to the chin only. If the systematic evaluation of facial symmetry has dental and skeletal midlines and vertical relationships of the maxilla normal and lower facial asymmetry is noted, then the asymmetry may be isolated to the chin. Measurement of the midsymphysis to the midsagittal plane is a logical indicator of chin asymmetry, but the parasymphyseal heights should also be measured when chin asymmetry is suspected (Figure 54-14). The frontal view is recommended, but a view from

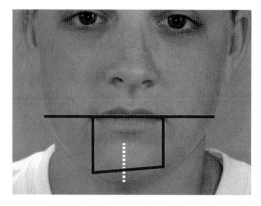

FIGURE **54-14** *Measurement of the midsymphysis to the midsagittal plane is a logical indicator of chin asymmetry, but the parasymphyseal heights should also be measured when chin asymmetry is suspected.*

the superior facial aspect (much like the evaluation of the mandibular dental midline) with the mouth closed also affords the clinician excellent visualization of the chin to the body of the mandible and the midsymphysis.

Maxillomandibular Asymmetry

Mandibular asymmetry is often accompanied by maxillary compensation, which is reflected clinically by a transverse cant of the maxilla. This means that evaluation of mandibular deformity should now include the possibility of maxillomandibular deformity. Transverse tilting of the maxilla may be detectable cephalometrically but is most evident during the macroesthetic examination (Figure 54-15). Clinically, one notes this, for example, as *right maxilla 4 mm more superior than left*. The transverse cant of the maxilla

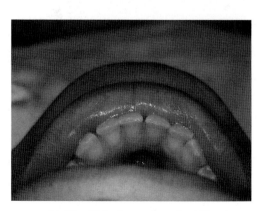

FIGURE **54-13** *If the lower dental midline is not coincident with the midsymphysis, it usually indicates a dental shift. However, chin asymmetry should also be considered.*

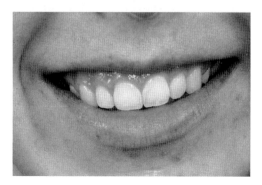

FIGURE **54-15** *Transverse tilting of the maxilla may be detectable cephalometrically but is most evident during the macroesthetic examination.*

is often determined by the relative difference in gingival show present at the level of the canine moving posterior at smile. Differentiation between the macro- and miniesthetic factors that are related to the transverse cant of the maxilla will be discussed later.

Macroesthetic Examination: Oblique View

The facial areas for macroesthetic examination, as investigated from the oblique view, can be summarized as follows:

- Midfacial
    Orbital position
    Nasal form
    Cheek/zygomatic form
- Lower facial
    Lip form
        Philtrum
        Vermilion
    Mandibular form
    Chin projection

The oblique view (Figure 54-16A) in the macroesthetic examination affords the surgeon and orthodontist another perspective for evaluating the facial thirds. With

regard to the upper face, the clinician may view the relative projection of the orbital rim and malar eminence. Orbital and malar retrusion is often seen in craniofacial syndromes. Cheek projection is evaluated in the area of the zygomaticus and malar scaffold. Skin laxity and atrophy of the malar fat pad in this area may actually be a characteristic of aging and therefore seen in the older orthognathic population.[16] This area can be described as deficient, balanced, or prominent. Nasal anatomy, which was described in the frontal examination, may also be characterized in this dimension.

Lip anatomy is also examined in the oblique and lateral views. The philtral area and vermilion of the maxillary lip should be clearly demarcated. The height of the philtrum should be noted as short, balanced, or excessive. Vermilion display should be termed as excessive, balanced, or thin.

The relative projection of the maxilla and mandible can be assessed in the oblique view. Midface deficiency can result in increased nasolabial folding, relaxed upper lip support, and altered columella and nasal tip support.

One of the greatest values of the oblique view is visualization of the body and gonial angle of the mandible as well as the cervicomental area. The patient in Figure 54-16A illustrates a desirable definition of the chin-neck anatomy. The patient in Figure 54-16B has a dolichofacial skeletal pattern with a steeper mandibular plane, not as esthetically pleasing as the previous illustration. The patient in Figure 54-16C demonstrates a brachyfacial pattern with an obtuse cervicomental angle secondary to submental fat deposition. Mandibular deficiency with associated dental compensation may produce lower lip eversion, excessive vermilion display, and a pronounced labiomental sulcus.

A characterization of mandibular form is also very important. The oblique view also demonstrates the effects of animation on the appearance of lip and chin projection. The patient in Figure 54-17A and B shows a moderate anterior divergence and facial concavity at rest, but during the smile, animation reveals an increased chin projection with excessive concavity.

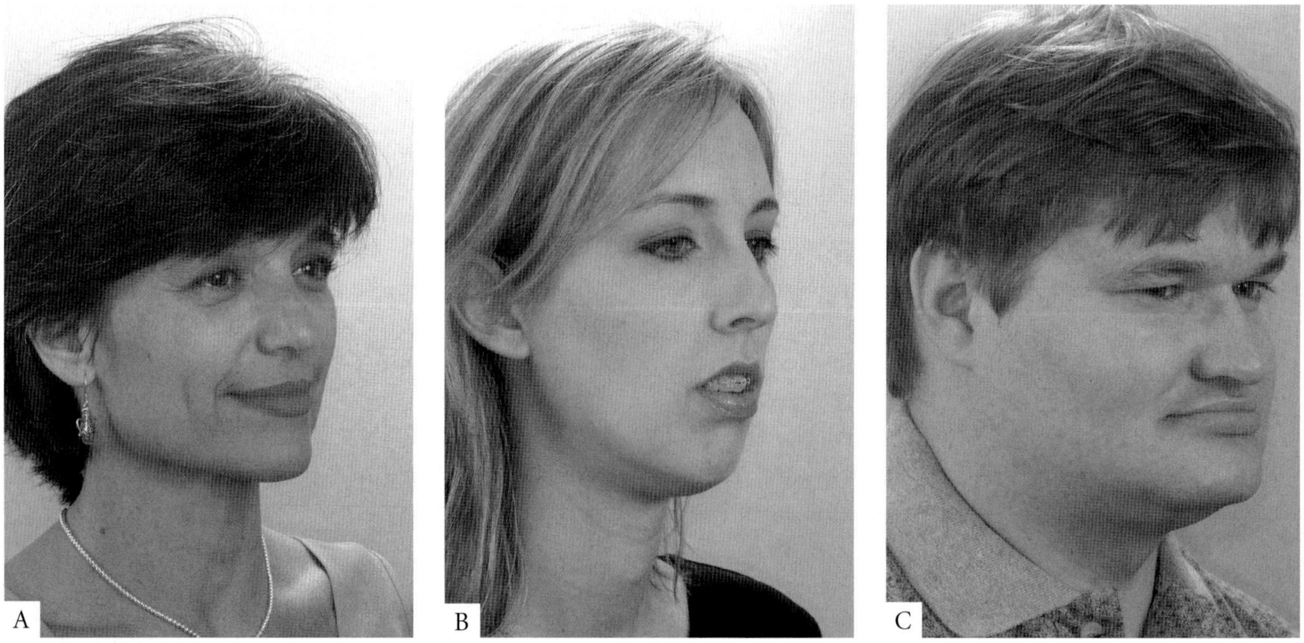

FIGURE 54-16 A, *Desirable definition of the chin-neck anatomy.* B, *A dolichofacial skeletal pattern with a steeper mandibular plane, not as esthetic as the previous illustration.* C, *A brachyfacial pattern with an obtuse cervicomental angle secondary to submental fat deposition.*

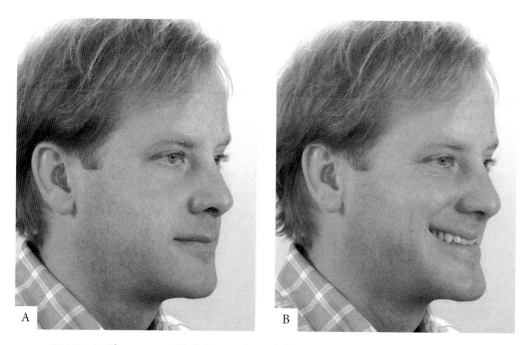

FIGURE 54-17 *A, The amount of facial concavity and chin projection at rest is within acceptable limits. B, When this patient animates, an excessive amount of chin projection and facial concavity is revealed.*

Macroesthetic Examination: Profile View

The facial areas for macroesthetic examination, as investigated from the profile view, can be summarized as follows:

- Lower facial
    - Maxillomandibular projection or facial divergence
    - Lip form
        - Size
        - Projection
        - Labiomental sulcus
    - Chin projection

The last view in the macroesthetic examination is the profile perspective. Natural head position is essential for accurate evaluation of profile characteristics. The patient should be instructed to look straight ahead and, if possible, into his or her own image in an appropriately placed mirror. The visual axis is what determines "natural head position." This axis very often, but not always, approximates the Frankfort horizontal plane. The classic vertical facial thirds should also be applied in profile view. An assessment of lower facial deficiency or excess should be noted.

The nasolabial angle describes the inclination of the columella in relation to the upper lip. The nasolabial angle should be in the range of 90 to 120° (Figure 54-18A).[17] The nasolabial angle is determined by several factors: (1) the anteroposterior position of the maxilla to some degree; (2) the anteroposterior position of the maxillary incisors; (3) vertical position or rotation of the nasal tip, which can result in a more obtuse or acute nasolabial angle; and (4) soft tissue thickness of the maxillary lip that contributes the nasolabial angle, where a thin upper lip favors a flatter angle and a thicker lip favors an acute angle.

The characterization of the lower face in profile (Figure 54-18B) is measured by the relative degree of lip projection, the labiomental sulcus, the chin-neck length, and the chin-neck angle. Maxillary and mandibular sagittal position can be described by means of facial divergence. The lower third of the face is evaluated in reference to the anterior soft tissue point at the glabella. Based on the position of the maxilla and mandible relative to this point, a patient's profile will be described as straight, convex, or concave, and either anteriorly or posteriorly divergent.

Lip projection is a function of maxillomandibular protrusion or retrusion, dental protrusion or retrusion, and/or lip thickness. The description of lip projection

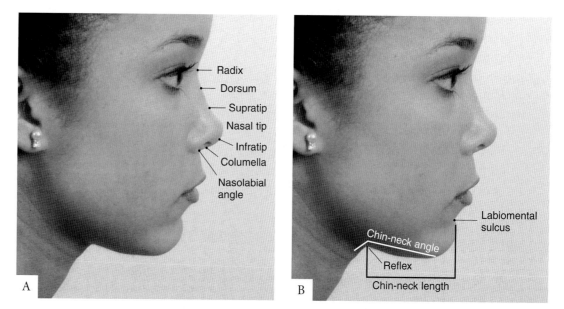

FIGURE 54-18 *A, The facial profile view. Superiorly, the radix of the nose is characterized by an unbroken curve that begins in the superior orbital ridge and continues along the lateral nasal wall. The nasal dorsum is made up of both bony and cartilaginous tissues. The nasal tip is described as the most anterior point of the nose, and the supratip is just cephalic to the tip. The columella is the portion of the nose between the base of the nose (subspinale) and the nasal tip. B, The characterization of the lower face in profile is measured by the relative degree of lip projection, the labiomental sulcus, the chin-neck length, and the chin-neck angle.*

should include pertinent information from any of the above sources. For example, a patient with lower lip protrusion may be maxillary (midface) deficient with dentoalveolar compensation including flared incisors and a thin maxillary vermilion display, or simply may have a thick lower lip that appears protrusive.

The labiomental sulcus is defined as the fold of soft tissue between the lower lip and the chin and may vary greatly in form and depth. The clinical variables that can affect the labiomental sulcus include (1) lower incisor position, where upright lower incisors tend to result in a shallow labiomental sulcus because of lack of lower lip projection, whereas excessive lower incisor proclination deepens the labiomental sulcus; and (2) vertical height of the lower facial third, which has a direct bearing on chin position and the labiomental sulcus. Diminished lower facial height will usually result in a deeper labiomental sulcus (just as in the overclosed full denture patient), whereas a patient with a long lower facial third has a tendency toward a flat labiomental sulcus.

Chin projection is determined by the amount of anteroposterior bony projection of the anterior, inferior border of the mandible, and the amount of soft tissue that overlays that bony projection. The amount of profile chin projection is measured by the distance from pogonion (or Pg, the most anterior point on the bony chin) to soft tissue pogonion' (or Pg', the most anterior point on the soft tissue profile of the chin) and is not particularly alterable by surgical means. In the adolescent, the amount of chin is directly correlated to the amount of mandibular growth that occurs because the chin point itself is borne on the mandible as it grows anteriorly.

The angle between the lower lip, chin, and R point (the deepest point along the chin-neck contour) should be approximately 90°. An obtuse angle often indicates (1) chin deficiency, (2) lower lip procumbency, (3) excessive submental fat, (4),

retropositioned mandible, and (5) low hyoid bone position.

Another important measure in this area is the chin-neck length and chin-neck angle. The angle, also termed the *cervicomental angle*, has been studied extensively in plastic surgery and orthognathic literature.[18] Studies report that a wide range of normal neck morphology exists, and that the cervicomental angle may vary between 105° and 120°, with gender being a major consideration. Age of the patient must be considered with regard to this area. Soft tissue "sag" due to the loss of skin elasticity during aging is a major cause of change in the cervicomental region. Weight gain is another important factor in the morphology of this area.

Miniesthetic Examination: Frontal View

The facial areas for miniesthetic examination, as investigated from the frontal view, can be summarized as follows:

- Vertical characteristics of the smile
  Lip-tooth-gingival relationships
  Gingival display on smile
    Excessive gingival display on smile
      Vertical maxillary excess
      Short philtrum height
      Excessive curtain
      Short clinical crown height
      Upright maxillary incisors
    Inadequate gingival display on smile
      Vertical maxillary deficiency
      Diminished curtain
      Short clinical crown height
      Flared maxillary incisors
- Transverse characteristics of the smile
  Arch form
  Buccal corridor
  Cant of the transverse occlusal plane

Vertical Characteristics *Lip-Tooth-Gingival Relationships* A key feature of vertical facial esthetic characteristics is the

relationship between the incisal edges of the maxillary incisors relative to the lower lip as well as the relationship between the gingival margins of the maxillary incisors relative to the upper lip. The gingival margins of the cuspids should be coincident with the upper lip, and the lateral incisors positioned slightly inferior to the adjacent teeth. It is generally accepted that the gingival margins should be coincident with the upper lip in the social smile. However, this is very much a function of the age of the patient, since children show more teeth at rest and gingival display on smile than do adults.[19]

Excessive Gingival Display on Smile The vertical characteristics of facial miniesthetics impact the relative amount of gingival display at rest and during animation. Gingival display is the amount of "gumminess" of the smile. Measuring the amount of gingival display on smile easily quantitates a "gummy" smile. The decision as to whether the amount of gingival display is an esthetic problem in which treatment is desirable is a personal choice. Orthodontists and oral and maxillofacial surgeons tend to see the "gummy" smile as an unesthetic characteristic, while laypersons attach importance only in the more extreme cases. The use of computerized graphic simulation of the frontal view of the smile is useful in counseling a patient and showing potential treatment changes. The individual is then able to guide the clinician and express opinions about what should and should not be corrected. Computer imaging not only provides the patient with a visual template for treatment but it also provides the clinician with a testing ground for treatment options. The patient in Figure 54-19A exhibits excessive gingival display on smile, secondary to vertical maxillary excess. The diagnosis of vertical maxillary excess is confirmed by the facial characteristics of a long lower facial third, lip incompetence,

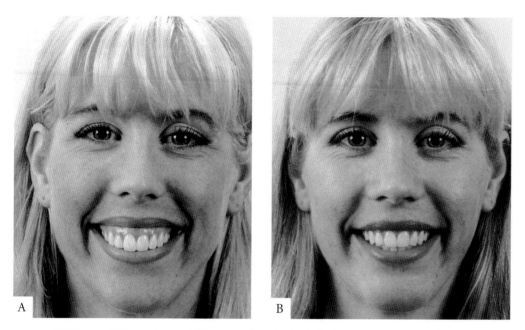

FIGURE **54-19**   A, *This patient exhibits excessive gingival display on smile, secondary to vertical maxillary excess. B, The actual post-treatment outcome.*

excessive incisor display at rest, and excessive gingival display on smile. Superior repositioning of the maxilla was performed with excellent facial proportions and smile esthetics (Figure 54-19B).

The patient in Figure 54-20A also exhibited excessive gingival display, but has normal vertical facial proportions. Her incisor crown height, however, is only 8 mm. The etiology of her "gummy" smile is not an orthognathic problem or an orthodontic problem but a cosmetic or periodontal problem. This diagnosis was confirmed and further visualized through computerized image modification (Figure 54-20B and C), simulating the crown-lengthening procedure. Orthodontic intrusion of maxillary incisors would have reduced gingival display but would also have adversely affected the smile arc with concomitant flattening. This case example emphasizes differential diagnosis of gingival display issues and it also emphasizes the optimization of unesthetic facial traits while preserving those positive facial esthetic attributes.

Transverse Characteristics   The three transverse characteristics of facial esthetics in the frontal dimension are (1) arch form,

(2) buccal corridor, and (3) the transverse cant of the maxillary occlusal plane.

Arch form plays a pivotal role in the transverse dimension. Recently, much attention has been focused on using broad square arch forms in orthodontic treatment and orthognathic surgical treatment. In cases in which the arch forms are narrow or collapsed, the smile may also appear narrow and therefore present inadequate transverse smile characteristics. An important consideration in widening a narrow arch form, particularly in the adult, is the axial inclination of the buccal segments. Cases in which the posterior teeth are already flared laterally are not good candidates for dental expansion. Upright premolars and molars allow for a more bodily transverse expansion of the buccal segments in both adolescent and adult patients, but are particularly important in the adult where sutural expansion is less likely. Orthodontic expansion and widening of a collapsed arch form can dramatically improve the appearance of facial esthetics and smile by decreasing the size of the buccal corridors and improving the *transverse smile dimension* (Figure 54-21A and B). The transverse smile dimension

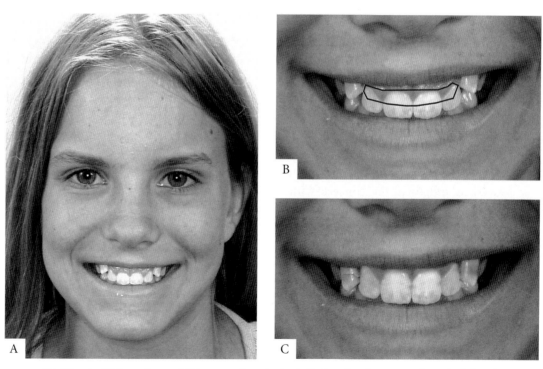

FIGURE **54-20**   A, *This patient exhibits excessive gingival display, but has normal vertical facial proportions. Her incisor crown height, however, is only 8 mm. The etiology of her "gummy" smile is not an orthognathic problem or an orthodontic problem but a cosmetic or periodontal problem. B and C, This diagnosis was confirmed and further visualized through computerized image modification, simulating the crown-lengthening procedure.*

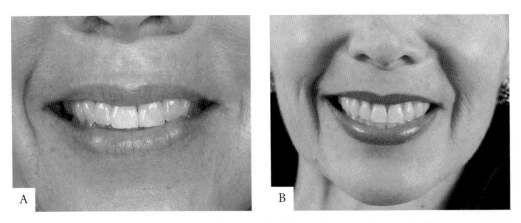

FIGURE **54-21**   A, *The transverse smile dimension in this patient was characterized by narrow arch form and excessive buccal corridor. In this adult, the axial inclinations of the molars and premolars were favorable for orthodontic expansion. B, The transverse smile dimension after orthodontic treatment.*

(and the buccal corridor) is related to the lateral projection of the premolars and the molars into the buccal corridors. The wider the arch form is in the premolar area, the greater would be the portion of the buccal corridor filled.

As alluded to in the previous cases above, arch expansion can have undesirable effects. Expansion of the arch form may fill out the transverse dimension of the smile, but two undesirable side effects may result and careful observation should be made to avoid these side effects wherever possible. First, the buccal corridor can be obliterated and create a "denture"-like smile. Second, when the anterior sweep of the maxillary arch is broadened, the smile arc may be flattened. Although it may not be possible to avoid these undesirable aspects of expansion, the clinician must make a judgment in concert with the patient as to what "trade-offs" are acceptable in the pursuit of the ideal facial esthetic outcome.

The last transverse characteristic of facial esthetics is the transverse cant of the maxillary occlusal plane. Transverse cant of the maxilla can be due to differential eruption and placement of the anterior teeth, and skeletal asymmetry of the skull base and/or mandible resulting in a compensatory cant to the maxilla. Intraoral images or even mounted dental casts do not adequately reflect the relationship of the maxilla to the smile. Only frontal smile visualization permits the orthodontist to visualize any tooth-related asymmetry transversely.

Smile asymmetry may also be due to soft tissue considerations such as an asymmetric smile curtain. In the asymmetric smile curtain, there is a differential elevation of the upper lip during smile, which gives the illusion of transverse cant to the maxilla. This smile characteristic emphasizes the importance of direct clinical examination in treatment planning the smile, since this soft tissue animation is not visible in a frontal radiograph or reflected in study models. It is not well documented in static photographic images, and is documented best in digital video clips.

Miniesthetic Examination: Oblique View

Miniesthetic examination from the oblique view involves two main areas:

*   Orientation of the palatal and occlusal planes
*   Smile arc

The oblique view of the smile reveals characteristics of the smile that are not obtainable on the frontal view and certainly not obtainable through any cephalometric analysis. The palatal plane may be canted anteroposteriorly in a number of

orientations. In the most desirable orientation, the occlusal plane is consonant with the curvature of the lower lip on smile (see discussion of *smile arc* below). Deviations from this orientation include a downward cant of the posterior maxilla, upward cant of the anterior maxilla, or variations of both.[20] In the initial examination and diagnostic phase of treatment, it is important to visualize the occlusal plane in its relationship to the lower lip.

The *smile arc* should be defined as the relationship of the curvature of the incisal edges of the maxillary incisors, canines, premolars, and molars to the curvature of the lower lip in the posed social smile. The ideal smile arc has the maxillary incisal edge curvature parallel to the curvature of the lower lip upon smile, and the term *consonant* is used to describe this parallel relationship. A *nonconsonant* or flat smile arc is characterized by the maxillary incisal curvature being flatter than the curvature of the lower lip on smile. Early definitions of the smile arc were limited to the curvature of the canines and the incisors to the lower lip on smile because smile evaluation was made on direct frontal view. The visualization of the complete smile arc afforded by the oblique view expands the definition of the smile arc to include the molars and the premolars (Figure 54-22).

Miniesthetic Examination: Profile View

The facial areas for miniesthetic examination, as investigated from the profile view, can be summarized as follows:

*   Overjet
*   Incisor angulation
        Upright maxillary incisors
        Flared maxillary incisors
        Retroclined mandibular incisors

The two miniesthetic characteristics visualized in the sagittal dimension are overjet and incisor angulation (Figure 54-23). Excessively positive overjet is one of the most

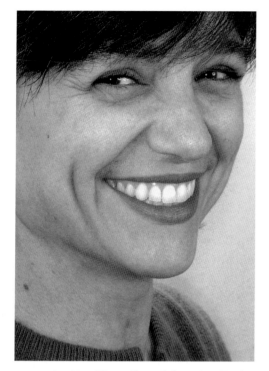

FIGURE 54-22 *The smile arc is best visualized in the oblique view, and should be defined as the relationship of the curvature of the incisal edges of the maxillary incisors, canines, premolars, and molars to the curvature of the lower lip in the posed social smile. The 45° view permits visualization of vermilion display, lip fullness, and turgor not readily seen in another view.*

recognizable dental traits to the layperson. Adolescents tend to label unflattering names such as "Andy Gump" and "Bucky Beaver" onto children unfortunate enough to have inherited this dentoskeletal pattern. How overjet is orthodontically corrected involves

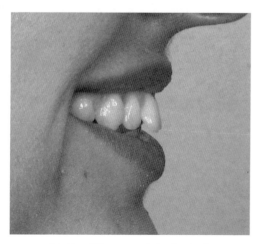

FIGURE 54-23 *The two miniesthetic characteristics visualized in the sagittal dimension are overjet and incisor angulation.*

macroelements such as jaw patterns and soft tissue elements such as nasal projection. Excessive positive overjet is not as readily perceived in the frontal dimension as it is in the sagittal dimension. Many Class II patterns have very esthetic smiles frontally, but not when the patient's smile is observed from the side. In Class III patterns, the same phenomenon may be true, in that the smile looks esthetic on frontal smile, but on the oblique or sagittal view, the overall appearance reflects the underlying skeletal pattern and dental compensation. The patient and parents have to decide with the clinician whether this is an acceptable outcome.

The amount of anterior maxillary projection also has great influence on the transverse smile dimension in the frontal view. When the maxilla is retrusive, the wider portion of the dental arch is positioned more posteriorly relative to the anterior oral commissure. This creates the illusion of greater buccal corridor in the frontal dimension. Overall, the sagittal cant of the maxillary occlusal plane in natural head position can influence the smile arc in the frontal dimension, affecting vertical characteristics. A negative cant of this plane will diminish the apposition of the incisal edges of the maxillary anterior teeth to the superior vermilion border of the lower lip at smile.

Dental Examination

The dental component of the clinical examination is the evaluation of any standing periodontal or cariogenic disease process and the assessment of the patient's occlusion. The areas for dental examination can be summarized as follows:

- Alignment
    Crowding
    Spacing
    Missing or supernumerary teeth
- Anteroposterior
    Angle classification
    Overjet
    Compensation
- Bite depth
    Anterior
    Posterior
    Compensation
- Transverse
    Compensation
- Functional occlusal issues
    Missing teeth and sequelae
    Occlusal interferences and parafunction

Intra-arch and interarch relationships are described in the categories of dental alignment, anteroposterior occlusion, and bite depth. Clinically, the patient's occlusion should be examined both in a static and dynamic sense.

The maxillary and mandibular dental arches are described as either well aligned, crowded, or spaced. The extent of crowding or spacing is usually noted in millimeters. Individual teeth are described by virtue of their spatial position and degree of rotation. Therefore, an incisor could be described as severely rotated and in linguoversion. Any congenitally missing, lost, or supernumerary teeth are noted. A description of teeth that have been severely worn or damaged due to trauma should be included.

In terms of the static occlusion, Angle's classification of the patient should be recorded. The Angle Class I relationship is such that the mesiobuccal cusp of the maxillary first molar should rest in the buccal groove of the mandibular first molar. The Angle Class II relationship exhibits a more anterior position of the mesiobuccal cusp of the maxillary first molar and the Angle Class III relationship exhibits a more posterior position of the mesiobuccal cusp of the maxillary first molar. The degree of incisor overjet that accompanies an anteroposterior discrepancy should also be noted.

Concepts of Incisor Compensation

Incisor compensation in the sagittal view is very important in planning the presurgical orthodontics, yet not fully recognized by both orthodontists and surgeons alike. In most cases of skeletal dysplasia, whether in the range of surgical or nonsurgical treatment, dental compensation is a common feature. The forms and expression of this compensation are as complex as the myriad of dentoskeletal problems that exist, but there are common patterns frequently encountered. In the diagnosis and proper treatment of these cases, the primary responsibility of the orthodontist is to recognize these compensations and eliminate or *decompensate* them. The range of which compensations are problematic is not concrete, so the surgeon and the orthodontist must decide how much compensation is acceptable and what is to be done for decompensation. Although we tend to think of these compensations as an anteroposterior consideration (incisor angulation problems), dental compensation can occur in all planes of space.

Class II and Class III Problems The classic pattern of compensation in Class II skeletal patterns is the proclination of the mandibular incisors and retroclination of the maxillary incisors. Conversely, Class III skeletal dysplasias often feature retroclination of the mandibular incisors and proclination of the maxillary incisors. The orthodontist must recognize these compensations and decide what degree of compensation is acceptable and what requires substantive treatment. For example, if lower incisor flare in the Class II patient is only moderate, what is the value of removing two mandibular premolars to upright the incisors? These decompensation decisions affect the treatment outcome in three basic ways: (1) inadequate incisor positioning can compromise buccal interdigitation; (2) incisor positioning can substantially affect the esthetic outcome; and (3) in certain types of functional problems such as obstructive sleep apnea syndrome, esthetic considerations have a lower priority compared to correction of the functional problem.

The effect of incisor angulation on buccal occlusal relationships was advanced and best expressed by Andrews.[21] In presurgical preparation for mandibular advancement, maxillary incisors that are not properly flared or mandibular incisors that are left overly flared may result in the following: (1) insufficient overjet to provide for adequate advancement of the mandible from the esthetic standpoint, and (2) the inability to achieve desired Class I buccal segments because the advanced nature of the lower incisor edge does not permit interdigitation of the buccal segments (Figure 54-24A and B). The appropriate amount of incisor angulation can be determined either through cephalometric investigation or by simply holding study models in a simulated Class I molar relationship.

Vertical Characteristics and Compensations *Bite Depth* The vertical component of the dental examination describes bite depth. A patient's anterior bite depth is the amount of maxillary incisor overbite relative to the mandibular incisors. Therefore, a patient can be described as having an anterior open bite, satisfactory bite (25 to 50% overbite), or an anterior deep bite. The posterior bite depth is usually characterized as being open, satisfactory, or collapsed. The latter is seen when the patient is missing unilateral or bilateral posterior dental units.

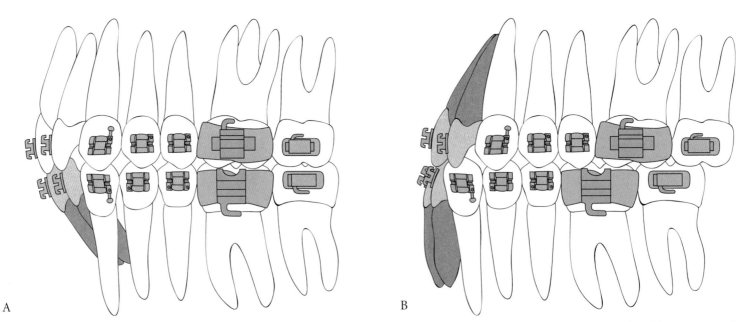

A   B

FIGURE **54-24**   A, *Inadequate decompensation in Class II correction makes Class I buccal segments not attainable because the flared lower incisors do not permit interdigitation of the posterior segments. B, Inadequate decompensation in Class III correction makes Class I buccal segments not attainable because the upright lower incisors or flared maxillary incisors do not permit interdigitation of the posterior segments.*

Curve of Spee Dental compensation in the vertical plane has to do with aberrations in the curve of Spee. The curve of Spee is measured by the arc extending from the cusp tips of the incisors posteriorly to the cusp tips of the molars in a sagittal view. Clinically, the study model can be placed on a flat surface and the cusp tips relative to that flat plane will give a rough estimate of the maxillary and mandibular curve of Spee. This is an important diagnostic feature of model analysis in recognizing potential pitfalls that may be encountered during orthodontic preparation for orthognathic surgery. For example, in a patient in whom the anterior segment is significantly superior (greater than 2 mm) to the posterior segment, failure to recognize this occlusal plane differential may result in orthodontic flattening prior to surgery and postsurgical relapse, resulting in anterior open bite.[22]

Transverse Compensations The Class II patient often has narrowing of the maxilla in response to the narrower portion of the mandible being placed in the broader portion of the maxillary arch. In the Class III patient, the maxillary posterior segments are often flared buccally in compensation for the wider portion of the mandible being placed into the narrower aspect of the maxilla. By holding the study models in a simulated Class I relationship, these compensations can be easily recognized (Figure 54-25).

Functional Occlusal Issues The last portion of the dental examination relates to dynamics of occlusal function. The clinician should ascertain whether the patient exhibits a discrepancy between maximum intercuspal position and retruded contact position in the anteroposterior dimension. In general, small differences exist in the vast majority of patients. Only large slides should be recorded. If the patient's dentition is mutilated the clinician should note the resultant occlusal compensa-

tions. Any supererupted teeth will create lateral and anteroposterior interferences. A history of bruxism or other parafunctional habits will affect orthodontic appliances and will impact on the type of retention used post-treatment.

Microesthetic Examination

The microesthetic portion of the clinical examination focuses on the morphology of tooth-to-tooth contacts and the surrounding intraoral tissues, summarized as follows:

- Dentogingival relationships
    Tooth form/tooth contact/gingival architecture

As a structural unit, the dentogingival complex is defined by the relationship of the teeth to the alveolar bone and surrounding gingival and masticatory mucosa. The factors that influence the appearance of the dentogingival complex are the patient's periodontal status and past history of disease, the proximal and occlusal contacts of the teeth, the shape of the individual teeth, and the type of gingival architecture.

An assessment of the patient's current periodontal status is exceedingly important from an orthodontic and surgical point of view. The clinician should take an accurate dental history in order to ascertain whether the patient has had any periodontal disease and related treatment. Clinically, the teeth should be examined for plaque accumulation and any supragingival calculus. Patients who cannot maintain a satisfactory level of oral hygiene are at risk for gingival inflammation, attachment loss, and caries during presurgical orthodontic treatment. Periapical radiographs combined with a panoramic radiograph will reveal alveolar architecture and any evidence of horizontal or vertical bone loss. Suspected periodontal defects should be probed and the depths recorded. The extent of attachment loss and degree of tooth mobility will influence tooth movement.

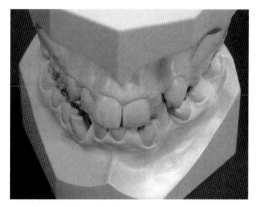

FIGURE 54-25 *Transverse problems are first diagnosed by holding the study models together in a simulated Class I relationship. The most commonly found transverse problem is that the maxilla is narrower than the mandible in cases similar to that of this patient who was being evaluated for Class II correction by mandibular advancement.*

Surgical treatment planning of the segmental Le Fort I osteotomy should consider gingival architecture in relation to maxillary segmentation. If the incisions are made mesial to the maxillary canines, the patient may lose the interdental papilla in between this tooth and the maxillary lateral incisor. By positioning the incisions distal to the maxillary canines, an obliterated papilla can be more easily camouflaged due to the convexity of the canine.

Computerized Cephalometric Prediction

For computer image prediction, a digital model of the cephalometric tracing must be entered into computer memory. It is important that the radiograph be obtained in natural head position, with the teeth lightly together and in retruded contact position and the lips relaxed. The details of the digital model vary among the several currently available software programs but the similarities are more impressive than the differences. The more points in the digital model, the greater the anatomic fidelity of that model. On the other hand, the more points that are digitized, the more time it takes to perform the digitization process.

A lateral image of the patient's profile, matching the cephalograms as closely as possible in head position and lip posture, must be captured and entered into the computer program (either directly via digital photography or by scanning a slide). Ideally, the radiograph and profile image would be taken simultaneously, although the hardware arrangement to do this does not yet exist.

The patient in Figure 54-26A presented for correction of a severe Class II dentofacial deformity. After clinical examination and diagnostic records, digital image integration and algorithmic projections are used for consultation with the patient.

After the records are gathered, the next step in the treatment planning is to superimpose the profile image and radiograph, with the hard and soft tissues matched to each other as closely as possible. Most programs use the profile as the major method of image coordination. Once the images are coordinated, any cephalometric analysis can be displayed, although in contemporary surgical planning, the goal of treatment is not what the analysis indicates.

At that point, a "treatment screen" (Figure 54-26B) provides the clinician with "handles" (the blue squares) by which selected sections of hard tissue can be moved (eg, the mandible, the maxilla, or maxillary incisor segment); the procedures similar to the use of templates and manual prediction. In this case illustration, surgical mandibular advancement is being contemplated. Dental compensation is present in the form of flared mandibular incisors, and decompensation is recommended to decompensate the dentition in order to increase the overjet, thus maximizing the magnitude of mandibular advancement. Simulation of lower first premolar extraction and lower incisor retraction is made on the treatment screen; the software applies its imbedded algorithms for profile prediction and creates a new line drawing of the profile (Figure 54-26C) reflecting the expected profile change after incisor decompensation. The algorithms may be ratios based on regressive equations and multiple correla-

tions. They are not the same in all programs: the quality of the algorithms is the major determinant of how well or poorly the predicted profile matches the actual change produced by the treatment. The quantitative table on the right of Figure 54-26C provides to the clinician the measurements of the movements made on screen calibrated to actual movements required clinically to achieve the projected change.

After decompensation movements are simulated, the mandible is advanced on the treatment screen to ideal overjet, and the software then "warps" the original profile image to fit the prediction line drawing, producing an image that conveys much more visual information to the clinician and patient than the line drawing (Figure 54-26D). As treatment is being planned, the amount of change is suggested until, within the limits of possible surgical change, it looks best; it is advantageous to include the patient in this process of adjusting the amount of change to provide an optimal outcome. In this case, a comparison image is generated so the patient may visualize the profile outcome expected with mandibular advancement (Figure 54-26E). The profile was judged to be improved but was still clearly chin deficient. Simulation of chin advancement is then performed (Figure 54-26F), not by using any cephalometric norm or predetermined value, but by simply using the facial outline as a guide. In other words, the chin is moved horizontally and vertically until it meets the approval of the patient. The projected final profile image is depicted in Figure 54-26G. The quantitative table reflects the exact movements in millimeters so that the surgeon and orthodontist have a precise plan for the amount of change needed to produce the desired result seen in Figure 54-26H. Presurgical planning using this methodology should eliminate "on-the-table" estimates of whether or not the patient needs "a bit more chin." It is ludicrous to make esthetic treatment decisions with the patient under general anesthesia,

horizontal, fully draped, paralyzed, and with a nasal tube in place.

An important consideration is the accuracy of the computer prediction process. Although it is far from perfect (some computer programs are more accurate than others), it is good enough to be clinically useful.[23–27] Chin predictions are usually quite accurate and those of the upper lip are reasonably good, whereas predictions of the lower lip can be problematic. As the data on which algorithms are based become more extensive, as different algorithms are applied when vertical and anterior changes occur, and as multiple regression equations replace simple ratios, accuracy can be expected to improve.[28]

It could be said that in this era of informed consent and bioethical decision-making, the patient should be actively involved in the process of computer prediction and treatment planning. Cultural and familial traits may be important to the patient. Surgeons and orthodontists tend to want to "optimize" all patients to the prevailing esthetic norm, which diminishes any ethnic variation in dentofacial appearance.

Synthesis of an Optimized Problem List

The data derived from the systematic clinical examination and analysis of patient records are synthesized into a diagnostic optimized problem list. Essentially there are two branches in the problem-solving tree: esthetics and function. Thus, the diagnostic problem list should be subdivided into the categories of macroesthetic problems, miniesthetic problems, microesthetic problems, and functional problems. All recognizable problems that are relevant to the patient's chief complaint should be rank-ordered. Lastly, each problem should be evaluated in terms of its therapeutic modifiability.

Conceptually and operatively, the orthodontist and surgeon have to visualize the desired solution to the specific problem and then assess whether the given solution will negatively impact some other dentofacial

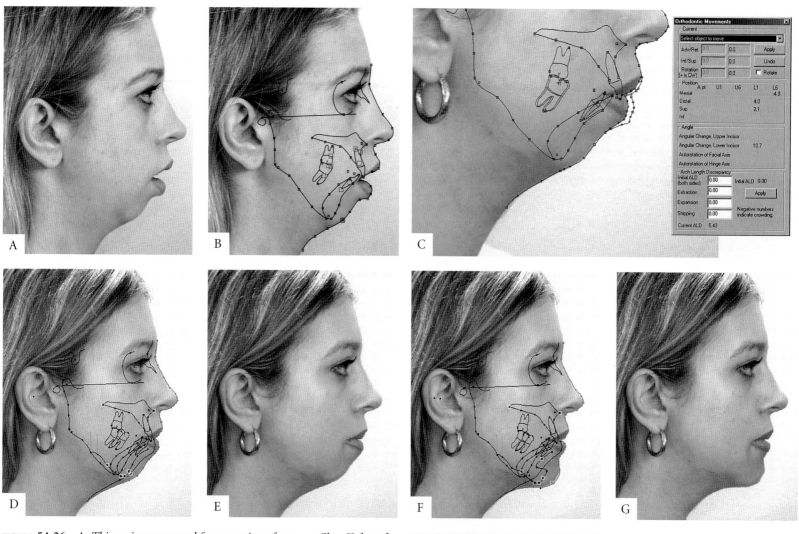

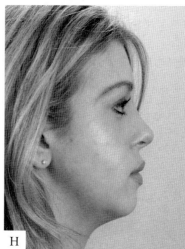

FIGURE **54-26** A, *This patient presented for correction of a severe Class II dentofacial deformity. B, A "treatment screen" provides the clinician with "handles" (the blue squares) by which selected sections of hard tissue can be moved (eg, the mandible, the maxilla, or the maxillary incisor segment); the procedures are similar to the use of templates and manual prediction. C, Simulation of lower first premolar extraction and lower incisor retraction is made on the treatment screen. The software applies its imbedded algorithms for profile prediction and creates a new line drawing of the profile reflecting the expected profile change after incisor decompensation. D, After decompensation movements are simulated, the mandible is advanced on the treatment screen to ideal overjet, and the software then "warps" the original profile image to fit the prediction line drawing, producing an image that conveys much more visual information to the clinician and patient than the line drawing. E, In this case, a comparison image is generated so that the patient may visualize the profile outcome expected with mandibular advancement. F, Simulation of chin advancement is then performed, not by using any cephalometric norms or predetermined value, but by simply using the facial outline as a guide. G, The projected final profile image. H, The actual treatment result.*

feature at the same time. The concept of facial optimization involves the preservation of as many positive elements as possible, while harmonizing those elements that fall short of the esthetic and functional needs of the patient. The problems that might exceed the limitations of treatment or perhaps have a poor therapeutic prognosis should be described. Informed consent and bioethical treatment of the surgical patient requires that the clinician explain the risk/benefit considerations of the proposed treatment strategy. The goal of the systematized clinical examination and optimized problem-oriented diagnosis is to record and analyze the data in such a way that the required treatment becomes implicit in the description of the problem.

References

1. Jacobson A. The proportionate template as a diagnostic aid. Am J Orthod 1979;75:156–72.

2. Jacobson A. Orthognathic diagnosis using the proportionate template. Oral Surg Surg 1980;238:820.

3. Jacobson A, editor. Radiographic cephalometry: from basics to videoimaging. Carol Stream (IL): Quintessence Publishing Co.; 1995.

4. Broadbent BH Sr, Broadbent BH Jr, Golden WH. Bolton standards of dentofacial developmental growth. St. Louis (MO): C.V. Mosby Co.; 1975.

5. Sonnesen L, Bakke M, Solow B. Malocclusion traits and symptoms and signs of temporomandibular disorders in children with severe malocclusion. Eur J Orthod 1998;10:543–59.

6. McNamara JA. Orthodontic treatment and temporomandibular disorders. Oral Surg Oral Med Oral Pathol Oral Radiol Endod 1997;83:107–17.

7. Sarver DM, Ackerman JL. About face — the re-emerging soft tissue paradigm. Am J Orthod Dentofacial Orthop 2000;117:575–6.

8. Sarver DM, Ackerman MB. Dynamic smile visualization and quantification: part 1. Evolution of the concept and dynamic records for smile capture. Am J Orthod Dentofacial Orthop 2003:124;4–12.

9. Sarver DM. Esthetic orthodontics and orthognathic surgery. St. Louis (MO): C.V. Mosby Co.; 1997.

10. Sarver DM. The smile arc — the importance of incisor position in the dynamic smile. Am J Orthod Dentofacial Orthop 2001;120:98–111.

11. Ackerman Jl, Ackerman MB, Brensinger CM, Landis JR. A morphometric analysis of the posed smile. Clin Orth Res 1998;1:1–11.

12. Ackerman MB. Digital video as a clinical tool in orthodontics: dynamic smile design in diagnosis and treatment planning. 29th Annual Moyers Symposium on Information Technology and Orthodontic Treatment. Vol 40. Ann Arbor (MI): University of Michigan Press; 2003.

13. Farkas LG, Munro JR. Anthropometric facial proportions in medicine. Springfield (IL): Charles C. Thomas Publisher Ltd; 1987.

14. Peck H, Peck S. A concept of facial esthetics. Angle Orthod 1970;40:284–317.

15. Mazur A, Mazur J, Keating C. Military rank attainment of a West Point class: effects of cadets' physical features. Am J Soc 1984;90:125–50.

16. Pessa JA. The potential role of stereolithography in the study of facial aging. Am J Orthod Dentofacial Orthop 2001;119:117–20.

17. Krugman ME. Photo analysis of the rhinoplasty patient. J Ear Nose Throat 1981;60:56–9.

18. Sommerville JM, Sperry TP, BeGole EA. Morphology of the submental and neck region. Int J Adult Orthod 1988;3:97–106.

19. Zachrisson BU. Esthetic factors involved in anterior tooth display and the smile: vertical dimension. J Clin Orthod 1998; 32:432–45.

20. Burstone CJ, Marcotte MR. The treatment occlusal plane. In: Problem solving in orthodontics: goal-oriented treatment strategies. Chicago (IL): Quintessence Publishing Co.; 2000. p. 31–50.

21. Andrews LF. Straight wire: the concept and the appliance. San Diego (CA): L.A. Wells Inc.; 1989.

22. Lo FM, Shapiro PA. Effect of presurgical incisor extension on stability of anterior open bite malocclusion treated with orthognathic surgery. Int J Adult Orthod Orthognath Surg 1998;13:23–34.

23. Sinclair PM, Kilpelainen P, Phillips C, et al. The accuracy of video imaging in orthognathic surgery. Am J Orthod Dentofacial Orthop 1995;107:177–85.

24. Upton PM, Sadowsky PL, Sarver DM, Heaven TJ. Evaluation of video imaging prediction in combined maxillary and mandibular orthognathic surgery. Am J Orthod Dentofacial Orthop 1997;112:656–65.

25. Syliangco ST, Sameshima GT, Kaminishi RM, Sinclair PM. Predicting soft tissue changes in mandibular advancement surgery: a comparison of two video imaging systems. Angle Orthod 1997;67:337–46.

26. Sameshima GT, Kawakami RK, Kaminishi RM, Sinclair PM. Predicting soft tissue changes in maxillary impaction surgery: a comparison of two video imaging systems. Angle Orthod 1997;67:346–54.

27. Kazandjian S, Sameshima GT, Champlin T, Sinclair PM. Accuracy of video imaging for predicting the soft tissue profile after mandibular set-back surgery. Am J Orthod Dentofacial Orthop 1999;115:382–89.

28. Peters DG. Lower lip changes in surgical correction of Class I malocclusion [Master's dissertation]. Chapel Hill (NC): University of North Carolina; 2001.

CHAPTER 55

Orthodontics for Orthognathic Surgery

Larry M. Wolford, DMD
Eber L. L. Stevao, DDS, PhD
C. Moody Alexander, DDS, MS
Joao Roberto Goncalves, DDS, PhD

Moderate to severe occlusal discrepancies and dentofacial deformities in late adolescents and adults usually require combined orthodontic treatment and orthognathic surgery to obtain optimal, stable, functional, and esthetic results. The basic goals of orthodontics and orthognathic surgery are to (1) satisfy the patients' concerns, (2) establish optimal functional outcomes, and (3) provide good esthetic results. To accomplish this the orthodontist and the oral and maxillofacial (OMF) surgeon must be able to correctly diagnose existing dental and skeletal deformities, establish an appropriate treatment plan, and properly execute the recommended treatment. The orthodontist is limited, to a great extent, by growth, and although the orthodontist can move teeth and, to some degree, the alveolar bone, he or she does not have any appreciable effect on the basal bone of the jaws. The orthodontist's role is to align the teeth relative to the maxillary and mandibular jaws. The OMF surgeon is responsible for surgically repositioning the jaw(s) and associated structures.

It is very important to listen to and understand the patients concerns. Empathetic listening from the first appointment and throughout the treatment will build trust, improve communication, and help provide a quality end result for all parties involved. Comprehensive analysis of the patient and the complete orthodontic records (cephalograms, pantomograms, photographs, dental models) are important for diagnosis and development of the presurgical orthodontic goals. Although detailed analysis of the patient's facial and jaw structures from a clinical and radiographic perspective are vitally important, the focus of this chapter will be the teeth and orthodontic considerations in preparation for orthognathic surgery. Other important factors in diagnosis, treatment planning, and outcomes, such as patient concerns, psychosocial factors, masticatory dysfunction, airway problems, speech difficulties, temporomandibular joint (TMJ) pathologies, and comprehensive orthognathic surgery work-up are discussed elsewhere in this book.

The normal values provided in this chapter are not absolutes for every patient because of individual size, morphologic variances, and racial and ethnic differences. They are provided as a guide to help the clinician evaluate his or her patient.

Establishing an all-inclusive diagnosis is paramount to developing a comprehensive treatment plan. The orthodontist must determine the orthodontic goals based on the pretreatment findings and on the projected treatment outcome. This chapter will first present orthodontic diagnostic information, followed by orthodontic treatment considerations.

Clinical and Dental Model Diagnosis

From an orthodontic standpoint, in evaluating the occlusion and dental factors, the clinical and dental model analyses correlated with the cephalometric analysis provide the most information for diagnosis and treatment planning. There are 12 basic evaluations that are helpful for these determinations.

1. Arch length: This assessment correlates the mesiodistal widths of the teeth relative to the amount of alveolar bone available and aids in identifying the presence of crowding or

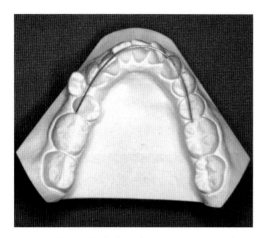

FIGURE 55-1 *Arch length assessment correlates the mesiodistal widths of the teeth relative to the amount of alveolar bone available and aids in identifying the presence of crowding or spacing. The curved wire illustrates ideal cuspid and incisor tip position relative to the basal bone.*

spacing. This helps determine if teeth need to be extracted or if spaces need to be either created or closed (Figure 55-1). Clinical and dental model assessment correlated to cephalometric analysis will aid in determining arch length requirements. Generally Class II patients will tend to have more crowding in the mandibular arch and less in the maxillary arch, whereas Class III patients may have spacing in the mandibular arch but a tendency for crowding in the maxillary arch.

2. Tooth-size analysis: This analysis relates the mesiodistal width of the maxillary teeth compared with the mandibular teeth. A tooth-size discrepancy (TSD) causes incompatibility of the dental alignment and can occur in the anterior teeth, premolars, and molars. Approximately 40% of patients with dentofacial deformities will have an anterior TSD affecting the anterior six teeth of the maxillary and mandibular arches (the mandibular arch is commonly too large compared with the maxillary arch), usually due to small maxillary lateral incisors. In such cases proper tooth alignment with all spaces closed often precludes the establishment of a good Class I cuspid-molar relationship with treatment. Instead, a Class II end-on cuspid-molar occlusal relationship may result. Occasionally the maxillary anterior six teeth may be too large for the mandibular anterior teeth, creating an excessive anterior overjet when in a Class I cuspid relationship. Determination of a TSD pretreatment will provide the opportunity to correct the TSD during the presurgical orthodontic phase of treatment. Explaining to the patient, before treatment, that small maxillary lateral incisors may need restorative bonding to maximize the quality esthetic and functional outcome is important, so that the patient is aware from the onset of the time and financial commitment necessary for treatment. The normal mesiodistal widths of each of the permanent teeth are recorded in Tables 55-1 and 55-2. Variations from the norm may create difficulties in the teeth fitting properly.

Bolton's analysis is a method to correlate the widths of the maxillary and mandibular anterior six teeth. Needle-point calipers can be used to measure each individual tooth, and successive holes punched into a tablet for each of the anterior six teeth for each arch. Then a measurement from the first to last holes will give the summation of mesiodistal widths of the anterior six teeth for each arch (Figures 55-2 and 55-3). The summation of the mesiodistal widths of the maxillary anterior six teeth measured at the contact level, divided into the combined width of the mandibular anterior six teeth, yields a value called

Table 55-1	Maxillary Mesiodistal Teeth Diameters						
	Central Incisor*	Lateral Incisor*	Cuspids*	First Bicuspids*	Second Bicuspids*	First Molars*	Second Molars*
Males	8.9 (0.59)	6.9 (0.64)	8.0 (0.42)	6.8 (0.47)	6.7 (0.37)	10.6 (0.56)	9.5 (0.71)
Females	8.7 (0.57)	6.8 (0.64)	7.5 (0.36)	6.6 (0.46)	6.5 (0.46)	10.2 (0.58)	8.8 (0.73)

Adapted from Moyers RE et al.[2] *Measurements in mm (SD).

Table 55-2	Mandibular Mesiodistal Teeth Diameters						
	Central Incisor*	Lateral Incisor*	Cuspids*	First Bicuspids*	Second Bicuspids*	First Molars*	Second Molars*
Males	5.5 (0.32)	6.0 (0.37)	7.0 (0.40)	6.9 (0.63)	7.2 (0.47)	10.7 (0.60)	10.0 (0.67)
Females	5.5 (0.34)	5.9 (0.34)	6.6 (0.34)	6.8 (0.70)	7.1 (0.46)	10.3 (0.74)	9.5 (0.59)

Adapted from Moyers RE et al.[2] *Measurements in mm (SD).

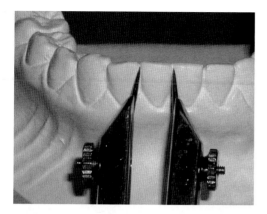

FIGURE **55-2** *Bolton's analysis. Needle-point calipers are used to measure each tooth at a contact-point level to aid in tooth-size analysis.*

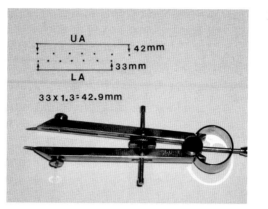

FIGURE **55-3** *Bolton's analysis. Successive holes are punched into a tablet for each of the anterior six teeth for each arch. Then measuring from the first hole to the last hole will give the summation of the mesiodistal widths of the anterior six teeth in each arch. Multiplying the summation of the mandibular anterior six teeth (LA) by 1.3 yields the calculated arch width for the maxillary anterior six teeth (UA). Subtracting the actual maxillary anterior arch width from the calculated width yields the tooth-size discrepancy.*

the intermaxillary (Bolton's) index. The average index (percentage) is 77.5 ± 3.5.[1] A simple conversion of this factor would be to measure the width of the mandibular anterior six teeth and then multiply that sum by 1.3. This results in a calculated ideal maxillary arch width. The difference between the calculated and the actual maxillary arch width values determines the TSD (see Figure 55-3). This evaluation is very helpful in determining presurgical orthodontic and surgical goals. TSDs can also occur in the premolar and molar areas (normally the same maxillary and mandibular teeth are similar in size) where the mandibular teeth may be significantly larger than the maxillary teeth.

The Bolton's analysis is not perfect and functions only as a guide in assessing the tooth-size compatibility of the anterior teeth because it does not take into consideration the labiolingual thickness of the incisors, the axial inclination of the teeth, or the thickness and prominence of the marginal ridges. A thin labiolingual dimension of the maxillary incisors may compensate for small TSDs, but thicker than normal dimensions or prominent marginal ridges may preclude a Class I cuspid relationship

even though the Bolton's index is normal. An accurate dental model orthodontic wax set-up may achieve a more accurate assessment.

3. Incisor angulation: This refers to the angulation of the maxillary and mandibular incisors relative to their respective basal bones. The dental models are correlated to the cephalometric analysis and the ideal axial inclination of the incisors determined (Figure 55-4). The incisor angulation analysis contributes to the determination of whether extractions are necessary, spaces need to be created or eliminated, and what mechanics are required to align and level the arches or segments of the arches. The key is to get the incisors in proper position and angulation over basal bone.

4. Arch width analysis: This refers to the evaluation of the intra-arch transverse widths between the maxillary and mandibular arches. The average maxillary and mandibular arch widths for adults are listed in Tables 55-3 and 55-4 (data from University of Michigan Caucasian study).[2] These averages are only guides and do not account for

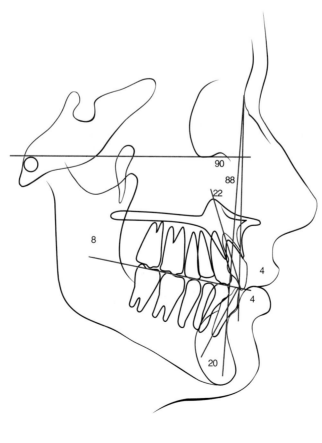

FIGURE **55-4** *Cephalometric analysis. Normal maxillary depth angle is 90° ± 3° and mandibular depth is 88° ± 3°. Normal occlusal plane angulation is 8° ± 4°. Normal maxillary incisor angulation to the nasion point A (NA) line is 22° ± 2° with the labial surface of the incisor being 4 mm ± 2 mm anterior to the NA line. Normal mandibular incisor angulation to the nasion point B (NB) line is 20° ± 2° with the labial surface of the incisor being 4 mm ± 2 mm anterior to the NB line.*

patient size, or racial or ethnic differences. However, from a practical standpoint a good way to analyze the arch width is to relate the models to the occlusal position that is to be achieved with the surgical correction and then assess the transverse relationship. For example, if a patient has a Class II occlusion, position the models in a Class I cuspid-molar relation and evaluate the transverse width relationship. Likewise, a patient with a Class III occlusion is evaluated by positioning the models into a Class I cuspid-molar relationship. When a Class II relationship is shifted to a Class I relationship, the maxilla may be narrow and require expansion. In some cases it may be indicated to evaluate the transverse relationship by placing the models into a Class II molar position to determine if a Class I cuspid and Class II molar relationship (this would require maxillary bicuspid extractions) would be best for that particular patient; this may be beneficial when there is significant crowding in the maxillary arch and no crowding in the mandibular arch. Transverse discrepancies will influence the presurgical orthodontics and dictate the surgical procedures required.

5. Curve of Spee: This evaluates the vertical position of the anterior teeth compared with the posterior teeth. This assessment can be determined by placing the occlusion of the maxillary dental model on a flat plane; the incisors should be about 1 mm above the flat plane (Figure 55-5A). Placing the occlusion of the mandibular dental model on a flat plane should see the mandibular incisors elevated 1 mm above the midbuccal teeth. A significant accentuated curve of Spee in the maxilla is usually associated with an anterior open bite and a reverse curve associated with an anterior deep bite. An accentuated curve of Spee in the mandible (Figure 55-5B) is commonly associated with an anterior deep bite and a reverse curve associated with an open bite. Accentuated or reverse curves of Spee will influence whether the curve in each arch requires correction, and if so, whether the correction will be achieved by orthodontics, with or without extractions, opening spaces, or by surgical intervention.

6. Cuspid-molar position: This identifies the angle classification and dental interrelationships. It is usually

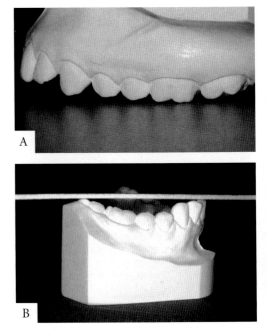

FIGURE 55-5   A, *This maxillary arch demonstrates an increased curve of Spee. B, An accentuated (increased) curve of Spee is seen in the mandibular arch.*

preferable to have a Class I cuspid-molar relationship as an outcome result; however, a Class II molar relationship is acceptable. A Class III molar relationship is less desirable because the mandibular first molar functions against the maxillary second bicuspid, but it may be indicated in some cases.

Table 55-3	Maxillary Arch Width*				
	Cuspids[†]	*First Bicuspids[†]*	*Second Bicuspids[†]*	*First Molars[†]*	*Second Molars[†]*
Males	32.3 (1.7)	36.7 (2.0)	41.5 (2.5)	47.1 (2.8)	52.3 (3.4)
Females	31.2 (2.45)	34.6 (3.2)	39.3 (2.2)	44.3 (2.3)	49.3 (2.8)

Adapted from Moyers RE et al.[2]
*All measurements at centroid.
[†]Measurements in mm (SD).

Table 55-4	Mandibular Arch Width*				
	Cuspids[†]	*First Bicuspids[†]*	*Second Bicuspids[†]*	*First Molars[†]*	*Second Molars[†]*
Males	24.8 (1.3)	32.8 (1.5)	37.6 (2.3)	43.0 (2.7)	49.0 (2.3)
Females	23.1 (2.0)	31.8 (1.4)	36.8 (1.3)	41.7 (2.3)	47.2 (2.1)

Adapted from Moyers RE et al.[2]
*All measurements at centroid.
[†]Measurements in mm (SD).

7. Tooth arch symmetry: This compares the left to right side symmetry within each arch. There may be a significant asymmetry within the arch, such as a cuspid on one side being more anteriorly positioned in the arch than the cuspid on the opposite side (Figure 55-6). This problem often occurs with a unilateral missing tooth. Also, vertical asymmetries can occur with individual teeth, sections of the dentoalveolus, or the entire dental arches, creating a cant in the transverse occlusal plane. Correcting these types of conditions may require special orthodontic mechanics, unilateral extraction or opening-up space, asymmetric extractions, and/or surgical procedures.

8. Curve of Wilson (buccal tooth tipping): This evaluates the mediolateral position of the occlusal surfaces of the maxillary (Figure 55-7) and mandibular posterior teeth. If the occlusal surfaces of the maxillary or mandibular posterior teeth are tipped too far buccally, it may be difficult to achieve a proper occlusal interdigitation relationship. In the presence of a transverse maxillary deficiency with preexisting increased curve of Wilson and posterior crossbites, it is very difficult, if not impossible, to correct the problem orthodontically, orthopedically, or even with surgically assisted rapid

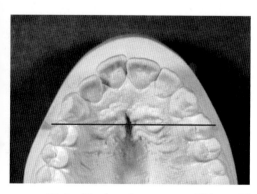

FIGURE 55-6 *Tooth arch symmetry. This model demonstrates that the cuspid on one side of the arch is significantly more anteriorly positioned in the arch compared with the cuspid on the opposite side.*

palatal expansion (SARPE). The curve of Wilson will usually get much worse with these mechanics. In these types of cases surgical expansion by multiple maxillary osteotomies may be indicated to decrease the curve of Wilson.

When the mandibular posterior teeth are tipped buccally, it is often related to macroglossia or habitual tongue posturing. Orthodontic lingual tipping of the posterior teeth is very difficult when macroglossia is present and will likely be unstable. A reduction glossectomy may be indicated before orthodontics in order to permit a more stable orthodontic result.

9. Missing, broken down, or restored teeth: These must be identified since they may influence treatment design. If a tooth is nonrestorable and requires extraction, it must be determined if the extraction space requires orthodontic closure or the space maintained for later dental reconstruction. In some cases it may be helpful to maintain the condemned tooth to improve stability during surgical alignment of the jaws or segments thereof, with removal postsurgery. Crowns on previously restored teeth may need to be redone post-orthodontics and -orthognathic surgery, since the crown anatomy may need to be changed for proper occlusion with the new dental relationships. Determination of salvageable teeth and restorative requirements are integral components in the planning and treatment of patients.

10. Ankylosed teeth: If undiagnosed, ankylosed teeth can have devastating effects on the presurgical orthodontics. Tooth ankylosis, the fusion of alveolar bone and cementum, results from damage to the periodontal ligament (PDL).

An ankylosed tooth may be identified by failure to move with orthodontic forces (Figure 55-8), failure of a tooth to erupt, submerged or incomplete tooth eruption (Figure 55-9), or lack of eruption of a tooth compared with adjacent teeth and alveolar bone growth. The most sensitive diagnostic test is percussion, where the ankylosed tooth has a high, clear, solid metallic sound. A normal tooth has a dull sound, being protected by the PDL. However, an erupted tooth with an impacted tooth directly against it will also have a solid sound to percussion. Normal multirooted teeth present a more solid sound than single-rooted teeth. Therefore, percussion testing should be compared with similar teeth (ie, test bicuspids against bicuspids, molars against molars, using both sides of the arch). An ankylosed tooth lacks

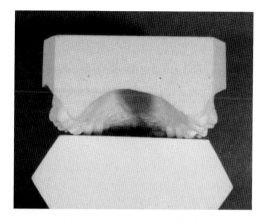

FIGURE 55-7 *Curve of Wilson. This evaluates the mediolateral position of the occlusal surfaces of the maxillary and mandibular posterior teeth.*

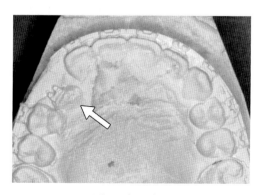

FIGURE 55-8 *This dental model shows a palatally displaced tooth, unresponsive to orthodontic mechanics, indicating probable ankylosis.*

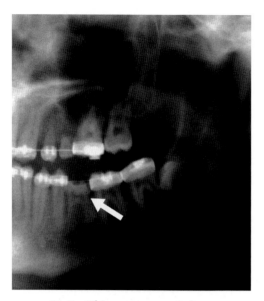

FIGURE 55-9 *This pantomogram demonstrates incomplete eruption of a primary tooth without a permanent successor, indicating ankylosis.*

mobility. Over 90% of ankylosed teeth are deciduous; most often the second molar followed by the first molar.[3] Ankylosed primary teeth are not susceptible to resorption by the follicle of the underlying permanent tooth and may result in its impaction.[3]

Ankylosed teeth can cause significant problems with jaw growth and development. Early ankylosis results in noneruption or partial eruption, resulting in incomplete development of the alveolar process.[4] Permanent teeth may be displaced from normal eruption pathways with resulting loss of alveolar bone height. The failure of an ankylosed tooth to erupt may allow adjacent teeth to drift and permit super-eruption of the tooth in the opposing arch. Ankylosed teeth do not respond to orthodontic forces and can create significant orthodontic problems when malaligned and tied into the orthodontic arch wire (Figure 55-10).[5] The ankylosed tooth functions as an anchor and in active uncontrolled orthodontics, will move adjacent teeth to align with its position, with subsequent development of an occlusal and possibly facial deformity.

11. Periodontal evaluation: This is very important, since preexisting periodontal pathologies could be exacerbated during orthodontic and orthognathic surgical treatments.[6] Factors that can adversely affect the health and outcome of the periodontal tissues as well as the orthodontics and orthognathic surgery include smoking, excessive consumption of alcohol or caffeine, habitual patterns such as bruxism and clenching, preexisting connective tissue/autoimmune diseases, diabetes, malnutrition, and other diseases that could affect the local tissue blood supply perfusion, and healing. Any pretreatment of acute or chronic periodontal disease should be addressed prior to the orthodontics and surgery. The lack of attached gingiva around the teeth (most commonly seen in the mandibular anterior arch) can cause gingival retraction, loss of bone, and loosening of teeth if orthodontics is initiated and the mandibular incisors are tipped forward (Figure 55-11). Gingival grafting may be indicated prior to orthodontics to provide attached gingiva so as to prevent these problems. Good communication between the periodontist, orthodontist, and OMF surgeon is of utmost importance.

Orthodontics can help prepare interdental osteotomy sites by tipping the roots of the adjacent teeth away from each other to increase the interosseous space between the roots. There have been a number of studies demonstrating that interdental osteotomies have a minimal effect on the periodontium when they are properly performed.[7–11] Having healthy stable dental tissues to work with during the orthodontics and surgery will maximize the periodontal outcome as well as the overall outcome. The failure to recognize preexisting periodontal pathology, identify risk factors, poor performance of surgery, and/or lack of attention to detail could result in significant periodontal problems as well as other problems that could compromise the final result.

12. Tongue assessment: An enlarged tongue (macroglossia) can cause dentoskeletal

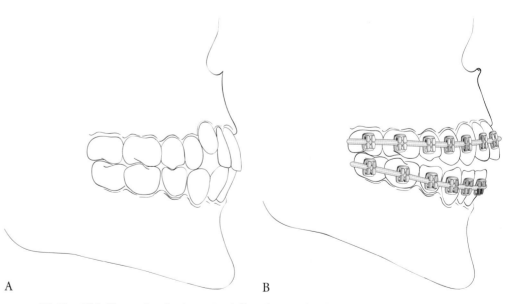

FIGURE 55-10 *This illustration depicts a partially submerged ankylosed maxillary cuspid (A). If tied into an active straight arch wire (B), the adjacent teeth will be orthodontically moved toward the ankylosed tooth, resulting in the development of a significant malocclusion.*

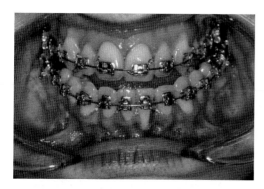

FIGURE **55-11** *Periodontal concerns. This patient had lack of attached gingiva prior to initiation of orthodontics and was left untreated, causing severe gingival retraction and loss of supporting bone. Gingival grafting should have been performed prior to initiation of orthodontics.*

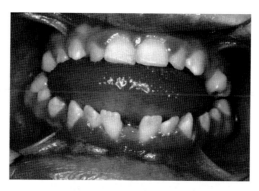

FIGURE **55-12** *Macroglossia. Some of the clinical features associated with macroglossia include anterior open bite, diastemata between the teeth, accentuated curve of Spee maxillary arch, and reverse curve of Spee mandibular arch.*

deformities, instability of orthodontic and orthognathic surgical treatments, and create masticatory, speech, and airway management problems. There are a number of congenital and acquired causes of true macroglossia, including muscular hypertrophy, glandular hyperplasia, hemangioma, lymphangioma, Down syndrome, and Beckwith-Wiedemann syndrome. Acquired factors include acromegaly, myxedema, amyloidosis, tertiary syphilis, cysts or tumors, and neurologic injury.[12] There are specific clinical and cephalometric features that may help the clinician identify the presence or absence of macroglossia, although not all of these features are always present. Specific clinical features include the following (Figure 55-12):

- Grossly enlarged, wide, broad, and flat tongue
- Open bite (anterior or posterior)
- Mandibular prognathism
- Class III malocclusion with or without anterior and posterior crossbite
- Chronic posturing of the tongue between the teeth at rest (rule out habitual posturing of a normal-sized tongue)
- Increased curve of Wilson of maxillary posterior teeth

- Reverse curve of Wilson of mandibular posterior teeth
- Accentuated curve of Spee in the maxillary arch
- Reverse curve of Spee in the mandibular arch
- Increased transverse width of maxillary and mandibular arches
- Diastemata with increased incisor angulation in the mandibular and/or maxillary arches

- Crenations (scalloping) on the tongue
- Glossitis (due to excessive mouth breathing)
- Speech articulation disorders
- Asymmetry in the maxillary or mandibular arches associated with an asymmetric tongue
- Difficulty eating and swallowing (severe cases)
- Instability in orthodontic mechanics or orthognathic surgical procedures that in normal circumstances would be stable
- Airway difficulties, such as sleep apnea, secondary to oral or oropharyngeal obstruction
- Drooling

Cephalometric radiographic features commonly seen with macroglossia (Figure 55-13) include the following:

- Tongue filling the oral cavity and extruding through an anterior open bite
- Mandibular dentoalveolar protrusion or bimaxillary dentoalveolar protrusion

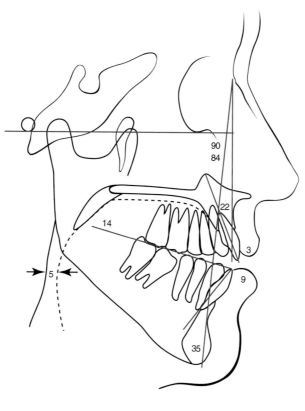

FIGURE **55-13** *Macroglossia. Cephalometric analysis shows mandibular dentoalveolar protrusion and overangulation of the mandibular anterior teeth. The tongue fills the oral cavity (dotted line) and the oropharyngeal airway is decreased (normal distance from posterior aspect of tongue to posterior pharyngeal wall is 11 mm).*

- Overangulation of the maxillary and mandibular anterior teeth
- Disproportionately excessive mandibular growth
- Decreased oropharyngeal airway
- Increased gonial angle
- Increased mandibular plane angle
- Increased mandibular occlusal plane angle

Most open bite cases are not related to macroglossia. In fact it has been established that closing open bites with orthognathic surgery will allow a normal tongue (which is a very adaptable organ) to re-adjust to the altered volume of the oral cavity, with little tendency toward relapse.[13,14] However, if true macroglossia is present with the open bite, then instability of the orthodontics and orthognathic surgery will likely occur, with a tendency for the open bite to return. Pseudomacroglossia is a condition where the tongue may be normal in size, but it appears large relative to its anatomic interrelationships. This can be created by (1) habitual posturing of the tongue; (2) hypertrophied tonsils and adenoid tissue displacing the tongue forward; (3) low palatal vault, decreasing the oral cavity volume; (4) transverse, vertical, or anteroposterior deficiency of the maxillary and/or mandibular arches decreasing oral cavity volume; and (5) tumors that displace the tongue. Pseudomacroglossia must be distinguished from true macroglossia because the methods of management are different.

Diagnostic List

Before a treatment plan can be properly developed, a diagnostic list of the existing problems is established based on patient concerns, and clinical, radiographic, dental model, and other indicated evaluations. This will include all findings relative to musculoskeletal and dental imbalances, occlusal problems, esthetic concerns, TMJ and/or myofascial pain problems, missing teeth, crowns, bridges, endodontically treated teeth (these teeth are sometimes ankylosed), periodontal problems, other functional disorders, as well as any other medical factors that may affect treatment outcomes. The treatment plan is formulated from the diagnostic problem list.

Presurgical Orthodontic Goals

The basic presurgical orthodontic goals are as follows:

- Align and position teeth over basal bone
- Avoid excessive intrusion or extrusion of teeth
- Decompensate teeth
- Avoid unstable expansion of the dental arches
- Avoid class II and class III mechanics (unless required for dental decompensation correction in the arches)
- Perform stable and predictable orthodontics

Relative to the position of the maxillary and mandibular incisors, the ideal presurgical orthodontic goals are as follows:

1. Position the long axis of the maxillary central incisors approximately 22° to the nasion point A (NA) line, with the labial surface of the incisors 4 mm anterior to the NA line relative to a normally positioned maxilla and normal occlusal plane angle (see Figure 55-4)
2. Position the long axis of the mandibular central incisors 20° to the nasion point B (NB) line with the labial surface of the incisors 4 mm anterior to that line relative to a normally positioned mandible and normal occlusal plane angle (see Figure 55-4)
3. Satisfy arch length requirements (crowding or spacing)

We have found that using the ideal position of the maxillary and mandibular incisors to the NA and NB lines, respectively (see Figure 55-4), is the most convenient and practical method to establish the presurgical orthodontic goals for the incisors. However, these presurgical orthodontic goals may be different if the occlusal plane angle is to be altered surgically. Removal of dental compensations is helpful before surgery so that maximum skeletal correction can be achieved. An exact orthodontic treatment plan, including the specific mechanics and anchorage requirements necessary to position the teeth to satisfy the presurgical orthodontic goals, must be developed and executed.

Initial Surgical Treatment Objective

The surgical treatment objective (STO), also known as a prediction tracing, is a two-dimensional visual projection of the changes in osseous, dental, and soft tissues as a result of orthodontics and orthognathic surgical correction of the dentofacial and occlusal deformity. The purpose of the STO is threefold: (1) establish presurgical orthodontic goals, (2) develop an accurate surgical objective that will achieve the best functional and esthetic result, and (3) create a facial profile objective which can be used as a visual aid in consultation with the patient and family members. A prediction tracing of the anticipated presurgical orthodontic dental movements is created by placing an acetate sheet on the original cephalometric tracing and retracing the teeth into the position they will be placed with the presurgical orthodontics, based on the goals and available mechanics (Figure 55-14A). The initial STO is then constructed with the teeth in their presurgical orthodontic final position.

The STO has significant importance in two phases of treatment planning: (1) the initial STO is prepared before treatment to determine the orthodontic and surgical goals; and (2) the final STO is prepared after the presurgical orthodontics are completed but prior to surgery to determine the exact vertical and anteroposterior skeletal and soft tissue movements to be achieved (Figure 55-14B). The

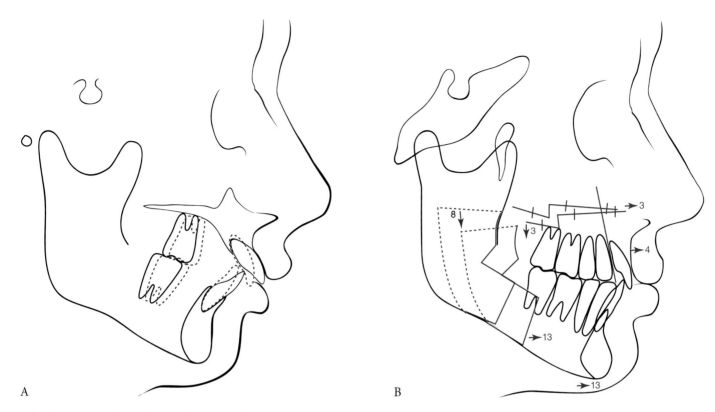

FIGURE 55-14 A, *Presurgical orthodontics. The orthodontic movements are traced on the acetate paper overlying the original lateral cephalometric tracing with the teeth in their predetermined, simulated positions. The solid lines, are the original position of the teeth. The dashed lines are the new position of the teeth following simulated extraction of four first bicuspids and orthodontic closure of the spaces. B, Surgical treatment objective (STO). This is an example of a completed final STO which shows the predicted outcome of the presurgical orthodontics and the anticipated surgical treatment. The arrows and numbers indicate the direction and millimeters of movement.*

STO is invaluable to the orthodontist and surgeon in establishing treatment objectives and projected results, acting as the *treatment plan blueprint.*

Definitive Interdisciplinary Treatment Plan

The definitive treatment plan is formulated based on the patient's concerns, clinical evaluation, radiographic analysis, dental model evaluation, initial STO, and other relevant evaluations. The general sequencing of the treatment that may be involved is described below.

Dental and Periodontal Treatment

Any indicated periodontal or general dental care related to maintaining teeth or improving dental health should be performed prior to orthodontics and surgical intervention. The objective is to maintain as many teeth as possible and stabilize the periodontium. Temporary crowns and bridges should be placed where necessary for the orthodontic and surgical phases of the treatment. Permanent crowns, inlays, and bridges should be constructed and inserted after the surgery and orthodontics have been completed. This gives the restorative dentist the opportunity to provide escapement grooves, cuspid protection, and incisal guidance for optimum function and esthetics. Initial periodontal management may include scaling and curettage, eliminating pockets, as well as gingival grafting to provide adequate attached gingiva. Occasionally, in patients with several missing teeth, osseointegrated implant placement prior to orthodontics and orthognathic surgery may provide anchorage for orthodontics and additional dental units to help in repositioning the jaw structures at surgery.

Presurgical Orthodontics

The orthodontist is responsible for positioning the teeth to the most desirable position over basal bone in preparation for surgery. The development of prescription brackets and straight wire orthodontic techniques has helped simplify orthodontics. Most prescription bracket systems are designed to tip the cuspid roots distally, creating some space between the roots of the lateral incisors and cuspids. In cases requiring segmentalization of the maxilla, this interdental space may be adequate through which to perform interdental osteotomies, but if inadequate, additional room can be created by tipping the lateral incisor roots mesially and the cuspids more distally. Bonded brackets are clean and eliminate interdental spacing problems created by circumferential bands. Bonded brackets with the currently available resins are quite adequate for orthognathic surgery procedures. However, inaccurate placement of the brackets on the teeth can result in undesired rotations, vertical discrepancies between teeth, malalignment of marginal ridges and labial surfaces of adjacent teeth, and unfavorable root positions. Careful placement of brackets is paramount in helping to achieve high-quality results.

Nickel-titanium or similarly shaped memory arch wires can be advantageous for many orthognathic cases to aid in presurgical orthodontic dental alignment goals. However, there are cases where shape memory wires could be detrimental, such as in an anterior open bite with an accentuated maxillary curve of Spee. The use of nickel-titanium wires or any type of straight wire in these cases can create unstable results such as extrusion of teeth and buccal tipping of the molars as a result of reciprocal forces. Stainless steel wires with compensating bends (Figure 55-15A) or sectional wires (Figure 55-15B) may be a better-controlled mechanical force in these types of cases. The type of arch wire and how long each is left in place is critical and must be carefully monitored by the orthodontist.

To follow are basic presurgical orthodontic factors that commonly must be addressed in preparing patients for orthognathic surgery.

It is important to avoid interarch class II mechanics (ie, class II elastics, growth appliances, TMJ "disk recapturing" splints, Herbst's appliances) unless they are specifically required during the presurgical orthodontics (ie, to correct arch asymmetry, decompensate mandibular arch with lingually inclined mandibular incisors). Long-term class II mechanics positions the mandibular condyle downward and forward in the fossa and may allow hypertrophy (thickening) of the TMJ bilaminar tissues (Figure 55-16). This same situation can occur in patients with a "Sunday" bite. In these situations, following surgical mandibular advancement, the bilaminar tissue will slowly thin out over time causing a slow relapse of the mandible toward a Class II relationship. In addition posturing the mandible forward for an extended time could result in foreshortening of the anterior articular disk attachments, increasing the risk of TMJ articular disk displacement postsurgery.

If a patient has been treated with long-term class II mechanics or has a "Sunday" bite, it may be an advantage to use light class III mechanics for a few months presurgery

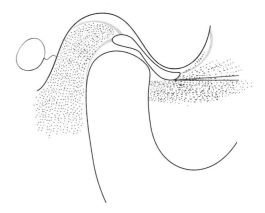

FIGURE **55-16** *Use of long-term class II mechanics, anterior repositioning splints, growth devices, or "Sunday" bite relationships can cause hypertrophy of the bilaminar tissue, positioning the condyle downward and forward in the fossa. Postsurgery, particularly with mandibular advancements, this tissue will slowly thin out, and the condyles will move posteriorly in the fossa causing a shift of the mandible and occlusion toward a Class II position.*

to eliminate the hypertrophied bilaminar tissue and to decompensate for any unstable orthodontics that may have been created. If the TMJ articular disk does become displaced, it would be better to have that occur before surgery because the articular disk can be surgically repositioned and stabilized with high predictability at the same time as the orthognathic surgery.[15–18] Attempts to recapture a TMJ displaced disk with splint therapy prior to surgery could be detrimental to the patient relative to outcome stability and pain. In most cases nonsurgical "recapturing" the disk procedures have proved clinically unsuccessful.

Treatment Options for Specific Orthodontic Problems

This section presents specific dental malrelationships and the orthodontic and surgical treatment options for consideration. Comprehensive assessment of the patient and developing treatment objectives will aid in selecting the appropriate treatment.

Adjustment for Tooth-Size Discrepancy

Usually TSDs occur because of small maxillary lateral incisors, making the combined

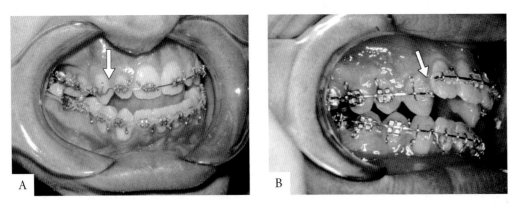

FIGURE **55-15**   A, *Compensating steps* (arrow) *have been placed in the orthodontic arch wire so that the anterior teeth are aligned at an elevated level compared with the posterior teeth to eliminate extrusion or intrusion of teeth that may otherwise result in unstable orthodontic movements. B, Sectioning the arch wire* (arrow) *is another approach to aligning teeth at separate independent levels to avoid extrusion or intrusion of teeth as seen in this maxilla. However, the use of sectional wires may decrease positional control of the teeth adjacent to the ends of the cut wire.*

mesiodistal width of the maxillary anterior six teeth too small to fit properly around the mandibular anterior six teeth, so that when the teeth are properly aligned, an end-on Class II cuspid relationship will result (Figure 55-17). If the Bolton's analysis indicates a significant TSD, presurgical orthodontic adjustments can usually correct the discrepancy and aid in providing a solid Class I cuspid relationship at surgery and in the final outcome. TSDs can also occur in the bicuspids and molars, with the maxillary teeth usually being too small compared with the mandibular teeth. The following are treatment options that can be used to correct TSDs.

Slenderizing Teeth (Interproximal Tooth Size Reduction)

This technique reduces the mesiodistal dimension of the involved teeth. Since most TSDs involve larger mandibular anterior teeth compared to the maxillary anterior teeth, slenderizing the mandibular anterior teeth can address the issue (Figure 55-18). Approximately 10 to 12% of the mesiodistal width can be safely removed from each tooth with 50% of the interproximal enamel remaining. Up to 3 mm of reduction can usually be safely achieved in the mandibular anterior

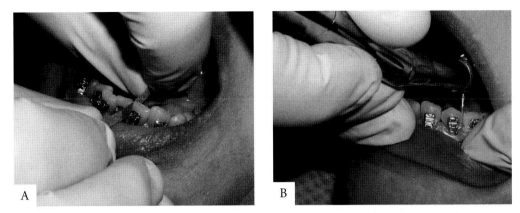

FIGURE 55-18 *Mandibular anterior teeth can be slenderized using (A) diamond strip or (B) thin cylindrical diamond bur to reduce the width of the teeth at the contact level. Spacing generated can then be closed with orthodontics.*

six teeth. Slenderizing the mandibular anterior teeth is an advantageous procedure, where the maximum width of the incisors is toward the incisor edge, particularly in the presence of crowding and/or overangulation of the mandibular incisors. It is not advantageous if the mandibular anterior teeth are decreased in angulation (lingual inclination), since closing the resultant spaces will further decrease the incisor angulation and may adversely affect esthetics and stability. This technique is not indicated when the contact points are positioned toward the gingiva, as this could result in tissue strangulation with loss of papilla and interdental bone, creating significant periodontal issues. In the rare case where the maxillary teeth are too large for the mandibular teeth, the maxillary teeth can be slenderized, but this is best used when the maxillary teeth are crowded and/or overangulated, and the individual crowns are wider than normal (see Table 55-1).

When TSDs occurs in the bicuspid and/or molar area, slenderizing the mandibular teeth will usually correct the problem, unless the slenderizing will cause excessive retraction of the mandibular anterior teeth. If this appears to be a potential outcome, then careful closure of the spacing by loosing (slipping) posterior anchorage (using mechanics that will

move the posterior teeth forward instead of the anterior teeth backward) may solve the problem. This approach may include class II mechanics to provide forward forces on the posterior teeth or moving one tooth at a time on each side. Dental implants placed adjacent to or posterior to the molars could provide stable anchorage to aid in applying the mechanics necessary to push the posterior teeth forward.

Creating Space In the Arch This can enlarge the circumference of the involved arch. Since TSDs are often related to small maxillary lateral incisors, opening space around the maxillary lateral incisors may be a logical approach. A simple technique involves placement of coil springs between the cuspids and lateral incisors and if needed between the lateral incisors and central incisors to open spaces (Figure 55-19). At the end of treatment the lateral incisors can be built up by bonding, veneers, or crowns. This technique can also be used in the mandibular arch when the mandibular anterior teeth are too small compared to the maxillary anterior teeth. In either arch this technique is most applicable when the teeth are decreased in angulation, since opening space will increase the axial inclination of the incisors. It may not be indicated when the maxillary or mandibular incisors are overangulated or crowded, as

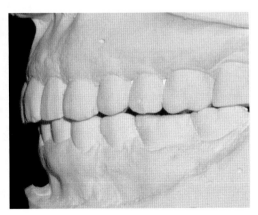

FIGURE 55-17 *This patient has well-aligned and leveled teeth in each arch. Maxillary lateral incisors are small creating a tooth-size discrepancy (TSD). Note that with the best possible fit, the patient has an end-on Class II occlusal relationship secondary to the TSD.*

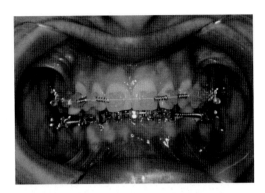

FIGURE **55-19** *Placing coil springs between the maxillary cuspids and lateral incisors as well as the lateral incisors and central incisors can open up spacing around the lateral incisors to correct a tooth-size discrepancy. Post-treatment, the lateral incisors can be built up by bonding, veneers, or crowns.*

the resultant increased angulation may be unstable and cause untoward periodontal changes. However, if there is significant crowding or overangulation of the incisors requiring extraction of bicuspids, during closure of the bicuspid spacing by retraction of the anterior teeth, space could be created around the lateral incisors.

When maxillary incisors are already overangulated, it is not feasible to open spaces during the presurgical orthodontics. In this situation performing interdental osteotomies between the maxillary cuspids and lateral incisors will permit opening space at surgery and the incisors can also be uprighted to decrease their axial angulation. A maximum 3 mm of spacing (1.5 mm on each side) can usually be acquired with this approach.

When the TSD occurs in the bicuspid or molar area, space can be opened around the maxillary bicuspids and/or molars to compensate for the tooth mass deficiency. Bonding, veneers, or crowns can then be placed to eliminate the created space.

Altering Axial Inclination of Incisors This technique can affect the labial circumference of the anterior teeth. Increased axial inclination slightly increases the arch length, and decreased axial inclination slightly decreases it. Application of this technique would result in

increasing the maxillary incisors' angulation above normal and decreasing the mandibular incisors' angulation below normal. This technique can accommodate small TSD differences, but may place the teeth in a compromised position relative to stability and esthetics.

Surgery can alter the axial inclination of the anterior teeth. In the maxillary arch, interdental osteotomies between the lateral incisors and cuspids, and in the mandibular arch anterior subapical osteotomies, will provide a means to alter axial inclination of the incisors.

Altering Mesiodistal Angulation of Maxillary Incisors Tipping the roots of the maxillary central incisors distally away from each other alters the position of the contact points, making the intercontact distance on each tooth slightly wider. This can only be used for small differences. However, it then usually requires recontouring of the distal aspect of the incisor edges and could cause a soft tissue void between the mesial contact points and gingival tissues ("the black triangle"), creating much concern for the patient. This technique is rarely recommended.

Extraction of Mandibular Incisor This technique should only be used for large TSDs (5 mm or more) and only if there is significant crowding and/or significant overangulation of the mandibular incisors. Removing a mandibular incisor usually creates a significant space (the width of the tooth), and closure of that space may significantly decrease the axial inclination of the mandibular incisors. In addition it may cause a decreased transverse width between the cuspids resulting in relative narrowing of both maxillary and mandibular arches. Extraction of a mandibular incisor may produce an increased overjet. If the patient has a good maxillary arch but mandibular crowding and overangulation, large TSD, and an end-on or slight Class III anterior

occlusion, the single mandibular incisor extraction may be the treatment of choice. An alternative in cases with large tooth-size discrepancies would be to slenderize the mandibular anterior teeth and create spacing around the maxillary lateral incisors.

A surgical alternative for a large TSD, when the teeth are not crowded and have good axial angulation, would be to extract the mandibular incisor and perform a vertical ostectomy through the mandible at the extraction site and rotate the segments together to eliminate the extraction space (Figure 55-20). This would prevent further decreased angulation of the incisors with subsequent orthodontics but may narrow the anterior aspect of the mandible.

Correct Overangulated (Proclined) and/or Crowded Maxillary Anterior Teeth

Overangulated and/or crowded maxillary anterior teeth are most commonly seen in patients with maxillary deficiency (hypoplasia). The following treatment methods can be used to correct this type of situation.

Slenderizing and Retraction This technique involves removal of tooth structure at the contact points and is applicable when there is a rare reverse TSD with the maxillary anterior teeth too large for the mandibular anterior teeth. Usually up to 3 mm of tooth structure can be safely removed from the contact area of the maxillary anterior six teeth with a margin of 50% of enamel remaining at the contact areas. However, this could make the maxillary incisors slightly smaller in size unless they are significantly oversized to begin with.

Extraction and Retraction First or second bicuspids can be extracted depending on the amount of crowding, the anchorage requirements, and the amount of retraction of the incisors necessary.

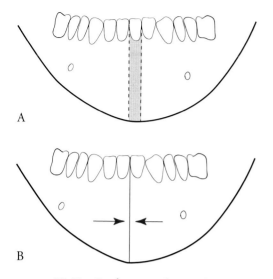

FIGURE 55-20 *In the case of a tooth-size discrepancy (TSD) ≥ 5 mm, in the presence of well-aligned teeth in proper angulation, the TSD can be managed by removing a mandibular central incisor and performing a vertical midline ostectomy (A) with closure of that space (B) and stabilization with a bone plate.*

Every 1 mm of incisor retraction will require 1 mm of space on each side of the arch. Therefore, if the orthodontic goal is to retract the maxillary incisors by 3 mm, then 6 mm of maxillary arch space will be required to accomplish this. Extracting first bicuspids will result in greater incisor retraction, whereas six multirooted posterior dental units (compared to six single-rooted anterior dental units) provide greater posterior anchorage. Extracting second bicuspids will result in less incisor retraction, whereas four posterior dental units (compared to eight anterior units) provide less posterior anchorage so that the posterior teeth will move forward a greater amount compared with first bicuspid extractions. The occlusal plane angle will also affect the posterior anchorage. Low occlusal plane angle cases will have greater posterior anchorage stability, even with second bicuspid extraction, than will high occlusal plane angle cases. High occlusal plane angle cases will have less posterior anchorage stability, even with first bicuspid extraction, than low occlusal plane angle cases. These factors are probably related to bite force influences. The amount of crowding may also influence which teeth to extract.

Distalizing Posterior Teeth   This objective can be accomplished using pendulum-type appliances, headgear, class II mechanics, or osseointegrated implants (ie, implants posterior to molars, zygomatic implants, palatal implants, or buccal cortex implants). Distalizing maxillary posterior teeth can be augmented with class II mechanics but should only be used short-term and discontinued several months prior to surgery to minimize postsurgical skeletal relapse potential that can occur with the use of long-term class II mechanics and the subsequent adverse effects on the TMJs. Another option is to distalize one tooth at a time on each side of the arch, beginning with the second molars (2 teeth moved against 12 anchor teeth). Another feasible approach is to use osseointegrated anchors to distalize the maxillary arch, with implants placed in either the zygoma buttress, posterior to second molars, or attached to the buccal cortex. The implants can be left submerged after orthodontic treatment is completed, or could require additional surgery for removal if not removed during the orthognathic surgery.

Anterior Maxillary Segmental Osteotomies   This technique permits uprighting of the anterior teeth but will cause the apical base of the segment to shift forward relative to the incisor edges unless teeth are extracted to reposition the incisal edges of the anterior teeth posteriorly. Careful assessment of the profile esthetics is necessary to determine if the patient can esthetically benefit from this change. The interdental osteotomies should be done between the lateral incisors and cuspids as this offers the best control in uprighting the segments (Figure 55-21) and also allows opening of space between the lateral incisors (up to 3 mm with 1.5 mm per side) that can be used for correction of crowding or TSD.

Maxillary Expansion by Orthodontics, Orthopedics (Rapid Palatal Expansion), and Surgically Assisted Rapid Palatal Expansion   These techniques will increase arch length and may allow retraction of the anterior teeth. However, they will also increase the curve of Wilson as the transverse width of the maxillary arch increases because the teeth will expand three times as much as the palate expands (Figure 55-22). In addition, with SARPE, the palate moves inferiorly. The expanded arches may not be as orthodontically stable, requiring long-term or permanent retention.

Correct Overangulated (Proclined) and/or Crowded Mandibular Anterior Teeth

Overangulated and/or crowded mandibular teeth occur most often with mandibular deficiency (hypoplasia). The following

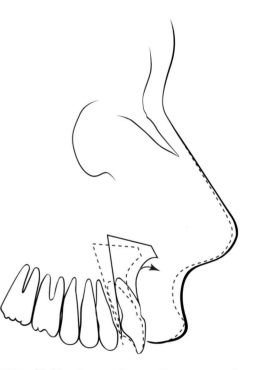

FIGURE 55-21 *An anterior maxillary segmental osteotomy can be used to upright the maxillary incisors. However, the dentoalveolus at the apical base will rotate anteriorly if no teeth are extracted. Since this may affect the position of the nose and upper lip, careful evaluation of facial esthetics is necessary to determine if this approach is appropriate. Dashed line represents the original position of the anterior maxilla, and the solid line represents the uprighted segment.*

treatment options can be used to correct these types of conditions.

Slenderizing and Retraction This technique involves removal of tooth structure at the contact points and is most applicable when there is a TSD with the mandibular anterior teeth being too large for the maxillary anterior teeth. Up to 3 mm of tooth structure can be safely removed from the contact areas of the mandibular anterior six teeth with a margin of 50% of enamel remaining at the contact areas. Subsequent retraction will decrease the axial inclination of the incisors providing that no major crowding is present.

Extraction and Retraction First or second bicuspids can be extracted depending on the degree of angulation, amount of crowding, the anchorage requirements, and the amount of retraction of the incisors necessary. Every 1 mm of incisor retraction will require 1 mm of space on each side of the arch. Therefore, if the orthodontic goal is to retract the mandibular incisors by 3 mm, then 6 mm of mandibular arch space will be required to accomplish this. Extracting first bicuspids will result in greater incisor retraction, whereas six multirooted posterior dental units (compared with six single-rooted anterior dental units) provide greater posterior anchorage. Extracting the second bicuspids will result in less incisor retraction, whereas four posterior dental units (compared with eight anterior units) provide less posterior anchorage, so that the posterior teeth will move forward a greater amount compared with first bicuspid extractions. The occlusal plane angle will also affect the posterior anchorage. Low occlusal plane angle cases will have greater posterior anchorage stability, even with second bicuspid extraction, than will high occlusal plane angle cases. High occlusal plane angle cases will have less posterior anchorage stability even with first bicuspid extraction than low angle cases. These factors are probably related to bite force influences. The amount of crowding may also influence which teeth to extract. If there is a large TSD ($\geq$ 5 mm), then extraction of a mandibular incisor could be considered.

Distalize Posterior Teeth The mechanics to accomplish this include intra-arch, inter-arch, extraoral, or implant mechanics. Class III mechanics (ie, elastics, headgear) can be used to distalize the mandibular teeth, but may increase loading on the TMJs and could initiate TMJ problems. Another option is to distalize one tooth at a time on each side of the arch, beginning with the second molars (2 teeth moved against 12 anchor teeth). However, this technique takes a lot of time. The placement of dental implants posterior to the molar teeth or in the posterior buccal cortex could facilitate retraction without appreciably increasing the load to the TMJs.

Anterior Mandibular Subapical Osteotomies This technique permits uprighting of the anterior teeth, but will cause the apical base of the segment to shift forward relative to the chin (Figure 55-23), unless teeth are extracted at the time of surgery to reposition the incisal edges of the anterior teeth posteriorly.

Bilateral Mandibular Body Osteotomies This technique will permit uprighting of the anterior teeth and forward rotation of the chin (Figure 55-24), unless teeth are extracted. Without extraction, bilateral body bone grafting will be required to provide bony continuity between the segments and facilitate healing. This technique would only be indicated if the chin is anteroposteriorly deficient before surgery.

Mandibular Symphysis Distraction Osteogenesis This technique, usually performed with a midline vertical osteotomy, will allow expansion of the dentoalveolus and widening of the mandibular arch,

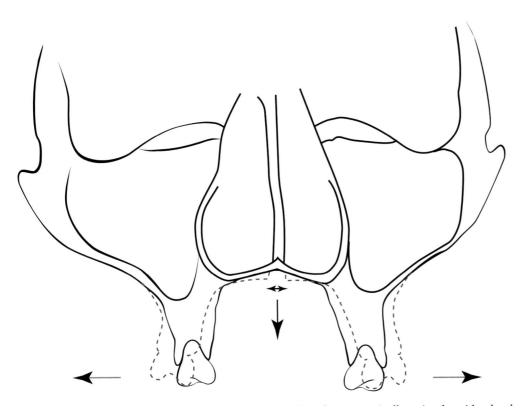

FIGURE **55-22** *Maxillary expansion by orthodontics, orthopedics, or surgically assisted rapid palatal expansion (SARPE) will cause an increase of the curve of Wilson. Even with SARPE, the occlusal surface will expand three times as much as the palate will expand, thus increasing the curve of Wilson. The palate will also move inferiorly.*

providing room to retract and/or align the teeth. This is an excellent treatment method to gain space for major arch length discrepancies. However, it is done as a prerequisite surgery to achieve the orthodontic goals prior to the major orthognathic surgery. Orthodontic preparation may be necessary prior to performing the midline vertical osteotomy. The roots of the central incisors (or the adjacent teeth, wherever the osteotomy is to be performed) must be tipped away from each other to make room for the interdental osteotomy. This can be accomplished by placing the mesial aspect of the bracket higher than the distal aspect on each of the central incisors. Placing a short segment straight arch wire will then tip the roots distally, creating space to safely perform the vertical interdental osteotomy (Figure 55-25). If a tooth-borne distraction device is used, orthodontic treatment on any other teeth should *not* be initiated until adequate healing of the distraction area has occurred (approximately 4 months from initiation of the distraction). Otherwise it may result in developing dental mobility and orthodontic instability, with the teeth expanding more than the basal bone. This can result in transverse dental

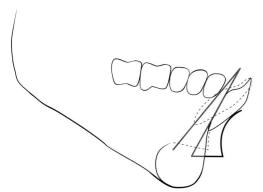

FIGURE 55-23 *The anterior mandibular subapical osteotomy can be used to upright the mandibular anterior teeth, causing the apical base of the segment to shift forward relative to the chin, if teeth (bicuspids) are not extracted at the time of surgery. This may or may not be a desired outcome. A chin augmentation may be required to achieve optimal esthetics.*

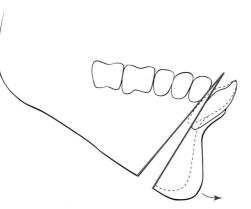

FIGURE 55-24 *Bilateral body osteotomies can be used to upright the mandibular anterior teeth, but the chin will rotate forward unless teeth are extracted. A gap created in the mandibular body area will require grafting unless teeth are extracted (first bicuspids) to allow the mandibular anterior teeth to move posteriorly, thus decreasing the forward movement of the chin.*

relapse postdistraction with less expansion of the dental arch than desired. Bone-borne devices are not affected by predistraction orthodontics.

Correct Underangulated (Retroclined) Maxillary Incisors

Underangulated maxillary incisors are most commonly seen in Class II Division 2 malocclusions or with missing teeth in the arch. The following approaches can be used to correct this type of condition.

Correct Crowding Crowding of the maxillary anterior teeth can accompany vertically inclined teeth. Therefore, correcting the crowding will increase the incisor angulation.

Open Space In Class I and Class II patients underangulated incisors may be present because of previous extractions (ie, bicuspids), congenitally missing teeth, previous trauma resulting in loss of teeth, or small maxillary anterior teeth (ie, small maxillary lateral incisors). Opening space in the bicuspid areas, if the problem exists there, can correct this problem and provide additional dental units for a more complete occlusal

result. The use of coil springs usually works well for this situation. If the problem is in the lateral incisor area, opening space can help correct the TSD as well as increase the incisor angulation (Figure 55-26).

Interarch Mechanics The use of class III mechanics (ie, elastics) can increase maxillary incisor angulation. However, the class III mechanics can be detrimental by overloading the TMJs.

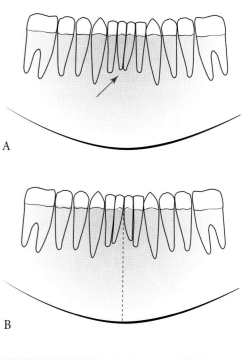

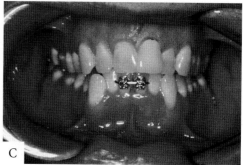

FIGURE 55-25 *Mandibular symphysis distraction osteogenesis. A, Often the incisor roots are very close together. B, Space must be created between the roots of teeth adjacent to the intended vertical osteotomy. C, Placing brackets on only the central incisors with the mesial aspect of the brackets higher than the distal aspect on each tooth and placing a short straight wire segment, will tip the roots distally away from each other, creating space to perform the vertical interdental osteotomy.*

Interdental Osteotomies An anterior maxillary subapical osteotomy or segmentalized Le Fort I osteotomy will permit rotation of the anterior teeth to increase their angulation. However, significant room must be created between the roots of the adjacent teeth (lateral incisors and cuspids) at the osteotomy areas. Since bone removal between the teeth may be required, there is an increased risk of damage to the adjacent teeth. If the maxilla requires surgical expansion, then segmentalization between the lateral incisors and cuspids will allow the anterior segment to rotate posteriorly between the expanded posterior segments with fewer requirements for bone removal, if required at all.

Correct Underangulated (Retroclined) Mandibular Incisors

Underangulated mandibular incisors are more commonly seen in patients with prognathic mandibles or with missing teeth. The following treatment methods can be used to correct this condition.

Correct Crowding Crowding of the mandibular anterior teeth often accompanies vertically inclined teeth. Therefore, correcting the crowding will increase the incisor angulation.

Open Space In Class I and Class II patients underangulated incisors may be present because of previous extractions, congenitally missing teeth, previous trauma resulting in loss of teeth, or small mandibular teeth. In Class III patients underangulated incisors may be present due to an excessive amount of alveolar bone compared with the size of the teeth. If bicuspids are missing, opening space in the bicuspid areas can correct this problem and provide additional dental units for a more complete occlusal result. The use of coil springs usually works well for this situation (see Figure 55-26).

Occasionally a mandibular incisor may be missing for various reasons. Viable options include opening appropriate space around the remaining three incisors and building up the crowns by bonding, veneers, or crowns. This technique works best if there is a TSD that is less than the width of the missing tooth. However, the maxillary dental midline will be in the center of a mandibular incisor. Another option would be to open space in the area of the missing tooth and then replace it with a dental implant or bridge. This technique may work best when there is no TSD with a full-size dental replacement.

Interarch Mechanics The use of class II mechanics (ie, elastics, Herbst's appliance) can increase mandibular incisor angulation. However, long-term class II mechanics can be detrimental to outcome stability and results, because of the potential untoward effects on the TMJs.

Interdental Osteotomies An anterior subapical osteotomy or bilateral anterior body osteotomies will permit rotation of the anterior teeth to increase their angulation. However, significant room must be created between the roots of the teeth adjacent to the osteotomy areas. Since bone removal between the teeth may be required, there is an increased risk of damage to the adjacent teeth.

Correct Excess Curve of Spee: Maxillary Arch

This condition is most often seen with anterior open-bite situations and high occlusal plane facial types. Careful assessment of the curve of Spee is important because using only orthodontic mechanics to correct this condition may not be very stable. An increased curve of Spee usually makes it difficult to get the occlusion to fit together. The condition can be addressed by the following treatment options.

Extruding Anterior Teeth Conventional orthodontics with straight wire techniques will tend to extrude the anterior teeth, and as a byproduct will tip the molars buccally, increasing the curve of Wilson. These dental changes may be unstable and fraught with relapse potential.

Intruding Midbuccal Teeth This is a very difficult technique, unless high-pull headgear or osseointegrated implants are used to provide intrusive forces. This would

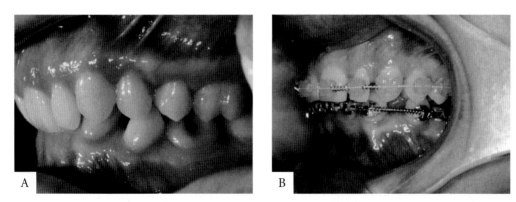

FIGURE 55-26 *Coil springs to open space. In some cases, "retroclined" incisors are a result of Division 2 malocclusion, crowding, missing dental units, or small teeth. If there is no significant crowding, spacing can be created by the use of coil springs that will tip the incisors forward. A, Small maxillary lateral incisors and missing mandibular bicuspids. B, The use of coiled springs is demonstrated to open up interdental spaces around the maxillary lateral incisor (to correct for an anterior tooth-size discrepancy) and in the mandibular first bicuspid area (to replace a missing dental unit and increase the angulation of the anterior teeth). The spaces around the maxillary lateral incisor can be eliminated by bonding, veneer, or crown. In the mandibular arch, the space can be eliminated by surgical ostectomy versus replacement of the missing dental unit by crown-and-bridge or osseointegrated implant and crown.*

require significant patient compliance and is not a commonly applied procedure.

Extraction and Retraction Extraction of maxillary first or second bicuspids with retraction will usually decrease the curve of Spee, providing the incisors are overangulated to begin with.

Orthodontic, Orthopedic, or Surgically Assisted Rapid Palatal Expansion with Retraction Expansion of the maxillary arch by any of these techniques will increase the arch length and allow some retraction of the anterior teeth. In late adolescence or adulthood, SARPE may provide better stability than the other two techniques. However, note that the curve of Wilson will increase because the expansion at the occlusal level compared with the palate will be a 3:1 ratio.[19]

Surgical Correction The maxilla can be orthodontically aligned in segments by aligning the four incisors at a different level, compared with the posterior teeth, to avoid extrusion, intrusion, and buccal tipping of teeth. Placing compensating vertical steps between the lateral incisors and cuspids (see Figure 55-15A) will accomplish alignment at different levels. For some cases the vertical positional difference may occur between the cuspids and bicuspids, or could occur asymmetrically on one side of the arch compared with the other side. The step in the arch would then be made between the appropriate teeth. Another technique to use involves cutting the arch wire into two or more segments and aligning groups of teeth in individual units (see Figure 55-15B). However, it may be more difficult to control rotations and root position, particularly of the teeth adjacent to the ends of the segmented wires, compared with using a continuous wire with compensating vertical steps. The arch can then be leveled surgically with a three-piece maxilla performing osteotomies between the lateral

incisors and cuspids. The three-piece Le Fort I osteotomy, with interdental osteotomies performed between the lateral incisors and cuspids, will permit repositioning of the anterior segment independent of the posterior segments (Figure 55-27). The anterior segment can be reoriented vertically and anteroposteriorly, and the axial inclination of the incisors can be changed to correct the curve of Spee and achieve the best interdigitation of the segments.

Correct Accentuated Curve of Spee: Mandibular Arch

An accentuated curve of Spee in the mandibular arch most often occurs in anterior deep-bite relationships.

Intruding Mandibular Anterior Teeth Intrusion mechanics can predictably inferiorly position mandibular anterior teeth approximately 2 mm. Beyond 2 mm the vertical relapse approaches 60%. With accentuated curves of Spee the contact area of the teeth will be at a different level

where the teeth are more narrow, below the normal contact level. Therefore, for every 1 mm of leveling of the mandibular arch, the mandibular incisor edges will move forward 0.6 mm to 1 mm as the contact points align. Any crowding of the arch will further contribute to flaring of the incisors. Intruding teeth will decrease the anterior mandibular vertical height and must also be taken into consideration so that the anterior mandibular height is not excessively shortened.

Extruding Midbuccal Teeth Extrusion of midbuccal teeth may be more stable than intrusion of anterior teeth. However, this technique is difficult to perform without special considerations. If the patient's malocclusion has the bicuspids and first molars in occlusion, extrusion will be virtually impossible. However, constructing a splint that will open the bite and engage only the mandibular anterior teeth and second molars, with the bicuspids and first molars out of contact with the splint, will permit extrusion

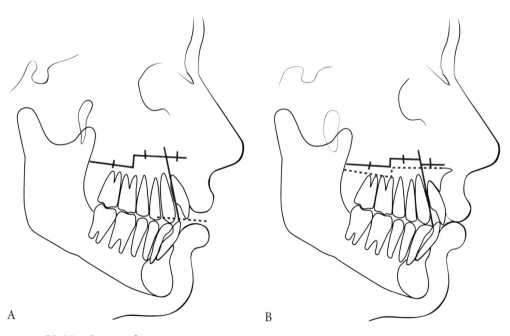

A   B

FIGURE 55-27 *Surgery for correcting an excessive curve of Spee. A, Aligning the maxilla in segments with the incisors at an elevated level compared with the posterior teeth will permit interdental osteotomies to be performed. B, Surgical leveling of the occlusal plane from a predictability and stability standpoint is superior to orthodontic means alone, particularly when no extractions are performed.*

of the midbuccal teeth. Another alternative would be to correct the accentuated curve of Spee after the mandible and occlusion are surgically repositioned, placing the incisors and molars into proper contact, and then extrude the midbuccal teeth postsurgery. With this approach the molars may tip distally and the arch may widen somewhat.

Interdental Osteotomies An anterior subapical osteotomy (Figure 55-28) or bilateral anterior body osteotomies (Figure 55-29) will permit downward repositioning of the anterior teeth, with very stable results when the surgery is properly performed. If the anterior vertical height of the mandible is excessive, then the subapical osteotomy would be indicated since it will shorten the anterior mandibular height by the amount that the incisors are lowered. Bilateral anterior body osteotomies would be indicated when the vertical height of the anterior mandible is normal or less, so that the anterior height remains unaltered while the curve of Spee is corrected.

Correct Reverse Curve of Spee: Maxillary Arch

Reverse curves of Spee are more commonly seen in Division 2 malocclusions and in vertical maxillary deficiencies with an anterior deep bite. The maxillary incisors are commonly in a decreased axial inclination. Crowding may or may not be present.

Correct Crowding or Division 2 Relations Eliminating crowding and Division 2 dental positions will tip the incisors forward, increasing the incisor axial angulation and decreasing the reverse curve of Spee. These movements will usually fill out the upper lip, but may decrease the maxillary tooth-to-lip relationship. Maxillary incisors may become intruded with a straight wire technique.

Extruding Midbuccal Teeth This technique is difficult if the midbuccal teeth are

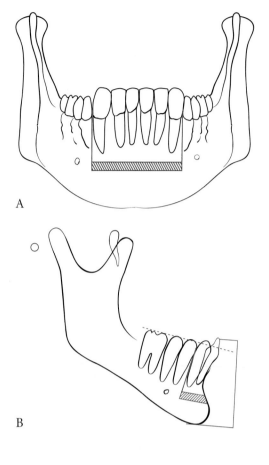

A

B

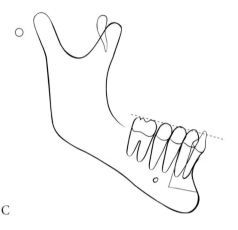

C

FIGURE 55-28 *Subapical osteotomy correcting an accentuated curve of Spee in the mandibular arch. A, This can be accomplished with a subapical osteotomy composed of two interdental osteotomies and a subapical ostectomy to set the anterior teeth inferiorly. B, C, This is indicated when the anterior mandibular height is greater than normal, as this technique will shorten the anterior mandibular height. This same basic technique can be used to elevate the segment to correct a reverse curve of Spee.*

in occlusion with mandibular teeth. However, the bite can be opened with a splint that affords contact on only the maxillary second molars and anterior teeth, with the maxillary midbuccal teeth out of contact with the splint. The midbuccal teeth (bicuspids and first molars) can then be extruded into position to improve the curve of Spee.

Open Spaces If the reverse curve of Spee is related to missing teeth or TSDs, then spaces can be opened to aid in increasing the axial inclination of the incisors and decreasing the reverse curve of Spee. These spaces can then be eliminated by bonding, crown and bridge, or dental implants and crowns.

Interdental Osteotomies Multiple maxillary osteotomies can be performed so that the maxilla can be repositioned in segments, enabling leveling of the arch. Presurgical orthodontics should be designed to align

the teeth at different vertical levels to facilitate the surgery and minimize orthodontic relapse potential. It is usually easiest and most applicable to make the osteotomies between the lateral incisors and cuspids. This may particularly be indicated when the maxilla must be repositioned anyway and maxillary expansion is also required. Performing a three-piece segmented maxillary osteotomy will then allow vertical alteration between the anterior and posterior segments to level the curve of Spee.

Correct Reverse Curve of Spee: Mandibular Arch

This condition is most commonly seen in patients with macroglossia, habitual tongue posturing, or tongue thrust, with an associated anterior open bite. The following techniques can be used to correct this type of condition.

Extruing Anterior Teeth Extrusion of anterior teeth may not be very stable long

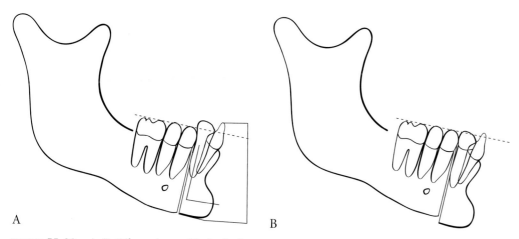

FIGURE 55-29   A, B, *Bilateral mandibular body osteotomies will permit leveling of the excessive curve of Spee without shortening the vertical height of the mandible and are indicated when the mandibular anterior dental height is normal or even slightly short vertically. This basic technique can also be used to correct a reverse curve of Spee by elevating the anterior segment.*

term, and without permanent retention, could result in re-intrusion and redevelopment of an anterior open bite.

Intrusion of Midbuccal Teeth   This is a difficult technique but may be accomplished with osseointegrated implants as anchors. However, it is not known if this would be stable long term.

Extract and Retract   If the mandibular incisors are significantly overangulated, with or without crowding, bicuspid extractions can be performed and the incisors retracted, which will decrease the reverse curve of Spee.

Bonding the Mandibular Anteriors   This technique can be used to level the arch by building up the incisors, increasing the crown height. However, care must be taken not to exceed a safe crown-root ratio and/or create an esthetic compromise.

Interdental Osteotomies   Anterior subapical (see Figure 55-28) or anterior bilateral mandibular body osteotomies (see Figure 55-29) can be used to elevate the anterior teeth. If the anterior mandibular height is short, then the subapical osteotomy can also be used to increase the anterior height of the mandible. If the anterior

mandibular height is normal, then the bilateral anterior body osteotomies will permit elevation of the anterior teeth while maintaining the anterior height of the mandible.

Anteroposterior Arch Asymmetry (Maxilla or Mandible)

Anteroposterior arch asymmetry, when the cuspid on one side of the arch is anterior to the cuspid on the opposite side of the arch, is fairly common in patients with dentofacial deformities. Arch asymmetries can be related to developmental abnormalities, missing teeth, or ankylosed teeth. Dental midlines may not align with the facial midline.

Extract Unilaterally   In some cases unilateral extraction and retraction will correct the problem. The decision must be made as to which tooth to extract. Extraction of a first bicuspid will allow greater anterior retraction compared with extracting a second bicuspid. This extraction would only be indicated if there were significant overangulation of the incisors, crowding, and/or significant midline dental shift.

Open Space Unilaterally   This technique would be indicated if a tooth is missing,

there is significant decreased angulation of the incisors, and/or the midline is significantly deviated to one side.

Interarch Mechanics   This technique can be effectively used by incorporating class II mechanics on one side and class III mechanics on the opposite side. Anterior cross-arch elastics can also be helpful. If only one arch is involved, then maximizing anchorage in the other arch is very important so that an asymmetry does not develop in the normal arch. Osseointegrated implants can be used as anchors to correct asymmetry in an arch without having to use interarch mechanics.

Osteotomies   Osteotomies can be used in the maxillary arch by segmentalization of the maxilla and advancing one side more than the other side. Osteotomies in the mandibular arch to correct arch asymmetry can become somewhat complex. Anterior subapical osteotomies with removal of a unilateral tooth can correct some large discrepancies (6 to 9 mm). However, the subapical osteotomy may need to be combined with ramus sagittal split osteotomies and a unilateral or bilateral body osteotomy, with or without extraction, to shift the occlusion into a symmetric position. These types of movements require a high degree of surgical skill, but can provide high-quality outcomes.

Divergence of Roots Adjacent to Interdental Surgical Sites

When interdental osteotomies are planned it may be necessary for the orthodontist to tip the adjacent tooth roots away from the area of the planned osteotomy to prevent damage to the teeth (Figure 55-30). If the roots are too close together, postsurgical periodontal problems may develop with possible loss of interdental bone and teeth. Creating interdental space between the roots significantly improves the margin of safety. This can be easily achieved by selective bracket placement. For the tooth mesial to the osteotomy, the bracket is slightly rotated so that the mesial aspect of the bracket is positioned slightly more gingivally compared with the distal aspect of the bracket (Figure 55-31). Conversely the distal tooth bracket is positioned so that the distal aspect of the bracket is placed slightly more gingivally compared with the mesial aspect of the bracket. With a straight wire technique the roots will diverge.

Postsurgically, periapical radiography may be necessary for the orthodontist to check for rebonding the adjacent teeth brackets to ensure proper root angulation at completion of treatment.

Extraction Versus Nonextraction

The decision to extract or not to extract can sometimes be difficult. There are a number of factors that may contribute to this determination.

Overangulated Anterior Teeth Excessive over-angulated anterior teeth may require extraction to set the teeth over basal bone. However, if the arch is to be expanded or teeth slenderized for TSD, for example, then extraction may not be necessary.

Crowding This is a common indicator, particularly with major crowding or overangulated teeth. However, if crowding is mild to moderate, widening of the arch or teeth slenderizing for TSD may eliminate the need for extraction.

Tooth-Size Discrepancy TSDs of significant magnitude may indicate the need for extraction, particularly if the TSD of the anterior mandibular teeth is 5 mm or greater and the mandibular incisors are overangulated and/or crowded, in which case a mandibular incisor extraction could be considered.

Curve of Spee Accentuated curves of Spee in the maxillary arch usually have overangulated maxillary incisors, and reverse curves of Spee in the mandibular arch usually have overangulated mandibular incisors. Extraction of bilateral first or second bicuspids and retraction will result in leveling of the arches. However, arch expansion, when indicated, may create enough room so that extractions are not necessary.

Arch Asymmetries With significant anteroposterior arch asymmetries, unilateral or bilateral asymmetric extractions (ie, first bicuspid on one side and a second bicuspid on the opposite side) may be indicated when there is coexisting crowding overangulated incisors, or midline shift.

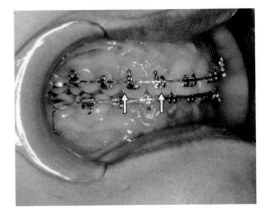

FIGURE **55-31** *Selective bracket placement can create adequate interdental space for osteotomies. On the tooth mesial to the osteotomy, slightly rotate the mesial aspect of the bracket gingivally, and on the distal tooth, slightly rotate the distal aspect of the bracket gingivally. A straight wire will then diverge the roots.*

Coordination of Maxillary and Mandibular Arch Widths

In some cases transverse arch width discrepancies can be corrected with stable and predictable orthodontic movements, but in other cases orthodontic correction may be very unstable and fraught with relapse. It must be determined whether to correct width problems by orthodontics, orthopedics, SARPE, or surgical expansion. Even with SARPE using a fixed device, the palate only expands approximately one-third the amount of the expansion that occurs at the occlusal level, thus increasing the curve of Wilson.[19] For example, if the maxilla is expanded with SARPE and the expansion at the occlusal level is 6 mm, then the expansion at the palatal level will only be 2 mm (see Figure 55-22). Patients with reverse curves of Wilson in the maxillary arch may benefit more from these techniques, but those with a pretreatment accentuated curve of Wilson may have unfavorable results, with subsequent difficulty getting the buccal cuspids to interdigitate. The following predictable changes will occur with maxillary arch expansion by orthodontic, orthopedic, or SARPE procedures.

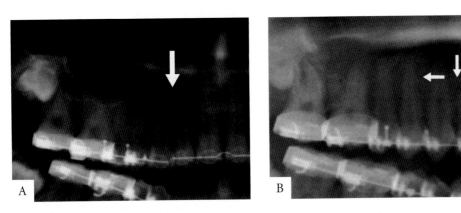

FIGURE **55-30** *Interdental osteotomies. A, Pantomogram demonstrating inadequate room between the roots of the lateral incisors and cuspids. Performing osteotomies with roots in this position could result in severe periodontal compromise and possible loss of teeth. B, Adequate spaces for interdental osteotomies can be created by selective bracket placement on the adjacent teeth.*

1. The bite may open anteriorly, particularly if the maxillary incisors have significant initial vertical inclination. If the maxillary incisors are overangulated, then the bite may deepen anteriorly as the spacing is closed.

2. Buccal tipping of the maxillary posterior teeth will increase the curve of Wilson, because the lingual cusps will move downward relative to the buccal cusps. This may make it very difficult to properly interdigitate the buccal cusps orthodontically. Therefore, these techniques are not recommended, especially when there is a preexisting accentuated curve of Wilson.

3. Long-term or perhaps permanent retention may be necessary to counterbalance the orthodontic relapse potential seen in a high percentage of these patients.

4. In late adolescent and adult patients, SARPE will likely be necessary to expand the maxilla orthopedically since the midpalatal suture is usually closed.

Surgical expansion of the maxilla at the time of the Le Fort I procedure using multiple segmentation of the maxilla, stabilization with bone plates and palatal or occlusal splints, and hydroxyapatite synthetic bone grafting in the palate and lateral maxillary walls can provide a good outcome. This technique when properly performed is very stable and eliminates the orthodontic relapse potential inherent with the other techniques.

Missing Teeth

Teeth can be missing from the arches for a number of reasons such as congenital absence, uneruption, previous orthodontic extractions, extractions for periodontal or dental pathology, and trauma. In some cases (ie, congenital absence of maxillary lateral incisors, previous inappropriate bicuspid extraction) opening space to accommodate replacement teeth may be indicated. This is most applicable when the incisors are decreased in angulation without appreciable crowding. If the incisors are already overangulated and/or crowding is present, then opening space orthodontically may be detrimental to stability and periodontal health. In this situation with missing maxillary lateral incisors, the cuspids can be used as lateral incisors, but may require considerable recontouring to esthetically and functionally conform to lateral incisor morphology. Although this cuspid substitution can work well for missing lateral incisors, it is done less frequently now that dental implants are so predictable and successful, thereby allowing the canine to be placed in its normal and more functional position.

When conditions permit, opening space for replacement teeth can be accomplished by appropriate mechanics to achieve the required space. Surgery can also be used to create spacing in some areas. In the mandibular arch, distraction osteogenesis can be used to create space. The missing teeth can then be replaced with dental implants, bridges, or partial dentures for example.

Correction of Rotated Teeth

Bracket placement and arch wire adaptation are the primary keys to correcting rotated teeth and it is usually best to achieve these corrections presurgery. However, if the malrotations do not interfere with the establishment of the desired dentoskeletal relationship, then the rotations can be corrected postsurgery. Severe rotations may require supracrestal fiberotomy to prevent relapse and improve permanent retention. This can often be done at the time of orthognathic surgery.

Management of Ankylosed Teeth

Treatment of ankylosed teeth depends on (1) whether the tooth is primary or permanent, (2) the surrounding dentition, (3) the eruption status, (4) tooth position and orientation, (5) the time of onset and diagnosis, (6) the age of the patient and, (7) the treatment goals.

Ankylosed Primary Tooth This can impede the development and eruption of the permanent successor. If a primary tooth has a permanent successor, treatment is immediate extraction followed by space maintenance until the permanent tooth erupts. If no permanent successor is present and the primary tooth ankylosis occurs at an early stage in jaw growth and development with submergence of the tooth eminent, treatment includes extraction and space maintenance.[20] If the ankylosis occurs late with no permanent successor, the occlusal and proximal contacts can be reestablished with restorative dentistry to provide esthetics and function with perhaps many years of service.[21]

It is important to diagnose and treat the ankylosed tooth before the adolescent growth phase. Retaining an ankylosed tooth during jaw growth leads to arrested development of the alveolar ridge. The severity of alveolar growth loss depends on the amount of facial growth left at the time that the ankylosis occurs. Timing the removal of an ankylosed tooth just at the start of the pubertal phase of adolescent growth may achieve the treatment objective of maintaining alveolar ridge height while allowing the tooth to remain long enough to act as a space maintainer and esthetic temporary.[22]

Ankylosed Permanent Tooth An unrecognized ankylosed permanent tooth tied into the arch wire can result in a significant malocclusion (Figure 55-32). There are several ways of treating the permanent ankylosed tooth. If ankylosis of the permanent tooth has an early onset during eruption, the tooth should be luxated, allowing for further eruption.[2] If repeated luxation proves ineffective, the tooth should be extracted to prevent submergence. If the onset of ankylosis occurs late in the normal eruption pattern, the tooth should be luxated. If the attempt is

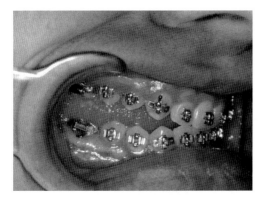

FIGURE 55-32 *An ankylosed first molar tied into the arch wire has prevented development of the alveolus and consequently created a significant posterior open bite.*

unsuccessful and the tooth does not submerge, it may be vertically restored on growth maturity. A composite build-up or crown can be added to a partially erupted ankylosed tooth to level and align the arch.[21] A deeply unerupted ankylosed tooth, primary or permanent, may be left undisturbed unless it is infected, alters the alveolar bone growth potential, or constitutes an immediate threat to the occlusion or adjacent teeth, or would impede the placement of an osseointegrated implant.[3]

Other treatment options include extraction followed by reimplantation, osseointegrated implant, or prosthetic replacement.[23] The patient's developmental age is very important in considering replacing an ankylosed tooth with an osseointegrated implant. The implant will have the same effect on growth of the alveolar ridge as the ankylosed tooth, and therefore should be considered for placement after alveolar growth is essentially complete.[24]

Proffit suggests surgical luxation of the tooth with extraction forceps disrupting the cementum-bone fusion followed by immediate orthodontic traction to move the tooth into position.[20] Luxation involves breaking the bony bridge of ankylosis without damaging the apical nutrient vessels. This procedure forms fibrous inflammation tissue in the reparative process. This tissue forms a false periodontal membrane, and tooth erup-

tion may resume. Orthodontic movement should begin immediately. Complications include possible crown, root, and alveolar fractures, loss of viability and vitality, as well as re-ankylosis. When an ankylosed tooth is impacted, a similar technique can bring an impacted tooth (usually canines) into the arch. Exposure involves surgical uncovering, application of orthodontic bonding, and tension forces applied to direct the tooth into occlusion. However, if the tooth becomes re-ankylosed, the orthodontic forces will intrude adjacent teeth.

Orthodontics for Surgical Management of Ankylosed Teeth   Presurgical orthodontics may be indicated to create adequate space (minimum of 2 to 3 mm) between the roots of the adjacent teeth to safely accommodate interdental osteotomies around the ankylosed tooth. Spacing is best assessed with pantomographic or periapical radiographs. The ankylosed tooth is left out of the arch wire, and all other teeth are properly aligned. If orthognathic surgery is required to correct a dentofacial deformity, the orthodontics are performed in the traditional manner, but the ankylosed tooth must remain out of the arch wire, unless it aligns well with one of the dental segments. Following surgery, orthodontic mechanics can be initiated immediately to help get the mobilized dental segment with the ankylosed tooth into the best possible position.

Osteotomy   Performing single-tooth osteotomies or sectional-arch osteotomies with mobilization of the segment will permit immediate repositioning of the ankylosed tooth (Figure 55-33), or facilitate repositioning by distraction osteogenesis.

In select cases where an ankylosed primary molar is present, without a successor, a treatment option is to remove the ankylosed tooth and eliminate the extraction space by performing a vertical body ostectomy in conjunction with a mandibular

ramus osteotomy and advance the posterior teeth and mandibular body forward (Figure 55-34). This eliminates the need for osseointegrated implants and extensive dental reconstruction.

Final Presurgical Preparation

As presurgical orthodontic treatment progresses, new diagnostic records (lateral cephalograms, pantomograms, dental models) are taken to determine the feasibility and timing of surgical procedures. This will also aid the orthodontist in identifying specific areas that may need to be addressed in completing the presurgical orthodontic goals (ie, sectional leveling of the arch

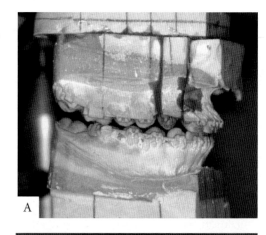

A

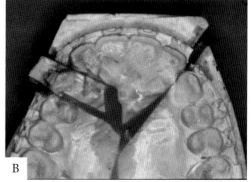

B

FIGURE 55-33 *Single-tooth osteotomies can be performed as isolated cases or they can be performed in combination with multiple maxillary osteotomies to allow individual movement of the dental osseous segments or application of immediate distraction osteogenesis to reposition the tooth properly. The case illustrated had an ankylosed maxillary right cuspid (see Figure 55-8) treated with segmental maxillary osteotomies including a single tooth segment containing the right cuspid (A, B)*

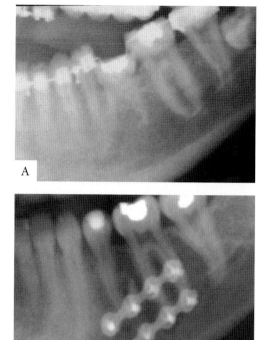

FIGURE 55-34 *A, B, An ankylosed submerged primary tooth without a permanent successor can be treated with extraction of the primary tooth as well as a vertical body ostectomy in conjunction with a mandibular ramus sagittal split osteotomy to advance the posterior teeth forward to eliminate the ankylosed tooth and associated space. This eliminates the need for an osseointegrated implant or crown-and-bridge work.*

segments, marginal ridge alignment, vertical dental alignment, buccal surface alignment, additional TSD correction).

During surgery the jaws are usually wired together once or twice, as each jaw is independently mobilized and stabilized with rigid fixation. To facilitate wiring the jaws together as well as providing a means of using postsurgical elastics if required, fixtures attached to the brackets or arch wires are usually necessary. Fixtures attached to the brackets are dependent on the manufacturer but may include ball hooks built onto the brackets, T pins, and K hooks, (Figure 55-35). Fixtures attached to the arch wire include crimped-on hooks and soldered pins (Figure 55-36). Hooks built onto the brackets are preferred, followed by the other

hooks placed on the brackets (T pins, K hooks). The least preferred are the hooks on the arch wire. The reason is that if post-surgery elastics are required for an extended time, the elastics and hooks on the arch wire will activate the arch wire, possibly creating unwanted orthodontic forces and movements (ie, tipping the crowns lingually and the roots buccally). This undesirable torquing occurs to a much lesser degree when the hooks are directly on the brackets.

When the maxilla or mandible are to be segmentalized, it may be better for the orthodontist to section the arch wire (see Figure 55-15B) and bend the ends inward at the predetermined osteotomy areas immediately prior to surgery, or the surgeon can cut the wire at surgery.

The best type of arch wire to place prior to surgery is a rectangular stainless steel wire that fills the bracket slot. For example, with an 18 slot, a 17×25 gauge wire is recommended, and for a 22 slot, a 21×25 gauge wire is indicated. This will help stabilize the individual dental units together as a whole arch or in segments when segmental surgery is required. The final wire should be placed 2 to 3 months prior to surgery.

Postsurgical Orthodontics

In preparation for the postsurgery orthodontic phase of treatment, the surgical stabilizing splint, if used, is usually removed 4 to 6 weeks postsurgery. If the palatal splint design is used and a large maxillary expansion has been performed, the splint can remain for a longer period and the postsurgical orthodontics can be performed around it. The maintenance of the splint will enhance the transverse stability and it can be left in for 2 to 3 months or longer if necessary. It can be made into a removable appliance.

If rigid skeletal fixation is used, active orthodontics involving changing the arch wires can usually resume 4 to 6 weeks post-surgery, when patients are usually comfortable enough to tolerate changing their arch

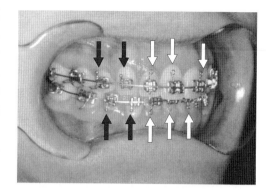

FIGURE 55-35 *Orthodontic hooks. Ball hooks built onto the brackets* (blue arrows) *provide the best stability. Other options include T pins and K hooks* (white arrows) *or other methods to provide attachments directly on the brackets.*

wires. The orthodontist can be fairly aggressive at finishing the occlusion because the osseous segments can still be moved slightly. The teeth move much more rapidly for the first few months post-surgery because there is an increased bony metabolism as a result of the surgery. The orthodontist can therefore accomplish in 1 to 2 weeks what would normally take 4 to 6 weeks to complete. Applying active mechanics at this early postsurgical orthodontic phase of treatment and booking the patient for a routine orthodontic follow-up 4 to 6 weeks later could result in uncontrolled excessive orthodontic movements, resulting in an unfavorable outcome.

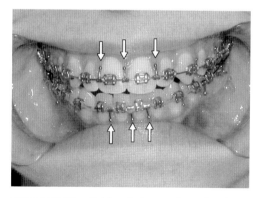

FIGURE 55-36 *Soldered pins on the arch wire or crimped hooks* (white arrows) *onto the arch wire can also be used but are not preferred because the use of postsurgical elastics will activate the arch wire, possibly creating unwanted orthodontic movements.*

For most cases the orthodontist should see the patient once a week for the first month, then every 2 weeks for the next 2 months for adjustments so that orthodontic changes can be closely monitored. At the initial appointments root positions are checked, loose brackets and bracket positions are evaluated and corrected, and new arch wires are placed if indicated. Interarch mechanics (ie, class II or III elastics, vertical elastics, and/or cross-arch elastics) can be applied as necessary to finalize the occlusion. Once the initial healing phase is completed (approximately 3 to 4 months postsurgery) and the occlusion is stable, the orthodontic appointment intervals can be extended to the more traditional time frame. The final positioning of the teeth usually takes from 3 to 12 months of postsurgical orthodontic treatment but could be longer depending on the postsurgical orthodontic requirements. Although reasonable stability from surgical healing occurs in approximately 3 to 4 months, the final postsurgical healing phase takes 9 to 12 months.

References

1. Bolton WA. The clinical application of a tooth-size analysis. Am J Orthod 1962;48:504–29.
2. Moyers RE, van der Linden FPGM, Riolo ML, McNamara JA. Standards of human occlusal development. The University of Michigan Ann Arbor (MI): The Center for Human Growth and Development; 1976. p. 53–94.
3. Alling CC III, Helfrick JF, Alling RD. Impacted teeth. Philadelphia (PA): WB Saunders Co.; 1993. p. 4.
4. Biederman W. The problem of the ankylosed tooth. In: Spengeman WG, editor. Dental clinics of North America. Philadelphia (PA): WB Saunders Co.; 1968. p. 409–24.
5. Jacobs SG. Ankylosis of permanent teeth: a case report and literature review. Aust Orthod J 1989;11(1):38–44.
6. Schultes G, Gaggl A, Karcher H. Periodontal disease associated with interdental osteotomies after orthognathic surgery. J Oral Maxillofac Surg 1998;56:414–7.
7. Wolford LM. Periodontal disease associated with interdental osteotomies after orthognathic surgery. J Oral Maxillofac Surg. 1998;56:417–9.
8. Dorfman HS, Turvey TA. Alterations in osseous crestal height following interdental osteotomies. Oral Surg Oral Med Oral Pathol 1979;48:120–5.
9. Shepherd JP. Long-term effects of segmental alveolar osteotomy. Int J Oral Surg 1979; 8:327–32.
10. Kwon H, Philstrom B, Waite DE. Effects on the periodontium of vertical bone cutting for segmental osteotomy. J Oral Maxillofac Surg 1985;43:953–5.
11. Fox ME, Stephens WF, Wolford LM, el Deeb M. Effects of interdental osteotomies on the periodontal and osseous supporting tissues. Int J Adult Orthod Orthogn Surg 1991; 6:39–46.
12. Wolford LM, Cottrell DA. Diagnosis of macroglossia and indications for reduction glossectomy. Am J Orthod Dentofac Orthop 1996;110:170–7.
13. Turvey TA, Journot V, Epker BN. Correction of anterior open bite deformity: a study of tongue function, speech changes, and stability. J Maxillofac Surg 1976;4:93–101.
14. Wickwire NA, White RP Jr, Proffit WR. The effect of mandibular osteotomy on tongue position. J Oral Surg 1972;30:184–90.
15. Wolford LM, Karras S, Mehra P. Concomitant temporomandibular joint and orthognathic surgery: a preliminary report. J Oral Maxillofac Surg 2002;60:356–62.
16. Wolford LM, Mehra P, Reiche-Fischel O, et al. Efficacy of high condylectomy for management of condylar hyperplasia. Am J Orthod Dentofac Orthop 2002;121:136–51.
17. Mehra P, Wolford LM. The Mitek mini anchor for TMJ disc repositioning: surgical technique and results. Int J Oral Maxillofac Surg 2001;30:497–503.
18. Wolford LM, Cardenas L. Idiopathic condylar resorption: diagnosis, treatment protocol, and outcomes. Am J Orthod Dentofac Orthop 1999;116:667–76.
19. Schwarz GM, Thrash WJ, Byrd DL, Jacobs JD. Tomographic assessment of nasal septal changes following surgical-orthodontic rapid maxillary expansion. Am J Orthod 1985;87(1):39–45.
20. Proffit WR. Contemporary orthodontics. St Louis (MO): C.V. Mosby Co.; 1986. p. 191–2, 352.
21. Williams HS, Zwemer, JD, Hoyt DJ. Treating ankylosed primary teeth in adult patients: a case report. Quintessence Int 1995;26:161–6.
22. Steiner DR. Timing of extraction of ankylosed teeth to maximize ridge development. J Endodont 1997;23:242–5.
23. Geiger AM, Bronsky MJ. Orthodontic management of ankylosed permanent posterior teeth: a clinical report of three cases. Am J Orthod Dentofac Orthop 1994;106:543–8.
24. Oesterle LJ. Implant consideration in the growing child. In: Higuchi KW, editor. Orthodontic applications of osseointegrated implants. Chicago (IL): Quintessence Publishing Co.; 2000. p. 133–59.

CHAPTER 56

Principles of Mandibular Orthognathic Surgery

Dale S. Bloomquist, DDS, MS
Jessica J. Lee, DDS

The development of mandibular osteotomies for correction of dentofacial deformities closely parallels the advancement of oral and maxillofacial surgery as a specialty more than any other group of surgical techniques. From Hullihen, who in 1849 was the first to describe a mandibular osteotomy, to Obwegeser, who developed the sagittal osteotomy of the vertical ramus, there has been dramatic progress in the techniques of mandibular osteotomies. After Obwegeser's original paper in German, and especially since his description of techniques in the English literature, orthognathic surgery has seen dramatic changes in use as well as refinement of the osteotomies. Although the development of osteotomy techniques is ongoing, it is the purpose of this chapter not only to describe the most commonly used surgical procedures for the mandible but also to emphasize the refinements in technique that have been the result of the most recent clinical as well as basic research.

History

Hullihen corrected a patient with anterior open bite and mandibular dentoalveolar protrusion with an intraoral osteotomy, very similar to what we now describe as an anterior subapical osteotomy (Figure 56-1).[1] His efforts did not seem to stimulate much interest, for it was almost 50 years later when Angle described a body osteotomy done by V.P. Blair (Figure 56-2A) for a patient with mandibular horizontal excess.[2,3] This technique, with minor modifications, was advocated until the 1970s. Since then the only major modifications in the body osteotomy that have occurred are a greater emphasis being placed on preserving the inferior alveolar nerve and a switch to an intraoral approach.

The horizontal osteotomy of the vertical ramus popularized by Blair (Figure 56-2B) was accomplished through an extraoral route.[4] As with many of the early mandibular procedures a horizontal bone cut was made above the lingula and was described for correcting both mandibular horizontal deficiency and horizontal excess. An intraoral technique was not suggested until Ernst discussed his procedure approximately 25 years later.[5] This method of correcting mandibular deformities was used for almost 60 years, but because of its lack of postoperative stability, it has fallen into disuse.

The subcondylar osteotomy (Figure 56-2C), a form of which was first reported by Limberg as an extraoral technique, has undergone relatively minor refinement to the intraoral vertical subcondylar osteotomy that is popular today.[6] There has, however, been a substantial number of osteotomy designs through the vertical ramus that begin in the sigmoid notch, which has led to some confusion in the

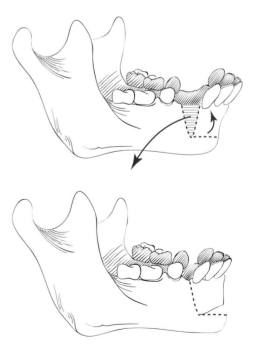

FIGURE 56-1 *Hullihen's mandibular subapical osteotomy. Adapted from Bloomquist DS. Principles of mandibular orthognathic surgery. In: Peterson LJ, Indresano AT, Marciani RD, Roser SM. Principles of oral and maxillofacial surgery. Vol 3. Philadelphia (PA): J.B. Lippincott Company; 1992. p. 1416.*

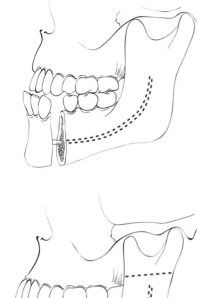

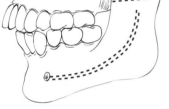

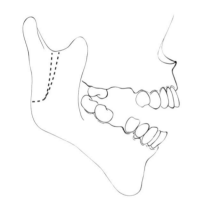

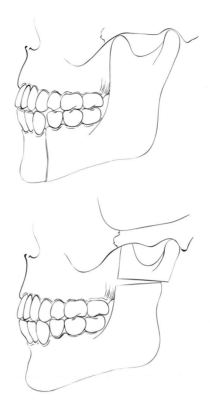

FIGURE **56-2** A, *Blair's body osteotomy.* B, *Blair's ramus osteotomy.* C, *Limberg's "oblique" osteotomy of the ramus. Adapted from Bloomquist DS. Principles of mandibular orthognathic surgery. In: Peterson LJ, Indresano AT, Marciani RD, Roser SM. Principles of oral and maxillofacial surgery. Vol 3. Philadelphia (PA): J.B. Lippincott Company; 1992. p. 1416.*

nomenclature of what is a fairly closely related group of osteotomies. The names that have been developed have generally been based on the length and direction of the cuts made in the posterior portion of the vertical ramus. The subcondylar osteotomy was used to describe the condylar neck osteotomies of Kostecka and of Moose.[7,8] Generally longer cuts that extended to the posterior border above the angle, such as described by Limberg, Thoma, and Robinson, were described as oblique osteotomies.[5–10] Shira, however, coined the term oblique sliding osteotomy for this particular surgery.[11] Finally Caldwell and Letterman described a vertical

osteotomy of the mandibular ramus that included a cut from the sigmoid notch to the inferior border in front of the angle of the mandible.[12] The cut was kept behind the foramen of the mandibular nerve, and a portion of the lateral cortex of the distal fragment was decorticated to allow a larger area of bone contact. Generally these latter two groups of osteotomies are now being called vertical osteotomies, but some semantic differences still persist. Specifically the terms vertical subcondylar osteotomies (VSOs) and vertical ramus osteotomies (VROs) are still used interchangeably in the literature. Primarily this type of osteotomy was designed for correc-

tion of mandibular horizontal excess of mandibular asymmetries, although Robinson described its use with a bone graft for horizontal deficiencies.[10]

The intraoral approach to the subcondylar osteotomies is relatively new, having first been described by Moose in 1964.[13] He approached the condylar neck medially with a straight bur. Winstanley suggested a lateral approach in 1968, but it was not until Hebert and colleagues described the use of a special oscillating saw that this approach became popular.[14,15]

A variation of the vertical subcondylar osteotomy was suggested by Wassmund in 1927 (Figure 56-3A), which is similar to what is now called the inverted **L** osteotomy.[16] Pichler and Trauner later suggested the use of bone grafts into the defect left by the advancement of the mandible.[17] Caldwell and colleagues further modified the inverted **L** by adding a horizontal cut just above the inferior border of the mandible to create what is now called the **C** osteotomy (Figure 56-3B).[18] The stated advantage of the **C** osteotomy was that the bone cut design made the use of a bone graft unnecessary. This advantage was further enhanced by the modification suggested by Hayes, with the splitting of the inferior limb sagittally so that more bone contact can be achieved.[19] A further interesting approach to this group of vertical ramus osteotomies done for horizontal mandibular deficiency is the modified **L** osteotomy described by Fox and Tilson.[20] They deleted the superior horizontal cut of the **C** osteotomy and instead extended the vertical cut to the sigmoid notch. Then the coronoid process was removed and added as a free graft into the defect resulting from the mandibular advancement.

The greatest development in osteotomies of the vertical ramus is the sagittal osteotomy, credited to Obwegeser and Trauner, but generally now used in a fashion modified from the original technique described in 1955.[21] Lane has been mentioned as the developer of a form of

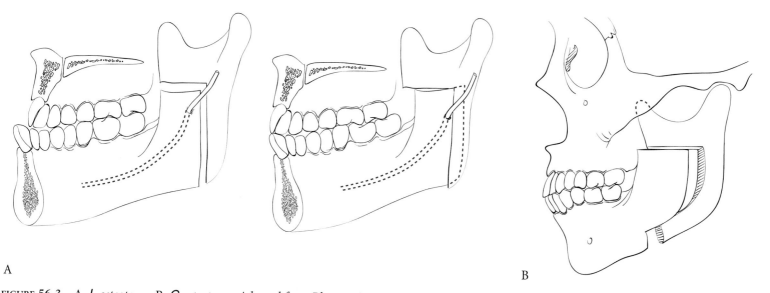

A   B

FIGURE **56-3** A, *L osteotomy*. B, *C osteotomy. Adapted from Bloomquist DS. Principles of mandibular orthognathic surgery. In: Peterson LJ, Indresano AT, Marciani RD, Roser SM. Principles of oral and maxillofacial surgery. Vol 3. Philadelphia (PA): J.B. Lippincott Company; 1992. p. 1417.*

the sagittal osteotomy, with parallel horizontal bone cuts made through the medial and lateral cortices of the vertical ramus (Figure 56-4).[22] The medial cut was made just above the lingula, with the lateral cut made just below it. This idea was expanded by Schuchardt before being refined and popularized by Obwegeser.[23] The major modifications in the osteotomy design were first made by DalPont with his vertical cut through the lateral cortex as well as the suggestion that the medial horizontal cut be extended only to a point above the

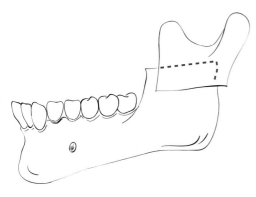

FIGURE **56-4** *Lane's osteotomy. Adapted from Bloomquist DS. Principles of mandibular orthognathic surgery. In: Peterson LJ, Indresano AT, Marciani RD, Roser SM. Principles of oral and maxillofacial surgery. Vol 3. Philadelphia (PA): J.B. Lippincott Company; 1992. p. 1417.*

lingula and not to the posterior border (Figure 56-5).[24] This latter technique shortens the split posteriorly, and as was further discussed by Hunsuck, decreases the trauma to the overlying soft tissue.[25] Many clinicians have offered suggestions for improving the sagittal osteotomy, but the only other major innovation to this technique has been the use of internal rigid fixation. Spiessl suggested the use of screws for fixation of the fragments in the sagittal osteotomy.[26] Although wire osseous fixation is still used by some surgeons, rigid internal fixation in some form has become the standard technique for the bilateral sagittal split osteotomy (BSSO).

Osteotomies of the mandibular body do not generally receive the same degree of attention as osteotomies of the vertical ramus, but they have undergone refinements and variations from the original anterior alveolar osteotomies of Hullihen and the body osteotomies of Blair. The first variation of Hullihen's procedure did not appear until 90 years after the original description, when Hofer demonstrated an anterior mandibular alveolar osteotomy to advance anterior teeth in correction of a mandibular dentoalveolar retrusion (Figure 56-6A).[27] Kole modified this procedure

by suggesting the use of bone grafts from the mental region to the defect caused by the rotation of the anterior dentoalveolar segment (Figure 56-6B).[28] Clinicians now

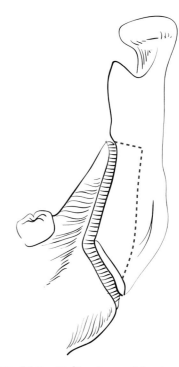

FIGURE **56-5** *DalPont's modification of the sagittal osteotomy. Adapted from Bloomquist DS. Principles of mandibular orthognathic surgery. In: Peterson LJ, Indresano AT, Marciani RD, Roser SM. Principles of oral and maxillofacial surgery. Vol 3. Philadelphia (PA): J.B. Lippincott Company; 1992. p. 1418.*

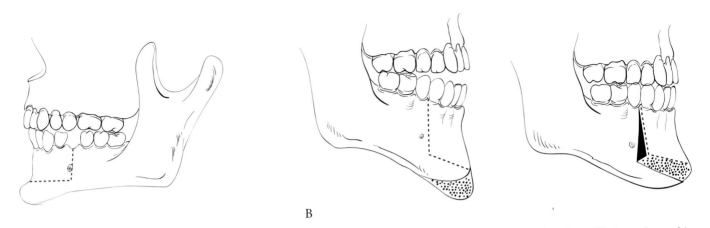

FIGURE **56-6**   A, *Hofer's subapical osteotomy.* B, *Kole's subapical osteotomy. Adapted from Bloomquist DS. Principles of mandibular orthognathic surgery. In: Peterson LJ, Indresano AT, Marciani RD, Roser SM. Principles of oral and maxillofacial surgery. Vol 3. Philadelphia (PA): J.B. Lippincott Company; 1992. p. 1418.*

employing Hofer's osteotomy generally use some form of bone graft in the alveolar defect if significant movement of the fragment is planned. Mandibular alveolar osteotomies have expanded in primarily two ways from Hofer's original procedure. Kent and Hinds initially presented the use of the single-tooth osteotomies of the mandible in 1971, and MacIntosh closely followed with his description of the total mandibular alveolar osteotomy in 1974.[29,30] This latter procedure continues to be popular, with minor variations being added by other clinicians.

Osteotomies of the body of the mandible have been described in almost every conceivable form, with the most durable advancements being the step osteotomy, initially described by Von Eiselberg in 1906 (Figure 56-7A), and the horizontal osteotomy of the symphysis described by Hofer in 1942 (Figure 56-7B).[31,32] The step osteotomy was originally described for treatment of mandibular horizontal deficiency, but it has been used in various forms for mandibular horizontal excess as well as asymmetry. The horizontal osteotomy of the symphysis has

also developed a large degree of versatility, with its use in various forms being suggested for almost any skeletal deformity of the bony chin.

Anatomic and Physiologic Considerations of Mandibular Surgeries

Vascular Supply

A major concern with surgery of the facial skeleton is the vascular supply of the bone segments. This was dramatically demonstrated by the explosion of orthognathic

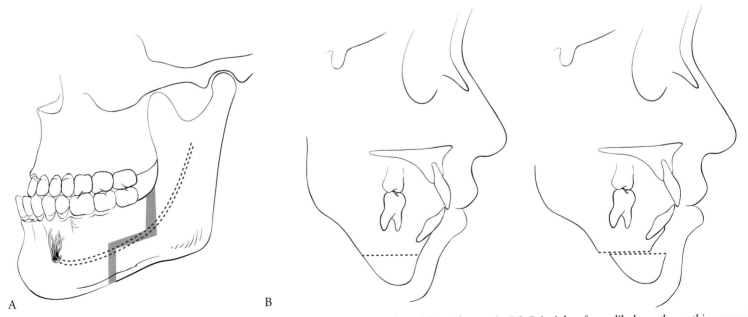

FIGURE **56-7**   A, *Von Eiselberg's step osteotomy.* B, *Hofer's horizontal osteotomy. Adapted from Bloomquist DS. Principles of mandibular orthognathic surgery. In: Peterson LJ, Indresano AT, Marciani RD, Roser SM. Principles of oral and maxillofacial surgery. Vol 3. Philadelphia (PA): J.B. Lippincott Company; 1992. p. 1419.*

surgery in the United States after Bell and Levy's studies of vascular effects of the osteotomies.[33] Although all of the techniques they looked at had been previously used in patients, there had not been any experimental evaluations of the physiologic basis for many of the procedures. Bell and Levy's work demonstrated that blood flow through the mandibular periosteum could easily maintain a sufficient blood supply to the teeth of a mobile segment, even when the labial periosteum was degloved. Blood flow from the periosteum was termed centripetal, to distinguish it from the blood flowing from endosteal vessels outward (centrifugal) that was associated with long bones. Previously clinicians felt that the inferior alveolar artery had a primary role in nourishing the mandible, but Bell and Levy demonstrated that there is also a sufficient blood supply from the surrounding soft tissues, even if the inferior alveolar artery was obstructed. More recent work in animals suggests that the blood supply to the body of the mandible under normal conditions comes almost entirely from the inferior alveolar artery.[34] However, when this source is obstructed, the peripheral blood vessels quickly take over for the anterior mandible. The posterior mandibular dentoalveolus, however, does not benefit from this kind of collateral blood supply, which calls into question the safety of posterior mandibular segmental alveolar osteotomies. Zisser and Gattinger showed pulpal necrosis in the molars of horizontal osteotomies done above the inferior alveolar nerve in the body of the mandible of dogs.[35]

The safety of combined mandibular osteotomies, such as ramal procedures and body osteotomies, has been a concern because of the predominant role of the inferior alveolar artery.[36] The fragility of the vascular supply to the mandibular alveolus engenders some concern over the common use of subapical osteotomies. Although their relative safety has been demonstrated by both animal studies and

substantial clinical experience, subapical osteotomies need to be carefully planned to ensure as large a vascular pedicle as possible.[33,37] Complications, such as pulpal necrosis, soft-tissue defects, and loss of teeth and bone, have demonstrated the delicate nature of the blood supply, especially when attempts at moving small dentoalveolar fragments are made. The effect of aging on the vascular supply to the mandibular body is an area about which very little information is known, particularly whether aging causes a switch from the centrifugal to centripetal blood supply. Bradley has demonstrated an apparent decreasing capacity of the inferior alveolar vessels that occurs with aging, but the impact of this effect on mandibular osteotomies is unknown.[38]

Osteotomy designs of the vertical ramus have profited by studies of the effect of surgery on vascular supply. The proximal segment of the vertical subsigmoid osteotomy maintains its blood supply through the temporomandibular joint capsule and the attachment of the lateral pterygoid muscle. However, the inferior tip of this fragment has undergone vascular necrosis in experimental studies.[39] This led to the suggestion that fewer problems may occur if the cut was made above the angle of the mandible.[39]

The importance of the periosteal blood supply as well as the endosteal supply in the vertical ramus has been explored by animal research.[40–43] When the medial pterygoid and masseter muscles are stripped, both blood flow and blood supply studies have demonstrated the possibility of avascular necrosis in the proximal segment. Comparisons of extensive muscle stripping of the vertical ramus against preservation of the masseter attachment have demonstrated a significant difference in the vascularity of the inferior portion of the proximal fragment. These studies of blood supply of the vertical ramus may be of value in predicting the vascular effects of the C or L osteotomies. However, resorp-

tion of the proximal fragment has not been reported in these particular bone cuts possibly because of the rarity of their use. However, given the available research, it is wise to minimize the periosteal and muscle attachment stripping on the medial surface of the proximal fragment with either the C or L osteotomy or any of their variations.

The last unanswered question concerning vascular supply in mandibular orthognathic surgery is the determination of a safe distance away from the apex of the teeth to make horizontal bone cuts. Many of the references to this question are based on research done in the maxilla.[44] From these early animal studies the pulpal blood supply of a tooth should not be affected if a cut was made at least 5 mm away from the apex of the tooth. Zisser and Gattinger, however, saw pulpal changes in dogs with some horizontal cuts that were made 10 mm away from the apex.[35] Whether these distances have any relevance to humans is presumptive. Clinically the incidence of tooth devitalization from horizontal subapical osteotomies is extremely low and it can be assumed that, for the most part, 5 mm is a good guideline. A cut made 10 mm from the apices, although allowing a greater safety margin, is often impractical because of other anatomic limitations. The greater distance from the apices of the teeth not only minimizes direct pulpal injury but increases the vascular pedicle to the mobile segment as well.

Nerves

The surgeon working around the face must be constantly aware of the nerve network that exists in this area. Fortunately, on approaching the mandible, these concerns can be narrowed to essentially two major nerves: the marginal mandibular branch of the seventh cranial nerve and the third division of the trigeminal nerve, most frequently one of its branches, the inferior alveolar nerve. The marginal mandibular branch is usually only at risk during extraoral procedures. Although trauma to this nerve has been reported to have occurred during intraoral approach, it is rare and for the mort part appears to be preventable. Avoiding damage to this nerve during extraoral approaches to the mandible is a major surgical goal; in most cases in orthognathic surgery it is achieved because soft tissue anatomy in patients undergoing the surgery has not been disturbed by disease or trauma. The techniques of these approaches are covered elsewhere in these book volumes as well as are the methods for minimizing the risks of damage to the marginal mandibular branch. Damage to the third division of the trigeminal is, however, a much-discussed problem in mandibular surgery. The course of the inferior alveolar nerve into the vertical ramus and then through the body of the mandible makes it extremely susceptible to damage from almost every mandibular surgical procedure. In most cases the surgeon's main goal relative to this nerve is to minimize the trauma because its avoidance is almost impossible. In the past surgeons stressed the importance of looking for and sometimes freeing up the nerve as it either entered or left the mandible before making osteotomies in the areas of the foramina. However, there is a trend toward avoiding this step, unless it is absolutely necessary to make the osteotomy as close to the nerve as possible. The simple act of exposing the nerve seems to increase the chance for postoperative sensory deficiency.

Often the debates on whether one mandibular osteotomy is preferable to another are primarily based on the potential of damaging the inferior alveolar nerve. This has resulted in many clinicians trivializing the damage found following a certain technique. Well-defined standards for both long- and short-term follow-up of nerve damage during mandibular procedures have been discussed[45]; however, in most papers these have not been used to evaluate sensory deficits. In addition very few controlled studies have been published com-

paring procedures; as a result not much can be said in support of any of the differing attempts to minimize nerve damage.

Studies looking at the loss of tooth sensibility from horizontal osteotomies below the dental apices, however, have been quite consistent. Most authors found a relatively high loss of response to pulp testing immediately after osteotomies, especially when teeth are close to a vertical osteotomy.[46–48] However, this loss may not correlate with actual loss of tooth vitality and, thus, either tooth loss secondary to an osteotomy or the need for endodontic therapy is very low.

The Muscle

Orthognathic surgery affects muscles in primarily two ways: it changes the length of a muscle or it changes the direction of muscle function. Effects of these changes are still not understood, although various authors have emphasized the importance of controlling muscular changes. The muscles commonly discussed in orthognathic surgery of the mandible have been the muscles of mastication and the suprahyoid group of muscles. Recent interest on the soft tissue effects of facial skeletal surgery has expanded interest to the other facial muscles. This latter group, however, has generally not been discussed relative to mandibular osteotomies, with the possible exception of the effect of the anterior mandibular osteotomies on the attachment of the mentalis muscle. The muscles of mastication, however, have received considerable attention, dating back to the early vertical ramus procedures. Research interest on the effects of altering these muscles concentrated either on their effect on the skeletal changes, especially relapse following mandibular osteotomies, or on the changes in function of these muscles.

Distraction of the superior fragment of a horizontal osteotomy of the vertical ramus following surgery was noted early by surgeons who used this technique.[49]

Evaluation of this procedure following correction of prognathism found a superior movement of the mandible in the gonial region as well as a downward and backward movement at the symphysis. This change, which was attributed to the forces of the pterygomasseteric sling, has received considerable attention, not only in mandibular setbacks done with osteotomies through the vertical ramus but also in mandibular advancements.[50–55] The apparent shortening of the vertical ramus has been noted in a number of studies, and in some a correlation has been demonstrated between this change and the posterior movement of the symphysis. The exact reason for the change in the gonion has not been clearly demonstrated. Kohn demonstrated the movement of this point inferoanteriorly in mandibular advancements by way of a measurement he termed the gonial arc (Figure 56-8).[54] Most investigators feel this represents distraction of the condyle from the fossa, and this

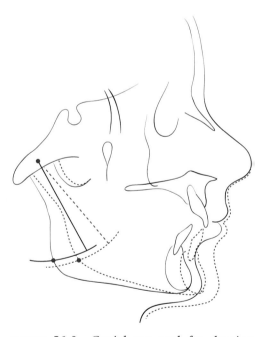

FIGURE **56-8** *Gonial arc used for showing condylar position change with a mandibular osteotomy. Adapted from Bloomquist DS. Principles of mandibular orthognathic surgery. In: Peterson LJ, Indresano AT, Marciani RD, Roser SM. Principles of oral and maxillofacial surgery. Vol 3. Philadelphia (PA): J.B. Lippincott Company; 1992. p. 1422.*

hypothesis was further supported by the migration of the gonion back during the postoperative period.[54,55] The long-term postoperative decrease in gonial arc was generally believed to be due to remodeling, especially resorption that occurred at the mandibular angle.[40,43] Especially in early studies, resorption could have accounted for this change because of the then-accepted technique of completely stripping muscle attachment from the proximal segment. However, in more recent studies in which minimal muscle stripping was done, a similar result has been noted.[56,57] Will and colleagues noted a condyle distraction followed by an "overshoot" in the resettling of the condyle in the fossa.[58] This change in condylar position may be due to either displacement of the disk within the joint or compression of the soft tissues of the joint by increased pressures secondary to the muscles of the pterygomasseteric sling.

The rotational change in the proximal segment of a mandibular osteotomy has been implicated in relapse by multiple clinicians who believe that the muscles of the pterygomasseteric sling reassert themselves after the surgery.[59,60] Therefore, there has been an emphasis on carefully repositioning the proximal segment close to its preoperative position. Unfortunately a correlation between mandibular ramus positioning and relapse in the case of mandibular advancements has never been demonstrated. There have been a few studies that have shown a relation between relapse of mandibular setback surgeries and the position of the vertical ramus.[61] It has been noted in these surgeries that the degree of clockwise rotation of the proximal fragment in a sagittal osteotomy seems to relate to the amount of forward relapse of the distal segment. Franco and colleagues theorized that a stretching of the medial pterygoid muscle as well as the elongation of the anterior fibers of the masseter and temporalis muscles from the clockwise rotation of the proximal seg-

ment both can contribute to relapse in lengthening the muscles of the pterygomasseteric sling.[61] This can result in a change in mandibular position as has been documented by Yellich and colleagues.[62] The degree to which this is active in orthognathic surgery remains unclear.

The contribution of the suprahyoid muscles to relapse in mandibular advancement surgery is equivocal, with many clinicians claiming an existence of this relationship. Ellis and Carlson demonstrated in monkeys that relieving the suprahyoid muscles from the symphysis of the mandible decreased the amount of relapse when the mandibles were advanced.[63] Clinical studies, however, have failed to show a relation between suprahyoid myotomies and relapse.[64,65] Animal studies have also demonstrated that adaptive changes occur in the connective tissues at the muscle-tendon and tendon-bone interfaces but only with large advancements.[66]

The belief, however unsubstantiated, that muscle pull in some way does affect the stability of mandibular osteotomies has led to a variety of recommendations. Historically the most common method advocated is the attempt at minimizing the change in muscle position and length. The cutting of muscle attachments, such as has been recommended for the suprahyoid group, has the potential for increasing morbidity. Without significant evidence that this is of much value, this additional surgery cannot be justified. However, there has been recognition that muscles and their attachments seem to adapt fairly quickly if the bone is held rigidly for a long enough time.[66,67] It is important to recognize that intermaxillary dental fixation does not provide a completely stable method of bone fixation, especially if the teeth have been under active orthodontic movement. Additionally the greatest amount of relapse of mandibular osteotomies seems to occur in the first 3 to 6 weeks after surgery. Whatever the causes of the instability during this time there

have been several techniques designed to provide increased stability for this initial period, to improve the stability of mandibular osteotomies. Primarily two techniques have been attempted: external supporting mechanisms and internal rigid fixation. The only external technique that has been of much value has been the wiring technique that has been termed skeletal fixation. With this procedure the bony skeletons are tied to one another, circumventing the periodontal ligaments of the teeth. This has been used with intermaxillary fixation, keeping the mandible immobilized for 6 to 8 weeks (Figure 56-9).[58,67,68] The alternative procedures of internal rigid fixation techniques using plates or screws will be discussed in the succeeding sections on the osteotomies.

Osteotomy Techniques

Vertical Ramus Osteotomies

Osteotomies in the vertical ramus have been the preferred technique for correcting developmental deformities of the mandible. This preference has increased with closer cooperation between orthodontists and

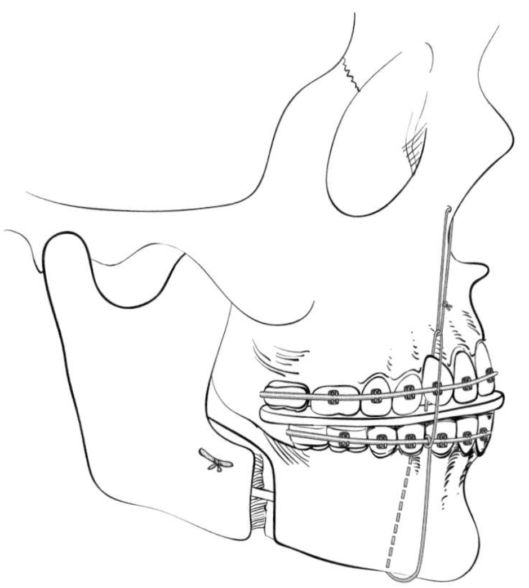

FIGURE **56-9** *Skeletal fixation used with maxillomandibular fixation or mandibular advancement. Adapted from Bloomquist DS. Principles of mandibular orthognathic surgery. In: Peterson LJ, Indresano AT, Marciani RD, Roser SM. Principles of oral and maxillofacial surgery. Vol 3. Philadelphia (PA): J.B. Lippincott Company; 1992. p. 1423.*

surgeons in treating dentofacial deformities. Most of the time the dental arch discrepancies can be orthodontically corrected, leaving the surgeon the responsibility for moving the coordinated dental arch into its new position, as dictated by functional and esthetic demands. Operations in the vertical ramus, therefore, have become almost automatically considered when the dental arch as a unit has to be moved. As previously noted there have been numerous techniques suggested for osteotomies of the ramus, but essentially three different procedures, with minor variations, have been accepted by the surgical community.

Vertical Subcondylar Osteotomies

Osteotomies extending from the sigmoid notch vertically behind the inferior alveolar nerve foramen to the inferior border or angle have had several different names, but generally, the VSOs seem to describe the procedure best (Figure 56-10). This osteotomy was initially done through an extraoral approach but with the development of small oscillating blades with a long shaft, the intraoral route has become preferred.

Indications   The VSOs have most commonly been limited to deformities requiring the mandible to be set back for mandibular horizontal excess or to be rotated for mandibular asymmetry. Robinson and Lytle have stated that this osteotomy can be used for mandibular advancement but generally this recommendation was not taken seriously because of the question of stability.[69] Hall and McKenna revived this indication for minor (2 to 3 mm) advancements.[70]

Techniques   When preparing for an intraoral VSO, one needs to closely evaluate the panoramic and lateral head films for the position of the inferior alveolar foramen relative to the posterior border of the mandible. The incision is made in the mucosa from midway up the anterior border of the ramus to the first molar area. The periosteum is reflected laterally to expose the entire ramus, with the exception of the condyle neck and coronoid tip. The posterior and inferior borders can be cleared of periosteum; muscle attachments at the angle are generally difficult to elevate and should be left to ensure blood supply to this area. A special retractor can be placed that

fits around the posterior border and, at the same time, retracts tissue laterally so that an oscillating saw can be used (Figure 56-11A).

The saw chosen should have a rounded blade that is set at an obtuse angle to the long shaft to facilitate the cut. The blade should be used first to score the proposed osteotomy line on the lateral cortex. This line is then closely checked for its position relative to the sigmoid notch, posterior border, and angle. The use of the so-called antilingula has been proposed as the landmark for the mandibular foramen, but has generally fallen into disfavor, both because of the difficulties with its identification and its lack of predictable relation to the foramen.[12,71,72] The cut should be made no more than 5 to 7 mm anterior to the posterior border at the anticipated level of the foramen, using the retractor as a guide to the posterior border.[73] The cut is carried through the medial cortex, starting in the middle of the ramus. It is carried superiorly to the sigmoid notch and then finished at the inferior border (Figure 56-11B). As the cut is completed, anterolateral tension is kept on the retractor so that the proximal fragment will be brought out laterally. A straight clamp can

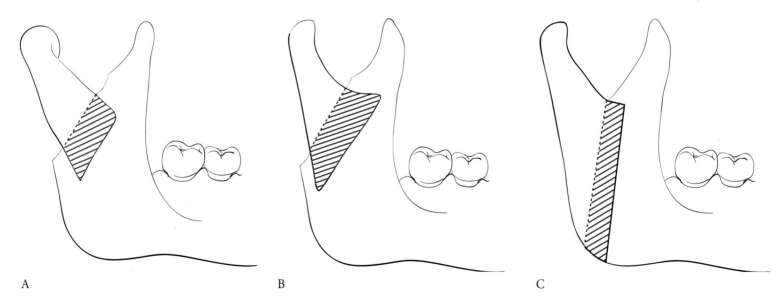

A   B   C

FIGURE 56-10   *Different lengths of the osteotomy in the vertical subcondylar osteotomies. Adapted from Bloomquist DS. Principles of mandibular orthognathic surgery. In: Peterson LJ, Indresano AT, Marciani RD, Roser SM. Principles of oral and maxillofacial surgery. Vol 3. Philadelphia (PA): J.B. Lippincott Company; 1992. p. 1423.*

be used to rotate the segment laterally after the cut is made and then to stabilize it while periosteum and muscle are stripped from the medial cortex down to the angle (Figure 56-11C). Again a small attachment is left at the angle to ensure a blood supply. This proximal fragment can be held forward and laterally by a small gauze pack while the opposite side is being completed. If the proximal fragment is lost medially, it usually can be brought into the field with the help of a small periosteal elevator that is inserted posteromedially at the level of the sigmoid notch while the distal fragment is being pulled forward. The mandibular dentition is brought into its new position after the completion of both osteotomies, as established by a preformed occlusal splint and stabilized with maxillomandibular fixation.

Attention is directed back into the wound and toward the placement and stabilization of the proximal fragment.

Wire osseous fixation is generally not needed, although advocated by some surgeons. Most important is the achievement of as broad a bone contact as possible, without displacing or rotating the condyle. Adjustment of the lateral cortex of the distal fragment may be performed with a straight fissure or small acrylic bur to permit the proximal fragment to lie as flat as possible against the vertical ramus. Care should be taken to ensure that the long axis of the proximal fragment does not differ appreciably from its preoperative position. After a thorough irrigation of the wound the mucosa is closed with a running stitch, using a resorbable suture. No drains or external dressings are placed, and the patient is left in fixation for 6 to 8 weeks. Postsurgical radiographs should be taken as soon as possible to confirm that the condyles have not been displaced. A small amount of forward and downward position of the condyle is common, and this gener-

ally resolves during the period of maxillomandibular fixation (Figure 56-12).

Submentovertex radiographs have been suggested to identify divergence of the posterior border. It has been suggested that an angle smaller than 130° produces such a significant surgical problem that this type of patient should be avoided and another technique used. The use of this radiograph as a criterion for choosing this technique has been questioned, but some still feel that it can be pursued to identify the more difficult cases.[73,74]

A large number of variations of the VSO have come in the osteotomy design. Oblique versions with the cut ending above the angle have been described by many clinicians, with the only apparent benefit being the relative ease in the technique.

Theoretically there should also be less chance of damaging the inferior alveolar nerve, but there has been no study to confirm this benefit. Interestingly the one

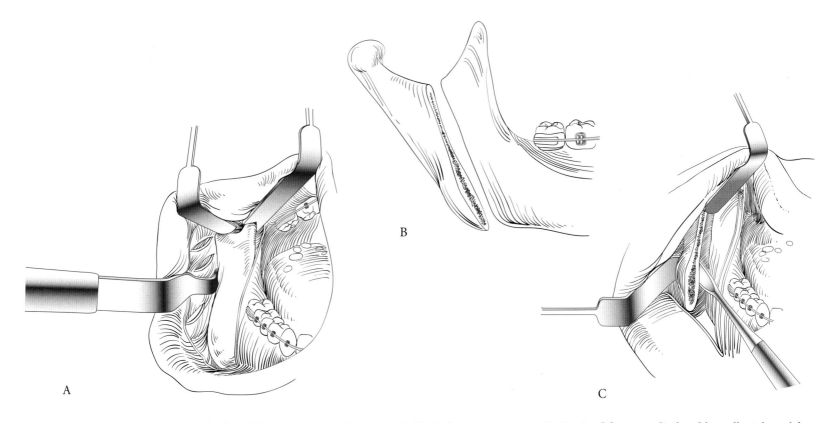

FIGURE 56-11 *The intraoral vertical subcondylar osteotomy. A, Exposure. B, Vertical ramus osteotomy. C, Proximal fragment displaced laterally. Adapted from Bloomquist DS. Principles of mandibular orthognathic surgery. In: Peterson LJ, Indresano AT, Marciani RD, Roser SM. Principles of oral and maxillofacial surgery. Vol 3. Philadelphia (PA): J.B. Lippincott Company; 1992. p. 1424.*

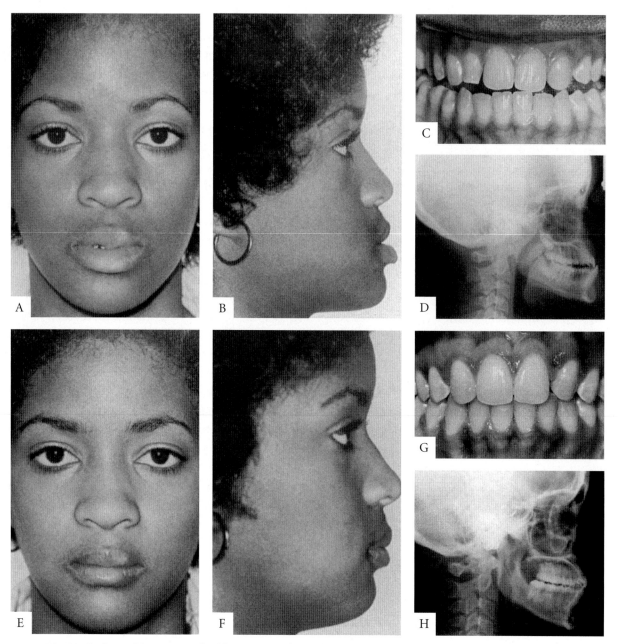

FIGURE **56-12** *Patient who was treated with an intraoral VSO for mandibular horizontal excess. A–D, Preoperative photographs and radiograph. E–H, Postoperative photographs and radiograph. Reproduced with permission from Bloomquist DS. Principles of mandibular orthognathic surgery. In: Peterson LJ, Indresano AT, Marciani RD, Roser SM. Principles of oral and maxillofacial surgery. Vol 3. Philadelphia (PA): J.B. Lippincott Company; 1992. p. 1426.*

potential drawback, that of decreased skeletal stability, appears not to be demonstratable.[75] In contrast with this shorter cut others have recommended that a larger portion of the inferior border be left with the proximal fragment, especially in the larger mandibular setbacks.[70] This permits a good attachment of the medial pterygoid muscle to be left at the mandibular angle, which has been

claimed to help seat the condyle in the fossa as the patient wakens from anesthesia. This variation, including the use of 8 weeks of fixation, is claimed to decrease one of the problems of the intraoral VSO, specifically that of condylar sag and the resulting open bite that can occur on the release of fixation. Unfortunately no clinical data have been reported that back this claim. The use of osseous wire fixation has

been advocated to ensure the seating of the condyle. Again no study comparing wire osseous fixation with no fixation has shown any advantage for the use of the wire.[76–78] This may be explicable in the intraoral procedures by the technical difficulties of wire placement. However, Ritzau and colleagues showed in an excellent prospective study that even from an extraoral approach, the position of the condyle in the fossa is not improved with the use of wire osseous fixation.[77]

The effect of the temporalis on relapse has led to other recommendations that include either stripping the temporalis attachment completely off the coronoid or cutting off the coronoid. The use of this latter coronoidotomy has been recommended by some clinicians for large setbacks, with a few using this modification routinely. The advantage of the coronoidotomy relative to prevention of relapse has not been studied, but the stability of the intraoral vertical subcondylar osteotomy (IVSO) with coronoidotomy, compared with the sagittal split osteotomy of the vertical ramus in mandibular setbacks, has been investigated and the IVSO seemed to be more stable.[79]

The use of the inverted L osteotomy is another way to neutralize the temporalis. This modification of the IVSO requires stripping of the medial periosteum to identify the lingula so that a horizontal cut can be made without increasing the risk of damaging the inferior alveolar nerve. A further modification of the inverted L osteotomy has been the use of rigid internal fixation. Although technically a difficult surgery it permits the early release from maxillomandibular fixation. Unfortunately there are no long-term studies on the stability of any of the inverted L techniques.

Alternative Techniques   The major variation of the described technique is the use of an extraoral approach. The soft tissue incision is similar to that commonly used for an external approach to a fracture of the mandibular angle, with an approximately 4 cm incision made 2 cm below the angle and the inferior border of the mandible (Figure 56-13A). A combination of sharp and blunt dissection is used to get to the inferior border of the mandible. Care is taken to avoid damaging the marginal mandibular branch of the facial nerve. After incising through the periosteum, the bone cuts are similar to those that have been described (Figure 56-13B).

The external approach has been advocated for large mandibular setbacks of greater than 10 mm, difficult asymmetries, or large vertical moves in patients with unusual facial structure. Except for the risk of the scar, the risks of this technique have been reported as being comparable with the intraoral technique.[50,80]

Complications *Stability* Postoperative change in skeletal and dental position following the use of a VSO in the treatment of mandibular horizontal excess has received much attention. Goldstein was the first to use serial cephalograms to evaluate the postoperative change of the mandible after surgical correction of the mandibular prognathism.[81] He noted the anterior relapse that has now been well documented. Poulton and colleagues recommended overcorrecting the mandibular setback by 2 mm to provide for the relapse they noted.[82] This amount of average relapse has surprisingly remained fairly consistent throughout the history of this technique, even though technical changes in procedures have been made.[80,83] Stella and colleagues noted that the variation in

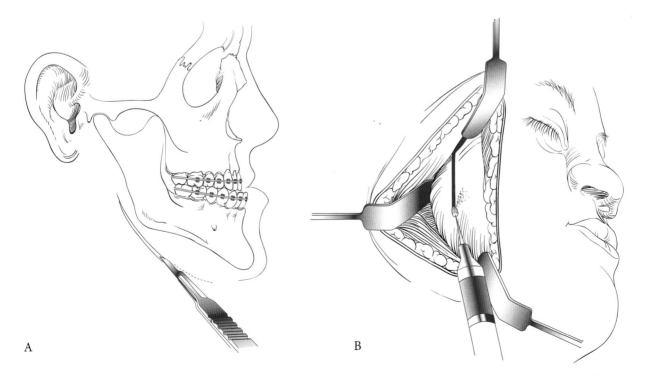

A   B

FIGURE **56-13**   *The extraoral vertical subcondylar osteotomy. Adapted from Bloomquist DS. Principles of mandibular orthognathic surgery. In: Peterson LJ, Indresano AT, Marciani RD, Roser SM. Principles of oral and maxillofacial surgery. Vol 3. Philadelphia (PA): J.B. Lippincott Company; 1992. p. 1428.*

the amount of relapse in mandibular set-backs was large and attempts at identifying controllable variables should be made.[84] They suggested that the proximal fragment rotation affects the short-term pogonion changes, although they did not present any corroborative research. The finding that the pogonion tends to move posteroinferiorly during intermaxillary fixation has been well documented.[52] This movement, later followed by the anterosuperior "relapse" that occurs after skeletal fixation wires, does seem to stabilize the initial movement but does not affect the long-term relapse.[50,51,56]

Vertical instability of the VSO develops soon after the release of intermaxillary fixation in many patients. This problem was initially attributed to the "condylar sag" seen on x-ray films taken soon after surgery.[73] Although condylar sag may be one cause of relapse, a major contributor seems to be insufficient time of fixation. The VSO is generally not considered an appropriate surgery for correction of anterior open bite. In Scandinavian countries, however, this surgical procedure has been successfully used for patients with mandibular horizontal excess and anterior open bite.[85]

Neural Damage   The chance of damaging the marginal mandibular branch of the facial nerve is one of the reasons given by several surgeons for avoiding the extraoral approach to the VSO. This concern, however, seems to be unsubstantiated, in that almost all of the clinicians reporting on the results of this approach have noted very little, if any, motor nerve damage. Damage to the inferior alveolar nerve, however, is a concern in using a VSO. The incidence of trauma to the inferior alveolar nerve at the time of surgery has been reported to vary from being "rare" to occurring 36% of the time.[70] Long-term sensory defects have also been reported to vary from none to 35%.[45,86] These apparent discrepancies can be explained by the differences in the sensitivity of the mea-

surement techniques; in addition there is a wide variation in the time after surgery during which the patients were tested. Other variables, such as whether the osteotomy was approached intraorally or extraorally as well as variations in the length of the cut, theoretically could affect the incidence of sensory problems, but comparison studies have not been done. From studies that have been done the incidence of damage to the inferior alveolar nerve is low with the VSO compared with the sagittal osteotomy.[86,87] The patient, however, should be warned that short-term sensory loss is a definite risk, and permanent neuropathy is possible.

Temporomandibular Joint Dysfunction
There has been interesting literature published on changes in tempromandibular joint function after a VSO. These have included a number of radiographic studies documenting positional change of the condyle relative to the fossa. Radiographically there is an initial downward and forward movement of the condyle, with a subsequent tendency to return to its preoperative position.[77,78,82] Sometimes a double contour of the condyle appears approximately 6 months postoperatively, which has been attributed to the condyle's remodeling after the surgery.[88] Remodeling of the glenoid fossa has also been documented.[78]

In one early review of 100 cases 6 patients were reported to have temporomandibular joint problems at 1 year after surgery.[89] A form of the VSO has been used to treat patients with temporomandibular pain and dysfunction. It appears that the VSO does not put the temporomandibular joint at any significant risk, and it may in fact be salutary for patients with temporomandibular joint dysfunction.[90–92]

Other Complications   Among the other reported complications of the VSO, vascular necrosis of the proximal segment

seems to be the most potentially devastating. The maintenance of some muscle attachment to the angles makes this possibility unlikely.

Inverted L and C Ramus Osteotomies

Osteotomy designs in the vertical ramus that include both the condyle and coronoid in the same segment have varied from Blair's simple horizontal osteotomy to the modified C osteotomy of Hayes. The horizontal osteotomy of the vertical ramus has generally fallen into disuse because of the substantial relapse potential, but many of the remaining suggested variations continue to have treatment value. The two procedures that seem to be the most popular are the inverted L and the C osteotomites. Both are generally approached extraorally, although intraoral variants are possible.[93] Clinical studies of either technique are rare, but those that exist seem to demonstrate reasonable success in correcting skeletal deformities with minimal complications.

Indications   The C osteotomy is generally reserved for treatment of horizontal mandibular deficiencies, with some authors suggesting that it can be used to close anterior open bite. The inverted L, however, has been used for the correction of most kinds of mandibular horizontal discrepancies, including anterior open bite. Generally advancements of the distal segment with either technique require bone grafting to ensure adequate bone union.

Techniques   The basic techniques for an extraoral approach to do a C and inverted L are the same, with the only modification being the inferior horizontal cut in the C osteotomy. For that reason the inverted L will be described first, with various modifications of the C discussed later. The patient is prepared and draped, such that access to both the mouth and the submandibular incision area can occur without contamination of the skin wound by oral organisms. This can be accomplished in a variety of ways, but most surgeons use a plastic drape with adhesive on one edge to separate the two areas. The external drapes should be arranged so that they allow turning of the head for access to the submandibular wounds as well as access to the mouth.

The submandibular incision is made 2 cm below the angle and inferior border of the mandible. The posterior portion is curved superiorly to follow the cervical skin line as well as to improve the access to the entire vertical ramus. Generally the incision is approximately 6 cm in length. Sharp dissection is used down through the platysma, and then blunt dissection is begun to minimize risk to the marginal mandibular branch of the facial nerve. The incision through the pterygomandibular sling and periosteum is made along the inferior border and is carried around the angle and up the posterior border about 2 cm. Periosteum and

attachments for the masseter are completely stripped off the lateral cortex of the vertical ramus up to the level of the sigmoid notch. Very little periosteum is stripped off the medial side, especially at the angle, to retain as much blood supply as possible to the proximal fragment. The posterior vertical osteotomy is made at least 7 mm in front of the posterior border and extends to a point of the inferior border just in front of the angle. The horizontal cut is made above the anticipated position of the inferior alveolar foramen (Figure 56-14A). As mentioned above with the VSO it is wise to have a good radiographic view of the ramus so that the position of this foramen can be more accurately located. The study by Reitzik and colleagues of the position of the foramen relative to the lateral landmarks is helpful to review to lessen trauma to the neurovascular bundle.[72]

Once the cuts are made the medial periosteum may have to be elevated from some of the distal fragment to allow its

advancement. Moist gauze is placed in the wound, and a similar procedure is done on the opposite side. After completion of the second side, drapes are pulled back and shifted such that the oral cavity can be entered to place the mandibular teeth into the new occlusal position and secured with maxillomandibular dental fixation. The surgeons who are involved in the intraoral fixation should change gloves and surgical gowns before the drapes are replaced so that the skin incisions can again be approached. The next step varies depending on the type of mandibular movement that occurred; however, the importance of maintaining the proximal fragment close to its preoperative position remains. If the distal segment is set back, then the proximal segment has to be overlapped laterally (Figure 56-14B). As described with the VSO some adjustments of the lateral cortex of the distal segment may be necessary to permit passive position of the proximal fragment as well as to provide a good area of bone contact. The use of some form of

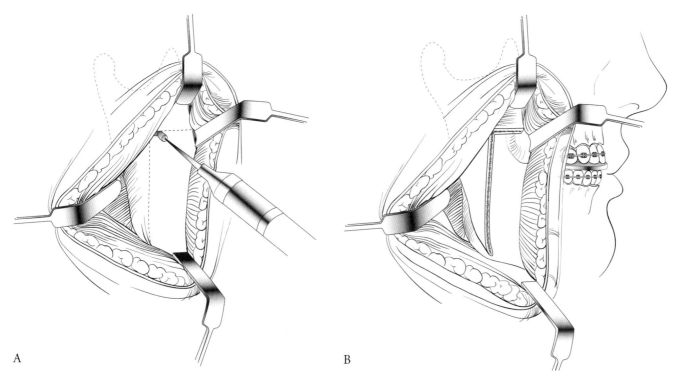

A   B

FIGURE **56-14** *The extraoral inverted* L *osteotomy. Adapted from Bloomquist DS. Principles of mandibular orthognathic surgery. In: Peterson LJ, Indresano AT, Marciani RD, Roser SM. Principles of oral and maxillofacial surgery. Vol 3. Philadelphia (PA): J.B. Lippincott Company; 1992. p. 1430.*

fixation is generally recommended, although the use of no interosseous fixation has been suggested.[93] The type of osseous fixation varies widely; however, rigid internal fixation with metal plates or mesh secured with screws has become more popular (Figure 56-15).[93] After irrigation the wound is closed in layers by whatever suturing method and material

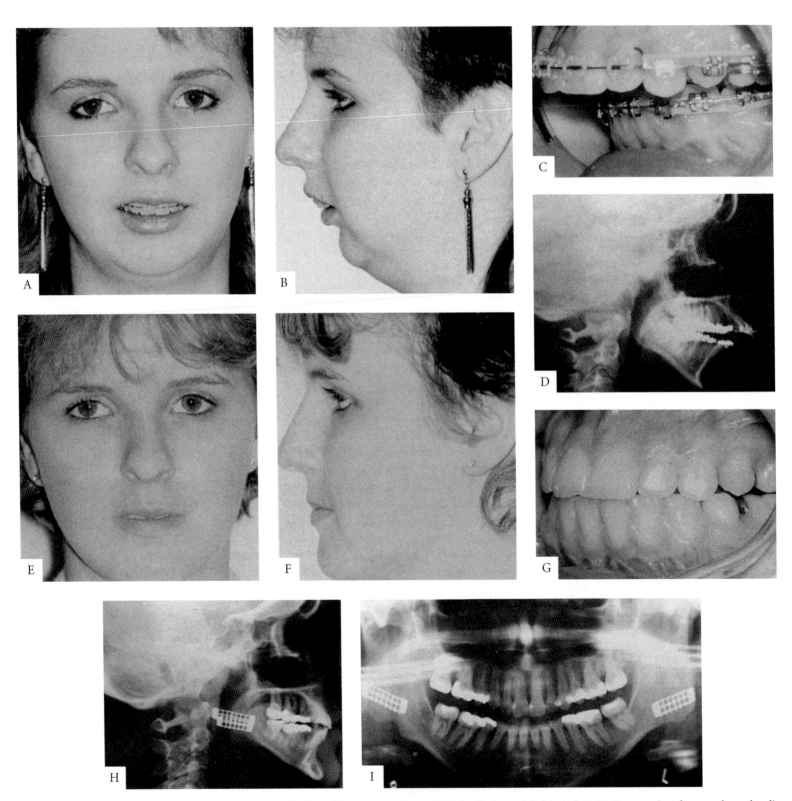

FIGURE 56-15   *Patient who was treated with an extraoral inverted L osteotomy (for mandibular horizontal deficiency). A–D, Preoperative photographs and radiograph. E–I, Postoperative photographs and radiograph. Reproduced with permission from Bloomquist DS. Principles of mandibular orthognathic surgery. In: Peterson LJ, Indresano AT, Marciani RD, Roser SM. Principles of oral and maxillofacial surgery. Vol 3. Philadelphia (PA): J.B. Lippincott Company; 1992. p. 1432–3.*

the surgeon prefers. Care should be taken to ensure hemostasis as the wound is closed. If there is any concern about hematoma formation a small drain should be placed. External pressure dressings are maintained for 24 to 48 hours. When the bone has been stabilized with wire fixation, maxillomandibular fixation is kept in place for at least 6 weeks and preferably 8 weeks.

Alternative Techniques The most commonly used variation of the previously mentioned technique is the **C** osteotomy. This technique was first described jointly by Caldwell and colleagues in an article reviewing their experiences with what they called a vertical **L** osteotomy.[18] They described a variation of their basic vertical **L** with the addition of a horizontal cut that extended forward from the vertical cut below the inferior alveolar canal (Figure 56-16A). This permitted a larger amount of bone contact when the mandible was advanced. They also realized the problems caused by advancing the coronoid process and recommended either cutting the coronoid loose (coronoidotomy) or including it with the proximal segment (**C** osteotomy). Arcing the inferior cut was suggested to permit increased bone contact as the distal segment was advanced (Figure 56-16B).[95] Unfortunately the proposed arc cannot always be made since the position of the neurovascular bundle may interfere. Sagittal splitting of the inferior limb of the **C** osteotomy was proposed both to increase the bone contact area when the mandible was advanced and to decrease the problem of "notching" of the inferior border (Figure 56-16C).[19] This latter problem, which is noticeable in some patients, is caused by the defect along the inferior border resulting from the advanced distal segment of the mandible. A further variation used to improve bone healing includes a bone graft taken from the lateral cortex of the distal segment and transferred back into the gap of the midramus area (Figure 56-16D). The coronoid

process has also been recommended as a free graft in to this defect.[20]

A further major modification of the described techniques is the use of rigid internal fixation.[94,96,97] The use of vitalium mesh with two screws in each fragment has been demonstrated as being effective, but any rigid plate with screws can be used to permit the early release of maxillomandibular dental fixation.

Complications The skeletal stability of the inverted **L** and its modifications,

unlike the VSO, seems to be technique-sensitive to the type of fixation used. Like stability studies for almost all aspects of orthognathic surgery, controlled clinical studies are nonexistent, and the comparison of techniques by a single institution, if reported, lacks sufficient numbers of patients to make valid conclusions. Farrell and Kent looked at inverted **L** and **C** osteotomies and reported skeletal relapse similar to what had been reported for the BSSO.[93] However, because there were different criteria for the use of these two

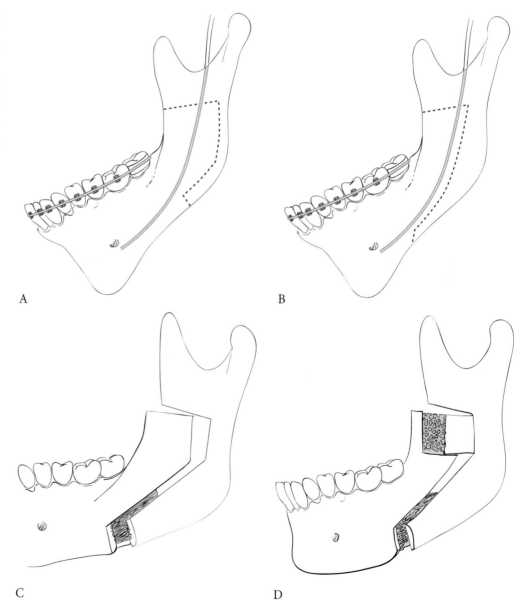

A B C D

FIGURE 56-16 *Different forms of the **C** osteotomy. Adapted from Bloomquist DS. Principles of mandibular orthognathic surgery. In: Peterson LJ, Indresano AT, Marciani RD, Roser SM. Principles of oral and maxillofacial surgery. Vol 3. Philadelphia (PA): J.B. Lippincott Company; 1992. p. 1434.*

types of osteotomies, comparisons between them are questionable. Greebe and Tuinzing compared the stability of mandibular advancement by way of an inverted L or a BSSO.[98] With only a few patients they did not show any difference between the groups, but they did claim that skeletal relapse was dependent on the ratio of posterior facial height to anterior facial height. The largest studies of the stability of the inverted L included the use of rigid internal fixation in patients who had the mandible advanced. These seem to demonstrate that the use of rigid fixation for this type of procedure is more stable than simple maxillomandibular fixation.[96,97] However, statements relative to stability of mandibular setbacks or the closure of open bites cannot be made, although a few authors seem to advocate these skeletal deformities as indications for the use of the inverted L osteotomy.[96,99]

The incidence of facial nerve damage has not been mentioned in any review of these techniques, although it can be inferred to be quite low, given the reports for the external approach to the VSO. The incidence of damage to the inferior alveolar nerve should be higher than the extraoral VSO because of the horizontal portions of the osteotomy, but Reitzik and colleagues reported only a 6% incidence of permanent anesthesia with inverted L osteotomies.[96] The incidence of unsightly scars, which many clinicians claim deters them from using this approach, is unknown with this group of osteotomies.

Bilateral Sagittal Split Osteotomy of the Vertical Ramus

The BSSO of the vertical ramus has in a relatively short time become the predominant orthognathic procedure of the mandible. Schuchardt is generally given credit for the use of an intraoral approach to what some call the "step" osteotomy of the vertical ramus.[23] Specifically he described parallel horizontal cuts through the cortex of the vertical ramus, the medial cut being placed above the lingula and a lateral cut being made about 1 cm below that. A split was then made between these two cortices, and the distal segment could then be advanced or set back. Lane evidently described a very similar procedure earlier, but it probably was done extraorally (see Figure 56-4).[22] The singular credit for improving on this osteotomy, as well as being its strongest advocate, belongs to Obwegeser, who together with Trauner in 1955 described a sagittal split of the vertical ramus.[21] This intraoral technique included the medial horizontal cut above the lingula, but the lateral horizontal cut was lower than Schuchardt's and extended to a point just above the angle, at least 25 mm below the lingual cortical cut (Figure 56-17A). A wide-splitting osteotome was then used to obtain a split between cortices, with care taken to preserve the inferior alveolar nerve and vascular bundle. This procedure was later slightly modified by Obwegeser by angling the lateral cut more toward the inferior border of the mandible (Figure 56-17B). The major modifications still in use today were suggested by DalPont.[24] The change commonly attributed to DalPont is the vertical cut through the lateral cortex behind the second molar. But he also suggested the use of a medial cut that extends just past the lingula so that the posterior split would occur in the mylohyoid groove instead of back at the inferior border. Multiple other modifications have been suggested, but surprisingly the present-day osteotomy remains very similar to that initially described by Obwegeser and DalPont.

Indications The BSSO has been advocated for almost every possible move that includes the entire horizontal ramus of the mandible.

Technique This osteotomy has had multiple variations suggested, as would be expected for such a popular procedure, but many of them are based on a surgeon's individual preference, and their effect on the outcome of the osteotomy is questionable. Therefore, only the basic procedures to be followed will be outlined, as well as the significant modifications that have been shown to affect the outcome or seem to have a good theoretical basis.

The incision is started on the anterior portion of the vertical ramus, midway between the occlusal planes. It is carried downward through the middle of the retromolar fossa to a point about 5 mm behind the second (or in some cases third) molar.

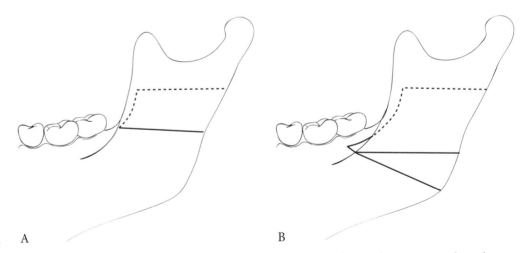

A   B

FIGURE 56-17 *Obwegeser's osteotomies of the ramus.* A, *Original cortical cuts.* B, *Later lateral cortex cuts. Adapted from Bloomquist DS. Principles of mandibular orthognathic surgery. In: Peterson LJ, Indresano AT, Marciani RD, Roser SM. Principles of oral and maxillofacial surgery. Vol 3. Philadelphia (PA): J.B. Lippincott Company; 1992. p. 1435.*

Then the incisions wind laterally and forward to a point distal of the first molar (Figure 56-18A). The incision should be kept lateral enough to allow easy closure of the wound with the teeth in fixation. The periosteum is reflected to expose the lateral cortex to the mandible down to the inferior border. The exposure should be limited posteriorly to maximize the blood supply to the proximal fragment; this usually means the exposure ends at about the antegonial notch. A lateral channel retractor can be placed at this time to assist in retraction as the periosteum is elevated from the retromolar area up the anterior border of the vertical ramus. Special periosteal strippers have been developed to assist this portion of the surgery. The attachment of the temporalis muscle can be tenacious, but it has to be removed to at least the level of the sigmoid notch to ensure adequate access for the medial cut. Most times this means stripping about a centimeter of the temporalis attachment off the anterior border of the coronoid. The periosteum is then elevated from the medial surface of the vertical ramus, starting at about the level of the sigmoid notch and extending back to the medial flare at the start of the condylar neck. Inferiorly the medial cortex is exposed to the lingula, with care being used to minimize trauma to the inferior alveolar nerve as it exits behind and below this point. The periosteal elevation can be extended inferoanteriorly along the internal oblique line to the distal of the second molar to allow better exposure of the osteotomy site. A variety of retractors are available for the protection of the medial soft tissue and nerve, but it is wise to choose one that permits as much visualization as possible while at the same time protecting the soft tissue (Figure 56-18B). Excessive medial retraction should not be done in order to minimize neural damage. It should be noted that no attempt is made to carry the exposure to the posterior border of the vertical ramus.

The osteotomy is started by making a horizontal bone cut through the medial cortex of the vertical ramus that extends from a point just posterior to and above the lingula to the anterior border. Anteriorly the cut is made about halfway through the ramus, but in the concavity above and behind the lingula it should be shallow to allow the posterior medial split to initiate in the mylohyoid groove (Figure 56-18C). Sometimes it is helpful to use a large round or acrylic bur to remove bone from the internal oblique ridge so that the depth of this concavity can be visualized. Occasionally at the level of this horizontal cut there is no significant cancellous bone to delineate the cortices. Here the use of a half thickness of the ramus is the most practical guideline for judging the depth of this cut.

The vertical cut through the buccal cortex is generally made just distal to the second molar and extends from the inferior border superiorly to the external oblique ridge. Sometimes the mandible is thin and the external oblique ridge ends at the distal buccal aspect of the second molar. In this case the superior aspect of the vertical cut should be posterolateral enough so that the roots of the second molar are not placed at risk. The cut should be as close to perpendicular to the inferior border as possible and extended just into cancellous bone. Caution must be used such that the cut is not taken any deeper because the inferior alveolar nerve can be just medial to the cortex.

The vertical and horizontal cortical cuts are connected, starting superiorly at the anterior border of vertical ramus and continuing down just inside the external oblique ridge to the vertical cut (Figure 56-18D). Again the cut is made into cancellous bone, when at all possible, with the superior part of this connection being as deep as possible, especially if there is no cancellous bone present. This will minimize the chance of an inadvertent fracture of the medial cortex. Difficulty is encountered often if a third molar is present and has been scheduled to be removed at the time of surgery. It is generally wise to plan for the mandibular third molars to be removed well in advance of the sagittal osteotomy since they can make the surgery more difficult. Experienced surgeons can remove the tooth and obtain a successful split, but almost all try to avoid this situation because it may increase the risk of an unplanned buccal or lingual cortical plate fracture and can make rigid fixation with the use of screws more difficult.

Techniques vary widely in how the split is accomplished. The method to be described is an attempt to be as universal as possible. First, steps are taken to ensure that the limits of the split occur as defined by the horizontal and vertical bone cuts. A narrow (4 mm) thin osteotome is driven along the horizontal cut and directed so that it cuts through the medial cortex above and behind the lingula. It is also used to ensure that the split at the base of the vertical cut is started through the midpoint of the inferior border. Many surgeons also use this type of thin osteotome to "step" along the connecting cut to help ensure that the split stays close to the lateral bone cortex. Traditionally wide-wedging osteotomes have been used to slowly complete the split. More often today a special spreading instrument is used along with a smaller osteotome to allow more control of the split. Generally the movement is initiated along the vertical cut and carefully extended posteriorly. The fine osteotome can be used to keep the split close to the lateral cortex. If the nerve is encountered it is carefully separated from the proximal fragment. The split along the inferior border can be difficult to control, and the judicious use of a thin osteotome will assist in this area. Finally as the posterior split through the medial cortex is made care should be used to prevent the split from continuing behind the mylohyoid fossa and starting up the neck of the condyle. The speed of the split often varies, depending on the elasticity of the bone. In older patients, in

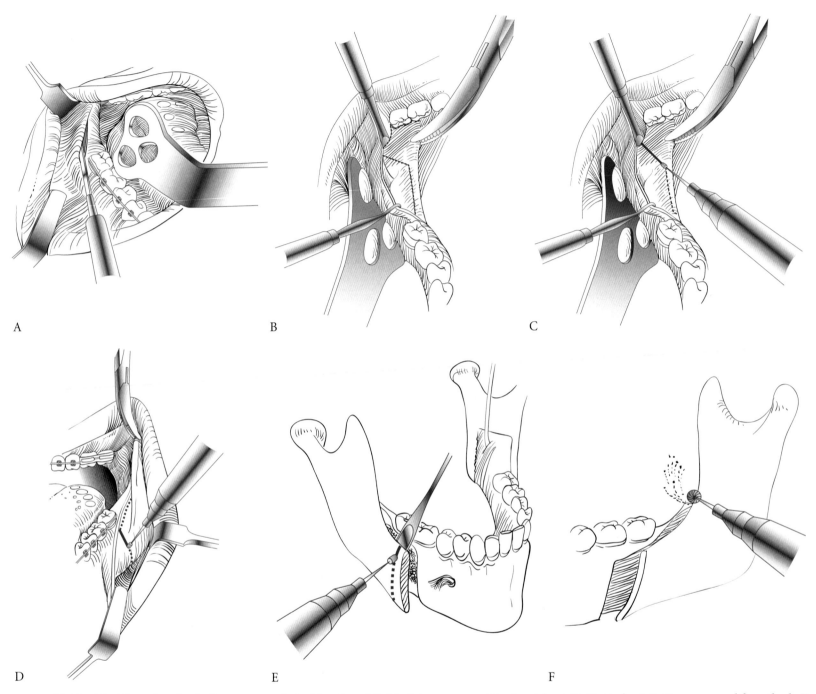

A

B

C

D

E

F

FIGURE 56-18   *The bilateral sagittal split osteotomy. A, Incision. B and C, Medial exposure and horizontal cut. D, Vertical cut. E, Bone removeal for setback. F, Bone removal for large adjustments. Adapted from Bloomquist DS. Principles of mandibular orthognathic surgery. In: Peterson LJ, Indresano AT, Marciani RD, Roser SM. Principles of oral and maxillofacial surgery. Vol 3. Philadelphia (PA): J.B. Lippincott Company; 1992. p. 1436–7.*

whom the bone is not as elastic, the split can occur very suddenly. Preventing inappropriate fractures is dependent on the care used not only in making the cortical bone cuts but also in ensuring that the splits occur as planned at the posterior aspect of the horizontal cut and along the inferior border.

Periosteum of the muscle attachment of the medial pterygoid is stripped off the proximal fragment to permit freedom of movement between the two fragments. If the mandibular teeth are scheduled to be moved posteriorly, either on one side when correcting an asymmetry or bilaterally for correction of horizontal mandibular

excess, an appropriate amount of bone is removed at this time from the anterior edge of the proximal fragment. The amount of removal can be based on model surgery or on the prediction tracings. On large setbacks, bone will need to be removed from the anterior edge of the vertical ramus to prevent this area from interfering with the patient's ability to clean the mandibular second molars (Figure 56-18E). Conversely in large advancements, bone sometimes has to be removed from the remaining portion of the anterior border of the vertical ramus of the distal segment just anterior to the lingula, to prevent encroachment of the segment against the tuberosity (Figure 56-18F). After the opposite side is split the mandible is moved into its new position and stabilized by maxillomandibular fixation. It is preferable that an occlusal splint be used to ensure accurate position of the mandible relative to the maxilla, based on the presurgical model surgery. It is rare that teeth occlude well enough that a splint is not needed.

The placement of osseous fixation is made at this point. As multiple techniques are possible, different options will be described in the following section "Alternative Techniques." After placement of osseous fixation, if rigid fixation is used, the maxillomandibular fixation is released, allowing the occlusion to be checked. The wounds are thoroughly irrigated and closed with the use of a resorbable running suture. No drains or external dressings are generally necessary (Figure 56-19).

Alternative Techniques There are many variations to the foregoing technique. In this section only the major ones will be discussed. The design of the osteotomy itself is an area that has received much attention, with each of these variations generally representing an attempt to decrease the incidence of one or more complications. There is very little supportive research for any of the modifications. Obwegeser was responsible for two variations, the first being his original design, in which the buccal cut was horizontal and parallel to the lingual cut through the cortex of the vertical ramus (see Figure 56-17A). This original technique was modified by making the lateral cortical cut at an angle to the medial cut so that the posterior portion of the osteotomy ended just above the angle (see Figure 56-17B).[100]

A popular modification of DalPont's vertical osteotomy is the continuation of this cut completely through the inferior border, which, according to its advocates, made the split easier.[59] This technique, however, makes the use of rigid fixation with screws difficult.[101] A few modifications have been suggested for the connecting cut, with the primary goal of allowing

better control of the proximal fragment. These modifications appear to be primarily personal preferences as there is no evidence that these changes improve the success of the procedure.

A major area of variation for the sagittal split osteotomy of the vertical ramus occurs in the use, or nonuse, of osseous fixation.[21,25,102,103] The original Obwegeser technique used wire through the superior lateral and medial cortices.[104] This technique, with minor variation, became the standard for the sagittal osteotomy until screw fixation became popular.[59] The use of circumandibular wire and inferior border wires have also been suggested as possibly better ways of controlling the proximal fragment.[105] No evidence exists that any of these wire techniques have an advantage for minimizing complications.[26]

Spiessl introduced the concept of using screws for the "rigid internal fixation" of the sagittal osteotomy.[26] Following its introduction in 1974 there was a slow acceptance of this method of osseous fixation. Currently there is little debate on the advantages of using rigid internal fixation. However, there exists a wide variety of methods and materials used. Initially the use of three 2.7 mm

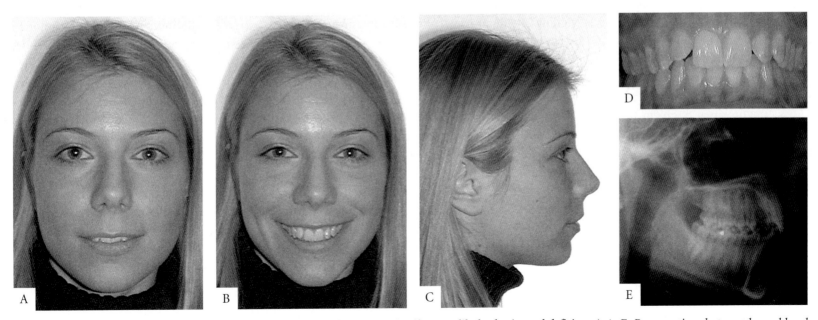

FIGURE **56-19** *Patient who was treated with bilateral sagittal split osteotomies (for mandibular horizontal deficiency). A–E, Preoperative photographs and head radiograph.* (CONTINUED ON NEXT PAGE)

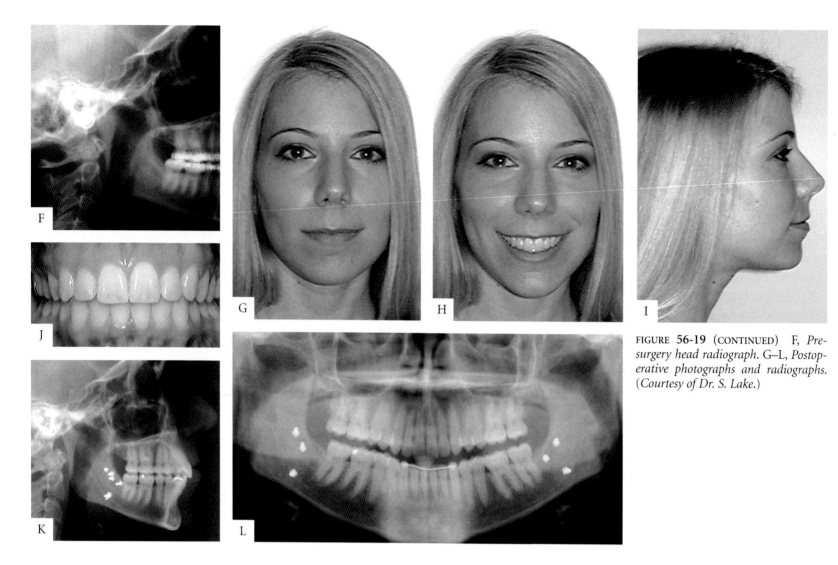

FIGURE 56-19 (CONTINUED) F, *Presurgery head radiograph. G–L, Postoperative photographs and radiographs. (Courtesy of Dr. S. Lake.)*

"lag" screws on each side was advocated. A lag screw is placed by drilling a "guiding" hole with a larger drill through the lateral cortex, followed by a smaller hole through the medial cortex that is threaded with the use of a tap. Lag screws are then used to fix the proximal fragment tightly to the distal fragment. Compression across the osteotomy site is felt to be important to speed the healing of the osteotomy as well as to ensure the stability of the mandible. Concern exists that compression may cause increased nerve damage and displacement of the condyles, with subsequent temporomandibular joint dysfunction.[106,107] An alternative technique, the position screw or bicortical screw, in which both cortices are tapped, has been advocated for stabilizing osteotomy segments.[100] This technique permits mainte-

nance of the gaps that may occur between the proximal and distal fragments, with no effort being made to compress the two segments together. Standardization of techniques does not exist in rigid fixation of the sagittal osteotomy as there are differences in screw sizes, number of screws, materials used, and whether plates are used across the osteotomy sites. Most of the research in the United States has centered on the use of three screws that are 2 mm in diameter. Direct comparisons of differing rigid fixation techniques are rare and do not demonstrate that any one technique is an advantage.[108–110] One exception was noted by Fujioka and colleagues, who found that there was more rotation through the osteotomy sites in patients with monocortical plate and screw fixation.[111]

The use of resorbable screws has been a recent addition to fixation techniques. First attempted in Finland, the screws are made from polyglycolic acid using different manufacturing techniques and formulas. Development of these self-reinforced polylactic/polyglycolic polymers that have reliable strength to withstand forces of mastication have made their use possible in orthognathic surgery. The obvious advantage of resorbable fixation is to obviate the need for future hardware removal, which has become important with patient concerns over the potential risks of any kind of permanent implants. The key features that are crucial in its application in orthognathic surgery are the material's rigidity and strength with an ability to resorb in a timely fashion. A few small studies have shown apparent stability of these resorbable implants comparable to the metallic fixation; however, some inherent problems with material handling and early fixation failures have been reported.[112–114] Suuronen and colleagues reported on the use of poly-L-lactic acid (PLLA) screws for fixation in BSSO, with no apparent malocclusion or skeletal relapse.[112] Harada and Enomoto and later Ferretti and Reyneke compared titanium and resorbable screws and noted no difference in healing between two groups and no statistically significant difference in skeletal relapse.[113,114] However, Harada and Enomoto's patients were placed in maxillomandibular fixation for a period ranging from 9 to 14 days following surgery.[112] Kallela and colleagues used self-reinforced PLLA (SR-PLLA) screws for mandibular osteotomies and no maxillomandibular fixation was used postoperatively.[115] Mean advancement was 4.57 mm at B point, and the mean relapse was 17%. In their 2-year follow-up study in 1999, the authors reported osteolytic changes seen around the resorbable screws in 27% of cases, and the screw canals remained as radiolucent shadows without bony filling. Turvey and colleagues reported their experience with resorbable fixation for 194 osteotomies of the maxilla and/or mandible.[116] Forty-three of the patients had a sagittal osteotomy with 2 mm screws placed on each side for fixation. They reported only one infection at a sagittal osteotomy site and one patient who exhibited abnormal masticatory pressures that resulted in loosening of the fixation. Acceptance of the routine use of resorbable fixation with the sagittal split is going to require long-term evaluations with well-designed studies comparing these materials to the metal hardware. The major potential risk of permanent metal fixation is the possibility of bone remodeling, causing the hardware to become noticeable and possibly irritating to the patient. Although not reported in the literature oral and maxillofacial surgeons have had experience with patients returning to have plates and screws removed simply because these implants have become noticeable. This problem has to be weighed against the still unexplored or unknown side effects of the resorbable materials. A good example of these unknowns is the precise time needed for total resorption and degradation of PLLA in human tissues, which is reported to range anywhere from 90 days to 5 years. Surgeons are going to have to closely follow the literature to determine the practicality of these new materials.

An interesting suggested modification in the BSSO technique is the purposeful changing of the rotational position of the proximal fragment to control the direction of mandibular growth. It has generally been recommended that the proximal segment be maintained as close as possible to its preoperative position. O'Ryan and Epker have further suggested that rotating the proximal fragment in a growing patient can change the vector of condylar growth and, thereby, influence the final mandibular position.[117] Studies have failed to support this contention.[118] Also there is concern in using a sagittal osteotomy in growing children, especially those requiring long advancement. Huang and Ross demonstrated what they felt to be a stoppage in mandibular growth and condylar resorption in growing patients in whom sagittal osteotomies were performed.[119] Whether this was a problem of the techniques used or a problem with performing surgery in such a young group of patients is unknown, but this effect has not been noted in any further literature.

A final modification of the BSSO is the concomitant use of a midsymphyseal osteotomy to allow for correction of width discrepancies in the dental arch. Although this procedure could be used with any of the ramal osteotomies, it has only been described with the sagittal osteotomies. First mentioned by Bell, it has become more practical with the use of rigid internal fixation.[120] A single four-hole plate across the bone cut, along with an intact orthodontic arch wire, provides sufficient stability.[121] Concerns of adverse effects on the temporomandibular joint and the periodontium were also shown to be insignificant.[122]

Complications *Stability* The stability of the sagittal osteotomy of the vertical ramus is the most studied complication in orthognathic surgery. Since the relapse patterns differ between mandibular advancements and setbacks, their particular causes most likely differ; however, many of the principles in preventing relapse may be the same. Whereas much of the research on mandibular advancement has been done in the United States, mandibular prognathism has generally received the greatest interest in the Scandinavian countries and the Far East. This highlights one of the major problems for surgeons attempting to decide on which techniques to use to minimize postoperative skeletal change. There are large variations in research techniques as well as surgical approaches that exist not only between surgical centers in different countries but also within the same country. Fortunately there is enough corroboration in the literature that some general statements can be made.

One of the most important findings made in the stability of mandibular osteotomies was that intermaxillary fixation does not prevent postoperative skeletal change. Although this is true of any type of mandibular osteotomy, it was first recognized in the evaluation of mandibular sagittal osteotomies. It is generally felt that soft tissue pressures and muscle pull are the major factors influencing relapse, especially in mandibular advancement.[52,53,122] However, early attempts at minimizing these effects, such as suprahyoid myotomies and external supportive devices, have not been shown to be effective.[64] Internal support techniques, however, have been shown to be effective. Before rigid fixation screws and plates were used, a type of internal support called skeletal fixation was shown to be effective in decreasing the down and back relapse pattern of mandibular advancements.[64] This fixation was usually used in addition to maxillomandibular fixation and consists of wires running from the piriform rim to circumandibular wires placed in the cuspid or molar areas (see Figure 56-9). Interestingly, Van Sickles noted a decrease in relapse in patients with large advancements when skeletal fixation was combined with rigid internal screw fixation.[123]

Other possible causes of relapse that have been implicated are patient's age, preoperative mandibular plane steepness, rotational position of the proximal fragment, amount of distal segment advancement, and the displacement of condyle from the fossa. The effect of mandibular plane steepness is somewhat controversial because of variable results reported in the literature, most of which looked at patients who had wire osseous fixation with intermaxillary fixation. Mobarak and colleagues did clearly find decreased stability in patients with steep mandibular plane angles when rigid internal fixation was used.[124] Of the remaining variables only the last two appear to be definitively supported by clinical studies as being important. In their multicenter study, Schendel and Epker found that displacement of the condyle from the fossa was a significant predictor of relapse.[64] This was further confirmed by Lake and colleagues, who also showed the relation between the amount of advancement and the amount of relapse.[55]

The final area that has been considered as possibly affecting relapse in both mandibular advancement and setback is the rigidity of the fixation across the osteotomy site. Early investigators felt that fixation across the osteotomy site may hinder the normal repositioning of the condyle in the fossa that occurs during maxillomandibular fixation.[103] Later studies showed that wire osteosynthesis was superior to no osseous fixation in frag-

ment position, and the incidence of relapse was less.[102] However, the search for a superior osseous wiring technique that would decrease relapse has not been successful, with most studies that looked at osseous wiring techniques being very consistent in finding a mean relapse of approximately 30%. The large range of individual relapses that does exist has led many surgeons to believe that there are multiple factors that influence relapse.

The use of rigid internal fixation techniques has become the preferred method for minimizing skeletal relapse in the BSSO. Spiessl together with Schmoker and colleagues first discussed the advantages of lag screws in mandibular sagittal split osteotomies. Their initial study of skeletal stability looked at mandibular setbacks, comparing the use of three 2.7 mm screws against wire fixation and one or two screws.[125] It was not until 1985 that Van Sickels and Flanary showed evidence that a similar rigid fixation technique provided increased stability in mandibular advancements.[126] Furthermore larger and longer studies have clearly shown the stability of using three bicortical screws for fixation of the sagittal osteotomy.[127–130] These studies have reported a mean relapse rate of between 0 and 8%. The majority of studies comparing rigid internal fixation techniques against the use of wire osseous fixation have also confirmed a significant difference in stability between the techniques.[131–135] Interestingly the only clinical study that evaluated the stability of osseous wire fixation versus rigid screw fixation on patients treated at the same center seemed to show a comparable long-term stability.[136] This study, however, reported an unusually high stability of the wire osseous fixation group and did nothing to dispute the stability of the screw fixation. The number of screws may very well influence the stability, although only Spiessl's original study demonstrated a difference.

Another common method for rigid internal fixation of the BSSO is the use of

miniplates with monocortical screws. Generally 2 mm systems are used with two screws placed on either side of the osteotomy.[137–140] Questions remain over the minimum number of screws necessary to prevent relapse and whether more or larger screws will improve stability in longer advancements. It has been shown that a single 2 mm screw does not seem to increase mandibular stability over wire osseous fixation, and thus it could be argued, in light of the previously reviewed research, that an increase in number or size of screws can result in more osseous stability.[130,141]

Nerve Damage The possibility of damage to the inferior alveolar nerve during the sagittal osteotomy has been well known since the technique was first described, but surprisingly the problem was minimized by early surgeons. Kole first mentioned a high incidence of sensory problems immediately after surgery for patients with sagittal osteotomies, but most clinicians claimed a very low incidence of long-term problems.[142,143] Walter and Gregg, during an objective study of sensory problems, noted a large incidence of long-term problems.[45] Since this first definitive study there has continued to be a variety of reported instances of both immediate postsurgical as well as chronic sensory disturbances.

Westermark and colleagues evaluated 496 sagittal osteotomies for possible correlations between neurosensory dysfunction and other variables, such as the age of the patient, mandibular movement, type of split technique and fixation, degree of intraoperative nerve encounter, and surgical skill.[144] Nerve dysfunction developed in 40% of the cases. The patient's age had a significant influence on the recovery of the neurosensory function as well as the severity of neurosensory disturbance. Intraoperative nerve encounter and nerve manipulation as well as surgical experience were also reported to have an effect on nerve dysfunction. Other variables had no significant effects on the incidence of neurosensory dysfunction. Ylikontiola and colleagues also found a statistically significant positive correlation between subjective neurosensory loss and the patient's age and, in addition, magnitude of mandibular movement and degree of manipulation of the nerve.[145]

A number of other clinical researchers have noted a significant relation between the patient's age and nerve recovery. This finding was noted early on by MacIntosh, who emphasized that he does not use this osteotomy for patients over age 40 years.[146] The only other interesting correlation was made by Van Sickels and colleagues who reported that patients with a concurrent genioplasty had a greater loss of sensation initially.[147] Unfortunately the wide variation in measurement protocols makes comparisons of these various reports difficult. This also makes difficult the evaluation of techniques that have been suggested to decrease the incidence of nerve damage.

White and colleagues pointed out that damage to the inferior alveolar nerve most likely occurs either during the medial retraction of the soft tissues and the nerve as it enters the canal or during the vertical bone cut.[148] Guernsey and DeChamplain felt that damage occurred during the splitting of the mandible and reported the problem of parts of the nerve staying in the proximal fragment after the split.[149] This has led some surgeons to recommend the use of a small flat (spatula) osteotome during the split, instead of the wide-splitting osteotome.[150] The fine osteotome is malleted carefully along the lateral cortex and cancellous bone junction. The nerve is exposed less often during the split by this technique, and consequently it has been assumed that this results in less sensory disturbances.[151,152] Unfortunately this technique has not been directly compared with any other, and the comparison of the occurrence of sensory disturbance between reports is impossible. Yoshida and colleagues and later Yamamoto and colleagues,

found that nerves that were close to the lateral cortex, as determined by radiographs, were more likely to have severe sensory alteration after surgery.[152,153] The deficits were also more likely to be present 1 year after surgery when the marrow space between the mandibular canal and the external cortical bone was 0.8 mm or less. Some authors feel that by making the vertical cut in the lateral cortex more posterior, a lower incidence of sensory problems occurs.[152,154] This has not been substantiated in comparison studies.

Another possible cause of sensory loss to the nerve may be due to the sharp bone irregularities of the proximal fragment or to compression of the nerve when the proximal fragment is positioned and fixed.[155,156] A round or acrylic bur can be used to remove any bone spicules as well as to widen and deepen the canal in the proximal fragment to prevent this effect. Care must be taken when working around the nerve so that instruments used during the osteotomy do not themselves cause direct damage. This concern was heightened with the use of screw fixation. Paulis and Steinhauser noted slightly higher incidences of long-term sensory loss in patients with rigid screw fixation compared with simple osseous fixation but statistics were not used and the significance of their numbers is highly suspect.[157] Nishioka and colleagues did a comprehensive study involving sensory loss after the use of screw fixation and found the incidence of inferior alveolar sensory loss to be high but well within the range of sensory loss reported by other well-designed objective studies.[158] Subsequently the effect of type of fixation on the neurosensory functional outcome was extensively studied by a number of authors using different methods of clinical testing.[159–162] Brush stroke detection was diminished to a greater extent in the rigid fixation group compared with the wire fixation group from 8 weeks through 2 years postoperatively; however, monofilament detection

did not show significant difference between types of fixation throughout the 2-year follow-up.[159] Despite a great number of studies on neurosensory disturbance following orthognathic surgery, the severity of inferior alveolar nerve injury is difficult to compare across different studies since there is lack of standardization as to which neurosensory tests were used, ways the tests were performed, and how the results were interpreted. Certain neurosensory tests are more sensitive in detecting sensory nerve deficit than others. Tests that evaluate patients' abilities to discriminate direction have been shown to be more sensitive indicators of trigeminal neurosensory impairment than other tests such as light touch detection. Westermark and colleagues used visual analog scale, light touch perception, and temperature testing and concluded that there is a good positive correlation with nerve dysfunction.[160] Alternatively, Chen and colleagues compared three methods of assessing neurosensory disturbance following BSSO: two-point discrimination, pressure-pain thresholds, and perceived sensation changes in specific facial regions.[161] The two-point discrimination test was consistent with patients' self-ratings of neurosensory problems using facial maps, but the pressure-pain test was the least sensitive to neurosensory changes. The frequency of the inferior alveolar nerve disturbance ranged from 10 to 94% depending on the test method and the test site used. In a well-controlled study by Nakagawa and colleagues, the occurrence of a long-lasting postoperative trigeminal sensory hypoesthesia was found to be dependent on the nerve involvement at the bone split interface, the manner of fixation, or the intraoperative handling of the tissue surrounding the nerve.[162]

Although the neurosensory function of the inferior alveolar nerve following sagittal split osteotomy has received a great deal of attention, very few studies have documented the incidence of lingual nerve dysfunction. Jacks and colleagues retrospectively reviewed the patient-reported incidence, duration, and perceived deficit associated with lingual nerve function.[163] In the BSSO patients 19% reported lingual nerve sensory changes of whom 69% reported a resolution of symptoms within a year and 88% reported altered daily activities. When compared with the inferior alveolar nerve, lingual nerve sensory changes occurred much less frequently and resolved more frequently and sooner, but they were associated with greater perceived deficits in patients' daily activities. Zuniga and colleagues were the first to report on studies performed to assess the effect of lingual nerve injury and repair on human taste perception.[164] Gent and colleagues later examined perceived taste intensity and taste quality identification on localized regions of the tongue after orthognathic surgery.[165] Lingual nerve function in taste perception was diminished at 1 to 2 months after surgery, likely due to impared chorda tympani nerve function, but it improved by 6 to 9 months after surgery.

Temporomandibular Joint Dysfunction

The incidence of temporomandibular joint dysfunction will be considered in two ways: first, the incidence of temporomandibular joint symptoms that are present after surgery compared with preoperative findings; and second, the change in mandibular range of motion. The latter may obviously not be related to temporomandibular joint dysfunction; on the other hand it has to be considered if evaluating the effects of the surgery on the temporomandibular joint. Unfortunately very few authors related these two areas when they reported on the effect of the sagittal osteotomy. Another factor that must be taken into account in evaluating the effects on the temporomandibular joint in any recent orthognathic surgery is the possible contribution of the orthodontics as provided in conjunction with the

surgery. There is still debate on how much orthodontics itself may help or cause temporomandibular joint dysfunction.

Similar to sensory loss the potential of the sagittal osteotomy causing temporomandibular joint dysfunction was recognized early in its use.[24] Reporting of the incidence of temporomandibular joint problems, however, has been highly variable, with most authors recording only the postoperative complaint without any reference to the preoperative condition. Some of the first reviews that did look at pre- and postoperative temporomandibular joint symptoms seemed to imply an increase in joint noises, but not in pain, following the sagittal osteotomy.[56,166,167] The use of rigid screw fixation was felt by some to cause an increase in temporomandibular joint problems.[168] This concern was highlighted by radiographic findings of condylar changes that occurred with rigid screw fixation. Kundert and Hadjianghelou demonstrated that this tendency occurred with both wires and screws but was greater with rigid fixation than with a wire osseous fixation technique.[106] In neither study was there a discussion of whether these changes had any clinical consequences. Hackney and colleagues found in their study of patients, in whom bicortical screw fixation with mandibular sagittal split was used for mandibular advancements, that little change in condylar position occurred, and there was no significant effect of the surgery on temporomandibular joint symptoms.[169] Paulis and Steinhauser compared preoperative and postoperative temporomandibular joint symptoms in two large groups who had either rigid screw fixation or wire osseous fixation of sagittal osteotomies.[157] They could find no difference in postoperative incidence between the two groups and in fact found a notable decrease in temporomandibular joint pain in both groups. The possibility that the sagittal osteotomy may benefit many patients with temporomandibular joint

symptoms was suggested by Martis and Karabouta.[170,171] He reported that only 11% of the patients who had temporomandibular joint symptoms before surgery had any symptoms after, whereas about 4% of the asymptomatic patients had problems after surgery. These results were better than but consistent with a study of all types of orthognathic surgery patients, which showed an improvement in a large percentage of patients, with relatively small risk for the asymptomatic patient.[172]

There is, surprisingly, a body of evidence in the literature that sagittal split osteotomy may have a beneficial effect on preexisting temporomandibular joint dysfunction. It is generally believed that temporomandibular joint dysfunction is found at a higher incidence in Class II patients compared with patients with Class I and III malocclusions. The use of the sagittal split osteotomy as an alternative to the mandibular condylotomy to treat patients with painful temporomandibular joint dysfunction has been proposed by some authors.[173] They suggest repositioning the proximal segment and increasing the joint space, both of which are thought to have an unloading effect on the highly innervated retrodiskal tissues. However, this is controversial and there has not been adequate research to confirm this impression.

Debate on rigid versus wire fixation relative to their effects on the temporomandibular joint has led to a number of studies. Most have shown that there is no significant difference in the incidence of temporomandibular joint symptoms between patients who have received rigid fixation versus wire osteosynthesis during sagittal split osteotomies.[174] Feinerman and Piecuch compared the temporomandibular joint outcomes of the miniplate with monocortical screw group versus the superior border wire fixation with maxillomandibular fixation group.[175] They found no demonstrable long-term differences between the two groups with respect to mandibular vertical opening, crepitance, and temporomandibular joint pain. In fact masticatory muscle pain and temporomandibular joint clicking improved with rigid fixation and worsened with nonrigid fixation.

The only negative report on the effects of BSSOs on the temporomandibular joint was submitted by Wolford and colleagues.[176] They evaluated changes in temporomandibular joint dysfunction in patients with presurgical temporomandibular joint internal derangement as well as the long-term stability of patients who underwent orthognathic surgery. Unlike other clinicians they observed the appearance of new or an aggravation of existing temporomandibular joint symptoms in a group of patients who were an average of 14 months postsurgery. Therefore, the authors recommended that surgical correction of preexisting temporomandibular joint pathology be considered, either preceding or simultaneous with the orthognathic surgery. In summary it appears that there is a low risk of worsening temporomandibular joint symptoms in patients who do have some form of temporomandibular joint dysfunction when using the BSSO. Conversely this osteotomy may result in improved symptoms in a greater number of patients. Unfortunately methods of predicting this outcome in individual patients have not been developed.

Mechanical displacement of the condyle out of its correct position has been implicated as a significant factor in postsurgical skeletal relapse after sagittal split osteotomy. For this reason, as well as in an attempt to minimize temporomandibular joint problems, a great deal of interest has been focused by early investigators on the issues of condylar position after sagittal split osteotomy.[177] There have been a myriad of technical notes on how to maintain the preoperative condylar position and use of different condylar repositioning devices, based on anecdotal reports of individual surgeon's experiences. Harris and colleagues examined factors influencing condylar position after sagittal split osteotomy fixed with rigid fixation.[178] The amount of advancement did not correlate with condylar displacement. Condyle angulation and superior-inferior movement did correlate somewhat with the amount of advancement. In addition Van Sickels and colleagues found that the condylar position was slightly different with rigid fixation versus wire osteosynthesis beyond 8 weeks postoperatively, but the ultimate position of the condyle was not different.[179] They found, as have many others, that the final condylar position was posterior and superior after a mandibular advancement. Renzi and colleagues specifically examined Class III patients without preoperative temporomandibular joint dysfunction; half of the patient population was treated with a condylar positioning device whereas the other half of patients was treated with manual control of condylar position.[180] The condylar repositioning device did not prevent the changes in condyle positions in all cases. Neither group had any skeletal or occlusal relapse or postsurgical temporomandibular joint dysfunction. However, the incidence of new onset of temporomandibular joint dysfunction in healthy individuals following orthognathic surgery is known to be low as previously mentioned, and this study only included patients without preoperative temporomandibular joint symptoms. Therefore, it is not surprising that the patients did not develop any postsurgical temporomandibular joint dysfunction. The clinical implication of condylar position in the healthy versus the preexisting temporomandibular joint dysfunction groups may be different; therefore, the true clinical significance of condylar position in exacerbation of temporomandibular joint symptoms remains an enigma.

Computed tomography (CT) has enabled clinicians to assess and quantify condylar position changes in three planes of space. Alder and colleagues reported that changes in condylar position occurred in all planes of space, but the most common postoperative condyle position was more lateral with increased condyle angle, the coronoid process was higher, and the condyle was again reported to be more superior and posterior in the fossa.[181] Rebellato and colleagues found in their study group that there was increased superior postsurgical movement of the condyles with increasing magnitudes of surgical advancement of the mandible.[182]

Magnetic resonance imaging (MRI) has revolutionized the examination of the temporomandibular joint, in that it allows not only the evaluation of condylar position but also provides information on the disk. Gaggl and colleagues reported clinical and MRI findings of the temporomandibular joint in Class II patients, preoperatively and 3 months postoperatively.[183] Clinically patients had improvements in joint pain and abnormal joint sounds such as clicking. The MRI showed displacement of the disk in 38 of the 50 joints preoperatively and in 28 postoperatively. No correlation was made between the change in disk position and improvement in temporomandibular joint symptoms, which is consistent with other MRI studies. Ueki and colleagues made interesting comparisons of the condylar and disk positions after BSSO and intraoral vertical ramus osteotomy (IVRO) and correlated these findings with temporomandibular joint symptoms postoperatively.[184] Fewer or no temporomandibular joint symptoms were reported by 88% of the patients who underwent IVRO and by 66% of patients who underwent BSSO. MRI study showed no change in anterior disk displacement after BSSO; however, improvement was seen in 44% of patients who underwent IVRO, at least in the early postsurgical period.

The effect of the sagittal osteotomy of the vertical ramus on mandibular range of motion has been extensively studied. Whereas Stacy found that patients who underwent mandibular setbacks with maxillomandibular fixation generally returned to presurgical limits within 9 months following surgery without any physical therapy, other authors have found very different results.[185] Storum and Bell found that without active physical therapy after the release of maxillomandibular fixation there was a decrease in the patient's ability to achieve preoperative opening when compared with patients who had an active rehabilitation program.[186] This latter study is consistent with most clinicians' experience, and some form of active physical therapy is recommended after release from maxillomandibular fixation. However, there is some evidence that rigid internal fixation that permits mandibular movement soon after surgery may result in a more rapid return to preoperative mandibular movement.[187] Nishimura and colleagues found that final postoperative mouth opening was not significantly influenced by the type of fixation.[188]

A final poorly understood temporomandibular joint complication is spontaneous resorption of condyles following sagittal osteotomies.[189] This is a process that may be different from standard relapse with the abnormal resorption being seen primarily in a specific group of patients—young females who have had a history of temporomandibular joint dysfunction before surgery and have undergone a mandibular advancement. Remodeling of the condyles is now accepted to occur after sagittal osteotomies, but fortunately only rarely has this condylar resorption resulted in significant clinical changes. Cutbirth and colleagues evaluated long-term condylar resorption after mandibular advancement stabilized with bicortical screws.[190] Large advancement and preoperative temporomandibular joint symptoms significantly correlated with long-term postoperative condylar resorption at the mean follow-up of 3 years. The amount of vertical resorption did not directly correlate with the amount of relapse seen between 6 to 8 weeks and

long term. Surprisingly there was an improvement in temporomandibular joint symptoms for the group as a whole and even among the group who developed condylar resorption. It should be noted, however, that it is often difficult to draw a line between normal condylar remodeling and condylar resorption. In the Cutbirth study, the authors arbitrarily established a parameter of less than 10% loss of height of the condyle to be considered as "normal remodeling."[190] Attempts to delineate the normal versus pathologic process are difficult, and may lead to an underestimation of the number of condylar resorptions that may occur.

Hoppenreijs and colleagues evaluated the long-term treatment results of 26 patients (23 women and 3 men) who developed progressive condylar resorption following orthognathic surgery.[191] The preoperative condylar configuration was noted in patients with deep bites to have more resorption on the superior aspect of the condyle, whereas patients with anterior open bites had resorption on the superior and anterior surfaces of the condyle. Thirteen patients were managed without surgery after the diagnosis of condylar resorption, and only 3 patients had Class I occlusion at the end of treatment. Thirteen patients underwent a second surgical correction, with 7 patients having satisfactory occlusal results. Four of the patients had relapse with a stable occlusion not requiring further treatment, and 2 patients had complete relapse requiring a third surgical procedure. It was suggested that without surgical intervention after condylar resorption, further resorption ceased after approximately 2 years. The authors speculated that either the mechanical loading during or after BSSO and/or the impediment of blood flow to the condylar segment and the temporomandibular joint capsule may play a role in the condylar resorption. However, the etiology for this process is still unclear, but it does seem to be self-limiting and the resulting

dental skeletal deformity can usually be successfully treated with further mandibular surgery.

Miscellaneous Complications A wide variety of other complications have been reported following the sagittal split osteotomy of the mandibular ramus. Early reviews of complications from this procedure noted some trouble with excess blood loss, postoperative airway compromise, large aseptic bone loss, and facial nerve damage. Greater experience and better instrumentation seem to have dramatically decreased the incidence of these problems. Bleeding is generally easily managed by direct or indirect pressure over the bleeding soft tissue and vessels. Lanigan and colleagues, reporting on a questionnaire sent to a large number of oral and maxillofacial surgeons, found only 21 cases of significant bleeding following mandibular osteotomies.[192] Suspected sources of bleeding included the inferior alveolar artery, facial artery, maxillary artery, and retromandibular vein. Management primarily included direct pressure packing or ligation of the vessel via the open wound. Extraoral approaches to gain access to the facial or external carotid artery can be ineffective due to the collateral circulation. Angiography with embolization is considered appropriate in cases of acute persistent postoperative arterial bleeding.

One group of problems that seems to persist is the inappropriate fracture in the proximal segment or the posterior lingual aspect of the distal segment. Good surgical technique minimizes these problems, and care used during the split is worth the effort, as correcting a "bad" split can be difficult. Fortunately the use of screws and plates does improve the chance of obtaining a satisfactory result, in light of an unexpected fracture, with minimum further morbidity to the patient.[193] It has been felt that one of the major risk factors predisposing to buccal cortex fracture is the presence of impacted third molars. Precious and colleagues retrospectively reviewed two groups of patients: one group with retained impacted third molars removed during BSSO and the other group with third molars having been removed at least 6 months before BSSO.[194] There was a 1.9% incidence of unfavorable fractures, and the majority of fractures occurred with the group who had the third molars removed at least 6 months before the BSSO. Mehra and colleagues reported 2.2% unfavorable fractures in 500 procedures.[195] They noted a larger percentage of unfavorable fractures in the patients with retained third molars (3.2% vs 1.2%). This finding is consistent with that of Reyneke and colleagues who found that the presence of unerupted third molars increased the degree of difficulty of BSSO, and all 4 (out of 139 patients) unfavorable fractures occurred in those patients with unerupted third molars present at the time of surgery.[196] Ideally third molars should be extracted at least 6 (preferably 9) months prior to the mandibular osteotomy, both to minimize unfavorable fractures and to allow optimal bony healing, especially when using internal rigid fixation.

Airway patency has become an area of concern to some clinicians, especially in the cases where the mandible is set back. Riley and colleagues reported two patients who were surgically treated for prognathism and later developed sleep apnea.[197] Kawamata and colleagues studied patients with mandibular prognathism who were treated with either sagittal split osteotomy or IVRO for mandibular setback.[198] Using three-dimensional CT images they quantified the airway space after surgery and found that the lateral and frontal widths of the pharyngeal airway had decreased by 23% and 11%, respectively. This reduction in airway dimension did not resolve at 1 year after surgery. However, in the longer postoperative period, a visible recovery of pharyngeal width was seen in some cases. These findings of the decreased airways sec-

ondary to mandibular setback have been confirmed by other investigators. Noteworthy, however, is that only one of these clinical studies had a reported incidence of a patient developing sleep apnea following orthognathic surgery. Therefore one should be cognizant of any physiologic and medical etiologic factors that may have contributed to the emergence of sleep apnea symptoms, rather than simply using the measurement of the posterior airway space following mandibular osteotomies as the sole means of predicting a new onset of sleep apnea disorders.

In general, the risk of infection seems to be low with the BSSO. In their clinical review of 700 consecutive cases of mandibular osteotomies, Bouwman and colleagues reported that screw removal due to infection was performed in 2.8% of cases.[199] Screw loosening occurred in the first postoperative week, which resulted in an occlusal discrepancy in four patients. Fifteen sides required one or more screws to be removed as a result of infection. In a large study of complications in orthognathic surgery, Acebal-Bianco and colleagues reported 36 infections out of 802 mandibular osteotomies (0.05%), but only 5 patients had hardware removed due to infections.[200]

Horizontal Ramus Osteotomies

Since Blair's first description of his osteotomy of the horizontal ramus, there have been a variety of osteotomy designs documented. Initially the surgeons used extraoral, or a combination of extraoral and intraoral techniques, but since the early 1950s the advocated approaches have primarily been intraoral. It is difficult to choose a representative technique for the body osteotomies because of the wide variations described as well as the relative infrequency of these techniques. Of the described procedures, the step osteotomy will be reviewed because of its versatility and its apparent common use in some centers.

Indications The largest limitation of body osteotomies is that the osteotomy has to be made through the dental alveolus and, thus, edentulous spaces are usually required. Because these osteotomies are made in front of the pterygomasseteric sling, some surgeons feel that the results are more stable and, therefore, prefer body osteotomies in the treatment of prognathism when there are already edentulous spaces. Other unusual mandibular abnormalities, such as asymmetries, may also be treated more appropriately with one of these forms of osteotomy.

With the step osteotomy the surgeon has to be concerned about the horizontal component of the "step," which often has to be made between the inferior alveolar nerve and the apices of the teeth. Sufficient room should therefore be available for this cut, unless the surgeon plans to externalize part of the inferior alveolar nerve so that the cut can be made at the level of or below the canal.

Technique An incision is made 4 to 5 mm below the level of the attached gingiva (enough tissue is left superiorly to permit later suturing) and is carried forward at this level until the cuspid, where it can be dropped down 5 mm and extended forward to the midline (Figure 56-20A). The periosteum is elevated inferiorly until the mental foramen is located and then the remainder of the periosteum is stripped to expose the area of the osteotomy. The attached gingiva is also carefully elevated in the area of the dental alveolar cut so that it can be protected during the osteotomy.

The vertical cut through the alveolus is made with either a saw or bur. A finger should be kept on the lingula to prevent the power instrument from penetrating the mucosa. When the surgical plan includes a mandibular setback, a block of bone needs to be removed to permit this movement. The distance between the parallel cuts necessary to remove the bone should be as close as possible to the planned setback, as determined by the model surgery. The vertical cuts are taken inferiorly to the level of the planned horizontal cut, which would be at least 5 mm below the dental apices. The inferior vertical cuts are then made, again using parallel cuts as necessary for a setback of the distal fragment. Finally the horizontal cut is made, preferably by a saw, to minimize bone removal and endangerment of the apices or the inferior alveolar nerve (Figure 56-20B).

The distal segment is related to the proximal segment with an occlusal splint and fixed with maxillomandibular fixation. If the mandible is set back any distance a wedge of attached tissue over the alveolar vertical osteotomy needs to be removed to permit the setback. This wedge should be narrower than the planned movement to allow tight mucosal contact. This eliminates the need for suturing in this area, which is often difficult, if not impossible. Osseous wire fixation can be placed at the inferior border or, if a rigid fixation technique is desired, straight four-holed plates with

monocortical screws can be placed above and below the nerve. With a rigid fixation technique the maxillomandibular wires can be cut and the segment's stability and position are checked before closure of the wound. The surgical sites are thoroughly irrigated and the mucosa is then closed with a resorbable suture. Maxillomandibular fixation, if used, is maintained for 6 to 8 weeks (Figure 56-21).

Alternative Techniques   There are multiple variations of body osteotomies. Generally the mucosal approaches are similar, although some surgeons prefer to make a cervical incision posterior to the mental foramen and then carry it below the attached tissue in the anterior symphyseal region. This approach unfortunately presents some difficulty in wound closure, especially if maxillomandibidar fixation is chosen.

One of the most difficult variations in the surgical approach occurs when there is a need for visualization or exteriorization

of the inferior alveolar nerve, if an osteotomy is planned through the canal. The easiest method for this is similar to that described by Epker.[201]

After the lateral surface of the mandible is exposed in the area of the planned osteotomies, parallel horizontal cortical cuts are made on either side of the anticipated route of the nerve. These cuts are extended beyond either side of the planned osteotomy, sufficient to permit adequate approach to the nerve, as well as to permit enough freedom of the nerve during stretching or compression that will occur with the planned segment movements. Perpendicular cuts are made just through the cortex at about 1 cm intervals (Figure 56-22). Starting with the forward cuts a thin sharp 4 mm osteotome is carefully used to start a cleavage line through the cancellous bone, preferably just below the cortex. As each individual section is broken away the medial aspect of the fragment needs to be checked to ensure that a nerve is not still attached to it. After all the small lateral cor-

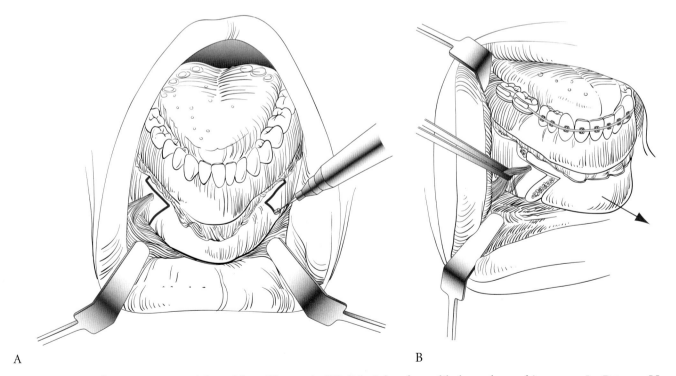

A

B

FIGURE 56-20   *The step osteotomy. Adapted from Bloomquist DS. Principles of mandibular orthognathic surgery. In: Peterson LJ, Indresano AT, Marciani RD, Roser SM. Principles of oral and maxillofacial surgery. Vol 3. Philadelphia (PA): J.B. Lippincott Company; 1992. p. 1444.*

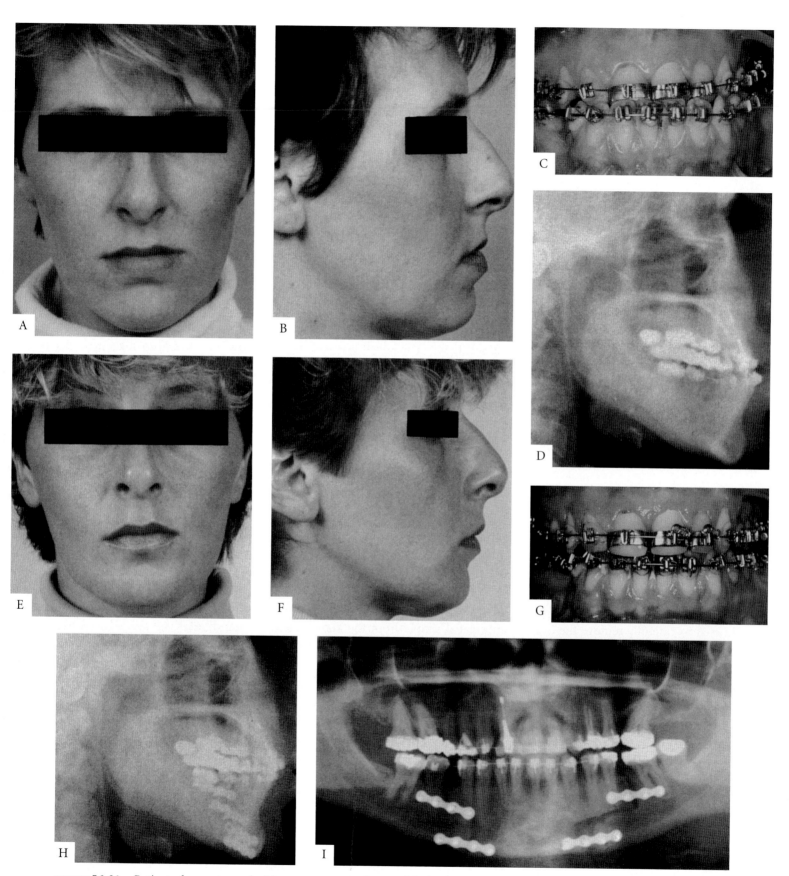

FIGURE **56-21** *Patient who was treated with a step osteotomy for mandibular horizontal excess. A–D, Preoperative photographs and radiograph. E–I, Postoperative photographs and radiographs. Reproduced with permission from Bloomquist DS. Principles of mandibular orthognathic surgery. In: Peterson LJ, Indresano AT, Marciani RD, Roser SM. Principles of oral and maxillofacial surgery. Vol 3. Philadelphia (PA): J.B. Lippincott Company; 1992. p. 1446–7.*

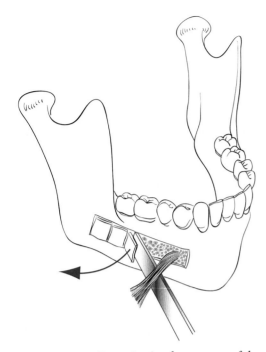

FIGURE 56-22   *Decortication for exposure of the inferior alveolar nerve and vessels. Adapted from Bloomquist DS. Principles of mandibular orthognathic surgery. In: Peterson LJ, Indresano AT, Marciani RD, Roser SM. Principles of oral and maxillofacial surgery. Vol 3. Philadelphia (PA): J.B. Lippincott Company; 1992. p. 1448.*

tical segments have been removed, often the nerve has been exposed and judicious use of a small surgical curette is all that is needed to remove any bone spicules over the nerve as well as carefully lift the nerve out of its canal. If cancellous bone is still covering the nerve, then a medium-sized round bur can be used to carefully remove the overlying bone. A small periosteal elevator or a surgical curette can be positioned in the lateral aspect of the canal when the nerve is exposed and the thin bur used to remove the remaining overlying bone. Following the visualization or exteriorization of the nerve the osteotomies can proceed as planned.

Although primarily used for distal fragment setback, the step osteotomy can be used for advancement. To accomplish that, a horizontal incision has to be made on the lingual side of the alveolus, posterior to the vertical alveolar bone cut. The mucoperiosteum below this cut can then be elevated to allow it to be stretched with the advance-ment. The lateral incision is designed to permit the labial tissue to be pulled lingual-ly, without tension, so that soft tissue closure can be done. Bone grafts are gener-ally used in the gaps created by the advancements, especially in the alveolar area, where prostheses may later be placed.

Sagittal osteotomies of the horizontal ramus have been described with either an extraoral or intraoral approach possi-ble.[202,203] In the intraoral approach the lin-gual exposure has to be increased to make the vertical cortical cut. This generally requires that the incision on the lingual side of the teeth be brought forward, close to the midline, so that retraction may occur without endangering the surround-ing soft tissue. The advantage of this type of osteotomy is that it allows the use of rigid internal fixation with bicortical screws, and generally a bone graft is not needed if the distal segment is advanced.

Complications   Reports of body osteoto-mies in the literature include mostly case histories; hence, there are few series report-ing an incidence of complications. The wide variety of techniques makes it impossible to make any definitive statements about body osteotomies. Therefore, this section will be primarily limited to the listing of the report-ed complications, many of which can be anticipated simply from the knowledge of the anatomy of the area.

Stability   One of the primary reasons given by surgeons for using a body proce-dure is the stability of the technique. San-dor and colleagues looked at relapse of the step osteotomy and found it to be very stable.[204] Most other authors have not strictly analyzed the results but claim a good long-term stability with their partic-ular technique.[205,206]

Neural Complications   Those studies that include reports of the incidence or duration of neurosensory damage report a high recovery ratio.[205,206] Unfortunately these studies are of questionable value because of the inadequate testing method. It can be expected, however, that immedi-ate postoperative sensory loss will be pre-sent after any of the body osteotomies, especially those that require visualization or exteriorization of the nerve. The inci-dence of devitalization of teeth on either side of the osteotomy, or of those teeth above the horizontal cut of the step osteotomy, is unknown, although it is probably similar to those reported with mandibular subapical osteotomies.

The increased potential of nonunion in body osteotomies has been discussed, but the incidence is unknown. The possi-bility of this occurring is probably very low if, as has been suggested, care is used in osteotomy design to ensure sufficient bone contact as well as in the provision of adequate fixation.

The possibility of periodontal defects does exist for osteotomies made close to the teeth where the surrounding soft tissue pedicle may be injured. As has been noted earlier the possibility of this occurring in midline osteotomies is low, but whether this can be related to other parts of the dental alveolus is doubtful.[207]

Subapical Osteotomies

There are essentially three types of mandibular subapical osteotomies: the anterior subapical, the posterior subapical, and the total alveolar osteotomy. Each has a place in orthognathic surgery and, there-fore, the indications and techniques of each shall be described individually. Their complications are similar; accordingly they will be discussed together in one section.

Anterior Subapical Osteotomy   *Indica-tions*   The subapical osteotomy has histor-ically been popular because of its versatility, and it has been used to move the anterior mandibular teeth and alveolus in almost every conceivable direction. The biggest concern of surgeons in this procedure is the potential of damaging teeth and, therefore, space must be present or made to permit a safe vertical cut in the dental alveolus.

Procedure If necessary, teeth are removed to permit the osteotomies or to provide space for the planned alveolar movement. The incision is started about 1 cm behind the planned vertical osteotomy and is carried forward about 4 to 5 mm below the attached tissue until reaching the cuspid, at which time it can be dropped down and carried to the midline to connect with an opposing incision. Periosteum is elevated, exposing the lateral cortex of the mandible, with care being used around the mental foramen as well as some attachments being left at the inferior border to ensure stability of the soft tissue chin. The attached tissue at the planned vertical osteotomy site needs to be elevated, and if posterior movement of the segment is anticipated, some of this tissue may have to be removed. As mentioned with the step osteotomy the width of the tissue removed should be less than the planned posterior movement to ensure adequate soft tissue contact.

The vertical osteotomies are made using parallel cuts when the posterior movement of the segment is planned. Good preoperative radiologic evaluation and planning will minimize the chance of damage to the inferior alveolar nerve. Most anterior subapical osteotomies are designed to include the cuspids and the incisors, which generally place the vertical cuts anterior to the mental foramen. Difficulties arise if the planned osteotomy includes extraction of the first bicuspid or if the cut is planned behind this point. The importance of being able to make the horizontal cut at least 5 mm below the teeth apices cannot be overemphasized. Not only the vitality of the teeth but the whole segment is affected by the level of the horizontal cut. If parallel horizontal cuts are planned to move the anterior segment apically, the superior cut is made first. The inferior cut is then made, and the segment of bone is removed without overly manipulating the dental alveolar segment and increasing the likelihood of injuring the soft tissue pedicle (Figure 56-23A). Beveling of the cut from anterior to posteroinferior will minimize the amount of bone to be removed and increase the size of the lingual pedicle. Usually, on trying to position the mobile dental alveolar segment to the rest of the mandible, further bone interferences are found. These exist primarily on the lingual cortex of the vertical cuts and care must be used in the rotation of the mobile segment to access this cortex. If possible a retractor should be placed between the bone and the thin lingual mucosa to minimize the soft tissue trauma.

After ensuring a good fit in the surgical splint the segment is stabilized by either wiring the splint to the teeth individually (Figure 56-23B) or by circumferential mandibular wires that can be combined with intermaxillary fixation. Osseous wires or plates with monocortical screws are rarely needed for stability but can be used if desired. Bone gaps caused by movement of the segment, especially by vertical movement necessary for the closure of an anterior open bite, should be grafted. The use of cortical bone from the symphysis, as advocated by Kole, has been popular because many patients with an anterior open bite have the long anterior face which can be improved by removal of the bone (Figure 56-23C).[28] The surgical site is then irrigated thoroughly and closed with resorbable sutures.

Posterior Subapical Osteotomy *Indications* The posterior subapical osteotomy has few indications, especially if orthodontics are available to the patient. Primarily it can be used as a correction of supereruption of posterior mandibular teeth or ankylosis of one or more posterior teeth. Abnormal buccal or lingual posi-

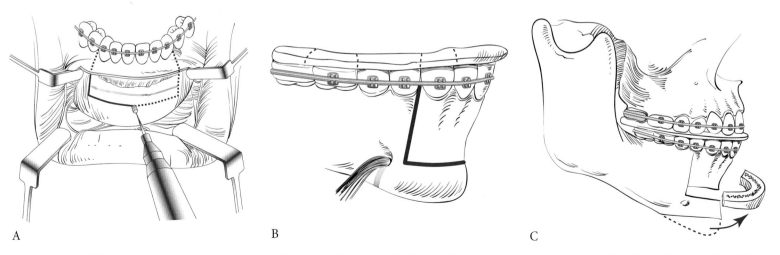

A   B   C

FIGURE **56-23** *The anterior subapical osteotomy. A, Osteotomy. B, Occlusal splint. C, Bone graft from chin for correction of anterior open bite (Kole). Adapted from Bloomquist DS. Principles of mandibular orthognathic surgery. In: Peterson LJ, Indresano AT, Marciani RD, Roser SM. Principles of oral and maxillofacial surgery. Vol 3. Philadelphia (PA): J.B. Lippincott Company; 1992. p. 1450.*

tion of these teeth can also be improved on when orthodontics is not feasible.[208]

Technique   The following technique is that of Peterson, who first described this osteotomy.[208] This procedure can be done under local anesthesia with sedation as well as with general anesthesia. An incision is started 3 to 4 mm laterally to the attached gingiva, beginning at the anterior border of the vertical ramus. This incision is made down into the bone and is carried forward to the cuspid. Periosteum is stripped superiorly and inferiorly sufficiently to expose the lateral cortex for the planned osteotomies (Figure 56-24). The osteotomy is outlined with a bur, based on the preoperative radiographic analysis of the length of the roots and the position of the nerve. The vertical cuts are made first through both cortices with a fine osteotome or thin saws. The horizontal cut is carried only through the buccal cortex, and a thick splitting osteotome is used to complete the osteotomy. Care is taken to

ensure that the nerve is not caught in the mobile segment and that appropriate bone adjustments are made to permit the planned movement. The segment is positioned and stabilized with an acrylic splint and wire. Grafting is used if a bone gap remains. The mucosa is closed with a running resorbable suture.

Alternative Techniques   Major modification of the foregoing technique would be appropriate if insufficient distance lay between the dental apices and the inferior alveolar nerve. In that situation the nerve can be externalized, as described previously, and a horizontal cut made through the canal. Periapical radiographs taken intraoperatively after the buccal horizontal cut will ensure that the osteotomies lie safely away from the teeth and nerve. This latter technique has been found to be useful, as a good visual angle is difficult with the posterior teeth. Also, with either of these techniques, the horizontal cut can be taken safely through the lingual cortex, which does away with the unpredictability of the lingual cortical fracture.

Total Alveolar Osteotomy

Indications   The total mandibular alveolar osteotomy, first described by MacIntosh and Carlotti, has limited application but can prove valuable in mandibular dental alveolar protrusion or retrusion.[209] It has also been advocated for the closure of anterior open bite when used with a bone graft.

Technique   An incision is started on the external oblique ridge of the base of the vertical ramus. The incision is carried down to bone and extends forward 4 to 5 mm below the attached gingiva. The incision can drop lower as the canine is passed and meets the contralateral incision at the midline. The periosteum is elevated to expose the lateral cortex, with care

used around the mental nerve, as well as leaving some attachment at the inferior border of the symphysis for the soft tissue chin. The vertical cut posterior to the last molar is made first and is taken down to the level of the planned horizontal osteotomy. As with the step osteotomies the horizontal cut needs to be well placed, based on periapical radiographs. If this cut cannot be made safely between the dental apices and the inferior alveolar nerve, then the nerve needs to be exteriorized or the cut placed below the nerve (Figure 56-25A). The horizontal cut can then be placed low enough to be away from dental apices as well as allowing a good vascular pedicle to the dental alveolus. The angle of the horizontal cut can be made to facilitate the segment movement; for instance, a flat cut permits the straight advancement of the segment without changing mandibular height, at the same time maintaining a large area of bone contact.

The mobile segment is related to the maxilla with an acrylic occlusal splint and intermaxillary fixation. Osseous fixation is achieved, with the lateral cortical wires being placed in the first bicuspid area. As with correction of an anterior open bite any bone gaps created are filled with graft material. The wound is thoroughly irrigated and closed with resorbable suture.

Technique Variations   Booth and colleagues suggested a variation of the total mandibular subapical osteotomy that combines the sagittal split osteotomy of the vertical ramus with the total mandibular alveolar osteotomy (Figure 56-25B).[210] This modification has a number of advantages over the original technique. First the osteotomy is made below the inferior alveolar nerve, thereby decreasing the risk of damaging the inferior alveolar nerve and the apices of the teeth, at the same time preserving much of the vascular supply to the mobile segment. Also the sagittal part of the osteotomy allows a larger bone contact area to assist in healing.

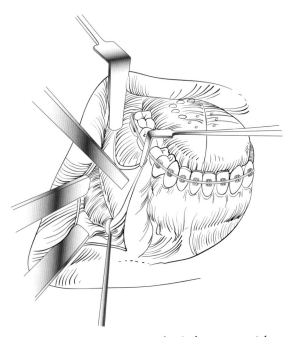

FIGURE 56-24   *The posterior subapical osteotomy. Adapted from Bloomquist DS. Principles of mandibular orthognathic surgery. In: Peterson LJ, Indresano AT, Marciani RD, Roser SM. Principles of oral and maxillofacial surgery. Vol 3. Philadelphia (PA): J.B. Lippincott Company; 1992. p. 1451.*

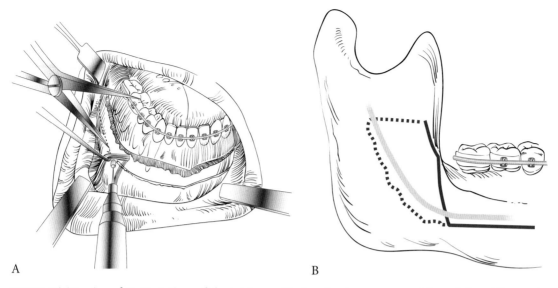

A   B

FIGURE **56-25**   A *and B, Variations of the total mandibular alveolar osteotomy. Adapted from Bloomquist DS. Principles of mandibular orthognathic surgery. In: Peterson LJ, Indresano AT, Marciani RD, Roser SM. Principles of oral and maxillofacial surgery. Vol 3. Philadelphia (PA): J.B. Lippincott Company; 1992. p. 1451.*

The total mandibular alveolar osteotomy can also be divided into interdental segments to correct axial inclination of teeth or to close the edentulous area. These modifications are not easily done with Booth's osteotomy but can be valuable as a variation of the original procedure.

Complications   The complications of all mandibular alveolar osteotomies will be considered together because of their similarities. Stability is often mentioned as one of the advantages of any of the alveolar osteotomies because of the minimal soft tissue forces generally placed on these areas. Unfortunately there have been very few studies to document this claim. Those that have been done question the stability of these segmental osteotomies. Theisen and Guernsey evaluated six patients who had anterior subapical osteotomies.[211] At 1 year after surgery, an average of 1 mm of movement of incisors was noted on lateral cephalograms. In contrast Kloosterman evaluated a much larger group and found a 30% recurrence of open bite after anterior maxillary osteotomies.[48]

Unlike segment stability, neurologic and vascular complications have received a lot of attention. Most of this evaluation has been directed at pulpal changes and not at peripheral inferior alveolar sensory loss or avascular bone loss. Both of these latter problems are recognized complications of mandibular subapical osteotomies, but there are no clinical studies noting their incidence.[28,36] Many authors report some incidence of sensory change of the lip but claim there have been no permanent problems; normal sensation returns in about 3 months.[209,211,212]

Clinical and animal studies of the effect of mandibular osteotomies on the pulp are numerous.[35,37,39,40] An early animal study did not note many vascular changes when a lingual vascular pedicle was maintained.[33] However, all subsequent studies have noted a significant decrease in blood flow, especially to the dental pulp.[213] Histologic studies of dental pulp after subapical osteotomies reveal some pulpal necrosis in most teeth.[35,214] Whether this is of clinical importance is questionable, as there were relatively few teeth in clinical series that required endodontics or that needed to be extracted.[47,48] It is likely that some pulpal necrosis occurs in greater numbers of teeth than are clinically obvious.[215] The only way the pulpal changes

have been assessed clinically is with "vitality testing." A change in pulpal nerve sensation obviously may not be related to a decrease in pulpal vascularity. However, the rate of recovery of sensory loss seems to give some measure of the trauma to the teeth. Early clinical studies seem to show that teeth in mandibular alveolar osteotomies fare better than their maxillary counterparts.[216] More recent and larger studies, however, have demonstrated the reverse.[47,48] One report found that approximately 40% of the teeth in the repositioned segment remain unreactive at 1 year.[47] This high incidence of pulpal trauma was attributed to technical errors during surgeries. The incidence of teeth requiring endodontics range from 1.5 to 10%. The teeth at greatest risk for damage are those in the mobile segment next to a vertical osteotomy. The teeth immediately posterior to the vertical cut are approximately equal in risk to the teeth in the center of the mobile segment.

Periodontal problems have been briefly mentioned by authors reviewing mandibular alveolar osteotomies.[48,211] The incidence and quantitative evaluations of soft and hard tissue loss have not been done, although individual cases of significant interdental bone loss have been noted. Periodontal problems are seen less frequently when the vertical cuts are made in extraction sites than when the cuts are attempted between teeth without extraction.[48]

Horizontal Osteotomy of the Symphysis

The horizontal osteotomy of the symphysis differs very little from that originally described by Hofer, except that the procedure is done intraorally.[32] The versatility of this procedure for skeletal deformities of the chin is impressive.

Indications This osteotomy with minor variations can be used to improve almost every conceivable skeletal abnormality of the chin. The technique is primarily used only for esthetic reasons. Therefore, its use depends on the patient's concern about appearance of this area of the face. Often the surgeon has to bring to the patient's attention the need for a genioplasty when other facial osteotomies are planned because of the impact that these osteotomies will have on chin prominence. The indications, therefore, are often made apparent by comprehensive treatment planning by the surgeon.

Technique The horizontal osteotomy of the symphysis is often done in conjunction with other major osteotomies and, thus, is frequently accomplished under a general anesthetic. However, it can be performed as a separate procedure on an outpatient basis under sedation and local anesthesia.

The mucosal incision is made on the labial side of the vestibule at about 1 cm above its depth and extends posteriorly to the first bicuspids. This incision is carried just below the mucosa to the depth of the vestibule and then angled directly to the labial cortex through the mentalis muscle (Figure 56-26A). Periosteum is elevated inferiorly to a point just below the intended level of osteotomy. Laterally the periosteum is elevated to the mental foramen and then extended posteroinferiorly to the inferior mandibular border. The extent of the posterior cortical exposure is generally determined by the position of the mental foramen and the vertical height of the mandible in this area. In many cases this means that it will end in about the first molar area.

No attempt is generally made to expose the mental nerve by releasing the soft tissue around it, primarily because the nerve can be small and friable, making inadvertent severing possible. The periosteal elevation behind the foramen is minimized to just that needed for placement of a narrow retractor and the saw blade or bur.

It is helpful at this point to inscribe a vertical mark (or marks) into the bone across the planned osteotomy site so that the transverse position of the inferior fragment can be more easily oriented after the osteotomy. The osteotomy cut is then made with a reciprocating saw (Figure 56-26B). The length and angle of the horizontal cut can have profound effects on postsurgical results. Further osteotomies or osteoplasties are made after mobilization of the lower segment. The stabilization of the segment in its new position can be made with cortical wires, circumandibular wires, or plates and screws. The wound is irrigated and closed in two layers (muscle and mucosa) with resorbable suture. Tape placed across the lip and chin is maintained for 24 to 48 hours to minimize hematoma formation as well as to help support the suture lines. Patients should be instructed not to pull their lip to minimize dehiscence of the wound.

Alternative Techniques The primary technique differences for the horizontal osteotomy center on the osteotomy design, and these design differences depend on the symphyseal deformity that is being corrected. Obwegeser concentrated on correction of horizontal deficiency of the chin when he described the basic procedure (Figure 56-27A).[100] He suggested that a midsagittal osteotomy of the inferior fragment may be helpful in preventing the prominence of the posterior ends of the fragment, relative to the body of the mandible, as the fragment is advanced (Figure 56-27B). A narrower chin point can also be obtained by taking a wedge of bone out from the lingual aspect of this cut (Figure 56-27C). The length of

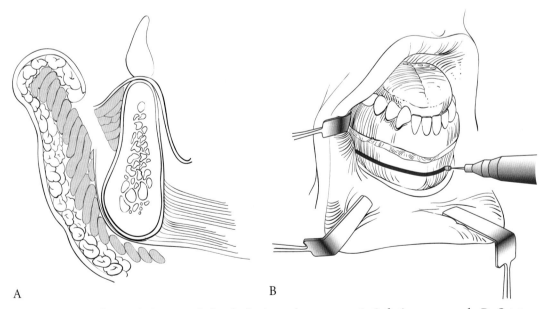

A   B

FIGURE **56-26**   *The surgical approach for the horizontal osteotomy. A, Soft tissue approach. B, Ostetomy. Adapted from Bloomquist DS. Principles of mandibular orthognathic surgery. In: Peterson LJ, Indresano AT, Marciani RD, Roser SM. Principles of oral and maxillofacial surgery. Vol 3. Philadelphia (PA): J.B. Lippincott Company; 1992. p. 1453.*

the cut posteriorly has important esthetic consequences. Most notably larger advancements require a larger cut to the first or second molar region. This permits a smoother line to the inferior border of the mandible. Overlapping an advanced inferior fragment on the lateral cortex of the symphysis allows both an increase in horizontal prominence as well as a decrease in the anterior mandibular vertical height (Figure 56-27D).[217] Larger advancements of the inferior fragment can be obtained by double or triple osteotomies, rotation of the fragment combined with a graft at the posterior gap, and bone graft between the symphysis and the fragment (Figure 56-27E–G).[218,219]

Horizontal chin excess is traditionally treated by moving the inferior fragment posteriorly.[220] Depending on the angle of the cut this will also increase facial height. Sometimes when this is done it is necessary to remove the posterior ends of the inferior fragment to prevent unsightly protrusions from the inferior border of the mandible (Figure 56-27H). When the patient has normal facial height, the plane of the osteotomy should parallel the Frankfort

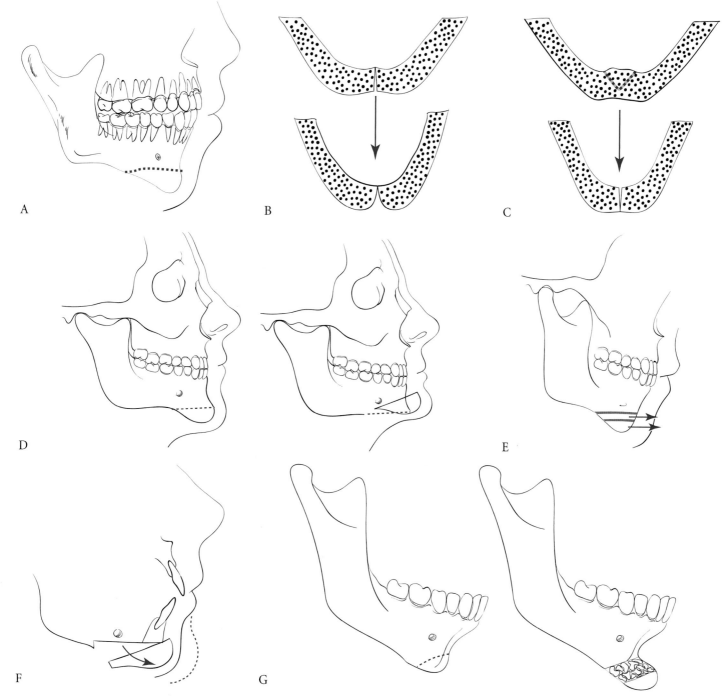

FIGURE **56-27** A–G, *Various forms of the horizontal osteotomy.* (CONTINUED ON NEXT PAGE)

horizontal or natural head position, if at all possible. The anterior chin projection can be reduced by using parallel or V-shaped osteotomies cut in a more vertical plane, with the middle segment removed (Figure 56-27I).

Vertical symphyseal excess can be reduced by removing the middle segment of bone when the plane of two parallel osteotomies is more horizontal (Figure 56-27J). These cuts, however, do not always need to be parallel and in fact should be designed to fit the particular structural problem. This design also permits the correction of a mild horizontal deficiency that is combined with a mild vertical excess (Figure 56-27K). This skeletal problem can also be corrected by making a single osteotomy more vertical and moving the segment anteriorly and forward (Figure 56-27L). Vertical symphyseal deficiency can be handled only by some type of interpositional material, with either bone grafts or implants (Figure 56-27M). Even the use of plates alone to hold the fragment in a lower position has been suggested (Figures 56-28 and 56-29).

The use of wires, screws, or plate and screws for the fixation of the inferior frag-

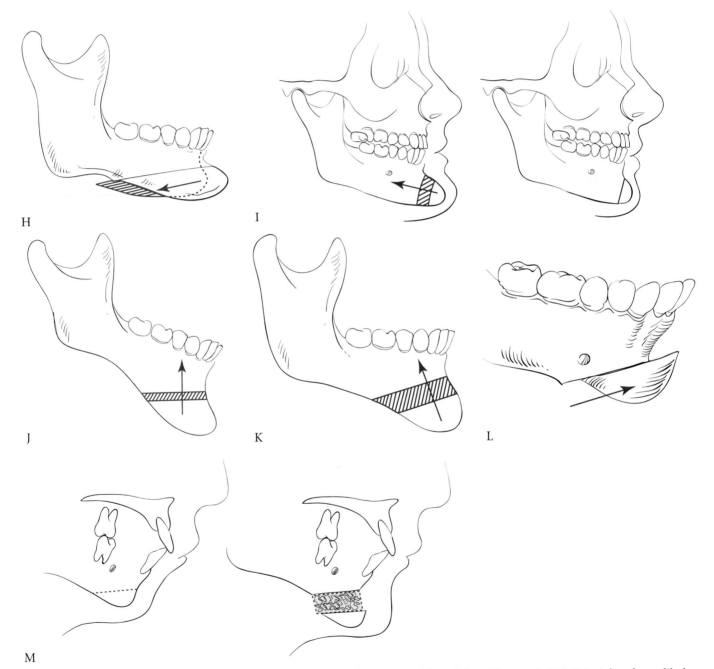

FIGURE 56-27 (CONTINUED) *H–M, Various forms of the horizontal osteotomy. Adapted from Bloomquist DS. Principles of mandibular orthognathic surgery. In: Peterson LJ, Indresano AT, Marciani RD, Roser SM. Principles of oral and maxillofacial surgery. Vol 3. Philadelphia (PA): J.B. Lippincott Company; 1992. p. 1454–5.*

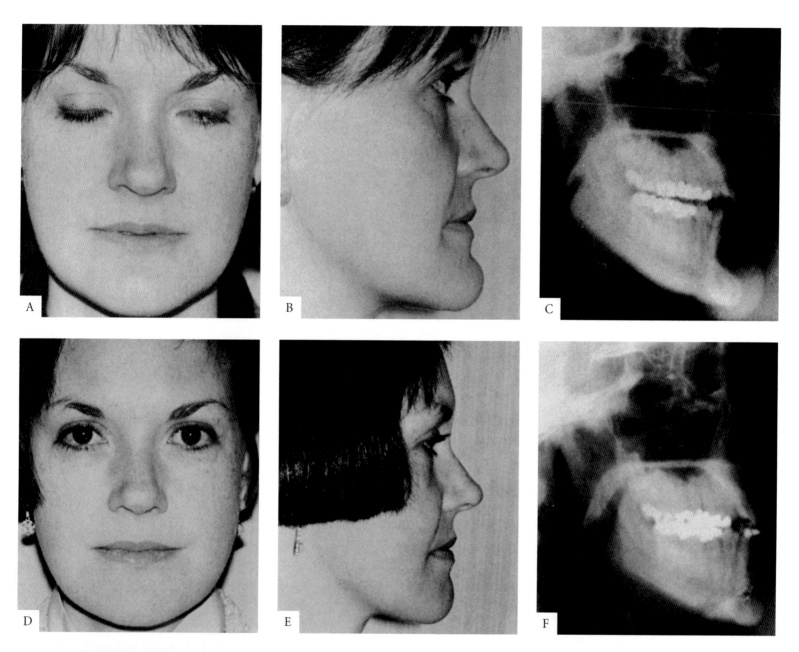

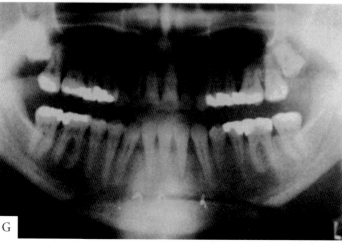

FIGURE **56-28** *Patient who was treated with a horizontal osteotomy for horizontal chin excess. A–C, Preoperative photographs and radiograph. D–G, Postoperative photographs and radiographs. Reproduced with permission from Bloomquist DS. Principles of mandibular orthognathic surgery. In: Peterson LJ, Indresano AT, Marciani RD, Roser SM. Principles of oral and maxillofacial surgery. Vol 3. Philadelphia (PA): J.B. Lippincott Company; 1992. p. 1456.*

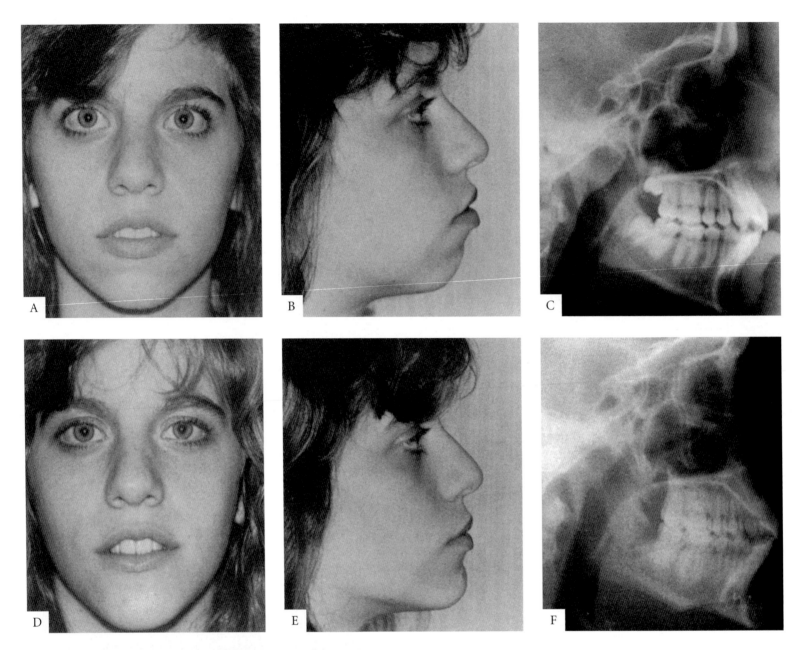

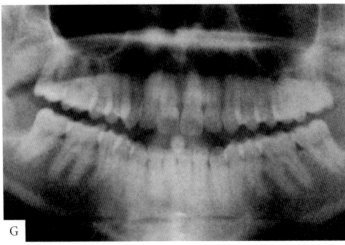

FIGURE 56-29   *Patient was treated with a horizontal osteotomy for horizontal chin deficiency. A–C, Preoperative photographs and radiograph. D–G, Postoperative photographs and radiographs. Reproduced with permission from Bloomquist DS. Principles of mandibular orthognathic surgery. In: Peterson LJ, Indresano AT, Marciani RD, Roser SM. Principles of oral and maxillofacial surgery. Vol 3. Philadelphia (PA): J.B. Lippincott Company; 1992. p. 1457.*

ment is still common. Precious and colleagues evaluated the changes that occur as the bone remodels following a horizontal osteotomy.[221] They recommended that the fixation take into account these changes, especially the positioning of rigid fixation such as plates. Plates along the superior border of the inferior fragment may become noticeable to the patient as the bone remodels.

Complications   The incidence of postoperative problems after a horizontal osteotomy of the symphysis is rarely mentioned. This may be because genioplasties are frequently done in conjunction with other osteotomies, which makes the attribution of various complications difficult. Most of the literature concerning genioplasties concentrates on the soft tissue response to the skeletal movement.

Reports of relapse after genioplasties are sparse and conflicting. Some clinicians report that there is essentially no relapse after a genioplasty, with a rounding of the sharp corners of the advanced segment occurring with time.[222–225] These studies, however, follow patients for only up to 1 year. Two other studies with follow-up of at least 1 year do seem to show some instability of the skeletal advancement.[226,227] The mean relapse with a genial advancement varies widely (2.6 to 30%). The one seemingly consistent finding is that much of the skeletal relapse occurs within the first year. As with stability studies of other osteotomies there exists a large variation in individual relapse, and no attempt has been made to identify the causes. However, there are probably many factors involved, including the magnitude of advancement. There have been no studies in the stability of this surgery in correction of other symphyseal deformities. Martinez and colleagues found that regeneration of the cortical thickness of the symphysis was significantly better in patients younger than 15 years of age.[224] They suggested that this may be beneficial if

further surgical advancement of the chin is to be considered.

The predictable possibility of sensory loss from this procedure has not been adequately evaluated. In one study it was noted that postsurgical sensory loss was found in all patients but was temporary, with normal sensation returning within 12 months.[228] Another study reported a 3.5% long-term incidence of sensory deficits following genioplasties. Other complications such as bone loss and infections have been reported, but small samples preclude any definitive statements on incidence.[229]

References

1. Hullihen SP. Case of elongation of the under jaw and distortion of the face and neck, caused by a burn, successfully treated. Am J Dent Sci 1849;9:157.
2. Angle EH. Double resection of the lower maxilla. Dent Cosmos 1889;40:635.
3. Blair VP. Report of a case of double resection for the correction of protrusion of the mandible. Dent Cosmos 1906;48:817.
4. Blair VP. Operations on the jaw bone and face. Surg Gynecol Obstet 1907;4:67.
5. Ernst F. Progenie. In: Kirshhner M, Nordmann O, editors. Die Chirurgie. IV. Berlin, Germany: Urban & Schwarzenberg; 1927. p. 802.
6. Limberg A. Treatment of open-bite by means of plastic oblique osteotomy of the ascending rami of the mandible.. Dent Cosmos 1925;67:1191.
7. Kostecka P. A contribution to the surgical treatment of open-bite. Int J Orthod 1934; 28:1082.
8. Moose SM. Surgical correction of mandibular prognathism by intra-oral subcondylar osteotomy. Br J Oral Surg 1964;39:172.
9. Thoma KH. Surgical treatment of the deformities of the jaws. Am J Orthod 1946;32:333.
10. Robinson M. Prognathism corrected by open vertical subcondylotomy. J Oral Surg 1958; 16:215.
11. Thoma KH. Oblique osteotomy of mandibular ramus — special technique for correction of various types of facial defects and malocclusion. Oral Surg 1961;14 Suppl 1:23.
12. Caldwell JB, Letterman GS. Vertical osteotomy in the mandibular rami for correction of prognathism. J Oral Surg 1954;12:185.
13. Moose SM. Surgical correction of mandibular prognathism by intraoral subcondylar osteotomy. J Oral Surg Anesth Hosp D Serv 1964;22:197.
14. Winstanley RP. Subcondylar osteotomy of the mandible and the intraoral approach. Br J Oral Surg 1968;6:134.
15. Hebert JM, Kent JN, Hinds EC. Correction of prognathism by an intraoral vertical subcondylar osteotomy. J Oral Surg 1970;28:651.
16. Wassmund M. Frakturen und luxationen des gesichtesschadels. 1927.
17. Pichler H, Trauner R. Lehrbuch der mund- und kieferchirurgie. Wien, Vienna;1948.
18. Caldwell JB, Hayward JR, Lister RL. Correction of mandibular retrognathia by vertical L osteotomy: a new technique. J Oral Surg 1968;26:259.
19. Hayes PA. Correction of retrognathia by modified "C" osteotomy of the ramus and sagittal osteotomy of the mandibular body. Oral Surg 1973;31:682.
20. Fox GL, Tilson HB. Mandibular retrognathia: a review of the literature and selected cases. J Oral Surg 1976;34:53.
21. Obwegeser H, Trauner R. Zur operationstechnik bei der progenie und anderen unterkieferanomalien. Dtsch Zahn Mund Kieferheilkd 1955;23:H1–2.
22. Hensel GC. The surgical correction of mandibular protraction, retraction, and fractures of the ascending rami. Int J Orthodont Oral Surg 1937;23:814.
23. Schuchardt K. Ein beitrag zur chirurgischen kieferorthopadie unter berucksichtigung ihrer bedeutung fur die behandlung angeborener and erworbener kieferdeformitaten Uei soldaten. Dtsch Zahn Mund Kiefer-hielkd 1942;9:73.
24. DalPont G. Retromolar osteotomy for the correction of prognathism. J Oral Surg Anesth Hosp D Serv 1961;19:42.
25. Hunsuck EE. Modified intraoral sagittal splitting technique for correction of mandibular prognathism. J Oral Surg 1968;26:250.
26. Spiessl B. Ostoesynthese abei sagittaler osteotomie nach Obwegeser/dal Pont. Fortschr Kiefer Gesichtschir 1974;18:145.
27. Hofer O. Die vertikale osteotomie zur verlangerung des einseitig verkurzten aufsteigenden unterkieferastes. Atschr Stomatol 1936;34:826.
28. Kole H. Surgical operations on the alveolar ridge to correct occlusal abnormalities. Oral Surg Oral Med Oral Pathol 1959;12:277.
29. Kent JN, Hinds EC. Management of dental facial deformities by anterior alveolar surgery. J Oral Surg 1971;29:13.
30. MacIntosh RB. Total mandibular alveolar osteotomy: encouraging experiences with an infrequently indicated procedure. J Maxillofac Surg 1974;2:210.
31. Von Eiselberg A. Uber plastik bei ektropium

des unterkeifers (progenie). Klin Wochenschr 1906;19:1505.

32. Hofer O. Operation der prognathie und mikrogenie. Dtsch Zahn Mund Kieferheilkd 1942;9:121.

33. Bell WH, Levy BM. Revascularization and bone healing after anterior mandibular osteotomy. J Oral Surg 1970;28:196.

34. Hellem S, Ostrup LT. Normal and retrograde blood supply to the body of the mandible in the dog. Int J Oral Surg 1981;10:31.

35. Zisser G, Gattinger B. Histologic investigation of pulpal changes following maxillary and mandibular alveolar osteotomies in the dog. J Oral Surg 1982;40:322.

36. Epker BN. Vascular considerations in orthognathic surgery. Oral Surg 1984;57:467.

37. Boc T, Peterson L. Revascularization after posterior mandibular alveolar osteotomy. J Oral Surg 1981;39:177.

38. Bradley JC. Age changes in the vascular supply of the mandible. Br Dent J 1972;132:142.

39. Bell WH, Kennedy JW III. Biological basis for vertical ramus osteotomies — a study of bone healing and revascularization in adult rhesus monkeys. J Oral Surg 1976;34:215.

40. Grammer FC, Meyer MW, Richter KJ. A radioisotope study of the vascular response to sagittal split osteotomy of the mandibular ramus. J Oral Surg 1974;32:578.

41. Bell WH, Schendel SA. Biologic basis for modification of the sagittal ramus split operation. J Oral Surg 1977;35:362.

42. Path MG, Nelson RL, Morgan PR, Meyer MW. Blood flow changes after sagittal split of the mandibular ramus. J Oral Surg 1977;35:98.

43. Grammer FC, Carpenter AM. A quantitative histologic study of tissue responses to ramal sagittal splitting procedures. J Oral Surg 1979;37:482.

44. Bell WH. Revascularization and bone healing after anterior maxillary osteotomy: a study using adult rhesus monkeys. J Oral Surg 1969;27:249.

45. Walter JM, Gregg JM. Analysis of postsurgical neurologic alteration in the trigeminal nerve. J Oral Surg 1979;37:410.

46. Hutchinson D, MacGregor AJ. Tooth survival following various methods of sub-apical osteotomy. Int J Oral Surg 1972;1:181.

47. Pepersack WJ. Tooth vitality after alveolar segmental osteotomy. J Maxillofac Surg 1973;1:85.

48. Kloosterman J. Kole's osteotomy: a follow-up study. J Maxillofac Surg 1985;13:59.

49. Ridell A, Soremark R, Lundberg M. Positional changes of the mandible after surgical correction of mandibular protrusion by horizontal osteotomy of the rami. Acta Odontol Scand 1971;29:123.

50. Tornes K, Wisth PJ. Stability after vertical subcondylar ramus osteotomy for correction of mandibular prognathism. Int J Oral Maxillofac Surg 1988;17:242.

51. Astrand P, Ridell A. Positional changes of the mandible and upper and lower anterior teeth after oblique sliding osteotomy of the mandibular rami. Scand J Plast Reconstr Surg 1973;7:120.

52. Poulton DR, Ware WH. Surgical-orthodontic treatment of severe mandibular retrusion. Am J Orthod 1971;58:244.

53. Poulton DR, Ware WH. Surgical-orthodontic treatment of severe mandibular retrusion (part II). Am J Orthod 1973;63:237.

54. Kohn MW. Analysis of relapse after mandibular advancement surgery. J Oral Surg 1978;36:676.

55. Lake SL, McNeill RNA, Little RM, West RA. Surgical mandibular advancement: a cephalometric analysis of treatment response. Am J Orthod 1981;80:376.

56. Smith GC, Moloney FB, West RA. Mandibular advancement surgery: a study of the lower border wiring technique for osteosynthesis. Oral Surg 1985;60:461.

57. Komiri E, Aigase K, Sugisaki M, Tanabe H. Skeletal fixation versus skeletal relapse. Am J Orthod Dentofac Orthop 1987;92:412.

58. Will LA, Joondeph DR, Hold TH, West RA. Condylar position following mandibular advancement: its relationship to relapse. J Oral Maxillofac Surg 1984;42:578.

59. Epker BN. Modifications in the sagittal osteotomy of the mandible. J Oral Surg 1977;35:157.

60. Komiri E, Aigase K, Sugisaki M. Cause of early skeletal relapse after mandibular setback. Am J Orthod Dentofac Orthop 1989;95:29.

61. Franco JE, Van Sickels JE, Thrash WJ. Factors contributing to relapse in rigidly fixed mandibular setbacks. J Oral Maxillofac Surg 1989;47:451.

62. Yellich GM, McNamara JA, Ungerleider JC. Muscular and mandibular adaptation after lengthening, detachment, and reattachment of the masseter muscle. J Oral Surg 1981;39:656.

63. Ellis E III, Carlson DS. Stability two years after mandibular advancement with and without suprahyoid myotomy: an experimental study. J Oral Maxillofac Surg 1983;41:426.

64. Schendel SA, Epker BN. Results after mandibular advancement surgery: an analysis of 87 cases. J Oral Surg 1980;38:265.

65. Bhatia SN, Yant B, Behbehanit I, Harris M. Nature of relapse after surgical mandibular advancement. Br J Orthod 1985;12:58.

66. Reynolds ST, Ellis E III, Carlson DS. Adapta-

tion of the suprahyoid muscle complex to large mandibular advancements. J Oral Maxillofac Surg 1988;46:1077.

67. Ellis E III, Reyolds S, Carlson DS. Stability of the mandible following advancement: a comparison of three postsurgical fixation techniques. Am J Orthod Dentofac Orthop 1988;94:38.

68. Ellis E III, Gallo JW. Relapse following mandibular advancement with dental plus skeletal maxillomandibular fixation. J Oral Maxillofac Surg 1986;44:509.

69. Robinson M, Lytle JJ. Micrognathism corrected by vertical osteotomies of the rami without bone grafts. Oral Surg Oral Med Oral Pathol 1962;15:641.

70. Hall HD, McKenna SJ. Further refinement and evaluation of intraoral vertical ramus osteotomy. J Oral Maxillofac Surg 1987;45:684.

71. Bereni B. Open subcondylar osteotomy in the treatment of mandibular deformities. Int J Oral Surg 1973;2:81.

72. Reitzik M, Griffiths RR, Mirels H. Surgical anatomy of the ascending ramus of the mandible. Br J Oral Surg 1976;14:150.

73. Hall HD, Chase DC, Payor LG . Evaluation and refinement of the intraoral vertical subcondylar osteotomy. J Oral Surg 1975;33:333.

74. Massey GB, Chase DC, Thomas PM, Kohn MW. Intraoral oblique osteotomy of the mandibular ramus. J Oral Surg 1974;32:755.

75. Tornes K. Osteotomy length and postoperative stability in vertical subcondylar ramus osteotomy. Acta Odontol Stand 1989;47:81.

76. Sund G, Eckerdal O, Astrand P. Changes in the temporomandibular joint after oblique osteotomy of the mandibular rami: a longitudinal radiological study. J   Maxillofac Surg 1983;11:81.

77. Ritzau M, Wenzel A, Williams S. Changes in condyle position after bilateral vertical ramus osteotomy with and without osteosynthesis. Am J Orthod Dentofac Orthop 1989;96:507. .

78. Sund G, Eckerdal O, Astrand P. Skeletal remodeling in the temporomandibular joint after oblique sliding osteotomy of the mandibular rami. Int J Oral Maxillofac Surg 1986;15:233.

79. Proffit WR, Phillips C, Denn C IV, Turvey TA. Stability after surgical-orthodontic correction of skeletal class III malocclusion. I: Mandibular setback. Int J Adult Orthodont Orthognath Surg 1991;6:7.

80. Nystrom E, Rosenquist J, Astrand P, Nordin T. Intraoral or extraoral approach in oblique sliding osteotomy of the mandibular ramus. J Maxillofac Surg 1984;12:277.

81. Goldstein A. Appraisal of results of surgical

correction of class III malocclusions. Angle Orthod 1974;17(3–4):59.

82. Poulton DR, Taylor RC, Ware WH. Cephalometric x-ray evaluation of the vertical osteotomy correction of mandibular prognathism. Oral Surg Oral Med Oral Pathol 1963;16:807.

83. Morrill LR, Baumrind S, Miller D. Surgical correction of mandibular prognathism. Am J Orthod 1974;65:503.

84. Stella JP, Astrand P, Epker BN. Patterns and etiology of relapse after correction of class III open bite via subcondylar ramus osteotomy. Int J Adult Orthod Orthogn Surg 1986;1:191.

85. Kahnberg KE, Widmark G. Surgical treatment of the open bite deformity: surgical correction of combined mandibular prognathism and open bite by oblique sliding osteotomy of the mandibular rami. Int J Oral Maxillofac Surg 1988;17:45.

86. Zaytoun HS, Phillips C, Terry BC. Long-term neurosensory deficits following transoral vertical ramus and sagittal split osteotomies for mandibular prognathism. J Oral Maxillofac Surg 1986;44:193.

87. Wang JH, Waite DE. Vertical osteotomy vs sagittal split osteotomy of the mandibular ramus: comparison of operative and postoperative factors. J Oral Surg 1975;33:596.

88. Hollender L, Ridell A. Radiography of the temporomandibular joint after oblique sliding osteotomy of the mandibular rami. Scand J Dent Res 1974;82:466.

89. Egyedi P, Houwing M, Juten E. The oblique subcondylar osteotomy: report of results of 100 cases. J Oral Surg 1981;39:871.

90. Bell WH, Yamaguchi Y, Poor MR. Treatment of temporomandibular joint dysfunction by intraoral vertical ramus osteotomy. Int J Adult Orthod Orthogn Surg 1990;5:9.

91. Upton LG, Sullivan SM. Modified condylotomies for management of mandibular prognathism and temporomandibular joint internal derangement. Clin Orthod 1990; 24:697.

92. Hu J, Wang D, Zou S. Effects of mandibular setback on the temporomandibular joint: a comparison of oblique and sagittal split ramus osteotomy. 2000;58:375.

93. Farrell CD, Kent JN. Evaluation of the surgical stability of 20 cases of inverted-L and C osteotomies. J Oral Surg 1977;3:239.

94. Reitzik M. Mandibular advancement surgery: stability following a modified fixation technique. J Oral Surg 1980;38:893.

95. Hawkinson RT. Retrognathia correction by means of an arcing osteotomy in the ascending ramus. J Prosthet Dent 1968; 20:77.

96. Reitzik M, Barer PC, Wainwright WM, Lim B. The surgical treatment of skeletal anterior open-bite deformities with rigid internal fixation in the mandible. Am J Orthod Dentofac Orthop 1990;97:52.

97. Barer PC, Wallen TR, McNeill RW, Reitzik M. Stability of mandibular advancement osteotomy using rigid internal fixation. Am J Orthod Dentofac Orthop 1987;92:403.

98. Greebe RB, Tuinzing DR. Mandibular advancement procedures: predictable stability and relapse. Oral Surg 1984;57:13.

99. Dattilo DJ, Braun TW, Sotereanos GC. The inverted L osteotomy for treatment of skeletal open-bite deformities. J Oral Maxillofac Surg 1985;43:440.

100. Obwegeser H. The surgical correction of mandibular prognathism and retrognathia with consideration of genioplasty. Oral Surg 1957;10:681.

101. Jeter TS, Van Sickels JE, Dolwick MR. Modified techniques for internal fixation of sagittal ramus osteotomies. J Oral Maxillofac Surg 1984;42:270.

102. Sandor GKB, Stoelinga PJW, Tideman H, Leenen RJ. The role of the intraosseous osteosynthesis wire in sagittal split osteotomies for mandibular advancement. J Oral Maxillofac Surg 1984;42:231.

103. Isaacson RJ, Kopytov OS, Bevis RR, Waite DE. Movement of the proximal and distal segments after mandibular ramus osteotomies. J Oral Surg 1978;36:263.

104. Obwegeser H. The indications for surgical correction of mandibular deformity by the sagittal splitting technique. Br J Oral Surg 1962;1:157.

105. Booth DF. Control of the proximal segment by lower border wiring in the sagittal split osteotomy. J Maxillofac Surg 1981;9:126.

106. Kundert M, Hadjianghelou O. Condylar displacement after sagittal splitting of the mandibular rami: a short term radiographic study. J Maxillofac Surg 1980;8:278.

107. Spitzer W, Rettinger C, Sitzman F. Computerized tomography examination for the detection of positional changes in the temporomandibular joint after ramus osteotomies with screw fixation. J Maxillofac Surg 1984;12:139.

108. Watzke IM, Tucker MR, Turvey TA. Lag screw versus position screw techniques for rigid internal fixation of sagittal osteotomies: a comparison of stability. Int J Adult Orthod Orthogn Surg 1991;6:19.

109. Bloomqvist JE, Isaksson S. Skeletal stability after mandibular advancement: a comparison of two rigid internal fixation techniques. J Oral Maxillofac Surg 1994;52:1133.

110. Bloomqvist JE, Ahlborg G, Isaksson S, Svartz K. A comparison of skeletal stability after mandibular advancement and use of two rigid internal fixation techniques. J Oral Maxillofac Surg 1997;55:568.

111. Fujioka M, Fujii T, Hirano A. Comparative study of mandibular stability after sagittal split osteotomies: bicortical versus monocortical osteosynthesis. Cleft Palate Craniofac J 2000;37:551.

112. Suuronen R, Laine P, Pohjonen T, Lindqvist C. Sagittal ramus osteotomies fixed with biodegradable screws: a preliminary report. J Oral Maxillofac Surg 1994;52:715.

113. Harada K, Enomoto S. Stability after surgical correction of mandibular prognathism using the sagittal split ramus osteotomy and fixation with poly-L-lactic acid (PLLA) screws. J Oral Maxillofac Surg 1997;55:464.

114. Ferretti C, Reyneke JP. Mandibular sagittal split osteotomies fixed with biodegradable or titanium screws: a prospective, comparative study of postoperative stability. Oral Surg Oral Med Oral Pathol Oral Radiol Endod 2002;93:534.

115. Kallela I, Laine P, Suuronen R, et al. Skeletal stability following mandibular advancement and rigid fixation with polylactide biodegradable screws. Int J Oral Maxillofac Surg 1998;27:3.

116. Turvey TA, Bell RB, Tejera TJ, Proffit WR. The use of self-reinforced biodegradable bone plates and screws in orthognathic surgery. J Oral Maxillofac Surg 2002;60:59.

117. O'Ryan F, Epker BN. Deliberate surgical control of mandibular growth: 1. A biomechanical theory. Oral Surg 1982;53:2.

118. Killiany DM, Johnston LE Jr. Surgical control of mandibular growth: test of a recent biomechanical hypothesis. Oral Surg 1986;62:500.

119. Huang CS, Ross RB. Surgical advancement of the retrognathic mandible in growing children. Am J Orthod 1982;82:89.

120. Bell WH. Augmentation of the nasomaxillary and nasolabial regions. Oral Surg Oral Med Oral Pathol 1976;41:691.

121. Alexander C, Bloomquist D, Wallen T. Stability of mandibular constriction with a symphyseal osteotomy. Am J Orthod Dentofac Orthop 1993;103:15.

122. McNeill RW, Hooley JR, Sundberg RJ. Skeletal relapse during intermaxillary fixation. J Oral Surg 1973;31:212.

123. Van Sickels JE. A comparative study of bicortical screws and suspension wires versus bicortical screws in large mandibular advancements. J Oral Maxillofac Surg. 1991;49:1293.

124. Mobarak KA, Espeland L, Rogstad O, Lyberg T.

Mandibular advancement surgery in high-angle and low-angle class II patients: different long-term skeletal responses. Am J Orthod Dentofac Orthop 2001;119:368.

125. Schmoker R, Speissl B, Gensheimer T. Functionally stable osteosynthesis and simulography in sagittal osteotomy of the ascending ramus: a comparative clinical study. Schweiz Monatsschr Zahnheilkd 1976;86:582.

126. Van Sickels JE, Flanary CM. Stability associated with mandibular advancement treated by rigid osseous fixation. J Oral Maxillofac Surg 1985;43:338.

127. Van Sickels JE, Larsen AJ, Thrash WJ. Relapse after rigid fixation of mandibular advancement. J Oral Maxillofac Surg 1986;44:698.

128. Van Sickels JE, Larsen AJ, Thrash WJ. A retrospective study of relapse in rigidly fixated sagittal split osteotomies: contributing factors. Am J Orthod Dentofac Orthop 1988;93:413.

129. Caskey RT, Turpin DL, Bloomquist DS. Stability of mandibular lengthening using bicortical screw fixation. Am J Orthod Dentofac Orthop 1989;96:320.

130. Knaup CA, Wallen TW, Bloomquist DS. Linear and rotational changes in large mandibular advancements using three or four fixation screws. Int J Adult Orthod Orthogn Surg 1993;8:245.

131. Douma E, Kuftinec MM, Moshiri F. A comparative study of stability after mandibular advancement surgery. Am J Orthod Dentofac Orthop 1991;100:141.

132. Mommaerts MY. Lag screw versus wire osteosynthesis in mandibular advancement. Int J Adult Orthod Orthogn Surg 1991;6:153.

133. Moenning JE, Bussard DA, Lapp TH, Garrison BT. A comparison of relapse in bilateral sagittal split osteotomies for mandibular advancement: rigid internal fixation (screws) versus inferior border wiring with anterior skeletal fixation. Int J Adult Orthod Orthogn Surg 1990;5:175.

134. Berger JL, Pangrazio-Kulbersh V, Bacchus SN, Kasczynski R. Stability of bilateral sagittal split ramus osteotomy: rigid fixation versus transosseous wiring. Am J Orthod Dentofac Orthop 2000;118:397.

135. Dolce C, Hatch JP, Van Sickels JE, Rugh JD. Rigid versus wire fixation for mandibular advancement: skeletal and dental changes after 5 years. Am J Orthod Dentofac Orthop 2002;121:610.

136. Watzke IM, Turvey TA, Phillips C, Proffit WR. Stability of mandibular advancement after sagittal osteotomy with screw or wire fixation: a comparative study. J Oral Maxillofac Surg 1990;48:101.

137. Rubens BC, Stoelinga PJW, Blijdorp PA, et al. Skeletal stability following sagittal split osteotomy using monocortical miniplate internal fixation. Int J Oral Maxillofac Surg 1985;17:371.

138. Lee J, Piecuch JF. The sagittal ramus osteotomy. Stability of fixation with internal miniplates. Int J Oral Maxillofac Surg 1992;21:326.

139. Abeloos J, Le Clercq C, Neyt L. Skeletal stability following miniplate fixation after bilateral sagittal split osteotomy for mandibular advancement. J Oral Maxillofac Surg 1993; 51:366.

140. Scheerlinck JP, Stoelinga PJ, Blijdorp PA, et al. Sagittal split advancement osteotomies stabilized with miniplate fixation. A 2–5 year follow-up. Int J Oral Maxillofac Surg 1994;23:127.

141. Bloomquist D. The use of a single lag screw in the mandibular sagittal osteotomy. Presentation at the AAO-ASOMFS Conference on Surgical Orthodontics; 1983; New Orleans, LA.

142. Kole H. Results, experience, and problems in the operative treatment of anomalies with reverse overbite (mandibular protrusion). Oral Surg 1965;19:427.

143. Behrman SJ. Complications of sagittal osteotomy of the mandibular ramus. J Oral Surg 1972;30:554.

144. Westermark SA, Bystedt H, von Konow L. Inferior alveolar nerve function after sagittal split osteotomy of the mandible: correlation with degree of intraoperative nerve encounter and other variables in 496 operations. Br J Oral Maxillofac Surg 1998;36:429.

145. Ylikontiola L, Kinnunen J, Laukkanen P, Oikarinen K. Prediction of recovery from neurosensory deficit after bilateral sagittal split osteotomy. Oral Surg Oral Med Oral Pathol Oral Radiol Endod 2000;90:275.

146. MacIntosh RB. Experience with the sagittal osteotomy of the mandibular ramus: a 13-year review. J Maxillofac Surg 1981;8:151.

147. Van Sickels JE, Hatch JP, Dolce C, et al. Effects of age, amount of advancement, and genioplasty on neurosensory disturbance after a bilateral sagittal split osteotomy. J Oral Maxillofac Surg 2002;60:1012.

148. White RP, Peters PB, Costich ER, Page HL Jr. Evaluation of sagittal split-ramus osteotomy in 17 patients. J Oral Surg 1969;27:851.

149. Guernsey LH, DeChamplain RW. Sequelae and complications of the intraoral sagittal osteotomy in the mandibular rami. Oral Surg 1971;32:176.

150. Fiamminghi L, Aversa C. Lesions of the inferior alveolar nerve in sagittal osteotomy of the ramus: experimental study. J Maxillofac Surg 1979;7:125.

151. Brusati R, Fiamminghi L, Sesenna E, Gazzotti A. Functional disturbance of the inferior alveolar nerve after sagittal osteotomy of the mandibular ramus: operating technique for prevention. J Maxillofac Surg 1981;9:123.

152. Yoshida T, Nagamine T, Kobayashi T, et al. Impairment of the inferior alveolar nerve after sagittal split osteotomy. J Craniomaxillofac Surg 1989;17:271.

153. Yamamoto R, Nakamura A, Ohno K, Michi KI. Relationship of the mandibular canal to the lateral cortex of the mandibular ramus as a factor in the development of neurosensory disturbance after bilateral sagittal split osteotomy. J Oral Maxillofac Surg 2002; 60:490.

154. Freihofer HP Jr. Probleme der behandlung der progenie durch sagittler spaltung der aufsteigenden unterkieferaste. Schweiz Monatsschr Zahnheilkd 1976;86:679.

155. Wolford LM, Bennett MA, Rafferty CG. Modification of the mandibular ramus sagittal split osteotomy. Oral Surg Oral Med Oral Pathol 1987;64:146.

156. Converse JM. Surgical treatment of facial injuries. In: Kazanjian VH, Converse JM, editors. Surgical treatment of facial injuries. Baltimore (MD): Williams & Wilkins; 1974.

157. Paulis GW, Steinhauser EW. A comparative study of wire osteosynthesis versus bone screws in the treatment of mandibular prognathism. Oral Surg 1982;54:2.

158. Nishioka GJ, Zysset ME, Van Sickels JE. Neurosensory disturbance with rigid fixation of the bilateral sagittal split osteotomy. J Oral Maxillofac Surg 1987;45:20.

159. Lemke RR, Rugh JD, Van Sickels J, Bays RA, Clark GM. Neurosensory differences after wire and rigid fixation in patients with mandibular advancement. J Oral Maxillofac Surg 2000;58:1354.

160. Westermark A, Englesson L, Bongenhielm U. Neurosensory function after sagittal split osteotomy of the mandible: a comparison between subjective evaluation and objective assessment. Int J Adult Orthod Orthogn Surg 1999;14:268.

161. Chen N, Neal CE, Lingenbrink P, et al. Neurosensory changes following orthognathic surgery. Int J Adult Orthod Orthogn Surg 1999;14:259.

162. Nakagawa K, Ueki K, Takasuka S, et al. Somatosensory-evoked potential to evaluate the trigeminal nerve after sagittal split osteotomy. Oral Surg Oral Med Oral Pathol Oral Radiol Endod 2001;91:146.

163. Jacks SC, Zuniga JR, Turvey TA, Schalit C. A retrospective analysis of lingual nerve sensory changes after mandibular bilateral

sagittal split osteotomy. J Oral Maxillofac Surg 1998;56:700.

164. Zuniga Jr, Chen N, Phillips CL. Chemosensory and somatosensory regeneration after lingual nerve repair in humans. J Oral Maxillofac Surg 1997;55:2.

165. Gent JF, Shafer DM, Frank ME. The effect of orthognathic surgery on taste function on the palate and tongue. J Oral Maxillofac Surg 2003;61:766.

166. Freihofer HPM Jr, Petresevic D. Late results after advancing the mandible by sagittal splitting of the rami. J Maxillofac Surg 1975;3:250.

167. O'Ryan F, Epker BN. Surgical orthodontics and the temporomandibular joint II: mandibular advancement via modified sagittal split ramus osteotomies. Am J Orthod 1983;83:418.

168. Buckley MJ, Tulloch JFC, White RP, Tucker MR. Complications of orthognathic surgery: a comparison between wire fixation and rigid internal fixation. Int J Adult Orthod Orthogn Surg 1989;4:69.

169. Hackney FL, Van Sickels JE, Nummikoski PV. Condylar displacement and temporomandibular joint dysfunction following bilateral sagittal split osteotomy and rigid fixation. J Oral Maxillofac Surg 1989;47:223.

170. Martis CS. Complications after mandibular sagittal split osteotomy. J Oral Maxillofac Surg 1984;42:101.

171. Karabouta I, Martis C. The TMJ dysfunction syndrome before and after sagittal split osteotomy of the rami. J Maxillofac Surg 1985;13:185.

172. Kerstens HCJ, Tuinzing DB, van der Kwast WAM. Temporomandibular joint symptoms in orthognathic surgery. J Craniomaxillofac Surg 1989;17:215.

173. Pruitt JW, Moenning JE, Lapp TH, Bussard DA. Treatment of painful temporomandibular joint dysfunction with the sagittal split ramus osteotomy. J Oral Maxillofac Surg 2002;60:996.

174. Flynn B, Brown DT, Lapp TH, et al. A comparative study of temporomandibular symptoms following mandibular advancement by bilateral sagittal split osteotomies: rigid versus nonrigid fixation. Oral Surg Oral Med Oral Pathol 1990;70:372.

175. Feinerman DM, Piecuch JF. Long-term effects of orthognathic surgery on the temporomandibular joint: comparison of rigid and nonrigid fixation methods. Int J Oral Maxillofac Surg 1995;24:268.

176. Wolford LM, Reiche-Fischel U, Mehra P. Changes in temporomandibular joint dysfunction after orthognathic surgery. J Oral Maxillofac Surg 2003;61:655.

177. Luhr HG. The significance of condylar position using rigid fixation in orthognathic surgery. Clin Plast Surg 1989;16:147.

178. Harris MD, Van Sickels JE, Alder M. Factors influencing condylar position after the bilateral sagittal split osteotomy fixed with bicortical screws. J Oral Maxillofac Surg 1999;57:650.

179. Van Sickels JE, Tiner BD, Keeling SD, et al. Condylar position with rigid fixation versus wire osteosynthesis of a sagittal split advancement. J Oral Maxillofac Surg 1999;57:31.

180. Renzi G, Becelli R, Di Paolo C, Iannetti G. Indications to the use of condylar repositioning devices in the surgical treatment of dental-skeletal class III. J Oral Maxillofac Surg 2003;61:304.

181. Alder ME, Deahl ST, Matteson SR, et al. Short-term changes of condylar position after sagittal split osteotomy for mandibular advancement. Oral Surg Oral Med Oral Pathol Oral Radiol Endod 1999;87:159.

182. Rebellato J, Lindauer SJ, Sheats RD, Isaacson RJ. Condylar positional changes after mandibular advancement surgery with rigid internal fixation. Am J Orthod Dentofac Orthop 1999;116:93.

183. Gaggl A, Schultes G, Santler G, et al. Clinical and magnetic resonance findings in the temporomandibular joints of patients before and after orthognathic surgery. Br J Oral Maxillofac Surg 1999;37:41.

184. Ueki K, Marukawa K, Nakagawa K, Yamamoto E. Condylar and temporomandibular joint disc positions after mandibular osteotomy for prognathism. J Oral Maxillofac Surg 2002;60:1424.

185. Stacy GC. Recovery of oral opening following sagittal ramus osteotomy for mandibular prognathism. J Oral Maxillofac Surg 1987;45:487.

186. Storum KA, Bell WH. The effect of physical rehabilitation on mandibular function after ramus osteotomies. J Oral Maxillofac Surg 1986;44:94.

187. Aragon SB, Van Sickels JE. Mandibular range of motion with rigid/non-rigid fixation. Oral Surg Oral Med Oral Pathol 1987;63:408.

188. Nishimura A, Sakurada S, Iwase M, Nagumo M. Positional changes in the mandibular condyle and amount of mouth opening after sagittal split ramus osteotomy with rigid or nonrigid osteosynthesis. J Oral Maxillofac Surg 1997;55:672.

189. Phillips RM, Bell WH. Atrophy of mandibular condyles after sagittal ramus split osteotomy: report of case. J Oral Surg 1978;36:45.

190. Cutbirth M, Van Sickels JE, Thrash WJ. Condylar resorption after bicortical screw fixation of mandibular advancement. J Oral Maxillofac Surg 1998;56:178.

191. Hoppenreijs TJ, Stoelinga PJ, Grace KL, Robben CM. Long-term evaluation of patients with progressive condylar resorption following orthognathic surgery. Int J Oral Maxillofac Surg 1999;28:411.

192. Lanigan DT, Hey J, West RA. Hemorrhage following mandibular osteotomies: a report of 21 cases. J Oral Maxillofac Surg 1991; 49:713.

193. Tucker MR, Ochs MW. Use of rigid internal fixation for management of intraoperative complications of mandibular sagittal split osteotomy. Int J Adult Orthod Orthogn Surg 1988;2:71.

194. Precious DS, Lung KE, Rynn BR, Goodday RH. Presence of impacted teeth as a determining factor of unfavorable splits in 1256 sagittal-split osteotomies. Oral Surg Oral Med Oral Pathol Oral Radiol Endod 1998;85:362.

195. Mehra P, Castro V, Freitas RZ, Wolford LM. Complications of the mandibular sagittal split ramus osteotomy associated with the presence or absence of third molars. J Oral Maxillofac Surg 2001;59:854.

196. Reyneke JP, Tsakiris P, Becker P. Age as a factor in the complication rate after removal of unerupted/impacted third molars at the time of mandibular sagittal split osteotomy. J Oral Maxillofac Surg 2002;60:654.

197. Riley RW, Powell NB, Guilleminault C, Ware W. Obstructive sleep apnea syndrome following surgery for mandibular prognathism. J Oral Maxillofac Surg 1987;45:450.

198. Kawamata A, Fujishita M, Ariji Y, Ariji E. Three-dimensional computed tomographic evaluation of morphologic airway changes after mandibular setback osteotomy for prognathism. Oral Surg Oral Med Oral Pathol Oral Radiol Endod 2000;89:278.

199. Bouwman JPB, Husak A, Putnam GD, et al. Screw fixation following bilateral sagittal ramus osteotomy for mandibular advancement: complications in 700 consecutive cases. Br J Oral Maxillofac Surg 1995;33:231.

200. Acebal-Bianco F, Vuylsteke PL, Mommaerts MY, De Clercq CA. Perioperative complications in corrective facial orthopedic surgery: a 5-year retrospective study. J Oral Maxillofac Surg 2000;58:754.

201. Epker BN. Dentofacial deformities. In: Integrated orthodontic and surgical correction. St Louis (MO): C.V. Mosby; 1986.

202. Beke AL, Yahner VB. Surgical correction of overbite and overjet with sagittal osteotomy of the mandibular horizontal ramus: report of case. J Oral Surg 1969;27:358.

203. Bloomquist DS. Mandibular body sagittal osteotomy in the correction of malunited edentulous mandibular fractures. J Maxillofac Surg 1982;10:18.

204. Sandor GK, Stoelinga PJ, Tideman H. Reappraisal of the mandibular step osteotomy. J Oral Maxillofac Surg 1982;40:78.

205. Keller EE, Hill AJ Jr, Sather AH. Orthognathic surgery: review of mandibular body procedures. Mayo Clin Proc 1976;51:117.

206. Nakajima T, Kajikawa Y, Ueda K, Hanada K. Sliding osteotomy in the mandibular body for correction of prognathism. J Oral Surg 1978;36:361.

207. Kavanaugh SH. Maxillary midline split surgery [dissertation]. Department of Orthodontics, University of Washington; 1985.

208. Peterson LJ. Posterior mandibular segmental alveolar osteotomy. J Oral Surg 1978;36:454.

209. MacIntosh RB, Carlotti AE. Total mandibular alveolar osteotomy in the management of skeletal (infantile) apertognathia. J Oral Surg 1975;33:921.

210. Booth DF, Dietz V, Gianelly AA. Correction of class III malocclusion by combined sagittal ramus and subapical body osteotomy. J Oral Surg 1976;34:630.

211. Theisen FC, Guernsey LH. Postoperative sequelae after anterior segmental osteotomies. Oral Surg Oral Med Oral Pathol 1976;41:139.

212. Pangrazio-Kulbersh V, MacIntosh RB. Total mandibular alveolar osteotomy: an alternate choice to other surgical procedures. Am J Orthod 1985;87:319.

213. Meyer MW, Cavanaugh GD. Blood flow changes after orthognathic surgery: maxillary and mandibular subapical osteotomy. J Oral Surg 1976;34:495.

214. Banks P. Pulp changes after anterior mandibular subapical osteotomy in a primate model. J Maxillofac Surg 1977;5:39.

215. Scheideman GB, Kawamura H, Finn RA, Bell WH. Wound healing after anterior and posterior subapical osteotomy. J Oral Maxillofac Surg 1985;43:408.

216. Johnson JV, Hinds EC. Evaluation of teeth vitality after subapical osteotomy. J Oral Surg 1969;27:256.

217. Converse JM, Wood-Smith D. Horizontal osteotomy of the mandible. Plast Reconstr Surg 1964;34:464.

218. Neuner O. Correction of mandibular deformities. Oral Surg Oral Med Oral Pathol 1973;36:779.

219. Fitzpatrick B. Reconstruction of the chin in cosmetic surgery (genioplasty). Oral Surg 1975;39:522.

220. Hinds EC, Kent JN. Genioplasty: the versatility of horizontal osteotomy. J Oral Surg 1969;27:690.

221. Precious DS, Armstrong JE, Morais D. Anatomic placement of fixation devices in genioplasty. Oral Surg Oral Med Oral Pathol 1992;73:2.

222. Scheideman GB, Legan HL, Bell WH. Soft tissue changes with combined mandibular setback and advancement genioplasty. J Oral Surg 1981;39:505.

223. Gallagher DM, Bell WH, Storum KA. Soft tissue changes associated with advancement genioplasty performed concomitantly with superior repositioning of the maxilla. J Oral Maxillofac Surg 1984;42:238.

224. Martinez JT, Turvey TA, Proffitt WR. Osseous remodeling after inferior border osteotomy for chin augmentation: an indication for early surgery. J Oral Maxillofac Surg 1999;57:1175.

225. Talebzadeh N, Pogrel MA. Long-term hard and soft tissue relapse rate after genioplasty. Oral Surg Oral Med Oral Pathol Oral Radiol Endod 2001;91:153.

226. Fitzpatrick BN. Genioplasty with reference to resorption and the hinge sliding osteotomy. Int J Oral Surg 1974;3:247.

227. McDonnell JP, McNeill RW, West RA. Advancement genioplasty: a retrospective cephalometric analysis of osseous and soft tissue changes. J Oral Surg 1977;35:640.

228. Hohl TH, Epker BN. Microgenia: a study of treatment results, with surgical recommendations. Oral Surg Oral Med Oral Pathol 1976;41:545.

229. Nishioka GJ, Mason M, Van Sickels JE. Neurosensory disturbance associated with the anterior mandibular horizontal osteotomy. J Oral Maxillofac Surg 1988;46:107.

CHAPTER 57

Maxillary Orthognathic Surgery

Vincent J. Perciaccante, DDS
Robert A. Bays, DDS

History

Orthognathic surgery of the maxilla was first described in 1859 by von Langenbeck for the removal of nasopharyngeal polyps.[1] The first American report of a maxillary osteotomy was by Cheever in 1867 for the treatment of complete nasal obstruction secondary to recurrent epistaxis for which a right hemimaxillary down-fracture was used.[2] Over the next 70 years numerous authors described osteotomy techniques that mobilized the entire maxilla for the treatment of pathologic processes.

In 1901 Le Fort published his classic description of the natural planes of maxillary fracture.[3] In 1927 Wassmund first described the Le Fort I osteotomy for the correction of midface deformities.[4] However, total mobilization of the maxilla with immediate repositioning was not performed until 1934 by Axhausen.[5] Separation of the pterygomaxillary junction was advocated by Schuchardt in 1942.[6] Moore and Ward in 1949 recommended horizontal transection of the pterygoid plates for advancement.[7] Willmar reported on over 40 cases treated this way and of severe bleeding in most, thereby abandoning this procedure in favor of separation at the pterygomaxillary junction.[8] Most of these techniques simply mobilized the maxilla to one degree or another, and then placed orthopedic forces on it to achieve the desired repositioning—a sort of unintentional distraction osteogenesis. These methods were associated with high levels of relapse.

In 1965 Obwegeser suggested complete mobilization of the maxilla so that repositioning could be accomplished without tension.[9] This proved to be a major advance in stabilization, as documented by Hogemann and Willmar, de Haller, and Perko, respectively.[10–12]

Anterior segmentalization of the maxilla was also addressed in the early descriptions, including those by Wassmund, by Cohn-Stock, and by Spanier.[4,13,14] Again, complete mobilization of the maxilla with vascular compromise was avoided, and multiple segments contributed to poor stability. Cupar, Kole, and Wunderer, respectively, reported more direct surgical access to these procedures with improved mobilization and maintenance of blood supply.[15–18] Posterior segmentalization of the maxilla was used by Schuchardt but it had limited stability also owing to incomplete mobilization.[19] Kufner improved on this technique by completely mobilizing the osteotomized segment prior to repositioning.[20] Logically, anterior and posterior segmental osteotomies were combined to accomplish total maxillary alveolar osteotomy for repositioning and segmental manipulation simultaneously.[21,22] Several forms of total maxillary osteotomies were described by Cupar, Converse and Shapiro, and Kole, respectively.[15,23,24] Willmar further established the stability of the Le Fort I osteotomy, and Bell and colleagues documented the overall superiority of the total down-fracture Le Fort I osteotomy for segmental and one-piece maxillary osteotomy.[8,25] Bone grafting to enhance stabilization was advocated by Cupar, Gillies and Rowe, and Obwegeser, respectively, who first advocated grafting in the pterygomaxillary fissure.[15,16,26,27] Interestingly, Willmar did not find a difference in stability with and without bone grafting in nonclefted cases.[8]

Early descriptions of the rigid fixation of maxillary osteotomies were published by Michelet and colleagues in 1973, Horster in 1980, Drommer and Luhr in 1981, and Luyk and Ward-Booth in 1985.[28–31] Since that time, many methods have been advocated for the rigid fixation of maxillary osteotomies. These have included bone plates, metallic mesh, pins, the rigid adjustable pin (RAP) system, and resorbable fixation.[32–34] Since these landmark papers, volumes have been written regarding a wide variety of technical factors, many of which reflect operator preference.

Basic Principles

Maxillary deformities may manifest in any of the three planes of space: sagittal, axial, and coronal. Patients displaying abnormal facial anatomy often exhibit elements of maxillary and mandibular deformities. Therefore, the clinician must recognize and be prepared to treat maxillary and midface deformities. Subjectively, patients with maxillary deformities often describe their problem in terms of the relative mandibular appearance. Patient expectations clearly demonstrate the importance of the chin in patient satisfaction.[35] This perceptual preoccupation with apparent mandibular excess or deficiency in the absence of a significant absolute mandibular abnormality may necessitate extensive consultation and guidance from the surgeon to assist the patient in recognition of the contribution made by the midface and maxilla to overall facial appearance. Similarly the patient may relate the importance of nasal prominence or deficiency in describing his or her chief complaint.

Scrutiny of physical characteristics, model surgery, and cephalometric analysis with prediction tracings will assist in obtaining a satisfactory treatment plan. These important diagnostic and treatment planning modalities are discussed extensively elsewhere in the text; however, model surgery is the most valuable tool in preparing for orthognathic correction of skeletal facial deformities. While model surgery is essential for immediate preoperative surgical simulation and splint construction, it may be even more important in early treatment planning. Prior to any orthodontic or surgical treatment, model surgery is the best method to determine the postoperative position of the *mandible* as well as the maxilla. No cephalometric prediction (computer generated or hand drawn) or photographic manipulation can reveal all of the three-dimensional and occlusal information gleaned from accurate model surgery. In the pretreatment state the teeth may not fit together perfectly during this preliminary model surgery, but orthodontics can be simulated to permit an accurate projection of the specific movements required of the maxilla and

mandible to achieve the desired results. The model measurements made at the time of this exercise should be exactly the same as those used for the actual preoperative model surgery (see below). Pretreatment model surgery is essential when contemplating maxillary surgery alone and very useful when planning two-jaw surgery. Pretreatment model surgery permits the *three-dimensional* evaluation of the maxilla and the mandible, whether the mandible is autorotated without surgery or also osteotomized.

Model Surgery, Reference Marks, and Intraoperative Positioning

The purposes of preoperative model surgery are to (1) mark the models to facilitate three-dimensional measurement of the pre- and postoperative positioning; (2) place the jaw models into the desired positions based on all of the database including three-dimensional clinical assessment (the most important), radiographic analysis, model studies and patient desires; (3) evaluate the feasibility of the planned surgical moves using the measurements and make necessary adjustments; (4) determine the vertical change that will be achieved at the time of surgery in such a way that it can be accurately duplicated intraoperatively; and (5) construct the surgical splint(s).

The following method has been used successfully for over 20 years by the senior author (RAB). The technique is based on three simple principles:

1. A measurement is made from a point above the osteotomy to a point below it at model surgery and intraoperatively. After the maxilla is moved the same superior point is used but the point on the maxilla has been moved along a predetermined plane. This creates a triangle defined by one superior point and two inferior points (pre- and postoperatively). This triangle can

be measured accurately on models and on the patient at surgery.
2. Central incisor vertical measurements can be made directly on the models.
3. If the measurements made on the models and at surgery have the same pre- and postoperative *differences*, the incisor vertical will be correct.

Centric relation mounted models are marked to record all possible surgical movements anteriorly and posteriorly (Figure 57-1). For the purpose of illustration Figure 57-1A and B demonstrate the measurements that are necessary for intraoperative control of the vertical position of the maxilla. The vertical measurements at the maxillary canines and first molars are the critical ones for use intraoperatively (see Figure 57-1C). The bilateral vertical measurements must be made from stable points on the top of the mounting ring, not just anywhere along the mounting ring (points A and P) to cusp tips. Gingival cuffs will be used intraoperatively (Figure 57-2) on the canines (point B) and first molars (point C). The maxillary model is then moved to the desired position, including vertical. The measurement of the vertical position of the incisor is made by placing the Boley gauge flat on the top of the mounting ring (parallel to the Frankfort horizontal) to the tip of the incisor (see Figure 57-1D). This vertical measurement of the maxillary central incisor is constantly controlled while the maxilla is positioned in all other planes of space (see Figure 57-2A). After the maxillary model has been fixed in the proper position, an imaginary triangle is created by points A, B, and B′ and by points P, C, and C′. The lines A–B and P–C are the preoperative vertical values and the lines A–B′ and P–C′ are the hypotenuses of the triangles and the postoperative vertical values (see Figure 57-2B). The *differences* between lines A–B and A–B′ and lines P–C and P–C′ are the important values. The absolute numbers are not.

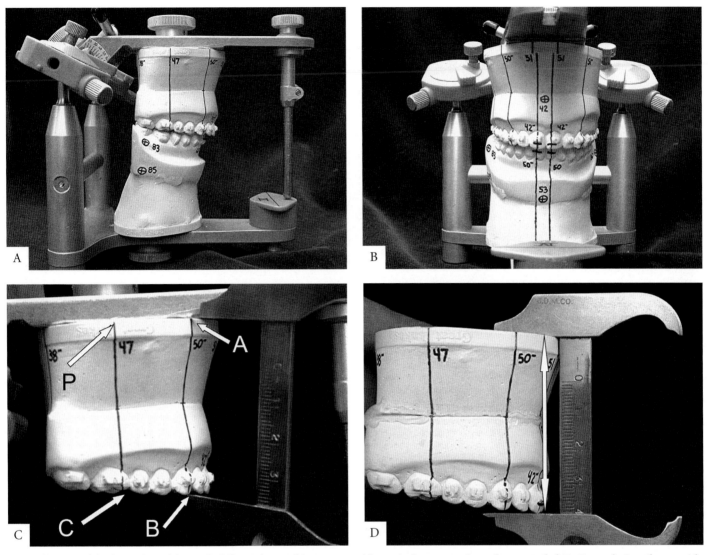

FIGURE **57-1** A, *Mounted models marked for orthognathic surgery with vertical preoperative values recorded.* B, *Frontal view shows midline markings that can be seen on either side of the pin when it is placed.* C, *Straight-line measurements are made from points* A *to* B *and points* P *to* C *on each side.* D, *Maxillary central incisor is measured perpendicular to the Frankfort horizontal, which is from the top of the mounting ring. (Note: This is not a straight point-to-point measurement, but a perpendicular to Frankfort one.)*

Intraoperatively marks are made above the proposed osteotomy sites in the piriform rims and the first molar/buttress areas (points A and P) (see Figure 57-2C). Measurements are made from point A to the gingival cuff of the canine (point B) and from point P to the first molar (point C). The gingival cuffs are used because the cusps will be hidden under the splint and the brackets may come loose during surgery. During maxillary positioning, lines A–B′ and P–C′ can be measured until the *difference* between lines A–B and A–B′ and lines P–C and P–C′ are as predicted by

the models (see Figures 57-2D and E). When this is accomplished the anterior vertical changes of the central incisors will be as they were on the models, so that no direct measurement of incisors is necessary. Usually the maxilla is repositioned anteroposteriorly and sometimes mediolaterally as it is moving vertically. This method of measurement is especially important when large anteroposterior or mediolateral moves are included.

Our experience and that of others has shown that external reference marks add nothing to the accuracy of vertical maxil-

lary positioning if the internal reference method is as outlined above.[36,37]

Surgical Anatomy

Osseous Structures

The body of the maxilla contains the maxillary sinus in its entirety, except rarely when the apex extends into the zygomatic bone.[38] The anterior surface of the maxilla is the anterolateral wall of the sinus. The infraorbital foramen is located at variable distances below the inferior orbital rim. Continuing inferiorly is the

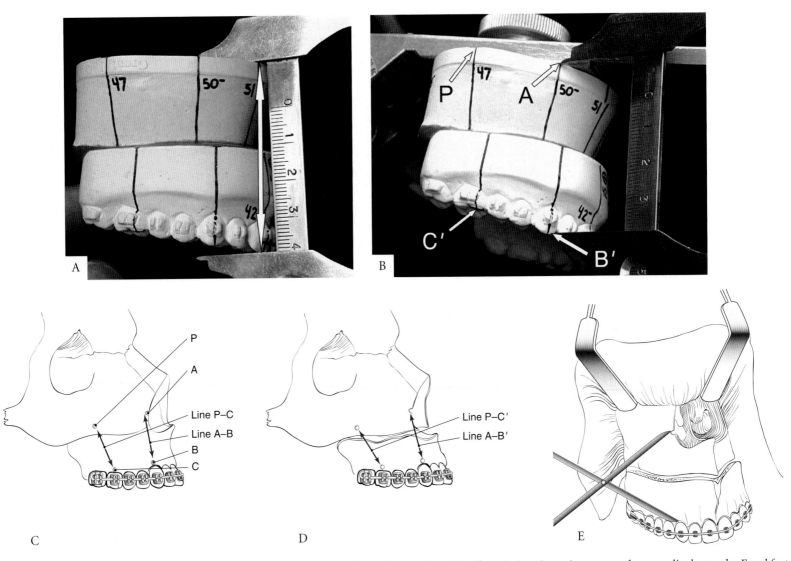

FIGURE 57-2   A, *Maxillary model has been moved into desired position including vertical. Maxillary incisor is again measured perpendicular to the Frankfort horizontal (ie, from the top of the mounting ring). B, Straight line measurements are made from points A to B′ and P to C′ bilaterally. C, At surgery, slots are made in the piriform rim and holes in the buttress to simulate points A and P bilaterally. The gingival cuffs of the canines and first molars represent points B and C. D, Following mobilization of the maxilla it is placed so that the* **differences** *between lines A–B and A–B′ are the same as they were on the models. Lines P–C and P–C′ can be used similarly. Note: If this is done precisely, the vertical change at the central incisors will be the same as it was on the models so that there is no need to make a direct measurement of the centrals. E, Illustration of measurement method at surgery.*

canine fossa lateral to the canine tooth. The anterior alveolar process of each maxilla surrounds the piriform aperture, and they unite in the midline to form the anterior nasal spine. This bony spine is the most anterior and inferior attachment for the mobile anterior cartilaginous nasal septum. An elevated sharp crest at the junction of the anterior and nasal surfaces of the maxilla, which forms the nasal floor, inclines this structure superiorly at the aperture. The body of the maxilla and its frontal process

form the superolateral boundary of the piriform aperture as a thin edge of bone (Figure 57-3).

In the midline the nasal crest of the maxilla articulates with the septal or quadrangular cartilage and vomer.[39,40] The septal cartilage rests in a central groove, which extends posterior to the anterior nasal spine. This articulation is flexible but strengthened by the perichondrium-periosteum continuity and interposed connective tissue. In the midline at the junction of the maxilla and the premaxilla is the incisive fossa, which

typically presents the openings of four canals through which the nasopalatine arteries and nerves are conducted.

The palate is formed by the palatine process of the two maxillas and the horizontal lamina of the palatine bones.[41] The transverse suture between the maxilla and palatine bones lies roughly 1 cm anterior to the posterior margin of the hard palate. At its lateral extent the suture widens into the greater palatine foramen, which is approximately 1 cm posteromedial to the second molar (Figure 57-4).

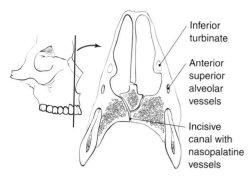

FIGURE **57-3** *Cross-sectional anatomy of the maxilla at the piriform rim.*

The greater palatine canal is formed similarly between the perpendicular laminae of the palatine and maxillary bones, which form the inferior lateral nasal wall. The inferior nasal concha also articulates with the maxillary and palatine components of the lateral nasal wall.

Posterolaterally the maxillary tuberosity is behind the third molar. Above this tuberosity the posterior superior alveolar foramina may be observed through which the nerves and vessels emerge. The pyramidal process of the palatine bone unites the two pterygoid plates of the sphenoid bone with each other and to the maxilla. The pterygomaxillary junction, formed by the palatine bone, ends superiorly in the pterygomaxillary fissure leading into the pterygopalatine fossa.[42,43] The foramen rotundum enters the posterior wall of the pterygopalatine fossa and the pterygoid or vidian canal. Medially the sphenopalatine foramen leads to the lateral nasal cavity posterior to the middle nasal concha of the ethmoid bone. Anteriorly the infraorbital and zygomatic nerves and infraorbital vessels run in the infraorbital canal, and inferiorly the descending palatine artery and greater palatine nerves course within the greater palatine canal.

Vascular Structures

Although numerous texts describe the anatomy of the intact maxilla, several aspects of maxillary blood flow remain in doubt following maxillary osteotomy.

The Le Fort I maxillary osteotomy had been performed for over 100 years before Bell first identified the exact nature of blood vessels in the osteotomized maxilla, which provided information regarding the viability to the pedicled maxilla.[44,45] It was obvious that even though the direct blood supply to the maxillary teeth and periodontium was interrupted, collateral circulation existed to perfuse the dental pulp and surrounding structures (Figures 57-5 and 57-6). This same circulation was also responsible for the survival of the rest of the maxilla; however, the exact nature of the various factors affecting maxillary perfusion is still not well documented or understood. Bell's studies revealed that saving the descending palatine arteries made little difference, indicating that a collateral vasculature existed, probably from the soft palate, which was adequate for maxillary perfusion. The down-fractured maxilla has a rich blood supply via the ascending pharyngeal artery and the ascending palatine branch of the facial artery.[46]

Bell also verified the revascularization of anterior maxillary osteotomies using the microangiographic technique.[45] Brusati and Bottoli performed revascularization studies similar to those of Bell and found quite different results.[47] They found

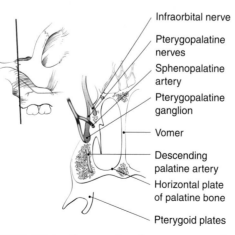

FIGURE **57-4** *Cross-sectional anatomy at the pterygomaxillary junction. Note the position of the greater palatine foramen and perpendicular plate of the palatine bone.*

Labels for Figure 57-4:
- Infraorbital nerve
- Pterygopalatine nerves
- Sphenopalatine artery
- Pterygopalatine ganglion
- Vomer
- Descending palatine artery
- Horizontal plate of palatine bone
- Pterygoid plates

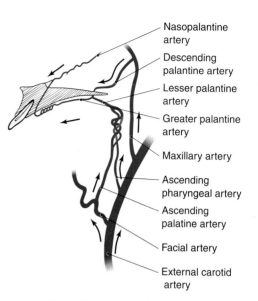

FIGURE **57-5** *Pathway of the ascending palatine, ascending pharyngeal, and descending palatine arteries as they continue into the greater palatine arteries.*

Labels for Figure 57-5:
- Nasopalantine artery
- Descending palantine artery
- Lesser palantine artery
- Greater palantine artery
- Maxillary artery
- Ascending pharyngeal artery
- Ascending palatine artery
- Facial artery
- External carotid artery

the tunneling technique to be superior in maintaining the blood supply, especially to the pulpal tissues, when compared with the labial pedicled anterior maxillary procedures.[17,18] This was just the opposite from the findings of Bell.[45] A possible explanation for this discrepancy is that Bell used monkeys whereas Brusati and Bottoli used dogs, which they claimed possess a more similar maxillary vasculature to that of the human.[48] The clinical significance of these differences is not clear to this day.

Revascularization does not necessarily represent blood flow, and therefore Nelson and colleagues used a radioactive microsphere technique to evaluate maxillary blood flow.[49] Unfortunately several variables were present in this study that make interpretation difficult. In none of the above-mentioned studies were the maxillas moved to a new position, which may represent the largest insult to the blood supply at the time of actual maxillary osteotomy. Additionally, in Nelson's study, severance of the descending palatine vessels was inadvertent and no ligation was performed.[49] This allowed bleeding to occur through the lacerated vessels and prevented a pressure head

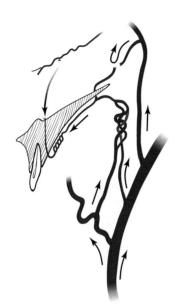

FIGURE 57-6 *Soft palatal, ascending pharyngeal, and ascending palatal vessels anastomose with the greater palatine artery. Major vessels have been sectioned and tied. The arrows signify direction of blood flow.*

from developing to maintain distal flow to the anterior maxilla. Also there were large differences in the preoperative microsphere values between animals such that postoperative comparisons were impossible. In other studies involving anterior maxillary osteotomies, Nelson and colleagues found no significant differences among three different techniques that were similar to the ones described by Brusati and Bottoli, plus a third procedure using only a palatal pedicle.[47,50] Although no statistical difference was seen, the palatal flap seemed to be slightly superior to the others. Again the same problems existed with this study as before, rendering conclusions impossible.

Soft Tissue Envelope of the Maxilla

The midfacial superficial fascia or subcutaneous tissue contains a variable amount of adipose tissue with the muscles of facial expression in its deep layer. This is tightly bound to bone except adjacent to the buccal fat pad and in the lower eyelids. Hollinshead divided the mimetic or facial muscles into five chief groups concerning the mouth, nose, orbit, ear, and scalp.[42] Of concern to the present discussion are the

muscles of the mouth and nose, which are innervated at their posterior inferior aspect by the facial nerve. They insert into the skin and most arise from periosteum of the facial skeleton.

The upper oral group of muscles radiates from their insertions near the corner of the labial commissure. From a horizontal to vertical orientation and inferior to superior the risorius, zygomaticus major and minor, and the levators (levator labii superioris alaeque nasi) insert and blend with the skin and orbicularis oris. The risorius does not arise from bone but originates from the superficial fascia over the parotid gland. The risorius, zygomaticus major, and zygomaticus minor elevate and retract the corner of the mouth and upper lip laterally. The superficial levator muscles and a third deeper one, the levator anguli oris, elevate the lateral upper lip. In addition the levator labii superioris alaeque nasi attaches to the skin and greater alar cartilage of the nose, thus lifting the ala and widening the naris.

The orbicularis oris is composed of many multidirectional fiber groups that blend with other surrounding facial muscles, encircle the mouth, originate from periosteum covering the roots of the canine teeth, insert laterally at the corner of the mouth, and pass at right angles to the encircling sphincter fillers connecting skin to labial mucosa. This diverse muscle draws the lips together, purses the lips, presses the lips against the teeth, and pulls the corners of the lips inward.

The buccinator arises from the mandible and maxilla and the pterygomandibular raphe, by which it is separated from the superior pharyngeal constrictor. The fibers pass forward and slightly inferiorly to blend with the orbicularis oris and attach to the mucosa and skin of the labial region. The buccinator flattens the cheek against the teeth.

Both Lightoller and Nairn place emphasis on the modiolus, which is the point at the lateral aspect and just superi-

or to the corner of the mouth where muscles of the oral group of the mimetic muscles converge.[51,52] The orbicularis oris and buccinator joined at the modiolus form a continuous muscular sheet on either side of the midline. The zygomaticus major, levator anguli oris, and depressor anguli oris (as a group referred to as "modiolar stays") immobilize the modiolus in any position. Additionally the marginal and peripheral parts of the orbicularis oris muscle are distinguished. The peripheral aspect of the muscle lies parallel with the inner labial mucosal surface, and the marginal part curls outward following the vermilion surface. As tension is expressed in the orbicularis oris, the marginal aspect of the muscle is thought to straighten and decrease vermilion exposure, thereby pulling the upper and lower lips toward each other and against the dentition.

The nasal group of facial muscles dilates and compresses the nares. The nasalis arises from the maxilla lateral and inferior to the ala. The transverse portion unites with the contralateral muscle over the dorsum of the nose. The alar part inserts into the greater alar cartilage. Thus, the two parts compress and dilate the nasal apertures respectively. The depressor septi muscle lies beneath the orbicularis oris and attaches to the base of the columella and posterior ala. Its action narrows the naris. The posterior and anterior dilator muscles are intrinsic muscles of the nose that course from the alar cartilages to the margin of the pads. The nasal mucoperiosteum is firmly fixed to the elevated piriform rim above the floor of the nose, to the lateral margin of the nasal aperture and the anterior nasal spine. The premaxillary wings that flare laterally from the anterior midline nasal crest provide an irregular attachment of the mucoperiosteum along the inferoanterior nasal floor.

The palate is covered by mucosa firmly adherent to the periosteum and containing mucous minor salivary glands. The mucosa is thin in the central palate and thickens toward the alveolar process. The palatine crest is a transverse elevation at the posterior border of the horizontal plate of the palatine bone that gives attachment to the tensor veli palatini muscle. The larger lateral pterygoid plate is the origin of the inferior head of the lateral and the medial pterygoid muscles. A small part of the medial pterygoid also arises from the maxillary tuberosity. The tensor veli palatini muscle curves around the hamulus, which is the inferior end of the medial pterygoid plate. From the hamulus the tensor muscle of the palate enters the soft palatal tissues. The tensor aponeurosis is an adherent connective tissue sheath continuous with the periosteum, which covers the posterior hard palate attaching laterally to the submucosal layer of the pharynx and the tensor veli palatini tendon.

Surgical Techniques

Soft Tissue Incision and Surgical Exposure of the Maxilla

Exposure of the anterior, lateral, and pterygomaxillary regions is most commonly achieved by incising horizontally through the buccolabial mucoperiosteum above the attached gingival margin at the level of the maxillary teeth apices (Figure 57-7A). The vestibular incision courses from the first molar to the contralateral first molar (Figure 57-7B). The parotid papilla is identified and retracted superolaterally during completion of the incision posteriorly. The incision can be made with electrocautery or steel as there have been no studies performed that show a difference between the two. After initial penetration of the mucosa the natural tendency to cut more superiorly with deeper penetration must be avoided. This is particularly important in the incisor area, as this would carry one into the nasal cavity.

The superior tissues are reflected subperiosteally, first at the piriform aperture margins (Figure 57-7C). Progressively more superior exposure lateral to the nasal

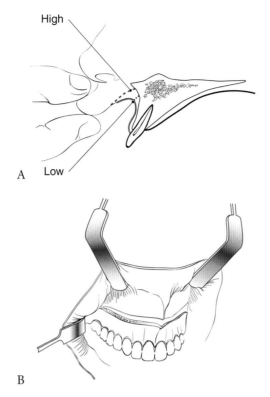

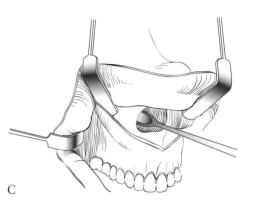

FIGURE 57-7 A, *The soft tissue incision for maxillary surgery. B, The circumvestibular incision extends from the area of the first molar to the same location on the opposite side. C, The nasal mucosa is elevated beginning on the superolateral surface of the piriform rim.*

aperture will expose the infraorbital nerve exiting from its foramen. Posterior reflection proceeding from the delineated infraorbital foramen reveals the zygomaticomaxillary suture, zygomatic buttress, and the most anterior aspect of the zygomatic arch. Inferiorly, with subperiosteal tunneling, the lateral aspect of the maxillary tuberosity and its junction with palatine bone and pterygoid plates of the sphenoid bone are identified. Care should be taken to direct this subperiosteal dissection inferiorly, toward the mucogingival junction, as it is carried back toward the pterygomaxillary fissure, to avoid vascular structures. Meticulous maintenance of the subperiosteal plane of dissection will prevent troublesome exposure of buccal fat pad tissue, which impairs visualization and retraction of soft tissue during subsequent osseous surgery. A retractor with a curvilinear end is placed in the pterygomaxillary junction to facilitate exposure. Attention should be paid to the placement of this retractor, as it too can be responsible for periosteal rents and exposure of the buccal fat.

Tissues inferior to the horizontal incision are elevated minimally. In areas of interdental osteotomies for segmentalization of the maxillary arch the inferior attached gingiva and periosteum are elevated conservatively, with a Woodson elevator, while retraction laterally is provided by skin hooks (Figure 57-8A). Since the alveolar osteotomy will be accomplished with thin osteotomes, osseous exposure requirements at the alveolar crest level are minimal.

When intersegmental movement will be great and may result in tearing of the gingival papilla, an alternative approach to the interdental region may be used. Additionally a wider exposure of alveolar bone is frequently needed when an osteotomy is to be performed in an edentulous or extraction space. In these situations a vertical mucosal incision at the line angle, one-tooth distant from the ostectomy site (Figure 57-8B), will facilitate wider exposure for osseous procedures. This incision should be used only when an anterior labial pedicle is maintained to maximize the labial vascular pedicle during multisegmental osteotomy.

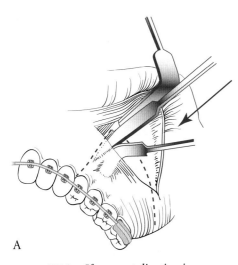

A

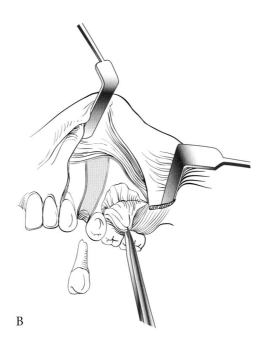

B

FIGURE 57-8 *If segmentalization is necessary, it is best to perform interdental osteotomies before horizontal osteotomies and down-fracture. A, Minimal exposure technique for interdental osteotomies. B, Vertical incision for interdental osteotomies.*

For one-, two-, and most routine three-piece maxillary osteotomies, a circumvestibular incision with minimal interdental exposure is preferred. For three-piece maxillary osteotomies that involve exceptionally wide expansion or extreme changes at the interdental site, four-piece maxillary osteotomies, and osteotomies in some ex-cleft patients, soft tissue incisions can be modified from second molar to first premolar to maintain an anterior labial pedicle (Figure 57-9). A midline vertical incision is placed to gain access to the midline of the maxilla.

Once the labial incisions are completed the nasal mucoperiosteum is elevated to complete soft tissue exposure of the osseous surgical site (see Figure 57-7C). Initial establishment of a subperiosteal dissection plane is imperative for completion of nasal tissue dissection without disruption of mucoperiosteal integrity. Because the nasal cavity is more voluminous inside the piriform rim than at the piriform aperture, the elevator should be held at an oblique angle to the surrounding maxillary bone adjacent to the nasal aperture. While maintaining the elevator tip against bone, the mucoperiosteum is

reflected from the nasal floor, lateral nasal wall, and nasal crest of the maxilla. The dissection should continue superiorly for a centimeter up the vertical nasal walls to prevent tearing during osteotomy or down-fracture of the maxilla, particularly at the superior reflections of the nasal floor medially and laterally. The anteroposterior depth of this soft tissue dissection is approximately 15 to 20 mm. The remaining posterior soft tissue is reflected more precisely after initial down-fracture of the maxilla.

Osseous Surgery

After recording the reference measurements as outlined earlier (see Figure 57-2), the osteotomy is performed. The design of the osteotomy will depend on the maxillary movement desired. Regardless of the design of the osteotomy the measurement marks are used as illustrated in Figure 57-2. Initially the basic horizontal osteotomy will be discussed and then alterations will be described for specific situations. *Segmentalization* of the maxilla may be necessary in certain cases. Specifics of this procedure will be discussed at the end of the basic horizontal technique. The lateral

maxillary osteotomy (Figure 57-10) is started at the greatest convexity of the zygomatic buttress because that is the easiest starting surface for the reciprocating saw. It is advanced anteriorly through the lateral piriform rim below the inferior turbinate while the nasal mucoperiosteum is retracted and protected using a periosteal elevator. For the basic maxillary osteotomy this horizontal osteotomy is parallel to the maxillary arch wire approximately coincident with the cut performed previously during model surgery. After the anterior osteotomy is completed, it is continued posteriorly by tapering inferiorly toward the pterygomaxillary junction. A thin reciprocating saw blade and copious irrigation are used for this osseous cut. The most posterior centimeter or so of the lateral wall can be cut with the same saw, but from inside out (Figure 57-11).

Next a nasal septal osteotome is directed slightly downward and posterior (Figure 57-12) beginning just above the anterior nasal spine while the anterior nasal mucoperiosteum is retracted. Proceeding posteriorly the osteotome is carefully maintained in the midline. The tendency toward superior deviation while separating the cartilaginous and vomerine septum from the nasal crest of the maxilla

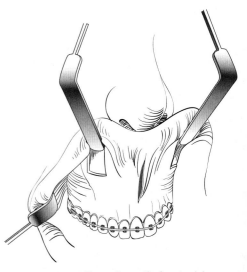

FIGURE 57-9 *Bilateral vestibular incisions are made from the first premolar to the second molar; shown with a midline vertical incision.*

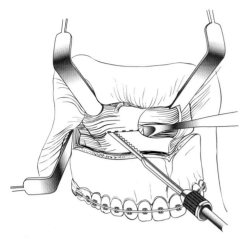

FIGURE 57-10 *Lateral wall osteotomy is begun at greatest convexity of the buttress and brought forward to the piriform rim with a periosteal elevator protecting the nasal mucosa and the endotracheal tube.*

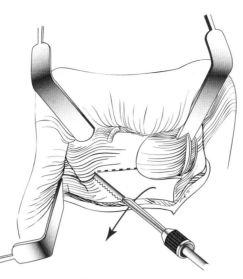

FIGURE 57-11 *The saw is then turned inside out and the osteotomy from the buttress to the pterygomaxillary junction is made angling downward as it goes posteriorly.*

necessitates maintenance of a slight downward inclination of the septal osteotome. The lateral nasal wall is severed using a thin osteotome directed posteriorly while medial retraction of the nasal mucoperiosteum is accomplished with a periosteal elevator. The osteotome is gently malleted posteriorly for a distance of approximately 20 mm to avoid premature injury to the descending palatine neurovascular bundle that resides in the lateral posterior nasal wall.

After the above osteotomies have been performed, the pterygoid plates are separated from the maxillary tuberosity (Figure 57-13) using a small sharp curved osteotome. This instrument is preferred over the traditional thick pterygomaxillary osteotome because the thin cutting edge limits fracture and promotes precise division of this bony junction.[53] The tip of the osteotome is directed as anteriorly, inferiorly, and medially as the tunneled buccal soft tissue allows. A finger placed palatal and posterior to the maxillary tuberosity will facilitate early verification of the complete separation of bone while avoiding trauma to the palatal vascular pedicle. The authors prefer to have this instrument sharpened before each case.

Downward pressure is placed on the anterior maxilla using the sharp hooks of a Senn retractor to facilitate initial down-fracture of the maxilla (Figure 57-14). If moderate pressure does not result in mobilization of the inferior segment, the completeness of the above osteotomies must be suspect. The cement spatula osteotome is used to ensure complete bony severance of the anterior lateral nasal wall and zygomaticomaxillary portions of the osteotomy. The curved osteotome is again placed into the pterygomaxillary junction, malleted gently, and then torqued to mobilize the maxilla. If no significant movement is detected, then the

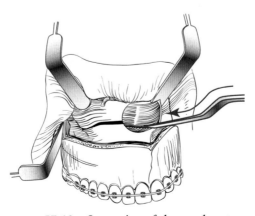

FIGURE 57-12 *Separation of the nasal septum from the septal crest of the maxilla with a special osteotome.*

osteotome may be stepped slightly superiorly, directed anteriorly, and malleted until the separation is complete.

When mobility occurs the nasal mucoperiosteum is elevated progressively more posteriorly until the posterior edge of the hard palate is encountered (see Figure 57-14). Portions of the pterygoid plates or perpendicular process of the palatine bone that resist fracture may be completely separated from the maxilla using an osteotome under direct visualization (Figure 57-15). The descending palatine neurovascular bundle is isolated, ligated, and divided.

Significant movement of the posterior maxilla can cause tensile forces on the descending palatine neurovascular components. Superior repositioning of the maxilla may also compress the exposed vessels and nerve between the inferior and superior osseous segments. Severe postoperative bleeding after Le Fort I maxillary osteotomy has been reported.[54–57] Attempts to preserve the neurovascular bundle may increase this possibility. Ligation and division of this structure has been shown to have no deleterious influence on perfusion or neurosensory function.[58,59] The bone of the perpendicular plate of the palatine bone surrounding the neurovascular bundle is

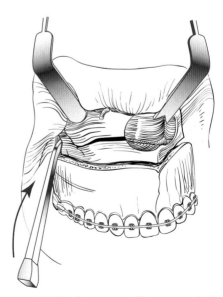

FIGURE 57-13 *Pterygomaxillary separation with a small sharp curved osteotome directed medially.*

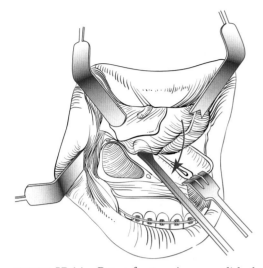

FIGURE **57-14** *Down-fracture is accomplished with a sharp-toothed Senn retractor, with simultaneous elevation of nasal mucoperiosteum.*

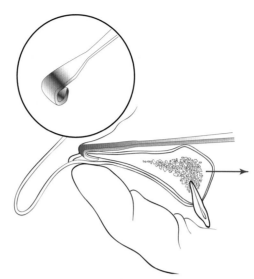

FIGURE **57-16** *Mobilization of the maxilla with a J stripper.*

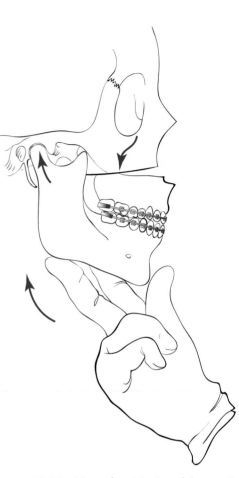

FIGURE **57-17** *Manual positioning of the maxillomandibular complex with condyles seated. Note the posterior pivot point that must be removed.*

carefully removed using a Woodson elevator, burs, and rongeurs, and the neurovascular bundle is ligated and divided (see Figure 57-15). After down-fracture, complete mobilization of the maxilla is the next objective. A **J** stripper normally used for periosteal elevation in sagittal osteotomies engages the posterior border of the midline nasal floor at the posterior nasal spine (Figure 57-16), and anterolateral pressure is

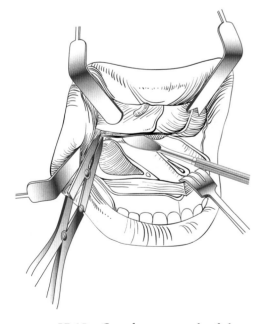

FIGURE **57-15** *Complete removal of bone around the perpendicular plate of palatine bone. The descending palatine artery is isolated, ligated, and divided.*

exerted to progressively increase mobility of the maxilla. The goal of these maneuvers is to move the maxilla into the approximate final position with only gentle digital pressure. After mobilization from the cranial base is completed, a reassessment of the surgical move is considered. Based on the movement planned any possible bony interferences posterior to the second molar must be removed before application of maxillomandibular fixation (MMF). When all possible interferences posterior to the second molar have been removed, the maxilla is wired to the mandible with the occlusal splint interposed.

We prefer to have the patient completely paralyzed during the period of maxillary positioning. Condylar positioning while rotating the maxilla and mandible is paramount to success. The physiologic position of the condyles is thought to be a superoanterior orientation relative to the glenoid fossae against the posterior slopes of the articular eminences, with the disk interposed between the condyle and the fossa. The surgeon must position the condyles of the maxillomandibular complex in this upward and forward direction prior to autorotation (Figure 57-17). The importance of this stage of the surgery cannot be overesti-

mated. The most likely points of unrecognized bony interferences are in the areas of the pterygoid plates, the maxillary tuberosities, and the perpendicular plate of the palatine bone. It is quite possible to rotate the maxillomandibular complex inappropriately while being unaware of a premature pivot point in these posterior bony areas (Figure 57-18A). This will result in Class II open bite discrepancy once the patient is released from MMF. If a significant period of MMF or training elastics is used postoperatively, this discrepancy may not become apparent for weeks or months (Figure 57-18B). Once these posterior interferences have been removed, the surgeon continues to rotate the entire complex around the temporomandibular joints until the appropriate vertical relationship is achieved as described above. The cartilaginous sep-

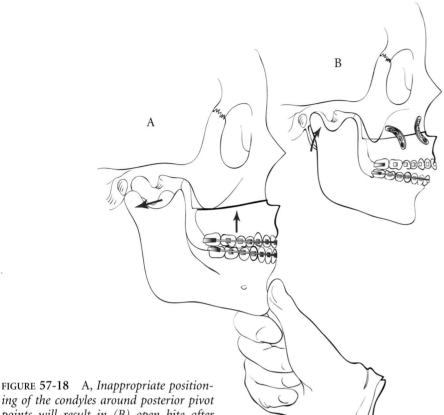

FIGURE **57-18** A, *Inappropriate positioning of the condyles around posterior pivot points will result in (B) open bite after release from maxillomandibular fixation.*

tum and vomer as well as the nasal crest of the maxilla are reduced in height equal to the planned movement of the maxilla. This may entail a submucous resection of the cartilaginous nasal septum to prevent buckling of the septum from pressure as the maxilla is repositioned. A groove can be fashioned in the midline of the nasal floor to accommodate the recontoured septum.

A portion of the inferior edge of the cartilaginous septum should be removed. The tendency is to remove too little because of the irregular inferior contact between septum and maxilla. Even if the maxilla is inferiorly positioned, buckling of the septum may occur because the cartilaginous septum extends anterior and inferior to the anterior nasal spine and therefore can be buckled as the maxilla moves forward even if there is some downward movement (Figure 57-19). All of the maxillary positioning has been predetermined by the model surgery and

splint construction, except for the vertical. As the maxilla is rotated upward around the condyles, bone is only removed at the point of contact, not a full wedge (Figure

57-20). This facilitates ideal bone-to-bone contact and avoids large gaps in between. Once the desired vertical relationship has been achieved based on the measurements described above, the maxilla should be fixed in position with internal rigid fixation. Sequentially eliminating only interfering osseous structures ensures optimal bone contact. This method is preferred over a wedge ostectomy.[60] Maxillomandibular fixation is removed and the mandible is rotated into the splint while held to the maxilla. If the occlusion is correct, the splint is removed and not left in place postoperatively.

Variations in the above basic osteotomy design may enhance osseous contact, facilitate bone graft placement, or aid fixation device application, and result in improved stability of the superiorly, inferiorly, or anteriorly repositioned maxilla. These variations will be described below as they apply to specific maxillary movements. To prevent septal deviation despite adequate bone and cartilage removal, it is often desirable to suture the nasal septum to the anterior nasal spine. This is done by drilling a hole through the anterior nasal spine and passing a 1-0 polyglycolic acid

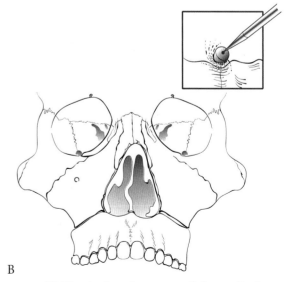

FIGURE **57-19** A, *Anterior aspect of the cartilaginous nasal septum extends anteroinferiorly to the anterior nasal spine. B, Pure horizontal advancement of the maxilla will buckle the septum unless adequate bony and cartilaginous relief is provided.*

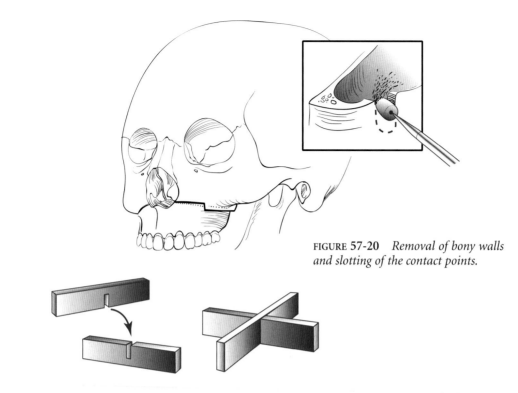

FIGURE **57-20** *Removal of bony walls and slotting of the contact points.*

suture through the hole and then through the cartilaginous septum (Figure 57-21). This will also prevent postoperative displacement of the septum during extubation or in the Post-anesthesia Care Unit.

Segmentalization

A wide range of permutations may be undertaken if segmentalization is needed. Three-piece maxillary osteotomy is perhaps the most common. The decisions regarding which of the many options will be used are made by pretreatment and preoperative model surgery. The need for extractions is also determined at this stage. If no extractions are necessary, interdental osteotomies can be safely made between parallel roots of the canines and laterals or canines and premolars. If extractions are decided on by the coordinated efforts of orthodontist and surgeon, they may be done early in treatment or during the osteotomy. A complete discussion of the indications and considerations that influence these decisions is covered elsewhere in this book. However, if there are no specific orthodontic reasons to extract teeth, it has been our experience that it is rarely necessary to extract just for the purpose of

surgery. The most common need for segmentalization is to widen the maxilla and adjust the angulations of the posterior maxillary segments. If the anterior six maxillary teeth fit well with the lower anterior teeth, the interdental osteotomy is performed between the canine and premolar teeth. This places the potential for a periodontal defect at the interdental osteotomy site more posteriorly in the mouth. But if the canines need to be widened along with the posterior segments, the interdental osteotomy is placed between canine and lateral incisor teeth. We prefer to make this osteotomy with a thin cement spatula osteotome while palpating palatally. The standard circumvestibular incision can be made with conservative tunneling from the incision inferiorly to the alveolar crest on the buccal surface of the maxilla. The osteotome is malleted through until palpated under the palatal mucosa (see Figure 57-8A). With care the osteotomy can be carried superiorly to the level of the horizontal maxillary osteotomy and medially to the horizontal surface of the palate. This should be done before any of the other maxillary osteotomies are done because the maxilla must be stable at the time of malleting. If teeth are to be extracted at the time of osteotomy, an alternative to tunneling is to lay a flap into the gingival sulcus for better access (see Figure 57-8B). However, if this is done, it is recommended that an anterior pedicle be retained for blood supply (see Figure 57-9).

Segmentalization using this or any other technique is more difficult when significantly altered osteotomy designs are used, such as high Le Fort I, II, or III. When the Z osteotomies (see below) are used, interdental segmentalization between canines and laterals is feasible, but more difficult if attempted between canines and premolars.

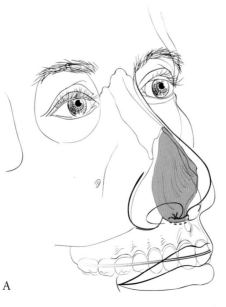

A

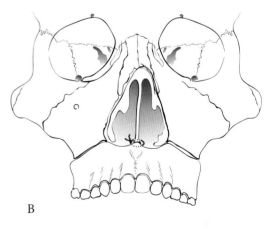

B

FIGURE **57-21** *A and B, To avoid septal deviation the cartilaginous septum should be sutured to the anterior nasal spine.*

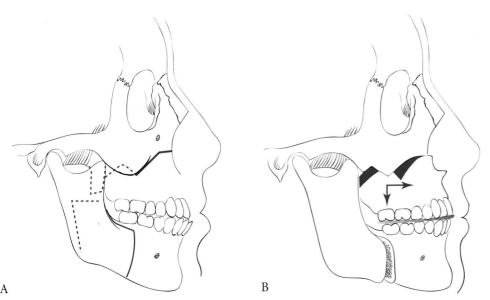

FIGURE 57-26   A, *A* **Z** *osteotomy with the posterior cut steeper than the anterior one to increase posterior facial height and to (B) rotate the maxilla downward and forward with adjustment to the occlusal plane.*

tuberosity just posterior to the second molar.[73,74] This will leave tuberosity bone attached to the pterygoid plates, which can be more safely removed. Dangers of the technique include damage to the greater palatine artery distal to its anastamosis with the lesser palatine.

Maxillary horizontal excess may also be addressed by anterior maxillary osteotomy when extractions are indicated or edentulous sites are present. These techniques are discussed in detail later in this chapter.

Stable Fixation for Maxillary Osteotomies

Rigid internal fixation with bone plates and screws has become the standard for maxillary stabilization. Although this technique has eliminated many of the early postoperative stability concerns, the technique is less forgiving than wire fixation. Therefore, intraoperative positioning is even more important. A wide variety of plating systems and sizes are available. Each surgeon will discover his or her preference, but 2.0 mm four-hole plates are used in most cases (Figure 57-31). These will require a little more effort for adaptation than lighter ones, but with

practice can be used just as accurately and with more stability. When used, these plates virtually eliminate postoperative plate fracture or mobility.

Specific Procedures

Total Maxillary Alveolar Osteotomy

The total maxillary alveolar osteotomy was designed to avoid some of the problems seen with the Le Fort I down-fracture

technique; however, it did not fare any better.[75] Purported advantages including improved nasal airway, improved stability due to better bony contact, improved ability to widen the maxilla, and better maxillary perfusion have not been realized.[75–81] In several thousand maxillary osteotomies over the past 20 years, we have not found a need for this procedure.

Anterior Maxillary Osteotomy

Numerous techniques have been used to accomplish the anterior maxillary osteotomy. The three major techniques involve the use of one of three vascular pedicles: labial (Figure 57-32), palatal (Figure 57-33), and a combination of these with vertical incisions in both (Figure 57-34). All of these can be successful, and when done properly have few complications; however, what scant literature exists would indicate that the palatal pedicle provides the best vascularity.[50]

Anterior maxillary osteotomies are generally used to treat horizontal maxillary excess when the posterior occlusion is correct or correctable by mandibular surgery. Commonly, anterior maxillary osteotomy with premolar extractions is used for bimaxillary protrusion in which both the anterior maxilla and the anterior mandible are to be retracted (Figure

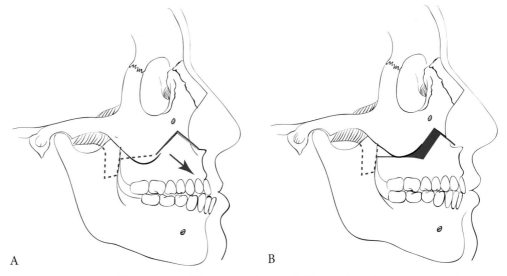

FIGURE 57-27   A, *A* **Z** *osteotomy with the posterior cut shallower than the anterior one to increase anterior facial height and to (B) rotate the maxilla down in the front and adjust the occlusal plane to a steeper angle.*

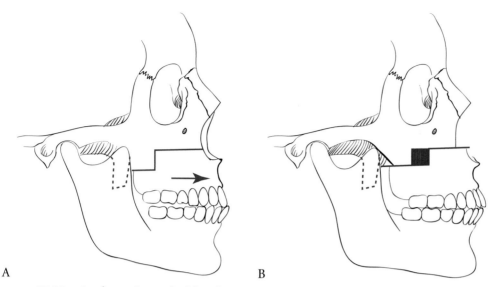

A   B

FIGURE 57-28   *An alternative method for advancement is to create a step (A) in the buttress and place a bone graft (B) in the step after repositioning.*

57-35). These procedures are also used for correction of anterior open bite. Occasionally anterior maxillary osteotomy may be coupled with mandibular advancement and anterior mandibular segmental surgery in patients with a severe curve of Spee.

Sequencing the work-up when both jaws are involved requires imagination, because the surgical procedures need to be done systematically so that the surgeon never loses orientation. There are two possible scenarios: (1) the posterior occlusion is not going to be changed because the posterior maxillary and mandibular teeth need not be moved, or (2) mandibular surgery will be performed thereby correcting the posterior occlusion. This a crucial difference because if the posterior occlusion is *not* going to be changed by surgery, then the models must be mounted in *centric occlusion*, not centric relation. If the posterior occlusion will be altered by mandibular surgery, then a new centric relation will be established by the surgery and model surgery can be done as usual. In the first case the maxillary anterior model is cut and repositioned to the best relationship against the uncut mandible in centric occlusion and the remaining maxillary dentition, and then a splint is constructed.

If mandibular surgery is to be done, two mandibular models are mounted, one mandibular model is cut, and the other is left intact to preserve the intermediate phase. The anterior maxilla and the mandible are cut and repositioned together to the final position and a final splint is made. The cut maxilla can then be articulated with the uncut mandible to establish the intermediate position and a second (intermediate) splint is made. The final splint will be wired to the maxilla for a postoperative period so there must be a separate intermediate splint that articu-

lates with the final splint and the mandibular teeth.

Particularly in segmental surgery the model surgery should simulate the actual surgery to provide a clear understanding of the three-dimensional movements necessary to the proper performance of the surgical procedure. Measurement marks should be made at the level of the interproximal spaces and the root tips. Marks should also be made on the palate at the root tips and the maxillary midline. If widening is to occur, transpalatal marks should also be used. The use of intermediate splints in segmental cases is a little different from their use in total arch cases. Since the posterior maxilla is not mobilized, the anterior maxillary positioning is more difficult and can be deceiving. For example, the anterior maxilla can fit into the splint and appear ideal until the mandible is rotated into occlusion. If the mandible does not arc into the ideal occlusion, it is possible that the anterior maxilla is tipped superiorly or inferiorly and must be adjusted. For this reason the mandible should not be wired into MMF but left free to rotate into the maxilla. At surgery, if the mandible is held into intermaxillary fixation during the fixation process for the anterior maxilla, it is possible to pull the condyles out of the fossae

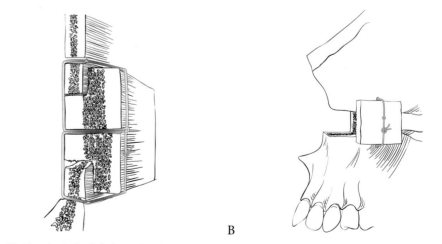

A   B

FIGURE 57-29   A, *A single hole is placed in the middle of the bone graft and a loop of 28-gauge stainless steel wire is placed through the hole from inside out. The two ends are divided, with one placed through the superior cranial base wall and the other through the inferior maxillary segment. Finally one end is passed through the loop and twisted to the other, much like an Ivy loop. B, Bone graft shown in place.*

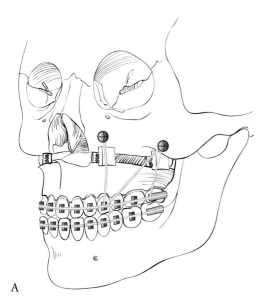

A

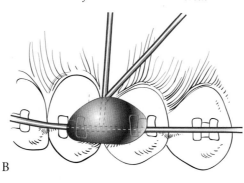

B

FIGURE **57-30** A, *Rigid adjustable pin system. A 0.045 inch orthodontic wire is fabricated on a skull preoperatively and adapted to the newly positioned maxilla intraoperatively so that the wire lies passively, close to the orthodontic appliances or arch bars. B, The acrylic cements the junction of the wire and the orthodontic appliances; the end of the wire is also covered.*

with a resultant malocclusion. Therefore, the splint must be ligated to the posterior maxilla first, and the anterior maxilla is then brought into the splint and ligated. If the mandible rotates into the desired occlusion, then the maxilla can be considered to be in the correct place and fixed accordingly. If mandibular surgery is required, it can be initiated at this time.

The choice of surgical technique is made on the basis of access and the areas that will be most difficult to visualize intraoperatively. For example, in cases of open bite in which no teeth are to be extracted, the anterior segment will be rotated clockwise downward after interdental osteotomies. Access to the interdental area, the midline of the palate, and the anterior nasal spine is not as critical as it is with other surgical movements. This procedure can be done with a circumvestibular incision or with bilateral horizontal incisions in the canine-molar regions and a vertical incision in the midline between the central incisors. On the other hand, if first premolars are to be extracted or have already been, and the anterior maxilla is to be retracted several millimeters, access to the midpalatal area is essential. The Wunderer technique, in which the palatal soft tissue is elevated posteriorly, gives great access to the palatal bony tissue, but care must be taken to preserve the labial soft tissue pedicle.[18] However, if superior repositioning is required, the access to the junction of the anterior nasal spine and the nasal septum is poor. A vertical incision can be made over the anterior nasal spine, but since this labial flap represents the total blood supply to the anterior maxilla, it is not recommended.

Our choice of procedures for most anterior maxillary osteotomies is a hybrid (see Figure 57-34). The labial incisions are made laterally as per Wunderer with a vertical midline incision to permit access to the anterior nasal spine–nasal septum. However, in place of a full palatal flap, circumdental incisions are made around the necks of the teeth on either side of the interdental osteotomies and a midline incision is made over the midpalatal suture with a small anterior Y if necessary. The Y should be anterior to the interdental bone cut and be as conservative as possible.

Fixation of anterior maxillary osteotomies is as varied as the surgical techniques.[82] Orthodontic arch wires and cast splints represent two of the extremes

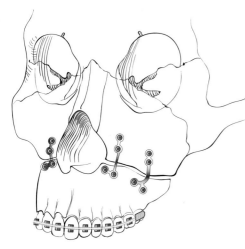

FIGURE **57-31** *Bone plating encompasses a wide variety of plates and screws, ranging from very rigid to very malleable. Generally 2.0 mm plates are used in the piriform rims and either 2.0 or 1.5 mm plates in the buttresses.*

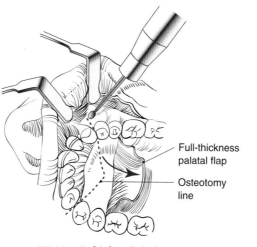

Full-thickness palatal flap

Osteotomy line

FIGURE **57-32** *Labial pedicle for anterior maxillary osteotomy; the palate is flapped open.*

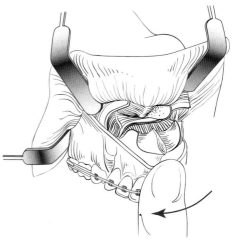

FIGURE **57-33** *Palatal pedicle for anterior maxillary osteotomy is created with a horizontal labial incision.*

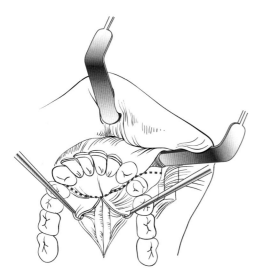

FIGURE **57-34** *A combination of labial and palatal pedicles can be used for an anterior maxillary osteotomy without extractions.*

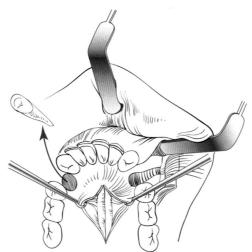

FIGURE **57-35** *Anterior maxillary osteotomy with first premolars extracted corrects maxillary excess, bimaxillary protrusion, and anterior open bite.*

in techniques used for fixation. Orthodontic appliances, if they are in place, are the handiest to use at least for part of the fixation. However, supplemental fixation may be desirable. An occlusal splint, with skeletal wire in the anterior nasal spine, is helpful in such cases, especially if tension on the free segment is expected. Small plates and screws can be carefully used to fixate the segment. Arch bars have been used and in certain cases may be appropriate, but a lower level of precision can be expected.

The most important guideline is that, at the time of surgery, the anterior maxilla must be mobile enough so that it does not require any significant pressure to move it into the desired position. Fixation can then be instituted by one of the many methods that will hold the segment in the proper position throughout the healing period. Maxillomandibular fixation is almost never required.

Posterior Maxillary Osteotomy

The posterior maxillary osteotomy and its modifications are rarely indicated today.[19,22,83–88] If open bite or transverse expansion is needed, the Le Fort I downfracture is much easier, quicker, and more predictable. Posterior maxillary osteotomy is usually indicated as a preprosthetic pro-

cedure to correct hypereruption of a posterior maxillary dentoalveolar segment. Meticulous model surgery is essential to visualizing the three-dimensional movements and in anticipating osseous interference of the segment. Periapical radiographs are useful for evaluating planned interdental and supra-apical osteotomy sites. Once again the models should be mounted in centric occlusion, not centric relation, unless the mandible is also going to be operated on.

Outpatient anesthesia can be used for isolated posterior segmental procedures. A high palatal vault permits palatal osteotomy transantrally beneath the nasal floor. The soft tissue incision is made horizontally in the maxillary buccal vestibule from the anticipated anterior interdental osteotomy site to the second molar (Figure 57-36). Mucoperiosteal dissection beneath the superior aspect of the incision exposes the lateral maxilla. The pterygomaxillary region is exposed and soft tissue retracted in a tunneling dissection. At the anterior interdental osteotomy site, conservative tunneling of the periosteum exposes the full vertical extent of the dentoalveolus. After retraction of the soft tissue with skin hooks and right-angle retractors, the buccal interdental osteotomy can be outlined

with a small fissure bur in a rotary handpiece or can be directly completed with a thin cement spatula osteotome.

A horizontal osteotomy is made approximately 5 mm above the roots of the teeth and connected with the anterior interdental cut (see Figure 57-36). The vertical interdental osteotomy should be completed first so that the segment is not mobile while using interdental osteotomes. The palatal osteotomy is accomplished with a small sharp curved osteotome directed at the juncture of the vertical alveolus and horizontal palatal shelf. The surgeon places a finger in the palatal mucosa to detect complete osseous sectioning while minimizing palatal mucosal trauma (Figure 57-37A and B). In cases with high palatal vaults the transantral cut is completed along the entire anteroposterior extent of the planned palatal osteotomy (see Figure 57-37B), except in the area of the descending palatal neurovascular bundle. Next the pterygomaxillary junction is separated with a chisel using a technique similar to that for a total maxillary osteotomy. Patients with low flat palatal vaults are more easily osteotomized through the nasal floor (Figure 57-37C).

The posterior dentoalveolar segment is down-fractured using digital pressure. Anticipated osseous interference may be

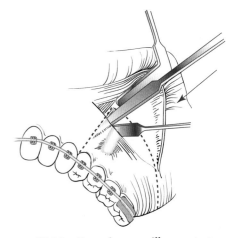

FIGURE **57-36** *Posterior maxillary osteotomy. Horizontal vestibular incision with tunneling access to the interdental papilla. The dashed line marks horizontal and interdental osteotomies.*

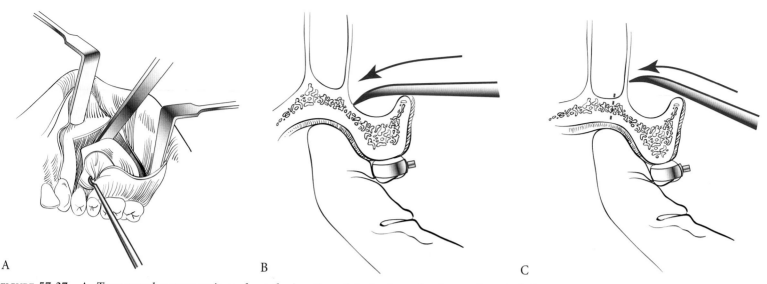

FIGURE 57-37 A, *Transantral osteotomy is made at the junction of the horizontal palate and vertical alveolar process. B, Approach for deep vaulted palates. C, Approach for flat shallow palates.*

removed using a bur or rongeur. Previously inaccessible medial and posterior walls of the mobile segment are addressed following mobilization and displacement of the posterior segment. Bone removal at the perpendicular plate of the palatine bone and mobilization should continue until the segment can be repositioned with minimal digital force (Figure 57-38). Final contouring is accomplished while holding the splint on the stable portion of the maxilla. The mandible is rotated into its dictated occluding position to ensure that no distortion of the splint has occurred. A slightly thicker splint and transpalatal acrylic or wire reinforcement will add rigidity to prevent inadvertent distortion of the posterior extension of the splint. The segment is ligated to the splint.

The repositioned posterior maxillary segment may be fixated with interosseous wire, suspension wire, stable pin fixation, or bone plates. Osseous grafts are rarely required but may be obtained from local regional sites. Additional stability is attained by luting the orthodontic arch wire back together with quick curing acrylic or by placing a rectangular arch wire across the interdental osteotomy site. Intermaxillary fixation is not required.

If the posterior segment is to be repositioned laterally or medially to any extent, added access is necessary. A midline palatal incision may be made and the palatal tissue reflected laterally (Figure 57-39). Careful dissection ensures the integrity of the greater palatine vasculature. This approach gives access to the sinus and nasal cavity. If the palatal vault is high, the osteotomy is usually carried through the sinus (see Figure 57-37B). If the alveolus is short and the palatal vault shallow, the osteotomy usually crosses the medial sinus wall and passes through the floor of the nose (see Figure 57-37C).

Surgically Assisted Rapid Palatal Expansion: History

The concept of correcting maxillary transverse width discrepancies originated in the United States in 1860 by Angell, who reported it in *Dental Cosmos*. Angell described a widening of the maxillary dental arch by opening the midpalatal suture.[89] The concept fell into disuse by American practitioners by the early 1900s. Haas re-introduced the concept in 1961 with rapid palatal expansion (RPE, also referred to as rapid maxillary expansion), appliances that effectively corrected arch width discrepancies.[90] In growing

children nonsurgical RPE results in opening of the midpalatal suture, but stability has been questioned. Timms and Moss, Haas, and Isaacson and Ingram have shown orthodontic RPE to result in alveolar bending, periodontal membrane compression, lateral tooth displacement, and tooth extrusion.[91–93] For those reasons Haas believed that overexpansion was very important. Even

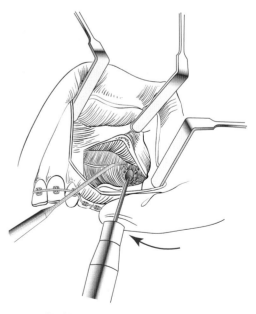

FIGURE 57-38 *Bone is removed at the perpendicular plate of the palatine bone using a transantral approach.*

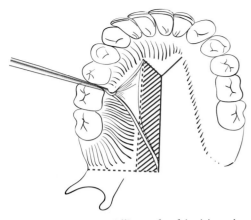

FIGURE **57-39** *A midline palatal incision gives access for the removal of bone as the posterior maxillary segment is moved medially.*

with 50% overexpansion, nonsurgical RPE has been associated with relapse and subsequent failure in adults, but has been relatively successful in children and adolescents.[91–93]

Although historically the midpalatal suture was thought to be the area of resistance to expansion, Isaacson and Ingram have shown that the major site of resistance is not the midpalatal suture but the remaining maxillary articulations.[93] Lines as well as Bell and Epker demonstrated that increased facial skeletal resistance to expansion was at the zygomaticotemporal, zygomaticofrontal, and zygomaticomaxillary sutures.[94,95] Wertz theorized that the resistance was due to the zygomatic arches.[96] Identification of these areas of resistance in the craniofacial skeleton stimulated the development of various maxillary osteotomies to expand the maxilla in conjunction with orthodontic appliances.[96] Published surgical techniques report the removal of the bony resistance of the maxilla in order to symmetrically expand the hemimaxillas with short-term orthopedic forces.[94,95,97–101] Lehman and colleagues have also demonstrated expansion with an RPE appliance.[97] Kennedy and colleagues reported a significant increase in the amount of lateral movement in animals that had osteotomies prior to orthodontic RPE.[98]

Reported results vary with technique and the timing of placement of an active orthopedic expansion device, but all note the expansion to be more stable than orthodontic RPE alone.

The role of surgery with RPE is to release the areas of resistance in the maxillas before RPE. Whether RPE will be done alone or in conjunction with surgery will depend on the patient's age and the condition of the midpalatal suture, but not the maxillomandibular relation. Lines found surgically assisted rapid palatal expansion (SARPE) to be extremely valuable in young patients (growing children) exhibiting maxillary collapse, maxillary retrusion, and pseudo-Class III malocclusions.[94]

SARPE is distraction osteogenesis of the maxilla in a transverse plane. The benefits of its use are gradual callous distraction that allows the soft tissues to accommodate, and greater long-term stability.

When maxillary expansion and total maxillary osteotomy are needed, two treatment regimens are possible: SARPE as a first stage followed by a one-piece maxillary osteotomy at a later date or multiple-piece maxillary osteotomy in the normal orthognathic sequence. The four factors that must be considered when determining which method is preferred are arch length discrepancy, arch morphology, vertical dimension, and ectopic eruption of posterior teeth.

Arch Length Discrepancy In cases of arch length deficiency, a SARPE increases arch circumference sufficiently, especially in the anterior, to permit alignment of crowded teeth and avoid extraction of premolars or excessive tipping of incisors. SARPE is also beneficial when minimal changes in the sagittal dimension are necessary because of the nasolabial angle and lip-to-tooth considerations.

Arch Morphology The majority of cases of transverse deficiency characteristically exhibit a narrow tapering arch form with

the discrepancy pronounced in the canine region. To achieve a functional occlusion, the intercanine width must be increased and the anterior segment flattened for a normal elliptical arch morphology. If nonextraction orthodontic therapy is desired, a SARPE is the treatment of choice. A three- or four-piece segmental maxillary surgical procedure may be less ideal, particularly because of potential periodontal problems and possible vascular compromise.

If the discrepancy is minimal and extraction of the first premolars is desired, a three-piece segmental maxillary procedure is indicated, but only after the canines are orthodontically moved posteriorly to provide an increased width. The inherent problem is relapse of the buccally displaced canines. This procedure is indicated if there is no transverse discrepancy in the canine region but significant constriction in the premolar-molar region.

Vertical Dimension The vertical dimension is of particular concern in patients who exhibit anterior open bites. Segmental orthodontics is suggested, with no attempt to level the arch, using a three- or four-piece maxillary procedure to level the arch and at the same time correct the bilateral absolute transverse maxillary deficiency.

Ectopic Eruption of One or Two Posterior Teeth If ectopic eruption is serious enough that it cannot be treated with orthodontic therapy, a segmental osteotomy with expansion may be done.

The stability of SARPE has been reported.[99,102] In one reported study on long-term stability of SARPE, the surgical results remained stable with only 6.4 to 7.5% relapse in the canine, premolar, and molar regions.[99] This stability exceeds that of multiple-piece Le Fort osteotomies.[100,102]

Surgically Assisted Rapid Palatal Expansion: Surgical Technique

Bilateral mucoperiosteal incisions are made from the piriform rims to zygomatic buttresses (Figure 57-40A). Bilateral osteotomies are then made from the piriform rims to low in the pterygomaxillary junction (see Figure 57-40A). A simple anteroposterior osteotomy from the piriform rim to the pterygomaxillary junction is suggested for SARPE. More complicated designs appear to be advantageous in two-dimensional drawings, but in fact are meaningless when applied to three-dimensional geometric structures such as the maxilla.[103] The theory put forth by Betts and colleagues shows a sloped cut from the piriform to the buttress.[103] The supposition is that as the maxilla is expanded, it will "ride down" this slope. This concept appears valid in a two-dimensional drawing; however, three-dimensionally, if the osteotomy is made flat from lateral to medial, as expansion occurs, then the bone at the piriform slides laterally over the flat surface lateral to it and the bone of the buttress slides laterally over the flat surface lateral to it. Therefore, if the lateral maxillary wall saw cuts are made straight in perpendicular to the midsagittal plane from lateral to medial, then the angulation of the cut from anterior to posterior does not affect the vertical position of the segments as they are expanded. This can be easily demonstrated on a dry skull.

Osteotomies are made of the anterior 1.5 cm of the lateral nasal wall because this is the thickest portion of the anterior nasal wall. Separation of the hemimaxillas is performed by driving a spatula osteotome between the central incisors parallel to the palate for approximately 1 to 1.5 cm (Figure 57-40B–D). The expansion device is turned until separation is noted between the central incisor teeth (Figure 57-41). Both segments are mobilized by prying until equal mobility is seen bilaterally. Mobilization is continued until approximately 1.5 to 2.0 mm is opened between central incisors.

Some authors recommend a subtotal Le Fort I osteotomy with a horizontal osteotomy, vertical midline osteotomy, and pterygoid and septal separation.[103] Shetty and colleagues demonstrated, with a photoelastic model, that the midpalatal and pterygomaxillary articulations were the primary anatomic sites of resistance to expansion forces.[104] The article by Shetty and colleagues in 1994 report performing only incomplete cuts of the lateral maxillary wall, from second bicuspid to second molar. It is unclear whether these findings would be as significant with complete cuts from the piriform to the pterygomaxillary fissure. Need for separation of the pterygomaxillary junction is therefore a point of debate. However, since our results have

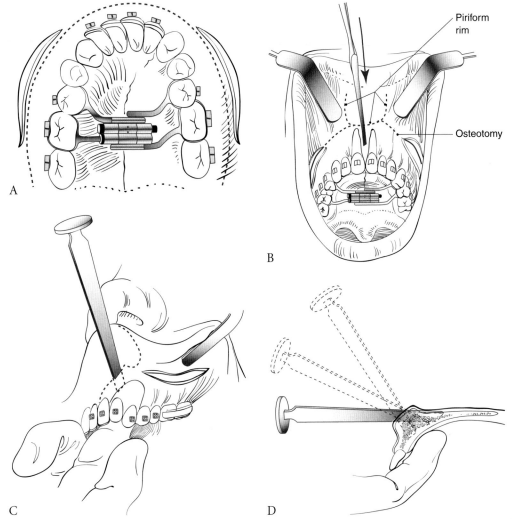

FIGURE **57-40** *Surgically assisted rapid palatal expansion. A, Bilateral horizontal mucoperiosteal incisions are made, followed by bilateral osteotomies from the piriform rims to pterygomaxillary junctions. B–D, Division of hemimaxillae is accomplished by inserting an osteotome in the midline.*

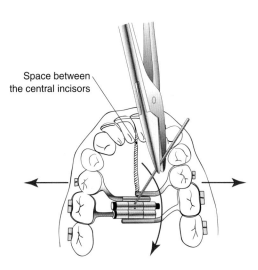

FIGURE **57-41** *Surgically assisted rapid palatal expansion. Expansion device is turned to separate hemimaxillas.*

shown minimal relapse without pterygo-maxillary disjunction, we do not perform this maneuver in most cases.[99]

If two sources of potential hemorrhage (manipulation of the pterygomaxillary junction and separation of the nasal septum from the nasal crest of the maxilla) are avoided, this procedure can be done as an office-based procedure, on an outpatient basis, and under intravenous sedation. Steroids are routinely used but antibiotics are not necessary. A 5-day postoperative rest period is observed, after which the expansion appliance is turned according to specific instructions until the desired expansion is achieved.

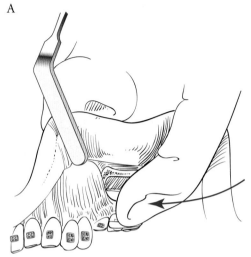

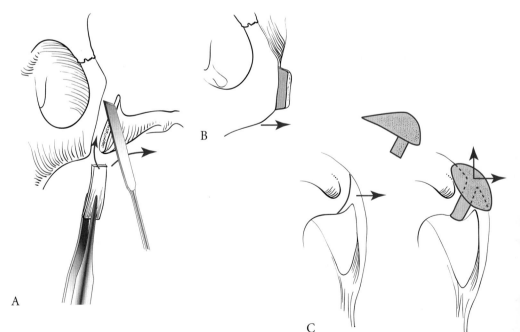

FIGURE **57-43** *Unilateral surgically assisted rapid palatal expansion. A, Segment is mobilized. B, Expander is activated until the desired expansion is achieved.*

Unilateral SARPE can be achieved by completing a vertical interdental osteotomy between the appropriate teeth and connecting that with a horizontal osteotomy extending posteriorly to the pterygomaxillary junction. If the entire hemimaxilla is to be mobilized, it is performed in the same way as described for a bilateral case, only unilaterally. If a widening of only the posterior part of the hemimaxilla is desired, the interdental osteotomy must be completed all the way to the midline suture (Figure 57-42). The segment is mobilized (Figure 57-43A) and expanded in the same manner as the bilateral procedure (Figure 57-43B).

Zygomatic Osteotomy

In patients with severe midface deficiency it may be favorable to enhance the prominence

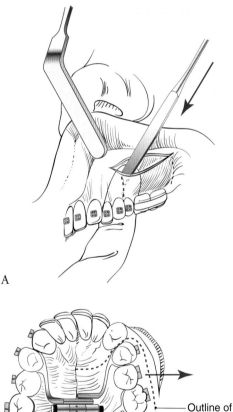

A

Outline of osteotomy

B

FIGURE **57-42** *Unilateral surgically assisted rapid palatal expansion. A, Osteotomy is driven to midpalatal suture. B, Horizontal osteotomy is completed in the same manner as bilateral osteotomy.*

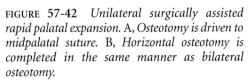

FIGURE **57-44** *Zygomatic osteotomy. A, Parasagittal vertical osteotomy cuts through the root of the zygoma. B, With out-fracturing and placement of graft material for transverse augmentation of the malar eminence. C, Mushroom-shaped graft placement for anteroposterior and transverse augmentation of the malar eminence.*

of the zygomas. Also, esthetically, high cheekbones have always been popular, and with a growing public awareness of surgical capabilities an increasing demand has surfaced for procedures to enhance this area. Numerous methods have been developed to augment the malar eminences, most involving grafts or implants. Autologous grafts are disappointing because of resorption and the need for a donor site. Allogeneic transplants such as lyophilized cartilage have been used with some success but are prone to migration. Presently our choice for malar augmentation is with alloplastic implants (porous polyethylene).

However, when alloplasts are contraindicated, the zygomatic osteotomy may be useful. The zygomatic osteotomy is approached through an intraoral incision. A reciprocating saw is used to make a parasagittal osteotomy through the zygoma just adjacent to the root of the structure (Figure 57-44A and B). This is done as close to the lateral orbital rim as possible. The zygoma is out-fractured gently so that an interpositional material can be placed to hold it in position. The interpositional material can be stabilized in any traditional method, since it is not difficult to fixate this area. This technique does not give anterior projection unless the interpositional material is fashioned to project forward (Figure 57-44C).

Modified Le Fort Osteotomies

Osteotomies that extend the traditional Le Fort I have been called by many names including modified Le Fort I, II, III; high Le Fort I; and pyramidal, middle, intermediary, quadrangular, and maxillary-malar-infraorbital osteotomies (Figure 57-45A–C). We have used them all and have described them previously.[105] This group of osteotomies is severely limited regarding expansion, and rotational and torquing movements. Therefore, with the success of porous polyethylene implants to the malar, infraorbital, lateral orbital, and paranasal regions, we rarely see a need for these more invasive osteotomies (Figure 57-46A–C).

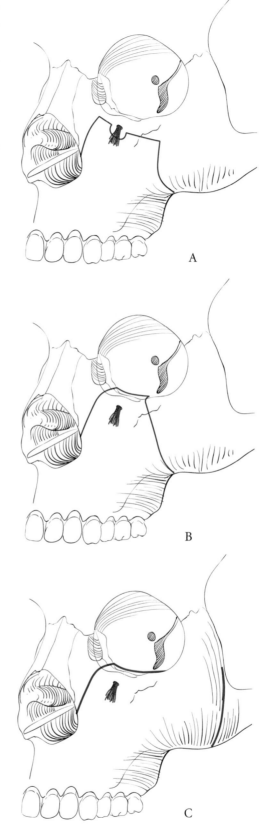

FIGURE **57-45** *Modified Le Fort I osteotomy. A, High Le Fort I below the infraorbital rims. B, Quadrangular Le Fort I extending into the orbital floor. C, Quadrangular Le Fort I including the lateral orbital rim and zygoma.*

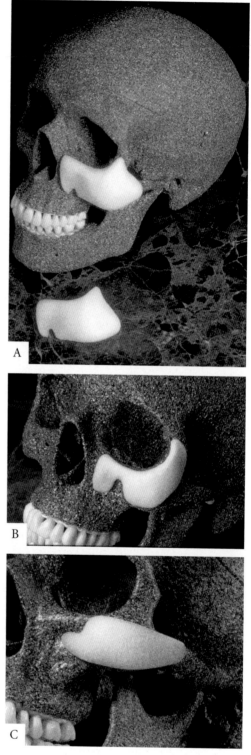

FIGURE **57-46** *Porous polyethelene implants. A, Infraorbital augmentation with the zygoma. B, Infraorbital augmentation with the zygoma and lateral orbital rim. C, Zygoma augmentation.*

References

1. von Langenbeck B. Beitrange zur Osteoplastik. In: Goschen A, editor. Die osteoplastische Resektion des Oberkierers. Deutsche Klinik. Berlin: Reimer; 1859.

2. Cheever D. Naso-pharyngeal polpus, attached to the basilar process of occipital and body of the sphenoid bone successfully removed by a section, displacement, and subsequent replacement and reunion of the superior maxillary bone. Boston Med Surg 1867;8:162.

3. Le Fort R. Fractures de la machoire superieure. Rev Chir 1901;4:360.

4. Wassmund M. Frakturen und Lurationen des Gesichtsschadels. Berlin; 1927.

5. Axhausen G. Zur Behandlung veralteter deslozieret verheilter Oberkieferbrunche. Dtsch Zahn Mund Kieferheilkd 1934;I:334.

6. Schuchardt D. Ein Beitrag zur chirurgeschen Kieferorthopadie unter Berucksichtigung ihrer Bedertung fur die Behandlung angeborener und erworbener Kieferdeformitaten bei Soldaten. Dtsch Zahn Mund Kieferheilkd 1942;9:73.

7. Moore F, Ward F. Complications and sequelae of untreated fractures of the facial bones and their treatment. Plast Surg 1949;1:262.

8. Willmar K. On Le Fort I osteotomy; A follow-up study of 106 operated patients with maxillo-facial deformity. Scand J Plast Reconstr Surg 1974;12 (Suppl 12):1–68.

9. Obwegeser H. Eingriffe an Oberkiefer zur Korrektur des progenen. Vol 75. Zahnbheilk; 1965. p. 356.

10. Hogemann K, Willmar K. Die Vorverlagerung des Oberkiefers zur Korrektur von Gebisanomalien. In: Schuchardt K, editors. Gesichtschir Hrsg. Stuggart: Thieme; 1967.

11. deHaller C. Ergebnisse ders operativin Vorbringens des Oberkiefers; 1969.

12. Perko M. Maxillary sinus and surgical movement of maxilla. Int J Oral Surg 1972; 1:177–84.

13. Cohn-Stock G. Die Chirugische-Immediatre-Julierung der Kiefer speziell die Chirurgische Behandlung der Prognathie. Vjischr Zahnheilk (Berlin) 1921;37:320.

14. Spanier F. Prognathie-Operationen Z zahnarytl. Orthop Munchen 1932;24:76.

15. Cupar I. Die Chirurgische Behandlung der Formund Stellungsveranderungen des Oberkiefers. Ost Z Stomat 1954;51:565.

16. Cupar I. Die Chirugische Behandlung def Formund Stellungsveranderungen des Oberkiefers. Buss Sc Cons Acad RPF Yougosl 1955;2:60.

17. Kole H. Surgical operations on the alveolar ridge to correct occlusal abnormalities. Oral Surg 1959;12:277.

18. Wunderer S. Erfahrungen mit der operatiren Behandlung hochgradiger Prognathien. Dtsch Zahn Mund Kieferheilkd 1963;39:451.

19. Schuchardt K. Experiences with the surgical treatment of deformities of the jaws: prognathia, micrognathia and open bite. In: Wallace AG, editor. Second Congress of International Society of Plastic Surgeons. Vol 73. London: E & S Livingstone; 1959.

20. Kufner J. Experience with a modified procedure for correction of open bite. In: Walker RV, editor. Transactions of the Third International Conference on Oral Surgery. Vol 18. London: E & S Livingstone; 1970.

21. West RA, McNeill RW. Maxillary alveolar hyperplasia, diagnosis and treatment planning. J Maxillofac Surg 1975;3:239–50.

22. Bell WH. Correction of skeletal type of anterior open bite. J Oral Surg 1971; 29:706–14.

23. Converse J, Shapiro H. Treatment of developmental malformation of the jaws. Plast Reconstr Surg 1952; 10:473.

24. Kole H. In: Reischenback, Kole, Brueckel, eds. Chir Kieferorthopadie. Leipzig: Barth, 1965.

25. Bell WH, Fonseca RJ, Kennedy JW, Levy BM. Bone healing and revascularization after total maxillary osteotomy. J Oral Surg 1975; 33:253–60.

26. Gillies J, Rowe N. L'osteotomie du maxillaire superieur envisagee essentiellement dans les cas de bec-de-lievre totale. Rev Stomat 1954;55:545.

27. Obwegeser HL. Surgical correction of small or retrodisplaced maxillae. The "dish-face" deformity. Plast Reconstr Surg 1969; 43:351–65.

28. Michelet FX, Deymes J, Dessus B. Osteosynthesis with miniaturized screwed plates in maxillo-facial surgery. J Maxillofac Surg 1973;1(2):79–84.

29. Horster W. Experience with functionally stable plate osteosynthesis after forward displacement of the upper jaw. J Maxillofac Surg 1980;8(3):176–81.

30. Drommer R, Luhr HG. The stabilization of osteotomized maxillary segments with Luhr mini-plates in secondary cleft surgery. J Maxillofac Surg 1981;9:166–9.

31. Luyk NH, Ward-Booth RP. The stability of Le Fort I advancement osteotomies using bone plates without bone grafts. J Maxillofac Surg 1985;13(6):250–3.

32. Edwards RC, Kiely KD. Resorbable fixation of Le Fort I osteotomies. J Craniofac Surg 1998;9(3):210–4.

33. Bays RA. Rigid stabilization system for maxillary osteotomies. J Oral Maxillofac Surg 1985;43:60–3.

34. Stringer DE, Boyne PJ. Modification of the maxillary step osteotomy and stabilization with titanium mesh. J Oral Maxillofac Surg 1986;44:487–8.

35. Olson RE, Laskin DM. Expectations of patients from orthognathic surgery. J Oral Surg 1980;38:283–5.

36. Ong TK, Banks RJ, Hildreth AJ. Surgical accuracy in Le Fort I maxillary osteotomies. Br J Oral Maxillofac Surg 2001;39:96–102.

37. Renzi G, Carboni A, Perugini M, Becelli R. Intraoperative measurement of maxillary repositioning in a series of 30 patients with maxillomandibular vertical asymmetries. Int J Adult Orthodon Orthognath Surg 2002;17(2):111–5.

38. Schaeffer J. The sinus maxillaires and its relations in the embryo, child and adult man. Am J Anat 1910b;10:313.

39. Klaff D. The surgical anatomy of the antero caudal portion of the nasal septum: a study of the area of the premaxilla. Laryngoscope 1956;66:995.

40. Cottle M, Loring RM, Fischer GG, Gaynon IE. The maxilla-premaxilla approach to extensive nasal septum surgery. Arch Otolaryngol 1958;68:301.

41. Hollinshead W. Anatomy for surgeons. 3rd ed. Philadelphia (PA): Harper and Row; 1982.

42. Hollinshead W. Textbook of anatomy. 3rd ed. Hagertown (MD): Harper and Row; 1974.

43. Sewall E. Surgical removal of the sphenopalatine ganglion. Ann Otol Rhinol Laryngol 1937;46:79.

44. Bell WH. Le Fort I osteotomy for correction of maxillary deformities. J Oral Surg 1975; 33:12–26.

45. Bell WH. Revascularization and bone healing after anterior maxillary osteotomy: a study using adult rhesus monkeys. J Oral Surg 1969;27:249–55.

46. Siebert JW, Angrigiani C, McCarthy JG, Longaker MT. Blood supply of the Le Fort I maxillary segment: an anatomic study. Plast Reconstr Surg 1997;100:843–51.

47. Brusati R, Bottoli V. Maxillary anterior segmentary osteotomy: experimental research on vascular supply of osteotomised segment. Fortschritte der Kiefer- und Gesichts-Chirurgie 1974;18:90–3.

48. Miller M, Christensen G, Evan H. Anatomy of the dog. Philadelphia (PA): WB Saunders; 1964.

49. Nelson RL, Path MG, Ogle RG, et al. Quantitation of blood flow after Le Fort I osteotomy. J Oral Surg 1977;35:10–6.

50. Nelson RL, Path MG, Ogle RG, et al. Quantitation of blood flow after anterior maxillary

osteotomy: investigation of three surgical approaches. J Oral Surg 1978; 36:106–11.

51. Lightoller G. Facial muscles J Anat (Lond) 1925;60:1.

52. Nairn RI. The circumoral musculature: structure and function. Br Dent J 1975;138:49–56.

53. Robinson PP, Hendy CW. Pterygoid plate fractures caused by the Le Fort I osteotomy. Br J Oral Maxillofac Surg 1986;24:198–202.

54. Lanigan DT, West RA. Management of postoperative hemorrhage following the Le Fort I maxillary osteotomy. J Oral Maxillofac Surg 1984;42:367–75.

55. Hemmig SB, Johnson RS, Ferraro N. Management of a ruptured pseudoaneurysm of the sphenopalatine artery following a LeFort I osteotomy. J Oral Maxillofac Surg 1987; 45:533–6.

56. Solomons NB, Blumgart R. Severe late-onset epistaxis following Le Fort I osteotomy: angiographic localization and embolization. J Laryngol Otol 1988;102:260–3.

57. Newhouse RF, Schow SR, Kraut RA. Price JC. Life-threatening hemorrhage from a Le Fort I osteotomy. J Oral Maxillofac Surg 1982;40:117–9.

58. Dodson TB, Bays RA, Neuenschwander MC. Maxillary perfusion during Le Fort I osteotomy after ligation of the descending palatine artery [comment]. J Oral Maxillofac Surg 1997;55(1):51–5.

59. Bouloux GF, Bays RA. Neurosensory recovery after ligation of the descending palatine neurovascular bundle during Le Fort I osteotomy. J Oral Maxillofac Surg 2000;58(8):841–5; discussion, 846.

60. Bell WH, Proffit WP. Maxillary Excess. In: Bell WH, Proffit WP, White RP, eds. Surgical correction of dentofacial deformities. Vol I. Philadelphia (PA): WB Saunders; 1980. p. 234–441

61. Reyneke JP, Masureik CJ. Treatment of maxillary deficiency by a Le Fort I downsliding technique. J Oral Maxillofac Surg 1985;43:914–6.

62. Bennett MA, Wolford LM. The maxillary step osteotomy and Steinmann pin stabilization. J Oral Maxillofac Surg 1985;43:307–11.

63. Kaminishi RM, Davis WH, Hochwald DA, Nelson N. Improved maxillary stability with modified Lefort I technique. J Oral Maxillofac Surg 1983;41(3):203–5.

64. Stringer DE, Boyne PJ. Modification of the maxillary step osteotomy and stabilization with titanium mesh. J Oral Maxillofac Surg 1986;4:487–8.

65. Bays RA. Maxillary osteotomies utilizing the rigid adjustable pin (RAP) system: a review of 31 clinical cases. Int J Adult Orthodont Orthognath Surg 1986;1:275–97.

66. Hedemark A, Freihofer HP Jr. The behaviour of the maxilla in vertical movements after Le Fort I osteotomy. J Maxillofac Surg 1978;6:244–9.

67. Epker BN, Fish LC, Paulus PJ. The surgical-orthodontic correction of maxillary deficiency. Oral Surg Oral Med Oral Pathol 1978;46:171–205.

68. Wolford LM, Hilliard FW. The surgical-orthodontic correction of vertical dentofacial deformities. J Oral Surg 1981;39:883–97.

69. Freihofer HP Jr. Results of osteotomies of the facial skeleton in adolescence. J Maxillofac Surg 1977;5:267–97.

70. Bell WH, Jacobs JD, Quejada JG. Simultaneous repositioning of the maxilla, mandible, and chin. Treatment planning and analysis of soft tissues. Am J Orthod 1986;89:28–50.

71. Persson G, Hellem S, Nord PG. Bone-plates for stabilizing Le Fort I osteotomies. J Maxillofac Surg 1986;14:69–73.

72. Wessberg GA, Epker BN. Intraoral skeletal fixation appliance. J Oral Maxillofac Surg 1982;40:827–9.

73. Dupont C, Ciaburro TH, Prevost Y. Simplifying the Le Fort I type of maxillary osteotomy. Plast Reconstr Surg 1974;54:142–7.

74. Trimble LD, Tideman H, Stoelinga PJ. A modification of the pterygoid plate separation in low-level maxillary osteotomies. J Oral Maxillofac Surg 1983;41:544–6.

75. Wolford LM, Epker BN. The combined anterior and posterior maxillary ostectomy: a new technique. J Oral Surg 1975;33:842–51.

76. Hooley J, West R. Vertical repositioning of total maxillary alveolus to compensate for "short upper lip." Second Congress of the Europe Association for Maxillofacial Surgery; 1974. [abstract]

77. Guenthner TA, Sather AH, Kern EB. The effect of Le Fort I maxillary impaction on nasal airway resistance. Am J Orthod 1984;85:308–15.

78. Turvey TA, Hall DJ, Warren DW. Alterations in nasal airway resistance following superior repositioning of the maxilla. Am J Orthod 1984;85(2):109–14.

79. Warren DW. A quantitative technique for assessing nasal airway impairment. Am J Orthod 1984;86:306–14.

80. Walker DA, Turvey TA, Warren DW. Alterations in nasal respiration and nasal airway size following superior repositioning of the maxilla. J Oral Maxillofac Surg 1988;46:276–81.

81. Moloney F, West RA, McNeill RW. Surgical correction of vertical maxillary excess: a re-evaluation. J Maxillofac Surg 1982;10:84–91.

82. Bays RA, Fonseca RJ, Turvey TA. Single arch stabilization devices for segmental orthog-

nathic surgery. Oral Surg Oral Med Oral Pathol 1978;46:467–76.

83. West RA, Epker BN. Posterior maxillary surgery its place in the treatment of dentofacial deformities. J Oral Surg 1972;30:562–3.

84. Sailer HF. [Routine methods in orthodontic surgery]. Revue d Orthopedie Dento-Faciale 1982;16:307–26.

85. Merville LC, Princ G, Postero-lateral expansion osteotomy of maxilla. A case report. J Craniomaxillofacial Surg 1987;15:20–3.

86. Bell WH, Turvey TA. Surgical correction of posterior crossbite. J Oral Surg 1974; 32:811–22.

87. Perko M. [Late surgical correction of tooth malpositions and jaw abnormalities in patients with clefts]. SSO: Schweizerische Monatsschrift fur Zahnheilkunde 1969;79:179–213.

88. Moloney F, Stoelinga PJ, Tideman H. The posterior segmental maxillary osteotomy: recent applications. J Oral Maxillofac Surg 1984;42:771–81.

89. Angell EH. Treatment of irregularities of the permanent adult tooth. Dent Cosmos 1860;1:540.

90. Haas A. Rapid expansion of the maxillary dental arch and nasal cavity by opening the mid palatal structure. Angle Orthod 1961;31:73.

91. Timms DJ, Moss JP. A histological investigation into the effects of rapid maxillary expansion on the teeth and their supporting tissues. Transact Europ Orthod Soc 1971:263–7.

92. Haas AJ. Long-term posttreatment evaluation of rapid palatal expansion. Angle Orthod 1980;50:189–217.

93. Isaacson R, Ingram A. Forces produced by rapid maxillary expansion: forces present during treatment. Angle Orthod 1964;34:256.

94. Lines PA. Adult rapid maxillary expansion with corticotomy. Am J Orthod 1975;67:44–56.

95. Bell WH. Epker BN. Surgical-orthodontic expansion of the maxilla. Am J Orthod 1976;70:517–28.

96. Wertz RA. Skeletal and dental changes accompanying rapid midpalatal suture opening. Am J Orthod 1970;58:41–66.

97. Lehman JA Jr, Haas AJ, Haas DG. Surgical orthodontic correction of transverse maxillary deficiency: a simplified approach. Plast Reconstr Surg 1984;73:62–8.

98. Kennedy JW III, Bell WH, Kimbrough OL, James WB. Osteotomy as an adjunct to rapid maxillary expansion. Am J Orthod 1976;70:123–37.

99. Bays RA, Greco JM. Surgically assisted rapid palatal expansion: an outpatient technique with long-term stability. J Oral Maxillofac Surg 1992;50(2):110–3; discussion 114–5.

100. Phillips C, Medland WH, Fields HW Jr.

Stability of surgical maxillary expansion. Int J Adult Orthod Orthognath Surg 1992;7(3):139–46.

101. Stephens C. An examination of the long-term stability of surgical-orthodontic maxillary expansion [dissertation]. Columbus (OH): Ohio State University; 1986.

102. Pogrel MA, Kaban LB, Vargervik K, Baumrind S. Surgically assisted rapid maxillary expansion in adults. Int J Adult Orthod Orthognath Surg 1992;7(1):37–41.

103. Betts NJ, Vanarsdall RL, Barber HD, et al. Diagnosis and treatment of transverse maxillary deficiency. Int J Adult Orthod Orthognath Surg 1995;10(2):75–96.

104. Shetty V, Caridad JM, Caputo AA, Chaconas SJ. Biomechanical rationale for surgical-orthodontic expansion of the adult maxilla. J Oral Maxillofac Surg 1994;52(7):742-9; discussion 750–1.

105. Bays RA, Timmis DP, Hegtvedt AK. Maxillary orthognathic surgery. In: Peterson LJ, et al, editors. Principles of oral and maxillofacial surgery. Philadelphia (PA): J. B. Lippincott; 1992. p. 1349–414.

CHAPTER 58

Management of Facial Asymmetry

Peter D. Waite, MPH, DDS, MD
Scott D. Urban, DMD, MD

In the 1960s surgical treatment of orthognathic deformities developed when satisfactory results were unobtainable by orthodontics alone. Mild cases of jaw deformities and malocclusion can sometimes be camouflaged by dental treatment and growth modification.[1] Severe malocclusion is often beyond the envelope of orthodontic treatment; therefore, surgical procedures of the maxilla and mandible have been developed. Just as some malocclusions are beyond orthodontics alone, some orthognathic deformities are beyond surgery directed at a single jaw, that is, the maxilla or the mandible. Although a single osteotomy might improve function and esthetics, bimaxillary surgery or double-jaw surgery is often indicated for large anteroposterior discrepancies, open bite, and most asymmetries.[2–5] As orthognathic surgery has been refined, it has become evident that some problems are beyond treatment of a single jaw. The novice might assume that single-jaw surgery is better—simple and less complicated—but the final outcome is often a compromise and unstable. Bimaxillary surgery allows a much greater degree of flexibility with regard to three-dimensional treatment.

In the 1960s and 1970s surgeons attempted to limit orthognathic surgery to one jaw, usually the mandible. Ramus osteotomies with maxillary osteotomies were complex, technically difficult, time consuming, unstable, and associated with higher morbidity.[6] It is impossible to correct a canted maxilla without adjusting the mandibular plane of occlusion. Even simple midline discrepancies resulting from unilateral tooth loss can be quickly improved by mild rotational changes in the facial skeleton.

This chapter focuses on the unique nature of asymmetric orthognathic deformities as an indication for bimaxillary surgery, which is really nothing more than a combination of two procedures. The most important aspect of bimaxillary surgery is not the ability to do simultaneous maxillary and mandibular procedures, but to understand the indications and treatment plan and how to maintain a stable reference during surgery.

Little has been written on orthognathic asymmetries as an indication for bimaxillary surgery. Poor treatment planning and poor surgical reference are common mistakes. Asymmetries require three-dimensional changes and complex skeletal movements with adjunctive soft tissue symmetry. The current discussion includes etiology amenable to orthognathic procedures, diagnostic imaging, treatment planning, and surgery.

Facial symmetry has a high correlation with attractiveness. Even a slight asymmetry is quickly noticed by the human eye. Greater degrees of asymmetry are correlated with clinical depression, neurosis, inferiority complex, poor self-esteem, and general poor-quality-of-life health problems.[7] Mandibular asymmetry is a significant dysfunction and difficult to correct.

Etiology

There are multiple causes of mandibular and facial asymmetry, but the differential can be separated into three classes: congenital, developmental, and acquired.[8,9] *Congenital* anomalies are conditions acquired during in utero development and can be further subdivided into malformations, deformities, and disruptions. Malformations are the result of an intrinsically abnormal developmental process in embryogenesis. Unilateral cleft lip is an example of a malformation.[9] Deformities are an abnormal form or position of a part of the body caused by a nondisruptive mechanical force during the fetal period.[9] Mandibular deformation may result from a prolonged sharply laterally flexed position of the head with the shoulder pressed against the mandible during late intrauterine growth. Disruptions are morphologic defects resulting from a breakdown of an otherwise normal developmental process.[9] Rare facial clefting and limb amputation from an amniotic band are good examples of disruption.[9] *Developmental* anomalies are conditions arising during postuterine growth through adulthood. *Acquired* anomalies are conditions arising from either trauma or pathology.

Congenital Anomalies

Hemifacial Microsomia

Hemifacial microsomia (HFM) is a craniofacial malformation of the first and second branchial arches presenting with asymmetric unilateral or bilateral hypoplasia of the orbit(s), maxilla, mandible, ear, cranial nerves, and soft tissue (Figure 58-1).[10] Current evidence supports the theory that hemifacial microsomia results from a defect in the proliferation and migration of embryonic neural crest cells.[11,12] Other theories have included hemorrhage of the stapedial artery during fetal development, which ultimately leads to impaired unilateral facial growth.[13,14] However, the true etiologic factors still remain unknown.

Two important factors need to be considered in the treatment planning of HFM: (1) the facial growth potential and/or restriction and its effect on surrounding structures and (2) the degree of hypoplasia involving the glenoid fossa, mandibular condyle, and ramus unit.[15,16] Classifying the extent of the HFM defor-

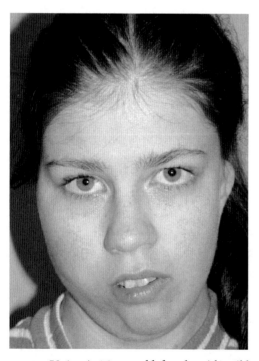

FIGURE 58-1 *A 16-year-old female with mild hemifacial microsomia type I. Note the canted maxilla, dental deviation, and facial asymmetry.*

mity can provide clarity in determining ideal reconstruction and accurate prognosis. The Pruzansky HFM classification,[17] modified by Kaban and colleagues,[18] currently provides a clinically useful framework to help guide the treatment plan based on the presence or absence of critical structures.[18,19]

HFM type I deformity can be summarized as a generalized mild hypoplastic state involving the muscles of mastication, the glenoid fossa, and the mandibular condyle and ramus unit. The temporomandibular joint (TMJ) functions with normal rotation and restricted translation. Patients present with mild mandibular retrognathia and facial asymmetry. Because there is satisfactory TMJ occlusal function and mild dysmorphology, surgical therapy is usually not indicated.

HFM type IIA deformity involves a hypoplastic cone-shaped condylar head. The condyle is located medial and anterior to a hypoplastic glenoid fossa. TMJ function is often satisfactory. Again, surgical intervention of the TMJ is usually not indicated.

HFM type IIB deformity involves a moderate to severe hypoplasia of the glenoid fossa, condyle, and mandibular ramus. Unlike the type IIA deformity, these patients have no articulation between the temporal bone and a condyle. However, manual manipulation reveals a posterior "stop" of the condyle contacting the glenoid fossa.[20]

A patient with HFM type III has a complete absence of the mandibular ramus and condyle. No manual condylar seating or posterior stop is present. These patients present with severe mandibular dysmorphology and often require TMJ surgical reconstruction (Figure 58-2).[20]

The treatment of HFM is controversial. The treatment philosophy of interceptive orthodontics and surgical treatment in growing children is based upon the theory that HFM is a progressive deformity.[15] Conversely, a treatment protocol based on

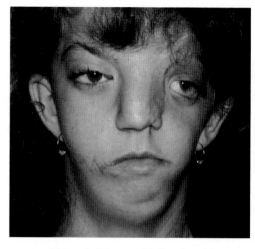

FIGURE 58-2 *A 14-year-old female with severe hemifacial microsomia type III, which is associated with facial clefting and a total absence of condyle.*

the theory that HFM is not progressive in nature is well described by Posnick.[16]

Cleft Lip and Cleft Palate

Patients with a cleft lip and cleft palate often present with a bilateral or unilateral midface deficiency resulting in augmentation and involving the paranasal, nasal, infraorbital, and zygomatic regions as well as the occlusal level.[21] However, the degree and location of maxillofacial growth deficiency in children with clefts is largely dependent on the location and type of cleft lip/cleft palate repair and the age of the child at the time of repair.[22–24] Most studies show that children with a repaired cleft lip/cleft palate have decreased vertical and horizontal maxillary growth and decreased vertical growth of the ramus and steep mandibular plane angle.[25–27] Ross has shown that approximately 25% of patients with a repaired cleft lip or cleft palate have a midface deficiency and class III malocclusion that require skeletal surgery.[28]

Plagiocephaly

Plagiocephaly is derived from the Greek word *plagios*, which refers to the twisted shape of the skull when viewed cranially-caudally. The etiology is often a unilateral synostosis of the coronal or lambdoid suture. Unilateral synostosis of the coronal suture results in an asymmetric parallelogram-shaped forehead and brow. The affected side is flattened, and the contralateral side may show compensatory bulging or bossing. In addition, synostosis of the coronal suture often indirectly affects the lower facial morphology. The root of the nose is deviated to the involved side, and the chin is often deviated to the side opposite of the flattened forehead. The mandible is normally developed but may exhibit secondary dysmorphology.[29,30]

Congenital Hemifacial Hyperplasia

Congenital hemifacial hyperplasia is a rare unilateral enlargement of the craniofacial soft and/or bony tissues. Although the term *hemihypertrophy* has commonly been used, it is inappropriate because the condition refers to hemihyperplasia.[31] Pollock and colleagues have hypothesized that the reason for the asymmetric facial development is abnormal neural crest migration.[32] Yoshimoto and colleagues have found increased proliferative activity of osteoblasts in a patient with congenital hemifacial hyperplasia and have hypothesized that fibroblast growth factor and its receptor signal transduction axis in osteoblasts may be selectively involved, lending to the progression of hemifacial overgrowth.[33]

Developmental Anomalies

Intrinsic Jaw-Growth Deformities

Facial Hemiatrophy   Facial hemiatrophy (Parry-Romberg syndrome) is characterized by a progressive unilateral facial loss of skin, soft tissues, cartilage, and bony tissue (Figure 58-3). Usually, the left side is affected rather than the right. Associated abnormalities include jacksonian epilepsy, cutaneous dyspigmentations, and ipsilateral alopecia.[31]

The syndrome usually starts during the first two decades of life and completes progression within 2 to 15 years.[34–36] The etiology of facial hemiatrophy remains largely unknown, but associations with Lyme disease, ablation of the superior cervical sympathetic ganglia, localized scleroderma, Rasmussen encephalitis, and systemic lupus erythematosus have been found.[37–41] Alterations in the peripheral trophic sympathetic system is one of the more emphasized theories.[31] Treatments have included silicone injections, alloplastic implants, microfat injections, and microvascular free tissue transfer.[42–44]

Hemimandibular Hyperplasia/Elongation   Another condition resulting in facial asymmetry is hemimandibular hyperplasia. Hemimandibular hyperplasia is characterized by a diffuse enlargement of the condyle, the condylar neck, and the mandibular ramus and body.[45] In 1986 Obwegeser and Makek described the deformity as hemimandibular hyper-

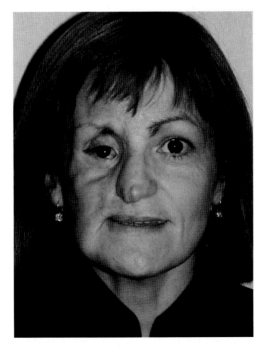

FIGURE **58-3**   *Right facial hemiatrophy (Parry-Romberg syndrome). At the time this photograph was taken, the patient had undergone skin and bone grafting.*

plasia or hemimandibular elongation.[46] In 1996 Chen and colleagues proposed that all cases of hemimandibular hyperplasia and hemimandibular elongation actually represent variations of condylar overgrowth.[47] They proposed that if condylar overgrowth is not arrested, it can progress into hemimandibular hyperplasia and hemimandibular elongation. In spite of the differences in nomenclature, no etiologic factor has been established. Condylar growth patterns can be evaluated by serial clinical comparisons, cephalometric tracings, and bone scanning with technetium 99m phosphate. However, no ideal method has been found to assess whether condylar overgrowth is "inactive." Therapy is guided by the patient's age and condylar growth activity. Treatment modalities have ranged from condylectomy to orthopedic maxillary management. However, strong consideration should be given to refraining from surgery until growth activity has ceased.[45]

Secondary Growth Deformities

Sternocleidomastoid torticollis is a condition thought to result from a birth trauma–induced hematoma of the sternocleidomastoid muscle that fibroses over time and leads to muscular contraction. However, the precise etiologic factors are still considered unknown. If the condition is not corrected with proper physiotherapy for the neck/sternocleidomastoid muscle or surgical therapy, malformed facial development may occur ipsilateral to the side affected by the torticollis.[48,49]

Duchenne's muscular dystrophy and cerebral palsy often result in areas of decreased muscle tone, which can affect the development of facial morphology by limiting the amount of bone formation at sites of muscle attachment and function. Consequently, facial asymmetry/dysmorphology can be a finding with Duchenne's muscular dystrophy and cerebral palsy.[50]

Acquired Facial Asymmetries

Condylar Trauma

A frequent cause of facial asymmetry in the growing child is trauma to the mandibular condyle (Figures 58-4 and 58-5).[51] Trauma-induced injury to the condyle can lead to a hemarthrosis, which can result in scarring and restricted translation of the condyle. Proffit and Turvey described this as a functional ankylosis or soft tissue extracapsular ankylosis.[52] Bony ankylosis of the condyle to the skull base can also occur from an intracapsular hemarthrosis.

Consequently, traumatic-induced scarring or bony ankylosis of the TMJ can result in relative degrees of restricted skeletal growth. In other words, the greater the degree of translational restriction, the greater the facial deformity. Thus, a frequently entertained question is whether open reduction and internal fixation of the condylar fracture are required to stabilize the condylar cartilaginous growth center. Studies in immature primates and children have revealed that the displaced condylar segment undergoes resorption and that a new condyle and the overlying cartilage are regenerated. Thus, there is nothing intrinsically important about the condylar head tissue as a mandibular

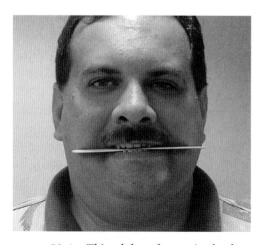

FIGURE 58-4 *This adult male sustained a fracture of the condyle as a teenager resulting in abnormal growth.*

growth center. Because the condylar head in children is generated spontaneously, the necessity of open reduction and internal fixation of the displaced condylar segment is eliminated. Moreover, the resulting scar and possible soft tissue and hard tissue restriction from open reduction could outweigh the benefits of surgical and anatomic condylar alignment. Thus, open reduction of condylar fractures in children should be avoided.[52–54]

Juvenile Idiopathic Arthritis

Facial asymmetry can be a finding in patients affected with juvenile idiopathic arthritis (JIA) of the TMJ.[55] JIA is a disease characterized by chronic inflammation of one or more joints affecting children up to the age of 18 years. The TMJ is frequently involved and can lead to facial growth disturbance including facial asymmetry.[55] TMJ involvement can be asymmetrical or asymptomatic and may not be evident clinically.[56,57] However, symptomatic TMJ involvement may not be associated with facial growth disturbances, and, conversely, facial growth disturbance may be present without TMJ symptoms.[56]

Both polyarticular- and pauciarticular-onset JIA have been found to have a negative impact on the form, function, and esthetics of the face; however, the effects are more pronounced with polyarticular JIA.[58,59] Characteristic facial features of patients with JIA include a small mandible, Class II malocclusion, and anterior open bite. Patients with polyarticular JIA with TMJ involvement tend to have small short faces with underdeveloped mandibles.[60]

Currently there is no effective therapeutic means to eliminate the progression of the disease and its effect on facial development; however, methotrexate therapy has been shown to minimize TMJ destruction and craniofacial dysmorphology in patients affected with polyarticular JIA.[61] Corticosteroids have been used in the treatment of JIA, but their therapeutic value is still controversial.

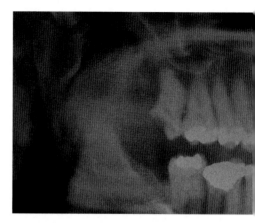

FIGURE 58-5 *Panoramic radiograph of the patient in Figure 58-4 demonstrates condylar asymmetry.*

Degenerative Joint Disease

Degenerative joint disease (DJD) is considered an end-stage result of progressive internal derangement of the TMJ. Usually, patients have bilateral involvement of the TMJ; however, unilateral involvement in not uncommon. The "wear and tear" effect of DJD on the TMJ results in condylar-glenoid erosion and decreased condylar ramus height. Clinically, patients often present with increasing preauricular crepitus, a limited mandibular range of motion, pain, and an anterior open bite.[62]

Clinical Assessment

Principles

The method of evaluating the patient with a dental facial condition begins with ascertaining the patient's chief complaint. Then, as the medical history of the present illness unfolds, the answers to pertinent questions regarding a history of facial trauma, arthritis, and congenital malformations, for example, are obtained.

A physical examination of the head and neck should include the following[63]:

1. Visual inspection of the entire face including facial subunits for symmetry
2. Palpation of the face to differentiate between soft and hard tissue defects

3. Comparison of dental and facial midlines with each other and with the central facial axis
4. Inspection for gonial angle symmetry and differences in antegonial notching
5. Analysis of the relationship between the upper lip and the maxillary central incisors
6. Inspection for malocclusion, occlusal canting, inclination of anterior teeth, dental crowning, open bites, maximal interincisal opening, and mandibular deviation with opening
7. Examination of the TMJ function

After the patient's chief complaint, history of present illness, past medical history, physical examination, radiographs and articulator mounted diagnostic casts have been obtained and evaluated, a problem list and corresponding treatment plan can then be constructed.

Radiography

Panoramic Radiographs The panoramic radiograph can provide information regarding the relative height of the mandibular condyle and ramus. Degenerative changes or asymmetric morphology can be identified with a comparative vertical measurement of the condylar head apex to the sigmoid notch base, and the sigmoid notch base to the mandibular angle.[63]

Posteroanterior Cephalometric Radiographs The posteroanterior cephalometric radiograph enables one to understand the extent of the deformity relative to the cranial base. By tracing soft and hard tissue features and then placing a true vertical and horizontal midline axis, one can visualize deviations of the dental and skeletal midline, occlusal cants, and vertical asymmetries.[63]

Lateral Cephalometric Radiographs A lateral cephalometric radiograph can provide clues of vertical differences by the lack of superimposition (eg, two separate radiographic mandibular inferior borders). However, to determine the relative significance of the differences in dentofacial superimposition, one must know whether the external auditory canals are level with the patient's natural head position. Only a single cephalometric ear rod should be used if the patient's auditory canals are not level.[63]

Computed Tomography

Computed tomography (CT) can provide two-dimensional localized views of the facial skeleton, or it can be developed further into three-dimensional views that can provide excellent detail necessary for the proper diagnosis and treatment of a complex facial dysmorphology (Figure 58-6).

Stereolithographic Modeling

Three-dimensional CT scans can provide information to allow the fabrication of an actual three-dimensional skeletal model. These models can help one make surgical predictions; however, because of their expense, these models are mainly used for complex dentofacial and craniofacial deformities.[64]

Technetium 99m Phosphate Bone Scans

Radionuclide skeletal scintigraphy has been shown to be a sensitive technique for identifying mandibular overgrowth in the patient with a facial deformity. However, scan findings are nonspecific and may be the result of a variety of bone and soft tissue abnormalities, including soft and hard tissue carcinomas, sarcomas, metastatic disease, hematologic disease, infections, inflammatory states, metabolic diseases, and trauma.[65] In patients with facial asymmetry mandibular overgrowth, nucleotide uptake is not symmetric bilaterally. In these cases, patients present with an increased nucleotide activity on the affected side. However, caution must be taken when evaluating an area of

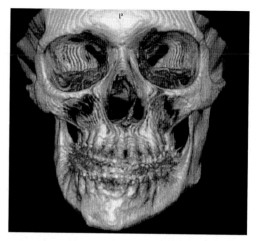

FIGURE 58-6 *Three-dimensional computed tomographic scan of asymmetric skull.*

increased uptake not to mistake condylar overgrowth for other conditions (ie, arthritis, TMJ disorders, trauma) that can mimic nucleotide uptake activity.[66] Additional techniques of fusing single-photon emission CT images to high-resolution structural CT images have been shown to provide a further precise anatomic delineation of bone activity.[67]

Surgical Treatment

Asymmetry may not always be obvious to the patient and family. Correct treatment begins with proper diagnosis. One should evaluate the face in all dimensions, carefully analyzing vertical and horizontal dimensions corresponding to facial subunits. Failure of the surgeon to recognize asymmetry until after surgery is often viewed by the patient as an excuse for poor treatment. In general, treatment planning of facial asymmetry is much the same as for any orthognathic case, except that more emphasis is placed on the frontal view.

Cephalometrics may be grossly inaccurate owing to ear rod positioning. Posteroanterior cephalometric radiographs are good simple screening tools but, standard computerized CT scans are much more accurate. CT data can be converted by computer-aided design/computer-aided manufacturing (CAD/CAM) imaging into an actual acrylic model. This model can be used for model surgery, implant fabrication, and distraction osteogenesis design.

Ultimately, the clinical examination is the most important diagnostic tool. Body posture, mannerisms, and hairstyle hide facial asymmetry and may mislead the treatment plan.

In a University of North Carolina study of 495 patients with facial asymmetry, the mandible was most often affected. Upper facial asymmetry was found only in 5%, but a chin deviation was present in 75% of all cases. Chin deviation is most often to the left, indicating a tendency for increased right-sided growth.[68] People notice chin deviation.

Delayed Treatment

Treatment of asymmetry in preadolescent children is extremely complex, and the results are not always predictable. Studies of growth modification with functional appliance have been problematic because of a various treatment designs with poor treatment group composition, poor control group composition, and difficulties with randomization. The topic is often discussed in orthodontic pediatric textbooks. Although noninvasive techniques do not harm the patient, most craniofacial asymmetry syndromes, condylar deformities, and traumatic injuries at an early age do require surgery. Bite-block therapy can be helpful in controlling the plane of occlusion but rarely prevents surgery. Bite-block therapy is mainly directed as an intervention for secondary growth deformities.

Maintenance of TMJ Function

Mild asymmetry in a growing patient with functional condyles should receive early interceptive orthodontics, and the patient should be allowed to finish growing before surgery is performed. Jaw movement is important following condylar fracture. Physical therapy and rehabilitation stimulates condylar and mandibular growth. Poor function results in a more asymmet-

ric mandible and secondary skull base. Asymmetry of the skull base correlates with maxillary midface asymmetry.

Post-traumatic mandibular hyperplasia is less frequently seen than growth retardation. Mandibular hyperplasia is usually apparent after adolescent growth, whereas delayed growth is often present early in life. Regardless of the true etiology, it is important to establish a surgical treatment plan with the most esthetic, functional, and stable result. Orthognathic asymmetries should be treated after growth is complete, and often require combined maxillary and mandibular surgery.

Orthodontic Considerations

Human facial symmetry has long been a critical factor for attractiveness. It is also well documented that true symmetry is not normal.[69,70]

For the average orthodontic patient, minor asymmetries become a concern only as an esthetic issue. Severe asymmetries often result in crossbite, malocclusion, cheek biting, poor mastication, condylar dysfunction, myositis, tendonitis, and chronic pain. From a diagnostic standpoint, patients with asymmetries differ from the typical orthodontic patient in several ways. The clinical examination and records should generate enough information to accurately diagnose and formulate the best possible treatment plan. This includes multiple photographs, lateral and posteroanterior cephalometric radiographs, and facebow-mounted dental models.[62–71]

Facial structures may be evaluated against a grid formed by the midsagittal plane and several perpendicular lines, according to the area being evaluated (eg, interpupillary, subnasal, stomion). A tongue blade or Fox plane can be used to determine whether a cant is present in the occlusal plane. Unilateral vertical maxillary excess and mandibular asymmetries are usually associated with an occlusal plane

cant.[63] This is why most asymmetries cannot be treated with single-jaw surgery.

Typical orthodontic diagnostic records rely heavily on a profile view. The lateral approach comes from the traditional diagnosis based on cephalometric radiographs; however, patients are more aware of their esthetic presentation from the frontal view. Additional diagnostic records may include a posteroanterior cephalometric radiograph, a submentovertex radiograph, and an accurate facebow transfer with casts mounted on a semiadjustable articulator.[65–73]

The orthodontic management of patients with asymmetries does not differ a great deal from that for a typical orthognathic patient. Good communication and a team approach during all phases of treatment are essential. Once the diagnosis and treatment plan are established, the presurgical orthodontic phase is initiated. Basic principles of presurgical orthodontics must be observed. All tooth movements that may compromise stability must be avoided, especially if the intended movement may be more easily accomplished with the movement of a bony segment during surgery, that is, transverse expansion. Dentoalveolar decompensation in the upper arch must take into account the postsurgical position of the upper incisor. Maxillary anteroposterior movements as well as posterior impactions have the greatest effect on the upper incisors with regard to anteroposterior positioning and torque, respectively. Dentoalveolar decompensations in the lower arch must observe the anatomic limits of the symphysis. One must observe that the morphogenetic pattern of patients with maxillomandibular discrepancies results in specific abnormal bony architectures. It is for this reason that cephalometric norms should not be used. There should be no compromise in the presurgical orthodontic treatment plan as it would severely limit the overall outcome. Do not hesitate to extract teeth if necessary. Impressions and early model surgery are helpful and confirm that the presurgical goals are correct and/or have been achieved. Common problems include improper buccal root torque in the upper arch, improper arch coordination (especially when anteroposterior movements are planned), and a lack of overjet (which would hinder placement of buccal segments in an ideal Class I occlusion).

The decision to extract teeth is often difficult. The first question that must be asked is whether there is severe crowding. The answer is based primarily on the planned position for the upper and lower incisors well positioned in basal bone. The upper incisors' relationships to the sella-nasion (SN) (104°), palatal plane (104°), and nasion-A point (NA) line (4 mm and 22°) are good indicators of whether these teeth need to be decompensated. It must be kept in mind that posterior impaction of the maxilla decreases the torque of the upper incisors. In addition, large unilateral vertical changes such as impaction downgrafting on one side also swing and rotate the midlines of the maxillary teeth. However, when this is anticipated, the upper incisors should be maintained slightly proclined. As a surgical objective, the position of the upper incisor and that of a point relative to the nasion perpendicularly can be used as reasonable cephalometric references. Therefore, dental crowding and the desired position for the upper incisors within basal bone of the maxilla ultimately determine the need for extractions. Upper second bicuspids are the teeth of choice for extraction when minimal incisor decompensation is required. Maxillary first bicuspids are extracted when the upper incisors require greater degrees of decompensation, such as in Class III malocclusions.

If mild crowding is present (up to 4 mm) and no dentoalveolar decompensation is needed, a nonextraction approach is acceptable, and some interproximal reduction may be required. If decompensation of the incisors is required, the cephalometric correction must be factored into the crowding assessment. For every 3° of change in the angle between the lower incisor and the mandibular plane, one must add or subtract 2.5 mm to the measured clinical crowding. In patients with Class II malocclusion, cephalometric correction most often adds to the clinical crowding since the lower incisor typically requires more upright positioning. In patients with Class III malocclusion, cephalometric correction usually alleviates crowding. In other words, cephalometric correction takes into account the goals for the lower incisor in the crowding assessment; moreover, it helps one decide which teeth should be extracted. When the measured crowding in the lower arch is moderate (5–9 mm), second bicuspids should be extracted. The result is the alignment and complete closure of the extraction sites. This should be achieved with the lower incisor in the ideal position. When crowding is severe (> 10 mm) after cephalometric correction, first bicuspids should be extracted to allow alignment and proper positioning of the lower incisor. The rationale is as follows: When two bicuspids are extracted, an average of 14 mm of space is created. If the total crowding is 10 mm including cephalometric correction, then 4 mm of space are left. These 4 mm are used by forward movement of the posterior teeth as lost anchorage during the alignment and retraction of the lower anterior tooth.

Maximum decompensation is often required with minimal clinical crowding, therefore requiring that the first bicuspid be extracted. If crowding exceeds 14 mm, extractions alone are not sufficient to alleviate crowding and achieve an ideal position for the lower incisors. Interproximal reduction may help to create another 3 to 4 mm of space.

Patients with hyperdivergent faces with an asymmetry require differential maxillary impaction. Such cases need a flattening of the curve of Spee on both arches prior to surgery. The curve of Spee is often different from left to right. Flattening this curve allows for maximum intercuspation to be achieved between the anterior teeth and bicuspids, with minimum posterior open bites. If the posterior maxilla is intentionally overimpacted when relapse is expected, the result is a posterior open bite, and no vertical elastics are placed distal to the bicuspids for the first 8 weeks after surgery. Intercuspation should be accomplished. In the patient with facial asymmetry, one side may be more open than the other. It is usually the hypoplastic side that remains slightly open, and teeth can be extruded postsurgically. An open bite of 2 mm is acceptable and sometimes desirable as settling and some relapse occur after surgery. After surgery no orthodontic forces should be in the direction of the potential surgical relapse.

Patients with hypodivergent asymmetric faces typically require mandibular advancement and an increase of the lower anterior facial height. The original malocclusion is often characterized by an excessive overbite, overjet, and curve of Spee. The upper curve of Spee should be flattened and the ideal position of the upper incisors achieved. The degree of curve of Spee may be different from side to side. No attempt should be made to level the lower curve of Spee because forward movement of the mandible to an ideal overbite and overjet automatically increases the lower facial height. If the lower mandibular plane angle has been maintained during advancement, this may result in a posterior open bite at the bicuspid or molars. The interocclusal space leads to leveling of the mandibular curve of Spee with minimal effort after surgery. A flexible braided wire is used in the lower arch as vertical intercuspation elastics are applied to extrude the lower posterior teeth. A class II or class III vector may be incorporated to achieve optimal occlusion. The upper arch should be stabilized by a heavy rectangular wire. Postsurgical orthodontic procedures usually are completed within 6 to 8 months of surgery if all other phases of treatment are successful. Vertical elastics may be directed by the orthodontist depending on the occlusion and the unique differences of the hyperplastic or hypoplastic side of the face. Severe orthognathic asymmetries are often difficult from an orthodontic standpoint owing to the presence of unilateral differences of a hyperplastic presentation and a contralateral hypoplastic dental compensation.

Surgical Approach and Techniques

In rare cases asymmetries may be treated in a single jaw. Generally, asymmetric growth causes compensation in the teeth, alveolus, and other jaw. Furthermore, this compensation is different from side to side and requires slightly different orthodontic mechanics. Facial asymmetry may be improved esthetically by an inferior border ostectomy, augmentation, and genioplasty. The esthetic impact of asymmetry involves both hard and soft tissue. The zygoma and periorbital and nasal structures may be asymmetric. Even adjacent soft tissues, such as the salivary glands, muscles, and adipose tissue, can be different in quantity from side to side. The patient should be well informed regarding the limitations and surgical expectations. Rarely can asymmetric deformities be corrected completely.

Most patients notice horizontal or transverse discrepancies more often than vertical asymmetries. Maxillary dental midline, chin, and nasal deviations are obvious clinically. Facial length is less apparent. In severe cases, such as hemifacial microsomia or other syndromes, soft tissue augmentation and even free vascularized tissue may be necessary.

The oral and maxillofacial surgeon should make a note of minor anatomic asymmetry. Orbital, nasal, and upper lip position; maxillary midline; smile arch; amount of gingival show per side; cheek mass; dimples; mandibular dental midlines; mandibular deviations on opening; TMJ articulation; translation; gonial angles; and cervical anatomy should be documented. The surgical procedure should be selected based on the etiology and a concern for stability. For example, when correcting a maxillary cant, vertical impaction is more stable than is vertical downgrafting. Often the discrepancy can be corrected by a combination of both impaction and downgrafting. Severe asymmetries with a short ramus height may require an extraoral inverted L osteotomy with bone grafting. This technique releases the mandibular sling and provides good access to the hypotrophic ramus, excellent bone grafting access, and accurate rigid fixation. Vertical changes of < 6 to 8 mm may be treated by intraoral sagittal split osteotomies. Rotational movements of the mandible produce proximal segment flaring on the advancing side and ramus collapse on the other. Proximal segment flaring may require modification (see Chapter 56, "Principles of Mandibular Orthognathic Surgery."). Some surgeons prefer a vertical oblique ramus osteotomy combined with a unilateral sagittal split ramus osteotomy. This combination surgery usually requires intermaxillary fixation, which may be beneficial in asymmetric cases. With current techniques, monocortical plate fixation can be achieved with a vertical ramus osteotomy. On the other hand, intermaxillary fixation is often necessary and even beneficial because alignment of the segments with rigid fixation is not always possible and the soft tissue pulls back to the original asymmetric position. A treatment plan should be established with an accurate clinical examination, cephalometric analysis, and model surgery. The surgical procedure should be executed efficiently, deftly, and with minimal morbidity. The aforementioned issues of relapse, stability, and mode of fixation should be established prior to surgery and discussed with the patient.

The first, and perhaps most important, treatment plan decision the surgeon encounters involves the upper incisor position. The choice of maxillary incisor position is key and essentially determines the three-dimensional position of everything else. The surgeon must correct maxillary incisor midlines, proclination, occlusal plane, smile arch, dental/gingival show, and lip support. An intermediate splint can be valuable in positioning the maxilla, assuming an accurate face-bow transfer and model surgery have been performed. One should not be a slave to an intermediate splint for it is only one method of aligning the asymmetry. Surgical experience and appreciation of esthetic symmetry are often more valuable.

The maxilla must be placed in the proper and most symmetric position. Consider the occlusion in relation to the unsplit mandible and ask yourself, Does that look reasonable according to the treatment plan? The maxillary position can best be measured using a combination of an external pin, Fox plane, lip position, and internal reference marks. The intermediate splint helps one place and hold the maxilla in the correct position during rigid fixation. The concept of an intermediate splint is based on proper condylar position. Functional condylar position in an awake upright person is not the same as it is in a supine paralyzed patient. Furthermore, asymmetric problems often originate from abnormal condylar (TMJ) disorders. Many patients with facial asymmetry do not have symmetric condylar rotation and therefore exhibit a great deal of muscular compensation with posturing. If an intermediate splint does not seem to position the maxilla properly in all three dimensions, the surgeon should consider other references for facial symmetry. Nothing can replace surgical experience. The mandible is usually cut first but is not split until after maxillary surgery and fixation. This prevents excessive force on the new maxillary position and seems to expedite the process. Some surgeons complete and fixate the mandibular osteotomy before maxillary surgery. This requires a predetermination of both mandibular and maxillary positions.

Mandibular ramus surgery is often difficult in cases of asymmetry because the ramus and body of the mandible are deformed and hypoplastic and the range of motion limited. Limited surgical access and a smaller soft tissue envelope create a difficult challenge. If the mandible is cut first but not split, the osteotomies are made and a moist sponge is placed while the maxillary surgery is completed. The mandible is later split and moved to the proper position with the maxilla and held in the proper occlusion by an occlusal wafer or splint with intermaxillary fixation. Rigid fixation of the mandible can be achieved with either bicortical position screws or monocortical plates, assuming the condylar position is correct. In large horizontal rotations of the mandible, bicortical screws cannot be placed as true compression screws (lag screws) without torquing the condyle. Modifications of the lingual cortical plate and selective grinding of the bone can be helpful in increasing the bony apposition. In most cases monocortical plates seem to provide adequate stability without compression of the nerve or torquing of the condyle.

Surgical mobilization is a key point in bimaxillary surgery. The mandible and maxilla should be free enough to be positioned passively without pulling the soft tissue. This is a significant point to be considered because the positioning can create a tight masseteric sling and limited periosteal tissue. If the segments are "stretched" into position, one cannot expect long-term stability. A balance between an excessive stripping of the vascularity and a restricted connective tissue envelope must be achieved. Therefore, in cases of severe hypoplastic asymmetry with only rudimentary condyle, one should consider condylar reconstruction

or extraoral procedures of the ramus. In some situations distraction osteogenesis may even be helpful in growing more bone and essentially expanding tissue.

Adjunctive simultaneous soft tissue procedures can be considered after successful positioning of the maxillomandibular dental component by secure rigid fixation. Alignment of the chin, nose, and malar complex should be performed after the functional anatomy of the maxilla and mandible is established. Simultaneous surgery has multiple advantages, but may not always be feasible.

The following case is an example of a patient with facial asymmetry resulting from trauma who required combination maxillary and mandibular surgery (Figure 58-7). She was a 20-year-old female with a chief complaint of difficulty eating and chewing; she had chronic myofascial pain and masticatory dysfunction. She had sustained a jaw fracture as a young child and had not received treatment. The young lady experienced gradual facial asymmetry and sought orthodontic treatment. Such a case cannot be treated properly with orthodontics alone; neither can it be corrected in a single jaw.

Her physical examination revealed a healthy young woman in no acute distress but with an obvious facial deformity. The basal view often better demonstrates the deformity, as does having the patient bite on a tongue blade (Figure 58-8). She was normocephalic (although she had a short face), asymmetric, and had deviation of the jaw to her right (Figure 58-9). The TMJ articulated and translated well without clicking or popping. The maximum incisal opening was 56 mm, with a deviation to the right. The mandibular midline was 7 mm to the right, the overjet was 5 mm, the overbite was 2 mm, and there was excessive lower dental show. She had a right buccal crossbite, an anterior crossbite, maxillary hypoplasia, a canted maxilla, and a short mandibular condyle (Figure 58-10).

The presurgical work-up included a three-dimensional CT scan, cephalometric and panoramic radiography, and facebow mounting for an accurate intermediate splint and model surgery (Figures 58-11–58-13). The Erickson table was used to measure the vertical change and to fabricate an intermediate splint to assist in positioning the maxilla from the stable mandible (Figures 58-14 and 58-15). The surgical plan was a Le Fort I advancement of 3 to 4 mm and a downgrafting of 4 to 5 mm on the right side (Figure 58-16). The osteotomy gap was bone grafted with

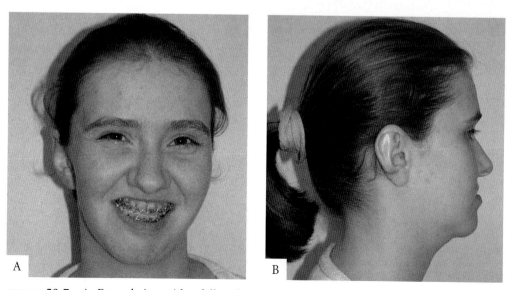

FIGURE 58-7 A, *Frontal view with a full smile.* B, *Later profile shows a midface deficiency and relative mandibular prognathism in spite of the old mandible fracture.*

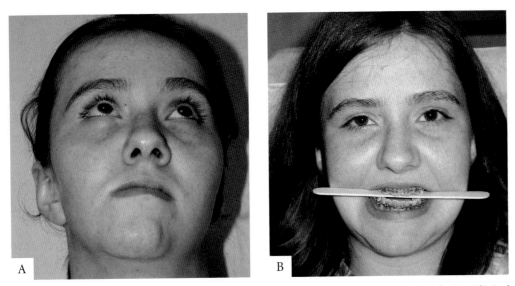

FIGURE **58-8**   A, *Basal view shows facial asymmetry and a chin deviation to the right.* B, *Clinical photograph of a tongue blade demonstrating the canted occlusal plane in relation to the orbital rim.*

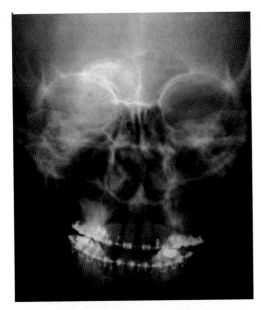

FIGURE **58-9**   *Cephalometric view showing a short right facial height.*

and careful clinical inspection from different perspectives are all valuable surgical skills in simultaneous jaw surgery for the patient with facial asymmetry. The unsplit mandible is also a key reference for determining the change in maxillary position. In this case, after the maxilla was correctly positioned and leveled, the mandible was split and set to the plane of occlusion. A bilateral sagittal split osteotomy of the mandible was cut prior to the Le Fort I procedure but was not split. This seems to be a common sequence for most surgeons. Consideration was given to a vertical oblique osteotomy on the left, but the rotation seemed favorable and the fixation more stable. Most patients with facial asymmetry are hypoplastic and need lower facial advancement not reduction. A horizontal geniotomy was performed to advance the chin point 4 mm and level the deviation. After the orthognathic phase of surgery, the tube was switched to the mouth by the transpharyngeal route. This technique is efficient and is commonly used for simultaneous rhinoplasty. A standard internal rhinoplasty was performed to narrow the nose, refine the tip, and reduce the dorsum. Often facial asymmetry affects multiple facial subunits. The nose may appear asymmetric or deviated in relation to the mouth and chin. Great

banked tibial bone that was mortised and fixated. This was determined with a model surgery to level the cant of the maxilla. A Steinmann pin was placed at the nasal bone for an external vertical reference. This technique is valuable in establishing the correct facial dimension. In addition, a Fox occlusal plane was used to evaluate the leveling of the maxilla in relation to the infraorbital rims during surgery (Figure 58-17). Multiple methods of evaluating symmetry are helpful in achieving a good result. Intermediate splints, internal/external reference marks,

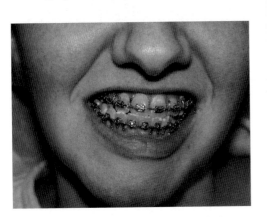

FIGURE **58-10**   *Clinical analysis of the teeth demonstrates an asymmetry and midline discrepancy.*

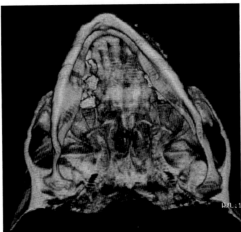

FIGURE **58-11**   *This three-dimensional computed tomogram clearly identifies the asymmetry.*

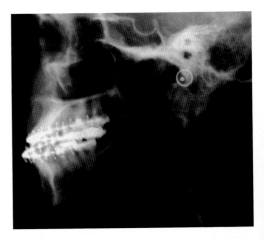

FIGURE **58-12**   *Lateral cephalometric view appears to show a prognathic jaw even though there is a history of a condylar fracture.*

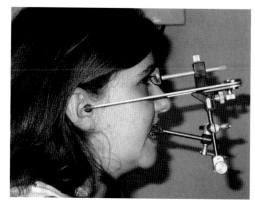

FIGURE **58-13** *A face-bow transfer is valuable but sometimes difficult in cases of severe asymmetry owing to an abnormal external auditory canal.*

attention must be given to creating middle face symmetry.

At 3 months the postoperative results were satisfactory and the patient was very happy (Figure 58-18). The occlusion was well aligned and finishing orthodontics were completed without difficulty. This case demonstrates well the principles discussed above.

An example of mild developmental asymmetry is demonstrated in the follow-

ing case. Such a case can be challenging for the orthodontist/surgical team because the orthodontic preparation may be different for right and left sides; the asymmetry is mild and it is tempting to undertreat the problem with single-jaw surgery. This patient was a 17-year-old female with an open bite and right laterognathia. She had posterior vertical maxillary excess mild crowding, Class III molar relation, dentofacial asymmetry, and a pseudomandibular prognathism (Figures 58–19 58–22). She complained of lip incompetence, difficulty chewing and biting food, nasal obstruction, and xerostomia. Her father had a history of mandibular prognathism and orthognathic surgery.

This patient denied previous trauma to her facial bones. The orbital rims were symmetric, but the right ear was slightly lower. The TMJs articulated well, and there was no myofascial pain. The mandibular midline was 4 mm to the right, as was the chin. She had 4 to 5 mm of gingival show with a high smile. There was no overjet and 4 mm of open bite. She had a mild transverse deficiency of the posterior maxilla.

The treatment plan began with an extraction of teeth no. 1, 16, 17, 18, 32, 4, 13, 21, and 28 prior to presurgical orthodontics. Orthodontics was performed to level alignment and to decompensate in

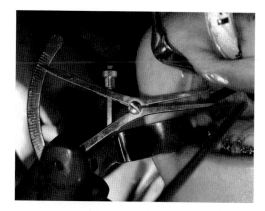

FIGURE **58-16** *Intraoperative measurement confirms the treatment plan and correct positioning as determined by the intermediate splint.*

preparation for a two-piece Le Fort I osteotomy, bilateral sagittal osteotomy, genioplasty, and rhinoplasty. Presurgical records included surgical mounted models, a face-bow transfer, and detailed radiographs. A CT scan was not obtained.

A sagittal split osteotomy was cut but not split until after the maxilla was positioned. The maxilla was impacted 4 mm posteriorly and widened by a segmental osteotomy between the central incisors. An intermediate splint was used to

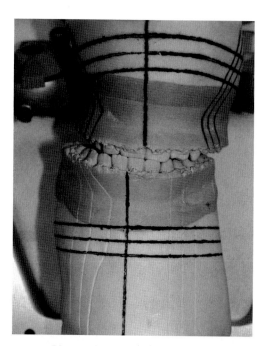

FIGURE **58-14** *Mounted dental models on an Erickson platform with reference marks help one determine the amount of change and fabrication of an intermediate splint. Note the amount of midline discrepancy.*

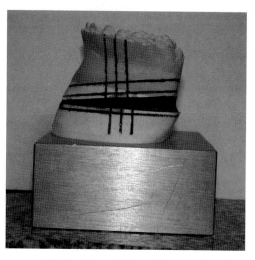

FIGURE **58-15** *Lateral view of mounted models.*

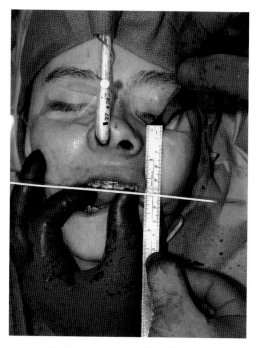

FIGURE **58-17** *A prosthetic Fox plane can be used as a final reference to evaluate the leveling of the maxilla in reference to the infraorbital rim.*

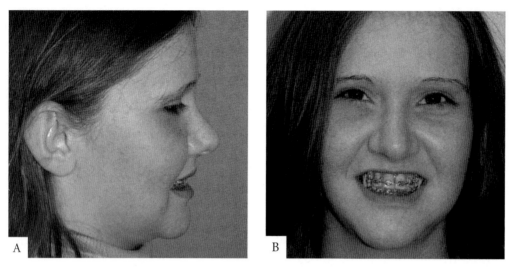

FIGURE **58-18**   A, *Postoperative lateral view with animation.* B, *Postoperative frontal view with animation.*

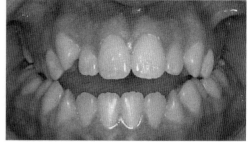

FIGURE **58-20**   *The frontal view of dentition demonstrates an open bite and midline asymmetry.*

position the maxilla. The maxilla was rigidly fixated with a resorbable mesh. Internal and external references were used to properly position the maxilla, as were the predetermined intermediate splint and model surgery. The mandible was then completed and rotated slightly by the sagittal split osteotomy. The chin point was moved to the left and advanced with a horizontal genioplasty. The endotracheal tube was changed to the oral route, and rhinoplasty performed to improve facial harmony and symmetry. The surgery was performed without complications.

The postoperative course was without complications. At 1 month the splint was removed and the occlusion was satisfactory (Figures 58-23 and 58-24). At 1 year the patient's occlusion was good, the open bite stable, and facial symmetry excellent (Figures 58-25–58-28).

Summary

Correction of orthognathic deformities often requires surgery of both the maxilla and the mandible. Combining osteotomies of the maxilla and the mandible is more complicated than single-jaw surgery and is perhaps associated with increased morbidity, but the surgical options and results are better. Double-jaw surgery does *not* result in twice the morbidity of single-jaw

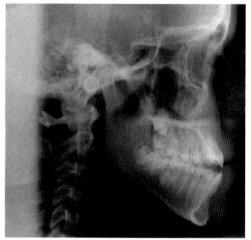

FIGURE **58-21**   *Initial cephalometric radiograph.*

surgery. The indications for bimaxillary surgery are severe deformities untreatable in one jaw, deformities of both jaws, unfavorable movement prone to relapse, and complex three-dimensional movements for which single-jaw surgery would be a functional/cosmetic compromise. Dentofacial asymmetry may develop from a primary cause but presents with secondary compensation in the hard and soft tissues of the face. Such asymmetry is a good indication for bimaxillary surgery.

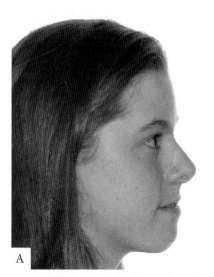

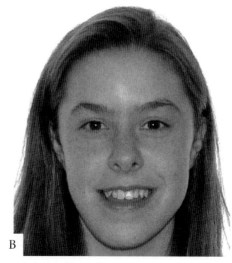

FIGURE **58-19**   A, *Initial lateral profile.* B, *Initial frontal view with smile.*

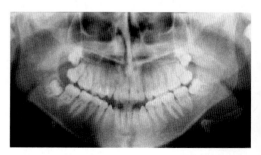

FIGURE **58-22**   *Initial panoramic radiograph.*

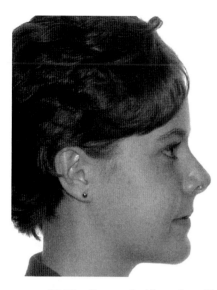

FIGURE **58-23**   *Postsurgical lateral profile.*

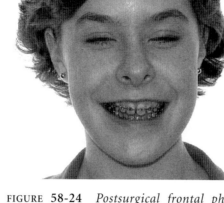

FIGURE **58-24**   *Postsurgical frontal photograph with smile.*

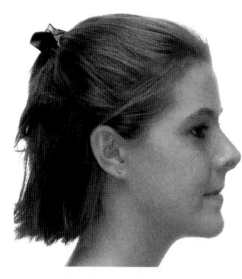

FIGURE **58-25**   *Final profile after surgery.*

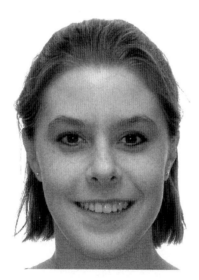

FIGURE **58-26**   *Final frontal view with smile after surgery. Note the facial symmetry.*

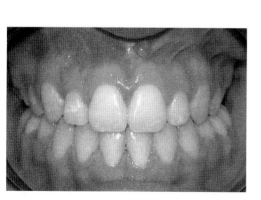

FIGURE **58-27**   *Frontal view of occlusion after surgery.*

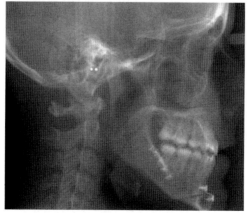

FIGURE **58-28**   *Cephalometric radiograph taken 1 year after surgery.*

Current surgical techniques have reduced the morbidity and length of stay in the hospital and have improved the outcome. This chapter presented combined maxillary and mandibular osteotomies with a special emphasis on asymmetries as an indication. The concept of comprehensive facial analysis and treatment was represented in the cases demonstrated. If correction of mild asymmetries is attempted with single-jaw surgery, the results are suboptimal and disappointing.

Acknowledgment

We would like to thank Dr. Andre Ferreira for orthodontic support.

References

1. Proffit W, White R, Savers D.Contemporary treatment of dentofacial dentoformity. St. Louis (MO): Mosby; 2003.
2. Bell WH, Condit CL. Surgical-orthodontic correction of adult bimaxillary protrusion. J Oral Surg 1970; 28:578–90.
3. Connole PW, Small EW. Combined maxillary and mandibular osteotomies: discussion of three cases. J Oral Surg 1971;29:572–8.
4. Epker BN, Wolford LM. Middle third face osteotomies: their use in the correction of acquired and developmental dentofacial and craniofacial deformities. J Oral Surg 1975;33:491–514.
5. Turvey TA. Simultaneous mobilization of the maxilla and mandible: surgical technique and results. J Oral Maxillofac Surg 1981;40:96–9.
6. Gross BD, James AB. The surgical sequence of combined total maxillary and mandibular osteotomies. J Oral Surg 1978;36:513–22.
7. Shackleford TK, Larsen RJ. Facial asymmetry as an indicator of psychological, emotional, physiological distress. J Pers Soc Psychol 1997;72:456–66.
8. Cohen MM Jr. The child with multiple birth defects. New York: Raven Press; 1982.
9. Cohen MM. Perspectives on craniofacial asymmetry 1. The biology of asymmetry. Int J Oral Maxillofac Surg 1995;24:2–7.
10. Gorlin RJ, Cohen MM, Levin LS. Syndromes of the head and neck. 3rd ed. New York: Oxford University Press; 1990.
11. Johnston MC, Bronsky PT. Prenatal craniofacial development: new insights on normal and abnormal mechanisms. Crit Rev Oral Biol Med 1995;6:368–422.
12. Seow WK, Urban S, Vafaie N, Shusterman S.

Morphometric analysis of the primary and permanent dentitions in hemifacial microsomia: a controlled study. J Dent Res 1998;77:27–38.

13. Poswillo DE. The pathogenesis of the first and second branchial arch syndrome. Oral Surg Oral Med Oral Pathol 1975;35:302–27.

14. Poswillo DE. Hemorrage in development of the face. Birth Defects 1975;11:61.

15. Kearns GJ, Padwa BL, Kaban LB. Hemifacial microsomia: the disorder and its surgical management. In: Booth PW, Schendel SA, editors. Maxillofacial surgery. St. Louis: Churchill Livingstone; 1999. p. 917–42.

16. Posnick JC. Hemifacial microsomia: evaluation and treatment. In: Craniofacial and maxillofacial surgery in children and young adults. Philadelphia: WB Saunders; 1999. p. 419–45.

17. Pruzansky S. Not all dwarfed mandibles are alike. Birth Defects 1969;1:120.

18. Kaban LB, Moses MH, Mulliken JB. Surgical correction of hemifacial microsomia in the growing child. Plast Reconstr Surg 1988;82:9–19.

19. Cousley RR, Calvert ML. Current concepts in the understanding and management of hemifacial microsomia. Br J Plast Surg 1997;50:536–51.

20. Vargervik K, Hoffman W, Kaban LB. Comprehensive surgical and orthodontic management of hemifacial microsomia. In: Turvey TA, Vig KW, Fonseca RJ, editors. Facial clefts and craniosynostosis: principles and management. Philadelphia: WB Saunders; 1996. p. 537–64.

21. Stella JP, Chaisresoahurnpon N, Epker BN. Diagnostic criteria for midface deficiency [abstract]. Cleft Palate-Craniofacial Association 1993;182:6.

22. Johnson GP. Craniofacial analysis of patients with complete clefts of the lip and palate. Cleft Palate J 1980; 17:17–23.

23. Fonseca RJ, Turvey TA, Wolford LM. Orthognathic surgery on the cleft patient. In: Fonseca RJ, Baker SB, Wolford LM, editors. Oral and maxillofacial surgery: cleft/craniofacial/cosmetic surgery. Vol 6. Philadelphia (PA): WB Saunders; 2000. p. 87–146.

24. Bishara SE. Cephalometric evaluation of facial growth in operated and non-operated individuals with isolated clefts of the palate. Cleft Palate J 1973;10:239–46.

25. Bardach J. The influence of cleft repair on facial growth. Cleft Palate J 1990;27:76–8.

26. Shaw WC, Dahl E, Asher-McDade C, et al. A six-center international study of treatment outcome in patients with clefts of the lip and palate. Part 5. General discussion and conclusions. Cleft Palate Craniofac J 1992;29:413–8.

27. Semb G. A study of facial growth in patients with unilateral cleft lip and palate treated by Oslo CLP team. Cleft Palate Craniofac J 1991;28:1–21.

28. Ross RB. Treatment variables affecting facial growth in complete unilateral cleft lip and palate. Cleft Palate J 1987;24:5–77.

29. Shin JH, Persing J. Asymmetric skull shapes: diagnostic and therapeutic consideration. J Craniofacial Surg 2003;14:696–9.

30. Kane AA, Lo LJ, Vannier MW, Marsh JL. Mandibular dysmorphology in unicoronal synostosis and plagiocephaly without synostosis. Cleft Palate Craniofac J 1996; 33:418–23.

31. Cohen MM. Perspectives on craniofacial asymmetry. IV Hemi-asymmetries. Int J Oral Maxillofac Surg 1995;24:134–41.

32. Pollock RA, Newman MH, Burdi AR, Condit DP. Congenital hemifacial hyperplasia: an embryonic hypothesis and case report. Cleft Palate J 1985;22:173–84.

33. Yoshimoto H, Yano H, Kobayushi K, et al. Increased proliferative activity of osteoblasts in congenital hemifacial hypertrophy. Plast Reconstr Surg 1998;102:1605–10.

34. Parry CH. Collections from unpublished papers. Vol 1. London: Underwood; 1825.

35. Romberg MH. Trophoneurosen. In: Klinische Ergebnisse. Berlin: A. Forstner; 1846. p. 75–81.

36 Stone J. Parry-Romberg syndrome: a global survey of 205 patients using the Internet. Neurology 2003;61:674–6.

37. Shah JR, Juhasz C, Kupsky WJ, et al. Rasmussen encephalitis associated with Parry-Romberg syndrome. Neurology 2003;61:395–7.

38. Stern HS, Elliott LF, Beegle PH. Progressive hemifacial atrophy associated with Lyme disease. Plast Reconstr Surg 1992; 90:479–83.

39. Moss ML, Crikelair GF. Progressive facial hemiatrophy following cervical sympathectomy in the rat. Arch Oral Biol 1959;1:254–8.

40. Rees TD. Facial atrophy. Clin Plast Surg 1976;3:637–46.

41. Roddi R, Riggio E, Gilbert PM, et al. Progressive hemifacial atrophy in a patient with lupus erythematosus. Plast Reconstr Surg 1994;93:1067–72.

42. Franz FP, Blocksma R, Brudage SR, et al. Massive injection of liquid silicone for hemifacial atrophy. Ann Plast Surg 1988;20:140–5.

43. Roddi R, Riggio E, Gilbert PM, et al. Clinical evaluation of techniques used in the surgical treatment of progressive hemifacial atrophy. Craniomaxillofacial Surg 1994;22:23–32.

44. Pisarek W. Reconstruction of craniofacial microsomia and hemifacial atrophy with free latissimus dorsi flap. Acta Chir Plast 1988;30:194–201.

45. Marchetti C, Cocchi R, Gentile L, Bianchi A. Hemimandibular hyperplasia: treatment strategies. J Craniofac Surg 2000;11:46–53.

46. Obwegeser HL, Makek MS. Hemimandibular hyperplasia—hemimandibular elongation. J Maxillofac Surg 1986;14:183–208.

47. Chen YR, Bendov-Samuel RL, Huang CS. Hemimandibular hyperplasia. Plast Reconstr Surg 1996;97:730–7.

48. Stassen LF, Kerwala CJ. New surgical technique for the correction of congenital muscular torticollis (wry neck). Br J Oral Maxillofac Surg 2000;38:142–7.

49. Chen CE, Ko JY. Surgical treatment of muscular torticollis for patients above 6 years of age. Arch Orthop Trauma Surg 2000;120:149–51.

50. Kiliaridis S, Katsaros C. The effects of myotonic dystrophy and Duchenne muscular dystrophy on the orofacial muscles and dentofacial morphology. Acta Odontol Scand 1998;56:369–74.

51. Proffit WR, Vig KW, Turvey TA. Fractures of the mandible condyle: frequently an unsuspected cause of facial asymmetry. Am J Orthod 1980;78:1–24.

52. Proffit WR, Turvey TA. Dentofacial asymmetry. In: Proffit WR, White RP, Sarver DM, editors. Contemporary treatment of dentofacial deformity. St. Louis: Mosby; 2003. p. 574–644.

53. Demianczuk AN, Verchere C, Phillips JH. The effect on facial growth of pediatric mandibular fractures. J Craniofac Surg 1999;10:323–8.

54. Pirttiniemi PM. Associations of mandibular and facial asymmetries—a review. Am J Orthod Dentofacial Orthop 1994;106:191–200.

55. Stabrun AE. Impaired mandibular growth and micrognathic development in children with juvenile rheumatoid arthritis. Eur J Orthod 1991;13:423–34.

56. Bazan MT. An overview of juvenile rheumatoid arthritis. J Pedod 1981;6:68–76.

57. Kjellberg H, Fasth A, Kiliaridis S, et al. Craniofacial structure in children with juvenile rheumatoid arthritis compared with healthy children with ideal or postnormal occlusion. Am J Orthod Dentofacial Orthop 1995;107:67–78.

58. Mericle PM, Wilson VK, Moore TL, et al. Effects of polyarticular and pauciarticular onset juvenile rheumatoid arthritis on facial and mandibular growth. J Rheumatol 1996;23(1):159–65.

59. Stabrun AE, Larheim TA, Hoyeraal HM, Rosler M. Reduced mandibular dimensions and

asymmetry in juvenile rheumatoid arthritis pathologic factors. Arthritis Rheum 1988;31:602–11.

60. Walton AG, Welburg RR, Thomason JM, Foster HE. Oral health and juvenile idiopathic arthritis: a review. Rheumatology 2000; 39:550–5.

61. Ince DO, Ince A, Moore TL. Effect of methotrexate on the TM joint and facial morphology in juvenile rheumatoid arthritis patients. Am J Orthod Dentofacial Orthop 2000;118:75–83.

62. Schellhas KP, Piper MA, Omlie MR. Facial skeletal remodeling due to temporomandibular joint degeneration: an imaging study of 100 patients. Cranio 1992; 10:248–59.

63. Hegtvedt AK. Diagnosis and management of facial asymmetry. In: Principles of oral and maxillofacial surgery. Philadelphia: JB Lippincott Company; 1992. p. 1400–14.

64. Sailer HF, Haers PE, Zollikofer CP, et al. The value of stereolithographic models for preoperative diagnosis of craniofacial deformities and planning of surgical corrections. Int J Oral Maxillofac Surg 1998;27:327–33.

65. O'Mara RE. Role of bone scanning in dental and maxillofacial disorders. In: Freeman M, Weissman HS, editors. Nuclear medicine annual. New York: Raven Press; 1985. p. 265–84.

66. O'Mara RE. Scintigraphy of the facial skeleton. Oral Maxillofac Surg Clin North Am 1992;4:51–60.

67. Strumas N, Antonyshyn O, Caldwell CB, Mainprize J. Multimodality imaging for precise localization of craniofacial osteomylitis. J Craniofac Surg 2003;14:215–9.

68. Severt TR, Proffit WR. The prevalence of facial asymmetry in the dentofacial deformities population at the University of North Carolina. Int J Adult Orthodon Orthognath Surg 1997;12:171–6.

69. Peck S, Peck L. Skeletal asymmetry in esthetically pleasing faces. Angle Orthod 1991; 61(1):43–8.

70. Burk PH. Stereophotogrammetric measurement of normal asymmetry in children. Hum Biol 1971;43:536–48.

71. Sutton PR. Lateral facial asymmetry methods of assessment. Angle Orthod 1968;38(1):82–92.

72. Cheney EA. Dentofacial asymmetry and their clinical significance. Am J Orthod 1961; 47:814–29.

73. Harvold E. Cleft lip and palate: morphologic studies of facial skeleton. Am J Orthod 1954;40:493–506.

CHAPTER 59

Soft Tissue Changes Associated with Orthognathic Surgery

Norman J. Betts, DDS, MS
Sean P. Edwards, DDS, MD

While few patients and clinicians question the functional benefits of orthognathic surgery, the esthetic results that accompany surgery of the bony foundation of the face are equally powerful, if not more so. It is therefore incumbent upon the surgeon to include a component of soft tissue changes in the surgical treatment plan while working to achieve a stable, functional dentoskeletal unit.

Fundamental to such treatment planning is a sound knowledge of the behavior of the soft tissues of the face in response to both orthodontic and surgical changes. Close collaboration between surgeon and orthodontist is essential for this to occur.

The soft tissue response to orthognathic surgery will be discussed in this chapter. In addition, the surgical procedures and techniques used to control the soft tissue changes will be presented and evaluated in order to help the surgeon understand, control, and maximize the beneficial aspects of the facial soft tissue response to surgery.

Historical Perspective

The orthodontic literature contains the origins of predicting changes in the soft tissues of the face following the treatment of dentofacial deformities. Orthognathic surgery initially was used to correct skeletofacial deformities and the resultant functional problems, often at the expense of the facial soft tissue esthetics. In time, a greater concern for the esthetic aspects of surgery developed, such that facial soft tissue prediction became an integral part of preoperative planning and postoperative outcome assessment.

Early studies produced average ratios, which related designated hard and soft tissue landmarks. The ratios were of use for predicting the response of the soft tissues to various skeletal and dental changes. These ratios are averages, however, and investigators realized that individual variability was significant. It was surmised that facial soft tissue response to orthodontics and surgery was multifactorial in nature. As a result, more elaborate statistical analyses were employed, with varying degrees of success, to elucidate the factors governing the soft tissue response to surgery. Consequently, prediction equations were developed that would help in preoperative surgical planning and postoperative outcome assessment.

Recently, much emphasis has been placed on developing procedures that assist the surgeon in controlling the soft tissue response to surgery. By using procedures such as the alar cinch suture and V-Y closure, the surgeon can minimize or eliminate unesthetic soft tissue changes and may optimize positive esthetic changes.

Facial Esthetics in Society

Physical appearance is critically important in our society.[1-3] Perception of oneself and the perceptions of others are both essential to self-esteem. The most significant aspect of one's self-image is facial appearance. As a result, dentofacial and skeletofacial deformities have a significant psychological and social impact on those afflicted. Further, the correction of these deformities can have an equally significant impact on self-esteem and personality.

General Considerations

Much has been written about soft tissue changes associated with orthognathic surgery, and each paper has its strengths and weaknesses. Variation in design, heterogeneity of study design, surgical technique, and patient populations do not allow for direct comparison. To make some objective comparisons between methodologically different studies, we identified a set of characteristics for the theoretically ideal study of the soft tissue changes associated with orthognathic surgery (Table 59-1). These criteria should help the reader to evaluate individual investigations. This technique for assessing the previous literature is helpful and should be considered for use in other areas of scientific investigation.[4]

Most of the studies dealing with this subject provide ratios of soft to hard tissue movement. Ratios are averages. Averages apply well to groups but often fail to account for individual variation within the group. Further, these ratios only describe the relationship of two specific points. It is highly improbable that consistently accurate predictions of soft tissue change can be accomplished with only simple correlations. The complex behavior of the facial soft tissue drape is much more realistically described by the interaction of several factors within the skeletal framework. This may explain some of the extreme variability that many authors have encountered.[5–9] At best, ratios serve to give a general appreciation of the expected outcome.[9] Some authors have stated that ratios are just as efficacious in predicting the soft tissue response to osseous surgery as multiple regression and stepwise regression analysis.[6,9] This may be a result of several factors such as lack of inclusion of important variables (eg, the method of soft tissue closure and osseous contouring) into their database; a mixed sample population (race, age, or sex); small numbers of patients; or inability to limit the sample to specific vectors of osseous movement.[4,6,8,9]

Recent investigations have shown improved predictive ability when patients were grouped by vector-specific movements of the osseous segments.[4,10]

Orthodontic Considerations

Tooth position and alveolar morphology result from the sum of applied forces during their development. These applied forces derive from the cheeks, lips, and tongue and parafunctional habits. Obviously, skeletal imbalances are accompanied by soft tissue imbalances. The result is dental compensation for skeletal malocclusions. Orthodontic correction of these compensatory changes will often result in a worsening of the malocclusion preoperatively, and the jaw-to-jaw discrepancy will appear clinically more severe.[11,12] Thus, initial treatment planning should consider these changes, and final surgical treatment plans should be based on records obtained as close to surgery as possible. When evaluating ratio studies, it becomes apparent that the position of the incisor teeth does not always accurately reflect the osseous movement. This is because of postoperative orthodontic tooth movement. The molar teeth or bony landmarks such as the anterior nasal spine (ANS) undergo less postoperative change and may more accurately describe the osseous surgical movement. Therefore, these landmarks should produce a more accurate ratio or prediction.[9]

Cephalometric Considerations

The use of a standardized cephalometric technique is essential to the study of this subject. The components of a standardized cephalometric technique are using the same cephalometer, with the same source-object and object-film distances, and positioning the patient in a natural head position with the teeth in centric relation and soft tissues in repose. The cephalogram obtained from the standardized cephalometric technique must allow visualization of the complete soft tissue profile. Relaxation of the soft tissues may be difficult to produce and reproduce. Relaxed lip posture is especially difficult to achieve in patients with excessive interlabial gap. Straining to close the gap by contracting the mentalis muscles flattens

Table 59-1   Theoretical Ideal Characteristics of a Study to Investigate the Soft Tissue Changes Associated with Orthognathic Surgery

1. Prospective
2. Adequate sample size
3. Randomized treatments (if treatments differ within the sample)
4. Nongrowing patients
5. No previous trauma to the osseous structures of the face
6. Exclusion of patients with congenital defects or syndromes (eg, cleft patients)
7. Elimination of the confounding effects of pre- and postoperative orthodontic tooth movement
8. Constant presence or absence of orthodontic appliances
9. Same cephalostat used for all cephalograms with identical source-subject and subject-film distances
10. Soft tissues in repose for all cephalograms
11. Superimposition of cephalograms on the nearest osseous structure not affected by surgery or on a stable reference line
12. Use of a tracing template to assist in landmark identification
13. Evaluation of both profile and full facial soft tissue changes, or 3-D analysis
14. No concomitant or prior soft tissue surgery
15. Exclusion of segmental surgical procedures
16. One vector of movement (or grouped in study)
17. No concomitant osseous surgery on another portion of the facial skeleton
18. Homogeneity of the soft tissue incisions and closure techniques
19. No hard tissue contouring (eg, recontouring of ANS)
20. Use of rigid osseous fixation
21. Uniform follow-up intervals
22. Follow-up time of at least 6 months (1 year is preferable)
23. Error analysis of measurement and landmark identification

ANS = anterior nasal spine.
Adapted from Betts et al.[4]

the labiomental fold and distorts the overall contour of the chin. It is important that patients be instructed to keep their lips in repose for the cephalogram.[13]

To minimize measurement error during cephalometric analysis, landmarks or planes approximating the structures being evaluated must be superimposed. This superimposition should be on landmarks not modified or changed during the surgical procedure.[9,14] Another contributing factor to measurement error is orthodontic tooth movement between the times of comparison. Orthodontic changes can be minimized by obtaining the preoperative cephalogram within a month of the planned surgical procedure,[6,9] and performing minimal postoperative orthodontics.[9] Also, the presence, or absence, of orthodontic appliances must be constant during the study period. The presence of orthodontic appliances influences lip posture, and their placement or removal will change the soft tissue drape.[4]

Landmark identification is simplified and becomes more accurate when templates are used.[9,10,14] This is especially valid for soft tissue landmarks.[11] Soft tissue landmarks are often arbitrary and located on gently curving contours. These landmarks can therefore move vertically over the surface of the tissue after surgically induced change.[8,12] If tracing templates are used, these points can be more accurately located.

Soft Tissue Considerations

The ability to predict the hard and soft tissue changes prior to an orthognathic surgical procedure is critical to the treatment planning process. With the refinement of surgical procedures and the advent of rigid fixation techniques, the surgeon is able to accurately reposition and retain the osseous components in a planned position. However, the change in soft tissue morphology after combined orthodontic and surgical therapy depends on several factors. These include surgical procedure,[6,15–19] method of wound closure,[6,9,15,16,18,19] the new spatial arrangement of the skeletal and dental elements,[19] the adaptive qualities of the soft tissues,[19] growth,[17,20] orthodontic vectors of tooth movement,[17,19] lip thickness,[5,6,17,21–23] lip tonus,[9] lip area, lip contact (competence), lip strength, interlabial gap, amount of overjet, amount of fatty tissue and musculature, and postoperative edema.[17]

Because of swelling, tissue redistribution, and functional adaptation, long-term follow-up is needed to assess soft tissue changes after surgical procedures. Most authors suggest that the soft tissues stabilize after 6 months.[15,17,19,21,22] Others suggest that at least 12 months are required.[11,24] Hack and colleagues found evidence of continued soft tissue settling several years after surgery.[25] Surgical technique and method of wound closure have been shown to affect soft tissue relationships.[6,9,15,16,18,19,26–28] For example, the horizontal incision in the upper labial vestibule commonly used to gain access to the maxilla for the Le Fort I osteotomy causes shortening of the lip with loss of vermilion and a decrease in lip thickness,[16] whereas vertical incisions with a tunneling approach and palatal flap for the same surgical procedure show minimal postoperative lip changes.[19] Betts and colleagues, investigating the soft tissue response to maxillary surgery, noted that soft tissue changes may be more affected by the type and position of the soft tissue incision and methods used in closure than by the surgically induced hard tissue change.[4]

Changes in facial esthetics and occlusion following orthognathic surgery depend highly on the stability achieved following surgery. Simply put, the soft tissue will mirror changes in the bony foundation should skeletal relapse occur.

Many authors have shown that thin lips move more predictably than thick lips.[5,6,10,17,22,23] Two theories have been advanced to explain this discovery. First, the actual bulk of a thick lip may have a tendency to absorb a large amount of bony advancement without a perceptible change in soft tissue contour. Second, "dead space" under the lip may absorb the first portion of a bony advancement before the soft tissue is affected (eg, with severe maxillary retrognathia).[5,6,10,17,22,23]

The general trend noted in the literature is that the horizontal changes in the soft tissues are often predictable, whereas the vertical changes are unpredictable. This may be because of smaller movements in the vertical plane and the use of soft and hard tissue landmarks better suited for horizontal assessment. Also, hard tissue change is less predictable and less stable in the vertical dimension.

The cephalometric landmarks shown in Figure 59-1 will be used to describe the relationships between the soft and hard tissue changes presented in the rest of this chapter.

Orthodontic Incisor Retraction

Most orthodontic changes will be reflected in changes in the position and posture of the lips. Early studies in the orthodontic literature stressed that the soft tissue profile was closely related to skeletal and dental structures.[29] More recent work has demonstrated that a direct relationship between hard and soft tissue changes may not always exist.[20,30] Simply put, the position of the lips is not solely determined by tooth position. The effects of growth and development, large ANB angle (angle formed by A point, nasion, and B point), positional relationship of the upper incisor on the lower lip (overbite and overjet), and adipose tissue are other factors that confuse the issue and may contribute to the great individual variability observed.[14,31]

The changes in the soft tissues associated with orthodontic incisor movements are seen in Table 59-2.

Review of the literature indicates that with incisor retraction, the upper lip rotates backward around subnasale,[18] with an associated reduction in the prominence of the lips relative to their adjacent sulci.[32]

Also, upper lip thickness increases with maxillary incisor retraction (1 mm with 3 mm of incisor retraction,[33] 1 mm with 1.5 mm of incisor retraction[34]). Correlation analysis discloses that upper lip response is related not only to the upper incisor retraction, but also to lower incisor movement, mandibular rotation, and the position of the lower lip.

The lower lip moves less predictably with retraction of the incisors than does the upper lip.[32] Several theories have been advanced to explain this phenomenon. Hershey has theorized that this is because the lower lip is much more self-supporting and not as dependent upon underlying incisor support.[32] Other investigators feel that this is explained by combined upper and lower incisor effects on the lower-lip positioning (note the –1:1 effect of upper incisor retraction to lower-lip retraction).[35] They feel that the upper teeth, not the lower, establish the curve of the lower lip. Therefore, if the upper incisor is retracted more than the lower incisor, the lower lip may displace more posteriorly than the lower incisor (–1.56:1,[35] –1.22:1[32]). Another theory is that many factors contribute to the final position of the lower lip. This theory is supported by correlation analysis, which indicates that mandibular rotation had a greater influence on lower lip response than did incisor movement. Stepwise regression analysis lends further support to this theory by revealing a complex interaction between dental movement, mandibular rotation, and the perioral soft tissues, as well as a complex relationship within the soft tissues themselves.

Maxillary Surgical Procedures

Most soft tissue change after Le Fort I surgery is manifested in the nasal and labial structures.[36–38]

Nasal Structures

Movement of the maxilla affects the lower aspect of the nasal dorsum.[5,6,21,36–39] The general trend is a widening of the alar base in all patients regardless of the vector of maxillary movement. An associated shortening of the columellar height, alar height and nasal tip projection has been observed, and the nasolabial angle decreases or remains constant in most cases (Figure 59-2).[4]

Different movements of the maxilla have distinct effects on the nasal and labial morphology (Table 59-3). Superior repositioning of the maxilla causes elevation of the nasal tip,[40,41] widening of the alar bases,[4,41] and a decrease in the nasolabial angle.[40] Inferior maxillary repositioning produces loss of nasal tip support, downward movement of the columella and alar bases, thinning of the lip, and an increase in the nasolabial angle. Anterior repositioning of the maxilla has a profound effect on the nose and upper lip, resulting in advancement of the upper lip, subnasale and pronasale, thinning of the lip,[16] widening of the alar bases, and an increase in the supratip break if the ANS is left intact.[8,36–38] The nasal tip advances approximately one-half the distance of subnasale.[21] This may be a result of widening at the alar base, which reduces nasal tip protrusion.[4]

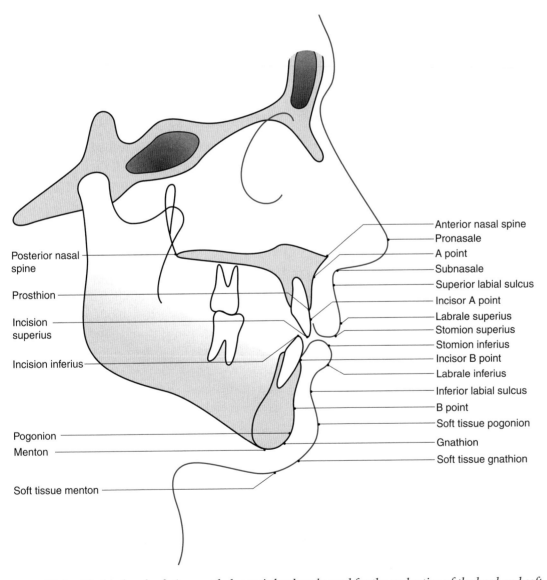

Posterior nasal spine
Prosthion
Incision superius
Incision inferius
Pogonion
Menton
Soft tissue menton

Anterior nasal spine
Pronasale
A point
Subnasale
Superior labial sulcus
Incisor A point
Labrale superius
Stomion superius
Stomion inferius
Incisor B point
Labrale inferius
Inferior labial sulcus
B point
Soft tissue pogonion
Gnathion
Soft tissue gnathion

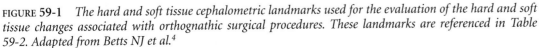

FIGURE 59-1 *The hard and soft tissue cephalometric landmarks used for the evaluation of the hard and soft tissue changes associated with orthognathic surgical procedures. These landmarks are referenced in Table 59-2. Adapted from Betts NJ et al.[4]*

Table 59-2	Soft Tissue Changes Associated with Orthodontic Tooth Movement		
Anatomic Structure	*Ratio*	*Orthodontic Movement*	*Author*
Superior sulcus (H)	−0.89:1	Upper incisor retraction	
Upper lip (H)	−0.87:1	Upper incisor retraction	
Lower sulcus (H)	−0.87:1	Lower incisor retraction	
Lower lip (H)	−0.93:1	Lower incisor retraction	
Lower lip (H)	−0.82:1	Upper incisor retraction	Bloom[*14]
Upper lip (H)	−0.34:1	Upper incisor retraction	
Lower lip (H)	−1.56:1	Lower incisor retraction	
Lower lip (H)	−1:1	Upper incisor retraction	Rudee[*35]
Upper, lower lips (H)	±0.75–0.9:1	Incisor protrusion or retraction	Robinson et al[*61]
Upper lip (H)	−0.5:1	Ls: Ia Upper incisor retraction	
Lower lip (H)	−1.22:1	Li: Ib Lower incisor retraction	Hershey , Smith[7]
Upper lip (H), increased nasolabial angle, no nasal change	−0.5:1	Maxillary incisor retraction	Proffit, Epker[18]
Upper lip (H)	−0.63:1	Ls: Upper incisor retraction	Rains, Nanda[101] Attarzadeh, Adenwalla[31]
Upper lip (H)	−0.4:1	Ls: Upper incisor retraction	
Lower lip (H)	−0.7:1	Li: Upper incisor retraction	Yogosawa[102]
Upper lip (H)	−0.44:1	Ls: Upper incisor retraction	
Lower lip (H)	−1.2:1	Li: Lower incisor retraction	Kasai[103]

*Includes growing patients.
H = horizontal; Ia = incisor A point; Ib = incisor B point; Li = labrale inferius; Ls = labrale superius.

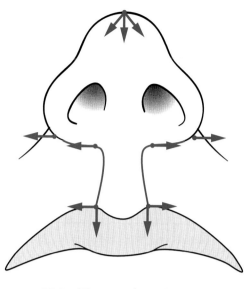

FIGURE 59-2   *The general trends of postsurgical changes in the nasal and labial soft tissues expressed in a nonvector format (the arrows are not specific for length, but are specific for direction). Generally, the alar base of the nose widened and the nasal tip decreased in height in relation to the adjacent soft tissues. The philtral columns of the lip widened and became longer, and the nasolabial angle decreased. Adapted from Betts NJ. Changes in the nasal and labial soft tissues after surgical repositioning of the maxilla. [master's thesis] Ann Arbor (MI): University of Michigan; 1990.*

Preoperative alar-base width of the nose is important in final postsurgical outcome. Narrow noses were observed to widen more at the alar base than did broad noses.[4,26] Important nasal changes have been documented as a result of rotation of the maxilla.[9,42] A counterclockwise rotation of the occlusal plane raises the nasal tip, while a clockwise rotation of the occlusal plane decreases the superior movement of nasal tip.[6,42]

Labial Structure

Maxillary surgery has a significant impact on upper lip morphology and position. The upper lip is attached to the nose and this prevents a 1:1 soft tissue change.[43] The upper lip widens and lengthens at the philtral columns after maxillary surgery.[4] Shortening of the upper lip with a loss of exposed vermilion can occur if a V-Y closure technique is not employed at the time of surgery.[16,28]

Anterior Segmental Repositioning

The soft tissue changes associated with the maxillary segmental setback osteotomy include an increase in the nasolabial angle because of posterior lip rotation around subnasale,[43–46] lengthening of the upper lip, decrease in interlabial gap,[46] and uncurling and retraction of the lower lip with associated decrease in the depth of the inferior labial sulcus (Table 59-4).[45]

Table 59-3	Nasal Effects of Maxillary Surgery				
Direction Maxillary Movement	*Alar Bases*	*Nasal Tip*	*Supratip Depression*	*Dorsal Hump*	*Nasolabial Angle*
Superior	Increase	Increase	Increase	Decrease	Decrease
Anterior	Increase*	Increase*	Increase*	Decrease	Decrease
Inferior	Inferior	Decrease	Decrease	Increase	Increase
Posterior	None	Decrease	Decrease	Increase	Increase

*Indicates a greater magnitude of change.
Adapted from O'Ryan F, Schendel S. Nasal anatomy and maxillary surgery. III. Surgical techniques for correction of nasal deformities in patients undergoing maxillary surgery. Int J Adult Orthodon Orthognath Surg 1989;4:157.

Table 59-4   Soft Tissue Changes Associated with Anterior Segmental Setback Osteotomy

Anatomic Structure	Ratio	Landmarks	Author(s)
Increased nasolabial angle			
Upper lip (H)	−0.68:1	Ls: Ia	Bell, Dann[69]
Upper lip (H)	−0.5:1	Ls: Is	Lines, Steinhauser[43]
Upper lip (H), increased nasolabial angle	−0.67:1		
Lower lip (H)	−0.3:1		Proffit, Epker[18]
Upper lip (H)	−0.43:1	Ls: Is	
Nasolabial angle	12.2°	Increase	Lew, et al[46]

H = horizontal; Ia = incisor A point; Is = incision superius; Ls = labrale superius.

Anterior Repositioning

Maxillary anterior repositioning has the greatest effect on the nose and upper lip. This movement precipitates advancement of the upper lip, subnasale, and nose,[6,36–38] slight shortening of the upper lip, thinning of the lip (approximately 2 mm),[10,36–38,47] widening of the alar bases,[36–38] and a deepening of the supratip depression if the ANS is left intact.[21,23,36–38,48] A progressive increase in the horizontal soft tissue displacement is seen from the tip of the nose to the free end of the upper lip.[37] A concomitant decrease in nasolabial angle is observed with only slight changes in the lower lip.[5,18] Leaving the ANS intact has a favorable effect on the forward displacement of the upper lip and especially the base of the nose (subnasale).[24] The ratios derived from previous investigations can be found in Table 59-5.

A significant difference between the ratio of horizontal change of upper incisor to vermilion border of the upper lip in previous studies (0.6:1)[6,21,22] compared with the ratio reported by Carlotti and colleagues (0.9:1)[48] is a result of the use of the alar cinch suture and V-Y closure during the surgical procedure. The ratio reduces with larger advancements because of soft tissue stretching.[48] If the ANS is left intact, the nasolabial angle may remain relatively unchanged. The nasal tip rises slightly so subnasale migrates forward along with the upper lip.[15]

Superior Repositioning

Superior repositioning of the maxilla causes elevation of the nasal tip,[21,36–38] widening of the alar bases (2–4 mm),[23,26,36–38] and a decrease in the nasolabial angle (Table 59-6).[36–38] These nasal changes occur without change in angulation of the upper lip.[6,8] The upper lip closely follows the movement of the maxillary incisor in the horizontal plane. The lip follows superiorly approximately 40% of the vertical maxillary change. This lip shortening is accentuated with combined anterior and superior maxillary movements.[23] The amount of vertical soft tissue change increases progressively from the nasal tip to stomion superius, with loss of vermilion if a V-Y closure is not used.[6,8] However, Phillips found that the vermilion border of the upper and lower lips decreased slightly in the lateral portion of the lip, even with a V-Y closure.[26] Interestingly, when superimposition is done on maxillary landmarks, the soft tissues of the lip migrate downward in relation to the maxilla. This may be because of the connection of the upper lip to the nose.[6,8]

Inferior Repositioning

Maxillary inferior repositioning produces loss of nasal tip support, downward repositioning of the columella and alar bases, thinning of the lip, and an increase in the nasolabial angle.[36–38] Lengthening and thinning of the upper lip is also observed.[18]

Posterior Repositioning

Maxillary setback procedures result in loss of nasal tip support because of posterior movement of the ANS and the bony support area around the piriform aperture.[37] The lip rotates posteriorly and superiorly about subnasale with increasing nasolabial angle[8,49] and thickens slightly (Table 59-7).[49]

Multidirectional Maxillary Movements

Most maxillary movements are multidirectional (anterior and superior, anterior and inferior, posterior and superior, posterior and inferior, etc). The expected soft tissue changes would be a combination of the expected changes from the pure vectors of movement (Figures 59-3–59-5).

Mandibular Surgical Procedures

Generally the soft tissues of the mandible follow the hard tissues closely. The exception is the lower lip. Because of its contact with the upper incisor and upper lip, its movement is often variable and unpredictable.

Anterior Segmental Posterior Repositioning

The lower lip follows the lower incisor posteriorly, which causes a flattening of the labiomental fold. There is less posterior displacement of the soft tissues as the chin is approached. No effective change is observed at the chin (Table 59-8).[43]

Anterior Repositioning

The soft tissue changes associated with mandibular advancement surgery are limited to the structures below the superior labial sulcus. There is little change in the upper lip[43,50–52] and none above the ANS.[53] The lower lip advancement is variable, and the lip often lengthens.[53] The lower labial sulcus and chin adhere to the bony structure of the mandible. Consequently, they follow the underlying osseous tissues closely, advancing more than the lower lip does (Figure 59-6). This leads to an opening of the labiomental

Table 59-5   Soft Tissue Changes Associated with Maxillary Advancement

Anatomic Structure	Ratio	Landmarks	Author(s)
Upper lip (H)	0.67:1	Ls: Is Cleft pts. removed ANS	Lines, Steinhauser [43]
Upper lip (H)	0.5:1	Ls: Is	
Upper lip (V)	0.3:1	Ls: Is	
Nasolabial angle	−1.2°:1	Nasolabial angle: Is	
Nasal tip (H)	0.28:1	Pn: Is	Dann, et al [5]
Nasal base (H)	0.57:1	Sn: A pt.	
Upper lip (H)	0.56:1	Ls: Is cleft pts	Freihofer [22]
Nasal base (H)	0.57:1	Sn: A pt.	
Nasal tip (H)	0.28:1	Pn: A pt. cleft pts	Freihofer [21]
Upper lip (H)	0.5:1		Proffit, Epker [18]
Nasal tip (H)	0.17:1	Pn: Ia	
Upper lip (H)	0.5:1	Ls: Is	Radney, Jacobs [8]
Nasal tip (H)	0.17:1	Pn: Ia	
Nasal base (H)	0.24:1	Sn: Ia	
Upper labial sulcus (H)	0.52:1	SLS: Ia	
Upper lip (H)	0.62:1	Ls: Ia	Mansour, et al [6]
Upper lip (H)	0.5:1	Ss: A pt.	
Upper lip (V)	−0.3:1	Ss: A pt.	Bundgaard, et al [42]
Upper labial sulcus (H)	0.8:1	SLS: A pt., alar cinch, V-Y closure	
Upper lip (H)	0.9:1	Ls: Is	Carlotti, et al [48]
Upper lip (H)	0.82:1	Ls: Is	
Upper lip (V)	−0.32:1	Ss: Is	
Nasal base (H)	0.51:1	Sn: A pt.	Rosen [23]
Nasal base (H)	0.3:1	Sn: A pt. (thick lip)	
Nasal base (H)	0.46:1	Sn: A pt. (thin lip)	Stella, et al [10]
Upper lip (middle) (H)	1:1	3-D analysis	McChance, et al [104,105]
Nasal base	1.25:1	3-D analysis	
Subnasale	0.63:1	Sn: A pt. cleft pts	Ewing, Ross [78]
Upper lip (H)	0.66:1	SLS: Is	
Nasal tip	0.36:1	Pn: Is	
Upper lip (H)	0.91:1	SLS: Is	
Upper labial sulcus (H)	0.38:1	SLS: A pt	
Nasal base (H)	0.60:1	Sn: ANS	Hack et al [25]
Upper Lip (H)	0.74	Ls: Is	
Upper labial sulcus (H)	0.76:1	SLS: A pt	Lin, Kerr [106]
Upper lip (H)	0.65:1	Ls: Is	Rosenberg, et al [27]

A pt. = A point; ANS = anterior nasal spine; H = horizontal; Ia = incisor A point; Is = incision superius; Ls = labrale
Pn = pronasale; SLS = superior labial sulcus; Sn = subnasale; Ss = stomion superius; V = vertical.

fold. As with maxillary and genial surgeries, the vertical changes are variable.

A correlation between the vertical change in menton and the angle and depth of the labiomental fold has been elucidated. As menton moves caudally, the angle opens and the depth decreases.[50]

Facial height is also affected by mandibular advancement. In low-angle, Angle Class II cases, facial height increases slightly with advancement, but in high-angle, Angle Class II cases, a large increase in facial height occurs with advancement. Further, soft tissue changes may be more pronounced with advancements in low-angle cases (Table 59-9).[54]

The position of the lower lip is affected by the upper incisor, the lower incisor, and its contact with the upper lip. The anterosuperior position of the upper one-half of the lower lip touches the upper incisor in Angle Class II, non-open-bite cases and is usually folded forward. As the mandible is advanced, the chin and lower labial sulcus come forward, but the superior portion of the lower lip does not, since it was already folded forward by its contact with the upper incisor. This causes an opening of the labiomental fold and may explain why the ratio of advancement at labrale inferius to the incisor inferius is reduced.[18,43,53] Consequently during treatment planning, the lower lip must be righted to a relatively normal position before it is advanced in order to approximate its true postsurgical position.

Dolce and colleagues, with 2 years of follow-up, suggest that these changes are more stable when rigid fixation techniques are employed.[55] Long-term, more horizontal relapse can be expected at the level of the lip and the lower labial sulcus than at the level of pogonion.[56] As Johnston[57] and Mobarak[54] point out, the lack of correlation between surgical hard tissue movements and the soft tissue changes long-term make prediction of lasting changes difficult to predict.

Posterior Repositioning

Mandibular setback surgery has no effects on subnasale or the tissues superior to subnasale. However, a slight posterior displacement of the upper lip, with lengthening,[18,58,59] and a slight increase in the nasolabial angle is observed.[60] The soft tissues follow the mandible posteriorly, with the chin following most closely, followed by the inferior labial sulcus and the lower lip. The lower lip shortens, becomes more protrusive by curling out, and the labiomental fold deepens and becomes more acute (Figure 59-7).[7,58–60] Vertical changes of the soft tissues of the lips are related to hard tissue vertical changes. During

Table 59-6   Soft Tissue Changes Associated with Maxillary Impaction

Anatomic Structure	Ratio	Landmarks	Author(s)
Upper lip (V)	–0.38:1	Ls: Is vertical maxillary excess	
Upper lip (V)	–0.51:1	Ls: Is bimaxillary protrusion	Schendel, et al [49]
Upper lip (V)	–0.4:1	Ss: Is	
Upper lip (V)	–0.3:1	Ls: Is	
Upper labial sulcus (V)	–0.25:1	SLS: Is	
Nose (V)	–0.2:1	Sn: Is	
Nose (V)	–0.16:1	Pn: Is (ANS removed)	Radney, Jacobs [8]
Upper labial sulcus (H)	0.76:1	SLS: Ia	
Upper lip (H)	0.89:1	Ls: Ia	
Nose (V)	–0.15:1	Pn: Pr	
Nasal base (V)	–0.28:1	Sn: Pr	
Upper lip (V)	–0.31:1	Ls:Pr	
Upper lip (V)	–0.42:1	SLS: Is	Mansour, et al [6]
Upper labial sulcus (V)	0.12:1	SLS: ANS	
Upper lip (V)	–0.06:1	Ls: ANS	
Upper lip (V)	–0.41:1	Ss: ANS	Sakima, Sachdeva [9]
Upper lip (V)	1.33:1	Ss: A pt (**V-Y** closure)	Rosenberg, et al [27]
Full face evaluation			
Greatest alar width	Average = 3.4mm	Full facial photographs	
Alar base width	Average = 2.7mm		
Decreased vermilion more lateral	Average l mm	V-Y closure	Phillips, et al [26]
Upper lip (middle) (H)	1:1	3-D analysis	McChance, et al [104,105]
Alar Base (H)	1.25:1	3-D analysis	
Nasal base (V)	0.29:1	Sn: ANS	Hack, et al [25]
Upper labial sulcus (V)	0.54:1	SLS: A pt	
Upper lip (V)	0.72:1	SLS: Is	

A pt. = A point; ANS = anterior nasal spine; H = horizontal; Ia = incisor A point; Is = incision superius; Ls = labrale superius; Me = menton; Pn = pronasale; Pr = prosthion; SLS = superior labial sulcus; Sn = subnasale; Ss = stomion superius; V=vertical.

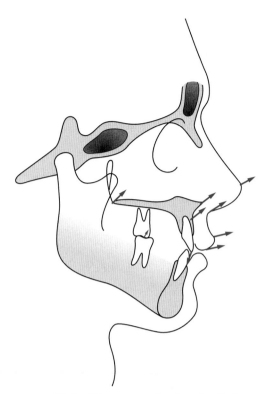

FIGURE **59-3**   *The average hard and soft tissue changes of the advancement, impaction group in vector format (arrows depict mean direction and mean amount of change). Note that the nasal tip elevates slightly, but subnasale advances more, effectively decreasing nasal tip protrusion. Adapted from Betts NJ. Changes in the nasal and labial soft tissues after surgical repositioning of the maxilla [master's thesis]. University of Michigan; 1990.*

superior mandibular repositioning, the lower lip becomes shorter, protrusive, and smaller in area. In contrast, with inferior mandibular repositioning, the lower lip becomes longer in area.[61] The vertical soft tissue changes correlate poorly with hard tissue movements (Table 59-10).[61] As with mandibular advancements, long-term soft tissue changes have been found to correlate relatively poorly with the initial surgical bony changes, though in the short term they do change predictably.[62]

Autorotation

During autorotation of the mandible, the soft tissues follow the osseous landmarks on approximately a 1:1 basis,[6,8] except the lower lip, which falls slightly lingual to the arc of rotation.[6,8,15] A slight increase in the labiomental angle is often observed,[6] as is a slight thickening of the lips as the vertical facial height decreases (Table 59-11).[43]

Table 59-7   Soft Tissue Changes Associated with Maxillary Setback

Anatomic Structure	Ratio	Landmarks	Author(s)
Upper lip (H)	–0.76:1	Ls: Incisor vertical maxillary excess	
Upper lip (H)	–0.66:1	Ls: Incisor bimaxillary protrusion	Schendel et al[49]
Upper lip (H)	–0.67:1	Ls: Is	
Upper labial sulcus (H)	–0.33:1	SLS: Is	
Nose (H)	–0.33:1	Sn: Is	
Nasolabial angle	Increase		Radney, Jacobs[8]

H = horizontal; Is = incision superius; LS = labrale superius; SLS = superior labial sulcus; Sn = subnasale.

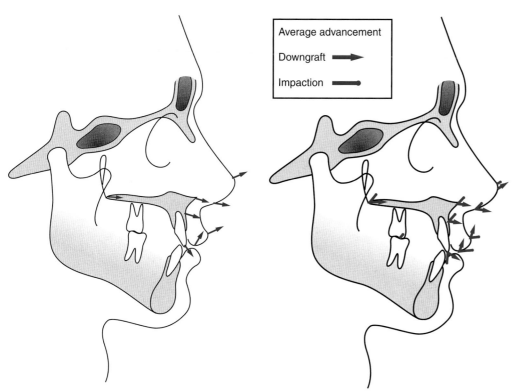

Average advancement

Downgraft ➡

Impaction ⟶•

FIGURE **59-4** *The average hard and soft tissue changes of the advancement, downgraft group in vector format (arrows depict mean direction and mean amount of change). Note that the nasal tip elevates slightly, but subnasale advances more, effectively decreasing the nasal tip protrusion. Adapted from Betts NJ. Changes in the nasal and labial soft tissues after surgical repositioning of the maxilla [master's thesis]. Ann Arbor (MI): University of Michigan; 1990.*

FIGURE **59-5** *Overlay of average hard and soft tissue changes of advancement, impaction and advancement, downgraft in vector format. Average advancement (see legend above) as defined by the mean direction and mean amount of change, is indicated by arrows (downgraft) and lines with dots (impaction). Note that subnasale moves in the direction of the anterior nasal spine and A point. Adapted from Betts NJ. Changes in the nasal and labial soft tissues after surgical repositioning of the maxilla [master's thesis] Ann Arbor (MI): University of Michigan; 1990.*

Genial Segment Surgical Procedures

The symphysis has been exposed both intraorally and extraorally for osteotomy of the inferior border of the mandible to advance, retract, widen, narrow, lengthen, or shorten the chin.[45] The majority of change seen after genioplasty is in the soft tissue of the chin, and less effect is seen in the labial sulcus and lower lip.[63] Early studies describing the soft tissue changes associated with genial surgery had several problems. They included few cases, related short-term results, and superimposed the cephalograms on the cranial base. Superimposition of the cephalograms should occur on the areas of the mandible not changed with surgery,[13,64,65] because concomitant maxillary and mandibular

surgery may invalidate chin measurements calculated from superimpositions on the cranial base.[66–68]

Anterior Repositioning: Bony

Early attempts at advancement genioplasty used nonpedicled free grafts or onlay bone

grafts. However, these procedures were later abandoned because of excessive resorption and poor predictability. Consequently, the surgical emphasis shifted to the horizontal osteotomy of the anterior mandible.

At first a degloving incision was used to expose the anterior mandible.[67,69,70] However, several investigators demonstrated that minimal soft tissue stripping gave a more predictable hard and soft tissue response because of less bone resorption of the advanced segment.[13,45,65,66,71,72] No bony remodeling of gnathion or menton was observed. However, bone resorption could be demonstrated near the osteotomy (the anterosuperior and posteroinferior aspects of the advanced genial segment).[66,67,69,70,72–74] Bony apposition occurred at B point and the inferior border osteotomy (Figure 59-8).[67] These same studies demonstrated that when the technique of minimal soft tissue stripping was used, the soft tissues followed the hard tissues closely without chin droop.[13,45,65,66,68] There was also a small but negligible effect on the labiomental sulcus,[66,68] an increase in submental length, an improved relationship of lower lip to tooth,[66] less soft tissue thinning,[68] and an improved neck-chin angle.

The soft tissue changes following horizontal advancement genioplasty depend on the magnitude and direction of the positional change of the genial segment, the design of the mucosal and osseous incisions, the amount of soft tissue stripping, and other concomitant jaw movements (Table 59-12).[13,66,67,69,70]

Table 59-8	Soft Tissue Changes Associated with Mandibular Anterior Segmental Osteotomy		
Anatomic Structure	*Ratio*	*Landmarks*	*Author(s)*
Lower lip (H)	−0.75:1	Li: Ii	Lines and Steinhauser[43]
Lower lip (H)	−0.67:1		
Chin (H)	No change		Proffit, Epker[18]
Lower lip (H)	−0.71:1	Li: Ii	Lew et al[46]

H = horizontal; Ii = incision inferius; Li = labrale inferius.

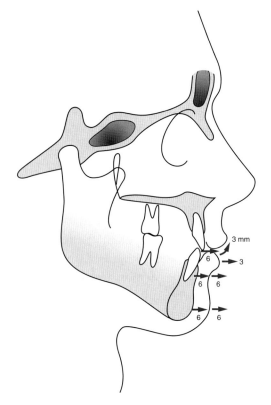

FIGURE **59-6** *Overlay of average hard and soft tissue changes of mandibular advancement in vector format. Generally the soft tissues follow the bony movements in a 1:1 ratio. Adapted from Betts NJ, Dowd KF. Soft tissue changes associated with orthognathic surgery. Atlas Oral Maxillofac Surg Clin North Am 2000;8:13–38.*

The advantages of osseous genial surgery are preservation of the normal chin contour,[75] improved predictability of the soft tissue response,[45] stability,[45,68] versatility,[45] and preservation of blood supply to osteotomized segments.[75]

Those patients who had both vertical reduction and advancement genioplasties showed slightly larger soft tissue advancement than those who had advancement genioplasty only (0.93:1 vs 0.81:1). This may be explained by bunching of the soft tissues. When the soft tissues are bunched (vertical reduction more than advancement), the soft tissues advance more than when the soft tissues are stretched (advancement only).[66,76]

Tulasne suggested that the overlapping bone flap genioplasty gives a more natural contour to the lower face and a better balance between the lower lip, chin, and submental

Table 59-9	Soft Tissue Changes Associated with Mandibular Advancement		
Anatomic Structure	*Ratio*	*Landmarks*	*Author(s)*
Lower lip (H)	0.62:1	Li: Ii	
Chin (H)	1:1	Pgs: Gn	Lines, Steinhauser[43]
Lower lip (H)	0.85:1	Li: Ii	
Lower labial sulcus	1.01:1	ILS: B pt.	
Chin (H)	1.04:1	Pgs: Pg	Talbott[51]
Lower lip (H)	0.75:1		
Chin (H)	1:1		Proffit, Epker[18]
Lower lip (H)	0.38:1	Li: Ii	
Lower labial sulcus (H)	0.97:1	ILS: B pt.	
Chin (H)	0.97:1	Pgs: Pg	
Chin (H)	0.97:1	Gns: Gn	
Chin (H)	0.87:1	Mes: Me	Quast, et al[11]
Lower lip (H)	0.56:1	Li: Ii	
Lower labial sulcus	1.06:1	ILS: B pt.	
Chin (H)	1.03:1	Pgs: Pg	
Chin (V)	0.93:1	Mes: Me	Mommaerts, Marxer[50]
Upper lip (H)	−0.02:1	Ls: Ii	
Lower lip (H)	0.43:1	Li: Ii	
Lower labial sulcus (H)	0.93:1	ILS: B pt.	
Chin (H)	0.94:1	Pgs: Pg	
Chin (H)	0.95:1	Gns: Gn	
Chin (H)	0.97:1	Mes: Me	Hernandez-Orsini et al[113]
Lower lip (H)	0.26:1	Li: Ii	
Lower labial sulcus (H)	1.19:1	ILS: B pt.	
Chin (H)	1.1:1	Pgs: Pg	Dermaut, De Smit[53]
Lower lip (H)	1.25:1	3-D analysis	
Chin (H)	1.25:1	3-D analysis	McChance[104,105]
Lower lip (H)	0.66:1	Li:Ii	
Lower labial sulcus (H)	0.88:1	ILS: B pt	
Chin (H)	1:1	Pgs:Pg	Thuer, et al[52]
Lower lip (H)	0.88:1	ILS:B pt	
Chin (H)	1:1	Pgs:Pg	Keeling, et al[56]
Lower lip (H)	0.8:1	Li:Ii	
Lower labial sulcus (H)	1:1	ILS:B pt.	
Chin (H)	1:1	Pgs:Pg	Ewing, Ross[78]
Lower lip (H)	0.6:1	Li:Ii (all faces)	
Lower labial sulcus (H)	0.86-0.95:1	ILS: B pt.	
Chin (H)	1-1.1:1	Pgs:Pg	
Menton	0.92-1.04:1	Mes:Me	Mobarak, et al[62]

B pt. = B point; Gn = gnathion; Gns = soft tissue gnathion;H = horizontal; Ii = incision inferius; ILS = inferior labial sulcus; Li = labrale inferius; Ls = Labrale superius; Me = menton; Mes = soft tissue menton Pg = pogonion; Pgs = soft tissue pogonion; V = vertical.

region than does the sliding genioplasty associated with a wedge ostectomy.[77] However, it is associated with a large amount of bony resorption, especially in adolescent patients.

Predictions of lower and genial soft tissue changes when a genioplasty is added

to a mandibular advancement are notoriously variable.[78] However, the use of rigid internal fixation for the mandibular advancement makes the soft tissue changes in the chin and lip more durable in the long term.[55]

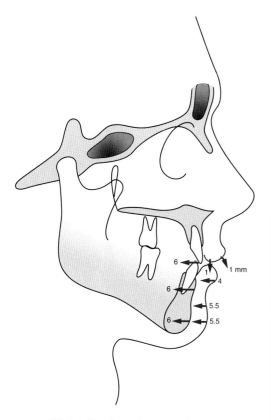

FIGURE **59-7** *Overlay of average hard and soft tissue changes of mandibular setback in vector format. The soft tissues of pogonion and B point move more predictably than labrale inferius. Adapted from Betts NJ, Dowd KF. Soft tissue changes associated with orthognathic surgery. Atlas Oral Maxillofac Surg Clin North Am 2000;8:13–38.*

Anterior Repositioning: Alloplastic

Early attempts at advancement genioplasty included the use of alloplastic implants. Unfortunately, long-term follow-up revealed several unforeseen complications. For this reason, advancement genioplasty with alloplastic implants has fallen out of favor. The disadvantages of alloplastic materials include resorption or deformation of the underlying symphyseal bone with possible devitalization of the mandibular anterior teeth,[12,18,47,79–81] migration of the implant,[45,69,79] extrusion of the implant,[79] infection (especially with Proplast),[45,69] and a less predictable soft tissue to hard tissue ratio.[45,69] In addition, alloplastic materials do not address excessive or reduced chin height.[69] Newer materials have been developed that reduce the incidence of these

Table 59-10 Soft Tissue Changes Associated with Mandibular Setback

Anatomic Structure	Ratio	Landmarks	Author(s)
Lower lip (H)	−0.69:1	Li: Pg	
Lower labial sulcus (H)	−0.93:1	ILS: Pg	Aaronson[60]
Lower labial sulcus (H)	approx. −1:1	ILS: B pt.	
Chin (H)	approx. −1:1	Pgs: Pg	Robinson et al[61]
Upper lip (H)	−0.2:1	Ls: Ii	
Lower lip (H)	−0.75:1	Li: Ii	
Chin (H)	−1:1	Pgs: Gn	Lines, Steinhauser[43]
Upper lip (H)	−0.2:1	Ls: Pg	
Lower lip (H)	−0.6:1	Li: Pg	
Chin (H)	−0.9:1	Pgs: Pg	Hershey, Smith[7]
Upper lip (H)	−0.2:1		
Lower lip (H)	−0.75–0.8:1		
Chin (H)	−1:1		Proffit, Epker[18]
Lower lip (H)	−0.93:1	Li: Ii	
Lower labial sulcus (H)	−.03:1	ILS: B pt	
Chin (H)	−.91:1	Pgs: Pg	Gjorup, Athanasiou[110]
Lower Lip (H)	−1:1	3-D analysis	McChance et al[104, 105]
Chin (H)	−1:1	3-D analysis	
Upper lip (H)	−0.32:1	Ls: Pg	
Lower lip (H)	−0.80:1	Li: Pg	
Chin (H)	−0.83:1	Pgs: Pg	Gaggl et al[111]
Lower lip (H)	−0.5:1	Li: Pg	Enacar et al[112]
Lower lip (H)	−1.02:1	Li: Ii	
Lower labial sulcus (H)	−1.09:1	ILS: B pt.	
Chin (H)	−1.04:1	Pgs: Pg	Mobarak et al[62]

B pt. = B point; Gn = gnathion; H = horizontal; Ii = incision inferius; ILS = inferior labial sulcus; Li = labrale inferius; Ls = labrale superius; Pg = pogonion; Pgs = soft tissue pogonion.

Table 59-11 Soft Tissue Changes Associated with Mandibular Autorotation

Anatomic Structure	Ratio	Landmarks	Author(s)
Chin (V)	−0.8:1	Pgs: Gn	Lines, Steinhauser[43]
Chin (H)	1:1		
Lower labial sulcus	1:1	ILS: B pt.	
Chin (H)	1:1	Pgs: Pg	Radney, Jacobs[8]
Lower lip (H)	0.75:1	Li: Ii	
Lower labial sulcus (H)	0.9:1	ILS: B pt.	
Chin (H)	0.86:1	Pgs: Pg	
Lower lip (V)	−0.93:1	Si: Is	
Chin (V)	−1.2:1	Mes: Me	Mansour et al[6]
Lower lip (V)	−1.03:1	Si: Me	
Lower lip (V)	−1.48:1*	Li: Me	
Inferior labial sulcus (V)	−1.05:1	ILS: Me	
Inferior labial sulcus (H)	0.61:1	ILS: Me	
Chin (H)	0.79:1	Pgs: Me	
Chin (V)	−0.98:1	Pgs: Me	Sakima Sachdeva[9]

*May represent uprighting of the lower lip due to a loss of contact with the upper incisor.
B pt. = B point; H = horizontal; ILS = inferior labial sulcus; Ii = incision inferius; Li = labrale inferius; Gn = gnathion; Me = menton; Mes = soft tissue menton Pg = pogonion; Pgs = soft tissue pogonion; Si = stomion inferius; V = vertical.

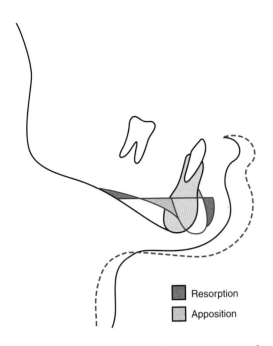

FIGURE **59-8** *Osseous resorption at pogonion and deposition at menton. Adapted from Polido WD, Bell WH. Long-term osseous and soft tissue changes after large chin advancements. J Craniomaxillofac Surg 1993;21:54–9.*

complications, making alloplastic augmentation a more viable option.

If alloplastic implants are used they should be placed subperiosteally, low on the inferior border below the mentalis muscle, and over dense cortical bone. See Table 59-13 for soft tissue changes with alloplastic chin implants. Alloplastic implants should not be used in the correction of severe deformities but can be used in patients with a mild to moderate deformity.[13,47,80] A periodic radiographic examination of the implant is recommended to monitor bony resorption.[47,81]

Posterior Repositioning

Early attempts at reducing horizontal excess of the genial segment of the mandible by bony recontouring caused very little improvement of the soft tissue profile.[64] This technique has been abandoned. The soft tissue changes associated with setback genioplasty are less well correlated with the orthal hard tissue movements than during advancement genioplasty (Table 59-14).

Reduction genioplasty is contraindicated in a patient with minimal or no labiomental fold. Flattening of the chin and elimination of the labiomental fold will

Table 59-12	Soft Tissue Changes Associated with Advancement Genioplasty		
Anatomic Structure	*Ratio*	*Landmarks*	*Author(s)*
Chin (H)	0.57:1	Pgs: Pg Ant. Sliding	Bell, Dann[69]
Chin (H)	0.75:1	Pgs: Pg H (some Multistep)	McDonnel et al[67]
Chin (H)	0.67:1		Proffit, Epker[18]
Chin (H)	approx. 1:1	H with broad soft tissue pedicle IVRO setback	Bell[14]
Lip (H)	0.44:1	Li: Pg H	Busquets, Sassouni[63]
Chin (H)	0.83:1	Pgs: Pg (some with ostectomy)	
Chin (H)	0.97:1	Pgs: Pg H with broad pedicle (IVRO setback)	Scheideman[68]
Chin (H)	0.85:1	H with broad pedicle	Bell, Gallagher[45]
Chin (H)	0.81:1	Pgs: Pg Advancement only, H sliding with broad pedicle	
Chin (H)	0.93:1	Pgs: Pg Advancement and vertical reduction, H sliding with broad pedicle, maxillary impaction	Gallagher et al[66]
Chin (H)	0.7:1	H	Epker, Fish[107]
Chin (H)	0.73:1	Pgs: Pg Overlapping, bone flap	Tulasne[75]
Chin (H)	0.97:1	Pgs: Pg H with broad pedicle	Park et al[65]
Chin (H)	1:1	Pgs: Pg	Krekmanov, Kahnberg[72]
Chin (H)	1.1:1	Pgs: Pg, BSSO+GP	Ewing, Ross[78]
Chin (H)	0.83:1	Pgs: Pg, H with broad pedicle and large advancements	Polido, Bell[108]

BSSO + GP = bilateral sagittal split osteotomy + genioplasty; H = horizontal; IVRO = intraoral vertical ramus osteotomy; Li = labrale inferius; Pg = pogonion; Pgs = soft tissue pogonion.

Table 59-13	Soft Tissue Changes Associated with Alloplastic Chin Implants		
Anatomic Structure	*Ratio*	*Landmarks*	*Author(s)*
Chin (H)	0.6:1	Pgs: Pg Silicone (unstable and cause resorption)	Bell, Dann[69]
Chin (H)	0.9:1	Pgs: Pg Proplast (resorption)	Dann, Epker[79]
Chin (H)	1:1		Proffit, Epker[18]

H = horizontal; Pg = pogonion; Pgs = soft tissue pogonion.

Table 59-14   Soft Tissue Changes Associated with Setback Genioplasty

Anatomic Structure	Ratio	Landmarks	Author(s)
Chin (H)	−0.33:1	Pgs: Pg ant. recontouring degloving dissection	Hohl, Epker[67]
Chin (H)	−0.75:1	Interpositional	Wessberg et al[109]
Chin (H)	−0.58:1	Pgs: Pg H with broad pedicle	Bell[13]
Chin (H)	−0.50:1	Pgs: Pg	Krekmanov, Kahnberg[72]

H = horizontal; sulcus; PG = pogonion; Pg ant. = pogonion anterior; Pgs = soft tissue pogonion.

result.[82] It is also important to realize that setback genioplasty will make undesirable changes in the neck-chin proportion. In a patient with a poor neck-chin proportion, this procedure is contraindicated.

Vertical Repositioning: Superior and Inferior

The soft tissues follow the hard tissues very closely in augmentation genioplasty. However, this is not the case for vertical reduction (inferior border ostectomy or sandwich ostectomy) genioplasty (Table 59-15).

Special Circumstances

Distraction Osteogenesis

Since its first use in the human mandible by McCarthy and colleagues, this surgical technique has exploded in popularity.[83] Its use does not lend itself well to soft tissue predictions of the sort used for orthognathic surgery for various reasons, and few efforts have been made in this regard. Difficulties derive from the fact that most patients are still growing when subjected to the technique, that the principle of gradual distraction of a bone is probably accompanied by a component of soft tissue growth, so-called distraction histogenesis, and that very little is known about the dimensional stability of these bony changes. Efforts in this regard have examined soft tissue profile changes associated with maxillary distraction.[84,85]

However, the technique allows for real-time adjustment of the change within the context of desired occlusion for most

applications, thereby not requiring precise predictions as for conventional orthognathic surgery. The topic will be of great interest, and the stability of the changes only more so as its use for the treatment of obstructive sleep apnea in adults becomes more prevalent.

Overall, the changes observed are comparable to those for maxillary advancement via the Le Fort I osteotomy with a decrease in midfacial concavity, increases in nasal tip projection, advancement of the lip, and closing of the nasolabial angle (Table 59-16).[84,85]

Bimaxillary Advancement Surgery for Obstructive Sleep Apnea

The 5-year incidence of obstructive sleep apnea (OSA) in adult populations in the United States has been estimated to be

7.5% for moderately severe cases and 16% for less severe cases.[86] While orthognathic surgery has traditionally been applied to correct stomatognathic deformities and dysfunction, it also has been shown to be a powerful tool in correcting obstructive sleep apnea.[87,88]

Little work has been done to describe the facial changes associated with this surgery, which differs from traditional orthognathic surgery in several ways. Patients presenting for maxillomandibular advancement surgery for OSA tend to be older, in their fourth and fifth decades of life.[89] They tend to be obese and have a thicker, laxer soft tissue envelope with which to "absorb" these bony changes. They will often present without skeletal imbalances that we traditionally seek to correct. Further, advancements of this sort are generally larger than those seen in the typical orthognathic surgery population, usually ranging from 10 to 12 mm. The goals of this surgery are very different. Here we seek to maximize the skeletal advancement to the benefit of the airway but often to the detriment of the soft tissue profile. Treatment planning then aims to minimize any untoward changes to the profile. Most patients seem to approve or be neutral with respect to their facial changes.[90] Prognathic patients are more likely to disapprove of

Table 59-15   Soft Tissue Changes Associated with Vertical Augmentation or Reduction Genioplasty

Anatomic Structure	Ratio	Landmarks	Author(s)
Augmentation			
Chin (V)	1:1	Interpositional	Wessberg et al[109]
Reduction			
Chin (V)	−0.25:1	Mes: Me, Inferior border, osteotomy, degloving dissection	Hohl, Epker[64]
Chin (V)	−0.26:1	Pgs: Pg H with broad pedicle	Park et al[65]
Chin (V)	−0.35:1	Mes: Me	Krekmanov, Kahnberg[72]
Chin (V)	−0.40:1	Mes: Me	Ewing, Ross[78]

H = horizontal; Me = menton; Mes = soft tissue menton; Pg = pogonion; Pgs = soft tissue pogonion; V = vertical.

Table 59-16   Soft Tissue Changes Associated with Maxillary Distraction Osteogenesis*

Anatomic Structure	Ratio	Landmarks	Author(s)
Nasal tip	0.53:1	Pn: ANS	
Superior labial sulcus (H)	0.96:1	SLS: A pt.	
Upper lip (H)	0.8:1	Ls: Is	Ko et al[85]
Nasal advancement	0.57:1	Pn: ANS	
Superior labial sulcus (H)	0.83:1	Sn: ANS	
Upper lip	0.71:1	Ls: ANS	Harada et al[84]

*All cleft patients.
A pt. = A point; ANS = anterior nasal spine; H = horizontal; Is = incision superius; Ls = labrale superius; Pn= pronasale; SLS = superior labial sulcus; Sn = subnasale.

their new profile.[90] Adjunctive measures such as ANS reshaping may help minimize upper lip and nasal tip rotation, but little can be done to minimize the effects of surgery at the chin (Table 59-17).

In terms of ratios of change in this population, only one study has been reported to date.[91] This overall lack of data does not permit a comparison to traditional orthognathic changes.

Poor Surgical Esthetic Results and Techniques of Soft Tissue Control

Maxilla

The secondary soft tissue changes found with maxillary surgery include widening of the alar bases,[36–38,48,92] upturning of the nasal tip, flattening and thinning of the upper lip,[19,36–38,48,92] downturning of the commissures of the mouth,[36–38,48,92] and opening of the nasolabial angle. These changes are similar to those found in the aging face and are generally perceived as unesthetic.[36–38] Other potentially unesthetic changes include loss of normal lip pout and a decrease in visible vermilion.[19,48,92]

Several investigators have suggested that the etiology of these soft tissue changes is attributable to three factors: (1) elevation of the periosteum and muscle attachments adjacent to the nose without adequate replacement, (2) postsurgical edema, and (3) increased bony support in advancement cases.[24,41]

The importance of muscle repositioning following superior repositioning of the maxilla was stressed by many investigators.[24,48,92,93] They state that the muscles detached during stripping of the periosteum required for maxillary surgery shorten and retract laterally. The muscles reattach in this position if they are not reapproximated at the time of surgery. The lateral movement of the muscles and subcutaneous tissues causes the alar base to flare and the upper lip to thin.

The loss of visible vermilion may be a result of other causes. These include a rolling under of the vermilion of the upper lip secondary to an incision made high in the vestibule with associated scarring and retraction[24,48,92] and inclusion of large amounts of tissue during closure.[24] This loss of vermilion is especially unattractive in those individuals with already thin lips[40] and is more pronounced with posterior and superior repositioning of the maxilla.

Postsurgical widening of the alar base after the maxillary Le Fort I procedure may be a favorable outcome in a patient with vertical maxillary hyperplasia and thin slit-like nares.[15] However, if a wide preoperative alar base is present, these same changes become undesirable,[24,41] especially with anterior or superior repositioning of the maxilla[94] (Figure 59-9A–D). Before techniques to control nasal width were developed, Bell and Proffit suggested that at the time of preoperative assessment, patients with a wide nose be warned that a rhinoplasty may be indicated.[40]

Techniques to Control the Soft Tissues

To control the soft tissue changes associated with maxillary surgery, the surgeon must first be aware of any preexisting deformity, the anticipated soft tissue adaptation to the surgical procedure being planned, and the importance of the effects of orofacial muscles on form, function, and esthetics. Once this has occurred the soft tissues can be manipulated to advantage by the surgeon.[4,93]

Several surgical techniques have been suggested to help control the detrimental soft tissue changes associated with maxillary surgery. They include the V-Y closure, the alar cinch suture, a combination of the alar cinch suture and the V-Y closure, contouring of the ANS, septum reduction, and the double V-Y closure.

Table 59-17   Soft Tissue Changes Associated with Maxillomandibular Advancement for OSA

Anatomic Structure	Ratio	Landmarks	Author(s)
Nasal tip (H)	0.16:1	Pn: Is	
Superior labial sulcus (H)	0.39:1	Sn: Is	
Upper lip (H)	0.80:1	SLS: Is	
Nasal tip (V)	0.16:1	Pn: Is	
Superior labial sulcus (V)	0.16:1	Sn: Is	
Upper lip (V)	0.16:1	SLS: Is	Louis et al[91]

H = horizontal; Is = incision superius; Pn = pronasale; SLS = superior labial sulcus; Sn = subnasale; V = vertical.

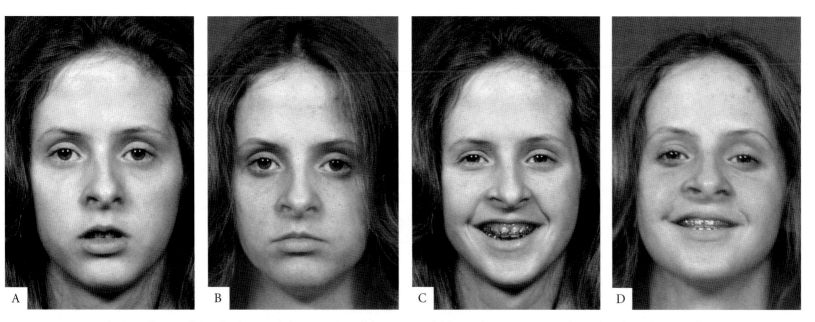

FIGURE 59-9   *Unesthetic widening of the alar base and downturning of the corners of the mouth in a patient with an already wide nose. This patient was treated with a maxillary procedure without an alar cinch or V-Y closure. A, Preoperative full facial view. B, Postoperative full facial view. C, Preoperative smiling full facial view. D, Postoperative smiling full facial view. Reproduced with permission from Betts NJ, Fonseca RJ. Soft tissue changes associated with orthognathic surgery. In: Bell WH, editor. Modern practice in orthognathic and reconstructive surgery. Vol 3. Philadelphia (PA): W.B. Saunders; 1992. p. 2197.*

V-Y Closure   There is always an anteroposterior thinning of the upper lip (especially with maxillary advancement) and a loss of vermilion (especially with maxillary impaction) unless a **V-Y** closure is used (Figure 59-10A–C).

The upper lip, when closed in a **V-Y** fashion, follows the hard tissues forward at more nearly a 1:1 ratio, with prevention of upper lip thinning and loss of the vermilion.[10,15,48,93]

The **V-Y** closure is accomplished during closure of the maxillary vestibular incision.

The mid portion of the incision is identified and retracted anteriorly with a single skin hook. One centimeter of the incision is closed in an anteroposterior direction. Using a separate suture mucosa, periosteum and interposed muscular tissue is engaged by the needle

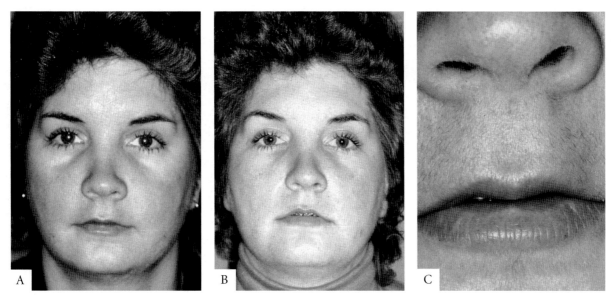

FIGURE 59-10   *Unfavorable change in the vermilion of the upper lip following maxillary impaction surgery in a patient with a preexisting thin vermilion. A, Preoperative state. Note preexisting minimal vermilion exposure. B, Postoperative state. C, Close-up view of the postoperative state. Note that the loss of vermilion is more pronounced in the lateral portions of the lip than in the medial portion. Reproduced with permission from Betts NJ, Fonseca RJ. Soft tissue changes associated with orthognathic surgery. In: Bell WH, editor. Modern practice in orthognathic and reconstructive surgery. Vol 3. Philadelphia (PA): W.B. Saunders; 1992. p. 2198.*

on either side of the incision and sutured in a continuous fashion. The superior aspect of the incision is gradually advanced toward the midline by taking smaller bites of tissue in the upper margin of the incision and larger bites in the lower margin (Figure 59-11A and B). Both sides of the incision are closed in a similar fashion to the midline suture. Often, following this type of closure, the lip will look rather full and short in the midline. Within the next several days, the lip will lengthen and become more normal in appearance.[93]

Alar Cinch   Collins and Epker identified patients who may develop undesirable nasal esthetic changes as those who have normal or wide frontonasal esthetics prior to surgery and will undergo a superior or anterior surgical repositioning of the maxilla.[94] These observations led to the development of techniques designed to control the alar base width after maxillary surgery. Bell and Proffit described adjunctive techniques to ensure an esthetic reconstruction of the alar base in maxillary impaction cases.[40] These included (1) reduction of the anterior extent of the piriform rim, (2) reduction of the ANS, and (3) trimming of the height of the anterior nasal floor. A different technique for correcting the flat and flaring nose was described by Millard.[95] This served as a model for the later development of the alar cinch techniques.[94] The original cinch suture was passed from the fibroadipose tissue on one side of the alar base to the other and was tied to a predetermined width (Figure 59-12A–E).

This technique was then modified to a figure-eight suture that was passed from lateral to medial, catching the fibroadipose tissue of the alar base (Figure 59-12F–H).[24,41] Schendel and Delarre suggest that the suture should be passed not through the fibroadipose tissue but through the transverse nasalis muscles of the nose.[92]

Past observations have suggested that the alar cinch suture does not control the alar base width[4,96] and may even cause fur-

ther widening of the alar base. Subsequently, another technique of alar cinch suturing was suggested. In this technique, a hole is placed in the ANS and the suture is passed through the soft tissues at the base of the nose and back to the ANS bilaterally and individually tied (Figure 59-12I–L).[15]

A measurement of the greatest alar width must be taken on the patient and

recorded in the chart preoperatively. This number should be available during surgery so that reference to it can be made at the time of nasolabial muscle reconstruction.

Combination of Alar Cinch and V-Y Closure   Several investigators indicated that the best control of the alar base in patients having maxillary superior or anterior repositioning could be achieved by using the V-Y closure and the alar cinch suture together.[15,36–38,41,92,93] Their objective was to quantify the alar base width changes with and without the alar base cinch suture. All patients had a V-Y closure. They

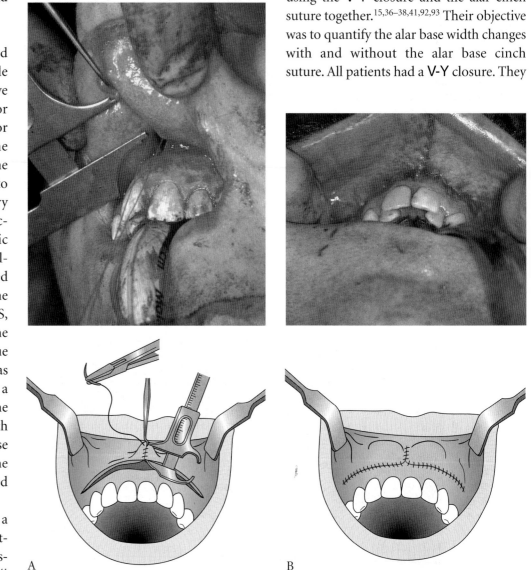

A   B

FIGURE **59-11**   A, *The* V-Y *closure is accomplished during closure of the maxillary vestibular incision. The midportion of the incision is identified and retracted anteriorly with a single skin hook. One centimeter of the incision is closed in an anteroposterior direction.* B, *Using a separate suture mucosa, periosteum and interposed muscular tissue are engaged by the needle on either side of the incision and sutured in a continuous fashion. The superior aspect of the incision is gradually advanced toward the midline by taking smaller bites of tissue in the upper margin of the incision and larger bites in the lower margin. Both sides of the incision are closed in similar fashion to the midline suture. Photographs reproduced with permission and illustrations adapted from Milles M, Betts NJ. Techniques to preserve or modify lip form during orthognathic surgery. Atlas Oral Maxillofac Surg Clin North Am 2000;8:71–9.*

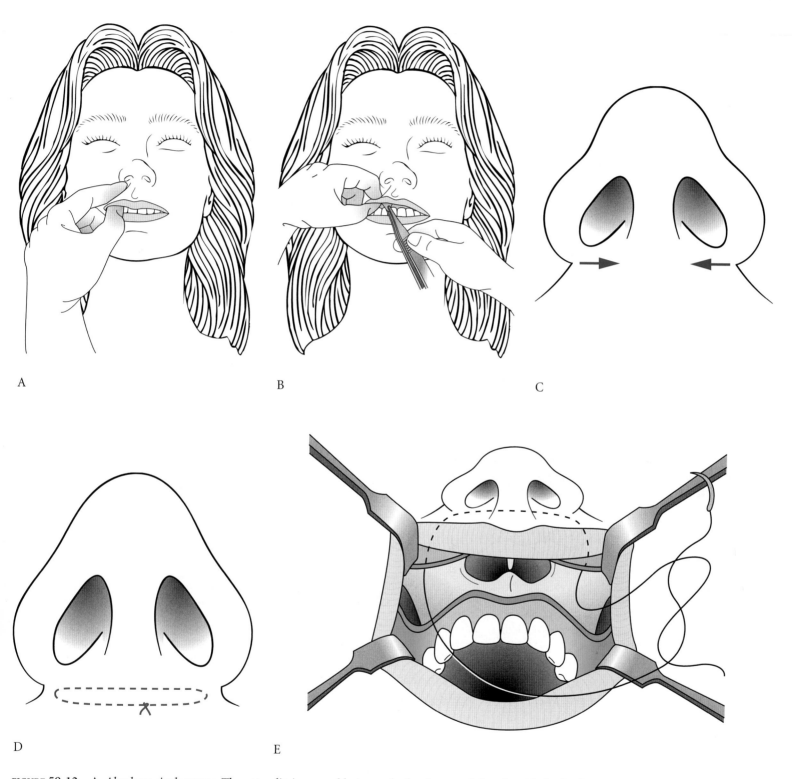

FIGURE **59-12** A, *Alar base cinch suture. The upper lip is grasped between the forefinger and thumb, with the forefinger placed directly on the junction of the ala with the face. B, The lip is inverted and the tissue lying over the forefinger is grasped with a forceps. The lip is released and the tissue grasped in the forceps is manipulated to ensure that the alar base moves properly. If appropriate movement is not observed, the process must be repeated until correct needle placement is ensured. C–E, A nonresorbable suture (ie, 2-0 Prolene) is passed from the fibroadipose tissue (or transverse nasalis muscle) on one side of the alar base to the other and is tied to a predetermined width.* (CONTINUED ON NEXT PAGE)

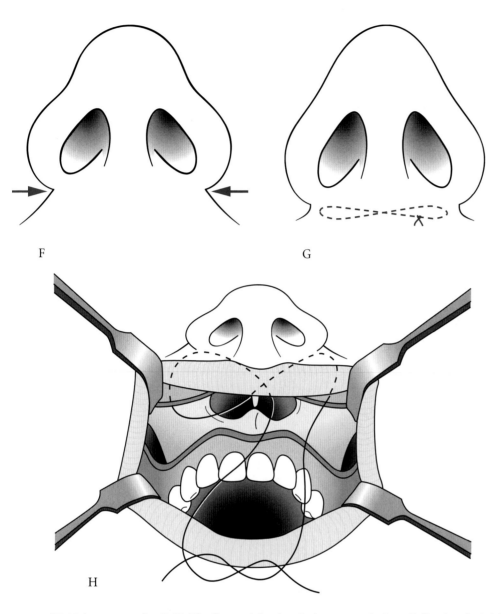

FIGURE **59-12** (CONTINUED) F–H, *The figure-eight alar cinch suture technique. Following the initial steps described above, the suture is passed in a lateral to medial direction through the fibroadipose tissue on one side, and in the identical fashion (lateral to medial direction) on the other side of the nose. It is then tied in the midline to a predetermined width.* (CONTINUED ON NEXT PAGE)

found that the alar bases widened in all patients and widening was lessened when the alar cinch suture was used. The alar base widened an average of 2.9% with the alar cinch suture and 10.8% without it.[41]

The effects of simultaneous placement of an alar cinch suture and a V-Y closure are successfully repositioning the lip muscles in a predictable manner,[93] preventing shortening of the lip in impaction cases,[41,93] maintaining the normal lip pout,[93] preventing loss of vermilion,[41,48,93]

maintaining the anteroposterior thickness of the lip,[41] decreasing the widening of the alar base,[41,48,93] and preventing drooping of the corners of the mouth[93] (Figure 59-13A–E). The ability of the figure of eight alar cinch suture combined with a V-Y advancement closure to reconstruct the patient to their preoperative soft tissue state was recently demonstrated in a prospective investigation with long-term follow-up. This study was performed in a surgical model (surgically assisted maxil-

lary expansion) that stressed the soft tissue closure technique and did not confound the soft tissue changes with vertical or anteroposterior vectors of maxillary movement. A figure-eight alar cinch suture combined with a V-Y advancement closure predictably reconstructed the patient's preoperative soft tissue state. Suturing the alar bases independently to the nasal septum (combined with a V-Y closure) was less effective but still superior to a V-Y closure alone.[97]

Contouring the ANS Reduction of the ANS is indicated in patients undergoing large advancements or impactions of the maxilla who already have good nasal tip projection (Figure 59-14).[21] The hard tissue changes in the position of the ANS affect primarily the soft tissue landmarks subnasale and pronasale.[4]

This technique should not be used in patients who have poor preoperative nasal tip projection. The nasal tip will rise if the ANS is left intact when advancing or impacting the maxilla. ANS reduction is also contraindicated in patients who are having a maxillary setback procedure. The result could lead to a "polybeak" deformity or drooping of the columella (Figure 59-15A–D).

Septoplasty The cartilaginous nasal septum should be reduced during maxillary impactions of greater than 3 mm to prevent postoperative deviation or buckling of the septum.[40,46] This is done by reflecting the septal perichondrium and removing the appropriate amount of cartilage from the inferior aspect of the nasal septum with a scissor or scalpel blade (Figure 59-16A and B). The same amount of septum should be removed as the maxilla is impacted. This technique can be combined with reduction of the maxillary nasal crest. Prudence must be exercised as overreduction of the septum can result in either a saddle nose deformity or a polybeak deformity depending on the location of the excessive cartilage resection.[15]

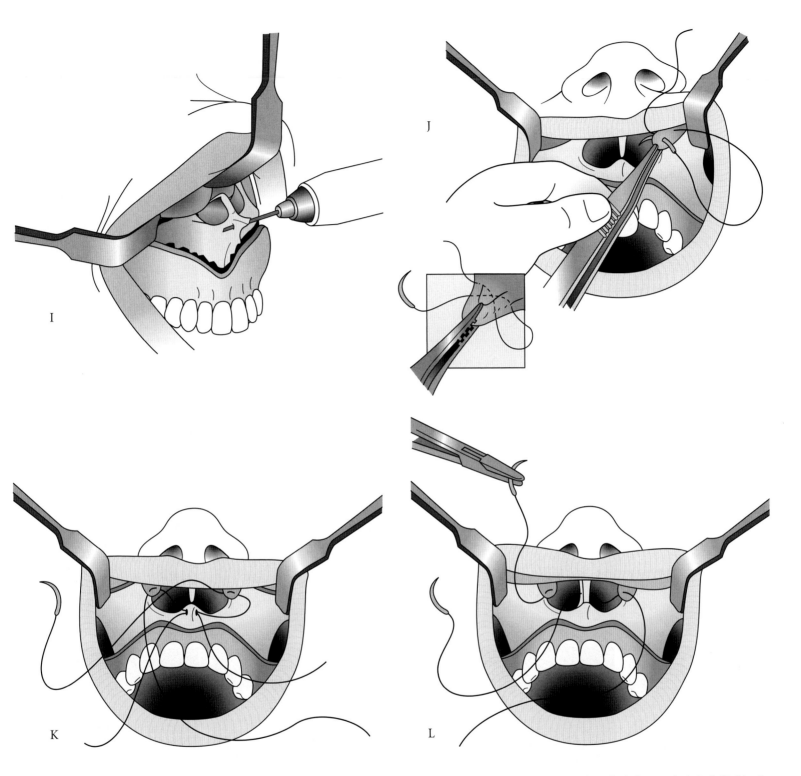

FIGURE **59-12** (CONTINUED)   I–K, *The dual-suture alar cinch technique. Before identifying the appropriate tissues described above, a hole is drilled in the ANS. Individual sutures are placed through the fibroadipose tissues, then through the hole below ANS and tied to a predetermined width for each nostril. L, Modification of this technique. Instead of the sutures being placed through the ANS, the individual sutures are passed through the anterior caudal septum. Adapted from Betts NJ. Techniques to control nasal features. Atlas Oral Maxillofac Surg Clin North Am 2000;8:53–69.*

Double V-Y Closure   The double V-Y closure was first proposed by Lassus for thickening of the thin lip (Figure 59-17A and B).[98] Hackney and colleagues com-pared muscle reorientation using an alar cinch suture in conjunction with a simple closure technique, a single V-Y closure technique, and a double V-Y closure tech-nique.[99] They observed that all three methods of closure yielded a significant increase in alar base width, and the dou-ble V-Y closure preserved the vermilion

FIGURE **59-13** *Favorable soft tissue changes after maxillary impaction surgery and mandibular autorotation in a patient with an already wide alar base by use of an alar cinch suture and a V-Y closure. A, Data from pre- and postoperative cephalograms. Patient 3.5 months preoperation at age 15 years, 4 months (solid line); patient at age 16 years, 1 month postoperation (dotted line). B, Pre- and C, postoperative full facial views. D, Pre- and E, postoperative smiling full facial views. F, Pre- and G, postoperative three-quarter views. H, Pre- and I, postoperative profiles. A adapted from and B–I reproduced with permission from Betts NJ, Fonseca RJ. Soft tissue changes associated with orthognathic surgery. In: Bell WH, editor. Modern practice in orthognathic and reconstructive surgery. Vol 3. Philadelphia (PA): W.B. Saunders; 1992. p. 2171–2209.*

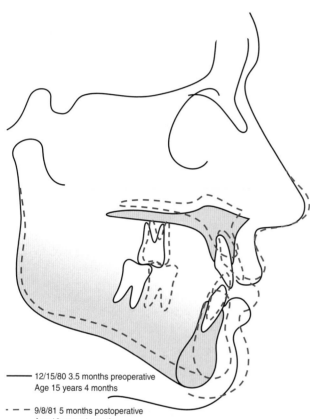

12/15/80 3.5 months preoperative
Age 15 years 4 months

- - - 9/8/81 5 months postoperative
Age 16 years 1 month

A

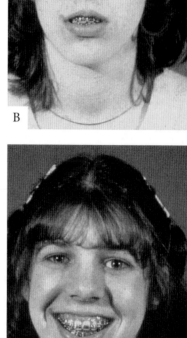

B

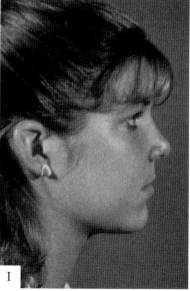

C

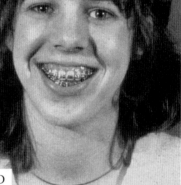

D

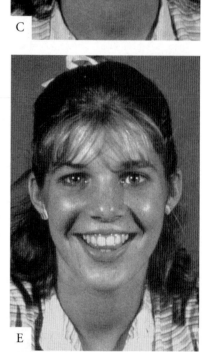

E

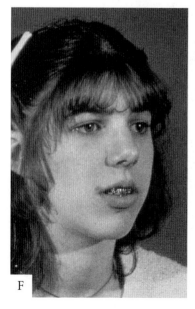

F

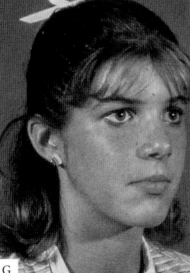

G

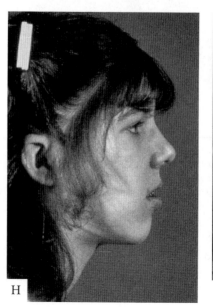

H

I

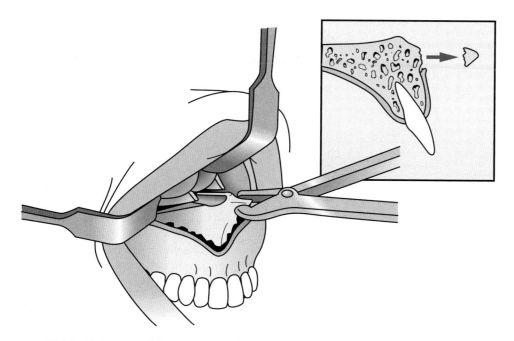

FIGURE 59-14   *Reduction of the anterior nasal spine during a maxillary osteotomy. This procedure is indicated in patients undergoing large advancements or impactions of the maxilla who already have good nasal tip projection. This procedure is contraindicated in patients who have poor preoperative nasal tip projection or are having a maxillary setback procedure. Adapted from Betts NJ. Techniques to control nasal features. Atlas Oral Maxillofac Surg Clin North Am 2000;8:53–69.*

Mandible

When contemplating a mandibular setback osteotomy the surgeon must carefully assess the patient's submentocervical morphology. If a patient has a short submental length and poor submentocervical proportion, mandibular setback may worsen this, resulting in a "double chin." If this complication is a possibility, the surgeon may elect to combine the mandibular setback procedure with an advancement genioplasty or submentocervical liposuction (if adipose tissue is present).

Chin

Incorrect planning, vestibular scarring, excessive detachment of soft tissue from the chin, suprahyoid myotomy, improper closure of the soft tissue incision, hematoma formation, genial remodeling, and excessive bone resorption may compromise the results of chin surgery.[66]

Bone resorption is related to the amount of soft tissue dissection and therefore is more pronounced in nonpedicled genioplasties.[69] Adolescent patients also have more bone resorption after genioplasty procedures.[77]

(especially in the lateral portion of the lip) with less variability than with the other two techniques of closure. The true indication for this procedure is the patient who preoperatively has a thin lateral vermilion.[100]

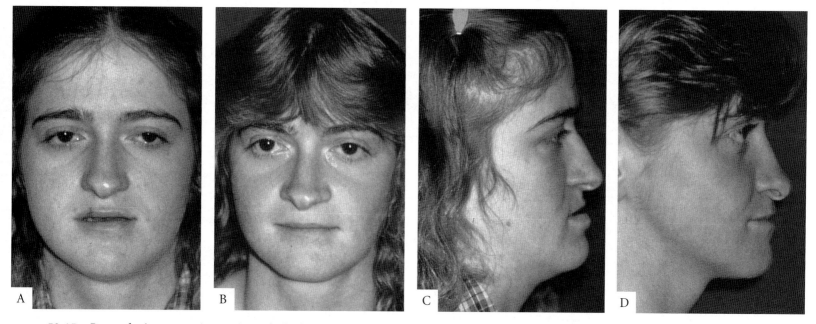

FIGURE 59-15   *Poor esthetic outcome in a patient who had overzealous reduction of anterior nasal spine (ANS) after a maxillary advancement procedure. A, Preoperative full facial view. B, Postoperative full facial view. C, Preoperative profile view. D, Postoperative profile view. Reproduced with permission from Betts NJ, Fonseca RJ. Soft tissue changes associated with orthognathic surgery. In: Bell WH, editor. Modern practice in orthognathic and reconstructive surgery. Vol 3. Philadelphia (PA): W.B. Saunders; 1992. p 2201.*

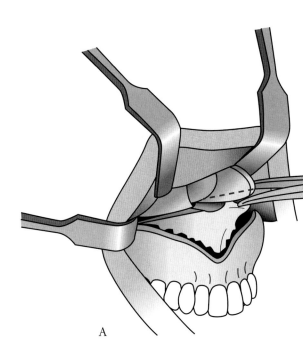

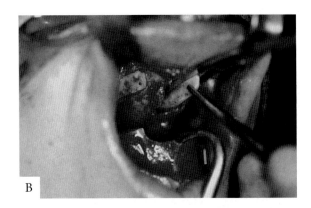

FIGURE **59-16** A, *Septal reduction during maxillary impaction osteotomy. The cartilaginous nasal septum should be reduced during maxillary impactions of greater than 3 mm to prevent postoperative deviation or buckling of the septum. This is done by incising the nasal mucosa and reflecting the septal perichondrium and removing the appropriate amount of cartilage with a scissor or scalpel blade. The same amount of septum should be removed as the maxilla is impacted. This technique can be combined with reduction of the maxillary nasal crest. B, Clinical example. A adapted from and B reproduced with permission from Betts NJ. Techniques to control nasal features. Atlas Oral Maxillofac Surg Clin North Am 2000;8:53–69.*

Chin ptosis or "witch's chin" (Figure 59-18A–C) is an unesthetic complication secondary to the degloving dissection of the chin or to lack of reattachment of the mentalis muscle at the time of surgery. This may lead to an inferior tissue slide causing excess interlabial incompetence and exposure of the lower teeth secondary to lower lip ptosis and redundant tissue in the submental area.[45,68,70]

Several investigators have demonstrated that using a procedure that minimizes soft tissue stripping may produce a more predictable hard and soft tissue response in the osteotomized segment.[44,45,65,66,68,71] Therefore, the surgeon should attempt to maintain as much soft tissue pedicle on the labial and lingual aspects of the mandible as possible. In addition to a predictable soft to hard tissue ratio, preservation of the soft tissue pedicle ensures a greater blood supply to the osteotomized segment, less bony resorption, and a decreased risk of infection.[64,71]

During closure, the mentalis muscles must be reapproximated to prevent ptosis of the chin. An incision out into the unattached tissues of the lip can help prevent postoperative wound dehiscence and facilitate muscle reapproximation.

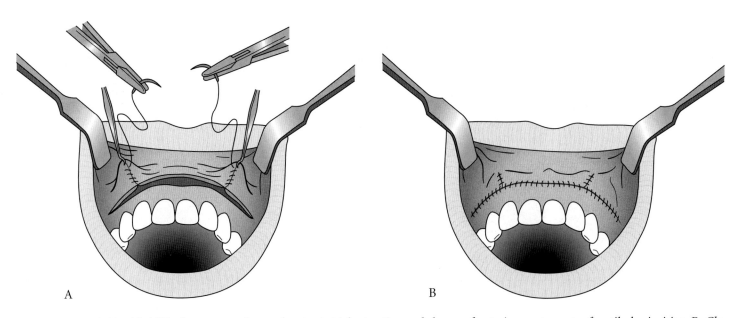

FIGURE **59-17**   A, *Double V-Y advancement closure showing initial retraction and closure of anterior components of vestibular incision. B, Closure completed. Adapted from Milles M, Betts NJ. Techniques to preserve or modify lip form during orthognathic surgery. Atlas Oral Maxillofac Surg Clin North Am 2000;8:71–9.*

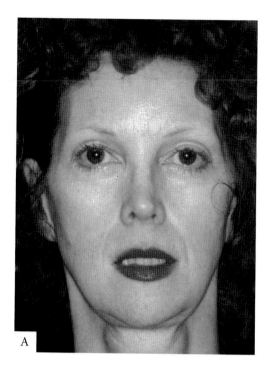

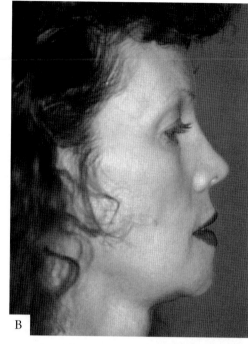

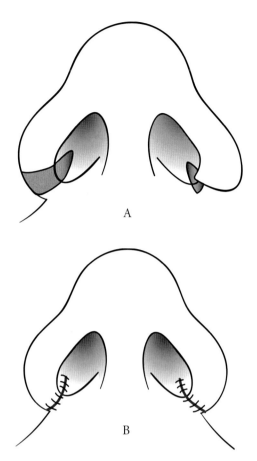

FIGURE 59-18 *Chin ptosis "witch's chin" after advancement genioplasty. Note the excessive show of the lower incisor in panels B and C. A, Full facial repose view. B, Profile view in repose. C, Close-up of the chin in repose. Reproduced with permission from Betts NJ, Fonseca RJ. Soft tissue changes associated with orthognathic surgery. In: Bell WH, editor. Modern practice in orthognathic and reconstructive surgery. Vol 3. Philadelphia (PA): W.B. Saunders; 1992. p. 2203.*

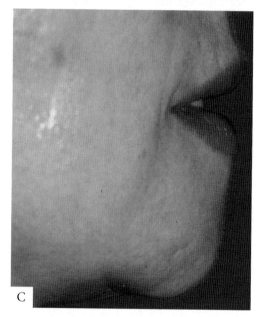

FIGURE 59-19 *Bilateral alar base wedge resections. A, Resected area of the alar base. B, The nostril area following suturing demonstrating narrowing of the width of the nostrils and nasal base. Adapted from Betts NJ. Techniques to control nasal features. Atlas Oral Maxillofac Surg Clin North Am 2000;8:53–69.*

A chin dressing fabricated from elastic tape should be placed at the end of the surgical procedure to stabilize the soft tissues and prevent hematoma formation. These dressings are typically worn for 5 to 7 days postoperatively.

Secondary Revision of Poor Surgical Results

The best method of treatment for a poor soft tissue outcome is prevention. The deformity should be recognized, the soft tissue effects of the surgical procedure should be anticipated, and the correct interceptive procedures instituted. However, if a secondary procedure is required, the same techniques described in the preceding sections can be used. Revision surgery is more difficult than control of the soft tissues at the time the original surgery because of scarring and change in normal anatomic relationships.[24,45] Rosen suggests that these secondary procedures be attempted only after the final soft tissue drape has been established and the residual defect has been identified.[23]

Other procedures for revising a poor surgical outcome are submental lipectomy, nasal wedge resection (Weir excisions) (Figure 59-19),[23] and rhinoplasty.

References

1. Dion KE, Berscheid E, Walster E. What is beautiful is good. J Pers Soc Psychol 1972;24:285.
2. Kalik M. Toward an interdisciplinary psychology of appearance. Psychiatry 1977;41:243.
3. Mathes E. The effects of physical attractiveness and anxiety on heterosexual attraction over a series of five encounters. J Marriage Fam 1975;37:769.
4. Betts NJ, Fonseca R, Vig P, et al. Changes in nasal and labial soft tissues after surgical repositioning of the maxilla. Int J Adult Orthodont Orthognath Surg 1993;8:7–23.

5. Dann JJ, Fonseca R, Bell WH. Soft tissue changes associated with total maxillary advancement: a preliminary study. J Oral Surg 1976;34:19–23.

6. Mansour S, Burstone C, Legan H. An evaluation of soft tissue changes resulting from LeFort I maxillary surgery. Am J Orthod 1983;84:37–47.

7. Hershey HG, Smith L. Soft tissue profile change associated with surgical correction of the prognathic mandible. Am J Orthod 1974;65:483–503.

8. Radney LJ, Jacobs J. Soft-tissue changes associated with surgical total maxillary intrusion. Am J Orthod 1981;80:191–212.

9. Sakima T, Sachdeva R. Soft tissue response to Le Fort I maxillary impaction surgery. Int J Adult Orthodon Orthognath Surg 1987;4:221–31.

10. Stella JP, Streater M, Epker BN, Sinn DP. Predictability of upper lip soft tissue changes with maxillary advancement. J Oral Maxillofac Surg 1989;47:697–703.

11. Quast DC, Biggerstaff R, Haley JV. The short-term and long-term soft-tissue profile changes accompanying mandibular advancement surgery. Am J Orthod 1983;84:29–36.

12. Robinson M. Bone resorption under plastic chin implants. J Oral Surg 1969;27:116–8.

13. Bell W. Correction of mandibular prognathism by mandibular setback and advancement genioplasty. Int J Oral Surg 1981;10:221–9.

14. Bloom L. Perioral profile changes in orthodontic treatment. Am J Orthod 1961;47:371.

15. Waite P. Simultaneous orthognathic surgery and rhinoplasty. Oral Maxillofac Surg Clin North Am 1990;2:339–50.

16. Ingersoll SK, Peterson L, Weinstein S. Influence of horizontal incision on upper lip morphology [abstract 360]. J Dent Res 1982;61:218.

17. O'Reilly M. Integumental profile changes after surgical orthodontic correction of bimaxillary dentoalveolar protrusion in black patients. Am J Orthod Dentofacial Orthop 1989;96:242–8.

18. Proffit WR, Epker B. Treatment planning for dentofacial deformities. In: Bell WH, White RP, editors. Surgical correction of dentofacial deformities. Philadelphia: WB Saunders; 1980. p. 183–7.

19. Tomlak DJ, Piecuch J, Weinstein S. Morphologic analysis of upper lip area following maxillary osteotomy via the tunneling approach. Am J Orthod 1984;85:488–93.

20. Subtelny J. A longitudinal study of the soft tissue facial structures and their profile characteristics, defined in relation to underlying skeletal structures. Am J Orthod 1959;45:481.

21. Freihofer HJ. Changes in nasal profile after maxillary advancement in cleft and non-cleft patients. J Maxillofac Surg 1977;5:20–7.

22. Freihofer HJ. The lip profile after correction of retromaxillism in cleft and noncleft patients. J Maxillofac Surg 1976;4:136–41.

23. Rosen H. Lip-nasal aesthetics following LeFort I osteotomy. Plast Reconstr Surg 1988; 81:171–82.

24. Wolford L. Lip-nasal aesthetics following LeFort I osteotomy [discussion]. Plast Reconstr Surg 1988;81:180.

25. Hack GA, de Molvan Otterloo J, Nanda R. Long-term stability and prediction of soft tissue changes after LeFort I surgery. Am J Orthod Dentofacial Orthoped 1993;104:544–55.

26. Phillips C, Devereux J, Camilla Tulloch JF, et al. Full face soft tissue response to surgical maxillary intrusion. Int J Adult Orthodon Orthognath Surg 1986;1:299–304.

27. Rosenburg A, Muradin M, van der Bilt A. Nasolabial esthetics after Le Fort I osteotomy and V-Y closure: A statistical evaluation. Int J Adult Orthodon Orthognath Surg 2002;17:29–39.

28. Filho HN, Goncales ES, Berrentin-Felix G, et al. Evaluation of facial soft tissues following surgically assisted expansion associated with the simple V-Y suture. Int J Adult Orthodon Orthognath Surg 2002;17:89–97.

29. Reidel R. An analysis of dentofacial relationships. Am J Orthod 1957;43:103.

30. Burstone C. Integumental contour and extension patterns. Angle Orthod 1959;29:93.

31. Attarzadeh F, Adenwalla T. Soft tissue profile changes concurrent with orthodontic treatment. Int J Orthod 1990;28:9–16.

32. Hershey H. Incisor tooth retraction and subsequent profile change in postadolescent female patients. Am J Orthod 1972;61:45.

33. Moss JP, McCance A, Fright WR, et al. A three dimensional soft tissue analysis of fifteen patients with class II division malocclusions after bimaxillary surgery. Am J Orthod Dentofacial Orthoped 1994;105:430–7.

34. Anderson JP, Joondeph D, Turpin DL. A cephalometric study of profile changes in orthodontically treated cases ten years out of retention. Angle Orthod 1973;43:324.

35. Rudee D. Proportional profile changes concurrent with orthodontic therapy. Am J Orthod 1964;50:421.

36. O'Ryan F, Schendel S. Nasal anatomy and maxillary surgery. I. Esthetic and anatomic principles. Int J Adult Orthodon Orthognath Surgery 1989;4:27–37.

37. O'Ryan F, Schendel S. Nasal anatomy and maxillary surgery. II. Unfavorable nasolabial esthetics following the LeFort I osteotomy.

Int J Adult Orthodon Orthognath Surg 1989;4:75–84.

38. O'Ryan F, Schendel S. Nasal anatomy and maxillary surgery. III. Surgical techniques for correction of nasal deformities in patients undergoing maxillary surgery. Int J Adult Orthodon Orthognath Surg 1989;4:157–74.

39. Proffit WR, Epker B, Ackerman JL. Systematic description of dentofacial deformities: the database. In: Bell WH, White RP, editors. Surgical correction of dentofacial deformities. Philadelphia: WB Saunders; 1980. p. 114–22.

40. Bell WH, Proffit W. Esthetic effects of maxillary osteotomy. In: Bell WH, White RP, editors. Surgical correction of dentofacial deformities. Philadelphia: WB Saunders; 1980. p. 368–70.

41. Guymon M, Crosby D, Wolford LM. The alar base cinch suture to control nasal width in maxillary osteotomies. Int J Adult Orthodon Orthognath Surg 1988;3:89–95.

42. Bundgaard M, Melson B, Terp S. Changes during and following total maxillary osteotomy (LeFort I procedure): a cephalometric study. Eur J Orthod 1986;8:21–29.

43. Lines PA, Steinhauser E. Soft tissue changes in relationship to movement of hard tissue structures in orthognathic surgery: a preliminary report. Journal of Oral Surgery 1974;32:891–6.

44. Bell WH, Brammer J, McBride KL, et al. Reduction genioplasty: surgical techniques and soft tissue changes. Oral Surg Oral Med Oral Pathol Oral Radiol Endod 1981; 51:471–7.

45. Bell WH, Gallagher D. The versatility of the genioplasty using a broad pedicle. J Oral Maxillofac Surg 1983;41:763–9.

46. Lew KKK, Loh F, Yeo JF. Profile changes following anterior subapical osteotomy in Chinese adults with bimaxillary protrusion. Int J Adult Orthodon Orthognath Surg 1989;4:189–96.

47. Freidland JA, Coccano P, Converse JM. Retrospective cephalometric analysis of mandibular bone absorption under silicone rubber chin implants. Plast Reconstr Surg 1976;57:144–51.

48. Carlotti AE Jr, Ashaffensburg P, Schendel SA. Facial changes associated with surgical advancement of the lip and maxilla. J Oral Maxillofac Surg 1986;44:593–6.

49. Schendel SA, Eisenfeld J, Bell WH, et al. Superior repositioning of the maxilla: stability and soft tissue osseous relations. Am J Orthod 1976;70:663–74.

50. Mommaerts MY, Marxer H. A cephalometric analysis of the long-term, soft tissue profile changes which accompany the advance-

ment of the mandible by sagittal split ramus osteotomy. J Craniomaxillofac Surg 1987;15:127–31.

51. Talbott J. Soft tissue response to mandibular advancement surgery [master's thesis]. Lexington (KY): University of Kentucky; 1975.

52. Thuer U, Ingervall B, Vuillemin T. Stability and effect on the soft tissue profile of mandibular advancement with sagittal split osteotomy and rigid internal fixation. Int J Adult Orthodon Orthognath Surg 1994;9:175–85.

53. Dermaut LR, De Smit A. Effects of sagittal split advancement osteotomy on facial profiles. Eur J Orthod 1989;11:366–74.

54. Mobarak KA, Espeland L, Krogstad O, Lyberg T. Soft tissue profile changes following mandibular advancement surgery: predictability and long term outcome. Am J Orthod Dentofacial Orthop 2001;119:368–81.

55. Dolce C, Johnson P, Van Sickels JE, et al. Maintenance of soft tissue changes after rigid versus wire fixation for mandibular advancement, with and without genioplasty. Oral Surg Oral Med Oral Pathol Oral Radiol Endod 2001;92:142–9.

56. Keeling SD, Labanc J, Van Sickels JE, et al. Skeletal change at surgery as a predictor of long-term soft tissue profile change after mandibular advancement. J Oral Maxillofac Surg 1996;54:134–44.

57. Johnston L. Discussion: skeletal change at surgery as a predictor of long-term soft tissue profile change after mandibular advancement. J Oral Maxillofac Surg 1996;54:145–6.

58. Weinstein S, Harris E, Archer SY. Lip morphology and area changes associated with surgical correction of mandibular prognathism. J Oral Rehabil 1982;9:335–54.

59. Fromm B, Lundberg M. The soft-tissue facial profile before and after surgical correction of mandibular protrusion. Acta Odontol Scand 1970;28:157–77.

60. Aaronson S. A cephalometric investigation of the surgical correction of mandibular prognathism. Angle Orthod 1967;379:251.

61. Robinson SW, Speidel T, Isaacson RJ, et al. Soft tissue profile change produced by reduction of mandibular prognathism. Angle Orthod 1972;42:227.

62. Mobarak KA, Krogstad O, Espeland L, Lyberg T. Factors influencing the predictability of soft tissue profile changes following mandibular setback surgery. Angle Orthod 2001;71:216–27.

63. Busquets CJ, Sassouni V. Changes in the integumental profile of the chin and lower lip after genioplasty. J Oral Surg 1981;39:499–504.

64. Hohl TH, Epker B. Macrogenia: a study of

treatment results, with surgical recommendations. Oral Surg Oral Med Oral Pathol Oral Radiol Endod 1976;41:545–67.

65. Park HS, Ellis E, Fonseca RJ, et al. A retrospective study of advancement genioplasty. Oral Surg Oral Med Oral Pathol Oral Radiol Endod 1989;67:481–9.

66. Gallagher DM, Bell W, Storum KA. Soft tissue changes associated with advancement genioplasty performed concomitantly with superior repositioning of the maxilla. J Oral Maxillofac Surg 1984;42:238–42.

67. McDonnel JP, McNeill R, West RA. Advancement genioplasty: a retrospective cephalometric analysis of osseous and soft tissue changes. J Oral Surg 1977;35:640.

68. Scheideman GB, Legan H, Bell WH. Soft tissue changes with combined mandibular setback and advancement genioplasty. J Oral Surg 1981;39:505–9.

69. Bell WH, Dann J III. Correction of dentofacial deformities by surgery in the anterior part of the jaws: a study of stability and soft tissue changes. Am J Orthod 1973;64:162–87.

70. Trauner RT, Obwegeser H. The surgical correction of mandibular prognathism and retrognathia with consideration of genioplasty. Part I. Surgical procedures to correct mandibular prognathism and reshaping of the chin. Oral Surg Oral Med Oral Pathol Oral Radiol Endod 1957;10:667.

71. Ellis E, DeChow P, McNamara JA Jr, et al. Advancement genioplasty with and without soft tissue pedicle: an experimental investigation. J Oral Maxillofac Surg 1984;42:637–45.

72. Krekmanov L, Kahnberg K. Soft tissue response to genioplasty procedures. Br J Oral Maxillofac Surg 1992;30:87–91.

73. Precious D, Armstrong JE, Morais D. Anatomic placement of fixation devices in genioplasty. Oral Surg Oral Med Oral Pathol Oral Radiol Endod 1992;73:2–8.

74. Ayoub AF, Stirrups D, Moos KF. Evaluation of changes following advancement genioplasty using finite element analysis. Br J Oral Maxillofac Surg 1993;31:217–22.

75. Converse JM, Wood-Smith D. Horizontal osteotomy of the mandible. Plast Reconstr Surg 1964;34:464.

76. Van Sickels JE, Tiner BD, Jones DL. Hard and soft tissue predictability with advancement genioplasties. Oral Surg Oral Med Oral Pathol Oral Radiol Endod 1994;77:218–21.

77. Tulasne J. The overlapping bone flap genioplasty. J Craniomaxillofac Surg 1987;15:214–21.

78. Ewing M, Ross R. Soft tissue response to mandibular advancement and genioplasty. Am J Orthod Dentofacial Orthoped 1992;101:550–5.

79. Dann JJ, Epker B. Proplast genioplasty: A retrospective study with treatment recommendations. Angle Orthod 1977;47:173–85.

80. Peled IJ, Wexler M, Ticher S, et al. Mandibular resorption from silicone chin implants in children. J Oral Maxillofac Surg 1986;44:346–8.

81. Robinson M. Bone resorption under plastic chin implants. Arch Otolaryngol 1972;95:30.

82. Bailey LJ, Collie F, White RP. Long-term soft tissue changes after orthognathic surgery. Int J Adult Orthodon Orthognath Surg 1996;11:7–18.

83. McCarthy JG, Schreiber J, Karp NS, et al. Lengthening of the human mandible by gradual distraction. Plast Reconstr Surg 1992;89:1–8.

84. Harada K, Baba Y, Ohyama K, Omura K. Soft tissue profile changes of the midface in patients with cleft lip and palate following maxillary distraction osteogenesis: a preliminary study. Oral Surg Oral Med Oral Pathol Oral Radiol Endod 2002;94:673–7.

85. Ko EW, Figueroa A, Polley J. Soft tissue profile changes after maxillary advancement with distraction osteogenesis by use of a rigid external distraction device: a 1 year follow up. J Oral Maxillofac Surg 2000;58:959–69.

86. Tishler PV, Larkin E, Schlutler MD, Redline S. Incidence of sleep-disordered breathing in an urban adult population: the relative importance of risk factors in the development of sleep-disordered breathing. J Am Med Assoc 2003;289:2230–7.

87. Riley RW, Powell N, Guillemenault C. Obstructive sleep apnea syndrome: a review of 306 consecutively treated surgical patients. Otolaryngol Head Neck Surg 1993;108:117–25.

88. Waite PD, Wooten V, Lachner J, et al. Maxillomandibular advancement surgery in 23 patients with obstructive sleep apnea syndrome. J Oral Maxillofac Surg 1989;47:1256–61.

89. Young T, Palta M, Dempsey J, et al. The occurrence of sleep-disordered breathing among middle-aged adults. N Engl J Med 1993;328:1230–5.

90. Li KK, Riley R, Powell NB, Guillemenault C. Patient's perception of the facial appearance after maxillomandibular advancement for obstructive sleep apnea syndrome. J Oral Maxillofac Surg 2001;59:377–80.

91. Louis PJ, Austin R, Waite PD, Matthews CS. Soft tissue changes of the upper lip associated with maxillary advancement in obstructive sleep apnea patients. J Oral Maxillofac Surg 2001;59:151–6.

92. Schendel SA, Delaire J. Facial muscles: form, function, and reconstruction in dentofacial deformities. In: Bell WH, White RP, editors. Surgical correction of dentofacial

deformities. Philadelphia: WB Saunders; 1980. p. 259–80.

93. Schendel SA, Williamson L. Muscle reorientation following superior repositioning of the maxilla. J Oral Maxillofac Surg 1983;41:235–40.

94. Collins PC, Epker B. The alar base cinch: a technique for prevention of alar base flaring secondary to maxillary surgery. Oral Surg Oral Med Oral Pathol Oral Radiol Endod 1982;53:549–53.

95. Millard D. The alar cinch for the flat flaring nose. Plast Reconstr Surg 1980;65:669–72.

96. Mack JA, Vizuette J, LaBanc J, et al. Three dimensional changes of the upper lip and nose following maxillary superior repositioning. Proceedings of the 68th Annual Meeting, American Association of Oral and Maxillofacial Surgeons. New Orleans (LA): WB Saunders;1986.

97. Betts NJ, Dalrymple D, Francioni SE. Two different alar cinch suturing techniques following surgically assisted rapid maxillary expansion (1 year data). J Oral Maxillofac Surg 1995;53 Suppl 4:82.

98. Lassus C. Thickening the thin lips. Plast Reconstr Surg 1981;68:950–2.

99. Hackney FL, Nishioka G, Van Sickels JE. Frontal soft tissue morphology with double V-Y closure following LeFort I osteotomy. J Oral Maxillofac Surg 1988;46:850–6.

100. Hackeny FL, Timmis D, Van Sickels JE. Esthetic evaluation of frontal labial morphology after double V-Y closure following LeFort I osteotomy. J Oral Maxillofac Surg 1989;47:1277–80.

101. Rains MD, Nanda R. Soft-tissue changes associated with maxillary incisor intrusion. Am J Orthod 1982:81:481–8.

102. Yogosawa F. Predicting soft tissue profile changes concurrent with orthodontic treatment. Angle Orthod 1990;60:199–206.

103. Kasai K. Soft tissue adaptability to hard tissues in facial profiles. Am J Orthod Dentofac Orthop 1998;113:674–84.

104. McCance AM, Moss JP, Fright WR, et al. A three-dimensional soft tissue analysis of 16 skeletal class III patients following bimaxillary surgery. Br J Oral Maxillofac Surg 1992;30:221–7.

105. Mchance AM, Moss JP, Fright WR, et al. A three-dimensional analysis of soft and hard tissue changes following bimaxillary orthognathic surgery in skeletal class III patients. Br J Oral Maxillofac Surg 1992;30:305–11.

106. Lin SS, Kerr JS. Soft and hard tissue changes in class III patients treated by bimaxillary surgery. Eur J Orthod 1998;20:25–33.

107. Epker BN, Fish LC. Definitive immediate presurgical planning. In: Epker BN, Fish LC, editors. Dentofacial deformities: integrated orthodontic and surgical correction. Vol. 1 St. Louis: CV Mosby; 1986. p. 103–27.

108. Polido WD, Bell WH. Long-term osseous and soft tissue changes after large chin advancements. J Craniomaxillofac Surg 1993; 21:54–9.

109. Wessberg GA, Wolford LM, Epker BN. Interpositional genioplasty for the short face. J Oral Surg 1980;38:584–90.

110. Gjorup H, Athanasiou AE. Soft tissues and dentoskeletal profile changes associated with mandibular setback osteotomy. Am J Orthod Dentofac Orthop 1991;100: 312–23.

111. Gaggl A, Schultes G, Karcher H. Changes in soft tissue profile after sagittal split ramus osteotomy and retropositioning of the mandible. J Oral Maxillofac Surg 1999; 52:542–6.

112. Enacar A, Taner T, Toroglus S. Analysis of soft tissue profile changes associated with mandibular setback and double jaw surgeries. Int J Adult Orthod Orthognath Surg 1999;14:27–35.

113. Hernandez-Orsini R, Jacobson A, Sarver DM, et al. Short-term and long-term soft tissue profile changes after mandibular advancements using rigid fixation techniques. Int J Adult Orthod Orthognath Surg 1989; 4:209–18

CHAPTER 60

Prevention and Management of Complications in Orthognathic Surgery

Joseph E. Van Sickels, DDS

Complications of orthognathic surgery can be divided into several broad and overlapping categories. Whether surgery of the maxilla or mandible is done, regional anatomy, amount of movement, number of segments needed, and type of fixation employed all influence the types of problems observed. Difficulties encountered can fall into one or more of the following areas: vascular, neural, infectious, fracture management, occlusal changes, joint dysfunction, dental, and miscellaneous complications.

The approach to complications used in this chapter is divided into two areas: prevention and management. Prevention can be summarized as preoperative evaluation and treatment planning. Many of the less than desired results can be traced to errors in preoperative clinical examination, models, or records. Patients with unusual anatomy may dictate departure from established treatment modalities, but their care should be planned in advance.

Vascular Complications

Hemorrhage in the Maxilla

Acute Injuries Severe hemorrhage has been documented with maxillary and mandibular surgery and can have both immediate and secondary effects.[1-7] Massive hemorrhage is rare whether acutely or in the postoperative period, but is possible with maxillary surgery. The vessels most at risk of injury during maxillary surgery are the internal maxillary artery, the posterior superior alveolar artery, and the greater palatine artery.

Massive blood loss can occur secondary to injury to the internal carotid artery and the internal jugular vein. When fracturing the pterygoid plates it is possible to fracture the base of the skull by vigorously manipulating chisels or directing chisels against the plates.[8,9] This can result in direct or indirect damage to major vessels in the neck or skull. When approaching maxillary surgery one should remember that vessels may be directly injured during osteotome placement or indirectly through shattering the pterygoid plates. Efforts should be made to properly direct osteotomes in the pterygoid plates and to down-fracture the maxilla without excessive force. If the maxilla is extremely difficult to mobilize, the posterior cut may be directed into the tuberosity and away from the pterygoid plates (Figure 60-1).[10] Patients who are undergoing a maxillary osteotomy to correct malposition of their maxilla following trauma may present special considera-

tions. The previous midface trauma may have resulted in fractures at the base of the skull. Manipulations to mobilize the maxilla may result in the osteotomy following the previous fracture lines.

Generally when brisk bleeding is encountered during surgery, the osteotomy should be completed, the maxilla down-fractured, and the site assessed for the bleeding source. Alternatively, the region may need to be packed to control blood loss, and then the osteotomy completed. The best opportunity to identify a

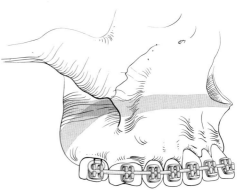

FIGURE 60-1 *The posterior cut is directed into the tuberosity behind the second molar when the maxilla is difficult to mobilize. Adapted from Van Sickels JE, Tucker MR. Prevention and management of complications in orthognathic surgery. In: Peterson LJ, Indresano AT, Marciani RD, Roser SM. Principles of oral and maxillofacial surgery. Vol. 3. Philadelphia (PA): JB Lippincott Company; 1992. p. 1466.*

bleeding vessel is when it is first cut. Ligature clips are applied or electrocautery is used if the vessel is easily seen. When hemorrhage obscures the field, packing followed by attempts to directly occlude the vessel should be attempted. The last option is to pack resorbable materials in the region under pressure, with tamponade of the bleeding source.

The carotid artery may be susceptible to both direct and indirect insult during the operation. Thrombosis of the internal carotid artery after orthognathic surgery may occur because of excessive extension of the head and neck.[11] Mortality associated with thrombosis of the internal carotid has been estimated at 40%, with an additional 52% of the patients being left with a serious neurologic deficit. Extension of the head and neck serves to stretch and partially fix the carotid artery against the cervical vertebrae, and contralateral rotation of the head results in further stretch of the artery. Positioning the patient in this manner places the internal carotid at risk for direct or indirect trauma.

Delayed Hemorrhage Delayed hemorrhage following a Le Fort I maxillary osteotomy may occur as early as the night of surgery to as late as 9 days postoperatively. The vessels most frequently involved are the greater palatine artery, the internal maxillary, and the pterygoid venous plexus of veins.[6]

Suggestions to reduce this type of injury include careful placement and orientation of the pterygomaxillary osteotome in the suture and angling the osteotomy inferior from the zygomaticomaxillary crest toward the pterygoid plates.[12] The mean distance from the most inferior junction of the maxilla and the pterygoid plates to the internal maxillary artery in the pterygopalatine fossa is 25 mm. With an average length of an osteotome of 15 mm, assuming normal anatomy, the margin of safety to separate

the entire pterygomaxillary junction is 10 mm. However, patients with dentofacial and craniofacial anomalies can have anatomic variation from these normative data. The internal maxillary artery and its branches are most vulnerable to damage in their course through the pterygopalatine fossa and fissure when the maxillary tuberosity is separated from the pterygoid plates with an osteotome.

The posterior superior alveolar and the greater palatine arteries may be severed during the Le Fort I procedure because they lie in the bony walls, although the posterior superior alveolar artery is not thought to present a significant problem for bleeding. It is generally recommended that the greater palatine arteries be preserved by gently removing bone that surrounds the vessels (Figure 60-2). However, if bleeding is encountered, the vessel should be ligated rather than letting it retract and bleed. Preserving the vessels maximizes the blood supply to segmented

maxilla and minimizes neural deficits to the palate.

There are several treatment options for the patient with postoperative hemorrhage after maxillary surgery, and they vary with the degree and severity of the bleeding. The most obvious sign of this type of problem is hemorrhage coming from both nares.[3] When a patient is initially seen with postoperative bleeding, intermaxillary fixation (IMF), if present, should be removed. The patient's general physical status should be assessed and appropriate bleeding and coagulation studies ordered. Abnormal parameters warrant correction and possible consultations. With a good light source present, the nose should be suctioned to reveal whether a bleeding site is arterial or venous in nature. If adequate assessment is not possible, the nose should be anesthetized and decongested with a local anesthetic and a vasoconstrictor. Local anesthetic injections in the nose and

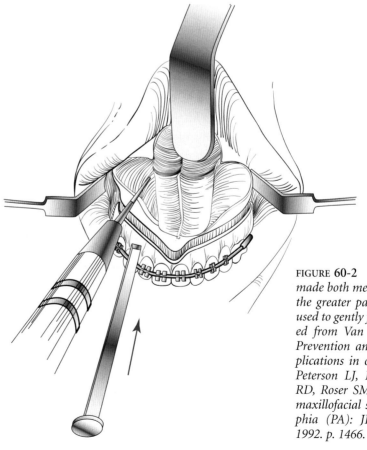

FIGURE **60-2** *Using a bur, a groove is made both medially and laterally up to the greater palatine artery. A chisel is used to gently fracture the bone. Adapted from Van Sickels JE, Tucker MR. Prevention and management of complications in orthognathic surgery. In: Peterson LJ, Indresano AT, Marciani RD, Roser SM. Principles of oral and maxillofacial surgery. Vol. 3. Philadelphia (PA): JB Lippincott Company; 1992. p. 1466.*

around the greater palatine foramen are helpful in stopping or slowing postoperative hemorrhage.

If the bleeding is minor in nature, it may be possible to treat the patient with bed rest. Anterior and posterior packing for 3 to 5 days combined with bed rest can be used for recurrent bleeding or for a patient not responding to initial therapy. For a patient who does not respond to these therapies or in whom the bleeding is severe or persistent, exploration of the surgical site and direct ligation or packing of problematic regions is suggested. An angiogram may be necessary. Additional operative techniques may be employed depending on clinical examination or angiographic findings. These include packing of the maxillary sinus and angiographic embolization of the specific vessel. Ligation of the external carotid artery might be considered in extreme emergencies; however, with collateral circulation, bleeding may still occur after this vessel is ligated.

Hemorrhage in the Mandible

Vascular Injury As with maxillary surgery, major vessels can be injured with mandibular procedures. Occlusion of the internal carotid has been described following a sagittal split osteotomy.[13] Major central nervous system morbidity can occur following this injury.

Vascular injuries are due to indirect trauma either through forceful placement of a retractor placed on the lingual surface of the ramus of the mandible or the use of a mallet and chisel on the medial aspect of the mandible. Medical and surgical management of carotid artery thrombosis is beyond the scope of this text. Prevention is relatively easy. Placement of retractors and chisels on the medial posterior aspect of the mandible should be used with caution. It is preferable to limit dissection and subsequent chisel placement just distal to the lingula.

Hemorrhage with Sagittal Split Osteotomy Early reports noted numerous incidences of excessive bleeding with the sagittal split osteotomy.[14] Vessels injured were the internal maxillary artery, the facial artery, and the inferior alveolar artery. These injuries were attributed to inexperience, excessive tissue stripping, and lack of sophisticated instrumentation. Excessive hemorrhage remains a problem with the sagittal split osteotomy although to a much lesser degree. In a series of 256 sagittal osteotomies the incidence of hemorrhage was 1.2% (3 cases).[15] This included 2 cases of injury to the inferior alveolar artery and 1 to the anterior facial artery.

Hemorrhage occurring secondary to vascular injury on the medial or lateral aspects of the mandible with a sagittal split osteotomy can be controlled in a number of ways. The simplest involves packing, clamping, or injecting epinephrine (1:100,000) into vessel walls. Caution should be used when applying electrocautery in close proximity to the inferior alveolar nerve. When necessary, bipolar cautery is suggested. Extraoral dissections to control bleeding sources are seldom necessary.

Hemorrhage with Other Ramal Procedures In a study of the intraoral vertical subcondylar osteotomies there was a low incidence of damage to the maxillary artery.[16] The masseteric artery may be injured by carrying a saw cut too far into the sigmoid notch. The inferior alveolar artery may also be injured with a vertical subcondylar osteotomy, which is usually caused by bringing the vertical cut of the ramus too far anteriorly to the posterior border of the mandible.

Access to the bleeding vessel is difficult given the approach. Fortunately in most instances, intraoperative bleeding along the ramal cut or in the sigmoid notch can be controlled by tamponade. Late sequelae such as an aneurysm may require embolization.

Loss of Vascularity

Segmental Procedures The results of vascular compromise vary between maxillary and mandibular procedures. Complications, ranging from fibrosis of pulpal tissues and periodontal defects to loss of segments, tend to increase with the number of segments. The most frequent cause of complications associated with the maxilla is interruption of the blood supply.[17] Additional causes may include lack of segment stabilization, patient factors, inadequate preoperative evaluations, poor follow-up, and multiple segments.[17] Patients who are heavy smokers or who have other systemic reasons for small vessel disease may mandate an altered treatment plan.

Several suggestions have been proposed to avoid vascular complications with segmental procedures. Preoperative planning to ensure adequate space between teeth, model surgery that minimizes the amount of bone removed, and careful examination of periapical radiographs prior to surgery are part of the planning that goes on prior to arriving in the operating room. Intraoperative management includes careful cutting between segments and the use of chisels and irrigated burs to complete cuts. These steps will minimize the amount of heat generated and decrease the chance of creating bone or tooth defects. Release of soft tissue adjacent to osteotomy sites and gentle mobilization of segments to avoid tearing and cutting of flaps is essential. Splints with palatal bars used for stabilization should not impinge on the palatal pedicle that serves as the major blood supply to maxillary segments. Special considerations must be given to the patient who has had previous palatal surgery or multiple segmental procedures or is a cleft palate patient. In these instances standard flap designs may not be adequate.

Complications such as periodontal defects, pulpal necrosis, and delayed union are more commonly seen in the anterior region of the mandible but may be associated with any segmental operation. Mandibular segmental procedures require detailed planning of soft tissue incisions and careful elevation of soft tissue pedicles. In order to minimize intraoperative complications, the vascular supply to involved segments must be optimized by designing as large a flap as possible to the involved segment, maintaining maximal soft tissue attachment to the segment to be mobilized, avoiding stripping the lingual mucoperiosteal pedicle, and making the bony cut as apical as possible to include as much muscle as possible.

Aseptic Necrosis   Major loss of soft and hard tissue of the maxilla is rare and is most often due to a compromised blood supply. This can be caused by a kinked pedicle in the palate or tearing of flaps. Isolated cases of loss of the entire maxilla or segments have been reported (Figure 60-3).[17] More subtle complications secondary to vascular

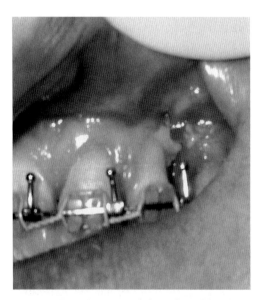

FIGURE 60-3   *Necrosis of the soft and hard tissues has occurred in the left lateral/cuspid region after a Le Fort I osteotomy. Adapted from Van Sickels JE, Tucker MR. Prevention and management of complications in orthognathic surgery. In: Peterson LJ, Indresano AT, Marciani RD, Roser SM. Principles of oral and maxillofacial surgery. Vol. 3. Philadelphia (PA): JB Lippincott Company; 1992. p. 1468.*

compromise range from flattening of the papilla and loss of the gingiva to periodontal defects in areas of osteotomy cuts.

Aseptic vascular necrosis of the proximal segment with a sagittal split osteotomy has been attributed to excessive stripping of the segments.[18] Loss of bone secondary to aseptic necrosis has resulted in disfigurement of patients. As early as 1974 Grammer and colleagues noted in animals the death of large areas of bone in the proximal fragment secondary to elevation of the mucoperiosteal pedicle.[19] They proposed that devitalized bone usually revascularized. However, when revascularization does not occur, a substantial loss of bone from the mandibular ramus can occur, especially in the gonial angle region. In 1977 Epker presented modifications of the sagittal split and discussed a technique in which the amount of dissection of the masseter was greatly decreased.[20] Adoption of this technique has greatly minimized the incidence of avascular necrosis after a sagittal split osteotomy. Rigid fixation of segments, which allows early revascularization, has also minimized the incidence of aseptic necrosis.

Early publications suggested that an advancement genioplasty could be done successfully by repositioning the lower border of the mandible as a free graft. However, when this is done, resorption of the advanced segment occurs to varying degrees and results in slight to almost complete loss of the genial segment. Leaving the lingual and the buccal pedicles intact minimizes resorption and gives a more predictable chin contour. Therefore, efforts should be made to preserve the largest pedicle possible. Large genial advancements may mandate more release of lingual soft tissue to achieve the desired results. However, with an adequate labial pedicle and rigid fixation, bone loss should not be appreciable.

The intraoral vertical subcondylar osteotomy is the mandibular procedure where the proximal segment is at most risk

due to release of periosteal attachments. One study reported 2 out of 42 patients with necrosis of the distal tip of the proximal segment.[21] The surgical technique involved stripping the entire lateral and medial surfaces of the mandible up to the mandibular neck. With more recent modifications of the technique where a pedicle of medial pterygoid muscle attached to the posterior and medial aspect of the proximal segment is maintained, necrosis of the proximal tip has not been a problem.[22]

Nonunion or Delayed Union of the Maxilla

Nonunion of the maxilla may be due to both local and systemic factors. The blood supply may be compromised by poor surgical planning or may be questionable because of previous surgery, as in cleft palate patients. Scarring in large advancements may make it difficult to passively reposition a maxilla. Patients may have parafunctional activity or excessive bite forces. In those patients in whom the maxilla has been moved superior and posterior, there may be insufficient bone interface to allow healing. Patients with systemic conditions that interfere with healing, such as diabetes and smoking, require individual case planning to minimize complications.

When an unstable maxilla is anticipated, bone plates may be combined with auxiliary forms of stabilization. In most cases this includes skeletal wires and a period of IMF from 1 to 6 weeks. With inferior positioning of the maxilla, bone plates and bone grafts can be combined with adjustable pins (Figure 60-4). When these are used the patient is not kept in IMF for more than 1 week. Bone gaps greater than 5 mm should be grafted. If the maxilla has good bone contacts in multiple regions, isolated defects may be filled with alloplastic material. Large bone gaps in multiple regions require autogenous grafts.

After surgery the major sign of a problem is mobility of the maxilla when the

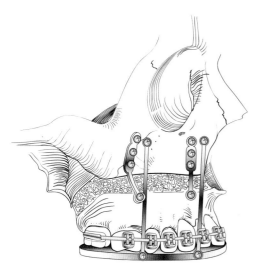

FIGURE 60-4 *The maxilla is inferiorly positioned using bone grafts, plates, and adjustable pins. Adapted from Van Sickels JE, Tucker MR. Prevention and management of complications in orthognathic surgery. In: Peterson LJ, Indresano AT, Marciani RD, Roser SM. Principles of oral and maxillofacial surgery. Vol. 3. Philadelphia (PA): JB Lippincott Company; 1992. p. 1469.*

patient occludes. Treatment of a mobile maxilla may be divided into early and late management. The use of IMF is controversial. If the patient is not in fixation a short period of fixation may help. On the other hand, if the patient is in IMF, removing it may allow consolidation. This is particularly important in the patient who has parafunctional activities. Additionally, flat plane splints may be used to distribute occlusal force more evenly. For minor problems selective occlusal equilibration may resolve premature contacts, contributing to movement of the maxilla. Patients should be placed on a soft diet. Heavy elastics should be discontinued, because with function they put intermittent strong forces on the maxilla. For patients with posterior relapse, light short class III elastics can help prevent further movement and may allow osseous consolidation. However, all elastics must be used judiciously as they may aggravate a problem. If a patient ends up with a minor Class III malocclusion, it is usually easier to manage than a nonunion maxilla.

Late management involves returning the patient to surgery for autogenous bone grafting and very rigid stabilization of the maxilla. This would include large bone plates, bone grafts, auxiliary techniques, and possibly alloplastic materials. Reoperation should be approached aggressively by completely mobilizing the maxilla and removing fibrous tissue.

Nonunion or Delayed Union of the Mandible

Nonunion or delayed union of the mandible may be due to avascular necrosis, insufficient bone contact, instability of the fixation appliances, or instability of bone fragments. It has been seen with sagittal split and vertical subcondylar osteotomies.

Vertical ramal osteotomies have special considerations, not only because a great deal of tissue may be stripped from the segments but also because the fragments may not lie in close apposition or be stabilized. Any large parafunctional movement of the jaws or trauma in the early phases after surgery may lead to nonunion (Figure 60-5).

Large advancements are of a greater concern than small advancements. For advancements of greater than 7 mm, additional plates may be needed to maintain stability (Figure 60-6). Alternatively, skeletal wires and a brief period of IMF have been shown to give increased stability.[23]

Delayed union of a sagittal split osteotomy can be treated by a period of IMF. Alternatively, the patient may need a second operation and additional plates or screws. Nonunion mandible following a vertical subcondylar osteotomy may be more of a problem with edentulous patients or when a very short vertical cut is used (Figure 60-7). A second operation, approaching the fragment from an extraoral approach to align and rigidly fix it, may be necessary.

Dental and Periodontal Injuries

Dental and periodontal injuries can be secondary to both vascular and nonvascular

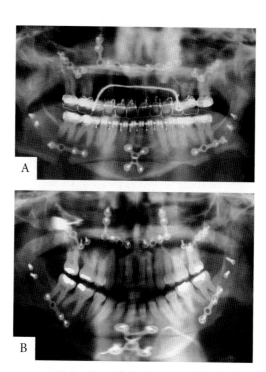

FIGURE 60-5 *A and B, Patient whose plates gave way 2 weeks after surgery when vigorous manipulation of her jaw was attempted.*

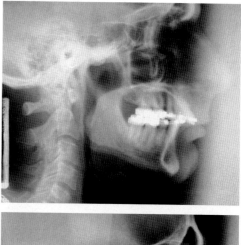
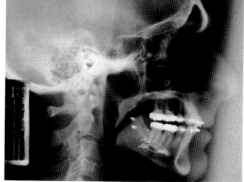

FIGURE 60-6 *Large advancement of the mandible with monocortical plates and bicortical screws.*

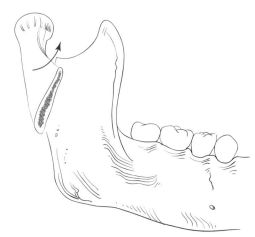

FIGURE **60-7** *Severe condylar rotation is common with a short subcondylar osteotomy. Adapted from Van Sickels JE, Tucker MR. Prevention and management of complications in orthognathic Surgery. In: Peterson LJ, Indresano AT, Marciani RD, Roser SM. Principles of oral and maxillofacial surgery. Vol. 3. Philadelphia (PA): JB Lippincott Company; 1992. p. 1470.*

causes and are most frequently related to planning or technical errors made at the time of surgery (Figure 60-8). Segmental procedures in the maxilla and mandible may cause a number of problems, including cut teeth, loss of teeth, need for postoperative root canals, and periodontal defects.

Preoperative orthodontic mechanics can be used to maximize a space between root apices in a planned osteotomy site.

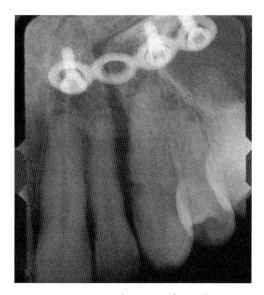

FIGURE **60-8** *Injured root surface adjacent to an interdental cut.*

Periapical radiographs should be studied to note the direction of the root apices. A minimum space of 3 mm is advocated when placing osteotomy cuts between teeth, and 5 mm is recommended above the apices to avoid injury to pulp.[24] Precise model surgery can greatly reduce the frequency of dentoalveolar injury. Surgery should be planned so that a minimal amount of bone is removed between segments. Manipulation and prying of segments should be done toward the apices of the teeth rather than at the gingival margin to minimize tears in the mucosa and subsequent periodontal defects. Segments should be tipped apart whenever possible. Copious irrigation of fine fissure burs should be used when cutting through the outer cortex in the maxilla. This is followed by gentle and progressive chisel placement in the region to separate the segments. When a bony palatal island is used, release of tissue should occur under the island rather than from the alveolar segments. After segments are gently separated, small amounts of bone may be judiciously removed. When larger wedges of bone are planned for removal, always remove less bone than was planned. When segments do not fit together, they can be gently trimmed. Defects seen following excessive removal of bone usually fill with scar tissue.

In the mandible it is necessary to cut both the buccal and lingual plates, leaving only a small amount of lingual cortical plate near the cervical portion of teeth to be separated by a chisel. Use of saws is recommended to cut through the mandible, with careful palpation on the lingual surface. Owing to the dense lingual cortex, chisels are much more dangerous in the mandible than in the maxilla where they could shatter the lingual cortex or tear the lingual pedicle region. For these reasons chisels should be used cautiously following a saw cut, and segments should be pried apart with minimal tapping through to the lingual surface.

Fistulas

Postoperative fistulas in the oronasal and oroantral regions generally result from soft tissue injury at the time of surgery. Fistulas have been reported with isolated segmental as well as total maxillary osteotomies.[25] This may occur as a result of rotary instruments, saws, or osteotomies that perforate the palatal mucosa at the time the segmental osteotomies are completed. Impingement of soft tissue in the segmental osteotomy site during segment repositioning and fixation may also result in tissue necrosis and fistula formation. Tearing of palatal mucosa at the time of attempted tissue stretching may also result in nonhealing defects. This is most common when a bony osteotomy is made in the midline of the maxilla while attempting to stretch the midpalatal tissue (Figure 60-9).

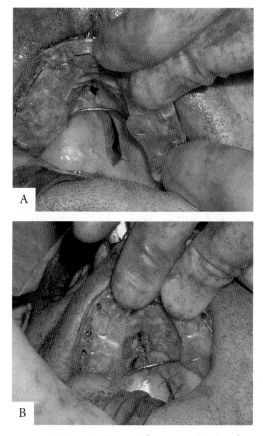

FIGURE **60-9** A, *Oronasal communication has been created during a Le Fort I osteotomy with palatal sectioning. B, Sutures placed at the time of surgery, with good oral hygiene, resulted in spontaneous closure at 8 weeks.*

Careful soft tissue manipulation at the time of surgery in an attempt to prevent tissue perforation is the best method for prevention of fistula formation. When expansion is needed, the palatal mucosa can be incised with two parallel incisions just medial to the greater palatine foramen; bony separation then occurs in the midpalatal area.[25] The tissue can stretch and expand in an area well away from the bony separation. An alternative technique involves making parasagittal cuts in the nasal floor immediately adjacent to the lateral nasal wall. The osteotomy can thus be made over tissue that is thicker and somewhat more elastic.[26] If a small tear is noted following a bony cut, care should be taken to release the palatal tissue from above prior to expansion of segments.

When a fistula is noted postoperatively, several measures can be pursued that may allow the fistula to close spontaneously. Preventing sinus or nasal infections is essential. This includes antibiotic therapy, decongestants, and nasal drainage. Construction of an appliance that will obturate the fistula without placing pressure on the overlying tissue will generally help in closure by reducing food contamination. Careful attention must be given to the construction of any appliance used to obturate a fistula in the immediate postoperative period. Excess pressure on the palatal mucosa may result in decreased vascularity, resulting in further loss of soft tissue and associated bone. If local measures, appropriate medical therapy, and fistula obturation have been unsuccessful, surgical closure of the fistula will be required.

When considering closure of a fistula, it is important to ensure that at least 6 months have elapsed to allow for revascularization of the maxillary segment. Carefully managed fistulas will continue to close for 8 to 12 weeks. If this therapy is not successful, a soft tissue flap should be raised from an area farthest from segments with the least potential for decreased vascularity. Timing varies, but the maxilla

should be revascularized by 6 months. If a large segment of the maxilla was involved in the initial hypovascular state, distant flaps should be considered. Choices include a buccal fat pad or a tongue flap, among others.

Management of Tissue after Vascular Compromise

Doppler flowmetry of the maxillary gingiva can be used to detect subtle decreases in the maxillary gingival blood flow following a Le Fort I osteotomy.[27] However, its use is limited to clinical studies at the present time. Clinically, blanched followed by cyanotic attached gingiva and adjacent free mucosa are early indications of vascular compromise following orthognathic surgery.[28] The overlying tissue can be an indicator of bony involvement. Three scenarios are possible: loss of vascularity to the soft tissue, whereupon the bone is perfused; loss of vascularity to the bone, whereupon soft tissue is perfused; and loss of vascularity to both the bone and soft tissue. If cyanosis is noted in the immediate postoperative period (hours to days after surgery), IMF, if present, should be released and the mouth inspected for kinked or constricted tissue. Splints must be carefully evaluated to identify areas of pressure on soft tissue by the appliance. If removal of IMF and relief or removal of splints is not helpful or the tissue is already necrotic, then supportive care is necessary to attempt to minimize the amount of bone loss. Loss of the soft tissue and exposure of the underlying bone is often what occurs. In severe cases this should be treated as an intraoral free graft. Meticulous irrigation should be performed several times a day with or without packing of the wound. Like all graft tissues it must be absolutely secure. Stability will allow some degree of revascularization. Hyperbaric oxygen therapy may be helpful to minimize bone loss while promoting neovascularization.

Reconstruction will vary and depend on the size of the resultant defect.

Nerve Injury

Sensory Injuries in the Maxilla

Sensory injuries in the maxilla have not been as thoroughly studied as those seen with mandibular surgery. With a carefully placed circumvestibular incision combined with gentle retraction, nerve injury is inconsequential and limited to the terminal branches of the infraorbital nerve. Recovery of sensation to the lip, cheeks, and nose usually occurs within 2 to 8 weeks.

Paresthesias secondary to damage of the sensory nerve supply to the teeth and mucosa are more common. Decreased sensation to the mucosa is transient and normal sensation commonly returns within 6 to 12 months. Although this is usually the case, patients will occasionally have permanent numbness intraorally on the palate and buccal gingiva. This is annoying, particularly if on the palate, as it can be burned by hot food. To preserve sensation to the palate, some authors feel that the greater palatine neurovascular bundle should be preserved.[28]

Failure of the teeth to respond to stimulation may also be temporary. However, permanent loss of response to electrical, hot, or cold stimulation is not unusual, and does not necessarily represent a tooth that needs endodontic therapy. The clinician must differentiate a nonvital tooth from one that does not respond to stimulation but has an intact blood supply. A tooth that shows periapical radiolucency on radiographs or a fistula upon examination is a candidate for root canal therapy.

Sensory Injuries in the Mandible

Sagittal Split Osteotomy Transections of the inferior alveolar nerve can occur during a sagittal split osteotomy.[29] The most likely time for this to occur is during the splitting process. When the segments are being separated, care should be taken to visualize the nerve. If the nerve is in the distal segment or encased in cortical bone, appropriate steps should be taken to release it. This may be as simple as releasing the nerve with an elevator from a medullar bone, or it may require additional bone cuts to release it from cortical bone. One study suggested that low body height of the patient and inferior position of the nerve may increase the risk for injury.[29] Repair of the nerve with one or more sutures placed in the epineurium has been recommended.[30] However, one large series had a 3.5% incidence of transection of the inferior alveolar nerve, which was anterior to or in the third molar region in all instances.[15] Nerve endings were approximated in 9 patients by positioning the segments but not suturing them. The length of follow-up for these patients was 2 to 5 years, and all of the patients had some return of sensation to the normal inferior alveolar nerve distribution. Whether this represented regeneration or new growth from the cervical plexus is unknown.

If the transection occurs at the vertical bony cut, immediate repair may be difficult. To expose more of the nerve in the distal segment a second cut anterior to the first is necessary. When excessive tension is present, the nerve may have to be exposed distally to the mental foramen to allow a tension-free repair. The need for such an extensive procedure needs to be weighed against other goals to be achieved with the surgery.

Injury to the inferior alveolar nerve in the absence of a transection is frequently associated with sagittal splitting of the mandibular ramus. Risk factors for an increased amount of neurosensory disturbance include the age of the patient, whether they have a genioplasty, and the amount of advancement.[31,32] Multiple techniques have been suggested to prevent these injuries, including osteotomy design, chisel placement, dissection technique, decompression of the lateral fragment,

and steroid use. Vigorous medial retraction may cause the inferior alveolar nerve to be compressed against the lingula and decrease intraoperative nerve conduction.[29,33] Retraction on the medial aspect of the mandible should be done carefully to avoid compression nerve injuries. The best place to make the lateral (vertical) cut is in the first and second molar region where the cortex is the thickest, the mandible is the thickest, and the nerve is furthermost from the lateral cortex.[15,34] Other suggestions have been made to prevent nerve injuries based on clinical experience, but no controlled studies have been done to prove whether one way is preferable to another.

Injury to the lingual nerve during a sagittal split osteotomy can occur but it is unusual.[35,36] The course of the lingual nerve near the medial surface of the mandible varies; therefore, any dissection on the lingual aspect of the mandible in the third molar region may temporarily or permanently injure this nerve.[37] As with inferior alveolar nerve injuries, lingual nerve injuries should be carefully followed and documented. If the nerve is visualized and has been transected, it should be repaired at the time of surgery.

Other Ramal Procedures Although vertical or oblique ramal osteotomies are frequently suggested as alternatives to a sagittal split osteotomy for horizontal mandibular excess, these procedures may also cause permanent injury to the inferior alveolar nerve. The incidence of permanent paresthesia following an intraoral vertical subcondylar osteotomy has ranged from 9 to 11%.[38,39] Endoscopic approaches to the ramus may have a different incidence of nerve injury, but experience with these techniques is limited.[40] The precise mechanism of injury to the inferior alveolar nerve is unclear and steps to prevent this complication require further study. The saw blade should follow the posterior border of the ramus until it reaches a point

well above the antelingual bulge on the lateral aspect of the mandible. Postoperative anesthesia should be carefully followed.

Motor Nerve Injury

Injury to the facial nerve is much more common with extraoral approaches than with intraoral surgery. However, there have been multiple reports of facial nerve injuries with sagittal split and vertical subcondylar osteotomies.[41–44] In one series that studied 1,747 cases of sagittal splits, the incidence was 0.26%.[43] The degree of injury varies from partial to total paralysis and is often seen following a setback of the mandible, but has been seen with a mandibular advancement.[42] The possible causes of injury are impingement of the nerve when the distal segment was moved back, fracture of the styloid process and subsequent displacement, and introduction of retractors behind the ascending ramus with impingement of the nerve. Most of the reported cases occurred with mandibular setbacks without use of the Hunsuck modification.[45] The most likely cause of nerve injury is pressure on the nerve trunk, either by the distal segment or by retractors placed behind the mandible (Figure 60-10). To prevent this problem a medial/ lingual split should be just distal to the inferior alveolar nerve when a sagittal split is used to set back the mandible. If a medial split extends to the posterior border, bone should be removed proximal to the lingula. Unfortunately the magnitude of setbacks causing this problem is unknown and probably varies with individuals. Care should be taken when retractors are placed behind the mandible on all ramus osteotomies.

When a facial paralysis occurs after surgery, there are a number of electrical tests that can be used to determine the depth of injury and subsequent therapy. Electroneurography, a study of peripheral nerve conduction, or electromyography, which is the detection and evaluation of electrical potentials from muscles,

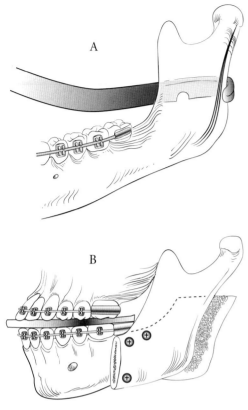

FIGURE 60-10 *Two possible causes of facial nerve injury with a sagittal split osteotomy. A, Retraction on the medial behind the ramus. B, Extension of the distal segment beyond the proximal segment. Adapted from Van Sickels JE, Tucker MR. Prevention and management of complications in orthognathic surgery. In: Peterson LJ, Indresano AT, Marciani RD, Roser SM. Principles of oral and maxillofacial surgery. Vol. 3. Philadelphia (PA): JB Lippincott Company; 1992. p. 1473.*

can be used.[46,47] It is important to distinguish between an injury that causes segmental demyelination and one that causes wallerian degeneration. With axonal interruption the ability to transmit an impulse is lost over a period of 5 to 7 days. When axonal degeneration occurs, the prognosis for complete recovery is poor. When this is noted, surgical exploration should be considered to rule out a laceration of the nerve. As long as the axon remains intact at the site of blockage, the nerve will continue to respond to stimulation distal to the blockage even though paralysis is present. Evoked eletromyography (EEMG), a test in which

the degree of muscle twitch elicited is recorded, has been used as a prognostic test.[48] If the response to EEMG remains greater than 25% at 5 days, the injury is mild and the prognosis is good.[48]

Clinical management of the patient during the paralysis can vary depending on the nerve branches and the type of nerve injury involved. When the patient has difficulty achieving eyelid closure, an eye patch and methylcellulose eye drops may be useful. Physical therapy such as heat, facial massage, and facial exercise performed twice a day have been suggested. Facial cream should be massaged into the skin around the eyes and mouth and over the midface, ideally using an electric vibrator. Exercises may consist of having the patient stand in front of a mirror to watch his or her face while raising the eyebrows, blowing the cheeks, and grinning. Even though no facial movement may be noted, intact nerve fibers will be activated and the exercise will help to maintain muscle tone. Electrical and mechanical stimulation may maintain muscle tone. Steroids had been given orally, intramuscularly, and intravenously for facial nerve paralysis.

Nasal and Sinus Considerations

Alterations in Nasal Form: Septum

Repositioning of the maxilla requires manipulation of nasal components and the maxillary sinus. As a result of these manipulations, alterations can occur with the internal nasal anatomy including position of the turbinates, nasal septum, and nasal valve. Adverse effects of maxillary osteotomies on the alar bases, nasal tip, supratip depression, and upper lip may result in an unesthetic postoperative facial appearance.[49–51]

The maxillary septum may be deviated prior to surgery, at the time of surgery, or during extubation. Hence the septum should be inspected prior to surgery and

at the time of surgery. During a Le Fort I maxillary surgery it is possible to align the septum at its inferior anterior caudal end. At surgery the septum is disarticulated from the entire maxilla. In particular, with impaction, the maxilla will encroach on the presurgical dimension of the nasal septum. Because of this movement, attention must be given to the positioning of the septum at the time of surgery. Failure to do so may result in septal deviation and obstruction, or in abnormal positioning of the columella and nasal tip.[50] There are several techniques for superior repositioning, including resection of an appropriate portion of the inferior aspect of the nasal septum or creating a groove in the superior aspect of the maxilla. In segmental osteotomies, creating a bony island with parasagittal palatal cuts may eliminate posterior superior pressure. However, it will not eliminate pressure from the anterior portion of the maxilla on the septum.

When septal deviation is recognized postoperatively, three choices for management should be considered (Figure 60-11). These include immediate manipulation, reoperation, or septoplasty at a later time. If appropriate management of the nasal septum was accomplished at the time of surgery but the nasal septum appears to be asymmetric, manipulation with an instrument placed within the nose on each side of the base of the nasal septum may allow for repositioning in the midline position (see Figure 60-11B and C). If rigid fixation has been used and the patient has no airway difficulties, short-term packing may be considered. If septal deviation is due to intraoperative management or if postoperative manipulation poses difficulty, immediate reoperation with further septal surgery may be indicated. If none of the previous approaches seems acceptable, and the patient does not have significant airway difficulty, the deviation can be reevaluated at a later date with consideration for a septoplasty through standard techniques.

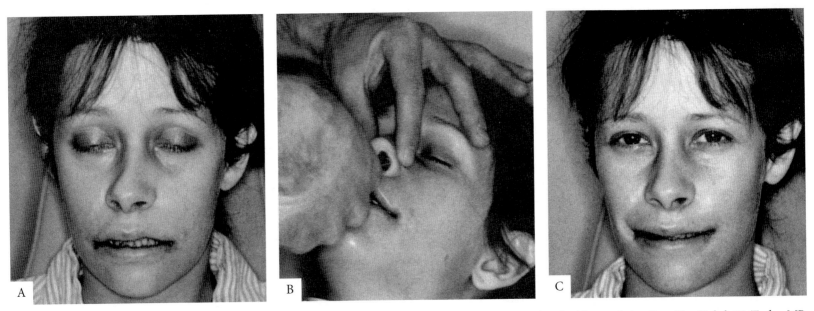

FIGURE 60-11   A, *Deviated septum initially after surgery. B, Manipulation. C, After manipulation.. Reproduced with permission from Van Sickels JE, Tucker MR. Prevention and management of complications in orthognathic surgery. In: Peterson LJ, Indresano AT, Marciani RD, Roser SM. Principles of oral and maxillofacial surgery. Vol. 3. Philadelphia (PA): JB Lippincott Company; 1992. p. 1475.*

Alterations in Nasal Form: Nasal Valve

An area of concern in maxillary surgery is alteration in internal nasal anatomy, nasal airway resistance, and breathing patterns as a result of maxillary surgery. Expansion of the maxilla with surgery has shown little change in the nasal airway. Some patients remain obligatory mouth breathers even after expansion.[52] Of greater concern is the possibility that superiorly repositioning the maxilla may decrease the nasal airway. Several studies have documented that the reverse is true.[53–55] Superior maxillary repositioning appears to increase nasal cross-sectional area, decrease nasal airway resistance, and increase nasal breathing. The explanation for this decrease in nasal airway resistance is most likely related to alteration in configuration of the nasal valve area.[53–55] The nasal valve is formed by the nasal septum, the floor of the nose, the soft tissue on the lateral aspect of the nose, and the caudal end of the upper lateral nasal cartilage. The increase in alar base width that results from elevating the soft tissues to expose the maxilla causes a slight widening of the nasal valve and thus reduces nasal airway resistance. Because this valve is at the smallest cross-sectional area of the nose, alterations in this area are likely to have a significant effect on nasal breathing whereas changes in much larger intranasal areas have little effect. This same phenomenon has been demonstrated in patients with cleft palates.[56]

Alterations in Nasal Form: Alar Base

In addition to the internal nasal changes, there are facial esthetic changes that may result from maxillary surgery. Failure to properly manage the nasal septum, paranasal musculature, and labial mucosa may result in undesirable facial esthetic results. Adverse changes in nasal and perioral configuration following maxillary surgery may include excessive alar base widening, increased prominence of the alar groove, upturning of the nasal tip (with an obtuse nasolabial angle), flattening and thinning of the upper lip, and downturning of the labial commissures.[50] These complications may also be compounded by internal deviation of the nasal septum or asymmetric positioning of the columella and nasal tip due to septal deviation. These types of problems are difficult to manage and are best treated by prevention. The need to control alar base width and the necessity of reconstruction of paranasal and perioral musculature have been previously described.[49]

Postoperative Sinus Symptoms

Postoperative complications related to the maxillary sinuses are primarily limited to infection, inadequate drainage, and open fistulas. Although many patients experience drainage and some sinus symptoms in the immediate postoperative period, true perioperative infections of the sinus area and long-term sinusitis are rare.[57,58] Between 2 and 6 months after surgery there will be normalization of the bony and soft tissue structures in over 55% of the patients.[58] However, at 6 months, 30% of the patients will show some latent mucosal borderline swelling.[58]

Despite the rarity of infections there are several potential causes of infections in the maxillary sinus area. The formation and retention of large blood clots in the sinus cavity is an obvious source of infection. Preoperative antibiotic prophylaxis with subsequent antibiotic levels present in the clot will help reduce infections from this source. Other potential causes of infection in the sinus are preexisting disease, dental infection secondary to trauma to the teeth, soft tissue ischemia and avascularity, and debris within the sinus. Foreign objects such as wires, bone plates, or screws are rarely, if ever, the isolated cause of a sinus infection and do not appear to cause a significant increase in the incidence of infection after maxillary surgery.[57]

Preoperative assessment of patients presenting for maxillary surgery should include a history and clinical examination, with careful attention to symptoms of any existing maxillary sinus infection. Evaluation of preoperative radiographs may provide some information regarding sinus pathology. Postoperative management of sinus infections should include appropriate antibiotic therapy verified by culture and sensitivity, decongestants, intranasal vasoconstrictors, and irrigation of patent fistulas if present. Generally sinus drainage can be managed within 10 to 14 days with these techniques. When a sinus infection is refractory to medical treatment, sinusoscopy should be considered. These patients should be managed in a manner similar to treatment for patients who have not had surgery.

Unanticipated Mandibular Osteotomy Fractures

Fragment Management

Fragment management, or more appropriately intraoperative management of unusual fragments, is a problem seen more frequently with mandibular procedures, especially sagittal split osteotomy. Additional segments may occur on either the proximal or distal fragments. The incidence of unfavorable fractures with a bilateral sagittal split is 1.9 to 2.2% with a slightly higher incidence when the third molars are present. [59,60]

These fractures may be in either the proximal or distal segment.

Intraoperative management of an inadequate split is that separation of the proximal and distal segments must first be completed. Intraoral management is the rule. A small or large fragment may have been fractured. Management will vary depending on the size and location of the fragment. It must first be determined where the fracture deviated from the desired split. Often it is necessary to remove the free segment to get access to the remaining mandible. Using a saw or a bur the intact mandible or segments are grooved so that a sagittal split can occur along the original planned lines. Chisels are used to complete the desired split. The key to management is to orient oneself to what is left. Once the split is successfully completed, the distal segment is advanced to its desired position. The position and size of the remaining fragments may make positioning of the condyle difficult. Segments are sequentially stabilized to the remaining fragments. An extraoral approach may be an option, but is usually not necessary. The following examples will illustrate management of various fractures.

Proximal Segment, Mandible Intact

The difficulty in managing segments depends on the location and size of the fractured pieces. A fragment may shear off the lateral aspect of the mandible, leaving the mandible intact. Whenever a buccal fragment shears off, the usual cause is an inadequate bone cut on the inferior border on the lateral vertical cut. The split must then be completed. This can be done by making a deep groove on the inferior border and connecting it with the previous groove coming down the external oblique ridge. By gently prying and, when necessary, cutting bone, the segments will be separated as originally planned. Placing the distal segment in occlusion, the free fragment should be stabilized with screws and

plates. In Figure 60-12 a buccal fragment has been fractured. The main portion of the mandible was intact before completion of the split. The segment is stabilized with a plate and screw osteosynthesis, as shown in Figure 60-13. Condylar position is not difficult to establish when a proximal segment is large enough to be positioned and overlapped with the distal segment in its new position. Bicortical screws can be used between the areas of contact of the two segments. With a small free fragment (as depicted) it is frequently easier to place a plate on it out of the mouth and then reattach it to the proximal segment.

Proximal Segment Split Complete

When the fragment occurs more superiorly, or there is a large advancement, such that there is no contact between the proximal and distal segments when placed into occlusion (Figure 60-14), a different approach must be taken. The condyle and coronoid are in one piece, simulating a horizontal osteotomy of the mandible,

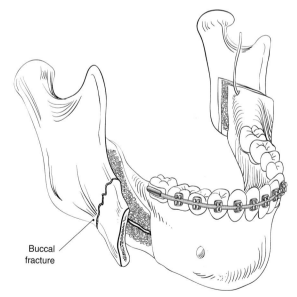

Buccal
fracture

FIGURE **60-12** *Buccal segment, fractured off. Adapted from Van Sickels JE, Tucker MR. Prevention and management of complications in orthognathic surgery. In: Peterson LJ, Indresano AT, Marciani RD, Roser SM. Principles of oral and maxillofacial surgery. Vol. 3. Philadelphia (PA): JB Lippincott Company; 1992. p. 1477.*

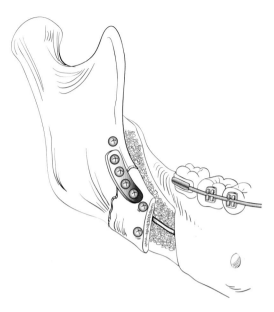

FIGURE **60-13** *A four-hole or larger plate is used to stabilize the free fragment to the proximal segment. Additional bicortical screws are placed to ensure stability of the complex. Adapted from Van Sickels JE, Tucker MR. Prevention and management of complications in orthognathic surgery. In: Peterson LJ, Indresano AT, Marciani RD, Roser SM. Principles of oral and maxillofacial surgery. Vol. 3. Philadelphia (PA): JB Lippincott Company; 1992. p. 1478.*

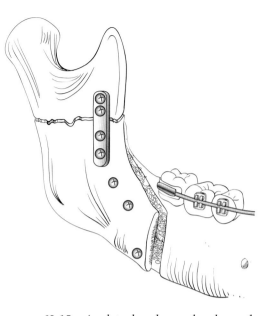

FIGURE **60-15** *A plate has been placed on the ascending ramus with additional bicortical screws placed between the proximal and distal segments. Adapted from Van Sickels JE, Tucker MR. Prevention and management of complications in orthognathic surgery. In: Peterson LJ, Indresano AT, Marciani RD, Roser SM. Principles of oral and maxillofacial surgery. Vol. 3. Philadelphia (PA): JB Lippincott Company; 1992. p. 1478.*

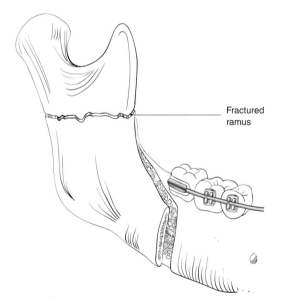

FIGURE **60-14** *The proximal fragment has a high or horizontal fracture. Adapted from Van Sickels JE, Tucker MR. Prevention and management of complications in orthognathic surgery. In: Peterson LJ, Indresano AT, Marciani RD, Roser SM. Principles of oral and maxillofacial surgery. Vol. 3. Philadelphia (PA): JB Lippincott Company; 1992. p. 1478.*

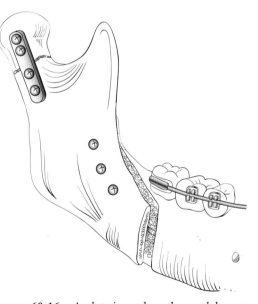

FIGURE **60-16** *A plate is used on the condylar segment with additional screws placed to stabilize the free fragment to the distal segment. Adapted from Van Sickels JE, Tucker MR. Prevention and management of complications in orthognathic surgery. In: Peterson LJ, Indresano AT, Marciani RD, Roser SM. Principles of oral and maxillofacial surgery. Vol. 3. Philadelphia (PA): JB Lippincott Company; 1992. p. 1479.*

with or without the angle as a separate fragment. Control of the condylar position is much more difficult. The large fragment that was sheared off should have a plate placed on it outside the mouth. It should be re-inserted and connected to the proximal segment (Figure 60-15). This usually requires two percutaneous incisions. Having done this the proximal segment is easier to manage and it can be united with the distal segment in its new position. This can be done with a series of plates or bicortical screws. Control of condylar position may be established by posterior, superior, and vertical pressure on the reunited proximal segment, followed by clamp placement prior to placement of bicortical screws, or by the use of a clamp on the coronoid process to stabilize the proximal fragment before screw placement.

The last case scenario is a fracture of the condyle with the coronoid and angle in a separate fragment. Here one must plate the condyle to the advanced reunited distal segment and use screws in other parts where there is overlap (Figure 60-16). Correct condylar positioning is extremely difficult to achieve in this environment. Through percutaneous incisions a plate is placed on the condyle. Using the plate as a handle, holes are drilled in the distal fragment and screws placed.

Lingual Segment Fracture

Fortunately, fractures of the lingual fragment occur less frequently than fractures of the buccal fragment. The underlying cause is frequently an impacted third molar or it may be secondary to wedging too high on the medial aspect of the mandible (Figure 60-17). To prevent this type of fracture it is wise to have third molars removed at least 9 months prior to surgery. When an unwanted fracture occurs, the split must be completed along the original planned osteotomy lines. As the free segment is not in the way when the split is completed, it is frequently possible to leave substantial vascular pedicle attached to it. The distal segment is placed into occlusion. The free fragment is manipulated to an anterior position and is fixed to the proximal segment by one or more bicortical screws. One or more plates or titanium mesh may be placed across the osteotomy site (Figure 60-18).

Excessive Lateral Displacement

Excessive lateral displacement can occur during a vertical subcondylar osteotomy. Depending on the geometry of the move, the proximal fragment or condylar segment may be displaced laterally or medially. The usual position is lateral to the main body of the mandible. Even with moderate flaring there is considerable remodeling possible and this is usually not a problem. Occasionally the proximal segment will be flared excessively. This can be remedied intraoperatively by removing a second wedge at the sigmoid notch region (Figure

60-19). Care must be taken in this region because the masseteric branch or the maxillary artery itself can be injured.

If excessive flaring is noted postoperatively, the segment may be manually repositioned, but if this does not succeed, reoperation is necessary.

Medial Displacement

In some cases of asymmetry the rotation may be such that the condylar fragment may be placed medially. Whether this will increase the incidence of nerve injury is unknown. Medial displacement rarely causes problems. A conceivable patient complaint is irritation of the pharynx. If this happens the medial fragment needs to be contoured or removed.

Proximal Segment Rotation

Lack of control of the proximal segment with a sagittal split osteotomy can have several effects that are both esthetic and

functional. Postoperation muscular pull is such that the proximal segment is pulled anterior and superior while the distal fragment is pulled posterior and inferior (Figure 60-20). Anterior superior rotation of the proximal segment may result in an unpleasant cosmetic result by flattening of the gonial angle and notching the inferior border of the mandible anterior to the angle. This causes a bulge in the cheek secondary to the position of the proximal fragment. The type of osteosynthesis used has been shown to affect the position of the fragment during surgery and in the initial postoperative period.[61]

Ideal management of a rotated proximal segment is prevention. Several positioning appliances have been presented to control the proximal segment during surgery.[62–64] Rigid fixation used without positioning appliances has shown minimal rotation of the proximal segment with surgery.[61] However, there is a tendency to

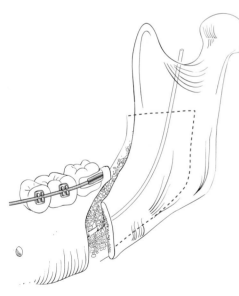

FIGURE 60-17 *A lingual split (distal segment) has occurred in the third molar region. Adapted from Van Sickels JE, Tucker MR. Prevention and management of complications in orthognathic surgery. In: Peterson LJ, Indresano AT, Marciani RD, Roser SM. Principles of oral and maxillofacial surgery. Vol. 3. Philadelphia (PA): JB Lippincott Company; 1992. p. 1479.*

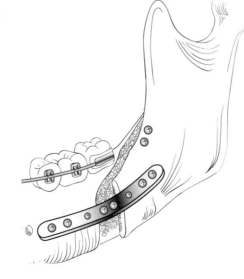

FIGURE 60-18 *Two bicortical screws are used to stabilize the free segment to the proximal segment. A plate can be used to stabilize the proximal segment to the distal fragment. Adapted from Van Sickels JE, Tucker MR. Prevention and management of complications in orthognathic surgery. In: Peterson LJ, Indresano AT, Marciani RD, Roser SM. Principles of oral and maxillofacial surgery. Vol. 3. Philadelphia (PA): JB Lippincott Company; 1992. p. 1480.*

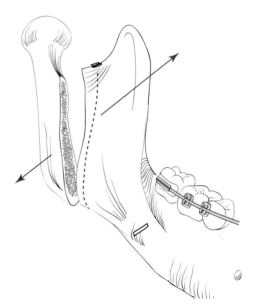

FIGURE 60-19 *Excessive flaring caused by bone contact at the sigmoid notch. This can be resolved by removing a wedge from the distal segment. Adapted from Van Sickels JE, Tucker MR. Prevention and management of complications in orthognathic surgery. In: Peterson LJ, Indresano AT, Marciani RD, Roser SM. Principles of oral and maxillofacial surgery. Vol. 3. Philadelphia (PA): JB Lippincott Company; 1992. p. 1481.*

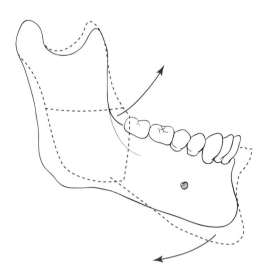

FIGURE **60-20** *Pull of the muscles of mastication on the proximal and distal segments. Adapted from Van Sickels JE, Tucker MR. Prevention and management of complications in orthognathic surgery. In: Peterson LJ, Indresano AT, Marciani RD, Roser SM. Principles of oral and maxillofacial surgery. Vol. 3. Philadelphia (PA): JB Lippincott Company; 1992. p. 1481.*

rotate the proximal segment medially and superiorly with large advancements.[65] This can result in an unesthetic effect for the patient, especially if there was any discrepancy in the height of the ramus prior to surgery (Figure 60-21). To date, the amount of rotation that will cause clinically significant decreases in muscle efficiency and unesthetic facial changes is unknown.

Excessive rotation of the proximal segment should be evaluated as to whether there are functional (decreased bite force, hypomobility) or esthetic (loss of the gonial angle) problems, or both. An esthetic problem seen in a patient with acceptable occlusal results may be treated by the use of an alloplastic implant. If the patient has an occlusal problem with esthetic considerations, the sagittal split can be redone (Figure 60-22). When these are combined with decrease in bite force and hypomobility, then reoperation must be combined with a vigorous postoperative physiotherapy program.

Most patients demonstrate decreased maxillomandibular opening compared with their preoperative state. The most dramatic decreases are seen after bilateral sagittal split osteotomies.[62] Temporomandibular mobility must be restored by postoperative physiotherapy. Ellis examined the range of mandibular motion after a sagittal advancement osteotomy in monkeys, when either IMF or rigid osseous fixation was used.[66] Animals that did not undergo IMF maintained a greater range of motion in the early postsurgical period and obtained preoperative mobility by 12 weeks postoperatively. Animals that underwent 6 weeks of IMF showed significant decreases in range of motion when compared to the rigid fixation group at each time period postsurgery. Several clinical studies have shown that whether IMF or rigid fixation is used, with postoperative physiotherapy, a normal or near-normal range of motion will return by 2 years after surgery.[61,67]

There are several potential causes of hypomobility in patients undergoing orthognathic surgery. Scar tissue induced by the surgery plays a major role. However, immobilization can compound the effects of surgical dissection and have adverse effects on the muscles, joints, and connective tissues. Immobilization by itself induces atrophy with a marked decrease in muscle fiber diameter. This problem may be compounded if the muscle is immobilized in a shortened position. In addition, following IMF, a series of degenerative changes occur in articular cartilage and synovial membranes.

Techniques that eliminate or minimize immobilization will probably decrease postsurgical hypomobility. Despite this it is strongly suggested that all patients have routine presurgical evaluation of muscle and joint function and a systematic rehabilitation regimen as part of their postsurgical program. Mandibular ramal procedures are potentially the most harmful to the surrounding tissue of the jaws. Mandibular advancements, in particular, are susceptible to postoperative hypomobility. If rigid fixation is used, mild self-directed physiotherapy beginning 1 to 2 weeks after surgery may suffice, consisting of instructions on active and passive exercises. When a patient's progress is limited or when surgery has been associated with longer periods of IMF, then more vigorous physical therapy is needed. If this is unsuccessful, intra-articular pathology may be responsible for the problem and additional steps may need to be taken to restore a normal range of motion.[68]

Temporomandibular Joint Dysfunction

Short-Term Disorders

Joint dysfunction in patients undergoing orthognathic surgery deserves careful preoperative examination. A number of patients presenting for orthognathic surgery will have muscular temporomandibular dysfunction.[69–71] Although a small percentage of patients will develop

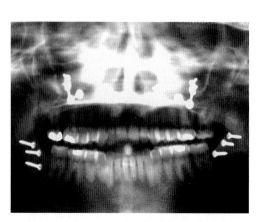

FIGURE **60-21** *Radiograph of short ramus.*

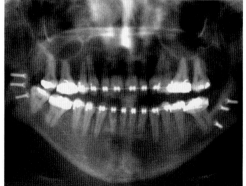

FIGURE **60-22** *Occlusal discrepancy.*

symptoms with surgery, the large majority will improve. Achieving a better functional relationship can help temporomandibular symptoms, but orthognathic surgery should not be offered as a cure for these problems. After surgery patients may have acute or gradual increases in temporomandibular symptoms. Acute exacerbations may be treated with anti-inflammatory medications and physical therapy. Gradual increases or chronic manifestations of temporomandibular problems are managed with standard protocols for these patients. Concern exists that with rigid fixation there will be a higher incidence of temporomandibular dysfunction compared with the use of wire osteosynthesis. Studies that have compared these two populations have not borne out these assumptions.[67,70]

Long-Term Disorders

Condylar resorption has been noted with and without orthognathic surgery. The cause of delayed relapse may be secondary to a number of factors including preexisting internal derangements. The role that surgery may play in these unusual cases is unknown. The incidence of condylar resorption or progressive condylar resorption ranges from 5 to 10% of the patients who undergo orthognathic surgery.[72–77] Patients who need large advancement of the mandible and who have preoperative temporomandibular symptoms are more likely to have this problem than those who have smaller advancements and no symptoms.[72,74] Condylar resorption has been noted 12 to 17 months after surgery.[76] Management includes splint therapy, with a possible role for medications.[76,77] Secondary surgery is unpredictable, with additional resorption possible in as many as 50% of cases.[76]

Unanticipated Maxillary Fractures

Whereas several reports have discussed management of additional fragments with mandibular osteotomies, little attention has been directed to maxillary surgery. With modified cuts of the maxilla, the bone leading to the zygomatic buttress (wing) may be thin and fractured (Figure 60-23). Management can be accomplished by using a plate to span the gap and then re-inserting the fragment (Figure 60-24).

Over- or underimpaction of the maxilla can occur at the time of surgery. This can be avoided with an external reference. One choice is to place a pin at nasion at the beginning of surgery. Intraoperative measurements will ensure that the maxilla is at the appropriate position at the end of surgery.[78] When the maxilla is under impacted, very few options exist. Plates, if present, may be removed and an attempt made to impact the maxilla with suspension wires in an outpatient environment. However, it is unlikely that this procedure will achieve the desired results. When the maxilla is overimpacted, it can rarely be successfully treated by multiple vertical elastics used in the early postoperative period. If unsuccessful, then a reoperation should be considered.

Postoperative Occlusal Discrepancies

Occlusal abnormalities may be related to a number of factors either in the preoperative, intraoperative, or postoperative phase of patient management. A review of cases of maxillary surgery suggests that the majority of discrepancies between what was desired and what was obtained can be traced to inaccurate preoperative records.[79]

Open Bites

Surgical Causes

Anterior open bites after surgery may be due to the technical difficulties seen with both the maxilla and mandible at the time of surgery. With the maxilla these include posterior interferences that are not recognized when the patient is in IMF. If the maxilla is fixed with condyles that are dislocated out of the glenoid fossa, when the

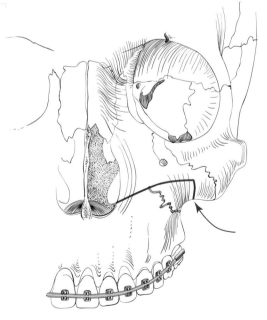

FIGURE **60-23** *"Wing" of the maxilla fractured off. Adapted from Van Sickels JE, Tucker MR. Prevention and management of complications in orthognathic surgery. In: Peterson LJ, Indresano AT, Marciani RD, Roser SM. Principles of oral and maxillofacial surgery. Vol. 3. Philadelphia (PA): JB Lippincott Company; 1992. p. 1483.*

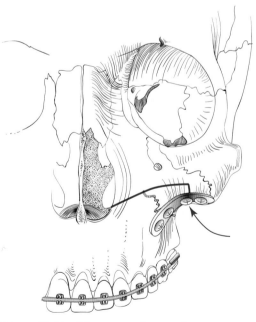

FIGURE **60-24** *Plate spans the gap; bone segment lies under the plate. Adapted from Van Sickels JE, Tucker MR. Prevention and management of complications in orthognathic surgery. In: Peterson LJ, Indresano AT, Marciani RD, Roser SM. Principles of oral and maxillofacial surgery. Vol. 3. Philadelphia (PA): JB Lippincott Company; 1992. p. 1483.*

patient is taken out of fixation, the occlusal discrepancy is usually recognized. Occasionally, however, it is not recognized until the next day. Depending on the severity of an open bite, the patient may have to be taken back to the operating room.

Open bites that occur after orthodontic appliances have been removed may be due to relapse of surgically or orthodontically treated transverse discrepancies. Surgical and orthodontic correction of severe transverse discrepancies have been noted to be unstable.[80] When relapse of the transverse discrepancy occurs, it is usually manifested by an anterior open bite. Management of late discrepancy will depend on its severity.

Dental or Orthopedic Causes

Open bites have been noted to recur years after treatment with both orthodontics and surgery.[80,81] Stability of orthodontic therapy varies depending on the orthodontic techniques used to treat an open bite.[82] Rotation of incisors that are flared with closure of an open bite may be no more problematic than for other tooth movements. When extrusion of teeth has occurred with orthodontic mechanics, the results are less predictable. Why this occurs is somewhat controversial. Extrusion may have increased sensitivity to external factors, such as the tongue and circumoral musculature. Lack of stability or recurrence of the open bite is therefore felt to be secondary to the continued presence of etiologic factors and failure of biologic adaptation. Measures taken to correct these problems may include orthodontic cribs or surgical techniques such as partial glossectomies.

Relapse of the Mandible

Relapse of the mandible following a bilateral sagittal split has been well documented in the literature, especially with larger advancements.[83–86] However, occlusal discrepancies can occur secondary to several reasons. Many of these occlusal discrepancies can be traced to the technical aspects of rigid fixation. Occlusal changes seen with rigid fixation may be secondary to condylar torque, condylar sag, or incorrect placement of the fragments at the time of surgery. This may result in anterior or posterior open bites or lateral shifts. Severe discrepancies may need to have a second operation. Minor discrepancies can be treated by early aggressive orthodontics. Posterior open bites of less than 3 mm can be treated with vertical elastics or orthodontic mechanics. Larger posterior open bites may have to be reoperated, with removal of the screws and replacement with either screws or wires. Anterior open bites represent failure to properly place the condyle or instability at the osteotomy site. IMF with anterior elastic traction may prevent reoperation when the cause is instability at the osteotomy site.

The preferred time to initiate therapy is as soon after surgery as the discrepancy is noted. Removal of the screws or plates in an outpatient environment at 3 weeks, coupled with elastic therapy, can sometimes correct some postoperative malocclusions. Failure to place the condyle in the fossa, either unilaterally or bilaterally, needs evaluation as to whether orthodontic therapy can correct the problem or if the surgery needs to be repeated. A lateral shift of the occlusion where the midline is off to one side is usually due to condylar torque at the time of surgery. When placing a clamp between the proximal and distal segments, the proximal segment should be observed for shifts or torque of the segment. If seen the fragments may need to be contoured or the clamp repositioned. After surgery a shift in the midlines secondary to torque of the segments may be treated by orthodontics or by reoperation. Small shifts of 1 mm or less can be managed by orthodontic mechanics. Larger ones may need a second surgery.

Relapse of a skeletal Class III occlusal condition upon release of IMF has been noted.[87–89] Several authors believe this can be caused by pushing the proximal fragment back during surgery. With the release of IMF the mandible rotates forward. To prevent this problem it has been suggested that the inferior border of the proximal and distal segments be aligned and that the medial sling be released.[88] Others disagree and feel that clockwise rotation of the proximal segment is not responsible for the relapse.[89] Additionally, the use of a monocortical plate on the proximal segment may provide a more stable result than that seen with bicortical screws (Figure 60-25). When this occlusal discrepancy is seen after surgery, short class III elastics can correct the problem if it is small. If the discrepancy is greater than 3 to 4 mm, a second operation is necessary.

Anterior Open Bite

As discussed above, an anterior open bite may be seen after a bilateral sagittal split osteotomy (Figure 60-26). This is usually due to a failure of the screws and/or plates placed at the time of fixation, or technical difficulties incurred at the time of splitting the segments with resulting edema in the joints which resolves with time. However, an anterior open bite is much more commonly seen in patients following an intraoral vertical ramus osteotomy upon

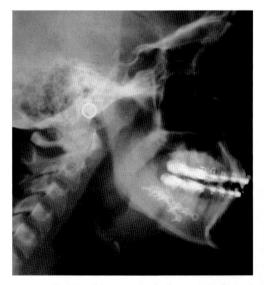

FIGURE 60-25 *Monocortical plate on the buccal surface of the proximal and distal segments.*

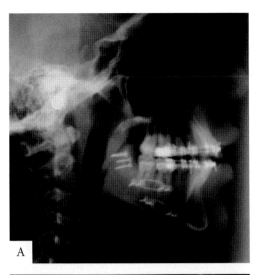

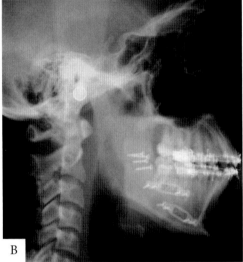

FIGURE **60-26** *Open bite following a bilateral sagittal split.* A, *At 24 hours.* B, *After 1 week.*

release of IMF.[90,91] Suggestions to prevent this problem from occurring include removing the coronoid process, placing skeletal wires, or using modified cuts of the ramus and 8 weeks of IMF.[91] Postoperative elastics have been used for 2 to 6 weeks when open bites have been noted.

Miscellaneous Occurrences

Endotracheal tubes have occasionally been cut during maxillary surgery. In some instances patients needed to be reintubated; in others packing around the endotracheal tube is sufficient.

Alar rim injuries are due to pressure on the rim from the nasotracheal tube. Care should be taken when wrapping the head so that there is no pressure on the tip of the nose or the forehead or ears.

Emphysema in the cervical and facial regions has been noted after a variety of procedures that are unrelated to orthognathic surgery. However, there are several reports of air in the soft tissues of the head, neck, and chest following Le Fort I osteotomies.[92] Subcutaneous emphysema of the cheeks is probably due to forceful blowing of the nose, which allows air into the surrounding tissues through the maxillary sinus. Forceful coughing can allow air to pass into the retropharyngeal space and into the mediastinum. Alternatively, rupture of a perivascular bleb or traumatic introduction of air through the cervical fascia is possible. Subcutaneous emphysema can be managed by observation, heat, and antibiotics. Therapy for pneumomediastinum consists of close observation, cardiac monitoring, intravenous fluids, and antibiotics. Chest tubes or drainage of the mediastinum may be necessary. Supplemental oxygen as well as pulmonary physiotherapy should be used.

Epiphora

Epiphora may be seen following a maxillary osteotomy and is frequently due to swelling of the nasal mucosa. Alternatively, the nasolacrimal duct may be injured when a concomitant turbinectomy is performed with an osteotomy. This is especially true if the bone cut along the medial wall of the sinus is high. Such tearing is infrequent and transient. Careful dissection and osteotomies around the medial aspect of the piriform aperture may decrease the incidence of this finding. Persistent tearing that does not decrease after 3 weeks may need to be addressed by a dacryocystorhinostomy.

Auriculotemporal Syndrome

The auriculotemporal syndrome, gustatory sweating, or Frey's syndrome is an unusual complication mainly of parotid surgery. After an injury to the auriculotemporal nerve, the symptoms are believed to be caused by a misdirected regeneration of parasympathetic fibers to denervated sweat glands. A number of authors have reported it occurring after extraoral vertical ramus osteotomies and bilateral sagittal split osteotomies.[93–96] Patients' symptoms occurred 3 months to 3 years after surgery.

Mild cases in which the patient may only have symptoms with spicy foods should be observed, because the symptoms may decrease with time. A variety of treatments have been suggested for more severe symptoms, including topical scopolamine and insertion of fascia lata or acellular human dermis matrix under the skin.[97] Topical scopolamine has a series of undesirable side effects. Recently there have been reports of the use of botulinum toxin as a successful treatment for this problem.[98,99]

Facial Scars

Although attempts are made to camouflage extraoral site incisions, unattractive facial scarring occasionally occurs. Egyedi and colleagues noted 6 undesirable scars in a group of 100 patients with extraoral incisions.[100] The criteria they used to determine what was attractive or unattractive are unknown. Percutaneous incisions of 2 to 4 mm seldom leave significant scars. More problematic is when the skin sticks to the underlying muscles. Scar revisions are usually able to improve on an existing scar. Intraoral management with the right instruments may obviate the need for most skin incisions.

Salivary Injuries

Injuries to the parotid gland can occur with extraoral procedures. Painless swelling, parotid sialoceles, and fistulas have been seen in the first week after surgery.[101] The treatment of sialoceles or salivary fistulas may include antisialogogues, pressure dressings, and aspiration from a nondependent point. Sialography is not recommended in the acute phases of these injuries, because it may create a fistula or increase its size. Resolution of a sialocele should be seen within 1 month with nonsurgical therapies. Failure of these more conservative therapies may be followed by more extensive surgical procedures.

References

1. Panula K, Finne K, Oikarinen K. Incidence of complications and problems related to orthognathic surgery: a review of 655 patients. J Oral Maxillofac Surg 2001; 59:1128–36.

2. Bradley JP, Elahi M, Kawamoto HK. Delayed presentation of pseudoaneurysm after Le Fort I osteotomy. J Craniofac Surg 2002; 13:746–50.

3. Lanigan DT, West RA. Management of postoperative hemorrhage following the Le Fort I maxillary osteotomy. J Oral Maxillofac Surg 1984;42:367–75.

4. Lanigan DT, Hey JH, West RA. Major vascular complications of orthognathic surgery: hemorrhage associated with Le Fort I osteotomies. J Oral Maxillofac Surg 1990;48:561–73.

5. Lanigan DT, Hey JH, West RA. Major vascular complications of orthognathic surgery: false aneurysms and arteriovenous fistulas following orthognathic surgery. J Oral Maxillofac Surg 1991;49:571–7.

6. Tiner BD, Van Sickels JE, Schmitz JP. Life threatening, delayed hemorrhage after Le Fort I osteotomy requiring surgical intervention: report of two cases. J Oral Maxillofac Surg 1997;55:91–3.

7. Lanigan DT, Hey J, West RA. Hemorrhage following mandibular osteotomies: a report of 21 cases. J Oral Maxillofac Surg 1991; 49:713–24.

8. Girotto JA, Davidson J, Wheatly M, et al. Blindness as a complication of Le Fort osteotomies: role of atypical fracture patterns and distortion of the optic canal. Plast Reconstr Surg 1998;102:1409–21.

9. Lanigan DT, Tubman DE. Carotid-cavernous fistula following Le Fort I osteotomy. J Oral Maxillofac Surg 1987;45:969–75.

10. Lanigan DT, Loewy J. Postoperative computed tomography scan study of the pterygomaxillary separation during the Le Fort I osteotomy using a micro-oscillating saw. J Oral Maxillofac Surg 1995;53:1161–6.

11. Brady SC, Courtemanche AD, Steinbok P. Carotid artery thrombosis after elective mandibular and maxillary osteotomies. Ann Plast Surg 1981;6:121–6.

12. Turvey TA, Fonseca RJ. The anatomy of the internal maxillary artery in the pterygopalatine fossa: its relationship to maxillary surgery. J Oral Surg 1980;38:92–5.

13. Sanni KS, Campbell RL, Rosner MJ, Goyne WB. Internal carotid artery occlusion following mandibular osteotomy. J Oral Maxillofac Surg 1984;42:394–9.

14. Behrman SJ. Complications of sagittal osteotomy of the mandibular ramus. J Oral Surg 1972;30:554–61.

15. Turvey TA. Intraoperative complications of sagittal osteotomy of the mandibular ramus: incidence and management. J Oral Maxillofac Surg 1985;43:504–9.

16. Tuinzing DB, Greebe RB. Complications related to the intraoral vertical ramus osteotomy. Int J Oral Surg 1985;14:319–24.

17. Lanigan DT, Hey JH, West RA. Aseptic necrosis following maxillary osteotomies: report of 36 cases. J Oral Maxillofac Surg 1990; 48:142–56.

18. Lanigan DT, West RA. Aseptic necrosis of the mandible: report of two cases. J Oral Maxillofac Surg 1990;48:296–300.

19. Grammer FC, Meyer MW, Richter KJ. A radioisotope study of the vascular response to sagittal split osteotomy of the mandibular ramus. J Oral Surg 1974;32:578–82.

20. Epker BN. Modifications in the sagittal osteotomy of the mandible. J Oral Surg 1977;35:157–9.

21. Hall HD, Chase DC, Payor LG. Evaluation and refinement of the intraoral vertical subcondylar osteotomy. J Oral Surg 1975;33:333–41.

22. Hall HD, McKenna SJ. Further refinement and evaluation of the intraoral vertical subcondylar osteotomy. J Oral Maxillofac Surg 1987;45:684–8.

23. Van Sickels JE. A comparative study of bicortical screws and suspension versus bicortical screws in large mandibular advancements. J Oral Maxillofac Surg 1991;49:1293–8.

24. Dorfman HS, Turvey TA. Alterations in osseous crestal height following interdental osteotomies. Oral Surg Oral Med Oral Pathol 1979;48:120–5.

25. Wolford LM, Rieche-Fischel O, Mehara P. Soft tissue healing after parasagittal palatal incisions in segmental maxillary surgery: a review of 311 patients. J Oral Maxillofac Surg 2002;60:20–5.

26. Turvey TA. Management of the nasal apparatus in maxillary surgery. J Oral Surg 1980; 38:331–5.

27. Dodson TB, Bays RA, Neuenschwander MC. Maxillary perfusion during Le Fort I osteotomy after ligation of the descending palatine artery. J Oral Maxillofac Surg 1997;55:51–5.

28. Epker BN. Vascular considerations in orthognathic surgery. II Maxillary osteotomies. Oral Surg Oral Med Oral Pathol 1984;57:473–8.

29. Teerijoki-Oksa T, Jaaskelainen SK, Forssell H, et al. Risk factors of nerve injury during a mandibular sagittal spit osteotomy. Int J Oral Maxillofac Surg 2002; 31:33–9.

30. Ziccardi VB, Assael LA. Mechanism of trigeminal nerve injuries. Atlas Oral Maxillofac Surg Clin North Am 2001;9:1–11.

31. Van Sickels JE, Hatch JP, Dolce C, et al. Effects of age, amount of advancement, and genioplasty on neurosensory disturbance after a bilateral sagittal split osteotomy. J Oral Maxillofac Surg 2002;60:1012–7.

32. Gianni AB, D'Orto O, Biglioli F, et al. Neurosensory alterations of the inferior alveolar and mental nerve after genioplasty alone or associated with sagittal osteotomy of the mandibular ramus. J Craniomaxillofac Surg 2002;30:295–303.

33. Jones DL, Wolford LM. Intraoperative recording of trigeminal evoked potential during orthognathic surgery. Int J Adult Orthodon Orthognath Surg 1990;5:163–74.

34. Rajchel J, Ellis E III, Fonseca RJ. The anatomic location of the mandibular canal: its relationship to the sagittal ramus osteotomy. Int J Adult Orthodon Orthognath Surg 1986;1:37–47.

35. Schendel SA, Epker BN. Results after mandibular advancement surgery: an analysis of 87 cases. J Oral Surg 1980;38:265–82.

36. Jacks SC, Zuniga JR, Turvey TA, Schalit C. A retrospective analysis of lingual nerve sensory changes after mandibular bilateral sagittal split. J Oral Maxillofac Surg 1998;56:700–4.

37. Miloro M, Halkias LE, Slone HW, Chakeres DW. Assessment of the lingual nerve in the third molar region using magnetic resonance imaging. J Oral Maxillofac Surg 1997;55:134–7.

38. Karas ND, Boyd SB, Sinn DP. Recovery of neurosensory function following orthognathic surgery. J Oral Maxillofac Surg 1990; 48:124–34.

39. Westermark A, Bystedt H, von Konow L. Inferior alveolar nerve function after mandibular osteotomies. Br J Oral Maxillofac Surg 1998;36:425–8.

40. Troulis MJ, Kaban LB. Endoscopic approach to the ramus/condyle unit: clinical applications. J Oral Maxillofac Surg 2001;59:503–9.

41. Sakashita H, Miiyata M, Miyamoto H, Miyaji Y. Peripheral facial palsy after sagittal split ramus osteotomy for setback of the mandible. A case report. Int J Oral Maxillofac Surg 1996;25:182–3.

42. Piecuch JF, Lewis RA. Facial nerve injury as a complication of sagittal split ramus osteotomy. J Oral Maxillofac Surg 1982;40:309–10.

43. de Vries K, Devriese PP, Hovinga J, van den Akker HP. Facial palsy after sagittal split osteotomies. A survey of 1747 sagittal split osteotomies. J Craniomaxillofac Surg 1993;21:50–3.

44. Motamedi MH. Transient temporal nerve palsy after intraoral subcondylar ramus osteotomy. J Oral Maxillofac Surg 1997;55:527–8.

45. Hunsuck EE. A modified intraoral sagittal splitting technique for correction of mandibular prognathism.1968;26:250–3.

46. Chow LC, Tam RC, Li MF. Use of electroneurography as a prognostic indicator of Bell's palsy in Chinese patients. Otol Neurotol 2002;23:598–601.

47. Gutmann L. Pearls and pitfalls in the use of electromyography and nerve conduction studies. Semin Neurol 2003;23:77–82.

48. May M, Klein SR, Blumenthal F. Evoked electromyography and idiopathic facial paralysis. Otolaryngol Head Neck Surg 1983; 91:678–85.

49. O'Ryan F, Schendel S. Nasal anatomy and maxillary surgery. I. Esthetic and anatomic principles. Int J Adult Orthodon Orthognath Surg 1989;4:27–37.

50. O'Ryan F, Schendel S. Nasal anatomy and maxillary surgery. II. Unfavorable nasolabial esthetics following Le Fort I osteotomy. Int J Adult Orthodon Orthognath Surg 1989;4:75–84.

51. O'Ryan F, Carlotti A. Nasal anatomy and maxillary surgery. III. Surgical techniques for correction of nasal deformities in patients undergoing maxillary surgery. Int J Adult Orthodon Orthognath Surg 1989;4:157–74.

52. Warren DW, Hershey HG, Turvey TA, et al. The nasal airway following maxillary expansion. Am J Orthod Dentofac Orthoped 1987; 91:111–6.

53. Walker DA, Turvey TA, Warren DW. Alterations in nasal respiration and nasal airway size following superior repositioning of the maxilla. J Oral Maxillofac Surg 1988;46:276–81.

54. Erbe M, Lehotay M, Gode U, et al. Nasal airway changes after Le Fort I impaction and advancement: anatomical and functional findings. Int J Oral Maxillofac Surg 2001;30:123–9.

55. Kunkel M, Hochban W. The influence of maxillary osteotomy on nasal airway patency and geometry. Mund Kiefer Gesichtschir 1997;1:194–8.

56. Gotzfried HF, Masing H. Improvement of nasal breathing in cleft patients following midface osteotomy. Int J Oral Maxillofac Surg 1988;17:41–4.

57. Bell CS, Thrash WJ, Zysset MK. Incidence of maxillary sinusitis following Le Fort I maxillary osteotomy. J Oral Maxillofac Surg 1986;44:100–3.

58. Kahnberg KE, Engstrom H. Recovery of maxillary sinus and tooth sensibility after Le Fort I osteotomy. Br J Oral Maxillofac Surg 1987;25:68–73.

59. Mehra P, Castro V, Freitas RZ, Wolford LM. Complications of the mandibular sagittal ramus osteotomy associated with the presence or absence of third molars. J Oral Maxillofac Surg 2001;59:854–8.

60. Precious DS, Lung KE, Pynn BR, Goodday RH. Presence of impacted teeth as a determining factor of unfavorable splits in 1256 sagittal split osteotomies. Oral Surg Oral Med Oral Pathol Oral Radiol Endod 1998;85:362–5.

61. Hatch JP, Van Sickels JE, Rugh JD, et al. Mandibular range of motion after bilateral sagittal split ramus osteotomy with wire osteosynthesis or rigid fixation. Oral Surg Oral Med Oral Pathol Oral Radiol Endod 2001;91:274–80.

62. Ellis E III. Condylar positioning devices for orthognathic surgery. Are they necessary? J Oral Maxillofac Surg 1994;52:536–52.

63. Helm G, Stepke MT. Maintenance of the preoperative condyle position in orthognathic surgery. J Craniomaxillofac Surg 1997; 25:34–8.

64. Merten HA, Halling F. A new condylar positioning technique in orthognathic surgery. Technical note. J Craniomaxillofac Surg 1992;20:310–2.

65. Harris MD, Van Sickels JE, Alder M. Factors influencing condylar position after the bilateral sagittal split osteotomy fixed with bicortical screws. J Oral Maxillofac Surg 1999;57:650–4.

66. Ellis E III. Mobility of the mandible following mandibular advancement and maxillo-mandibular or rigid internal fixation: an experimental investigation in *Macaca mulatto*. J Oral Maxillofac Surg 1988;46:118–23.

67. Feinerman DM, Piecuch JF. Long-term effects of orthognathic surgery on the temporomandibular joint: comparison of rigid and non-rigid fixation methods. Int J Oral Maxillofac Surg 1995;24:268–72.

68. Van Sickels JE, Tiner BD, Alder ME. Condylar torque as a possible cause of hypomobility after sagittal split osteotomy. Report of three cases. J Oral Maxillofac Surg 1997; 55:398–402.

69. De Boever AL, Keeling SD, Hilsenbeck S, et al. Signs of temporomandibular disorders in patients with horizontal mandibular deficiency. J Orofac Pain 1996;10:21–7.

70. Rodrigues-Garcia RC, Sakai S, Rugh JD, et al. Effects of major class II occlusal correction on temporomandibular signs and symptoms. J Orofac Pain 1998;12:185–92.

71. Panula K, Somppi M, Finne K, Oikarinen K. Effects of orthognathic surgery on temporomandibular joint dysfunction. A controlled prospective 4 year follow-up study. Int J Oral Maxillofac Surg 2000;29:183–7.

72. Cutbirth M, Van Sickels JE, Thrash WJ. Condylar resorption after bicortical screw fixation of mandibular advancement. J Oral Maxillofac Surg 1998;56:178–82.

73. Hwang SJ, Haers PE, Zimmermann A, et al. Surgical risk factors for condylar resorption after orthognathic surgery. Oral Surg Oral Med Oral Pathol Endod 2000;89:542–52.

74. Scheerlinck JP, Stoelinga PJ, Blijdorp PA, et al. Sagittal split advancement osteotomies stabilized with miniplates. A 2–5 year follow-up. Int J Oral Maxillofac Surg 1994;23:127–31.

75. Hoppenreijs TJ, Freihofer HP, Stoelinga PJ, et al. Condylar remodeling and resorption after Le Fort I and bimaxillary osteotomies in patients with anterior open bite. A clinical and radiological study. Int J Oral Maxillofac Surg 1998;27:81–91.

76. Hoppenreijs TJ, Stoelinga PJ, Grace KL, Robben CM. Long-term evaluation of patients with progressive condylar resorption following orthognathic surgery. Int J Oral Maxillofac Surg 1999;28:411–8.

77. Arnett GW, Milam SB, Gottesman L. Progressive mandibular retrusion-idiopathic condylar resorption. Part II. Am J Orthod Dentofac Orthop 1996;110:117–27.

78. Nishioka GJ, Van Sickels JE. Modified external reference measurement technique for vertical positioning of the maxilla. Oral Surg Oral Med Oral Pathol 1987;64:22–3.

79. Jacobson R, Sarver DM. The predictability of maxillary repositioning in Le Fort I orthognathic surgery. Am J Orthod Dentofac Orthop 2002;122:142–54.

80. Profitt WR, Turvey TA, Phillips C. Orthognathic surgery: a hierarchy of stability. Int J Adult Orthodon Orthognath Surg 1996; 11:191–204.

81. Burford D, Noar JH. The causes, diagnosis and treatment of anterior open bite. Dent Update 2003;30:235–41.

82. Beane RA. Nonsurgical management of the anterior open bite: a review of options. Semin Orthod 1999;5:275–83.

83. Dolce C, Van Sickels JE, Bays RA, Rugh JD. Skeletal stability after mandibular advancement with rigid versus wire fixation. J Oral Maxillofac Surg 2000;58:1219–8.

84. Dolce C, Hatch JP, Van Sickels JE, Rugh JD.

Rigid versus wire fixation for mandibular advancement skeletal and dental changes after 5 years. Am J Orthod Dentofac Orthop 2002;121:638–49.

85. Blomqvist JE, Ahlborg G, Isaksson S, Svartz K. A comparison of skeletal stability after mandibular advancement and use of two rigid internal fixation techniques. J Oral Maxillofac Surg 1997;55:568–74.

86. Moenning JE, Bussard DA, Lapp TH, Garrison BT. Comparison of relapse in bilateral sagittal split osteotomies for mandibular advancement: rigid internal fixation (screws) versus inferior border wires with anterior skeletal fixation. Int J Adult Orthodon Orthognath Surg 1990;5:175–82.

87. Proffit WR, Phillips C, Turvery TA. Stability after surgical-orthodontic corrective of skeletal Class III malocclusion. 3. Combined maxillary and mandibular procedures. Int J Adult Orthodon Orthognath Surg 1991;6:211–25.

88. Franco JE, Van Sickels JE, Thrash WJ. Factors contributing to relapse in rigidly fixed mandibular setbacks. J Oral Maxillofac Surg 1989;47:451–6.

89. Costa F, Robiony M, Sembronio S, et al. Stability of skeletal Class III malocclusion after combined maxillary and mandibular procedures. Int J Adult Orthodon Orthognath Surg 2001;16:179–92.

90. Proffit WR, Phillips C, Dann C IV, Turvey TA. Stability after surgical orthodontic correction of skeletal Class III malocclusion. I. Mandibular setback. Int J Adult Orthodon Orthognath Surg 1991;6:7–18.

91. Tornes K, Wisth PJ. Stability after vertical subcondylar ramus osteotomy for correction of mandibular prognathism. Int J Oral Maxillofac Surg 1988;17:242–8.

92. Nannini V, Sachs SA. Mediastinal emphysema following Le Fort I osteotomy: report of a case. Oral Surg Oral Med Oral Pathol 1986;62:508–9.

93. Berrios RJ, Quinn PD. Frey's syndrome: a complication after orthognathic surgery. Int J Adult Orthodon Orthogn Surg 1986;1:219–24.

94. Kopp WK. Auriculotemporal syndrome secondary to vertical sliding osteotomy of the mandibular rami: report of a case. J Oral Surg 1968;26:295–6.

95. Tuinzing DB, van der Kwast WA. Frey's syndrome. A complication after sagittal splitting of the mandible. Int J Oral Surg 1982;11:197–200.

96. Guerrissi J, Stoyannoff J. Atypical Frey syndrome as a complication of Obwegeser osteotomy. J Craniofac Surg 1998;9:543–7.

97. Sinha UK, Saddat D, Doherty CM, Rice DH. Use of AlloDerm implant to prevent Frey syndrome after parotidectomy. Arch Facial Plast Surg 2003;5:109–12.

98. Eckardt A, Kuettner C. Treatment of gustatory sweating (Frey's syndrome) with botulinum toxin A. Head Neck 2003;25:624–8.

99. Restivo DA, Lanza S, Patti F, et al. Improvement of diabetic autonomic gustatory sweating by botulinum toxin type A. Neurology 2002;59:1971–3.

100. Egyedi P, Houwing M, Juten E. The oblique subcondylar osteotomy: report of results of 100 cases. J Oral Surg 1981;39:871–3.

101. Dierks EJ, Granite EL. Parotid sialocele and fistula after mandibular osteotomy. J Oral Surg 1977;35:299–300.

Orthognathic Surgery in the Patient with Cleft Palate

Timothy A. Turvey, DDS
Ramon L. Ruiz, DMD, MD
Katherine W. L. Vig, BDS, MS, D Orth
Bernard J. Costello, DMD, MD

The estimated incidence of orofacial clefts involving the lip and palate in the United States is approximately 1 to 2 per 1,000 births or approximately 1 in 700 live births.[1] The average cost of rehabilitation of a child born with an oral cleft is estimated at approximately $100,000 (US). The occurrence rate of infants born with a cleft lip and/or palate is influenced by race and gender, and the cost varies by the number of procedures and interventions performed.

Care for an infant born with an orofacial cleft begins with primary surgical repair of the lip followed by the palate and continues in defined and appropriate stages to late adolescence, at which point public funding is usually discontinued. The burden of care assumed by the patient and family in the indirect costs of time off from work/school and transportation by the caregiver is not to be underestimated, and it is often inadequately equated with the financial or direct costs of treatment.

The interdisciplinary approach to the management of patients with a cleft lip and/or palate and other craniofacial anomalies requires careful coordination and communication; a cleft palate team establishes a patient-centered approach

that follows critical pathways.[2–5] The timing and sequencing of care is critical because of the interaction of facial growth with the development of the dentition. Clefts of the maxilla, especially the unilateral cleft lip and palate, are associated with a skeletal maxillary deficiency in the transverse, anteroposterior, and vertical dimensions. The dysmorphology in all three dimensions has been attributed to scar tissue following the primary repair of the lip during the first 6 months of life and the palatal repair, which is performed typically at 12 to 18 months. Clefts of the maxilla, both unilateral and bilateral, have been considered to have an intrinsic growth deficiency of skeletal, soft tissue, and dental components. However, in those children who have unrepaired clefts early in childhood, relatively normal occlusal relationships are established compared with those relationships in children who are surgically repaired in the first 2 years of life. This latter group is characterized by anterior and posterior dental crossbites, midface sagittal deficiency, and associated vertical overclosure.[6] Because the cleft involves the dentoalveolus and occurs owing to the lack of fusion of the primary

palate during embryogenesis, the dental lamina may also be involved, with consequences of extra teeth such as supernumerary teeth, malformed and misplaced teeth, or an absence of teeth in the cleft site. Normal biologic variation is the result of phenotypic variation, which allows one individual to be distinguished from another by facial appearance. Therefore, dental malocclusions may occur on all skeletal patterns, but in the population with a cleft lip and palate, the pathogenesis of clefting is superimposed on the individuals' inherited facial pattern. Additionally, facial clefts are associated with over 300 syndromic conditions,[7,8] so a patient may have syndromic or nonsyndromic facial cleft; this distinction and diagnosis is confirmed by the geneticist on the team.

Asymmetry is a typical facial characteristic and is one of the stigmas associated with unilateral orofacial clefts. Cleft patients typically express concerns about their facial appearance, but they also have problems with communication because their speech is affected. This is partially because the velopharyngeal mechanism is inadequate to close off the oropharynx from the nasopharynx, resulting in hypernasality and a lack of intelligibility of the phonetic components.

The severity of the skeletal aspect of the malocclusion and facial asymmetry determines the surgical/orthodontic approach. Mild discrepancies may be camouflaged by the orthodontic dentoalveolar compensation. However, during adolescence the compensation for the skeletal discrepancy may be outgrown; orthognathic surgery is the treatment of choice for patients in their late teens. Because growth prediction is not an exact science, an anterior crossbite corrected in the mixed dentition frequently reestablishes following the pubertal growth spurt and adolescent growth.

The purpose of this chapter is to discuss the surgical and orthodontic correction of the cleft in dysmorphic faces. The focus is on patients with cleft lip and palate who would benefit from bone grafts in the early mixed dentition, and maxillary advancement with contour bone grafting in adolescence when growth of the nasomaxillary complex has stabilized. The successful correction of these secondary skeletal deformities frequently requires treatment protocols that include orthognathic surgery in conjunction with the final phase of orthodontic treatment. Patients with a cleft lip and palate benefit from staged and coordinated procedures to achieve optimal results. These include bone-graft construction of the cleft maxilla and palate in the mixed dentition phase of development, and orthognathic surgery to correct the midface deficiency in adolescence. These procedures are designed to be only stages in the process of reconstruction and rehabilitation.

Timing and Sequencing of Bone Grafting the Cleft Maxilla and Palate

An understanding of craniofacial growth and development is critical in timing both surgical and orthodontic interventions. In bone grafting, dental development is more important than is the chronologic age of the patient. The decision for determining orthodontic expansion to detect the dental crossbite, as a presurgical phase of orthodontics, depends on the root development of the unerupted canine. If the lateral incisor is developing on the posterior side of the cleft, a bone graft needs to be performed early to allow eruption to the cleft site. Seminal papers defined the age for secondary alveolar bone grafting, which is now a well-accepted procedure after primary lip and palate repair.[9,10] They divided the timing into early, 2 to 5 years of age; intermediate, 6 to 15 years of age; and late, 16 years to adult. A retrospective interdisciplinary study reported the outcome of bone grafts to the cleft maxilla relative to radiographic and periodontal parameters; as well, it stated that the closure of fistulas and the eruption of the canine through the bone-graft site suggested high success in age-appropriate patients.[11] A longitudinal retrospective study provided evidence for the timing and sequencing of the surgical and orthodontic treatment, using cancellous bone harvested from the iliac crest and the stage of development of the unerupted canine, typically between 9 and 11 years of age.[12] Contemporary opinion considers this intermediate time frame to have the greatest benefits and the least risk in compromising midface skeletal and dental growth and development.

Benefits of bone grafting include the following:

- Bone is provided into which the unerupted teeth adjacent to the cleft may erupt or be moved orthodontically. The timing and sequencing of the bone graft is determined by the position of the teeth adjacent to the cleft, their root development, and their stage of eruption, rather than the chronologic age of the patient.
- Supernumerary or malformed teeth may be removed at the time of the surgical placement of the bone graft into the cleft site. Patent oronasal fistulas either in the palate or the nasolabial vestibule are closed. Fistula closure is achieved by using a three-layered closure technique with the grafted bone sandwiched between the two soft tissue planes.
- The grafted bone provides support and elevation of the alar base in the defect and improves nasal and lip symmetry.
- Because there is continuity of the maxilla, the restorative dentist has the opportunity to provide a more esthetic and hygienic prosthetic replacement, even if teeth are missing. The placement of implants into bone grafts is successful and is a contemporary alternative to a bridge or removable appliance.
- In repaired bilateral clefts of the lip and palate, the placement of bone grafts bilaterally in the cleft sites stabilizes the premaxilla while providing bone into which the adjacent unerupted teeth may erupt.

Through efforts to determine the optimal timing of treatment, several controversies have arisen related to the age of the patient, the type of bone graft, the site from which the graft is harvested, and the optimal timing of orthodontic expansion of the maxilla in relation to the surgical placement of the bone graft.[12]

The surgical technique for bone grafting the cleft maxilla and palate involves a three-layered closure with autogenous cancellous bone graft sandwiched between the nasal floor and the oral mucosa. An incision is made around the cleft to preserve the fixed gingiva to circumscribe the fistula (Figure 61-1). The tissue is then elevated from the bone on both sides of the cleft in the subperiosteal plane to the level of the anterior nasal spine and the lateral piriform rim. The tissue is elevated, inverted, and sutured to form a reconstructed nasal floor (Figure 61-2). Fresh cancellous bone is then condensed in the cleft defect and over the hypoplastic bone edges of the cleft (Figure 61-3). Oral tissue is either rotated or advanced to close over the bone grafts (Figures 61-4–61-6).

Timing of Midface Advancement Surgery in Adolescents

Biologic and psychosocial concerns govern the decision for the timing of surgical maxillary advancement. It is always prudent to delay surgery of the nasomaxillary complex until growth has stabilized and the peak velocity of somatic growth has passed. This improves the predictability and long-term stability of treatment and reduces the risk that surgical-orthodontic correction will be outgrown. The optimal time for surgical correction of the skeletal discrepancy is when the patient is physically and psychologically prepared. Patients need to appreciate the relevance of facial growth and development and the consequences if surgical correction is

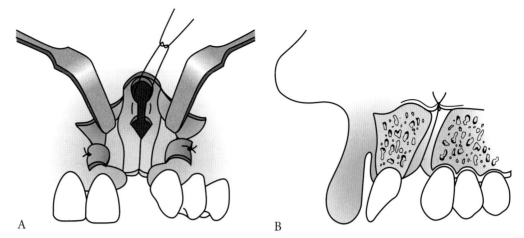

FIGURE **61-2** A, *The tissues lining the cleft are elevated to the nasal cavity to construct a floor. B, Closure of the nasal lining is accomplished with a horizontal mattress suture to evert the edges toward the nasal side. Adapted from Turvey TA, Vig KWL, Fonseca RJ. Surgical management. In: Facial clefts and craniosynostosis: principles and management. Philadelphia (PA): W.B. Saunders Company; 1996. p. 413.*

undertaken prior to maturation. Another biologic consideration regarding the timing of surgery is the eruption of the permanent dentition. Delaying surgery until the canine and second molars have erupted minimizes the risk of endodontic requirements and displacement of the second molars. Third molars can usually be removed at the time of maxillary surgery, and their presence should not be a major concern. Patients, parents, and treating doctors participate in the decision regarding when to proceed with surgery; the approach should be patient centered and evidence based with regard to the risks, costs, and benefits. Patient autonomy in the decision should be given the highest priority in orthognathic surgery. This requires that patients be in late adolescence to understand the consequences of the decision and be able to rationalize the expectations for the outcome.

Adolescents are under enormous pressures to conform to their peers. At no other time in life is an individual exposed to concerns about their self-image and physical attractiveness with such additional pressure of peer criticism of appearance differences. Many adolescent patients with clefts are subjected to ridicule about their facial appearance, and

this is accompanied by low self-esteem and impaired socialization. Social withdrawal is another issue resulting from the pressures felt by adolescents, especially those with facial disfigurement. Although counseling can help, the patient must still

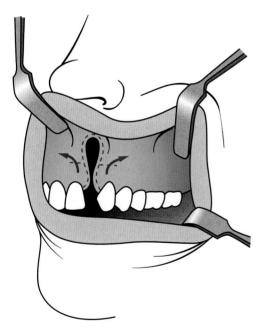

FIGURE **61-1** *Outline of the incision to prepare the cleft site for bone grafting. The fixed gingival tissues are preserved and sutured back. Adapted from Turvey TA, Vig KWL, Fonseca RJ. Surgical management. In: Facial clefts and craniosynostosis: principles and management. Philadelphia (PA): W.B. Saunders Company; 1996. p. 412.*

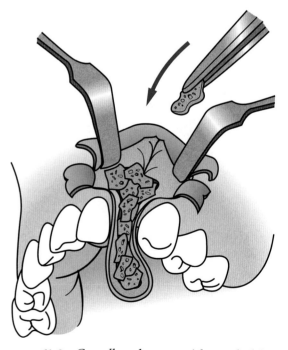

FIGURE **61-3** *Cancellous bone particles packed into the defect must extend from the nasal rim to the alveolar crest. Adapted from Turvey TA, Vig KWL, Fonseca RJ. Surgical management. In: Facial clefts and craniosynostosis: principles and management. Philadelphia: W.B. Saunders Company; 1996. p. 415.*

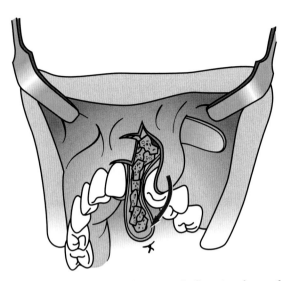

FIGURE **61-4** *A buccal mucosal flap is elevated, maintaining a wide and thick anterior base. The flap is then rotated to cover the defect. Adapted from Turvey TA, Vig KWL, Fonseca RJ. Surgical management. In: Facial clefts and craniosynostosis: principles and management. Philadelphia (PA): W.B. Saunders Company; 1996. p. 417.*

cope with the disfigurement; however, this may be improved with surgery.

Improving facial appearance by addressing the skeletal disproportion often

results in dramatic and complementary changes. Patients typically perceive these changes positively—the changes send a clear message that someone cares about them and is sensitive to their concerns. An improvement in self-concept and image in patients with a cleft lip and/or palate usually follows surgical correction of the midface deficiency and skeletal disproportion. Patients' perception of their quality of life is an important consideration and should not be overlooked in the timing of surgery. However, care should be taken in the psychosocial assessment to identify unrealistic expectations and to recognize those patients who use the stigmas as an excuse for dependency. Identification of these individuals prior to surgery is not easy; interdisciplinary management should include the involvement of a psychologist on the cleft palate team.

The decision to proceed with surgery prior to maturation may result in additional surgery being needed once growth is complete. This need is tempered by the reduced morbidity of repeat surgeries in contemporary settings. The postoperative course for facial skeletal surgery has become more comfortable and convenient for the patient since the technologic

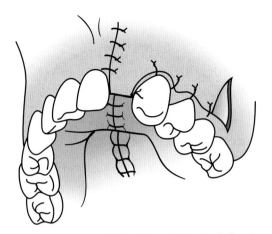

FIGURE **61-6** *A sliding buccal gingival flap is elevated from around the teeth and advanced forward, leaving the posterior defect to granulate. Adapted from Turvey TA, Vig KWL, Fonseca RJ. Surgical management. In: Facial clefts and craniosynostosis: principles and management. Philadelphia (PA): W.B. Saunders Company; 1996. p. 419.*

advancements of bone plates and screws have essentially replaced the need for intermaxillary fixation. The contemporary use of steroids and antibiotics has controlled swelling and infection, and alternatives to homologous blood transfusion (autologous blood banking and the use of recombinant erythropoietin) are effectively employed. Impatient surgeons or orthodontists should not rationalize early skeletal surgery prior to maturation for their own convenience. Final decisions regarding the timing of surgery should recognize the wishes of patients and parents, and the orthodontists and surgeons should provide the information needed to make an informed decision.

Presurgical Counseling

Patients born with a congenital facial malformation are psychologically different from those patients with acquired dentofacial deformities, who tend to be more prone to neuroticism.[13] Patients with a cleft have had their problem since birth and have adapted to multiple changes from their previous surgical procedures. Many patients with orofacial clefts have experienced the disappointment of previous

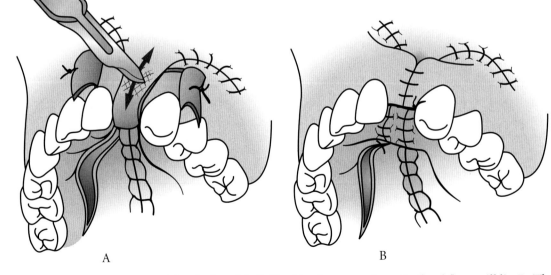

A   B

FIGURE **61-5** A, *The rotated flap is de-epithelialized in the areas where the fixed flaps will lie.* B, *The fixed gingiva is then secured to the flap and around the margins of the teeth. Adapted from Turvey TA, Vig KWL, Fonseca RJ. Surgical management. In: Facial clefts and craniosynostosis: principles and management. Philadelphia (PA): W.B. Saunders Company; 1996. p. 417.*

surgical soft tissue revisions that were expected to erase the scar on the lip and correct the nasal asymmetry. However, unrealistic expectations of skeletal surgery should be identified before the surgical intervention, and the patient should be referred for counseling.

Skeletal surgery does not erase the lip scar, but it does provide an opportunity to improve the skeletal support for the soft tissue drape. It can help improve the symmetry of the lip and nasal base and also support the nasal tip. Skeletal support may reduce the stigmas of midface deficiency associated with the cleft defect so that soft tissue revisions may not be needed or desired. The scar commonly falls on a flat unsupported position of the lip and becomes obvious. Often, appropriate skeletal support moves the scar to an area of greater curvature, which reflects light differently and results in a less conspicuous scar. Therefore, patients should be counseled that the skeletal surgery sets the stage for future definitive lip and nasal revisions.

Orthognathic Surgery for the Cleft Patient

In contemporary cleft team settings, most patients with clefts of the maxilla undergo bone grafting at a developmentally appropriated time in the mixed dentition stage. When midface advancement surgery is planned later in adolescence, it is a relatively straightforward procedure. For those patients who have not benefited from previous bone grafts, the situation is more complex. In both circumstances the general principles of flap design for maxillary advancement, ensuring adequate perfusion to the mobilized maxilla, are of paramount importance. A cleft maxilla differs because of the absence of tissues, and multiple surgical procedures are needed to repair and close defects. Perfusion of the mobilized maxilla is dependent on vessels coming from the overlying soft tissues, predominantly the palatal tissues. In cleft patients this tissue is commonly scarred and fibrot-

ic; therefore, care must be exercised when designing the incision to perform the osteotomy. With few exceptions, almost all patients can be treated with a Le Fort I osteotomy via the circumvestibular incision and a down-fracture approach. For those with severe palatal scarring, who have previously undergone an island palatal repair, and those with bilateral clefts of the maxilla, an anterior buccal pedicle should be left on the mobilized maxilla to maintain adequate perfusion. Technically, this is a more challenging operation.

The circumvestibular incision is made from the zygomaticomaxillary buttress to the opposite side, high in the mucobuccal fold (Figure 61-7). Subperiosteal dissection exposes the entire lateral wall of the maxilla from the nose to the pterygoid plate and from the alveolus, above the roots of the teeth, to the inferior orbital rim. The broad exposure permits excellent visualization of all osteotomies. At the time of mobilization, this incision permits the maxilla to be down-fractured and entirely pedicled to the palatal tissues and the remaining buccal tissues below the incision. Good visualization and ease of mobilization are the major advantages of this approach. Hemorrhage control is performed with direct visualization, usually by the ligation of vessels.

When an anterior buccal pedicle remains, the operation is technically more difficult (Figure 61-8). Visualization is reduced, and mobilization by down-fracturing is not possible. Mobilization of the midface is achieved by in-fracturing, combined with anterior traction. For most patients with a cleft palate, the area of greatest resistance to mobilization of the maxilla is the vertical portion of the palatine bone, located in the posteromedial aspect of the maxillary sinus. The bone is thick and access is limited, especially when down-fracturing is not possible. Compounding this is the presence of the greater palatine vessels, which descend from the sphenopalatine fossa to the pos-

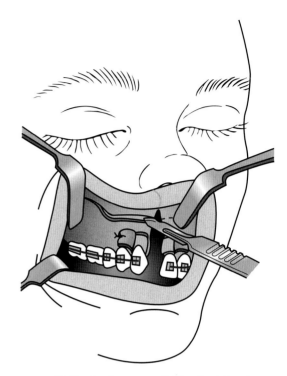

FIGURE **61-7** *A circumvestibular incision is used when a Le Fort I down-fracture is performed. The incision is made high on the zygomaticomaxillary buttress to ensure adequate perfusion to the anterior maxilla. Note that the attached gingiva around the teeth on both sides of the cleft is reflected and preserved. The remaining tissue lining the cleft walls is later incised and reflected palatally or buccally, depending on where it is needed for closure (see Figure 61-11B). Adapted from Turvey TA et al.*[15]

terior maxilla (Figure 61-9). The vessels, which run through the canal in this bone, are prone to rupture during mobilization. Hemorrhage control is limited—packing and the use of a vasoconstrictor (epinephrine 1:100,000) are usually effective.

The surgical technique employed for both of these approaches has been described in detail previously, and interested readers are referred to more detailed sources.[14]

Residual oronasal fistulas are common in patients whose maxillas have not been bone grafted previously. An incision design should permit simultaneous closure of oronasal fistulas. Of key importance is the construction of a nasal floor, which is created by using the tissues lining the fistulas (Figures 61-10–61-12).

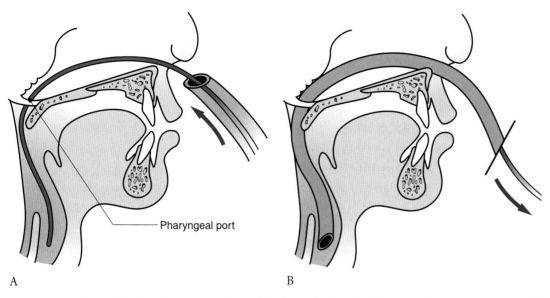

A   B

FIGURE **61-8**   A *and* B, *A catheter passed nasally through the velopharyngeal ports serves to guide the nasoendotracheal tube past the pharyngeal flap. Adapted from Turvey TA et al.*[15]

Creativity and care are the important elements in surgery to correct midface deficiency in patients with clefts. Since the skeleton is always asymmetric in cleft patients, it is crucial that the osteotomy is designed for maximum improvement of esthetics (Figure 61-13). If an adequate

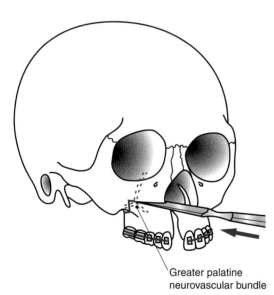

FIGURE **61-9** *A small osteotome is tapped through the lateral nasal wall posteriorly toward the perpendicular part of the palatal bone. At this point the resistance increases because this part of the lateral nasal wall thickens. The greater palatine neurovascular bundle descends through this region and is at risk. Adapted from Turvey TA et al.*[15]

improvement cannot be obtained by an osteotomy alone, onlay bone grafting to enhance skeletal support and shape should be considered. Sometimes even subtle differences between osteotomy designs on the cleft side reflect positive soft tissue changes.

Adequate mobilization is a key factor for success when performing midface osteotomies in the presence of a cleft. The scarring and thickness of bone (particularly in the vertical part of the palatine bone) are two major obstacles. The posteromedial aspect of the maxillary sinus is unusually thick in cleft patients, and it must be cut or fractured to permit adequate mobilization. This is usually accomplished with a small osteotomy tapped along the lateral nasal walls (see Figure 61-9). Failure to weaken these structures prior to mobilization may result in an unfavorable fracture extending to the skull base or orbit. Blindness has been reported following Le Fort I osteotomies in cleft patients, and an inadvertent fracture in this area is the suspected cause.[15] If excessive forces are required to mobilize the maxilla, repeated use of the osteotomy to further weaken the structure is advisable prior to beginning mobilization.

It is often tempting to segment the maxilla of patients with a cleft to improve

occlusal relationships. However, segmenting the maxilla in this population should be undertaken with caution, considering the compromised vascularity and scarring of the tissues. Accepting posterior crossbites and other occlusal compromises may be judicious, rather than risking necrosis of a segmental osteotomy. A contemporary goal of cleft care is to eliminate and/or reduce the need for prosthetic management. Closing dental spaces with segmental osteotomies is an effective way to achieve this goal. Additionally, this maneuver results in more soft tissue availability to create an intact nasal lining. Although opening the space with segmental osteotomies is possible, it requires bone grafts and a rotation of soft tissues to close the defects. Except in extreme salvage circumstances, dental space opening should be avoided (Figures 61-14 and 61-15).

Bone Grafting with Maxillary Advancement

There are three important reasons to use bone grafts in patients with a cleft when performing midface advancement. First,

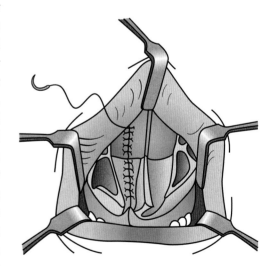

FIGURE **61-10** *The mucosa lining the cleft alveolar region is elevated from the nasal side and pushed orally, where it is sutured on both the palatal and buccal sides. The bone edges of the cleft must be adequately exposed for successful reconstruction. The nasal mucosa is also closed primarily. Adapted from Turvey TA et al.*[15]

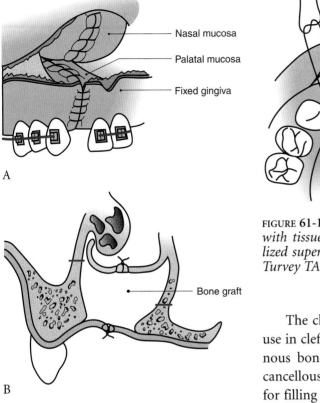

A

B

FIGURE **61-11** A, *Buccal view demonstrating the tissues lining the cleft elevated, pushed orally, and sutured on the oral side.* B, *Deeper view into the cleft demonstrating the closure of the oral and nasal tissues and the pocket for the bone graft. Adapted from Turvey TA et al.[15]*

the bone graft can be wedged into the defects in the lateral maxillary walls; this helps to maintain the position of the maxilla during healing. Second, the bone graft also encourages bone healing and reduces the risks of fibrous union. The third reason to use bone grafts in midface advancement is to contour the middle face. In patients with a cleft, the midface is not just retruded, it is also malformed. Thus, altering the skeletal morphology is important for esthetic enhancement. Augmentation of the cheek projection, infraorbital regions, paranasal regions, nasal bridge, or chin is commonly employed at the time of midface advancement. These maneuvers are helpful and easily performed at the time of surgery, and their importance should not be underestimated.

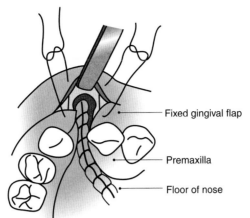

FIGURE **61-12** *The nasal floor is constructed with tissues lining the cleft that are mobilized superiorly and sutured. Adapted from Turvey TA et al.[15]*

The choice of bone-graft material for use in cleft surgery is always fresh autogenous bone. Cancellous bone or corticocancellous blocks are generally reserved for filling defects in the alveolus or lateral

maxillary walls. The authors' preference for bone grafts to contour the middle face is split-thickness calvaria. For the chin a pedicled bone graft from the inferior border of the mandible is always employed.

Bone Grafting of the Cleft Maxilla and Palate

Cancellous grafts can generally be condensed into cleft defects and are self-retained. Block grafts or onlay grafts should always be secured with a screw to promote healing, reduce resorption, and the risk of infection.

There are multiple bone donor sources, including the ilium, cranium, tibia, mandible, and ribs. Although harvesting bone requires more surgical time and has associated morbidity, the predictability of the result easily justifies its use. There is no autogenous bone substitute that has the same success in patients with a cleft as does fresh autogenous bone. The morbidity of

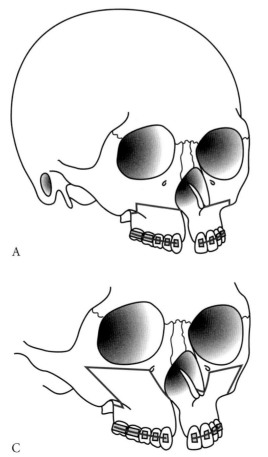

A

B

C

FIGURE **61-13** *The design of the lateral maxillary osteotomy is determined by the patient's esthetic needs.* A, *The classic low-level cut.* B, *A higher-level cut approaching the infraorbital rims.* C, *A modification used when enhancement of the cheek prominence is desired. When the options shown in Figures B and C are used, there is risk of fracturing these buttresses because the bone is thin. Repair is possible with microplates. Adapted from Turvey TA et al.[15]*

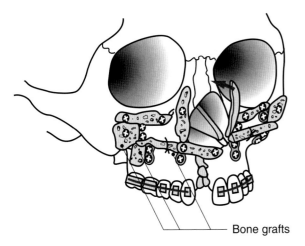

FIGURE 61-14 *Onlay bone grafts are positioned and secured with screws. Wires are occasionally necessary to prevent displacement of the inlaid bone grafts into the sinus. Adapted from Turvey TA et al.[15]*

bone harvest can be reduced with a good surgical technique and should not be an excuse for using bone alternatives.

Stabilizing the Operated Maxilla

The development of more rigid fixation devices permits improvement of results of cleft skeletal surgery. Originally, stainless steel plates and screws and, later, titanium systems were used instead of the traditional stainless steel wires to secure the position of the maxilla. The many benefits of using more rigid fixation include a reduced time for intermaxillary fixation and better assurance of the position of the midface during healing. A single disadvantage of the use of metallic bone plates and screws is a reduced ability to manipulate tooth-bearing segments with elastic traction during the postoperative period to correct the occlusal result.

Velopharyngeal Considerations

One of the complexities of the cleft malformation involves the function of the velopharyngeal sphincter. Under normal circumstances, sealing the nasal cavity from the oral cavity occurs by a simultaneous elevation of the soft palate and contraction of the lateral pharyngeal walls to produce closure of the nasopharynx from the oral cavity. In many patients with a repaired cleft palate, the velopharyngeal mechanism is fragile and the patient has learned to overcome a short or scarred immobile palate by compensating and recruiting adjacent structures. Passavant's bar (a hypertrophy of tissue in the posterior pharyngeal wall) is a result of a compensatory effort that many patients with a cleft develop to overcome the deficit and inadequacy of velar movement.

Forward displacement of the maxilla in patients without a cleft is well tolerated, and these patients have adequate compensatory reserve to overcome the change in position of soft palate. A minority of patients with a cleft are not able to tolerate even small degrees of maxillary displacement, and the velopharyngeal function may deteriorate, affecting the patient's speech and communication ability.[16] This potential risk should be evaluated before maxillary-advancement surgery, and patients should be appropriately counseled. In patients with a cleft, the occurrence of velopharyngeal inadequacy following midface advancement is infrequent and additional surgical procedures are usually unnecessary. Almost all patients with a cleft experience hypernasality immediately following surgery. Fortunately, this gradually resolves with time, and most patients return to their baseline speech by 6 months after surgery. It is prudent to delay subsequent surgery to reduce nasality for at least 6 months following maxillary advancement. This allows natural compensation to occur and permits bone healing to proceed without introducing more scarring, which may contribute to relapse.[17]

An interesting observation in some patients with pharyngeal flaps who do not have velopharyngeal adequacy prior to midface advancement is an improvement of nasal speech after surgery. Although sibilant distortions secondary to malocclusion are expected to improve, reduction of hypernasality after maxillary advancement is paradoxic. The explanation of this occurrence is the altered dynamics of the sphincter that result after

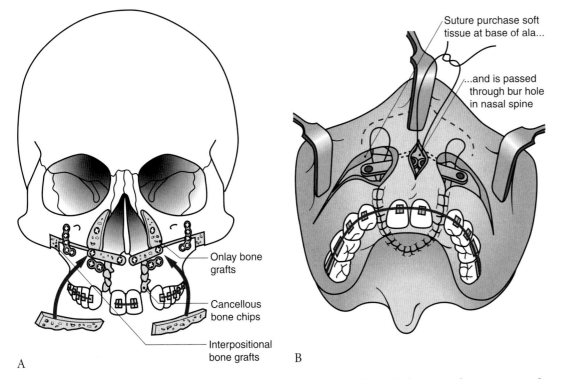

FIGURE 61-15 *A and B, The premaxilla is secured with bone grafts, which are used to construct the inferior piriform rim. These grafts are tunneled under the buccal flaps and screwed to the nasal spine anteriorly and to the lateral maxilla posteriorly. Adapted from Turvey TA et al.[15]*

surgery. Apparently, stretching the flap and its positional change improve the dynamics of the velopharyngeal mechanism so that improved speech occurs in some patients. This observation is not predictable, and patients must be cautioned appropriately.

When a pharyngeal flap is in place and maxillary advancement is undertaken, the flap should be removed only if it does not permit adequate mobilization of the maxilla. When the flap is in place, nasal intubation can be difficult; the anesthesiologist must be prepared to use endoscopic assistance with endotracheal tube insertion (see Figure 61-8).

References

1. Murray JC, Daack-Hirsh S, Buetow KH, et al. Clinical and epidemiological studies of the cleft lip and palate in the Philippines. Cleft Palate Craniofac J 1997;34:7–10.

2. Christensen K. Methodological issues in epidemiological studies in oral clefts. In: Wyszynski D, editor. Cleft lip and palate. Oxford: Oxford University Press; 2002.

3. Lidral AC, Vig KWL. The role of the orthodontist in the management of cleft lip and palate. In: Wyszynski D, editor. Cleft lip and palate. Oxford: Oxford University Press; 2002.

4. Washington Department of Health. Cleft lip and palate: critical elements of care: Washington: Washington Department of Health; 1997.

5. American Cleft Palate–Craniofacial Association. Parameters for the evaluation of treatment of patients with cleft lip/palate or other craniofacial anomalies. Cleft Palate Craniofac J 1993;30 Suppl:4.

6. Mars M, Houston WJB. A preliminary study of facial growth and morphology in unoperated male unilateral cleft lip and palate subjects over 13 years of age. Cleft Palate J 1990;27:7–10.

7. Cohen MM Jr. Syndromes with cleft lip and palate. Cleft Palate J 1978;15:306–28.

8. Cohen MM Jr, Bankier A. Syndrome delineation involving orofacial clefting. Cleft Palate J 1991;28:119–20.

9. Boyne PJ, Sands NR. Secondary bone grafting of alveolar and palatal clefts. J Oral Surg 1972;30:87.

10. Boyne PJ, Sands NR. Combined orthodontic-surgical interaction in the management of residual palato-alveolar cleft defects. Am J Orthod 1976;70:21.

11. Turvey TA, Vig KWL, Moriarty J, Hoke J. Delayed bone grafting in the cleft maxilla and palate: a retrospective multidisciplinary analysis. Am J Orthod 1984;86:244–56.

12. Bergland O, Semb G, Abyholm FE. Elimination of the residual alveolar cleft by secondary bone grafting and subsequent orthodontic treatment. Cleft Palate J 1986;23:175.

13. Phillips C, Proffit WR. Psychosocial aspects of dentofacial deformity and its treatment. In: Proffit WR, White RP, Sarver DM. Contemporary treatment of dentofacial deformity. St. Louis (MO): Mosby; 2003. p. 70–91.

14. Vig KWL, Turvey TA, Fonseca RJ. Orthodontic and surgical considerations in bone grafting in the cleft maxilla and palate. In: Facial clefts and craniosynostosis: principles and management. Philadelphia (PA): W.B. Saunders; 1996.

15. Turvey TA, Vig KWL, Fonseca RJ. Maxillary advancement and contouring in the presence of cleft lip and palate. In: Facial clefts and craniosynostosis: principles and management. Philadelphia (PA): W.B. Saunders; 1996.

16. Lo LJ, Huen KF, Chen YR. Blindness as a complication of LeFort I osteotomy for maxillary disimpaction. Plast Reconstr Surg 2002;109:688–98.

17. Mason RA, Turvey TA, Warren DW. Speech considerations with maxillary advancement procedures. J Oral Surg 1980;38:752.

CHAPTER 62

Distraction Osteogenesis

Suzanne U. Stucki-McCormick, MS, DDS

Distraction osteogenesis (DO), a useful technique to generate bone and soft tissue, can be applied to craniofacial reconstruction, including orthognathic surgery, cleft lip and palate reconstruction, a new mandibular condyle regeneration, a dentoalveolar unit reconstruction for dental implants and transport DO for discontinuity defects.

Regardless of the surgical site, adherence to the following basic Ilizarov principles is the key to surgical success[1]:

1. Osteotomy of the bone site with minimal periosteal stripping
2. Latency period: 3, 5, or 7 days, depending on the surgical site
3. Distraction rate: 1.0 mm per day (0.5–2.0 mm)
4. Distraction rhythm: continuous force application is best, yet device activation bid is more practical and allows for better patient compliance
5. Consolidation: until a cortical outline can be seen radiographically across the distraction gap, usually 6 weeks

The distraction technique involves creating an osteotomy in an area adjacent to an area of bone deficiency. Applying slow tension forces separates the bony edges, which creates a regenerate chamber from which the new bone and soft tissues are formed (Figure 62-1). This regenerate chamber may be large and wide, with abundant blood supply from the overlying muscle and skin, as in mandibular distraction. Conversely, the distraction gap may be small, with thin mucosal coverage, as in dentoalveolar distraction for dental implants. The local periosteal blood supply and the size of the distraction segment influence the treatment plan decisions; in fact, for small bone segment distraction, the rate of distraction may need to decrease to 0.5 to 0.7 mm per day. However, for sagittal distraction of the mandible whereby the bone segments overlap, the distraction rate should increase to 2.0 mm per day. I recommend modifying the Ilizarov principles in each individual, based on the size of the distraction bone segment and the regional blood supply (Table 62-1).

Initially, the regenerate chamber is filled with a fibrous matrix that ossifies from the periphery centrally.[2] The distraction gap shape and the resultant new DO bone are influenced by the vector of distraction and the rate of distraction. Altering the vector of distraction during active DO will correspondingly alter the three-dimensional shape of the regenerate chamber and the resultant new DO bone (Figure 62-2). If the distraction rate is too rapid, then the regenerate chamber will be hourglass shaped, and the new DO bone will be thinned centrally.

The osteotomy location can affect the shape of the regenerate chamber and the final new bone. If the osteotomy is created in an area of thin bone stock, then the

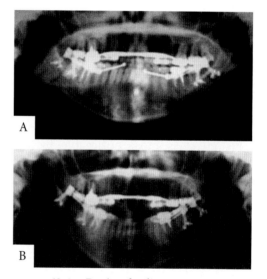

FIGURE 62-1 *During the distraction process the bony edges of the osteotomy (A) are separated slowly over time to create an initial radiolucent regenerate chamber (B), which has the size and shape of the native bone.*

regenerate chamber will thin and assume the shape of the native bone. In treatment planning and during surgery, it may be necessary to adjust the osteotomy site, placing the bone cut in an area of maximum bone thickness to create a large and robust regenerate chamber (Figure 62-3).

Until the distraction gap ossifies completely, the regenerate chamber is influenced by the local muscle pull. As distraction proceeds, the regenerate chamber becomes enlarged and is filled initially with a weak fibrous matrix. Simultaneously, the local muscles that are attached to the DO site are stretched. The stretched

Table 62-1 Distraction Protocol			
Distraction	*Latency (d)*	*Rate (total) (mm/d)*	*Rhythm*
Mandible	5	1.0	bid
Maxilla	5	1.0	bid
Alveolus/implant	5–7	0.5–0.7–1.0	bid
Transport	5–7	1.0	bid
Condyle: transport	5–7	1.0	tid, qid
Mandible: children	3–5	1.0–2.0	bid
Mandible: sagittal	5–7	2.0	bid
Transport: neck dissection	7–10	0.5–1.0	bid
Transport: XRT	7–10	0.5	bid

bid = twice a day; qid = four times a day; tid = three times a day; XRT = external beam radiation therapy.

muscles tend to return to their original sarcomeric length, pulling on the regenerate chamber and on the intervening immature bone matrix, causing an alteration of the vector of DO and displacement of the distraction segment in the direction of the muscle (Figure 62-4). This effect is most noticeable by the action of the temporalis and the mylohyoid musculature. Vector control maneuvers, including the use of surgical guides, orthodontic appliances, and interim partial dentures with a portal for DO device access, help to maintain and adjust the vector of distraction.[3]

Clinicians may use the fibrous matrix nature of the regenerate chamber to their advantage to mold the regenerate into the proper orientation and location, including distraction of a segment outside the normal anatomic periosteal plane. Specifically, clinicians may mold the regenerate at any time in the distraction process—during active DO and at the end of DO.

During active distraction, the regenerate is molded by altering the vector of the distractor. Some DO devices have mechanical hinges that allow the clinician to adjust the vector of distraction. This is done easily in an office setting, often using local anesthesia, if necessary. If performing a significant (≥ 3 mm) molding move or vector change, then I recommend that a short (1 to 3 days) latency is observed prior to commencing with the distraction protocol. This allows for healing of the disrupted microvasculature and osteoid matrix within the regenerate chamber that the vector change produced. A longer latency (2 to 4 days) is recommended if the bone segment is small, as in dentoalveolar distraction for dental implants.

Perform regenerate molding at the end of active distraction to help guide the bone segment into its final position.[4] After only 3 weeks of consolidation, remove the distractor prematurely, and reposition the segment to its final position. Use traction orthodontic elastics to guide the segment to its final position and to hold the segment in this position until final ossification occurs. At the time of device removal, however, the segment may be repositioned

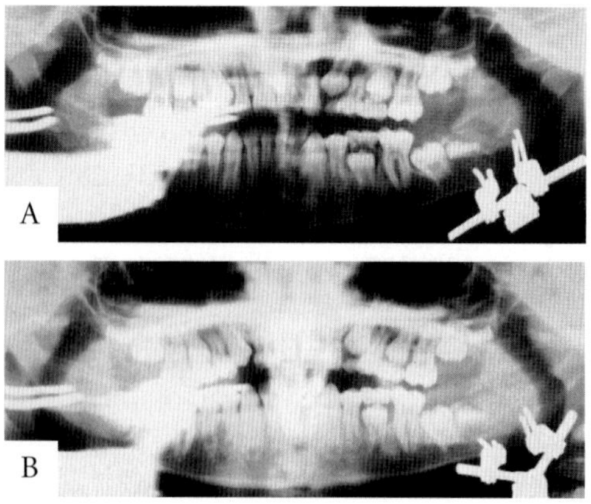

FIGURE 62-2   *Initially the distraction vector is linear (A). Once 5 mm of regenerate chamber has been created, the distractor can be adjusted, altering the vector of distraction, which correspondingly alters the three-dimensional shape of the new bone (B).*

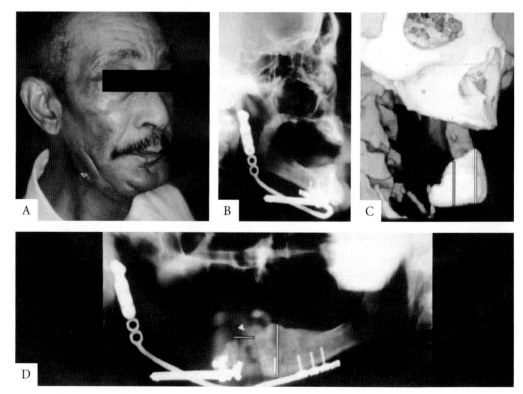

FIGURE 62-3   *For transport distraction to create a new mandible (A, B), the osteotomy should be placed in an area of maximal bone stock (C, D) to create a robust regenerate chamber.*

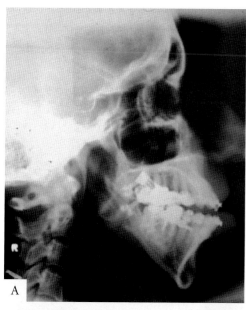

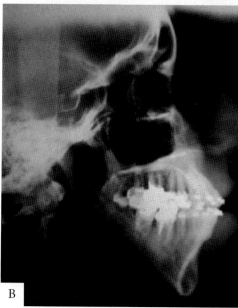

FIGURE 62-4 *During the final stages of distraction osteogenesis, the weak regenerate chamber is under the influence of local muscle pull. A, Here the mylohyoid created an open bite, which was counteracted by orthodontic elastics. B, Using callous manipulation with orthodontic elastics, the open bite was closed.*

manually and held in place with rigid fixation plates and screws.

Perform "dancing" of the distraction segment if a discrepancy occurs in planned distraction amounts, such as bilateral mandibular advancement for asymmetries.[5] Initially, both segments are advanced at the planned distraction rate.

When the larger, less asymmetric side reaches its final position, the segment becomes the dancing side, advancing the DO segment in the morning then turning it back the same amount in the evening. In the meantime, the lesser more asymmetric segment continues to be advanced at the planned rate until it catches up with the contralateral side. Carry out any final adjustments to the mandibular positioning when the asymmetry has been corrected by advancing or dancing the two sides as needed (Figure 62-5).

As with orthognathic surgery, treatment planning for distraction osteogenesis includes predicting the amount and trajectory of the planned bone movement. Although the DO device may be activated 1.0 mm per day, this does not translate to 1.0 mm of bone advancement per day. The amount of actual bone movement is always less than the distance that is indicated on the distraction device, therefore the clinician monitors the patient's progress closely, including radiographs.

The surgical approach and technique are similar to orthognathic surgery. When locating and positioning the bone cut, also consider the placement and orientation of the distraction device. Mark the planned osteotomy. Then, create a corticotomy, verifying the ability to place the distractor in the proper orientation. Make the screw fixation holes for the distraction device, and remove the device. The corticotomy is then converted atraumatically to an osteotomy, and the distraction device is fixated into place. The device is activated to ensure impedance-free advancement of the distraction segments.[6] Remove any bony interferences, and return the device to its closed neutral position. Prior to initial device orientation and placement, activate the distractor 1.0 to 2.0 mm. Thus, after the osteotomy and the device are secured into place, the DO device can be "closed" 1.0 to 2.0 mm, reducing and minimizing the initial distraction gap created by the bone cut.

Mandibular Distraction

For patients with craniofacial microsomia, mandibular distraction of the affected side is a useful technique for generating both bone and soft tissue. The surgical approach is similar to a sagittal osteotomy. Create a bone cut in the ramus of the mandible on the affected side above the lingua along the ramus to the posterior border of the mandible above the gonial angle. Position the distractor, and convert the corticotomy to an osteotomy, after which the distraction device is secured. Intraoral distractors are preferred to external devices to decrease scarring. Compared with a completely submerged device, DO devices in which the distraction mechanism is intraoral yet extramucosal allow the clinician to monitor the distractor directly without the need for radiographs. In addition, removal of the device is facilitated if the distraction mechanism is extramucosal. The vector of distraction is calculated based on the trajectory of the bone segment and on the local anatomy, including bone stock, tooth buds and/or roots, and position of the inferior alveolar nerve. Achieve chin point correction by vertical distraction of the ramus (Figure 62-6).[7]

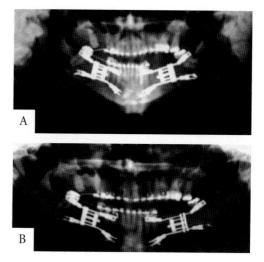

FIGURE 62-5 *To correct asymmetry the devices are initially distracted by the same amount (A), then using "disk dancing," the regenerate chamber can be advanced or returned to bring the segment into proper position (B).*

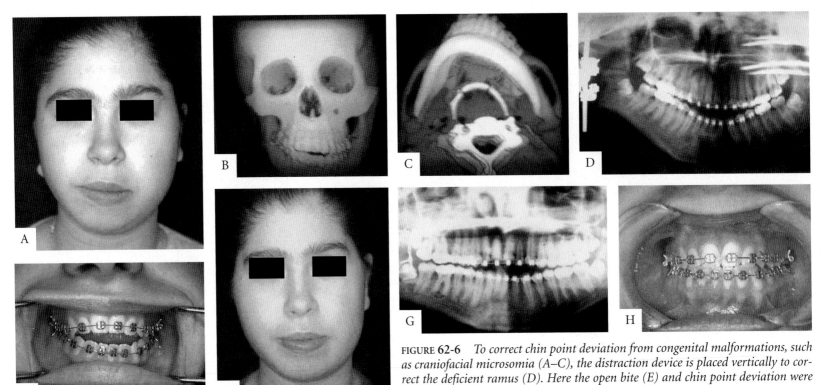

FIGURE 62-6   *To correct chin point deviation from congenital malformations, such as craniofacial microsomia (A–C), the distraction device is placed vertically to correct the deficient ramus (D). Here the open bite (E) and chin point deviation were corrected (F–H).*

The distraction process continues 1.0 mm per day until the mandibular asymmetry is corrected. I recommend age-dependant overcorrection to compensate for the decreased growth potential of the genetically affected side.[8] Remove the distractor when a cortical outline can be seen radiographically (Figure 62-7). Perform mandibular distraction for all Pruzansky-Mulliken classifications of craniofacial microsomia (Figure 62-8).[9]

Mandibular distraction plays a unique role for infants with airway compromise, as a consequence of micrognathia.[10,11] Early distraction of the body of the mandible bilaterally has shown promise for improving airway volume and in decreasing airway resistance, leading to early decannulation or avoidance of a tracheotomy.[12,13]

For large mandibular advancements or for patients with a history of temporomandibular joint disorders, DO is a useful treatment alternative. Use a modification of the classic sagittal split technique for such cases.[5] As the proximal and distal segments overlap, the distraction rate is increased to 2.0 mm per day (0.5 mm qid [4 times a day]). Further, create a groove in the superior aspect of the horizontal bone cut above the lingual to allow for impedance-free rotation of the proximal segment during DO (Figure 62-9). Ideally, the distractors are placed parallel to the midsagital plane of the mandible, although this is not always achieved.[14,15] Class II orthodontic elastics are placed to "unload" the temporomandibular joint. At the time of surgery, place a maxillary occlusal surgical guide that extends to one-half of the occlusal surface of the maxillary second molar, with the final occlusion indexed. As distraction proceeds, guide the mandible into the proper occlusion using light elastics. Sagittal distraction of the mandible appears to provide condylar axis stability and has minimal deleterious effects on the temporomandibular joint.[5]

Mandibular Widening

DO, a useful tool to create space for severe mandibular crowding, is often combined with maxillary transverse widening and surgically assisted palatal expansion (Figure 62-10).[16] For the mandible, make a vestibular incision similar to a genioplasty, approach the mandible, and score the planned osteotomy site. Create the osteotomy in the corpus of the mandible with a bur or a saw. Perform the interdental osteotomy with fine chisels in a tunneling technique, reducing the periosteal stripping, being careful to avoid encroaching on or injuring the periodontal ligament of the teeth in the osteotomy line. The tissue type in the osteotomy site is the template for DO. Consequently, if the osteotomy is positioned completely in the bone, bone will be created. If the osteotomy encroaches on periodontal ligament tissues, the distraction gap fills with bone and moderate amounts of periodontal ligament-like tissues, leading to a pseudo-union.[17] For the central incisors that are extremely crowded, carry out the interdental osteotomy laterally between less crowded teeth; namely, the lateral incisor and the cuspid. Create a horizontal step 5 mm below the roots of the incisor teeth, and make the main osteotomy of corpus of mental region vertically in the midline.

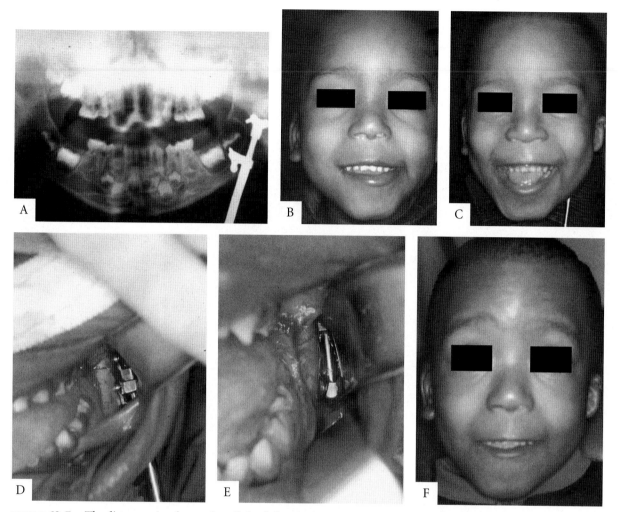

FIGURE 62-7 *The distractor is advanced until the deformity is corrected (A–C). Initially, osteotomy (D) produces a radiolucent regenerate chamber (A) that ossifies with time (E), at which point the distractor is removed (F).*

The distractor of choice is placed. Most distractors are tooth and bone borne. Distractors that are solely bone borne tend to produce a V-shaped regenerate chamber, with more widening at the level of the alveolus and less widening at the level of the inferior border.

After a 5- to 7-day latency, distraction proceeds at 1.0 mm per day. Be sure to apply slow incremental distraction forces; DO forces generated during mandibular widening may translate to the mandibular condyle.[18] Minimal in nature, these forces cause mild adaptive bony changes that are well tolerated. Nevertheless, monitor patients closely for any complaints of preauricular pain or limitation of motion, which would indicate altering the 1.0 mm per day DO protocol from 0.5 mm twice daily to 0.25 mm four times daily device activation.

After DO, the surgeon may place a plastic pontic tooth in the gap between the central incisors to stabilize the teeth and to prevent their central migration.[19] To prevent migration of the teeth into the DO gap, include these teeth in the orthodontic arc wire, with the possible placement of a light spring. Remove the distractor once a cortical outline can be seen on the radiograph. Place a lingual arch to help stabilize the new transverse dimension.

Simultaneous Maxillary and Mandibular Distraction

Patients who have craniofacial microsomia often have maxillary hypoplasia and a concomitant occlusal cant toward the affected side. Using mandibular DO during the primary or mixed dentition phase often autocorrects the maxillary occlusal cant (Figure 62-11). If the maxillary molar teeth are present in full occlusion or if the patient is in permanent dentition, then a concomitant maxillary distraction, along with the mandibular distraction, may be indicated.[20,21] The surgeon performs a corticotomy at the Le Fort I level, including pterygoid disjunction, taking care to avoid the unerrupted tooth buds or roots during the bone cut. The maxilla is loosened but not down-fractured. Orthodontic elastics (8 oz) are then applied bilaterally, with increased elastic traction on the affected side to guide the maxilla to its proper orientation during the DO process (Figure 62-12). Elastic traction that results in max-

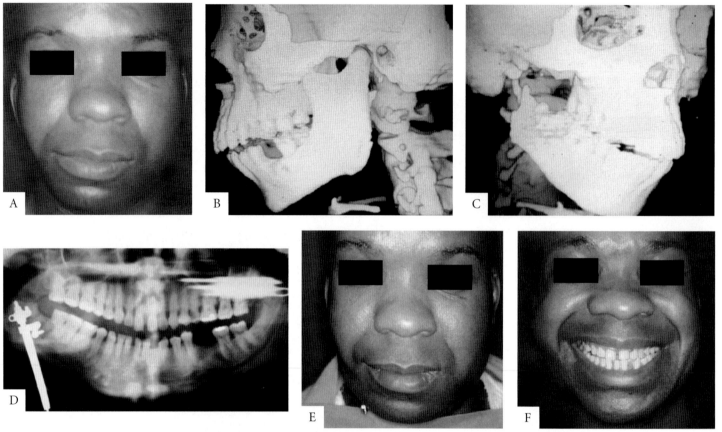

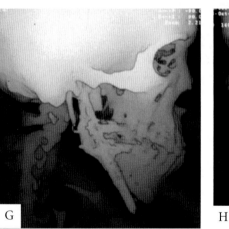

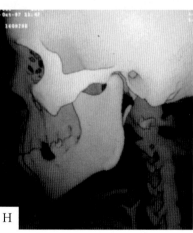

FIGURE **62-8**   *This patient with grade III craniofacial microsomia (A–C) successfully underwent ramal distraction (D–F) to correct his deformity (G, H).*

illomandibular fixation (MMF) is not required to guide the maxilla along with the mandible during DO.[22]

Maxillary Distraction

Likewise, use DO for maxillary advancement. This technique is especially useful for patients with large advancements or in patients postpalatoplasty for cleft lip and palate whose scarring causes inadequate tissue or difficulty in moving the maxilla.[23,24] The surgical approach is sim-

ilar to conventional orthognathic surgery, with the osteotomy at the Le Fort I level. The maxilla is freed but not completely down-fractured. If the maxilla is inadvertently completely down-fractured, then loosely place a suspension suture (2-0 polydioxanone suture) in the bone across the bone gap at the level of the first molar tooth and the zygomatic buttress to help stabilize and prevent inferior tipping of the posterior maxilla. The distractors are pre-bent to

facilitate device placement. The zygomatic buttress region is a good point for device fixation. Ideal trajectory would locate the two distractors that are parallel to each other and the midsagittal plane. Achieving this congruity is much more difficult in the maxilla owing to local anatomy, device design, and location of the osteotomy, limiting device placement and orientation. Ensure that the resultant moment arm of the two distractors will not cancel each other as the distractors

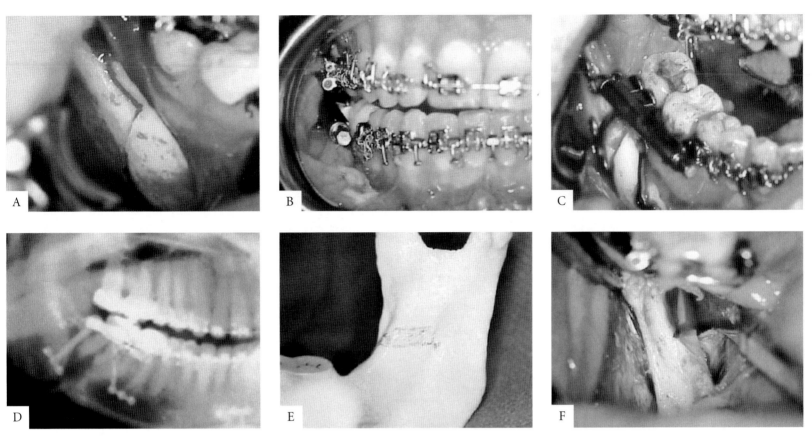

FIGURE 62-9   A–D, *Classic sagittal split osteotomy technique can be modified to allow for mandibular advancement. E, F, The horizontal bone cut is modified to allow for impedance-free advancement during distraction osteogenesis. (Courtesy of Dr. J.J. Moses.)*

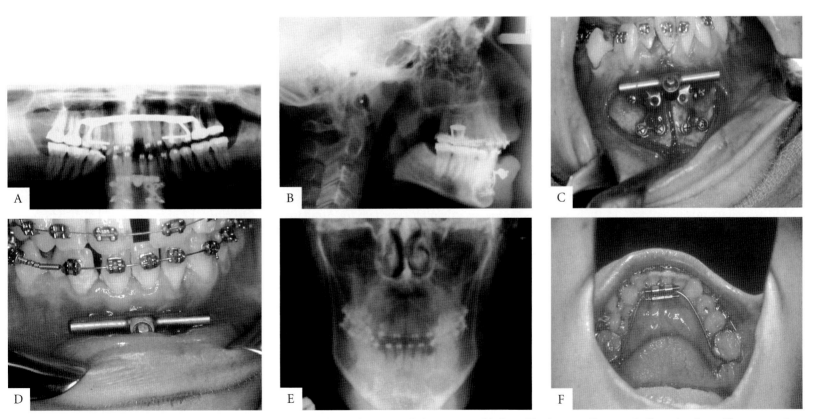

FIGURE 62-10   A, B, *Patients with narrow arch forms and dental crowding are aided using mandibular widening as well as surgically assisted maxillary expansion. C, D, Bone-borne devices can be placed into the vestibule. E, F, The resultant increase in transverse dimension can be stabilized with a lingual orthodontic appliance.*

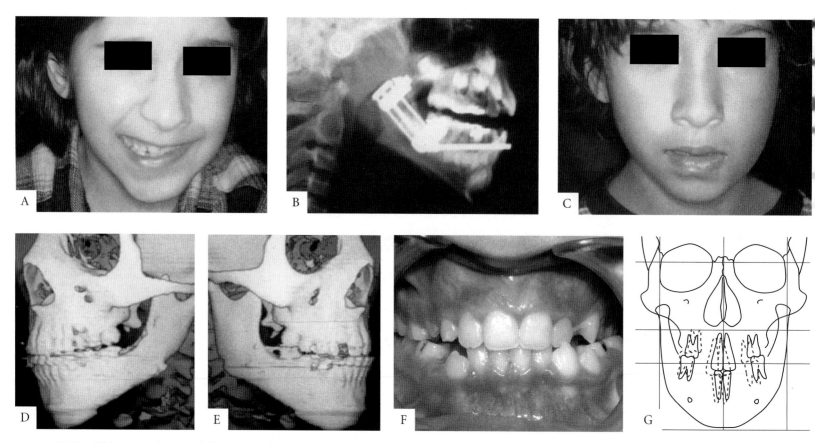

FIGURE 62-11   *This patient in mixed dentition with significant occlusal cant (A) underwent mandibular distraction using a submerged device (B) to correct the deformity (C). The neomandible (D) mimics the native mandible (E) in size and form. The mandible was overcorrected with the dental midline distracted one-half tooth toward the contralteral side (F). The maxillary occlusal cant was autocorrected as the mandible was placed in the proper position and with the eruption of the permanent teeth (G).*

reach their maximal length. Use anterior traction elastics to guide the maxilla to its proper position. Put an intravenous tubing that is cut to size over the two ends of the distraction device activation rods to prevent lip ulcers (Figure 62-13).

Expanding the soft tissue envelope is often the rate-limiting step in large maxillary advancements. In these patients (> 8 to 10 mm advancement) or for those who have palatal scarring, the use of an external halo frame is indicated. Although a bit cumbersome and unsightly, the external frame can produce significant and dramatic maxillary advancements (Figure 62-14). The surgery is similar to conventional orthognathic surgery. Perform a high Le Fort or stepped osteotomy, if indicated. Secure the device below the height of contour of the skull; otherwise, the halo may dislodge vertically.

Active DO requires careful observation, as the center of rotation of the maxilla is at the level of the roots of the maxillary first molar.[25] Left unchecked, the maxilla will be distracted anteriorly and superiorly, creating an open-bite malocclusion. Using the external halo frame, adjust the arms vertically to allow the maxilla to advance in a downward and forward vector. Similarly, to allow for correction of a maxillary asymmetry, the arms of the halo device can be differentially activated (ie, 0.5 mm on one side and 1.0 mm per day on the other (see Figure 62-14). Once the ossification of the distraction site is complete (ie, until the maxilla is stable to palpation, usually in 5 to 6 weeks or when radiographic evidence of a cortical outline is seen), the halo device is removed in the office without the need for rigid fixation of the maxilla. Occasionally, prior to complete ossification of the site, the patient

may request to have the halo removed. The device is removed with concomitant placement of rigid fixation plates.

Maxillary Segmental Distraction

In patients who have a wide alveolar cleft, perform a segmental osteotomy in the lesser segment, advancing it via distraction to close the alveolar defect.[26] The bone cut is usually located between the bicuspid and the molar teeth of the lesser segment (Figure 62-15). In the same way, place the bone cut in the greater segment between the incisor and the cuspid teeth to distract the gap closed from either one or two directions. Use of orthodontic appliances and the arch wire allows the distraction segment to follow the curvature of the maxillary arch. During post-distraction, place an orthodontic spring on the arch wire, paralleling the regenerate chamber to

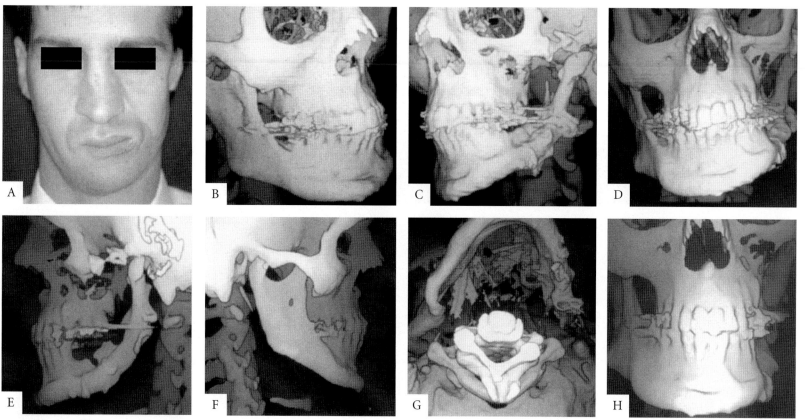

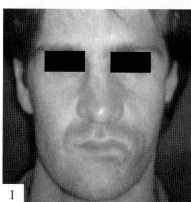

FIGURE **62-12** *For adults in permanent dentition (A), the occlusal cant involves not only the dentoalveolar unit but also the piriform rim and affected paranasal areas (B–D). As this patient had a previously placed costochondral graft, which was the site of the distraction, the neomandible has the same size and shape of the original bony template of the costochondral graft (E), rather than the contralteral side (F). The chin point deviation and occlusal cant to the level of the zygoma are best seen in the frontal and submentovertex views (D,G). Postdistraction, the mandibular chin point is brought to the midline. A concomitant Le Fort I osteotomy is performed at the time of distraction osteogenesis surgery and the maxilla is brought down with the mandible using orthodontic elastics. Note the correction of the occlusal cant and piriform rim and zygomatic buttress regions (H). This is reflected in the soft tissue changes (I).*

help hold the segment in proper orientation. In 1 to 2 weeks after distraction ossification, move the bicuspid and cuspid teeth orthodontically back to their correct position into the ossified DO bone, leaving the anterior dentoalveolar unit for implant reconstruction or for final periosteoplasty and smaller bone graft, if indicated. This segmental distraction is a form of transport DO.

For patients who have congenital agenesis of the premaxilla or who experience traumatic loss of the dentoalveolar unit,

anterior maxillary segmental distraction is indicated (Figure 62-16). Use tunneling techniques to perform the anterior osteotomy, making the horizontal bone cut parallel to the occlusal plane to facilitate segment advancement along a horizontal vector (Figure 62-17). Bilateral distractors are placed, and distraction proceeds after a 5-day latency at a rate of 1.0 mm per day. Anterior traction elastics aid in the forward thrust of the segment. The distractors are removed once a bony outline can be seen radiographically and

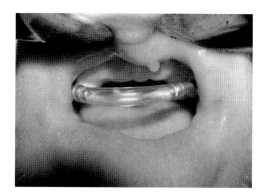

FIGURE **62-13** *An intravenous tubing can be placed over the free end of maxillary distractors to avoid lip ulcers. The tubing is removed to activate the device then reapplied.*

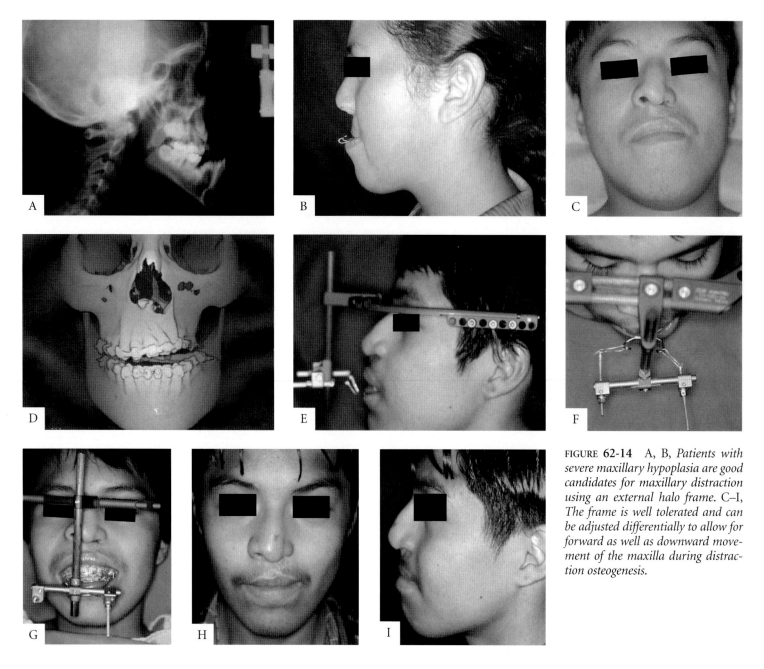

FIGURE **62-14**   A, B, *Patients with severe maxillary hypoplasia are good candidates for maxillary distraction using an external halo frame. C–I, The frame is well tolerated and can be adjusted differentially to allow for forward as well as downward movement of the maxilla during distraction osteogenesis.*

once the segment is stable. The distractors can be removed prior to complete ossification (3 to 4 weeks) to mold the regenerate or at the patient's request. Position rigid fixation plates at the time of device removal. Resorbable rigid fixation plates are useful for this purpose; the site will ultimately undergo dental implant reconstruction.

Transport Distraction Osteogenesis

The power of DO is that both bone and soft tissues are regenerated. Transport distraction involves creating a transport disk in the bone stump, adjacent to a discontinuity defect or a resection site. The transport disk is then advanced 1.0 mm per day as the distraction gap increases in size to span the discontinuity defect (Figure 62-18).[27] The resultant regenerate chamber will have the same size and shape of the transport disk. Careful treatment planning is necessary to plan the site of the osteotomy, thus determining the shape of transport disk and regenerate (Figure 62-19). Occasionally, a tooth may need to be sacrificed to allow for osteotomy placement in an optimal position.

Both external and submerged devices have been used for transport DO. Three points of fixation are required for transport DO: (1) in the proximal stump, (2) in the distal site, and (3) in the transport disk. Use a rigid fixation plate as a substitute for the three points of fixation along with a conventional distractor. The rigid fixation plate also acts as a guide for the transport disk during distraction (see Figure 62-18). Once the transport disk reaches the docking site, the segment is held in neutral fixation until a cortical outline is seen in the regenerate. At the time of

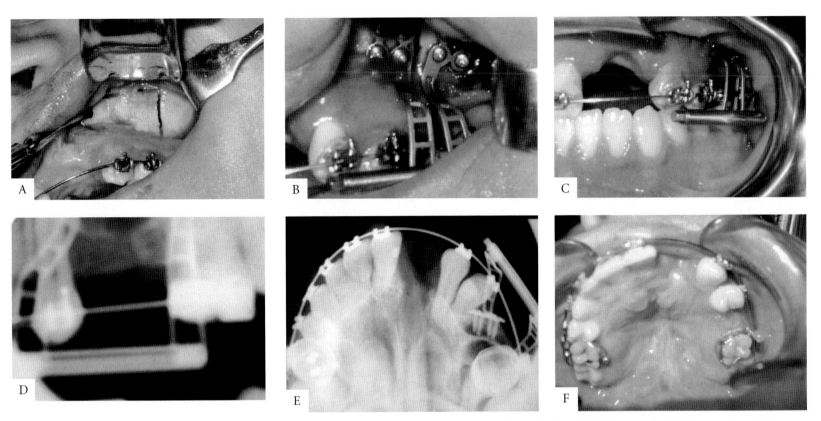

FIGURE **62-15** *Segmental distraction can be performed for focal bone and soft tissue deficiencies such as alveolar cleft defects. A–C, The bone cut is made between the molar and bicuspid teeth and the orthodontic wire acts as a guide during distraction osteogenesis. D–F, A new dentoalveolar unit is formed and the cuspid and bicuspid teeth can be moved back into proper position orthodontically post-distraction osteogenesis.*

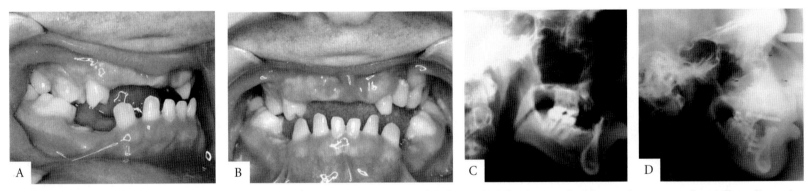

FIGURE **62-16** *Patients with anterior maxillary congenital deformities including anodontia (A, B) are treated with anterior segmental maxillary distraction osteogenesis (DO) and concomitant posterior mandibular DO widening (C, D).*

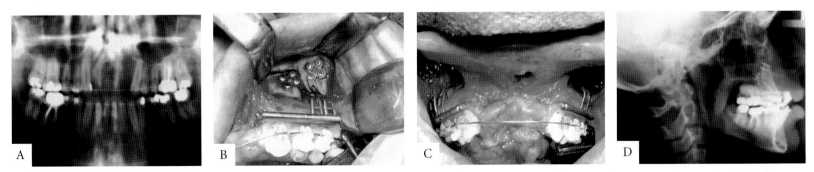

FIGURE **62-17** *A, Patients with traumatic avulsion of the premaxillary segment can be treated with segmental anterior distraction osteogenesis. B, The bone cut is made parallel to the occlusal plane and the distractors placed via a tunneling technique (Courtesy of KLS Martin L.P., Jacksonville, FL). C, D, A flat plane occlusal splint is inserted to allow for impedance-free maxillary advancement.*

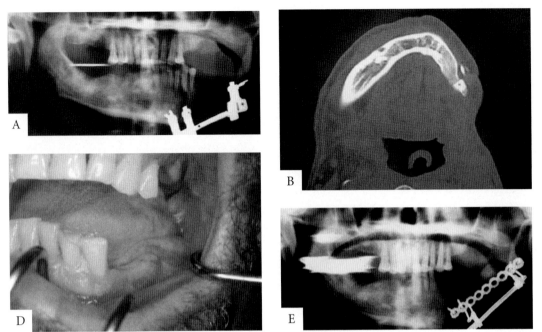

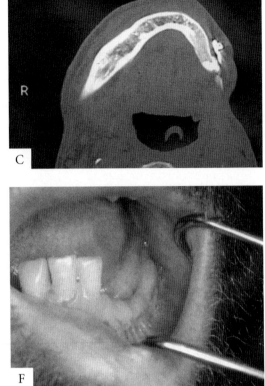

FIGURE **62-18** *Transport distraction osteogenesis brings bone and soft tissue into a defect by creating a transport disk (A), which is distracted to span the gap creating new bone that is similar in shape to the native mandible (B, C). D, All tissues are created, including mucosa. E, The technique can be combined with a submerged device and a rigid fixation plate to stabilize the discontinuity defect. F, The hemimandible can be successfully reconstructed.*

distractor removal, the surgeon may need to position a small bone graft between the transport disk and the docking site because the transport disk becomes rounded and encased with a fibrocartilagenous cap. Obtaining osseous union necessitates removal of this intervening fibrocartilagenous cap.

During active DO, monitor the patient closely to rule out soft tissue dehiscence. Occasionally the leading edge of the transport disk can migrate through the soft tissue. The suggested local wound-care measures include antibiotics and antimicrobial mouth rinses. A blood supply that is compromised (eg, a patient status post-radiation therapy) indicates disk dancing until the dehiscence site closes.

Symphyseal reconstruction can be difficult because the regenerate chamber tends to assume a straight line, rather than follow and maintain the curvilinear shape.[28] Use molding devices, including an intraoral surgical guide, to facilitate and maintain the shape of the regenerate chamber (see Figure 62-19).[29] Viewed

from above, the dentoalveolar unit assumes an arcuate form. Viewed from below, the mandible assumes five lines: two body regions, two parsymphyseal regions, and one symphyseal region. Thus, plan for five linear distraction vectors to reconstruct the mandible (Figure 62-20).

One alternative treatment plan calls for the creation of a large transport disk (1.5 to 3.0 cm) advanced in a linear fashion until the junction of the next linear segment.[28] The disk is held in neutral fixation for a few days or weeks until early ossification occurs. Subsequently, the disk is divided into two segments, with one-half of the original transport disk held in place to the reconstruction plate. The other one-half becomes a new transport disk reoriented in the proper vector, which, after a 3- to 5-day latency, is advanced by distraction in the new trajectory (see Figure 62-20).

Transport distraction has been used successfully either in primary reconstruction at the time of bone resection or in secondary reconstruction. For primary

reconstruction, the devices are placed at the time of resection. If a concomitant neck dissection is done, then the latency period should be increased to 7 days. For secondary reconstruction, limited surgical dissection is advocated. As the soft tissue bed may be heavily scarred, the distraction rhythm may need to be altered to four times a day rather than twice a day to allow incremental stretching of the overlying soft tissues. Tension within the overlying soft tissue may cause daily "relapse" by

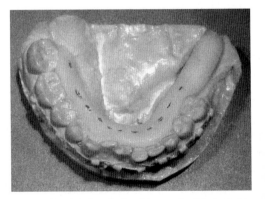

FIGURE **62-19** *Surgical guides can be fabricated to help maintain the curvilinear shape of the regenerate during transport distraction osteogenesis.*

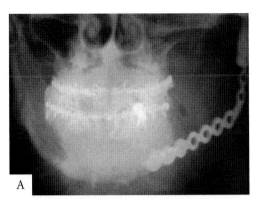

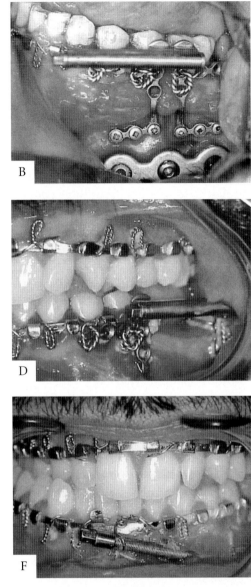

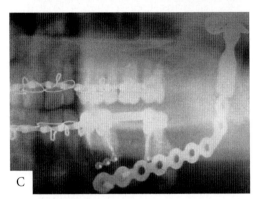

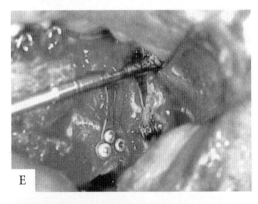

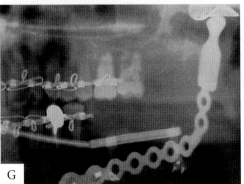

FIGURE **62-20**   *During transport distraction osteogenesis (DO), the mandible can be divided into five linear segments. Transport DO can be performed sequentially (A–C). Sectioning the transport disk to advance the segments (D–G). (Courtesy of Dr. J.J. Moses.)*

apy. The distraction rate is reduced to 0.5 mm per day, and the overlying soft tissues are carefully monitored.

DO can be used in conjunction with conventional reconstructive techniques (eg, microvascular flaps). One concern, however, is that the donor bone, such as a fibula, may not have the ideal form post-mandibular reconstruction for implant placement and prosthetic reconstruction. Use distraction as a secondary technique to obtain ideal height and width for implant reconstruction.[33] The technique is similar to that for DO of an atrophic mandible for dental implants.

Transport Distraction to Generate a Neocondyle

During transport DO, the transport disk becomes rounded and covered by a fibrocartilagenous cap. This cap is removed to ensure osseous continuity in mandibular reconstruction. Use this fibrocartilagenous cap to reconstruct a neocondyle.[34–36] Create a reverse **L** osteotomy in the ramus of the mandible from the sigmoid notch behind the lingua to 1.0 to 1.5 cm above the inferior border of the mandible (Figure 62-21). The distractor is oriented vertically, almost parallel to the posterior border of the ramus, to guide the transport disk into the fossa, creating a neocondyle. In the same way, the segment can be overdistracted to increase posterior vertical ramal height and to reestablish the gonial angle. For bilateral cases, a coranoidectomy prevents rotation of the proximal segment from temporalis muscle pull during the DO process.

In patients who have bony ankylosis, carry out a gap arthroplasty concomitantly with the distraction surgery (Figure 62-22). As the neocondyle assumes the form of the fossa, it is important to surgically shape the new fossa well in all three planes of space during the gap arthroplasty portion of the procedure. Distraction is initiated after a 5-day latency period and proceeds until the transport disk reaches the glenoid fossa.

exerting a counterforce on the transport disk. Transport DO has been used to successfully create a neomandible in patients who have had post-resection radiation therapy.[30,31] Although predistraction hyperbaric oxygen therapy is appropriate, it is not mandatory. During active distraction, neovascularization has occurred.[32] Use transport DO to reconstruct a neomandible without hyperbaric oxygen ther-

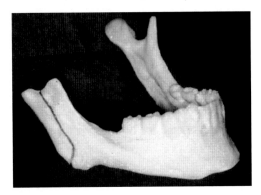

FIGURE 62-21 *A reverse L osteotomy is performed in the ramus of the mandible for condylar transport distraction osteogenesis.*

The patient will remark that they can feel pressure as the articulation of the condyle and fossa is reestablished. This is confirmed radiographically. The DO device is held in neutral fixation until a cortical outline is viewed in the regenerate chamber near the angle of the mandible.

Patients with condylar resorption (idiopathic, degenerative, and rheumatoid arthritis) experience a loss of posterior vertical height and an anterior open bite as a consequence of the resorptive process of the condyle. The slow applica-

tion of force over time via DO to generate new bone is ideally suited to patients requiring mandibular advancement who have a history of temporomandibular joint involvement. Using the same osteotomy, the ramus is over distracted, creating an edge-to-edge Class III profile (Figure 62-23). Remove the distractors after 3 weeks of osseous consolidation, and mold the regenerate using orthodontic elastics to rotate the mandible counter clockwise and to close the open bite. Elastic maxillomandibular fixation is not required to mold the regenerate. Insert a maxillary splint to decrease the load on the temporomandibular joints. Likewise, instruct patients to wear the molding elastics in intervals, allowing other time intervals for free mandibular movement (ie, 4 hours in elastics and 3 hours off). Monitor patients closely, and if the patient complains of preauricular discomfort or limitation of motion, adjust the regenerate molding protocol.

Regardless of the etiology, all patients undergoing condylar transport DO are in active physical therapy during the entire DO

process and are also instructed about at-home physical therapy exercises. Success of the transport DO technique to create a neo-condyle depends on mandibular motion.

Alveolar Distraction Osteogenesis for Dental Implants

Bone grafting techniques for alveolar ridge reconstruction prior to dental implant reconstruction are well established. For cases requiring greater than 4 to 5 mm, apply vertical height augmentation, or if the overlying soft tissue may not support osseous augmentation, alveolar DO is a useful treatment alternative.[37–39]

Carry out a vestibular incision to approach the site. Minimal periosteal stripping is advocated as the transport disk is small. Carefully create the bone cut, using a saw or bur for the horizontal cut, and use chisels at the alveolar crest, sparing the lingual or palatal periosteum. The distractor is adapted to the site. Apply the distractor to the outer cortical surface of the regenerate chamber or place with a central activation pin extending transosseously (Figure 62-24). Once placed, activate the distractor

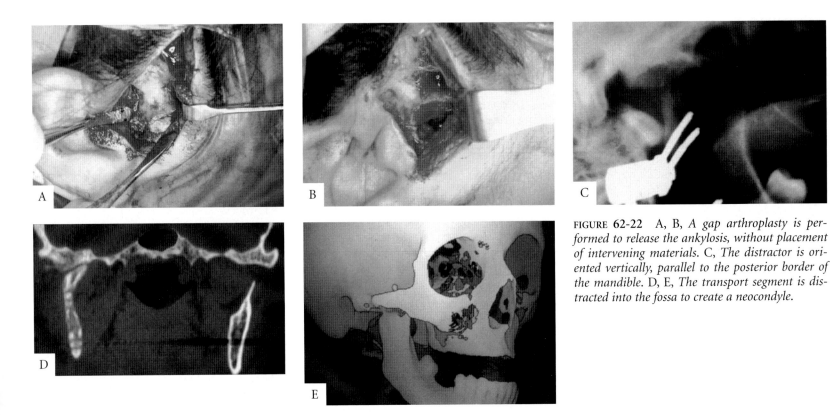

FIGURE 62-22 A, B, *A gap arthroplasty is performed to release the ankylosis, without placement of intervening materials.* C, *The distractor is oriented vertically, parallel to the posterior border of the mandible.* D, E, *The transport segment is distracted into the fossa to create a neocondyle.*

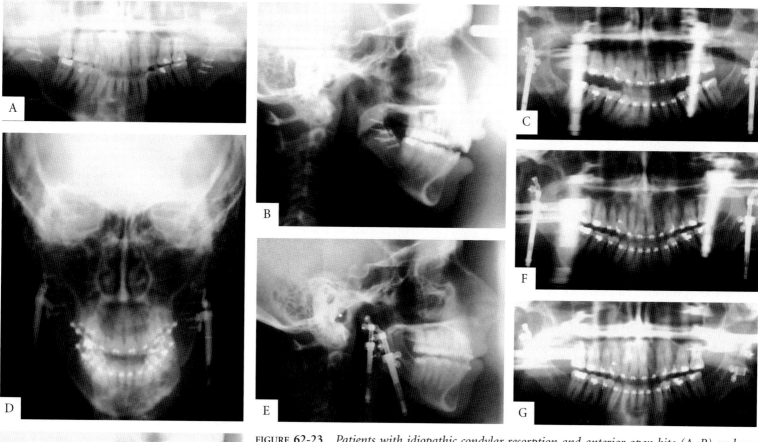

FIGURE 62-23 *Patients with idiopathic condylar resorption and anterior open bite (A, B) undergo bilateral ramal distraction osteogenesis (C, D) to correct the vertical height loss. Initially the mandible is distracted into Class II occlusion (E, F), the distractor is removed after 3 weeks of consolidation, and elastics are used to guide the mandible into proper occlusion (G, H).*

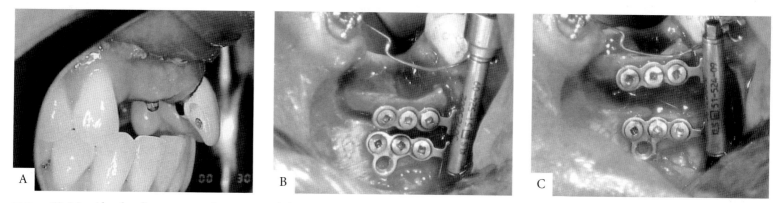

FIGURE 62-24 *Alveolar distractors are interosseous (A) or extraosseous (B). C, After device application the distractor is activated to ensure impedance-free moment of the segment. The transport disk is then returned to the closed position.*

to check for impedance-free movement of the distraction segment. Remove any bony interferences. The wound is closed and after a 3- to 5-day latency, the distractor is activated up to 0.7 to 1.0 mm per day. The distraction disk is small; thus, a rate of 0.5 to 0.7 mm per day is advocated if the blood supply to the segment is compromised. Distraction proceeds until the desired amount of bone is obtained. Often the segment is overdistracted to a position above the alveolar crest of the adjacent teeth. During implant placement, the excess crestal bone can be sculpted and contoured using a periodontal bur that produces an esthetic implant site. The segment is held in place to allow for ossification. Some authors recommend 8 weeks of ossification, whereas others recommend 12 weeks prior to implant placement.[37,39] Initially, the regenerate chamber is radiolucent. This decreases with time, but the generate chamber will continue to be less radio-

dense for up to 1 year post-distraction. Applying platelet rich plasma (PRP) into the distraction gap at the time of initial distraction surgery may increase DO bone ossification.[40]

Both interosseous and extraosseous distraction devices work well; however, they have some drawbacks. Devices placed on the outer cortical surface may cause slight buccal resorption of the outer cortex, requiring a "patch graft" at the time of device removal. Placing a guided bone regeneration (GBR) membrane next to the bone below the distraction device will also act to decrease this buccal resorption.[41] Devices that are placed transosseously result in fibrous tissue in-growth around the central distraction pin. This tissue is removed at the time of the device removal but can limit immediate implant placement. Dental implants may be placed at the time of distractor removal or at 1 month later. Second-stage implant place-

ment allows the soft tissues to mature and facilitates treatment planning for ideal implant placement. Place implants to span the regenerate chamber, including a portion of the distal osteotomy site.

Vector control is paramount with small-segment distraction, such as DO for dental implants. The small bone segments are under local muscle pull, especially the mylohyoid. Vector control devices, including orthodontic appliances and interim treatment partials with an access hole for the DO device activation rod, are useful to help guide the distractor into place (Figure 62-25). Callus manipulation as previously described may be performed under local anesthesia to re-direct the proper path of distraction. New alveolar DO devices that incorporate hinges allow the clinician to redirect the vector during active distraction (Figure 62-26).[42,43]

Local osseous anatomy can influence distraction device placement. The fixation plates of an extraosseous device may require bending to make the distraction pin more vertical and to optimize the ideal vector. Placing the device flush directly on the bone surface can direct the bone segment in an inappropriate direction, as is the case with the atrophic anterior maxilla and mandible (Figure 62-27). Similarly, to ensure proper device trajectory, the central pin hole of an intraosseous device may require angling more buccally than along the central axis of the alveolus. The fixation plates may need altering that takes into account the local anatomy, including the mental nerve and piriform rim regions. In fact, place the extraosseous device in a cantilever fashion with the central portion of the device offset (Figure 62-28).

Knife-edge ridges can be a difficult problem. Distracting the alveolus in a straight vertical direction will produce an increase in height but a narrow bone stock. Perform differential distraction by performing the lingual cut incompletely, allowing the lingual site to act as a "hinge."[44,45] The

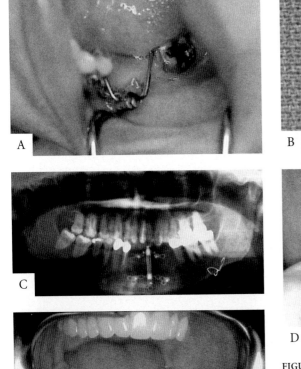

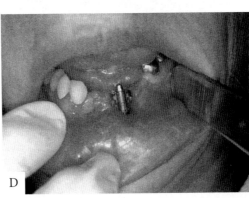

FIGURE 62-25 *Vector control devices include: orthodontic devices (A), treatment partials with access holes (B), and occlusal splints with pontic teeth (C–E).*

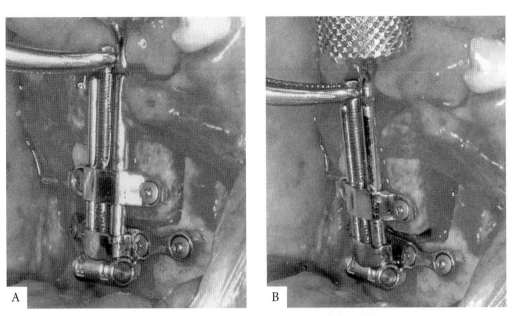

A   B

FIGURE 62-26   A *and* B, *Alveolar distraction devices with internal hinges allow for vector adjustment during active distraction osteogenesis. (Courtesy of Dr. M. Robinoy.)*

62-30).[45,46] Distraction proceeds with the anterior portion of the distraction segment rotating and hinging around the distal fixation plate to differentially increase the anterior region.

Use distraction to reconstruct atrophic edentulous maxillas and mandibles. The technique is the same. One device is placed in the midline, and the vector is adjusted to distract the bone segment up and buccally. To avoid fracture of the atrophic mandible, modify the bone cut to a trapezoidal shape. Rounding the internal corners of the osteotomy eliminates local inherent stresses, which have been associated with mandibular fractures.[47] For severely atrophic cases, place a reconstruction plate, in conjunction with the distraction devices, at the time of the osteotomy.[48]

Complications

Most complications associated with the distraction technique are iatrogenic and

device is placed, and distraction proceeds as usual. The hinge motion allows the buccal wall to be initially distracted differentially more than the lingual; specifically, the buccal site "opens" to create a flat crestal surface suitable for implants (Figure 62-29).

Posterior saddle deformities of the mandible are also problematic. The curve of Spee dictates that straight vertical distraction results in generating more bone in the retromolar region. To alleviate this

problem, make an L-shaped bone cut adjacent to the remaining teeth, and use a monocortical miniplate to fixate the posterior-most portion on the bone cut (Figure

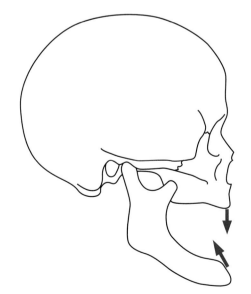

FIGURE 62-27   *Placing the extraosseous distractor flush on the native bone will produce a poor trajectory to the vector.*

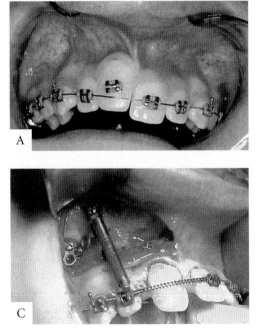

A

C

FIGURE 62-28   A, *Distraction osteogenesis (DO) was performed prior to extraction of this malpositioned, ankylosed, previously hopelessly avulsed tooth.* B, *DO prior to extraction facilitated proper crestal bone and gingival height.* C, D, *The DO device is placed lateral to the transport disk in a cantilever fashion to optimize bone stock for device placement.*

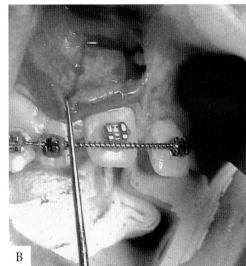

B

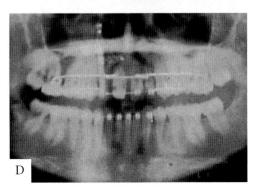

D

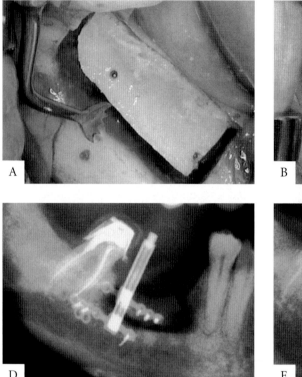

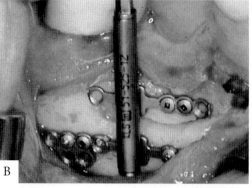

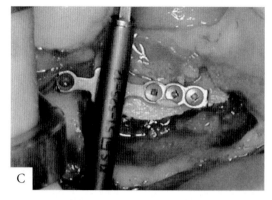

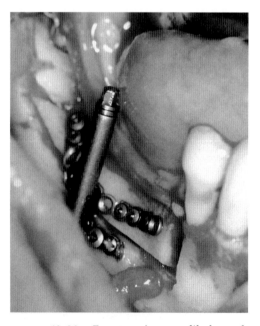

FIGURE 62-29   A, *Differential osteotomy of knife-edge ridges allows the flat buccal surface to become the crest of the ridge after distraction osteogenesis. B, The distractor is placed with the vector oriented vertically and slightly lingually. C–E, The bone cut is incomplete on the lingual site and acts as a hinge. (Courtesy of Dr. M. Robiony.)*

FIGURE 62-30   *For posterior mandibular saddle deformities, an L-shaped osteotomy is performed in the alveolus with a monocortical miniplate placed at the distal tip acting as a hinge. (Courtesy of Dr. G. Milessi.)*

easily managed.[49,50] Inaccurate planning may lead to poor vector trajectory of the bone segments. Molding the regenerate can alleviate this problem. Careful follow-up is mandatory during the entire distraction process, including the time of post-distraction ossification. During this latter time period, the regenerate chamber is fully extended and is most under the influence of local muscle pull. Also, the period of post-distraction ossification is the best time to easily mold the regenerate.

Wound dehiscence problems can occur. Local wound care, including antibiotics and antimicrobial mouth rinses, alleviates this problem. Disk dancing can be performed to allow the local wound site to heal after which DO can begin. Occasionally, however, the distractor fixation screw heads become visible, but this is not a concern. Overdistracting the segment can compensate for potential crestal bone loss from screw-head exposure.

References

1. Ilizarov GA. The principles of the Ilizarov method. Bull Hosp Joint Dis 1988;48:1–16.
2. Karp NS, McCarthy JG, Schreiber JS, et al. Membranous bone lengthening: a serial histologic study. Ann Plas Surg 1992;29:2.
3. Herford A, Audia F, Stucki-McCormick SU. Alveolar distraction osteogenesis and vector control—a preliminary report. In: Arnaud E, Diner PA, editors. Proceedings 3rd International Meeting on Craniofacial DO; 2001 Jun 14–16; Paris, France. Bologna (IT): Monduzzi; 2001.
4. Hoffmeister B, Marcks CH, Wolff KP. The floating bone concept in intraoral distraction. J Craniomaxillofac Surg 1998;26 Suppl 1:76–81.
5. Moses JJ. Sagittal distraction of the mandible: a technique for nerve preservation and condylar axis stability. Proceedings 4th International Congress of Osteogenesis of the Facial Skeleton; 2003 Jul 2–5; Paris, France. Bologna (IT): Monduzzi; 2003.
6. Watzinger F, Wanschitz F, Rasse M, et al. Computer-aided surgery in distraction osteogenesis of the maxilla and mandible. Int J Oral Maxillofac Surg 1999;28:171–5.
7. McCarthy JG, Stelnicki EJ, Grayson BH. Distraction osteogenesis of the mandible: a ten-year experience. Semin Orthod 1999;1:3–8.
8. Grayson BH, Stucki-McCormick SU, Santiago PE. Vector of device placement and trajectory of mandibular distraction. J Craniofac Surg 1998;8:473–80.
9. Stucki-McCormick SU, Fox R, Mizrahi R. Distraction osteogenesis for congenital mandibular deformities. Atlas Oral Maxillofac Surg Clin North Am 1999;7:85–110.
10. Perlyn CA, Schmelzer RE, Sutera SP, et al. Effect of distraction osteogenesis of the

mandible on upper airway volume and resistance in children with micrognathia. Plast Reconstr Surg 2002;109:1809–18.

11. Denny A, Kalantarian B. Mandibular distraction in neonates: a strategy to avoid tracheostomy. Plast Reconstr Surg 2002;109:896–904.

12. Woodson BT, Hanson PR, Melugin MB, Gama AA. Sequential upper airway changes during mandibular distraction for obstructive sleep apnea. Otolaryngol Head Neck Surg 2003;128:142–4.

13. Smith KS. Pediatric sleep apnea and treatment with distraction osteogenesis. Ann R Australas Coll Dent Surg 2000;15:163–7.

14. Cope JB, Yamashita J, Healy S, et al. Force level and strain patterns during bilateral mandibular osteodistraction. J Oral Maxillofac Surg 2000;58:171–89.

15. Cope JB, Samchukov ML, Cherkashin AM, et al. Biomechanics of mandibular distractor orientation: an animal model analysis. J Oral Maxillofac Surg 1999;57:952–64.

16. Contasti G, Guerrero C, Rodriguez AM, Legan HL. Mandibular widening by distraction osteogenesis. J Clin Orthod 2001;35:165–73.

17. Bell WH, Gonzalez M, Samchukov ML, Guerrero CA. Intraoral widening and lengthening of the mandible in baboons by distraction osteogenesis. J Oral Maxillofac Surg 1999;57:548–63.

18. Kewitt GF, Van Sickels JE. Long-term effect of mandibular midline distraction osteogenesis on the status of the temporomandibular joint, teeth, periodontal structures, and neurosensory function. J Oral Maxillofac Surg 1999;57:1419–26.

19. Guerrero CA, Bell WH, Contasti GI, Rodriguez AM. Intraoral mandibular distraction osteogenesis. Semin Orthod 1999;5:35–40.

20. Molina F. Combined maxillary and mandibular distraction osteogenesis. Semin Orthod 1999;5:41–5.

21. Padwa BL, Kearns GJ, Todd R, et al. Simultaneous maxillary and mandibular distraction osteogenesis with a semiburied device. Int J Oral Maxillofac Surg 1999;28:2–8.

22. Moses JJ, Vega L. Sagittal distraction of the mandible. In: Arnaud E, Diner PA, editors. Proceedings 3rd International Meeting on Craniofacial DO; 2001 Jun 14–16; Paris France. Italy. Bologna (IT): Monduzzi;2001.

23. Polley JW, Figueroa AA. Rigid external distraction: its application in cleft maxillary deformities. Plast Reconstr Surg 1998;102:1360–74.

24. Cohen SR. Midface distraction. Semin Orthod 1999;5:52–8.

25. Ahn JG, Figueroa AA, Braun S, Polley JW. Biomechanical considerations in distraction of the osteotomized dentomaxillary complex. Am J Orthod Dentofacial Orthop 1999;116:264–70.

26. Liou EJ, Chen PK, Huang CS, Chen YR. Interdental distraction osteogenesis and rapid orthodontic tooth movement: a novel approach to approximate a wide alveolar cleft or bony defect. Plast Reconstr Surg 2000;105:1262–72.

27. Costantino PD, Buchbinder D. Mandibular distraction osteogenesis: types, applications, and indications. J Craniofac Surg 1996;7:404–7.

28. Guerrero CA, Gonzalez M. Intraoral bone transport by distraction osteogenesis in mandibular reconstruction. In: Arnaud E, Diner PA, editors. Proceedings 4th International Congress of Osteogenesis of the Facial Skeleton; 2003 Jul 2–5; Paris, France. Bologna (IT): Monduzzi; 2003.

29. Herford AS. Use of a plate guided distraction device for transport distraction osteogenesis of the mandible. In: Arnaud E, Diner PA, editors. Proceedings 4th International Congress of Osteogenesis of the Facial Skeleton; 2003 Jul 2–5; Paris, France. Bologna (IT): Monduzzi; 2003.

30. Stucki-McCormick SU, Fox R, Mizrahi R, Erickson M. Transport distraction: mandibular reconstruction. Atlas Oral Maxillofac Surg Clin North Am 1999;7:65–84.

31. Gantous A, Phillips JH, Catton P, Holmberg D. Distraction osteogenesis in the irradiated canine mandible. Plast Reconstr Surg 1994;93:164–8.

32. Aronson J. Temporal and special increases in blood flow during distraction osteogenesis. Clin Orthop Rel Res 1994;301:124–31.

33. Klesper B, Lazar F, Siessegger M, et al. Vertical distraction osteogenesis of fibula transplants for mandibular reconstruction – a preliminary study. J Craniomaxillofac Surg 2002;30:280–5.

34. McCarthy JG, Stelnicki EJ, Mehrara BJ, Longaker MT. Distraction osteogenesis of the craniofacial skeleton. Plast Reconstr Surg 2001;107:1812–27.

35. Stucki-McCormick SU, Fox RM, Mizrahi RD. Reconstruction of a neocondyle using transport distraction osteogenesis. Semin Orthod 1999;5:59–63.

36. Piero C, Alessandro A, Giorgio S, et al. Combined surgical therapy of temporomandibular joint ankylosis and secondary deformity using intraoral distraction. J Craniofac Surg 2002;13:401–10.

37. Chin M. Distraction osteogenesis for dental implants. Atlas Oral Maxillofac Surg Clin North Am 1999;7:41–63.

38. Jensen OT, Cockrell R, Kuhike L, Reed C. Anterior maxillary alveolar distraction osteogenesis: a prospective 5-year clinical study. Int J Oral Maxillofac Implants 2002;17:52–68.

39. Block MS, Gardiner D, Almerico B, Neal C. Loaded hydroxylapatite-coated implants and uncoated titanium-threaded implants in distracted dog alveolar ridges. Oral Surg Oral Med Oral Pathol Oral Radiol Endod 2000;89:676–85.

40. Robiony M, Polini F, Costa F, Politi M. Osteogenesis distraction and platelet-rich plasma for bone restoration of the severely atrophic mandible: preliminary results. J Oral Maxillofac Surg 2002;60:630–5.

41. Millisi W, Millisi-Schobel G. Alveolar distraction osteogenesis of the mandible. In: Arnaud E, Diner PA, editors. Proceedings 4th International Congress of Osteogenesis of the Facial Skeleton; 2003 Jul 2–5; Paris, France. Bologna (IT): Monduzzi; 2003.

42. Zechner W, Bernhart T, Zauza K, et al. Multidimensional osteodistraction for correction of implant malposition in edentulous segments. Clin Oral Implants Res 2001; 12:531–8.

43. Stucki-McCormick SU, Moses JJ, Robinson R, et al. Alveolar distraction devices. In: Jensen, editor. Alveolar distraction osteogenesis. Carol Stream (IL): Quintessence Publishing Co. Inc; 2002. p. 41–58.

44. Chin M. Alveolar distraction osteogenesis with endosseous devices in 175 cases. In: Arnaud E, Diner PA, editors. Proceedings 3rd International Meeting on Craniofacial DO; 2001 Jun 14–16; Paris, France. Bologna (IT): Monduzzi; 2001.

45. Stucki-McCormick SU, Moses JJ. Vertical alveolar distraction of the posterior mandible. In: Jensen, editor. Alveolar distraction osteogenesis. Carol Stream (IL): Quintessence Publishing Co.; 2002. p. 89–94.

46. Millesi G, Klug C, Millesi W, et al. Vertical distraction osteogenesis in the mandible combined with L-shaped osteotomy and guided bone regeneration. Cranio-maxillo-facial distraction. Graz (AU): University of Graz; 2002.

47. Hidding J, Lazar F, Zoller JE. The Cologne concept on vertical distraction osteogenesis. In: Arnaud E, Diner PA, editors. Proceedings 3rd International Meeting on Craniofacial DO; 2001 Jun 14–16; Paris, France. Bologna (IT): Monduzzi; 2001.

48. Hidding J, Lazar F, Zoller JE. Initial outcome of vertical distraction osteogenesis of the atrophic alveolar ridge. Mund Kiefer Gesichtschir 1999;3 Suppl 1:79–83.

49. Garcia AG, Martin MS, Vila PG, Maceiras JL. Minor complications arising in alveolar distraction osteogenesis. J Oral Maxillofac Surg 2002;60:496–501.

50. Grayson BH, Santiago PE. Treatment planning and biomechanics of distraction osteogenesis from an orthodontic perspective. Semin Orthod 1999;5:9–24.

CHAPTER 63

Surgical and Nonsurgical Management of Obstructive Sleep Apnea

B. D. Tiner, DDS, MD
Peter D. Waite, MPH, DDS, MD

Sleep and dreaming have been sources of mystery and fascination since biblical times. Sleep consists of inevitably recurring episodes of readily reversible relative disengagement from sensory and motor interaction with the environment.[1] The function of sleep remains a mystery, and only in recent years has there been research into specific symptom complexes and causes of sleep disorders. In 1979 the Association of Sleep Disorders Center and the Association for the Psychophysiological Study of Sleep published the first classification of sleep and arousal disorders.[2]

Modern sleep research became possible in 1924 when Hans Berger, a German psychiatrist, described the recording of human electroencephalography.[3] Loomis and colleagues in 1935 published a quantitative description of the four levels of sleep based on electroencephalogram (EEG) characteristics.[4,5] The historic discovery of a cyclic phase of sleep characterized by rapid conjugate eye movements was made by Aserinsky and Kleitman in 1953.[6] Subsequent studies confirmed this to be a very active phase of sleep that correlated closely with dreaming.[7]

Normal Sleep Stages

Normal sleep architecture includes both quiet sleep (nonrapid eye movement [non-REM] sleep) and active sleep (rapid eye movement [REM] sleep). Non-REM sleep consists of four stages which are based largely on the original criteria of Loomis and colleagues.[4,5] Stage 2 predominates and comprises 45 to 50% of total sleep time. The four stages of non-REM sleep represent progressively deeper sleep marked by the increasing appearance of high-amplitude slow waves in stages 3 and 4, which are collectively known as delta sleep. Non-REM sleep is characterized by a general slowing of all levels of activity. Progression through all four stages of non-REM sleep usually occurs rapidly after sleep onset. REM sleep occurs after non-REM sleep has been established, and the first REM period normally occurs after 70 to 90 minutes of non-REM sleep. The average duration of a period of REM sleep is about 20 minutes. The initial REM period of the night is usually very brief, but subsequent REM periods become longer. During an average night of REM/non-REM cycle progression, 4 to 6 REM periods normally occur at intervals of 60 to 90 minutes. REM sleep occupies about 20 to 25% of total sleep time in a healthy young adult. REM sleep EEG patterns look very similar to those seen during the wakeful state. Generalized skeletal muscle atonia (except for the ocular muscles) and absence of reflexive activity are other features unique to REM sleep. Marked physiologic changes also occur during REM sleep. Temperature, blood flow, and oxygen use in the brain are increased. Heart rate, blood pressure, and respiration show dramatic fluctuations and increase in average rate.

During sleep the control of respiration is influenced by two systems: the metabolic control system and the behavioral control system.[8] The influences of hypoxia and hypercarbia on ventilation are the predominant components of the metabolic control system of respiration. This system predominantly controls respiration during non-REM sleep. The behavioral control system governs respiration during voluntary activities, such as swallowing or speaking, and may suppress the ventilatory response to metabolic stimuli. During REM sleep, the effects of hypoxia and hypercarbia on ventilation are much less than during non-REM sleep, and the behavioral control system may predominate. With a blunted response to hypoxia and hypercarbia, irregular respirations, and decreased skeletal muscle tone of the upper airway muscles during REM sleep, an episode of partial or complete airway obstruction with apnea or hypopnea may occur.

Sleep Apnea Syndrome

The sleep apnea syndrome is a disorder characterized by abnormal breathing in sleep and sleep fragmentation. At least 30 episodes of apnea occur during 7 hours of nocturnal sleep in these patients. Apnea is defined as the cessation of airflow from the nostrils and mouth for at least 10 seconds. These apneic episodes can result in hypoxemia, hypercarbia, systemic and pulmonary hypertension, polycythemia, cor pulmonale, bradycardia, and cardiac dysrhythmias. Sudden death has occurred in patients with sleep apnea. Throughout the night the alternating episodes of apnea and arousal from sleep may occur as frequently as 400 to 600 times, with each typical apnea episode lasting 15 to 60 seconds. These episodes can amount to as much as 50% of a night's sleep. The frequent disruption results in symptoms similar to sleep deprivation. These include excessive daytime sleepiness, fatigue, depression, personality changes, and impotence. These dysfunctional symptoms are common primary complaints and are often the reason people seek treatment.

Epidemiologic data suggest that sleep apnea syndrome may be quite common, particularly in its milder forms. In fact, obstructive sleep apnea is the second most common sleep disorder, insomnia being the most common. A 1993 Sleep Commission Report estimated that 20 million Americans have sleep apnea, with the majority being undiagnosed and untreated.[9] The exact prevalence is unknown, but sleep apnea syndrome may affect up to 2 to 3% of adult males.[8] In certain populations the prevalence may be as high at 10%. Most patients are diagnosed after age 40, but sleep apnea can occur at any age. There is a strong male predilection, with men outnumbering women by up to 8 to 1 until menopause. This implies a hormonal influence. The cost for diagnosis and treatment of this sleep disorder accounts for over $50 million (US) in hospital bills each year. Overall, sleep disorders and sleepiness cost the United States economy a minimum of $15.9 billion (US) in direct costs each year.[10]

Classification

Central sleep apnea, obstructive sleep apnea, and mixed sleep apnea are the variations of apnea that occur in the syndrome. In central sleep apnea, respiratory muscle activity ceases simultaneously with airflow at the mouth and nostrils.[11] This disorder is found in patients with central nervous system (CNS) insufficiency that affects the outflow of neural output from the respiratory center to the diaphragm and other muscles of respiration. CNS disorders associated with central sleep apnea include brainstem neoplasms, brainstem infarctions, bulbar encephalitis, bulbar poliomyelitis, spinal surgery, cervical cordotomy, and primary idiopathic hypoventilation.

Patients with central sleep apnea have been treated with some success by using respiratory-stimulating drugs such as theophylline, progesterone, and acetazolamide. In severe central apnea, modalities of treatment have included phrenic nerve pacemaker implantation to ensure regular respiration during sleep and nocturnal mechanical ventilation with a negative pressure ventilator for more severe cases. There are no simple and convenient methods of treatment for mild central apnea.

The most common type of sleep apnea by far is obstructive. This is characterized by sleep-induced obstruction of the upper airway that results in cessation of airflow with preservation of respiratory effort, respiratory center drive, and diaphragmatic contraction.[11]

Mixed sleep apnea is a combination of central and obstructive apnea. This pattern begins with an episode of central apnea with no airflow detectable at the mouth and nostrils and no respiratory muscle activity. The pattern ends with an episode of obstructive apnea with only cessation of airflow at the mouth and nostrils.[11]

Differential Diagnosis

Profound hypersomnolence is a characteristic feature of both sleep apnea and narcolepsy; hence, they are often confused. However, unlike sleep apnea, narcolepsy affects both sexes equally, with most patients experiencing the onset of symptoms around or shortly before puberty.[12] The first symptom to appear with narcolepsy is usually excessive daytime somnolence (EDS). The sleep attacks can range from mild to severe and are characterized by the sudden onset of overwhelming sleepiness that lasts 30 seconds to 20 minutes. Following brief naps, the narcoleptic usually feels refreshed and relatively free from disturbing symptoms for up to 2 hours. Serious accidents, marital discord, and the inability to hold jobs frequently result from these sleep attacks. Another feature of narcolepsy is the abrupt loss of muscle control (cataplexy). Attacks can be particularly disabling, because they are characteristically precipitated by emotional experiences such as laughter, anger, or excitement. Additional associated symptoms of narcolepsy include sleep paralysis and hypnagogic hallucinations. Sleep paralysis is the skeletal muscle atonia of REM sleep persisting into the awake state. Hypnagogic hallucinations are REM sleep imagery occurring while falling asleep. Patients are sometimes misdiagnosed as schizophrenic if hypnagogic hallucinations are prominent.

Diagnosis of narcolepsy is made by documenting sleep-onset REM periods during a nocturnal polysomnography.[12] In normal sleep REM sleep is usually not seen until about 70 to 90 minutes into sleep. The clinical features of narcolepsy probably represent abnormal manifestations of REM sleep.

Treatment modalities for narcolepsy include behavioral therapies, CNS stimulants, tricyclic antidepressants, or monoamine oxidase inhibitors (only in resistant cases) and L-tryptophan.[13]

Other disorders that may be confused with sleep apnea syndrome include sleep-related abnormal swallowing syndrome, gastroesophageal reflux, depression, alcohol or drug dependence, and sleep-related nocturnal myoclonus.

History of Obstructive Sleep Apnea Syndrome

Obstructive sleep apnea has a remarkably short history considering the incidence and disabling symptoms of the syndrome. Burwell and colleagues published the first description of the syndrome in 1956.[14] Their report compared an obese, somnolent, polycythemic patient with the sleepy red-faced boy, Joe, in the Charles Dickens novel *The Posthumous Papers of the Pickwick Club* (1837). However, Burwell and colleagues did not link their patient's excessive daytime sleepiness to nocturnal sleep fragmentation. In 1966, Gastaut and colleagues were the first investigators to demonstrate repeated apneas in pickwickian patients during sleep.[15] They correctly attributed the excessive daytime somnolence in these patients to nocturnal sleep fragmentation caused by repeated apneas.

The misdiagnosis of narcolepsy in patients with sleep apnea and the general skepticism of excessive daytime somnolence as a valid clinical sign are the two main reasons sleep apnea syndrome was overlooked for so long.

Clinical Manifestations

Sleep apnea patients present with a variety of symptoms and clinical manifestations. Patients with obstructive sleep apnea most often complain of EDS. The patients may experience serious social, economic, and emotional problems from the EDS associated with this disorder. The uncontrollable desire to sleep may predispose the patients to occupational or automobile accidents.

Almost all patients or their bed partners give a history of heavy, loud snoring which has usually been present for several years before the EDS was noted. The snoring is produced from the passage of air through the oropharynx causing vibrations of the soft palate. Typically the snoring is interrupted periodically by apneic episodes that last 30 to 90 seconds. Bed partners usually describe an episode in which the snoring stops and the patient seems to stop breathing for a period of time. A loud snort followed by a hyperventilation usually signals an end to the apneic episode.

Other common presenting complaints are morning headaches and nausea that result from the hypercarbia which develops with the hypoventilatory episodes. Depression, personality changes, and intellectual deterioration may also develop.

The systemic hypertension that is a common finding in obstructive sleep apnea may be related to the catecholamine release triggered by the systemic hypoxemia. In more advanced severe cases, pulmonary hypertension, polycythemia, and cor pulmonale may develop and become life threatening. However, most patients do not manifest these disturbances because their ventilation during wakeful periods is sufficient to prevent these complications of chronic hypoxia.

A prominent sinus dysrhythmia is commonly associated with the apneic episodes. The extent of bradycardia is directly proportional to the severity of the oxygen desaturation. The greatest degree of cardiac slowing occurs in obstructive apneas in which a Müller maneuver is performed. Increased vagal efferent tone mediates the bradycardia.

The development of severe and life-threatening medical complications from the apneic events clearly depends on the frequency, duration, and degree of hypoxemia and associated hypertensive response.

Physical Findings

A major feature of obstructive sleep apnea is obesity. The increased body weight correlates with increased frequency of apnea and the severity of hypoxemia. However, the morbidly obese, somnolent, hyperventilating patient with cor pulmonale represents only a small number of sleep apnea patients. Lower BMI (body mass index) patients with obstructive sleep apnea often have more abnormal cephalometrics than obese people.[16,17]

Obstruction can occur at a number of points in the airway. Physical examination of these patients may reveal hypertrophy of the tonsils or adenoids, retrognathia, micrognathia, macroglossia, deviation of the nasal septum, a thick short neck, or tumors in the nasopharynx or hypopharynx. Both primary and secondary medical conditions are associated with obstructive sleep apnea, owing to their effects on the upper airway anatomy. These may include temporomandibular joint disorders, myxedema, goiter, acromegaly, and lymphoma.

Most patients with classic obstructive sleep apnea have no identifiable craniofacial anomaly. However, there does appear to be a significant subpopulation of sleep apnea patients with craniofacial anomalies.[18,19] Lowe and colleagues found several alterations in craniofacial form in subjects with obstructive sleep apnea that may reduce the dimensions of the upper airway and subsequently impair stability of the upper airway.[20] A sample of 25 adult male patients with moderate to severe obstructive sleep apnea showed a posteriorly positioned maxilla and mandible, a steep occlusal plane, overerupted maxillary and mandibular teeth, proclined incisors, a steep mandibular plane, a large gonial angle, increased upper and lower facial heights, a posteriorly placed pharyngeal wall, and an anterior open bite in association with a long tongue.[20] Bacon and colleagues evaluated 32 patients with sleep apnea by cephalometry and demonstrated an anteroposterior shortening of the cranial base, a posterior facial compression with narrowing of the pharyngeal airway, and an increased lower facial height.[18] Rivlin and colleagues reported on nine obstructive sleep apnea patients with posterior displacement of the mandible.[21] The number of apneas correlated with the total posterior displacement.[21]

Diagnosis

Physical Examination

A diagnostic evaluation includes a thorough history and physical examination, fiberoptic endoscopy, radiologic evaluation, and polysomnography. Little additional information can be gained from routine laboratory tests. Except in severe cases, pulmonary function tests, electrocardiogram (ECG), arterial blood gases, and chest radiographs are often normal during wakefulness in sleep apnea patients.

Other diagnostic tests that may aid in evaluating sleep apnea patients include a complete blood count (CBC), serum electrolytes, and thyroid function tests. Secondary polycythemia may be revealed by a CBC, and nocturnal carbon dioxide retention may be reflected by increased bicarbonate levels. Hypothyroidism, a contributing cause of sleep apnea, may be identified from thyroid function studies.

After a complete history is obtained from the patient and his or her bed partner, a complete clinical examination of the mouth, nasal, pharyngeal, and laryngeal areas is performed. The emphasis of the clinical examination should be the identification of anatomic abnormalities that may contribute to or produce obstruction during sleep. The nose is examined for a deviated nasal septum and enlargement of the turbinates. Micrognathia, retrognathia, and macroglossia may be noted in examination of the oral cavity. Occasionally masses or tumors in the nasopharynx or hypopharynx may be noted. In the pharynx, adenotonsillary hypertrophy, a long soft palate, a large base of the tongue, and excess pharyngeal mucosa are potential causes of obstruction. The larynx is examined for vocal cord webs and paralysis of the vocal cords. Obstructive sleep apnea patients may present with any combination of these anatomic abnormalities.

After topically anesthetizing the nasal cavity and pharynx, a fiberoptic endoscope is introduced through the nose. In sequential fashion the nasopharynx, oropharynx, hypopharynx, and larynx are examined. The appearance and position of the soft palate, base of tongue, and lateral pharyngeal walls are evaluated. Changes in the position of the base of the tongue such as forward movement with protrusion of the mandible are noted. The appearance of the pharyngeal airway and degree of pharyngeal wall collapse is noted while the patient performs a modified Müller maneuver. To accomplish this maneuver the patient attempts to inspire with the mouth and nose closed. Increased negative pressure in the pharynx will demonstrate the point of collapse.

Cephalometric Examination

A lateral cephalogram is routinely obtained in the radiologic evaluation of sleep apnea patients (Figure 63-1). Cephalometric analysis is performed to identify any skeletal and soft tissue abnormalities that may exist. The advantages of cephalometry are its easy access, low cost, and minimal radiation exposure. However, it should be recognized that there are obvious limitations of evaluating a three-dimensional area with a two-dimensional lateral cephalometry.

Mandibular or maxillary position can be evaluated by a number of methods including the SNA and SNB angles. Patients with skeletal deficiencies are more likely to have obstruction at the base of the tongue or at the level of the soft palate. Riley and colleagues determined that obstructive sleep apnea patients had an inferiorly positioned hyoid bone, a longer-than-normal soft palate, and a narrowing at the base of the tongue.[22,23] The position of the hyoid bone is determined by drawing a perpendicular line from the mandibular plane (MP) through the hyoid bone (H). The mean MP-H distance for normal subjects is 15.4 ± 3 mm (see Figure 63-1). The position of the hyoid bone is important because it serves as a central anchor for the muscles of the tongue and thereby partly determines tongue position. Soft palate length is measured from a line drawn from posterior nasal spine (PNS) to the tip of the soft palate shadow (P). The mean PNS-P distance in normal subjects is 37 ± 3 mm. Posterior airway space is determined by a line drawn from point B through the gonion (Go) intersecting the base of the tongue and the posterior pharyngeal wall. Figure 63-2 demonstrates change in posterior airway spaces following maxillomandibular advancement. Mean posterior airway space in normal subjects was determined to be 11 ± 1 mm. Lower face height is measured from the anterior nasal spine (ANS) to the menton (Me). There is no absolute value for this measurement in obstructive sleep apnea patients. However, some studies have

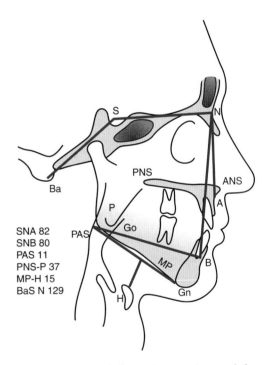

FIGURE **63-1** *Cephalometric screening used for initial evaluation of patients with obstructive sleep apnea syndrome. A = A point; ANS = anterior nasal spine; B = B point; Ba = basion; Gn = gnathion; Go = gonion; H = hyoid; MP = mandibular plane; N = nasion; P = palate; PAS = posterior airway space; PNS = posterior nasal spine; S = sella; SNA = sella-nasion–A point; SNB = sella-nasion–B point. Adapted from Tiner BD, Waite, PD. Surgical and nonsurgical management of obstructive sleep apnea. In: Peterson LJ, Indresano AT, Marciani RD, Roser SM. Principles of oral and maxillofacial surgery. Vol. 3. Philadelphia (PA): J.B. Lippincott Company; 1992. p. 1535.*

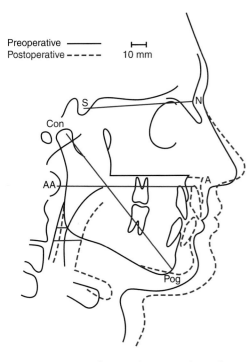

Preoperative ———
Postoperative - - - -   ⊢——⊣ 10 mm

FIGURE 63-2 *Change in posterior airway space following maxillary and mandibular advancement. A = A point; AA = anterior edge of atlas; Con = condylion; N = nasion; Pog = Pogonion; S = sella. Adapted from Tiner BD, Waite, PD. Surgical and nonsurgical management of obstructive sleep apnea. In: Peterson LJ, Indresano AT, Marciani RD, Roser SM. Principles of oral and maxillofacial surgery. Vol. 3. Philadelphia (PA): J.B. Lippincott Company; 1992. p. 1536.*

shown an increased lower face height and a shortened cranial base with obstructive sleep apnea patients.[18]

Computed Tomography

Computed tomography (CT) is an alternative to cephalometry and has been used to provide a quantitative assessment of the upper airway at various levels. With three-dimensional CT reconstructions, Lowe and colleagues found obstructive sleep apnea patients with larger tongue surface areas and smaller airway surface areas.[24] Haponik and colleagues found significantly decreased cross-sectional areas of the nasopharynx, oropharynx, and hypopharynx in obstructive sleep apnea patients when compared with control subjects by using CT scanning.[25] Some authorities feel that the airway can only be assessed by a CT scan. However, Riley and colleagues compared patients who

had three-dimensional CT scans and found a statistically significant correlation between the posterior airway space (PAS) measured on the lateral cephalogram and the volume of the pharyngeal airway measured on CT scans.[23,26] Waite and Villos demonstrated by helical CT analysis that maxillomandibular advancement increases both anteroposterior and lateral dimension of the airway at all levels from nasopharynx to hyoid.[27] Many studies are currently being done to determine the effects of patient position and changes in airway. A cephalogram and a CT scan are static evaluations at a fixed time of a dynamic system and they should be viewed as only part of the overall evaluation of the patient.

Polysomnography

Nocturnal polysomnography remains the gold standard for establishing the diagnosis of sleep apnea, quantitating its severity, and determining the success of treatment modalities. The study is performed in a sleep laboratory and the patient's sleep is monitored overnight. At least 4 hours of total sleep time must be recorded for a diagnostic study. The components of the polysomnogram include the EEG, electro-oculogram (EOG), electromyogram (EMG), and electrocardiogram (ECG, lead V_2). Sleep staging and architecture are determined by the EEG, EOG, and EMG tracings. Potentially lethal cardiac dysrhythmias are detected by the ECG. Oxygen saturation is measured by ear oximetry. A 5% or greater decrease in arterial oxygen saturation from baseline is significant during episodes of apnea or hypopnea. Respiratory effort and breathing pattern are measured using respiratory inductive plethysmography or by measuring intrathoracic pressure changes with an esophageal balloon catheter. The distinction between an episode of central apnea and obstructive apnea is made by correlating airflow at the nose and mouth with movement of the abdominal and thoracic respiratory muscles. Central apnea occurs

if both airflow and respiratory muscle movement stop simultaneously. An episode of obstructive apnea occurs when airflow at the mouth and nose ceases but respiratory muscles in the abdomen and thorax continue to move dysfunctionally.

Of particular interest are the number of respiratory events (apneas and hypopneas), the number of oxygen desaturations below 90%, and the lowest oxygen desaturation. The respiratory disturbance index (RDI) can be calculated from these data:

$$RDI = \frac{Apneas + Hypopneas}{Total\ sleep\ time} \times 60$$

An RDI greater than 5 is considered abnormal and an RDI greater than 20 is considered clinically significant, because EDS usually does not occur below this level. Obstructive sleep apnea also becomes clinically significant when oxygen desaturation events fall below 85%.

Site of Obstruction

Following a complete presurgical evaluation, each patient is grouped according to the site of obstruction: type I, oropharynx; type II, oropharynx and hypopharynx; type III, hypopharynx. In a review of 40 obstructive sleep apnea patients, Riley and colleagues found the majority of patients had a type II obstruction (soft palate and base of tongue).[28]

The mandible, base of tongue, hyoid, and pharyngeal wall are intimately related by their muscular and ligamentous attachments. The mandible is related to the base of the tongue by the genioglossus muscle. The tongue, through multiple muscular and connective tissue attachments, is related to the hyoid bone and to the mandible in such a way that retraction of the mandible results in a narrowing of the airway and posterior movement of the tongue. Compensatory mechanisms exist in non-sleep apneic patients to prevent occlusion of the airway. However, in sleep apneic patients, these mechanisms do not exist or are unable to compensate adequately.

Obstruction of the upper airway is primarily prevented by the action of the pharyngeal dilating muscles contracting in phase with respiration. Reduced muscle tone is normal and prominent during REM sleep. However, obstructive sleep apnea patients may have a significant reduction in muscle activity during non-REM sleep so that the pharynx becomes narrower and airway resistance increases. In patients with abnormal skeletal development the reduction in size of the resting airway may predispose them to upper airway obstruction during sleep.

The patency of the upper airway is determined by a balance between the pharyngeal musculature and the negative oropharyngeal pressures that are generated from resistance to airflow in the nasopharynx. Because the airway of obstructive sleep apnea patients is unstable even at rest, any structural narrowing of the airway will eventually hinder the muscular component of the balance. Collapse of the airway in obstructive sleep apnea is primarily a result of high intraluminal negative pressures associated with hypotonic pharyngeal wall musculature and disproportionate anatomy in either the oropharynx or hypopharynx or both. Disproportionate anatomy includes any combination of large base of tongue, long soft palate, narrow mandibular arch, shallow palatal arch, or retrognathic mandible.

Medical Treatment

Once the diagnosis has been confirmed, the treatment approach for sleep apnea is determined by the severity of the physiologic derangements and the predominant type of apnea. Regardless of the predominant type of apnea present, all patients should be cautioned that certain drugs may precipitate or exacerbate obstructive sleep apnea. Alcohol and other central nervous system depressants have been shown to aggravate sleep apnea and even to precipitate apnea and oxygen desaturations in normal persons.[29]

Weight loss and nasal continuous positive airway pressure are the initial modes of therapy that should be initiated in obese patients with moderate obstructive sleep apnea. A study of 16 patients who lost an average of 20 kg showed fewer apneas, reduced oxygen desaturations, and less daytime sleepiness than a control group of patients who did not lose weight.[30] Many patients can relate weight gain in preceding years to an increase in severity of their obstructive sleep apnea symptoms. Unfortunately weight loss by dietary measures is seldom sustained, and obstructive sleep apnea symptoms recur with weight gain. Riley and colleagues found that 47 of 50 obstructive sleep apnea patients who were between 20 and 100% overweight at the time of diagnosis had regained all the weight they had initially lost 5 to 7 years later.[31]

The role of oxygen therapy in the treatment of sleep apnea is controversial. In a study by Motta and Guilleminault, the administration of oxygen increased the duration of apneic episodes and led to worsening of acidosis and hypercarbia during both REM and non-REM sleep.[32] It is unknown how many of their patients had chronic obstructive lung disease. Other studies have shown that supplemental oxygen therapy consistently reduced the severity of oxygen desaturation and decreased the frequency of apnea.[33,34]

The combined experience of these reports suggests that oxygen therapy limited to a flow rate of 2 L/min can be used safely in most obstructive sleep apnea patients and will produce beneficial effects on respiration. The dangers of profound hypoxemia are greater than the concerns of prolonged apnea, acidosis, and hypercarbia. The effects of oxygen therapy on a patient with severe airway obstruction or chronic respiratory acidosis should be monitored with oximetry or polysomnography.

Several drugs have been used in the treatment of obstructive sleep apnea syndrome with variable results. The carbonic anhydrase inhibitor acetazolamide stimulates respiration by producing a metabolic acidosis. This drug reduced the number of apneas and decreased the severity of oxygen desaturations in a group of patients with central sleep apnea.[35] However, in several cases, acetazolamide given to patients with mild obstructive sleep apnea produced more frequent obstructive apneas of longer duration.[36] Therefore, acetazolamide is probably not indicated in the management of obstructive sleep apnea syndrome.

Some patients with obstructive sleep apnea benefit from the respiratory stimulant effect of progesterone, especially those with the obesity-hypoventilation syndrome.[37–40] Progesterone increases alveolar ventilation and improves oxygenation, but its effect on frequency of apnea is limited. Major side effects that limit its long-term use include decreased libido, alopecia, and impotence.

The tricyclic antidepressant protriptyline is the most effective and best studied drug for the treatment of obstructive sleep apnea.[41] In a study of 12 patients, Smith and colleagues showed a reduction in apnea frequency and oxygen desaturation during non-REM sleep, in addition to a decrease in REM sleep.[42] Protriptyline produces its beneficial effect by a preferential stimulation of upper airway muscle tone and by decreasing the percentage of time spent in REM sleep, thereby reducing the more severe REM-related apneas. Anticholinergic side effects such as dry mouth, constipation, urinary retention, and impotence are frequent and limit its use.

Oral Appliances

The use of a variety of prosthetic devices is another approach to treatment. The nasopharynx and the posterior tongue are the two anatomic areas of concern. Insertion of a nasopharyngeal airway has been used to prevent upper airway occlusion at the level of the soft palate.[43] The American Sleep Disorders Association recommends that oral appliances may be used in patients with primary snoring, mild obstructive sleep apnea, or in patients with moderate to severe obstructive sleep apnea who refuse or are intolerant of nasal continuous positive airway pressure. The Food and Drug Administration has granted market clearance for 32 oral appliances for snoring but only 14 of these have received market clearance for treatment of snoring and obstructive sleep apnea (Table 63-1).[44] Common side effects of oral appliance therapy include excessive salivation, xerostomia, soft tissue irritations, transient discomfort of the teeth and temporomandibular joint (TMJ), and temporary minor occlusal changes. Uncommon, more serious complications include permanent occlusal changes and significant TMJ discomfort.

Removable anterior repositioning splints have been used somewhat successfully to temporarily advance the mandible while passively bringing the tongue forward with it.[44–46] The optimal amount of forward movement is between 50 and 75% of the patient's maximum protrusive distance. An important design feature of these devices is that the appliance must maintain the mandible in the forward position while the patient is asleep. Bear and Priest used a mandibular anterior repositioning splint to determine whether surgical advancement of the mandible would have any lasting and positive effect on a patient's obstructive sleep apnea.[47]

A tongue-retaining device (TRD) that pulls the tongue forward without moving the mandible forward has also been used successfully in some patients with mild to moderate obstructive sleep apnea.[48,49] The TRD functions by placing the tongue into a cup or bubble positioned between the anterior teeth. Surface adhesion holds the tongue in place and the appliance requires that the patient's jaw remains partially open. One disadvantage of the TRD is that the tongue is not always held forward because surface tension of the tongue in the bubble is lost after a time. The TRD and mandibular anterior repositioning splints both force nasal breathing, which can be difficult for patients with inadequate nasal airways.

Arguably, the most researched oral appliance is the Klearway titratable appliance developed by Alan Lowe, DMD, PhD, at the University of British Columbia, Canada. It features a maxillary and mandibular component connected with an adjustable screw mechanism (Figure 63-3). The components are made of a thermoactive acrylic resin that is slightly soft at body temperatures and very compliant at high temperatures. This property decreases major tooth discomfort and considerably increases retention in those patients who have lost a significant number of teeth. A unique feature of the Klearway appliance is that it permits both lateral (1 to 3 mm) and vertical (1 to 5 mm) jaw movement during sleep which reduces the risk of TMJ and jaw muscle discomfort. This movement also facilitates oral breathing in patients with nasal airway obstruction. The screw mechanism of the appliance allows for an 11 mm anterior movement of the mandible with a total of 44 incremental steps of 0.25 mm. In a study of 38 patients with moderate to severe obstructive sleep apnea by Lowe and colleagues, the Klearway appliance reduced the RDI to less than 15 per hour in 80% of the moderate group and in 61% of the severe group.[50] The Klearway appliance is marketed worldwide by Great Lakes Orthodontic Ltd., Tonawanda, NY, USA.

Another commonly used and effective oral appliance is the Herbst appliance, which is an anterior mandibular positioning device. It consists of two full-coverage clear acrylic components snapped onto the maxillary and mandibular teeth connected with two rod and tube attachments that allow vertical opening, protrusion, limited lateral movement, and no retrusive movement. It is used only at night and advances the mandible 5 to 7 mm or at least 75% of the patient's maximum protrusive distance. A study by Clark and colleagues on 24 patients with mild to severe obstructive sleep apnea patients using the Herbst appliance showed a significant improvement in the RDI after 4 months of appliance use in 58% of the subjects on the post-appliance polysomnogram.[51]

Another disadvantage of oral appliances is the need to wear them nightly. As with any device, compliance has been shown to be a problem with oral appliances. If appliance therapy is successful,

Table 63-1 Food and Drug Administration Approved Oral Appliances for the Treatment of Obstructive Sleep Apnea	
Appliances	*Manufacturer*
Adjustable PM Positioner	Jonathan A. Parker, DDS
Elastic Mandibular Advancement, Triation (EMA-T)	Frantz Design, Inc.
Elastic Mandibular Advancement	Frantz Design, Inc.
Elastomeric Sleep Appliance	Village Park Orthodontics
Equalizer Airway Device	Sleep Renewal Inc.
Herbst	Orthodontics, SUNY at Buffalo
Klearway	Great Lakes Orthodontics, Ltd.
NAPA	Great Lakes Orthodontics, Ltd.
OSAP	Snorefree, Inc.
PM Positioner	Jonathan A. Parker, DDS
Silencer	Silent Knights Ventures, Inc.
Sleep-In Bone Screw System	Influence Inc.
SNOAR Open Airway Appliance	Kent J. Toone, DDS
Thornton Oral Appliance	W. Keith Thornton, DDS

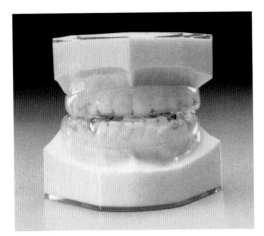
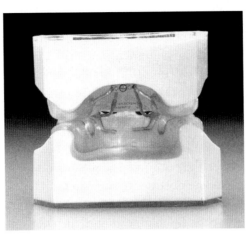

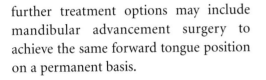

FIGURE **63-3**   *Klearway oral appliance.*

further treatment options may include mandibular advancement surgery to achieve the same forward tongue position on a permanent basis.

Continuous Positive Airway Pressure

Continuous positive airway pressure (CPAP) through the nose has been shown to be quite successful in treating a broad range of obstructive sleep apnea patients and is presently the most successful nonsurgical treatment.[52–54] The nasal CPAP is administered while the patient is asleep by means of a tight-fitting mask that is connected to a compressor. A CPAP of 7 to 15 cm of water acts as a pneumatic splint of the upper airway and prevents passive collapse of soft tissues during respiration. Stimulation of mechanoreceptors of the genioglossus muscle leading to increased airway tone has also been suggested as a mechanism of action. Sullivan and colleagues were the first to report the successful treatment of sleep apnea with nasal CPAP in 1981.[55] In most cases this therapy is effective in eliminating apneas and hypopneas, improving arterial oxygen saturations, reducing or eliminating excessive daytime sleepiness, and eliminating sleep disruption and fragmentation. CPAP may be combined with surgery and weight loss, or it may be used as a sole form of therapy. Although initially recommended for short-term relief of sleep apnea, the use of nasal CPAP for long-term care of patients has increased over the past few years. In recent years bilevel positive airway pressure (Bi-PAP) systems that allow independent regulation of inspiratory and expiratory pressures and the newest modification in CPAP systems, Auto-CPAP, have been used to more effectively treat obstructive sleep apnea and increase tolerance and compliance.[56,57] Auto-CPAP units adjust the CPAP throughout the night rather than delivering one fixed pressure. Optimal CPAP is delivered to the patient adjusting for positional changes, alcohol or sedative effects, sleep–state-dependent changes (REM vs non-REM), and the effects of upper airway infections or congestion. Bi-PAP ($2,500) and Auto-CPAP ($1,600) systems are more expensive than traditional CPAP ($600 to $800) systems.

Despite the uniform success of this therapy, patient compliance remains a problem. Compliance rates at 12 months have been reported as low as 54%.[58] The average nightly use of CPAP is 4.8 hours and the rate of use is usually determined in the first week of use. Overall approximately one-third of patients love CPAP, one-third struggle with CPAP but eventually tolerate it, and one-third hate CPAP and never use it. Patient dissatisfaction results from nasal dryness and congestion, sore throat, dryness of the skin and eyes, claustrophobia, and the inability to tolerate the noise, dis-

comfort, or mask. Careful patient selection and follow-up are essential if nasal CPAP is selected as a treatment modality.

Surgical Treatment

Surgery has been the primary form of therapy for obstructive sleep apnea. To be successful the surgical procedure must either bypass the obstructive area or prevent collapse of the soft tissues in the upper airway at the obstruction. Many patients and surgeons tend to view surgical treatment of obstructive sleep apnea as a quick and permanent cure. However, a clear definition of what constitutes a cure is lacking in the literature. This problem often makes a determination of the efficacy of individual surgical procedures difficult. Only objective data obtained from a postoperative polysomnogram can be accepted as proof of efficacy for surgical procedures. Currently the procedures used in the surgical treatment of obstructive sleep apnea include tracheostomy, nasal surgery, uvulopalatopharyngoplasty, and several orthognathic surgical procedures. Selection of the individual procedure is determined by the severity of the sleep apnea, the presence of a maxillofacial skeletal deficiency, the site of the obstructive segment, and the presence of morbid obesity.

Tracheostomy

Tracheostomy was the first efficacious surgical procedure for treating obstructive sleep apnea, performed by Kuhlo and colleagues in 1969.[59] It is almost 100% curative in relieving the signs and symptoms of obstructive sleep apnea because it bypasses all the potential obstructive sites in the upper airway. After tracheostomy there is a rapid and striking reduction in daytime somnolence and a marked improvement in sleep architecture due to a major reduction in the frequency of arousals. Sinus dysrhythmias, bradycardia, pulmonary hypertension, hypoxemia, and apnea all improve dramatically with the procedure. Tracheostomy clearly is an effective surgical treatment for patients with obstructive apnea.

The disadvantages of a permanent tracheostomy can have a devastating effect on sleep apnea patients. Almost all patients experience psychological depression from the social and medical problems associated with a lifelong tracheostomy. The tracheostomy leaves the patient esthetically disfigured and exposes the patient to common local complications such as bleeding, infection, pain, and granulation tissue formation. Patients are also at increased risk for the more serious complications of tracheal stenosis or erosion into an adjacent blood vessel. Because of these disadvantages and complications, a permanent tracheostomy should be reserved for severe cases of obstructive sleep apnea with significant cardiovascular symptoms. Simmons and colleagues have suggested that tracheostomy should be the primary therapy for all patients who spend substantial time in severe oxygen desaturations below 50% and for those who have life-threatening cardiac dysrhythmias during sleep apnea.[60] Tracheostomy may also be used as an interim treatment until adjunctive procedures to reconstruct the upper airway are completed.

Nasal Surgery

Significant obstruction in the nasal cavity has been shown to cause excessive daytime sleepiness, sleep fragmentation, hypopneas, and periodic breathing during sleep.[61] In most patients with moderate to severe obstructive sleep apnea, nasal obstruction is not the major contributing factor. The obstruction may be due to a deviated nasal septum, nasal polyps, or enlargement of the turbinates. In these patients septoplasty, nasal polypectomy, or turbinectomies are usually helpful only as adjunctive surgical procedures in the treatment of obstructive sleep apnea. Unless the obstruction in the nasal cavity is severe, surgical correction usually will not yield any significant improvement on a repeat polysomnography.

Uvulopalatopharyngoplasty

The oropharynx and soft palate can cause significant airway obstruction during sleep. At least 10% of persons over the age of 40 years snore regularly and significantly. Loud and intermittent snoring is found in almost all patients with obstructive sleep apnea. In many cases habitual snoring is present for many years before sleep apnea is diagnosed. Ikematsu followed a large number of habitual snorers over several years and found that 91% of these patients had decreased oropharyngeal dimensions and longer soft palates and uvulas than normal subjects.[62] He was able to eliminate their snoring by surgically excising the excessive soft tissue in the palatal folds and partially excising the uvula.

With minor modifications, Simmons and colleagues and Fujita and colleagues popularized the uvulopalatopharyngoplasty (UPPP) for the treatment of obstructive sleep apnea.[60,63] The procedure was designed to eliminate oropharyngeal obstruction by performing a tonsillectomy and adenoidectomy, excising the uvula, removing redundant lateral pharyngeal wall mucosa, and resecting 8 to 15 mm along the posterior margin of the soft palate.

The surgical technique of UPPP varies to some degree by patient and surgeon, but the basic goal is to shorten the palate and widen the posterior airway space (Figure 63-4). A mucosal incision is created with electocautery on the anterior surface of the soft palate. The dissection is frequently carried laterally to include the palatine tonsil. The tonsillar bed is coagulated and hemostasis achieved. Palatal muscle is excised and mucosa from the nasopharynx is pulled forward for primary closure. Multiple interrupted resorbable sutures are placed. If the tonsil is removed, the mucosa of the anterior fauces pillar is closed to the posterior fauces pillar. This attempt to remove redundant pharyngeal

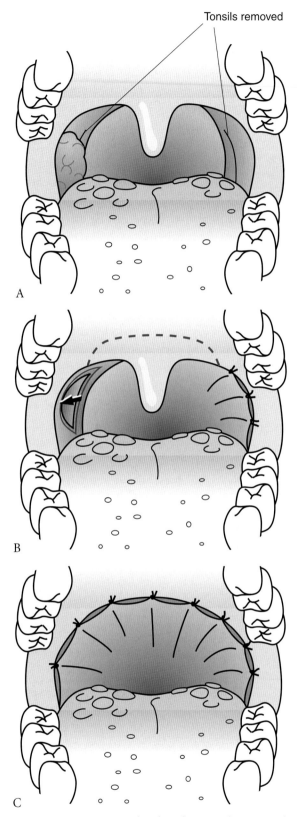

FIGURE 63-4 *A–C, Uvulopalatopharyngoplasty. Tonsils and uvula are removed and the anterior pillar is closed to the posterior pillar. Adapted from Tiner BD, Waite, PD. Surgical and nonsurgical management of obstructive sleep apnea. In: Peterson LJ, Indresano AT, Marciani RD, Roser SM. Principles of oral and maxillofacial surgery. Vol. 3. Philadelphia (PA): J.B. Lippincott Company; 1992. p. 1540.*

tissue and stretch or tighten the posterior pharyngeal wall results in constriction. In addition, frequently by shortening the soft palate, the width of the soft palate is thickened, as demonstrated cephalometrically. Lymphoid tissue from the tonsillar fossa can be removed separately or in conjunction with the uvula (Figure 63-5). The amount of velum to be excised is determined by the location of palatal competence and closure of the nasopharynx. These can be estimated or identified during nasopharyngoscopy. Palatal incompetence can occur but usually is of minimal concern if the patient swallows carefully. Pain with swallowing usually lasts for several weeks.

UPPP results in symptomatic improvement in the patient and eliminates habitual snoring in almost all cases. However, reports show that significant objective improvement on the postoperative polysomnogram ranges only from 41 to 66%.[58,60,64,65] This procedure only eliminates the obstruction at the level of the soft palate and does not address obstructions occurring in the hypopharyngeal and base

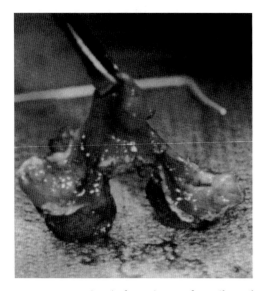

FIGURE 63-5 *Surgical specimen of tonsils and uvula. Reproduced with permission from Tiner BD, Waite, PD. Surgical and nonsurgical management of obstructive sleep apnea. In: Peterson LJ, Indresano AT, Marciani RD, Roser SM. Principles of oral and maxillofacial surgery. Vol. 3. Philadelphia (PA): J.B. Lippincott Company; 1992. p. 1541.*

of tongue areas. Many patients have more than one site of obstruction. If UPPP is performed when the presurgical evaluation demonstrates obstruction localized to the soft palate–tonsil area, then the success rate of the surgical procedure approaches 90% treating obstructive sleep apnea.[23,26]

Complications from UPPP are related to changes in palatal function. Permanent velopharyngeal incompetence occurs in approximately 5% of patients and is more common during the first 2 months postoperatively. Patients experience occasional reflux of liquids into the nose and mild nasal air escape during speech. However, hypernasal speech and changes in the quality of the patient's speech are usually not seen. Simmons and colleagues reported a 5 to 10% rate of minor wound infections that resolved with antibiotics.[64] Palatal stenosis is definitely a risk with this operation and occurs in about 1% of patients. It occurs more frequently with excessive resections of the posterior tonsillar pillars and injudicious use of electrocautery. Postoperative pain after UPPP is significant, and narcotic analgesia should be used with caution to prevent sedation-induced exacerbation of obstructive sleep apnea. Postsurgical deaths have resulted from the combination of pharyngeal edema and narcotic use.

Laser-Assisted Uvulopalatoplasty

In the late 1980s Dr. Yves-Victor Kamami (Paris, France) designed a procedure to reshape and recontour the soft palate under local anesthesia with a CO_2 laser to treat snoring and selected patients with obstructive sleep apnea syndrome.[66] He originally named the procedure "laser resection of the palatopharynx" or LRPP. Initially the procedure was accomplished in four or five sessions spaced at monthly intervals. Over time the procedure evolved into a one-stage technique for most patients. It consisted of two paramedian vertical incisions placed lateral to the uvula extending up toward the junction of the

hard and soft palates for 2 to 3 cm. A second horizontal incision was placed just under the roof of the uvula leaving a small uvula to prevent centripetal scar formation. Over a 5-year period, Kamami treated 63 obstructive sleep apnea patients with this technique. The RDI was reduced by more than 50% in 55 patients that were classified as successful responders. The RDI improved from 41.5 to 16.9 for the average responder, and for the entire group the average RDI improved from 41.3 to 20.3.

In the early 1990s in the United States, Dr. Yosef Krespi modified the procedure and renamed it "laser-assisted uvulopalatoplasty" or LAUP. He initially used the procedure to treat loud habitual snoring. In a study of 280 patients treated in the office under local anesthesia, 84% were cured with an average of 2.7 sessions.[67] Overall results for obstructive sleep apnea patients treated with LAUP are far less encouraging, with an average successful surgical response of 52.2%.[68] Based on these findings the current main indications for LAUP include loud habitual snoring, upper airway resistance syndrome, and mild obstructive sleep apnea (apnea index < 20). All snoring patients who elect to undergo LAUP should be evaluated for obstructive sleep apnea preoperatively and again postoperatively if obstructive sleep apnea was previously diagnosed. If not, then the patient and surgeon may be lulled into a false sense of security by eliminating the snoring without eliminating the undiagnosed obstructive sleep apnea, potentially increasing patient morbidity and mortality.[69]

The most common complication following LAUP is a moderate to severe sore throat. Patients experience pain 8 to 10 days after surgery and reach their peak pain intensity on the fourth or fifth postoperative day. Pain control is achieved with oral analgesics and anesthetic gels. The risk for velopharyngeal insufficiency is low since the procedure is frequently done in stages and the surgeon has the opportunity to evaluate speech and soft palate function after each session. Patients are also at low risk for bleeding and infection. The great majority of patients can eat, drink, and speak almost immediately and can resume full activities the following day.

Orthognathic Surgery Procedures

Various orthognathic surgical procedures have been described for the treatment of obstructive sleep apnea. The majority of patients have airway obstruction at the level of the soft palate and at the base of the tongue (type II obstruction). Orthognathic surgical procedures can change the size of the airway in several regions. Mandibular advancement and genial advancement probably work by changing the position of the mandible and hyoid bone with subsequent effects on the genioglossus and hyoglossus muscles. Obstructive sleep apnea patients with identifiable craniofacial anomalies can clearly benefit from a variety of these procedures.

Mandibular Advancement Total mandibular advancement was the first orthognathic surgical procedure used in the treatment of obstructive sleep apnea. Kuo and colleagues in 1979 and Bear and Priest in 1980 reported complete reversal of sleep apnea symptoms in patients with horizontal mandibular deficiency treated by mandibular advancement.[47,70] More recently Alvarez and colleagues reported the successful treatment of an edentulous patient with sleep apnea by mandibular and genial advancement.[71]

A bilateral sagittal ramus osteotomy is usually the procedure of choice for total mandibular advancement. The amount of advancement is determined preoperatively from the orthognathic surgery database. Adjunctive orthodontic treatment is frequently necessary to obtain the desired occlusion and to eliminate dental compensations that would otherwise limit the amount of advancement. After advancement with the standard surgical technique, the fragments are rigidly fixed with screws or bone

plates. For large advancements of 7 mm or more, long-term stability is enhanced with a 5- to 7-day course of maxillomandibular fixation and skeletal suspension wires. In advancements of 6 mm or less, maxillomandibular fixation is usually not necessary.

The exact reason for how mandibular advancement improves obstructive sleep apnea is not clearly known, but the suspected effect is the pulling of the tongue forward off the pharyngeal wall. This effect is created by anteriorly moving the insertion of the genioglossus and geniohyoid muscles. If this were the only factor, then anterior chin procedures would be equally effective as total mandibular procedures. Variations of geniotomies have been designed to maximally pull the tongue muscles forward.

Genial Advancement A rectangular osteotomy apical to the teeth but maintaining the inferior border of the mandible allows the genial tubercles with their muscular attachments to be maximally advanced with minimal cosmetic change (Figure 63-6). A modified vestibular mucosal incision is made in the anterior mandible. Periosteum is reflected down to the inferior border. An oscillating saw is used to make parallel horizontal cuts that include the genial tubercle. The osteotomy is designed in a shape similar to a drawer so that it can be pulled outward with the genial muscles. The bone must be broad enough cuspid tocuspid to be rotated 90° and set on top of the buccal cortex. The outer cortical and cancellous bone of the rectangle can then be removed and the inner cortex rigidly fixed with bone screws. Any hemorrhage from the cancellous bone should be controlled.

This procedure does not change the esthetic chin or advance the anterior belly of the digastric muscle, which may be helpful in suspending the hyoid. In contrast to this procedure a horizontal sliding geniotomy does advance the genial tubercles and the anterior belly of the digastric muscle.

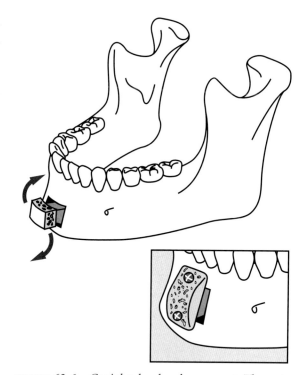

FIGURE **63-6** *Genial tubercle advancement. The outer table of symphysis is removed and the inner table is secured with 2 mm screws. Adapted from Tiner BD, Waite, PD. Surgical and nonsurgical management of obstructive sleep apnea. In: Peterson LJ, Indresano AT, Marciani RD, Roser SM. Principles of oral and maxillofacial surgery. Vol. 3. Philadelphia (PA): J.B. Lippincott Company; 1992. p. 1542.*

Genial Advancement with Hyoid Myotomy and Suspension In 1984 Riley and colleagues described an alternative technique in which an inferior mandibular osteotomy and an associated hyoid myotomy and suspension were used in the treatment of obstructive sleep apnea (Figure 63-7).[72] This technique is similar to a horizontal mandibular osteotomy, which is commonly used for advancement genioplasty. The osteotomy is designed to include the genial tubercle on the inner cortex of the anterior mandible where the genioglossus muscle attaches. Repositioning the anteroinferior segment of the mandible forward with the attached genioglossus muscle theoretically pulls the tongue forward and improves the hypopharyngeal airway. In conjunction with the osteotomy, the body and greater cornu of the hyoid are isolated

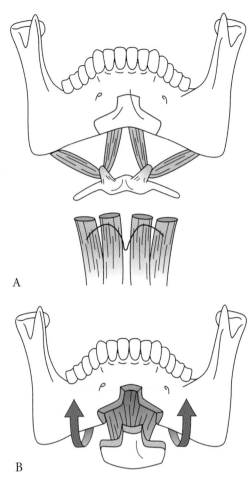

A

B

FIGURE 63-7 *Inferior mandibular osteotomy and hyoid myotomy. A, Omohyoid, sternohyoid, and thyrohyoid muscles released (see Figure 63-8 for more detail on muscular relationships). B, Inferior segment is advanced anteriorly and locked on the anterior mandible. Adapted from Tiner BD, Waite, PD. Surgical and nonsurgical management of obstructive sleep apnea. In: Peterson LJ, Indresano AT, Marciani RD, Roser SM. Principles of oral and maxillofacial surgery. Vol. 3. Philadelphia (PA): J.B. Lippincott Company; 1992. p. 1543.*

through a submental incision. The infrahyoid muscles are transected, taking care to remain on the hyoid bone at all times to avoid injury to the superior laryngeal nerves (see Figure 63-7A). This allows the hyoid bone to be pulled anteriorly and superiorly. Strips of fascia or nonresorbable suture are passed around the body of the hyoid and attached to the intact portion of the anterior mandible to complete the hyoid suspension.

In 1989 Riley and colleagues published a review of 55 patients with obstructive sleep apnea who were treated with inferior mandibular osteotomy and hyoid suspension.[73] Forty-two patients had obstruction at both the oropharynx and hypopharynx and received concomitant UPPP and inferior mandibular osteotomy with hyoid myotomy and suspension. The remaining 6 patients were determined to have obstruction localized to the base of the tongue and underwent the osteotomy and hyoid suspension only. All patients were reevaluated 6 months following surgery by polysomnography. Thirty-seven patients (67%) were considered to be responders to surgery based on the polysomnogram results. Genioglossus advancement ranged from 8 to 18 mm with a mean of 13 mm. All responders to surgery showed significant improvement in their RDI and oxygen desaturation events. Eighteen patients (33%) were considered nonresponders and failed to show significant improvement by polysomnography. The presence of preexisting chronic obstructive pulmonary disease was found to be a determining factor in increasing the risk of failure.

In 1994 Riley and colleagues reported on a new modified technique for hyoid suspension that fixed the hyoid to the thyroid cartilage instead of the anterior margin of the mandible.[74] When this modified technique was performed with inferior mandibular osteotomy, in lieu of the original hyoid suspension technique, the surgical response rate (with or without UPPP) was raised to 79.2%. The 5 nonresponders in this study of 24 patients achieved postoperative RDI values close to levels at which they would have been considered surgical responders.

Long-term follow-up of these patients has shown that the indication for this procedure is limited. Patients with normal pulmonary function, normal skeletal mandibular development, the absence of obesity, and moderate obstructive sleep apnea are candidates for treatment with inferior mandibular osteotomy with hyoid myotomy and suspension.

The most serious reported complication from a hyoid suspension has been severe aspiration in one patient, in which the thyrohyoid membrane was totally sectioned.[28] Other complications have included wound infections, transient sensory disturbances of the mental nerve, and mandibular fracture. An advantage to hyoid suspension is that it circumvents the need for maxillomandibular fixation and does not affect the occlusion.

Maxillomandibular Advancement   Combined advancement of the maxilla and mandible with or without hyoid suspension is the most recent and efficacious surgical procedure for the treatment of obstructive sleep apnea. The surgical technique includes a standard Le Fort I osteotomy in combination with a mandibular sagittal split osteotomy for advancement of the maxilla and mandible. A concomitant inferior mandibular osteotomy with or without hyoid myotomy and suspension, as previously described, is also performed. This surgery may result in a significant facial change, which is most often favorable (Figures 63-8 and 63-9). Several authors have described the use of maxillomandibular advancement (MMA) in treating large series of obstructive sleep apnea patients.[75-80] In a series of 23 patients, Waite and colleagues performed a high sliding horizontal geniotomy without the hyoid myotomy and suspension.[75] All patients were reevaluated by polysomnography at 6 weeks postoperatively. The surgical success with MMA was 65% based on a postsurgical RDI of less than 10. Riley and colleagues reported the largest series of obstructive sleep apnea patients treated with MMA in which 98% (89 of 91) were successfully treated based on a postoperative RDI of less than 20 with at least a 50% reduction in the RDI compared to the preoperative study.[76] It should be noted that 67 of the 91 patients (74%) did not receive phase 1 therapy based on their two-phase protocol for reconstruction of the upper

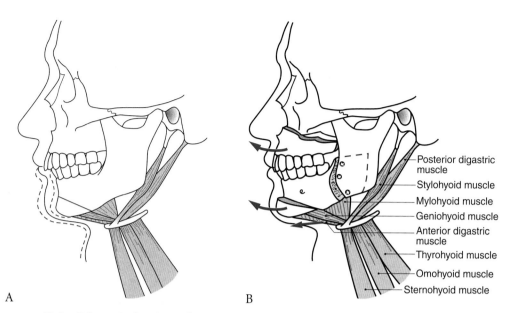

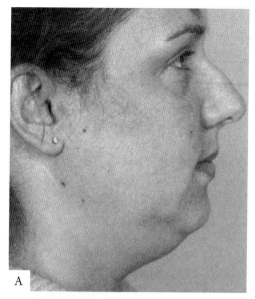

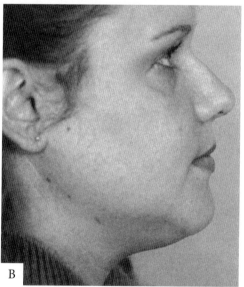

FIGURE **63-8** *Schematic drawings of preoperative (A) and postoperative (B) two-jaw advancement, genial advancement, and hyoid suspension. Adapted from Tiner BD, Waite, PD. Surgical and nonsurgical management of obstructive sleep apnea. In: Peterson LJ, Indresano AT, Marciani RD, Roser SM. Principles of oral and maxillofacial surgery. Vol. 3. Philadelphia (PA): J.B. Lippincott Company; 1992. p. 1544.*

airway. Despite this, the MMA was labeled a phase 2 procedure. In 1997, Hochban and colleagues reported a 98% success rate on 38 obstructive sleep apnea patients consecutively treated with a 10 mm MMA as the primary surgery, without any adjunctive procedures.[77] Their criteria for success were based on the more rigid postoperative RDI of less than 10. Patient selection for MMA was based on subjective symptoms of excessive daytime sleepiness, an RDI of greater than 20, and specific craniofacial characteristics determined cephalometrically. Only 2 patients who were morbidly obese were treated surgically. Based on their excellent results the authors concluded that a stepwise algorithm of staged surgical procedures was not justified. In a series of 50 obstructive sleep apnea patients consecutively treated with MMA, Prinsell reported a 100% success rate based on a postoperative RDI of less than 15, an apnea index (AI) of less than 5, or a reduction in the RDI and AI of greater than 60%.[78] In this series occasional concomitant nonpharyngeal procedures and an anterior interior mandibular osteotomy were accomplished with the MMA as a sin-

gle-stage operation. In 1999 Lee and colleagues proposed a three-stage protocol for the surgical treatment of obstructive sleep apnea patients.[79] All 35 patients in their series had type II obstruction with collapse at the oropharyngeal and hypopharyngeal areas. Stage 1 reconstruction consisted of a UPPP and inferior sagittal osteotomy with genioglossus muscle advancement, or an anterior mandibular osteotomy. If stage 1 was unsuccessful, then patients advanced to stage 2, which consisted of MMA with rigid fixation. A hyoid myotomy and suspension was the sole component of stage 3 reconstruction. Based on postoperative polysomnography, 69% (24 of 35) were considered surgical respondents based on an RDI of less than 20. Of the 11 stage 1 failures, 3 elected to proceed to stage 2 reconstruction with MMA. All patients who underwent MMA had a postoperative RDI of less than 10, indicating a 100% response rate. No patient required stage 3 reconstruction. Bettega and colleagues treated 51 consecutive obstructive sleep apnea patients according to the Stanford two-step surgical procedure.[80] Forty-four patients had phase 1 surgery with a success

FIGURE **63-9** *Preoperative (A) and postoperative (B) photographs of a patient with obstructive sleep apnea syndrome who underwent two-jaw surgery with a genial advancement. Reproduced with permission from Tiner BD, Waite, PD. Surgical and nonsurgical management of obstructive sleep apnea. In: Peterson LJ, Indresano AT, Marciani RD, Roser SM. Principles of oral and maxillofacial surgery. Vol. 3. Philadelphia (PA): J.B. Lippincott Company; 1992. p. 1545.*

rate of 22.7% (10 of 44). Twenty patients underwent MMA as part of phase 2 in the protocol. Of these, 75% (15 of 20) were considered to be surgical responders based on a postoperative RDI of less than 15 and at least a 50% reduction in the RDI. Of the 5 failures, 3 had postoperative RDIs of less than 20.

The PAS consistently increases with maxillomandibular advancement. However, there is no direct relationship between the gain in PAS and the remission of sleep apnea. MMA is effective for patients who have obstruction at the base of the tongue. This surgical treatment is the most efficacious procedure for expanding the pharyngeal airway and improving or eliminating obstructive sleep apnea. It remains the best current alternative to tracheostomy.[81] Indications for this procedure include severe mandibular deficiency (SNB < 74°), morbid obesity, severe obstructive sleep apnea (RDI > 50, oxygen desaturations < 70%), hypopharyngeal narrowing, and failure of other forms of treatment.[82] The success rate of MMA appears to increase when adjunctive procedures such as UPPP, partial glossectomy, septoplasty, or turbinectomies are included in the treatment plan. This lends support to the theory that most obstructive sleep apnea patients have multiple levels of obstruction.

Adjunctive orthodontic therapy is usually indicated in patients selected for MMA. Presurgical orthodontics improves the postoperative occlusion and eliminates preexisting dental compensations that would otherwise limit the amount of advancement. Maximum advancement of the facial skeleton and maintenance of a functional occlusion and acceptable esthetics are the goals of surgical-orthodontic correction.

The osteotomies are rigidly fixed with miniplates and bicortical screws (Figure 63-10). With large advancements (> 7 mm), skeleton suspension wires and a short course of maxillomandibular fixation (1 wk) can be used to reduce surgical relapse. Potential complications of MMA include surgical relapse, nonunion, bleeding, malocclusion, infection, unfavorable changes in facial appearance, and permanent or temporary sensory disturbances of the inferior alveolar and infraorbital nerves.

The long-term skeletal stability of MMA has been shown to be quite good.

Louis and colleagues showed a mean relapse of 0.9 ± 1.8 mm among 20 maxillary advancement patients who underwent MMA for obstructive sleep apnea.[83] The mean follow-up period was 18.5 months (range 6 to 29 mo). When the patients were divided into three groups reflecting small (6 mm or less), medium (7 to 9 mm), and large (10 mm or more) advancements, there was no statistical difference in the measured relapse among the groups. Rigid fixation was achieved with four miniplates and no bone grafts were used in any of the maxillary advancements. Nimkarn and colleagues reported on 19 obstructive sleep apnea patients who underwent MMA with simultaneous genioplasty and found relatively stable long-term (> 12 mo) surgical stability of the maxilla and mandible.[84] Maxillary and mandibular advancement was stable over the long term in both the vertical and horizontal planes. With the exception of gonion in the vertical plane, there was no statistically significant correlation between the amount of surgical advancement and the amount of postsurgical instability.

Mandibular Setbacks   In a small number of patients, a mandibular setback procedure can be the initiating factor in the development of obstructive sleep apnea. Riley and associates reported on two women who developed obstructive sleep apnea syndrome after mandibular osteotomies for correction of Class III malocclusion and skeletal prognathism.[85] Neither patient had any symptoms of sleep apnea prior to surgery. Postoperatively both patients began to snore loudly. Evaluation by polysomnography confirmed the presence of obstructive sleep apnea syndrome. A comparative examination of the preoperative and postoperative lateral cephalograms of each patient showed a more inferiorly positioned hyoid bone and a narrowing of the pharyngeal airway as a result of the mandibular setback procedure.

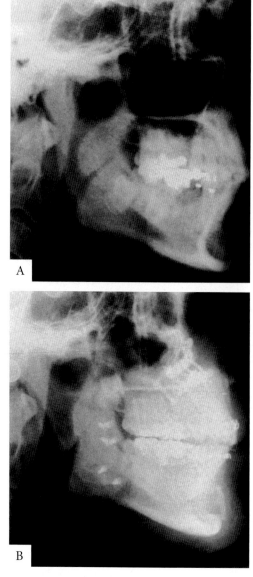

FIGURE **63-10**   *Preoperative (A) and postoperative (B) radiographs of a two-jaw surgery and genial tubercle advancement for sleep apnea. Reproduced with permission from Tiner BD, Waite, PD. Surgical and nonsurgical management of obstructive sleep apnea. In: Peterson LJ, Indresano AT, Marciani RD, Roser SM. Principles of oral and maxillofacial surgery. Vol. 3. Philadelphia (PA): J.B. Lippincott Company; 1992. p. 1546.*

In an attempt to identify those patients potentially at risk for obstructive sleep apnea, all patients who are planned for mandibular setback procedures should be questioned preoperatively and postoperatively about the presence or absence of snoring, excessive daytime sleepiness, or observed apneas during sleep. Although the vast majority of patients who undergo

Table 63-2 Results of Maxillomandibular Advancement for Obstructive Sleep Apnea

Results	RDI	Desaturation*	No. of Patients	Percent of Total
Excellent	≤ 10	0	20	28.2
Good	≤ 10	≤ 20	26	36.6
Satisfactory	≤ 10	> 20	15	21.1
Poor	> 20	> 20	10	14.1

Maxillomandibular advancement surgery results for 71 obstructive sleep apnea syndrome patients classified by polysomnography.
RDI = respiratory disturbance index.
*Number of oxygen desaturations below 90%.

mandibular setbacks are able to adapt to the changes in the skeletal and muscular apparatus, there is a subset of patients who may be at risk for developing overt signs of obstructive sleep apnea following mandibular setbacks.

Summary

Because the obstructive sleep apnea syndrome is a complex disorder, the type of treatment selected should be tailored to the individual patient based on the relative risks and benefits of the therapy and the severity of the disease. Although a subset of the patients who present with obstructive sleep apnea have an identifiable craniofacial anomaly, care must be used in choosing a simple mechanistic therapy. The success of the chosen therapy should be evaluated both subjectively and objectively. There is no clear agreement on what constitutes a cure of sleep apnea. Most authors use the RDI in assessing severity of disease and success of treatment. However, all agree that the potentially significant physiologic consequences that can be life threatening result from hypoxemia. In some cases patients after treatment have no oxygen desaturations below 90%, but in terms of RDI they are considered not cured and are deemed treatment failures.

A more reasonable approach would be to define the concept of success in terms of excellent, good, fair, and poor and to avoid using the term "cured" in assessing treatment outcomes. These terms could be quantitatively approached assigning low-est oxygen desaturation and RDI parameters to each one. In Table 63-2 the results of 71 patients treated by maxillomandibular advancement are assessed by these criteria. In managing patients with severe sleep apnea, a "cure" is seldom achieved with a single surgical or medical treatment (tracheostomies excluded). However, maxillomandibular advancement may significantly improve a patient to the point that nonsurgical therapies are more efficacious, if needed at all.

References

1. Schmidt HS. Disorders of sleep and arousal. In: Gregory I, Smeltzer DJ, editors. Psychiatry essentials of clinical practice. Boston (MA): Little, Brown & Co.; 1983. p. 343.
2. Association of Sleep Disorders Center. Diagnostic classification of sleep and arousal disorders. 1st ed. Prepared by the Sleep Disorders Classification Committee. Sleep 1979;2:1.
3. Berger H. Uber das elektrenkephalogramm des menschen. Arch Psychiatr Nervenkr 1929;87:527.
4. Loomis AL, Harvey EN, Hobart GA. Potential rhythms of the cerebral cortex during sleep. Science 1935;81:597.
5. Loomis AL, Harvey EN, Hobart GA. Further observations on the potential rhythms of the cerebral cortex during sleep. Science 1935;82:199.
6. Aserinsky E, Kleitman N. Regularly occurring periods of eye motility and concomitant phenomena during sleep. Science 1953;118:273.
7. Freemon FR. Sleep research: a critical review. Springfield (IL): Charles C. Thomas; 1972.
8. Waldhorn RE. Sleep apnea syndrome. Am Fam Physician 1985;32:149.
9. National Commission on Sleep Disorders Research. Wake up America: a national sleep alert. Washington (DC): Government Printing Office; 1993.
10. Sher AE. Treating obstructive sleep apnea syndrome: a complex task [editorial]. West J Med 1995;162:170–2.
11. Bornstein SK. Respiration during sleep: polysomnography. In: Guilleminault C, editor. Sleep and waking disorders: indications and techniques. Menlo Park (CA): Addison-Wesley; 1982. p. 183.
12. Baker TL. Introduction to sleep and sleep disorders. Med Clin North Am 1985;69:1123.
13. Roth B. Narcolepsy and hypersomnia. Basel: S. Karger AG; 1980.
14. Burwell CS, Rubin ED, Whaley RD, et al. Extreme obesity associated with alveolar hypoventilation: a pickwickian syndrome. Am J Med 1956;21:811.
15. Gastaut H, Tassinari CA, Duron B. Polygraphic study of the episodic diurnal and nocturnal (hypnic and respiratory) manifestations of the pickwick syndrome. Brain Res 1966;2:167.
16. Partinen M, Quera-Salva MA, Jamieson A. Obstructive sleep apnea and cephalometric roentgenograms: the role of anatomic upper airway abnormalities in the definition of abnormal breathing during sleep. Chest 1988;93:1199–205.
17. Tsuchiya M, Lowe AA, Pae EK, Fleetham JA. Obstructive sleep apnea subtypes by cluster analysis. Am J Orthod Dentofacial Orthop 1992;101:533–42.
18. Bacon WH, Krieger J, Turlot J-C, Stierle JL. Craniofacial characteristics in patients with obstructive sleep apnea syndrome. Cleft Palate J 1988;25:374.
19. Lyberg T, Kogstad O, Ojupesland G. Cephalometric analysis in patients with obstructive sleep apnea syndrome. J Laryngol Otol 1989;103:287.
20. Lowe AA, Santamaria JD, Fleetham JA, Price C. Facial morphology and obstructive sleep apnea. Am J Orthod 1986;90:484.
21. Rivlin J, Hofstein V, Kalbfleisch J, et al. Upper airway morphology in patients with idiopathic obstructive sleep apnea. Am Rev Respir Dis 1984;129:355.
22. Riley R, Guilleminault C, Herran J, Powell N. Cephalometric analyses and flow-volume loops in obstructive sleep apnea patients. Sleep 1983;6:303.
23. Riley R, Guilleminault C, Powell N, Simmons FB. Palatopharyngoplasty failure, cephalometric roentgenograms, and obstructive sleep apnea. Otolaryngol Head Neck Surg 1985;93:240.
24. Lowe AA, Gionhaku N, Takeuchi K, Fleetham JA. Three-dimensional CT reconstruction

of tongue and airway in adult subjects with obstructive sleep apnea. Am J Orthod Dentofacial Orthop 1986;90:364.

25. Haponik EF, Smith PL, Bohlman ME, et al. Computerized tomography in obstructive sleep apnea. Am Rev Respir Dis 1983; 127:221.

26. Riley RW, Powell N, Guilleminault C. Current surgical concepts for treating obstructive sleep apnea syndrome. J Oral Maxillofac Surg 1987;45:149.

27. Waite RD, Villos G. Surgical changes of posterior airway spaces in obstructive sleep apnea. Oral Maxillofac Surg Clin North Am 2002;August.

28. Riley RW, Powell NB, Guilleminault C. Maxillary, mandibular, and hyoid advancement for treatment of obstructive sleep apnea: a review of 40 patients. J Oral Maxillofac Surg 1990;48:20.

29. Wiggins RV, Schmidt-Nowara WW. Treatment of the obstructive sleep apnea syndrome. West J Med 1987;147:561.

30. Smith PL, Gold AR, Meyers DA. Weight Loss in mild to moderately obese patients with obstructive sleep apnea. Ann Intern Med 1985;103:850.

31. Riley RW, Powell NB, Guilleminault C, Nino-Mucia G. Maxillary, mandibular, hyoid advancement: an alternative to tracheostomy in obstructive sleep apnea syndrome. Otolaryngol Head Neck Surg 1986;94:584.

32. Motta J, Guilleminault C. Effects of oxygen administration in sleep-induced apneas. In: Guilleminault C, Dement WC, editors. Sleep apnea syndrome. New York (NY): Alan R. Liss; 1978. p. 137.

33. Martin RJ, Sanders MH, Gray BA, et al. Acute and long-term ventilatory effects of hyperoxia in the adult sleep apnea syndrome. Am Rev Respir Dis 1982;125:175.

34. Smith PL, Haponik EF, Bleecker ER. The effects of oxygen in patients with sleep apnea. Am Rev Respir Dis 1984;130:958.

35. White DP, Zwillich CW, Pickett CK, et al. Central sleep apnea: improvement with acetazolamide therapy. Arch Intern Med 1982;142:1816.

36. Sharp JT, Druz WS, D'Souza V, et al. Effect of metabolic acidosis upon sleep apnea. Chest 1985;87:619.

37. Lyons HA, Huang CT. Therapeutic use of progesterone in alveolar hypoventilation associated with obesity. Am J Med 1968;44:881.

38. Sutton FD, Zwillich CW, Creagh CE, et al. Progesterone for outpatient treatment of pickwickian syndrome. Ann Intern Med 1975;83:476.

39. Orr WC, Imes MK, Martin RJ. Progesterone

40. Strohl KP, Hensley MJ, Saunders NA, et al. Progesterone administration and progressive sleep apneas. JAMA 1981;245:1230.

41. Brownell LG, West P, Sweatman P, et al. Protriptyline in obstructive sleep apnea: a double-blind trial. N Engl J Med 1982;307:1037.

42. Smith PL, Haponik EF, Allen RP, et al. The effects of protriptyline in sleep-disordered breathing. Am Rev Respir Dis 1983;127:8.

43. Afzelius LE, Elmquist D, Hougaard K, et al. Sleep apnea syndrome: an alternative to tracheostomy. Laryngoscope 1981;91:285.

44. Lowe AA. Oral appliances for sleep breathing disorders. In: Kryger M, Roth T, Dement W, editors. Principles and practice of sleep medicine. 3rd ed. Philadelphia (PA): W.B. Saunders Co.; 2000. p. 929–31.

45. Clark GT. Management of obstructive sleep apnea with dental appliances. Calif Dent Assoc J 1988;16:26.

46. Soll BA, George PT. Treatment of obstructive sleep apnea with a nocturnal airway-patency appliance. New Engl J Med 1985; 313:386.

47. Bear SE, Priest JH. Sleep apnea syndrome: correction with surgical advancement of the mandible. J Oral Surg 1980;38:543.

48. Cartwright RD, Samelson CF. The effects of a nonsurgical treatment for obstructive sleep apnea: the tongue-retaining device. JAMA 1982;248:705.

49. Clark GT, Nakano M. Dental appliances for the treatment of obstructive sleep apnea. J Am Dent Assoc 1989;118:611.

50. Lowe AA, Sjoholm CF, Ryan JA, et al. Treatment, airway and compliance effects of a titratable oral appliance. Sleep 2000;23:172–8.

51. Clark GT, Arand D, Chung E, Tong D. Effect of anterior mandibular positioning on obstructive sleep apnea. Am Rev Respir Dis 1993;147:624–9.

52. Sullivan CE, Issa FG, Berthon-Jones M, et al. Home treatment of obstructive sleep apnea with continuous positive airway pressure applied through a nose-mask. Bull Eur Physiopathol Respir 1984;20:49.

53. Issa FG, Sullivan CE. The immediate effects of continuous positive airway pressure treatment on sleep pattern in patients with obstructive sleep apnea syndrome. Electroencephalogr Clin Neurophysiol 1986;63:10.

54. Klein M, Reynolds LG. Relief of sleep-related oropharyngeal airway obstruction by continuous insufflation of the pharynx. Lancet 1986;1:935.

55. Sullivan CE, Issa FG, Berthon-Jones M, et al. Reversal of obstructive sleep apnea by continuous positive airway pressure applied through the nares. Lancet 1981;1:862.

56. Laursen SB, Dreijer B, Hemmingsen C, Jacobsen E. Bi-level positive airway pressure treatment of obstructive sleep apnea syndrome. Respiration 1998;65:114–9.

57. Meurice J, Marc I, Series F. Efficacy of auto-CPAP in the treatment of obstructive sleep apnea/hypopnea syndrome. Am J Respir Crit Care Med 1996;153:794–8.

58. Katsantonis GP, Schweitzer PK, Branham GH, et al. Management of obstructive sleep apnea: comparison of various treatment modalities. Laryngoscope 1988;98:304.

59. Kuhlo W, Doll E, Franck MD. Erfolgreiche behandlung eines pickwick-syndroms ddurch eine dauertrachealkanuele. Dtsch Med Wochenschr 1969;94:1286.

60. Simmons FB, Guilleminault C, Silvestri R. Snoring, and some obstructive sleep apnea, can be cured by oropharyngeal surgery. Arch Otolaryngol 1983;109:503.

61. Heimer D, Scharf S, Lieberman A, et al. Sleep apnea syndrome treated by repair of deviated nasal septum. Chest 1983;84:184.

62. Ikematsu T. Study of snoring, 4th report: therapy. J Jap Otorhinolaryngol 1964;64:434.

63. Fujita S, Conway W, Zorick F, et al. Surgical correction of anatomic abnormalities in obstructive sleep apnea syndrome: uvulopalatopharyngoplasty. Otolaryngol Head Neck Surg 1981;89:923.

64. Simmons FB, Guilleminault C, Miles LE. The palataopharyngoplasty operation for snoring and sleep apnea: an interim report. Otolaryngol Head Neck Surg 1984;92:375.

65. Guilleminault C, Hayes B, Smith L, et al. Palatopharyngoplasty in obstructive sleep apnea syndrome. Bull Eur Physiopathol Res 1983;19:595.

66. Kamami YV. Outpatient treatment of sleep apnea syndrome with CO_2 laser: laser-assisted UPPP. J Otolaryngol 1994;23:395–8.

67. Krespi YP, Pearlman SJ, Keidar A. Laser-assisted uvula-palatoplasty for snoring. J Otolaryngol 1994;23: 328–34.

68. Terris DJ, Wang MZ. Laser-assisted uvulopalatoplasty in mild obstructive sleep apnea. Arch Otolaryngol Head Neck Surg 1998;124:718–20.

69. Sher AE. Update on upper airway surgery for obstructive sleep apnea. Curr Opin Pulm Med 1995;1:504–11.

70. Kuo PC, West RA, Bloomquist DS, et al. The effect of mandibular osteotomy in three patients with hypersomnia sleep apnea. Oral Surg 1979;48:385.

71. Alvarez CM, Lessin ME, Gross PD. Mandibular advancement combined with horizontal

advancement genioplasty for the treatment of obstructive sleep apnea in an edentulous patient. Oral Surg 1987;64:402.

72. Riley R, Guilleminault C, Powell N, et al. Mandibular osteotomy and hyoid bone advancement for obstructive sleep apnea: a case report. Sleep 1984;7:79.

73. Riley RW, Powell NB, Guilleminault C. Inferior mandibular osteotomy and hyoid myotomy suspension for obstructive sleep apnea: a review of 55 patients. J Oral Maxillofac Surg 1989;47:159.

74. Riley RW, Powell NB, Guilleminault C. Obstructive sleep apnea and the hyoid: a revised surgical procedure. Otolaryngol Head Neck Surg 1994;111:717–21.

75. Waite PD, Wooten V, Lachner J, et al. Maxillomandibular advancement surgery in 23 patients with obstructive sleep apnea syndrome. J Oral Maxillofac Surg 1989; 47:1256.

76. Riley RW, Powell NB, Guilleminault C. Obstructive sleep apnea syndrome: a review of 306 consecutively treated surgical patients. Otolaryngol Head Neck Surg 1993;108:117–25.

77. Hochban W, Conradt R, Brandenburg U, et al. Surgical maxillofacial treatment of obstructive sleep apnea. Plast Reconstr Surg 1997;99:619–26.

78. Prinsell JR. Maxillomandibular advancement surgery in a site-specific treatment approach for obstructive sleep apnea in 50 consecutive patients. Chest 1999;116:1519–29.

79. Lee NR, Givens CD, Wilson J, Robins RB. Staged surgical treatment of obstructive sleep apnea syndrome: a review of 35 patients. J Oral Maxillofac Surg 1999; 57:382–5.

80. Bettega G, Pepin JL, Veale D, et al. Obstructive sleep apnea syndrome fifty-one consecutive patients treated by maxillofacial surgery. Am J Respir Crit Care Med 2000;162:641–9.

81. Riley RW, Powell NB, Guilleminault C. Obstructive sleep apnea syndrome: a surgical protocol for dynamic upper airway reconstruction. J Oral Maxillofac Surg 1993;51:742–7.

82. Prinsell JR. Maxillomandibular advancement surgery for obstructive sleep apnea syndrome. J Am Dent Assoc 2002;133:1489–97.

83. Louis PJ, Waite PD, Austin RB. Long-term skeletal stability after rigid fixation of Lefort I osteotomies with advancements. Int J Oral Maxillofac Surg 1993;22: 82–6.

84. Nimkarn Y, Miles PG, Waite PD. Maxillomandibular advancement surgery in obstructive sleep apnea syndrome patients: long-term surgical stability. J Oral Maxillofac Surg 1995;53:1414–8.

85. Riley RW, Powell NB, Guilleminault C, Ware W. Obstructive sleep apnea syndrome following surgery for mandibular prognathism. J Oral Maxillofac Surg 1987;45:450–2.

Part 9

FACIAL ESTHETIC SURGERY

CHAPTER 64

Blepharoplasty

Heidi L. Jarecki, MD
Mark J. Lucarelli, MD
Bradley N. Lemke, MD

Current blepharoplasty techniques were at least two thousand years in the making. Reports from as early as AD 25 to 35, such as *De Re Medica* by Roman encyclopedist and philosopher Aulus Cornelius, demonstrated appreciation of upper eyelid skin excision in the treatment of upper eyelid disorders.[1] Early descriptions of surgery involving eyelid reconstruction by Carl Ferdinand von Graefe, often regarded as the founder of modern plastic surgery, in 1818, and Johann Karl George Fricke, a student of von Graefe's, in 1829, represent the first reported uses of the term blepharoplasty.[1,2] A.W. Sichel first accurately described "herniated orbital fat" in 1844.[1] Sidney Fox originated the term dermachalasis in 1952 to describe age-associated excess in eyelid skin.[2]

Cosmetic surgery was not embraced until the early twentieth century when Charles Conrad Miller penned the first book dedicated to cosmetic surgery in 1907 entitled *Cosmetic Surgery: The Correction of Featural Imperfections.*[1] Shortly thereafter Frederick Kolle published a text on plastic and cosmetic surgery in which he detailed the value of preoperative eyelid skin marking to determine the proper amount to excise during surgery.[2] The value of preoperative and postoperative photography was introduced in 1926 by Parisian A. Suzanne Noël, one of the first female pioneers in cosmetic surgery.[2] These landmark contributions spawned current blepharoplasty techniques, which continue to be further refined and optimized to achieve superior functional and cosmetic results.

Blepharoplasty is frequently performed either as an adjunctive procedure or as a freestanding operation. A 2002 American Academy of Cosmetic Surgery (AACS) survey reported 27,503 blepharoplasty surgeries performed by AACS members, making blepharoplasty the tenth most frequently performed cosmetic procedure in the United States (K. Rybarczyk, personal communication, January 2003). Common indications for blepharoplasty are dermatochalasis, blepharochalasis, orbital septum weakness with resultant fat pad herniation, hypertrophic orbicularis oculi muscle, eyelid laxity with malposition, and other adnexal abnormalities (ie, herniated lacrimal gland, varicose veins, eyelid skin lesions). Dermatochalasis is simply an excess of eyelid skin, often the result of age- or ultraviolet (UV)-associated decreases in collagen and changes in elasticity and composition of the dermis and epidermis.[3] Recurrent angioedema of the eyelid results in characteristic laxity, fullness, and episodic edema known as blepharochalasis. Acquired blepharoptosis indicates a drooping eyelid that usually results from disinsertion of the aponeurotic insertion of the levator palpebrae superioris into the upper eyelid. Blepharoptosis may be present in the setting of dermatochalasis or blepharochalasis. Orbital septal weakness is evident when "bulges," which represent herniation of orbital fat, are present in the eyelids. A hypertrophic orbicularis oculi muscle presents as a horizontal prominence of the lower eyelid immediately beneath the palpebral margin. Eyelid laxity may manifest as ectropion, canthal angle alterations, and epiphora.

The ensuing chapter is intended as a survey of important information for the blepharoplasty surgeon to consider. On completion of the chapter the surgeon should understand pertinent anatomy, be able to identify good blepharoplasty candidates, be capable of developing a surgical plan, and understand the major complications and how to avoid them. This information should serve as a springboard to direct the surgeon in routes of appropriate inquiry.

Anatomy

A thorough understanding of the topography of the upper two-thirds of the face is requisite for successful eyelid surgery. Eyelids should not be viewed in isolation but rather in context of the relationship to the eyebrow above and midface below.

Forehead and Eyebrow

Understanding the normal or idealized brow position is important during evaluation for blepharoplasty.[4,5] In general men tend to have lower flatter brows at the level of the superior orbital rim. The typical female brow rests 1 cm above the superior orbital rim and peaks between the lateral corneal limbus and lateral commissure, creating a higher and gently arched appearance. Figures 64-1 and 64-2 demonstrate the typical position of the female and male brow, respectively, in youth. Women frequently alter eyebrow position and shape by epilating eyebrow hair so as to approximate the more idealized arched brow.

The eyebrow provides vertical support to the upper eyelid, contributing to the architecture of the eyelid. Eyebrow position is significantly influenced by the elevators and depressors of the brow as well as underlying connective tissue attachments. The frontalis muscle, which originates within the galea aponeurotica, is the main elevator of the eyebrow. The corrugator supercilii, depressor supercilii, procerus, and orbicularis oculi depress the medial brow, whereas the orbicularis muscle is the main lateral brow depressor. Corrugator contraction compresses the medial eyebrows toward the midline with slight depression, forming vertical or oblique

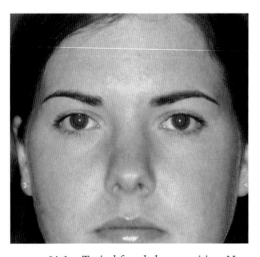

FIGURE **64-1** *Typical female brow position. Note the relationship of the brow relative to the superior orbital rim.*

glabellar furrows. Contraction of the procerus depresses the glabella, creating horizontal rhytids across the dorsum of the nose. Depressor supercilii contraction causes medial eyebrow depression and formation of oblique glabellar furrows. At its insertion point into the eyebrow the frontalis muscle interdigitates with the orbicularis oculi muscle.

Beneath the frontalis lies the eyebrow fat pad, a structure composed of loose fibrous septae with fat-filled interseptate spaces. The eyebrow fat pad is continuous inferiorly with the filmy areolar posterior orbicularis fascia on the undersurface of the orbicularis muscle.[6] On the underside of the eyebrow fat pad, dense connective tissue attachments fasten the superficial muscle plane to the supraorbital ridge, thereby supporting the medial one-half to two-thirds of the eyebrow.[6] Similar attachments for the lateral third of the brow are lacking, thus explaining the preferential ptosis of the temporal brow with aging.[6] In addition the elevating frontalis muscle does not extend to the lateral-most portion of the eyebrow, further contributing to temporal brow ptosis.

The eyebrow provides vertical support to the anterior upper eyelid structures below, therefore ptosis of the eyebrow increases the amount of apparent upper eyelid tissue. Failure to appreciate the contribution of eyebrow ptosis to upper eyelid dermatochalasis may result in excessive eyelid skin removal, further exacerbation of inferior brow displacement, and an inability to close the eyelids. With mild temporal brow ptosis as the only brow position abnormality, more eyelid skin can be removed laterally during blepharoplasty to provide a satisfactory result. With more severe eyebrow and forehead ptosis, consideration of eyebrow and forehead lifting is important.

Midface

Comprising the area from the inferior orbital rim to the mouth, the midface pos-

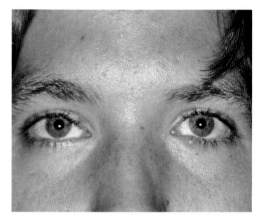

FIGURE **64-2** *Typical male brow position. Note that relative to the female brow the male brow position is lower and flatter.*

sesses structures and landmarks important to the planning of a successful lower lid blepharoplasty. Nasojugal and malar folds separate the thin lower eyelid skin from the thicker skin of the cheek. The superficial musculoaponeurotic system (SMAS) is a fibrous fascial network interconnecting the muscles of facial expression, which acts as a force distributor of facial muscle contractions to the skin to allow for facial expression.[7] The SMAS divides the subcutaneous fat into two layers and possesses fibrous septae connecting to the dermis. The orbitomalar and zygomatic ligaments provide connections between the periosteum and dermis.[8,9]

In youth the eyelid cheek contour is a smooth single convexity from the tarsus inferiorly to the cheek. With age numerous soft tissue and skeletal changes occur in the eyelid and midface. The orbital septum weakens permitting orbital fat prolapse, orbital rim exposure, and a prominence of the cheek. Inferolateral aging-associated descent of the orbicularis oculi muscle can also disrupt the eyelid cheek contour.[10] Descent of the malar fat pad contributes substantially to midfacial ptosis.[11,12] Anatomic studies demonstrate attenuation or abnormal inferior displacement of the subcutaneous insertions of the orbitomalar, masseteric cutaneous, and zygomatic ligaments in the setting of midfacial ptosis.[12,13] Important changes of the maxilla, as described by Pessa and colleagues, also contribute to midfacial aging.[14,15]

Ocular Adnexa

The eyelid margin is traditionally divided into anterior and posterior lamellae. The anterior lamella is composed of the skin, orbicularis oculi muscle, muscle of Riolan, and glands of Zeis and Moll, whereas the posterior lamella is composed of the palpebral conjunctiva, tarsal plates, and associated meibomian glands. A cross-section of the upper and lower eyelid structures demonstrates the composition of the anterior and posterior lamellae (Figure 64-3). The anterior and posterior lamellae are divided by the orbital septum, a structure occasionally referred to as the middle lamella.

Eyelid Skin *Thickness* Eyelid skin possesses a minimal subcutaneous fibroadipose layer and an attenuated dermis, contributing to its status as the thinnest skin in the body. Subcutaneous fat is completely absent in the pretarsal area. An abrupt transition to thicker skin with a correspondingly more dense fibroadipose layer is encountered near the orbital rim. Care must be taken to minimize surgical incisions laterally beyond the thin eyelid skin as scar appearance may markedly differ. The eyelid skin of Asians tends to be slightly thicker than that of Caucasians primarily due to a thicker dermis and subcutaneous fat.[16]

Aging Skin Changes Aging skin changes, such as pigmentary aberrations (dyschromia) and wrinkling (rhytids), result from a combination of UV-induced photodamage, mechanical forces from gravity, and facial muscle contraction and altered chemical environment.[3] Decreases in the synthesis of Type I collagen have been demonstrated in aged human eyelid skin.[17]

Eyelid Topography *Fissure Heights, Upper Eyelid Crease* The adult vertical interpalpebral fissure measures 9 to 12 mm,

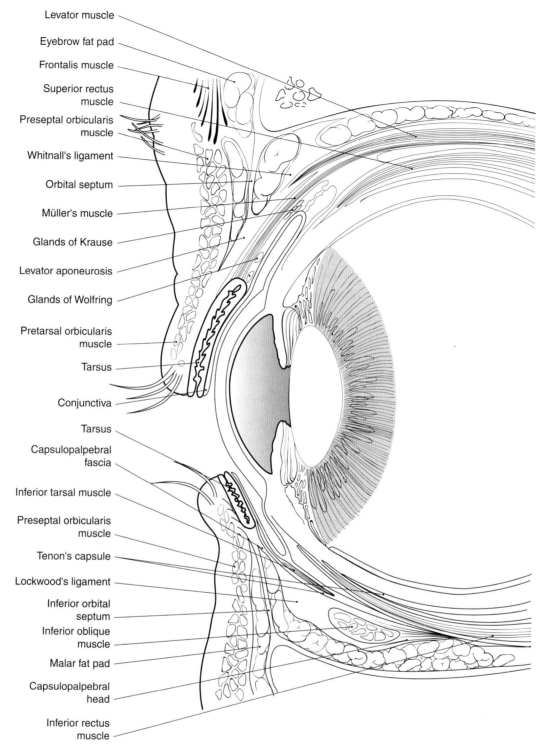

FIGURE **64-3** *Cross-sectional view of the structures composing the upper and lower eyelid. Adapted from Kikkawa DO and Lemke BN.*[41]

whereas the horizontal interpalpebral fissure is 28 to 30 mm. With age the horizontal fissure shortens by approximately 10%.[18] The lateral canthal angle lies 1 to 2 mm superior to the medial canthal angle,

giving the youthful eye a subtle lateral inclination. The apex of the upper eyelid margin rests slightly nasal to the pupil at the level of limbus in children and 1.0 to 2.0 mm below the limbus in adults, yielding a margin reflex distance of 4 to 5 mm. The lower eyelid margin peaks inferiorly directly beneath the pupil. Figure 64-4 demonstrates the normal upper and lower eyelid position. As depicted in Figure 64-5 dermal and conjoined fascia attachments of the levator palpebrae superioris aponeurosis form the upper eyelid crease, an important anatomic and surgical landmark often used as an incision site.[6,19,20] Position of the upper eyelid crease varies with age, gender, and, to some degree, ethnicity.[21] The youthful eyelid crease is approximately one-third of the distance from the eyelid margin to the lower edge of the brow.[22] Elevation of the upper eyelid crease may signify disinsertion or attenuation of the levator muscle attachments due to age-related lipid infiltration. Concomitant upper lid blepharoptosis is commonly present in the setting of an elevated upper lid crease. In general upper eyelid creases in Caucasian females are 9 to 10 mm above the upper lid margin, whereas in Caucasian males they are 7 to 8 mm above the upper lid border. A cross-sectional study demonstrated upper lid crease heights lower than traditionally purported values, although small sample size and variation in measuring technique may account for the inconsistency.[21] Upper eyelid crease position in African Americans has not been documented extensively in the literature, although clinical experience suggests a position similar to that found in Caucasians.

Asian Upper Eyelid In individuals of Asian ethnicity three main variations of upper eyelid crease anatomy exist: single eyelid, low eyelid crease (inside-fold type of crease), and double eyelid with lid crease parallel to lid margin (Figure 64-6).[16,23–25] In patients with a single eyelid or low eyelid crease the levator aponeurosis fuses with the orbital septum near the eyelid margin below the supratarsal border, creating an essentially absent or low upper lid crease.[16] In the Asian double eyelid the level of fusion of the orbital septum with the levator aponeurosis is higher than in the Asian single eyelid.[16] Aside from the orbital septum fusion site, thicker fat layers and a lower primary insertion of the levator aponeurosis to the upper eyelid skin contribute to the characteristic topography of the Asian eyelid.

Lower Eyelid Crease The lower eyelid crease, formed by connective tissue fibers extending anteriorly from the capsulopalpebral fascia into the subcutaneous tissues, is less prominent than its upper eyelid counterpart and is often most noticeable in children.[26] The lower lid crease begins medially 4 to 5 mm inferior to the lower lid margin and slopes inferiorly as it proceeds laterally.

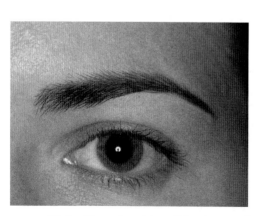

FIGURE **64-4** *Normal position of the upper and lower eyelids.*

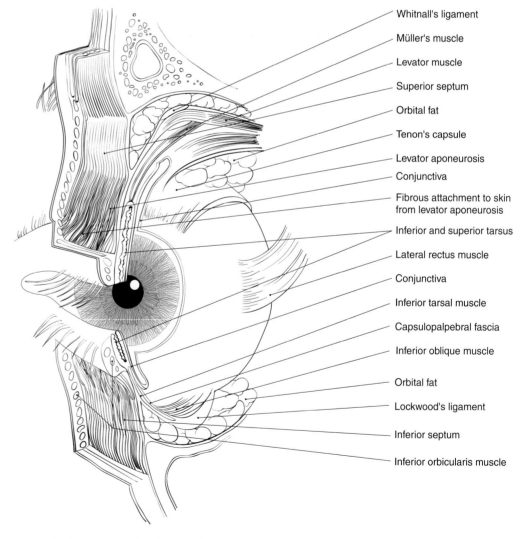

Whitnall's ligament
Müller's muscle
Levator muscle
Superior septum
Orbital fat
Tenon's capsule
Levator aponeurosis
Conjunctiva
Fibrous attachment to skin from levator aponeurosis
Inferior and superior tarsus
Lateral rectus muscle
Conjunctiva
Inferior tarsal muscle
Capsulopalpebral fascia
Inferior oblique muscle
Orbital fat
Lockwood's ligament
Inferior septum
Inferior orbicularis muscle

FIGURE **64-5** *Cross-sectional view of the dermal and conjoined fascial attachments of the levator aponeurosis responsible for lid crease formation. Adapted from Lemke BN and Lucarelli MJ.[111]*

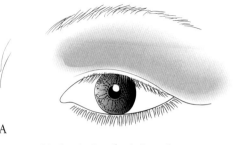

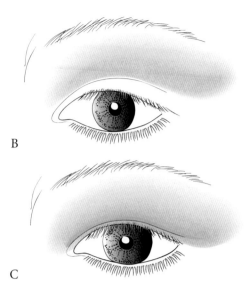

FIGURE **64-6** *Artist depiction demonstrating three common variations of the upper eyelid crease in Asians. A, Single eyelid with absence of crease. B, Low eyelid crease with inside fold type of crease. C, Double eyelid with parallel crease. Adapted from Chen WP.*[24]

ders.[28] The tarsal plates taper convexly medially and laterally to conform to the globe (Figure 64-8). Within the tarsal plates are the meibomian glands, holocrine sebaceous glands responsible for the lipid layer of the tear film. The meibomian glands are branched acinar glands with long central ducts opening at the eyelid margin just posterior to the gray line. There are approximately 25 glands in the upper eyelid and 20 in the lower eyelid.

Eyelid Connective Tissue   *Orbital Septum*

The orbital septum, an anatomic boundary between the eyelids and orbit, is a multil-amellar layer of dense connective tissue arising from the arcus marginalis, a thickened white fibrous line on the periosteum of the bony orbital margin.[27] The orbital septum forms the anterior boundary of the orbit. Medially the septum splits to cover the posterior aspect of Horner's muscle and adhere to the lacrimal fascia, inserting on the posterior lacrimal crest and anterior lacrimal crest, respectively. Laterally the septum inserts anteriorly on the lateral canthal ligament and posteriorly on Whitnall's tubercle of the lateral orbital rim. In the upper eyelid the orbital septum joins the levator aponeurosis 2 to 5 mm above the superior tarsal

border.[27] In the lower lid the septum fuses with the inferior tarsal border after joining the lower lid retractors 4 to 5 mm inferior to the tarsus.[26] A cadaver demonstration with artist's depiction of the orbital septum is shown in Figure 64-7. Orbital septal strength varies among individuals and with age. Attenuation of the septum allows for anterior orbital fat prolapse.

Tarsus   Composed of dense fibrous tissue the tarsal plates contribute structural integrity to the eyelids. Approximately 1.0 to 1.5 mm thick the tarsal plates measure approximately 25 mm in length and range from 10 to 12 mm in height in the upper lid and 3 to 5 mm in the lower lid, with no difference noted between gen-

Medial and Lateral Canthal Ligaments

The medial and lateral tarsal borders are firmly attached to the orbital rims via the fibrous medial and lateral canthal ligaments, respectively (see Figure 64-8). The medial canthal ligament is more complex anatomically due to its often tripartite attachment as well as its relationship with the lacrimal system. The anterior arm inserts onto the maxillary bone, anterosuperior to the lacrimal crest. The posterior arm attaches to the posterior lacrimal crest in a fanlike fashion and may partially fuse with the posterior surface of the lacrimal sac. The superior arm inserts onto the orbital process of the frontal bone, contributing to the formation of the lacrimal sac fossa roof.[29] The lateral canthal ligament inserts on the zygomatic bone at Whitnall's tubercle 1.5 mm inside the lateral

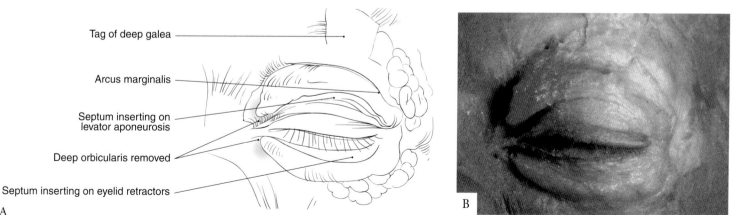

Tag of deep galea

Arcus marginalis

Septum inserting on levator aponeurosis

Deep orbicularis removed

Septum inserting on eyelid retractors

A

B

FIGURE **64-7**   A *and B, Cadaver demonstration of the orbital septum after removal of the forehead and eyelid musculature. A adapted from and B reproduced with permission from Lemke BN and Della Rocca RC.*[112]

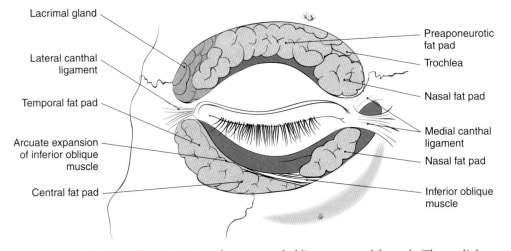

FIGURE 64-8 *Skeletonized anterior view of tarsus, canthal ligaments, and fat pads. The medial canthal ligament possesses a complex tripartite attachment. Adapted from Kikkawa DO and Lemke BN.[41]*

orbital rim and serves as both a stabilizer of the lids and a mobilizer of the lateral canthal angle via attachments to the lateral rectus check ligaments.[30,31] Whitnall's tubercle is a key surgical landmark as it is the site of lateral lid attachment when performing a canthopexy. Approximately 2 mm of temporal movement of the lateral canthal angle is afforded on lateral gaze due to the fusion of the lateral rectus check ligaments with the lateral canthal ligament.[30]

Whitnall's Superior Transverse Ligament
The junction of the levator muscle and levator aponeurosis is encircled by a transverse fibrous condensation known as Whitnall's superior transverse ligament, a supporter of the superior anterior eyelid. Although originally thought to serve as a check ligament for the levator, Whitnall's ligament has also been postulated to function as a suspender providing vertical support for the orbit (Figure 64-9).[32,33] Whitnall's ligament inserts superomedially within the orbit on the frontal bone behind the trochlea and superolaterally near the frontozygomatic suture after attaching to the posterior fibers of the lacrimal gland capsule.[34] During ptosis surgery Whitnall's ligament is a key landmark, often corresponding to the transition from levator muscle to aponeurosis.

Lockwood's Ligament The lower lid counterpart to Whitnall's ligament is Lockwood's ligament, a product of the conjoined fascia of the inferior rectus and inferior oblique. Inserting on the medial and lateral canthal ligaments as well as the bony orbital rim, Lockwood's ligament serves as a suspensory sling for the inferior anterior orbit. Lockwood's ligament is strongest anterior to the inferior oblique muscle.[26]

Eyelid Musculature *Orbicularis Oculi* Part of the anterior lamella of the upper eyelid, the orbicularis oculi is a ring-shaped superficial sphincter muscle that can be thought of in three concentric portions: pretarsal, preseptal, and orbital. Figure 64-10 demonstrates the orbicularis oculi muscle in the setting of the superficial facial muscles. Adherent to the tarsus the pretarsal orbicularis requires sharp dissection for isolation. Posterior to the preseptal orbicularis, a thin fibrofatty inferior extension of the eyebrow fat pad, the postorbicularis fascia facilitates dissection of the preseptal orbicularis from the orbital septum. The peripheral-most orbital orbicularis covers the orbital rims. Together the pretarsal and preseptal orbicularis comprise the palpebral orbicularis, responsible for reflexive eyelid closure. The clinical implication of the palpebral orbicularis' function is evident in the postoperative period when the reflexive blink response is temporarily decreased as a result of preseptal orbicularis removal in the blepharoplasty skin muscle flap. The patient must be reminded to blink fully and frequently during postoperative healing to adequately moisten the cornea. Orbital orbicularis contraction produces forceful voluntary eyelid closure. The orbicularis has firm attachments to under-

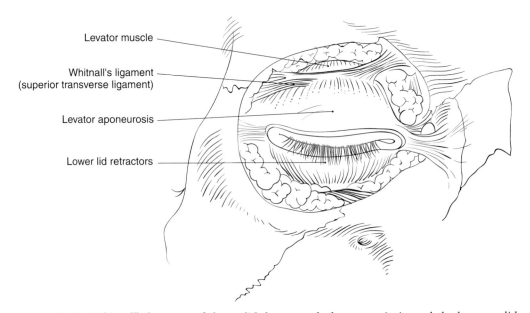

FIGURE 64-9 *Whitnall's ligament of the eyelid, levator palpebrae superioris, and the lower eyelid retractors. Adapted from Nerad JA.[76]*

lying structures at the lateral palpebral raphe, medial canthal region, and upper and lower eyelid retractor insertions. The muscle of Riolan, a small portion of the orbicularis separated from the pretarsal orbicularis fibers by the cilia, creates the gray line of the lid margin. The lacrimal (Horner-Duverney) muscle, formed by the deep pretarsal head of the orbicularis as it inserts on the posterior lacrimal crest and lacrimal fascia, is thought to play a role in lacrimal outflow, although the exact nature of its function is controversial.[35] Contraction of the lacrimal muscle results in medial and posterior movement of the lower eyelid with the blink.

Levator Palpebrae Superioris

The levator palpebrae superioris, the main retractor of the upper eyelid, arises from the lesser wing of the sphenoid deep in the bony orbit, coursing anteriorly above the superior rectus muscle and forming an aponeurosis with several important bony, dermal, and tarsal attachments. As mentioned above, the dermal and conjoined fascial attachments of the levator aponeurosis are responsible for the superior lid crease location (see Figure 64-9).[19,20]

Müller's Muscle

Müller's muscle, a sympathetically innervated minor retractor of the upper lid arising from the undersurface of the levator palpebrae superioris muscle, inserts into the superior tarsal border. Shortening of this muscle from the posterior aspect may be performed as an adjunct ptosis repair during blepharoplasty.[36–38] Approximately 2 mm of upper lid lift are provided by contraction of Müller's muscle, practically evidenced by the mild upper lid lift experienced with a rush of sympathetic excitation (ie, during the fight-or-flight response).

Lower Eyelid Retractors

The lower lid counterparts of the levator and Müller's muscles are the capsulopalpebral fascia and the inferior tarsal muscle, the retrac-

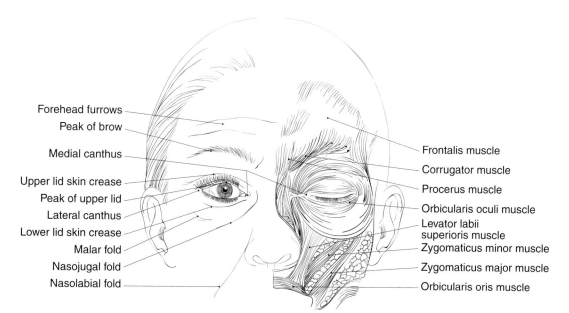

FIGURE **64-10** *Selected musculature of the eyelid. Orbicularis oculi in the setting of the superficial facial muscles. Adapted from Nerad JA.*[76]

tors of the lower lid (see Figure 64-9). The terminal fibers of the inferior rectus muscle give rise to a fibrous extension known as the capsulopalpebral head of the inferior rectus which splits to encompass the inferior oblique muscle, forming the inferior tarsal muscle and the capsulopalpebral fascia.[26] These layers fuse anterior to the inferior oblique muscle, forming Lockwood's suspensory ligament, the analog to Whitnall's ligament of the upper lid. Continuing anteriorly the lower lid retractors insert on Tenon's fascia, the inferior tarsal border, and the orbital septum at a level 4 to 5 mm below the tarsal border.

Eyelid Fat Pads *Orbital Relations*

In the anterior orbit, distinct fat compartments can be identified, although the majority of the anterior orbital fat pads remain continuous with posterior orbital fat (Figure 64-11).[39] This continuity prompted concern that excessive traction on orbital fat was responsible for orbital hemorrhage complicating blepharoplasty with fat removal.[40] Most surgeons implicate faulty hemostasis of fat pads, rather than traction, as the cause of postblepharoplasty orbital hemorrhage. Careful hemostasis is essential when performing eyelid fat removal.

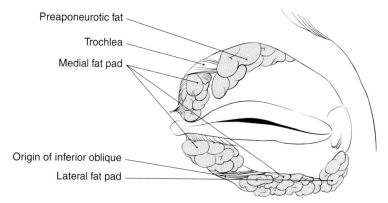

FIGURE **64-11** *Artist rendition of the eyelid fat pad. Adapted from Lemke BN and Della Rocca RC.*[112]

Aging Changes In the youthful face, orbital fat is held in check by a hearty orbital septum. Weakening of the septum associated with aging, chronic allergic swelling, or medical problems resulting in fluid retention (ie, hypo- or hyperthyroidism) may permit anterior prolapse of orbital fat, resulting in steatoblepharon. Aging may also cause atrophy of eyelid fat, creating a superior sulcus deformity. Dietary deficiency alone, however, has not been shown to result in orbital fat loss.[41]

Upper Eyelid Fat Pads The upper eyelid contains central and medial fat pockets anterior to the levator muscle and aponeurosis. Immediately posterior to the orbital septum lies the yellow central or preaponeurotic fat, which is not continuous with posterior orbital fat. Medially and inferior to the trochlea is the firmer and more pale fibrous medial fat pad.[39] Manipulation of the medial fat pad often requires placement of additional anesthesia into the fat pad itself, as more superficial anesthesia will not adequately infiltrate this structure. Laterally the superior anterior orbit houses the lacrimal gland. Orbital fat does not herniate in the lateral upper eyelid. Care must be taken to avoid removal of lacrimal tissue when fat pad excision is intended. Inspecting for color difference between the pink lacrimal gland and yellow fat is helpful in differentiation. Note that lacrimal gland prolapse may occur as an involutional change or in association with thyroid orbitopathy, making the position of the gland more anterior than usual.

Lower Eyelid Fat Pads The lower lid contains medial, central, and lateral fat pads, which may prolapse separately. Between the medial and central compartments resides the arcuate expansion of the inferior oblique muscle. Care must be taken to avoid damage to the inferior oblique muscle during lower lid blepharoplasty as vertical or torsional diplopia will result.

Eyelid Vasculature *Arteries* The eyelid vascular supply is rich, allowing for excellent healing and infection resistance, while mandating the surgeon to be cognizant of vascular relationships to avoid excessive bleeding. Both internal and external carotid arteries contribute to eyelid blood supply via the ophthalmic artery and the facial and infraorbital arteries, respectively (Figure 64-12). The facial artery becomes the angular artery in the medial canthal region and then perforates the orbital septum to anastomose with branches of the ophthalmic artery medial and anterior to the lacrimal sac. Arising from the maxillary artery the infraorbital artery travels within the infraorbital sulcus and canal to emerge from the infraorbital foramen and aid in arterial supply of the lower lid. The ophthalmic artery terminates in the lacrimal, frontal, supraorbital, supratrochlear, and nasal arteries.

Several anastomotic networks, known as arcades, exist in the eyelids. The peripheral arcade of the upper lid lies superior to the tarsus and directly anterior to Müller's muscle, supplying the superior aspect of the upper lid and superior conjunctival fornix. The marginal arcades of the upper and lower lids lie 2 to 4 mm from the eyelid margin, directly anterior to the tarsi. A peripheral arcade may be present in the lower lid, although it is less well developed.[41]

Veins The eyelid venous supply possesses deep and superficial anastomoses. The facial vein, the principal vein of the eyelids, forms a deep anastomosis with the superior ophthalmic vein via the supraorbital vein and a second deep anastomosis with the deep pterygoid plexus via the deep facial vein. Both anastomoses are potential routes for cavernous sinus spread of superficial infection.

Lymphatics Recent anatomic studies demonstrate the lymphatic system of the upper and lower eyelids to consist of superficial subcutaneous and deep pretarsal plexuses.[42] Using lymphoscintigraphy to characterize drainage pathways, parotid lymph node drainage from the upper eyelid, medial canthus, and lateral lower eyelid was shown.[43] Similar studies demonstrated medial and central lower

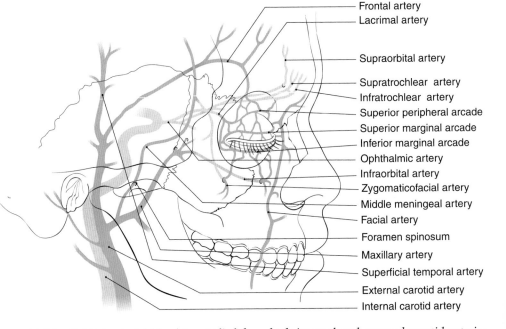

— Frontal artery
— Lacrimal artery
— Supraorbital artery
— Supratrochlear artery
— Infratrochlear artery
— Superior peripheral arcade
— Superior marginal arcade
— Inferior marginal arcade
— Ophthalmic artery
— Infraorbital artery
— Zygomaticofacial artery
— Middle meningeal artery
— Facial artery
— Foramen spinosum
— Maxillary artery
— Superficial temporal artery
— External carotid artery
— Internal carotid artery

FIGURE **64-12** *Orbital arterial blood is supplied from both internal and external carotid arteries. Adapted from Kikkawa DO and Lemke BN.*[41]

eyelid drainage to the submandibular lymph nodes and a dual drainage of the central upper eyelid to both submandibular and parotid nodes.[43]

Innervation *Motor* Cranial nerve VII, the facial nerve, supplies motor innervation for all the facial muscles (Figure 64-13). The facial nerve arises from the pons, eventually dividing into temporal, zygomatic, buccal, mandibular, and cervical branches. The temporal branch innervates both frontalis and orbicularis oculi, whereas the zygomatic and buccal divisions also contribute in an overlapping fashion to innervation of the orbicularis oculi.[44]

The levator palpebrae superioris receives motor innervation from the terminal branches of the superior division of cranial nerve III, the oculomotor nerve, which travels within the muscle cone and enters the superior rectus inferiorly 15 mm from the orbital apex and subsequently enters the levator. Müller's muscle is sympathetically innervated by postganglionic fibers that arise in the superior cervical ganglion, enters the cavernous sinus surrounding the internal carotid artery, and subsequently joins nerve branches to enter the orbit.

Sensory Sensory innervation of the eyelids is via the ophthalmic and maxillary divisions of the trigeminal nerve (cranial nerve V), which give rise to the lacrimal, frontal, and nasociliary nerves, and the infraorbital, zygomatic, sphenopalatine, and posterosuperior alveolar nerves, respectively (Figure 64-14). The lacrimal nerve courses superotemporally to supply the lacrimal gland, conjunctiva, and lateral upper lid and send an anastomotic branch to the zygomaticotemporal nerve. The frontal nerve divides into supraorbital and supratrochlear branches near the orbital rim. The supraorbital nerve exits the orbit via a notch or foramen in the superior orbital rim to provide sensation for the majority of the forehead and scalp. The

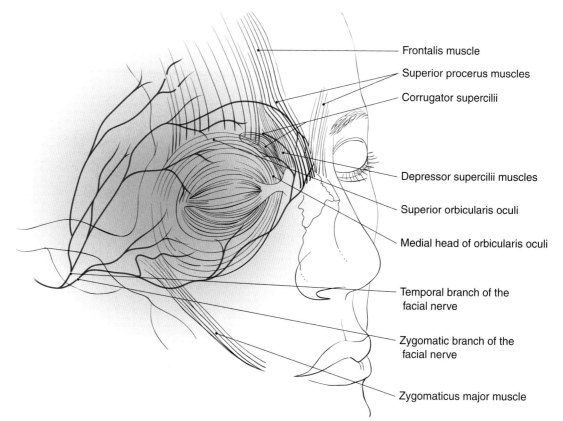

FIGURE **64-13** *Anatomy of cranial nerve VII, the source of motor innervation for the face. Adapted from Knize DM.*[113]

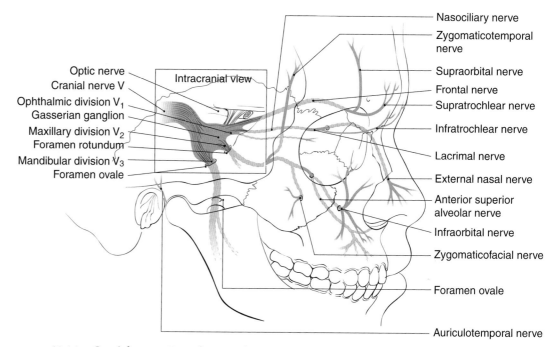

FIGURE **64-14** *Cranial nerves V_1 and V_2 supply sensory innervation to the periorbital region. Adapted from Kikkawa DO and Lemke BN.*[41]

supratrochlear nerve, exiting the orbit lateral to the corrugator muscle, conveys sensory input from the bridge of the nose and medial aspect of the upper eyelid and forehead.[45,46] The nasociliary nerve gives rise to the anterior and posterior ethmoidal nerves, the long ciliary nerves to the globe, and a sensory root to the ciliary ganglion and terminates as the sensory root to the infratrochlear nerve.[41] Emerging from the infraorbital foramen the infraorbital nerve supplies the skin and conjunctiva of the lower eyelid, nasal skin and septum, and upper lip skin and mucosa via the inferior palpebral, lateral nasal, and superior labial nerve terminal branches, respectively. The zygomatic nerve divides into the zygomaticofacial and zygomaticotemporal nerves. The former travels along the inferolateral orbit, traversing the zygomaticofacial foramen before innervating the cheek skin, whereas the latter exits the orbit to the temporal fossa and supplies the lateral forehead.

Lacrimal System and Tear Film Composition   *Lacrimal Glands*   The lacrimal gland, incompletely divided by the lateral horn of the levator into orbital and palpebral lobes, lies in a shallow depression of the superotemporal frontal bone. In the superior and inferior conjunctival fornices are the accessory lacrimal glands of Krause and Wolfring.

Lacrimal Drainage System   The lacrimal drainage system is diagrammed in Figure 64-15. The upper and lower lid puncta lie 8 and 10 mm lateral to the tear sac, respectively, and are normally well apposed to the globe. Initially vertical for 2 mm the canaliculi make a 90° turn and travel 8 mm within the orbicularis muscle just beneath the lid margin to join, forming the common canaliculus. The common canaliculus then joins the lacrimal sac, which is found within the bony lacrimal fossa. Ten percent of the population lacks a common canaliculus, and the canaliculi simply lead to the lacrimal sac. The nasolacrimal duct drains beneath the inferior turbinate into the inferior meatus.

Tear Film Composition   The precorneal tear film is comprised of three layers:

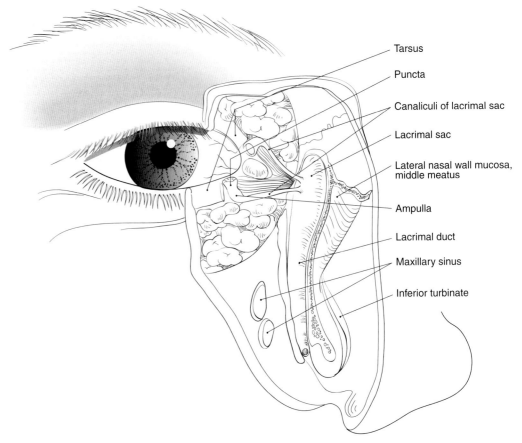

FIGURE 64-15   *The lacrimal system of the eyelid. Adapted from Lemke BN and Lucarelli MJ.*[111]

mucin, aqueous, and lipid. The inner mucin layer, produced by conjunctival goblet cells, stabilizes the tear film while lubricating the corneal surface. Accessory and main lacrimal glands account for the middle aqueous layer, the thickest portion of the tear film. The most superficial lipid layer, secreted by the meibomian glands and glands of Zeis and Moll, further stabilizes the tear film and prevents evaporation. Reflex tearing prompted by emotion or an ocular irritant is produced by the main lacrimal gland. Deficiency of any component of the tear film leads to dry eye symptoms.

The tear layer must be regularly redistributed by the eyelid blink mechanism to maintain ocular surface comfort and integrity. Postoperative lessening of the magnitude and frequency of the blink may temporarily elicit dry eye symptoms in predisposed individuals. Blepharitis, conjunctivitis, and corneal irritation symp-

toms are also amplified by this temporary postblepharoplasty eyelid dyskinesia.

Patient Evaluation: History

Eliciting the Chief Concern

Whether primarily cosmetic or functional, patient selection for blepharoplasty requires careful consideration of history elements, physical features, and patient expectations as well as investigation into potential clinical pitfalls. The blepharoplasty surgeon must thoroughly explore the goals of the patient. Patients needing a functional blepharoplasty owing to severe dermatochalasis often describe frontal headache or fatigue from frontalis contraction, impairment of superior visual field, or a need to raise the chin or use manual elevation of the brow or lids to enhance vision. Symptoms are frequently exacerbated by fatigue and are generally worse in the evening (ie, while reading in downgaze

The labeled structures in the figure are: Tarsus, Puncta, Canaliculi of lacrimal sac, Lacrimal sac, Lateral nasal wall mucosa, middle meatus, Ampulla, Lacrimal duct, Maxillary sinus, Inferior turbinate.

before bedtime). Patients may relate needing to raise their lid skin to see better. Patients seeking cosmetic blepharoplasty may lament they "look tired all the time" or describe a sagging change in their lid and eyebrow position compared with the lid and brow position of their youth. Documentation of lid effect on patient quality of life is valuable. Information on the impact on occupation, hobbies, driving, and other activities of daily living is essential both for better understanding of the patient's goals and for third party reimbursement.

The patient is encouraged to demonstrate the problem areas while looking at a handheld mirror. Patients are also asked to bring old photographs that reveal eyebrow position at an earlier age. Asian blepharoplasty candidates are encouraged to present photographs demonstrating the desired upper eyelid crease type. Some surgeons use computer modeling programs to illustrate possible results to patients. An immediate demonstration of the effect of eyebrow elevation or the impact of aging can be achieved through use of digital photography of the patient with comparison to prior photographs.

In functional and cosmetic patients, especially in the latter group, expectations must be well defined. Ideal cosmetic candidates can describe which physical parameters they find problematic. It is helpful to have the patient point out, either in a mirror or a photograph, the objectionable features. Vague complaints or withdrawal from the decision-making process often predict inadequate understanding and unrealistic expectations. The issues under discussion should be those of the surgical candidate, not issues generated by others. An open patient-physician relationship and thorough dialogue remain key building blocks to a successful surgical outcome.

Important History Elements

Historic questions on the initial evaluation are designed to clarify the patient's issues while identifying factors that can alter treatment or contraindicate blepharoplasty. A complete past ocular history, including documentation of contact lens use or intolerance, tearing abnormalities, dry eye history, and previous surgery, as well as a thorough past medical history are necessary. Any history of dry eye symptoms, such as ocular scratchiness, blurred vision, foreign body sensation, or pain, should be investigated, as blepharoplasty may aggravate these symptoms. Ophthalmology consultation should be considered. Epiphora, ocular irritation with ambient wind, or current use of artificial tears all raise the possibility of postoperative dry eye symptoms. Keratoconjunctivitis sicca or cicatricial conjunctival disease should make the surgeon wary of proceeding with blepharoplasty.

Prior facial, and especially lid and brow, surgeries should be discussed. If upper eyelid blepharoplasty has been previously performed and the patient complains of a persistent skin fold, evaluate the eyebrow position to rule out forehead ptosis. Similarly the appearance of medial fat pad fullness can be mimicked by medial eyebrow ptosis. A descended eyebrow fat pad or a prolapsed lacrimal gland may also be mistaken by the patient as "residual upper eyelid fat" for which a secondary upper lid procedure is sought. The patient is shown their upper eyelid appearance with the forehead supported in the normal position. If a significant effect is noted the patient must compromise on the final blepharoplasty result or accept concomitant forehead lifting. Previously performed lower blepharoplasty may leave the patient desiring more fat removal, treatment of an accentuated nasojugal fold, skin laxity or deformity, eyelid malposition, or a lateral canthal deformity. A surgeon performing a transcutaneous lower blepharoplasty reenters the muscle later with an increased risk of postoperative lid retraction.

Although rare with blepharoplasty given the thin nature of the eyelid skin, the possibility of hypertrophic scar formation should be discussed, especially with higher Fitzpatrick skin types.[47] The possibility of pigmentary change of the surgical wound should also be addressed. Any history of periocular trauma should be explored as to the timing and nature of the injury.

Clinical course and physiologic stability should be documented in patients with thyroid eye disease, as eyelid retraction associated with thyroid ophthalmopathy may worsen after poorly executed blepharoplasty. Eyelid retraction, eyelid edema, and any herniated fat measurements in patients with thyroid disease should be stable for at least 6 months prior to consideration of surgery.[48] Excessive proptosis in patients with thyroid eye disease is generally treated with orbital decompression prior to any eyelid surgery. Patients with thyroid orbitopathy often exhibit persistent eyelid fat herniation, eyebrow fat pad hypertrophy, and a glabellar grimace (Figure 64-16).

A full medication history should be documented, especially the use of aspirin, nonsteroidal anti-inflammatory medications, anticoagulants, homeopathic herbal

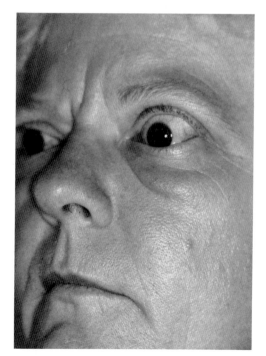

FIGURE 64-16 *Patient displaying features characteristic of thyroid orbitopathy.*

preparations, and vitamin E, as patients will need to discontinue these medicines preoperatively for 1 to 2 weeks. Warfarin is generally held for 4 days preoperatively. Inquiry regarding cigarette, alcohol, and illicit drug use should be made as the former may influence skin quality and healing and the latter two may affect the patient's ability to complete postoperative care.

Physical Examination

The preoperative physical examination of a patient requesting blepharoplasty focuses on eyelid function (ocular protection, tear film distribution, and clearance of the visual axis) as well as structure and regional anatomy that may necessitate adjunctive procedures for a superior result.

The Eyebrow Examination of the forehead and eyebrow seeks to define brow position as a contributor to apparent upper lid skin redundancy. Findings may be demonstrated to the patient with a mirror. Eyebrow position below the supraorbital rim yields a T-type configuration to the nasal-eyebrow angle, whereas the youthful female brow position creates a Y-type nasal-eyebrow angle configuration.[46] Measuring the distance from the central inferior eyebrow to the inferior corneal limbus while the patient is in primary gaze can aid in identification of patients with brow ptosis. A value less than 22 mm, especially in women, may warrant consideration of brow elevation as an adjunctive procedure.[48] Quantitative grading of brow ptosis can be obtained by placing a millimeter ruler vertically over the eyebrow and measuring the difference in millimeters between current location and ideal position when the eyebrow is elevated by the clinician's finger. Performing the measurement over the medial, central, and lateral brow is beneficial to quantify brow ptosis, which is often segmental. Adjunctive brow elevation must be considered if more than mild brow ptosis is present.

Upper Eyelid The skin quantity, quality, and resilience are important in determining the amount of skin to excise and use of adjunctive procedures. With the patient's eyes closed and gentle elevation of the brow to smooth out the upper eyelid skin, an objective measurement of the amount of eyelid skin can be obtained. Generally 18 to 21 mm of eyelid skin is retained during upper lid blepharoplasty.[4] Eyelid skin should be examined for dermatopathology (ie, eczema), inflammation, pigmentary inconsistencies, and prior surgical scars. Any suspicious skin lesions suggestive of neoplasia should be documented and dealt with prior to surgery. Rhytids should be assessed. Orbital fat herniation, manifested as lid fullness, can be appreciated in the medial and central upper lid by palpation. Fullness in the lateral upper lid may signify lacrimal gland prolapse, which may necessitate repositioning during blepharoplasty.

The upper eyelid crease is identified by gently lifting the eyebrow and asking the patient to look down, then slightly up, and then down again while inspecting upper lid skin for a dynamic crease that retracts with slight upgaze. Static eyelid skin creases may or may not reflect this dynamic infolding produced by levator muscle activity. The distance from the central upper lid crease to the upper lid margin is normally 9 to 11 mm in women and 7 to 8 mm in men, except for the aforementioned variation in Asian eyelid crease location. Greater values than expected may indicate levator aponeurosis disinsertion and possible blepharoptosis. Lesser values may indicate preaponeurotic fat pad incursion into the pretarsal space. Lid crease reformation may be considered when desired.

It is critical that the upper eyelid position, evaluated with the forehead relaxed, be assessed preoperatively in the blepharoplasty candidate and that the measurements be recorded in the chart. The margin reflex distance (MRD), the distance from the middle of the pupil to the upper lid margin, is determined by shining a penlight in the patient's eyes to obtain a pupillary light reflex while the patient is in primary gaze. Should the patient's upper lid ptosis preclude visualization of the light reflex, the lid should be raised until the reflex is seen and the number of millimeters of lift needed is recorded as a negative value. A normal MRD is 4 to 4.5 mm (Figure 64-17). Care must be taken to distinguish between genuine lid ptosis and severe dermatochalasis wherein the draped skin obscures the light reflex. An MRD greater than 5.5 mm and superior scleral show are indicative of upper lid retraction. Investigation of possible thyroid disease should be considered. Upper eyelid position with the eyelids gently closed should be inspected for lagophthalmos (incomplete lid closure), which may herald dry eye symptoms if greater than 2 mm. Special attention to lagophthalmos is warranted in patients who have undergone prior blepharoplasty.

Levator palpebrae superioris function is key to upper lid position and should be objectively measured. While holding a vertical millimeter ruler lateral to the greatest diameter of the palpebral fissure, the upper lid margin is measured in extreme downgaze and extreme upgaze. Care must be taken to immobilize the brow so as to avoid the influence of frontalis recruitment. Repeating the measurement several times is useful to obtain an average, which is recorded. Lid lag, evidenced by lack of

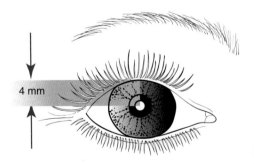

FIGURE **64-17** *The margin reflex distance measures the distance between the center of the pupil and the margin of the upper eyelid. Adapted from Putterman AM.[48]*

smooth pursuit of the upper lid margin with the superior corneal limbus while the patient moves from upgaze to downgaze, can alert the examiner to possible thyroid disease. The presence of excessive upper lid laxity, upper lash ptosis, and papillary conjunctivitis in a patient with ocular irritation and injection suggests floppy eyelid syndrome. Lash ptosis is an altered trajectory of the lashes whereby cilia project inferiorly rather than anterosuperiorly. If floppy eyelid syndrome is suspected, examination findings will confirm abnormally easy distraction of the upper lid off the ocular surface. Horizontal tightening of the upper eyelids, performed by lateral shortening and re-insertion of a tarsal strip within the orbital rim, may be indicated.

The eyelid margin should be inspected. Evidence of blepharitis, such as collarettes along the lashes, thickened lid margins, and plugged meibomian glands, should be noted and lid hygiene (ie, warm washcloth soaks with gentle baby shampoo eyelid cleansing) prescribed to resolve the blepharitis prior to surgery.

Lower Eyelid Careful skin examination is equally as important in the lower eyelid area as in the upper lid. Rhytids, especially "crow's feet," should be noted, as prominence may necessitate adjunctive topical retinoic acid, chemical peels, laser resurfacing, and botulinum toxin A injections. Assessing for extra lower lid skin is best performed in upgaze. The pinch test uses an angled forceps, such as a Brown-Adson, to grasp a redundant fold of lower lid skin without altering lid position while the patient is in upgaze with his or her mouth open (to allow for maximal necessary excursion of lower lid skin). The amount of skin grasped approximates the amount to excise. Orbital fat prolapse is noted in the medial, central, and lateral lower lid. Facile differentiation of orbital fat from edema is achieved by gentle ballottement of the upper eyelid; fat herniation will result in distinct anterior movement of the

fullness whereas edema will not. Hypertrophied orbicularis muscle is most prominent when the patient smiles.

Lower lid position can be quickly assessed by examining the lower eyelid margin position relative to the inferior corneoscleral limbus. Any inferior scleral show in primary gaze is objectively measured from the inferior corneoscleral limbus to the lower eyelid margin, or using the margin reflex distance-2 (MRD_2), the distance from the pupillary light reflex to the lower lid margin in primary gaze. Together the MRD and MRD_2 compose the palpebral fissure height. Normally the lower lid rests at or slightly above the inferior corneal limbus. An increased MRD_2 raises concern of lower lid retraction from thyroid ophthalmopathy, lower lid laxity, mechanical forces, or cicatricial causes. A hypoplastic maxilla causing decreased prominence of the inferior orbital rim may contribute to postoperative susceptibility to lower lid retraction and ectropion.

Abnormal lower lid position and rounding of the lateral canthal angle often result from lower lid laxity. Laxity is assessed by distraction and the snap-back test. By gently grasping the lower lid centrally, the lid is distracted off the globe anteriorly. Normal distraction is less than 6 mm. Greater distraction suggests laxity. To perform the snap-back test the lower lid is pulled inferiorly and released while the patient refrains from blinking. A normal lid returns to the globe quickly with one or fewer blinks. A lax lid requires several blinks to resume its former position and may remain inferiorly displaced and everted, indicating ectropion. Laxity of the lateral canthal tendon is the most common cause of lower lid laxity. The ability to displace the punctum greater than 2 mm laterally indicates laxity of the medial canthal tendon.[49] Lower lid horizontal tightening procedures should be performed at the time of blepharoplasty surgery for the lax lower lid to prevent postoperative ectropion and recreate the

youthful, slightly elevated, well-defined lateral canthal angle.

Midface Architecture Midfacial ptosis, festoons, and malar mounds are important aspects to note on evaluation, as separate procedures are necessary to address these concerns. Midfacial ptosis encompasses a host of changes caused by attenuation of the subcutaneous portions of the orbitomalar, masseteric cutaneous, and zygomatic ligaments, including soft tissue inferior migration of the lower eyelid structures, cheek, and midface, as well as concomitant prominence of the nasolabial fold (Figure 64-18).[12] When attenuation of the lower lid orbicularis oculi and laxity of orbicularis attachments to deep fascia develop, the orbicularis may sag or form redundant folds known as festoons.[50] Several levels of festoons have been described including pretarsal, preseptal, orbital, and malar, and composition varies to include one or more of the following: skin, muscle, suborbicularis fat,

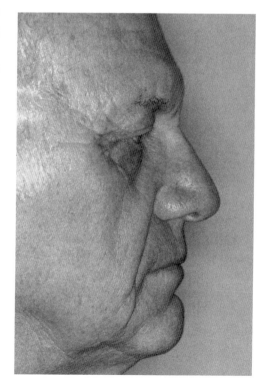

FIGURE **64-18** *Profile of a patient with descent of the cheek prominence characteristic of midfacial ptosis.*

and herniated orbital fat.[50] Malar mounds, projections of skin and fat in the area of the malar eminence, are areas of altered inferior orbital orbicularis fibers that allow abnormal communication between subdermal and suborbicularis fat.[50] Malar mounds often prove challenging to resolve.

Lacrimal Secretion and Ocular Surface Evaluation Dry eye symptoms are frequent following blepharoplasty, and preoperative evaluation of the lacrimal system may direct surgical intervention and patient education, thereby avoiding significant morbidity. The tear meniscus, tear break-up time, Schirmer testing, and/ or fluorescein corneal staining are often used. The tear meniscus may be measured using a thin cross-sectional beam of light of a slit lamp biomicroscope focused on the patient's lower lid. The beam height is changed to match the height of the tear meniscus on the lower lid. Normal values are approximately 0.2 to 0.3 mm. The tear break-up time test requires instillation of 2% fluorescein dye on the cornea and examination with a cobalt blue light. The patient is asked to blink once and then refrain from blinking. Any loss of the tear film continuity (evidenced as a streaky dry spot and color change from green to blue) in less than 10 seconds is considered abnormal. The tear break-up test measures tear stability, which is largely due to the lipid component of the tear film. The Schirmer tests, the gold standards for lacrimal testing, quantify the aqueous tear secretory component. After blotting the inferior cul de sac and palpebral conjunctiva, a bent filter paper strip (ie, a Schirmer strip), is placed in the lateral third of the lower eyelid with the strip notch at the eyelid margin such that the strip proceeds anteriorly. The room lights are dimmed to avoid reflex tearing. The strip is removed after 5 minutes and the amount of strip wetting measured. Topical anesthesia is

generally used in the basic secretion test, which indicates basal tear secretion. The normal value is approximately 15 mm. Tear hyposecretion is indicated with 5 to 10 mm of wetting and less than 5 mm suggests dry eye. Interpalpebral corneal and conjunctival staining with fluorescein (Figure 64-19) is characteristic of keratitis sicca, while inferior corneal staining suggests exposure keratopathy or blepharitis.[51,52] The extent of evaluation for dry eye varies among surgeons and often from patient to patient with the same surgeon.[53] There is controversy in the literature regarding the most appropriate evaluation, although the general consensus is that historic and physical examination elements suggestive of dry eye warrant more thorough evaluation and an especially conservative blepharoplasty.[54–56] Patient education should stress the role of ocular lubrication.

One of the important ocular surface protective mechanisms is the Bell's phenomenon, or the normal "rolling back" of the eyes with lid closure. This may be tested by asking the patient to tightly close their eyes while the examiner manually opens the lids to assess corneal position. A poor Bell's phenomenon indicates a risk of postoperative corneal exposure and irritation.

Corneal sensation is another key aspect of ocular surface protection. It may be tested by touching a wisp of cotton to the peripheral cornea while the patient is in upgaze. A blink response is normal. Patients who wear contact lenses or who have undergone refractive surgery may have decreased corneal sensation.[57–59] Individuals seeking cosmetic corneal surgery often seek cosmetic blepharoplasty.

Ocular Motility Evaluation Diplopia may result spontaneously after blepharoplasty or be due to iatrogenic injury of the superior or inferior oblique muscles. A baseline evaluation of extraocular motility is therefore warranted. Using a muscle light or the examiner's finger, the patient is

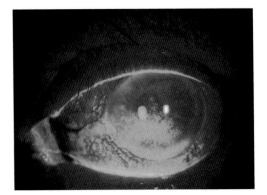

FIGURE **64-19** *Punctate staining of the cornea typical of keratitis sicca.*

directed to look in the nine positions of gaze: superotemporal, superior, superonasal, lateral, medial, inferotemporal, inferior, inferonasal, and straight ahead. Any ocular motility deviations should be evaluated prior to surgery. Patients with thyroid ophthalmopathy having impaired ocular motility are generally recommended to have their strabismus surgery prior to any eyelid surgery.

Visual Acuity A vital sign of ocular function, the best-corrected visual acuity of both eyes, should be documented prior to surgery. If visual acuity is subnormal, ophthalmologic evaluation is especially important. In addition postoperative visual complaints can be more accurately assessed when the baseline visual acuity has been recorded. Visual decline postoperatively may be wrongly attributed to blepharoplasty if preoperative visual acuity has not been documented.

Ancillary Studies

Both visual field testing and photography aid in demonstrating preoperative changes in visual function and appearance. Visual field testing is necessary for patients wishing to determine insurance benefits for surgery.

Visual Field Evaluation Peripheral visual field testing is performed to document visual field loss, usually of the superior field, due to upper eyelid dermatochalasis or blepharoptosis. Several different perimeters may be used, such as the automated Humphrey or manually operated Goldmann perimeter or tangent screen. Perimetry is performed with the patient's eyelid unaltered and repeated with the eyelid skin or ptotic lid elevated.

Photographic Documentation Preoperative photography is key when performing eyelid surgery. Documentation of preoperative appearance serves as a benchmark from which postoperative change can be determined and is a valuable reference when initially unforeseen postoperative complications arise. Minimum photographs recommended include frontal primary, upgaze and downgaze, and lateral views. Discussion of photographic specifics is beyond the scope of this chapter and the reader is referred to alternate texts for a more complete discourse.[60]

Anesthesia

The majority of blepharoplasty surgery is performed in an outpatient surgical environment or an office procedure room, under local anesthesia, with or without intravenous sedation. Oral anxiolytics such as diazepam are often employed when intravenous sedation is not used. Adjunctive procedures performed at the time of blepharoplasty may warrant general endotracheal anesthesia, and the anesthesia and sedation needs may vary on an individual basis.

The blepharoplasty surgeon should be familiar with topical and local infiltrative anesthesia options. Commonly used topical ocular anesthetics include the ester-type compounds, proparacaine (0.5%) and tetracaine (0.5%). Commonly used local infiltrative anesthesia choices are all amides and include lidocaine (0.5 to 2.0%), mepivacaine (1 to 2%), and bupivacaine (0.25 to 0.75%). Lidocaine and mepivacaine have an onset of action from 3 to 6 minutes and a comparable duration of action (120 minutes) when epinephrine

is mixed with lidocaine. Bupivacaine has a slower onset of action (10 minutes) and a longer duration of action (8 to 12 hours). Epinephrine is added to promote hemostasis through vasoconstriction and slow absorption, thereby prolonging duration of the anesthetic and increasing the maximum safe anesthetic dosage. No additional therapeutic benefit is gained by adding concentrations of epinephrine greater than 1:100,000. A mixture of 2% lidocaine with 1:100,000 epinephrine and 0.5% bupivacaine with epinephrine allows for rapid onset of prolonged anesthesia. Overdose toxicity of the amide-type anesthetics manifests as mild hypertension and tachycardia, lightheadedness, mild agitation, and confusion. Severe toxicity is marked by seizures, coma, respiratory depression, bradycardia, ventricular dysrhythmias, and asystole. Maximal doses based on milligram per kilogram and total daily dose are 7 mg/kg and 500 mg for lidocaine with epinephrine, 4.5 mg/kg and 300 mg for lidocaine without epinephrine, and 7 mg/kg and 1,000 mg for mepivacaine. Bupivacaine daily dose should not exceed 175 mg and maximal daily dose with epinephrine is 225 mg.

Hyaluronidase, an enzyme that degrades the polysaccharide hyaluronic acid, may be added to local anesthetics to aid in anesthetic diffusion and tissue permeability. Duration of anesthetic action is decreased when hyaluronidase is used concomitantly.

Sodium bicarbonate has been advocated as a local anesthetic adjunct to reduce the discomfort associated with anesthetic infiltration.[61] A base, sodium bicarbonate, partially neutralizes the acidic nature of local anesthetics with epinephrine, thereby decreasing the irritation that the acidic anesthetic pH induces.

Anesthesia injection is performed from the temporal aspect with the needle bevel up. Keeping the needle as parallel as possible to the eyelid skin and carefully stabilizing the patient's head during injec-

tion guard against inadvertent globe penetration. Injection sites are placed within the skin area to be excised, thereby allowing removal of the occasionally produced microhematomas. Milking the injected fluid medially aids in minimizing the number of sites injected. Injection depth is at the level of the orbicularis muscle.

Upper Eyelid Blepharoplasty

Preoperative Concerns

On the day of surgery, review of the surgical plan and examination of the patient in an upright position are helpful.

Once in the operating room, skin incision lines are marked with a methylene blue surgical marking pen prior to skin preparation or immediately thereafter. The former has the advantage of allowing full view of the patient's face during the marking process and providing several minutes of anesthesia infiltration while the surgeon is scrubbing for the surgery and the patient is being draped. Injection prior to surgical marking is not recommended unless the surgeon waits for the injected volume to diffuse as the injected volume may influence placement of surgical marks. The patient's periocular area should be thoroughly prepared with a 5% povidone-iodine or pHisoHex solution. Care should be taken to not allow pHisoHex solution to contact the corneal or conjunctival surfaces. Irrigate the ocular surface well if contact occurs. Care must be taken to avoid removing the surgical marking during preparation if marking is performed prior to the prep. Topical ocular anesthesia drops (ie, proparacaine or tetracaine) are instilled onto the ocular surface and a protective corneal contact may be inserted.

Surgical marking requires that the patient be supine with the surgeon intermittently elevating the brow manually so as to flatten any redundant upper eyelid skin. If the brow is not elevated, erroneously high surgical marking may result. Special care is taken to provide vertical traction on the pretarsal skin to remove any redundancy as the inferior incision is designed. The initial surgical mark extends from the punctum to the lateral canthus and lies along the upper eyelid crease or where the intended lid crease will be. The location of the upper eyelid crease should be measured with calipers to confirm proper placement of the inferior aspect of the incision. In women the initial surgical mark is generally 8.5 to 10 mm above the superior lid margin centrally. The corresponding value in men is 7 to 8 mm. The crease may be designed 0.5 mm lower than ultimately desired as vertical traction will stretch the skin somewhat and provide desired lash eversion. Surgical marking in the Asian patient varies from these values and will be discussed below. The superior surgical mark is placed next. Approximately 18 to 21 mm of upper eyelid skin should be left after the intended skin is removed. Care should be taken to avoid confusing epilated inferior eyebrow skin for true eyelid skin. Excessive skin removal will result in difficulty with eyelid closure and impair ocular surface protection. Excessive skin removal might also preclude future correction of eyebrow or forehead ptosis. The upper and lower surgical marks are connected in a curvilinear manner (Figure 64-20). To test the adequacy of lid skin remaining, the upper and lower marks should be approximated using a pinching technique with forceps. The forceps should grasp all excessive skin without altering the closed eyelid margin. Slight elevation of the eyelashes with the pinch may be desired. Any opening of the lids during medial, central, and lateral pinch assessment should warrant modification of intended incision lines.

Local anesthesia is next injected subcutaneously into the skin intended for removal. Gentle pressure may be used to diffuse the injected fluid.

Excision of the Skin-Muscle Flap After sufficient anesthesia infiltration has occurred and a corneal protector has been placed on the operative eye if desired, the eyelid skin is held taut for the incision. Careful traction perpendicular to the incision site can be provided by the surgical assistant. A no. 15 Bard-Parker blade, straight iris scissors, carbon dioxide (CO_2) laser, electrosurgical microdissection needle, or radiosurgical unit is used to incise the skin and orbicularis muscle along the previously placed surgical marks.

The skin-muscle flap is next dissected off the orbital septum by elevating the lateral aspect of the flap superiorly with forceps while the assistant provides perpendicular traction at the superior and inferior margins of the flap. A gentle painting motion is used, with care to avoid violating the orbital septum. The edges of the flap should be angled at approximately 45° to avoid a bulky muscular ridge when the edges are reapproximated during closure. Angulation of the edge is especially important temporally where the muscle layer is thicker. Hemostasis should be achieved with cautery after flap dissection and, if no fat excision is planned, the skin can be closed at this point.

Fat Debulking Upward traction is used to lift the orbital septum prior to opening the septum in the superomedial aspect with Westcott scissors, electrosurgical microdissection needle, or CO_2 laser. The septal opening is extended laterally to comprise the full width of the flap. The herniated orbital fat pads should be evident medially and centrally. Color as well as location can be helpful in differentiation, as the medial fat pad is a more pale lemon color as opposed to the brighter yellow central fat pad. The connective tissue capsule overlying the medial fat pad is opened. Gentle ballottement of the globe through the upper lid aids in herniating the fat through the incised capsule. The medial fat pad may require additional anesthetic injection to facilitate comfort during manipulation. The fat is gently grasped with straight forceps and teased out, then clamped at the base exiting the capsule. Cautery is used to separate the fat from the clamp. Care should be taken to achieve excellent fat pad hemostasis as postoperative bleeding may contribute to the rare but vision-threatening complication of orbital hemorrhage. Herniation of the central or preaponeurotic fat pad is addressed in a similar fashion by incising the overlying capsule, teasing out the fat, and clamping and cauterizing the herniated fat.

Over the last decade emphasis has been placed on removing less fat during both upper and lower blepharoplasty. In male blepharoplasty patients, fat excision should be especially judicious as the superior sulcus in men is generally more full than in women and excessive fat excision may feminize appearance by creating an unnaturally hollow-appearing superior sulcus. With a bilateral upper eyelid blepharoplasty, attention should be directed toward leaving rather than resecting symmetric amounts of fat. Alternatively fat may be thermally sculpted to improve the eyelid contour.

Lacrimal Gland Prolapse A fullness to the lateral upper eyelid may suggest prolapse of the orbital lobe of the lacrimal gland, which is seen as a pink to tan firm lobulated structure intraoperatively after the septum is opened. Care should be taken not to resect lacrimal gland tissue as postoperative dry eye may result. Repositing the prolapsed lacrimal gland in the lacrimal gland fossa should be easily achieved. Difficulty in repositing may suggest a neoplastic or infiltrative process and warrant a biopsy. A double-armed 5-0 polypropylene suture may be used to refixate the prolapsed gland to the orbital roof periosteum.[62,63]

Eyelid Crease Reformation and Skin Closure Reformation of the upper eyelid crease seeks to establish a connection between the levator aponeurosis and the orbicularis oculi muscle. In most instances

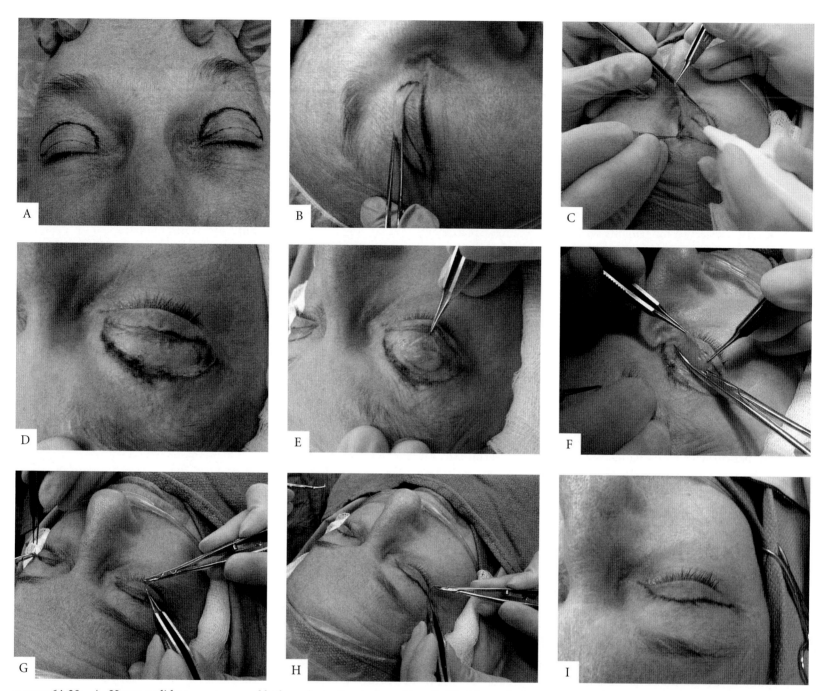

FIGURE **64-20** A, *Upper eyelid transcutaneous blepharoplasty. Surgical marking.* B, *Pinching technique to assess adequacy of amount of remaining lid skin.* C, *Dissection of the skin-muscle flap.* D, *Completion of skin-muscle flap dissection showing intact orbital septum.* E, *Opening of the orbital septum.* F, *Fat pad debulking.* G, *Closure of the orbicularis.* H, *Closure of the skin.* I, *Completed result.*

the inferior tissues are sufficiently adherent posteriorly such that a lid reformation suture may not be required. Prior to eyelid crease reformation, meticulous hemostasis should again be checked. Reformation is performed using buried interrupted sutures with an intermediate duration absorbable suture (ie, polyglactin) passed through both upper and lower orbicularis edges and the

levator aponeurosis at the level of the top of the tarsus. Care should be taken to achieve symmetric upper lid creases bilaterally.

The orbicularis is next approximated with several buried interrupted sutures of 7-0 polyglactin or a similar suture material. Placement of these interrupted sutures should allow facile reunion of the upper eyelid skin edges with a smooth contour.

Redundant skin causing cutaneous standing defects should be excised using Burow's triangle technique. The skin is closed using 6-0 fast-absorbing gut suture in a running fashion, beginning medially and progressing laterally. Alternative suture options for skin closure include nylon, polypropylene, or silk, although sutures that are not absorbable require removal approximately 5 to 7 days postoperatively. Greater duration of suture retention is required if CO_2 laser resurfacing is performed concomitantly with blepharoplasty. Skin closure sutures should have only minimal tension. Recent evidence suggests the tissue adhesive octyl-2-cyanoacrylate is a viable alternative to sutures.[64] Several key steps of transcutaneous upper eyelid blepharoplasty are shown in Figure 64-20.

Transconjunctival Upper Lid Blepharoplasty   Reserved for patients with isolated medial fat pad herniation and minimal or no wrinkling of the upper eyelid skin is the transconjunctival approach, which is relatively new.[65,66] The transconjunctival approach is a valuable one for patients in whom a noticeable scar would be unavoidable with the transdermal approach (ie, young patients), patients who have residual medial fat pad prominence after traditional upper lid blepharoplasty, or as an adjunct to a brow lift and periorbital laser for periorbital rhytids. Patients with severe blepharoptosis, dermatochalasis or prominent upper lid asymmetry are not candidates for this approach.[65]

After instilling tetracaine on the corner of the operative eye a corneal protective lens is inserted. Local anesthesia is next injected into the medial aspect of the upper fornix. A Desmarres retractor is used to expose the upper lid palpebral conjunctiva. An incision is made 3 to 4 mm above the upper tarsal margin, and medial dissection toward the contralateral parietal bone is carried out using angled scissors. Once the connective tissue of the medial fat pad is opened the fat protrudes outward. The fat is next gently grasped, clamped, and cauterized at the excision base. When fat excision is complete the lid is released without closure of the incision site.[65,67]

Asian Upper Eyelid Blepharoplasty   Originally described in 1896 by the Japanese physician M. Mikamo, the double eyelid procedure creates a superior palpebral crease in Asian patients with single eye-

lids.[68] This frequently performed cosmetic procedure seeks to create a defined crease parallel to the eyelid margin or an arcing crease that begins at the medial canthal area and gradually fans away from the lid margin laterally.[69] Consideration of the patient's facial features should guide surgical planning of the lid crease.[70] Because lid crease asymmetry is the most frequent complication, careful surgical planning and marking are critical to ensure proper crease placement.[71]

The patient is prepared in the manner described for a transcutaneous blepharoplasty. The lower surgical mark, which indicates the final desired crease location, should be 5 to 8 mm from the ciliary margin, thereby approximating the superior tarsal margin.[24] Vertical tarsal height can be ascertained by lid eversion. The lower surgical mark shape depends on whether a parallel or arcing crease is planned.[24] The amount of skin excised, as determined by the superior surgical mark, should be conservative. The skin-muscle flap is next dissected. A suborbicularis fat pad may be encountered, which can be carefully excised to reveal the orbital septum.[16] The orbital septum is next gently opened to allow for any necessary preaponeurotic fat pad treatment and to access the levator aponeurosis. Two options are frequently employed for lid crease creation, which requires an adhesion between the skin and levator aponeurosis. Direct suturing of the pretarsal orbicularis to the levator aponeurosis is accomplished via multiple small interrupted sutures that incorporate bites of the levator aponeurosis and the pretarsal orbicularis in the area of the desired final lid crease. A running suture would then be used to close the skin. Alternatively the skin edges can be directly sutured to the levator aponeurosis by picking up the lower skin edge, incorporating a small bite of levator aponeurosis in the desired crease location, and finishing by passing through the upper skin

edge. Placing several such sutures can fix the crease location and the remainder of the skin incision can be closed using sutures performed in a running fashion.[24] Figure 64-21 depicts the latter variation in Asian eyelid crease reformation.

Lower Eyelid Blepharoplasty

Selection of Approach   Blepharoplasty of the lower eyelid can be approached via an anterior transcutaneous or a posterior transconjunctival approach depending on the abnormalities to be addressed. The traditional transcutaneous route provides excellent visualization of lower lid fat pads and allows for excision of excessive skin, hypertrophic orbicularis muscle, and herniating fat. The risk of lower lid malposition, however, is not insignificant using an

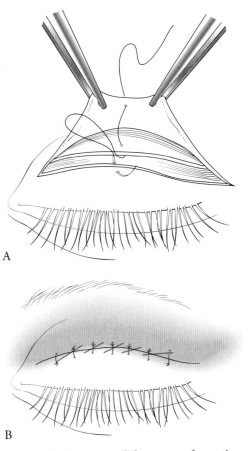

FIGURE **64-21**   *Asian lid crease reformation. A, Direct suturing of the orbicularis to the levator aponeurosis. B, A continuous suture is used to approximate wound edges. Adapted from Chen WP.[24]*

anterior approach. The transconjunctival approach carries a significantly lower risk of postoperative lower lid malposition and does not create an external scar. The transconjunctival approach is ideal in the setting of isolated fat herniation with minimal skin redundancy. The darkly pigmented patient predisposed to altered pigmentation or scar formation may also be a good transconjunctival blepharoplasty candidate. Patients with thyroid eye disease, who are prone to lower eyelid retraction, are potential posterior blepharoplasty candidates provided enough lid laxity is present to allow conjunctival access. Adjunctive procedures such as chemical peels, CO_2 laser skin resurfacing, or pinch skin excision are commonly performed in association with transconjunctival lower lid blepharoplasty. These adjunctive procedures have expanded the lower lid pathologies successfully treated by the transconjunctival approach to include most patients.[72]

Presence of lower eyelid laxity calls for an adjunctive horizontal lower lid tightening procedure at the time of lower eyelid blepharoplasty. Failure to perform such a procedure heightens the risk of lower lid retraction, lateral canthal abnormalities, and inferior scleral show.

Transcutaneous Approach An infraciliary surgical mark is drawn approximately 1.5 mm beneath and parallel to the lower lash line extending from the punctum to the lateral canthus. Temporal to the lateral canthus the mark is continued laterally within a preexisting "laugh line" for approximately 5 mm. Care should be taken to avoid an inferiorly sloping termination of the incision as an unnatural surgical scar will result. Subcutaneous anesthesia is next injected and the patient is prepared for surgery in a similar manner to that described for upper eyelid blepharoplasty.

A no. 15 Bard-Parker blade, CO_2 laser, microdissection needle, or other incising instrument is used to make the skin incision. A 4-0 silk traction suture

may be placed through the skin, orbicularis, and superficial tarsus to aid in upward displacement of the lower eyelid. Subcutaneous dissection is carried out taking care to minimize trauma to the pretarsal orbicularis. Next the orbicularis is incised below the inferior tarsal border with Westcott scissors or other appropriate instrument for the full length of the incision. A skin and muscle flap is dissected inferiorly toward the orbital rim. Excellent hemostasis should be obtained with judicious use of cautery. The orbital septum is next opened with Westcott scissors where it overlies the lower eyelid fat pads. The fat pad capsules are subsequently incised beginning with the lateral fat pad, which is the more difficult compartment to visualize. Gentle ballottement of the globe is used to aid in fat prolapse. The herniated fat is grasped, clamped, and excised. Meticulous hemostasis of fat is essential to avoid retrobulbar hemorrhage. Conservative fat resection is recommended, as over-resection results in a hollow appearance rather than a youthful one. The central and medial fat pads are debulked as needed in a similar fashion. Fat removal is compared bilaterally for symmetry.

A horizontal tightening procedure is indicated in nearly all cases of anterior approach lower lid blepharoplasty. The lateral tarsal strip procedure is a secure time-honored method of resuspending the lower eyelid but requires opening of the lateral commissure.[73] Alternative procedures addressing lower lid laxity include suspension of the lateral retinaculum and canthal-sparing lateral canthopexy.[74,75]

The skin and muscle flap are draped over the edge of the lid margin while the lid is not held in traction and the patient is looking upward and opening his or her mouth. These latter maneuvers simulate the lower eyelid's maximally extended position and aid in preventing excessive skin removal.[72] The redundant skin and muscle flap is drawn superolaterally,

marked with a surgical marking pen, and subsequently excised. A conservative approach to skin and muscle excision is crucial to prevent postoperative lower lid malposition. Rarely should more than 2 to 3 mm of the skin muscle flap be excised in total.[72] Special care should be taken to avoid creating lateral canthal rounding by not removing excessive skin laterally. Suturing the muscle flap to the zygomatic periosteum prior to excision of excess skin and orbicularis muscle may provide better appreciation of final tissue location and permit modifications prior to permanent tissue alteration. If hypertrophic orbicularis was earlier noted, a strip of orbicularis muscle should be excised in the affected area prior to closure of the skin. The muscle is later closed with interrupted buried absorbable suture (ie, 7-0 polyglactin). Alternatively, should greater support be desired, the muscle may be anchored to the zygomatic periosteum, if not already performed. The skin is closed with a running 6-0 fast-absorbing gut suture proceeding from the medial to lateral aspect. Figure 64-22 demonstrates several of the important aspects of transcutaneous lower eyelid blepharoplasty.

Transconjunctival Approach Formal marking is not performed for transconjunctival lower eyelid blepharoplasty, although marking the herniating fat pads may be of benefit.[76] Topical anesthesia is instilled onto the ocular surface and a corneal protective contact is inserted. Local anesthesia is injected subcutaneously in the central lower lid just beneath the lashes and into each fat pad. The skin is next prepared with 5% povidone-iodine or pHisoHex as in the previously described fashion.

The inferior palpebral conjunctiva is exposed using a Desmarres retractor or a 4-0 silk traction suture placed through the skin, orbicularis, and superficial tarsus in the central lower eyelid. The traction suture may be placed through the

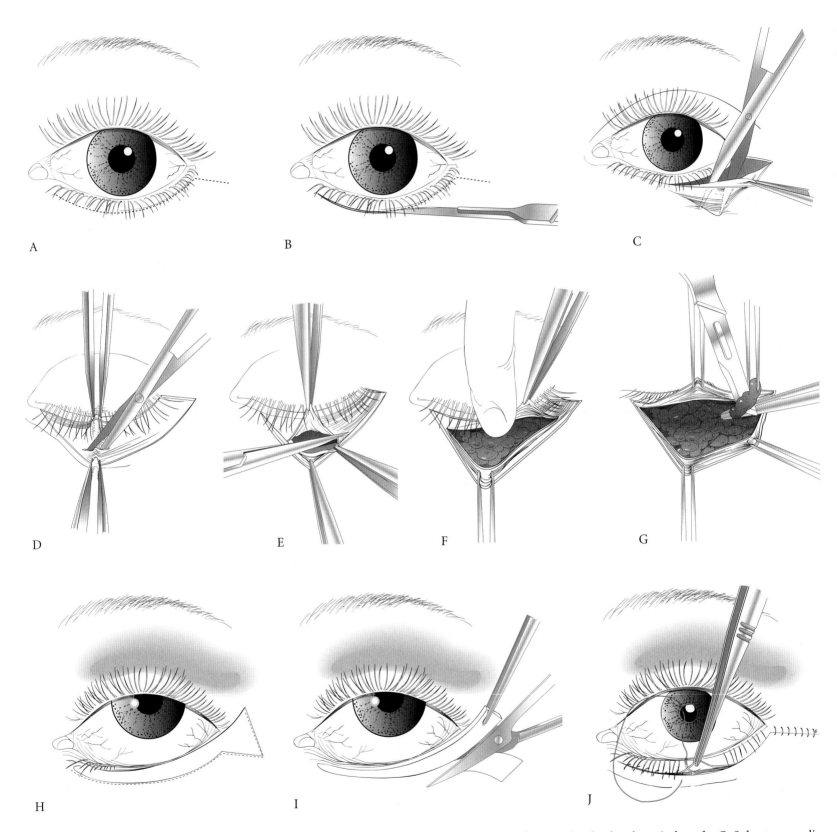

FIGURE 64-22 *Transcutaneous lower eyelid blepharoplasty. A, Surgical marking. B, Skin incision along previously placed surgical marks. C, Subcutaneous dissection. D, Orbicularis incision beneath the inferior tarsal border. E, Extension of orbicularis incision to achieve full length of skin incision. F, Gentle globe ballottement to expose herniated fat after orbital septal incision. G, Herniated fat treatment after incision of overlying fat pad capsule. H, Determination of redundant skin and orbicularis. I, Excision of redundant tissue. J, Skin closure after orbicularis fixation and orbicularis closure. Adapted from Putterman AM.[48]*

inferior conjunctiva and lower lid retractors and fixed superiorly to aid in exposure. An incision through the conjunctiva and the lower eyelid retractors is made approximately halfway from the inferior border of tarsus and the inferior fornix. The incision is extended medially beneath the punctum and laterally nearly to the lateral canthus. The lower lid is next retracted anteriorly and inferiorly to facilitate isolation of the three fat pads, which are further defined by blunt dissection through the capsulopalpebral fascia. The inferior oblique muscle should be identified between the central and medial fat pads. Care should be taken to avoid aggressive or sharp dissection that may induce injury to the muscle. Fat removal or sculpting is next performed beginning with the lateral fat pad. As described above gentle ballottement of the globe aids in orbital fat prolapse. The herniating fat is carefully grasped and excised. Some surgeons favor clamping the fat during excision. Meticulous hemostasis is essential during fat pad excision. After fat pad debulking the anterior border of the fat pads should be flush with the inferior orbital rim. Overzealous fat pad excision risks a postoperative hollow appearance.

The superior traction suture is removed prior to closing the conjunctiva. Complete hemostasis should be confirmed before closure is attempted. The conjunctiva and lower eyelid retractors are reapproximated with two or three buried interrupted sutures of 6-0 or 7-0 polyglactin or other suture. Several important aspects of transconjunctival lower eyelid blepharoplasty are demonstrated in Figure 64-23.

Skin Pinch Excision Transconjunctival lower lid blepharoplasty does not address excess lower lid skin, making skin pinch excision a useful adjunct for small amounts of excess lower lid skin. Significant excessive lower lid skin is identified using the aforementioned pinch test. Local anesthesia is next injected and the pinch

test is performed again, taking care to place the tine of the forceps within a pre-existing skin fold and create a pinched off ridge of tissue to be removed. The redundant skin is then excised using curved scissors. The skin is closed using 6-0 fast-absorbing gut suture in a running fashion.

Lateral Canthopexy A time-honored procedure for lateral canthopexy is the lateral strip procedure, which entails determining the amount of horizontal excess of lower eyelid (part of which is used as the tarsal strip), dividing the lower lid of the strip at the gray line, and removing the anterior lamella, conjunctiva, cilia, and lid margin–associated glands.[73] Desired lower lid position is determined and a suture on a semicircular needle is used to fasten the tarsal strip to the periosteum inside the lateral orbital rim at a level to yield the optimal postoperative lower lid location and apposition of lower eyelid to the globe. A canthal reformation suture is passed through the gray line of the upper eyelid and the tarsal strip to recreate the lateral canthal angle. The orbicularis is closed using buried interrupted absorbable suture. Fast-absorbing gut suture is used to close the skin.

Midfacial Rejuvenation Standard lower eyelid blepharoplasty does not address midfacial aging changes often present in the blepharoplasty patient. Hamra proposed an arcus marginalis release procedure to recreate the contour of the youthful lower lid and cheek.[77] The procedure entails creating a skin-muscle flap, incision of the arcus marginalis at the orbital rim, and removal of a portion of the inferior orbital septum, with subsequent reposition and fixation of the orbital fat over the orbital rim.[77] A transconjunctival approach to the arcus marginalis with similar transposition of orbital fat has recently been advocated.[78] Elevation of the soft tissue of the midface by suture plication using transcuta-

neous, subperiosteal, transconjunctival, and supraperiosteal routes has also been described.[79,80]

Steinsapir recently reported the use of a hand-carved expanded polytetrafluoroethylene orbital rim as both a site for resuspension of the midfacial soft tissues and a mechanism to compensate for lost midface volume.[81]

Postoperative Management

Postoperative instructions seek to limit edema and ecchymosis and prevent postoperative bleeding.

Ice-cold compresses are placed over the operative site immediately on arrival in the postoperative recovery area. These compresses should be used continuously for 36 to 48 hours after the procedure with cessation only for dining and bathroom breaks. After 48 hours warm compresses may be used for comfort and to hasten resolution of edema. Up to 4 weeks should be allowed for resolution of bruising, although the majority of patients note limited discoloration beyond 1 week. Complete resolution of edema may require several weeks.

During the first 48 to 72 hours minimal physical activity is recommended. Patients should remain supine with approximately 30 degrees of head elevation provided by pillows or a recliner. Walking and low impact activities can be resumed after postoperative days 2 to 3, although refraining from strenuous physical activity for the first week postoperatively is strongly recommended. During weeks 2 and 3, activity may gradually be increased. In general most patients require 1 to 2 weeks off from work including the operative day. For patients with physically intense occupations, longer time away is required.

Application of a combination antibiotic and steroid ointment to any dermal incision site is recommended. Keeping the absorbable sutures moist allows for their timely dissolution. A typical schedule includes three times per day application for

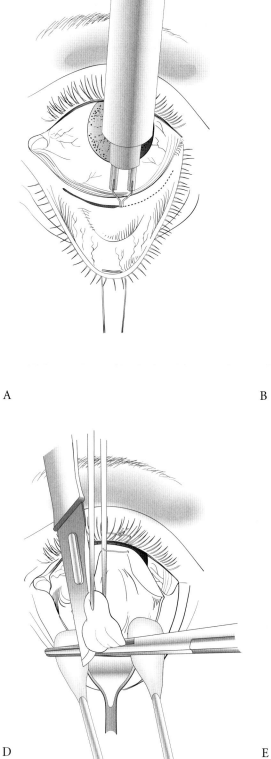

A

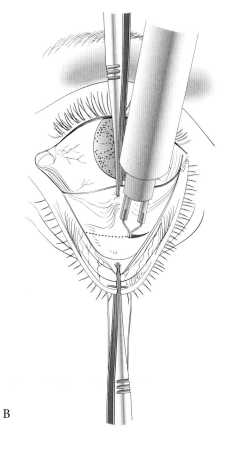

B

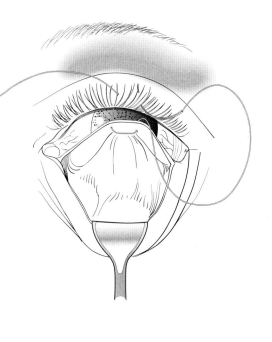

C

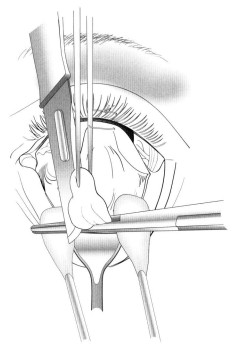

D

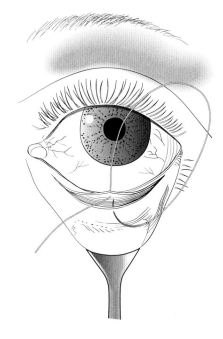

E

FIGURE **64-23** *Transconjunctival lower eyelid blepharoplasty. A, Incision through conjunctiva. B, Incision through lower eyelid retractors. C, Placement of a superior traction suture. D, Treatment of herniating orbital fat. E, Reapproximation of the conjunctiva after reapproximation of the lower eyelid retractors. Adapted from Putterman AM.[48]*

the first week, with taper to twice daily application in the second week and application four times daily in the third week. Transconjunctival incision sites should be lubricated with an antibiotic ointment in a similar schedule. Application of makeup to the incision sites should be deferred 1 week.

Postoperative pain is usually not a significant concern. Nonetheless a prescription for several tablets of a low potency opioid and acetaminophen combination analgesic may be provided. Acetaminophen should be sufficient for the majority of patients. Routine aspirin and nonsteroidal anti-inflammatory drug use can be resumed several days postoperatively. Warfarin may be restarted on the day after surgery. Excessive postoperative discomfort should be investigated as it may herald an orbital hemorrhage or other complications.

The patient is advised to trim short loose absorbable skin sutures. Care should be taken to avoid rubbing the incisions or vertically stressing the incisions with digital traction when attempting to open the eyes. The buried absorbable sutures may occasionally be palpated postoperatively as small nodules along the incision for as long as 5 to 6 weeks. Occasionally these buried sutures may surface and require trimming.

Follow-up evaluation 1 week postoperatively is typical, with additional visits scheduled as needed. Postoperative photography is typically obtained approximately 4 months after the procedure.

Management of Complications

Complications following blepharoplasty are either cosmetic, functional, or vision-threatening. The majority of complications can be readily prevented by clear preoperative communication, careful preoperative and intraoperative measurements, and meticulous surgical technique. Prior to pursuing surgery all the major possible complications should be discussed with the patient.

Complications of Upper Eyelid Blepharoplasty

Inadequate Skin Excision A common postoperative cosmetic concern, inadequate skin excision manifests as a second fold superior to the upper eyelid crease. Previously unrecognized eyebrow ptosis may contribute to the appearance of excess skin, especially laterally, and should therefore be assessed. When a true excess of upper lid skin is present, careful additional resection of skin and orbicularis is indicated. In general revision blepharoplasty should be delayed for several months to allow resolution of edema.

Excessive Skin Excision Overzealous removal of upper eyelid skin may result in cosmetic as well as functional concerns. Patients may describe a tight sensation in their lids, demonstrate lagophthalmos, or display symptoms and signs of exposure keratitis. Like most complications, excessive skin excision is best prevented as subsequent management is challenging. Lid massage, consisting of vigorous downward massage on the anterior tarsal surface, instituted 1 to 2 weeks postoperatively, can resolve mild cases. The patient is advised to blink fully and use artificial tears during the day and ophthalmic ointment at night. More significant over-resection of skin may require full-thickness skin grafting, commonly performed after 6 months to allow for more complete wound healing. Retroauricular skin is frequently used as a graft site for eyelid reconstruction. Care must be taken to properly thin the graft. If possible the graft placement should be superior to the lid incision to lessen cosmetic impact.

Lid Crease Asymmetry Raising an inferior lid crease is easier than lowering an excessively high crease; therefore, unless the higher crease; is abnormally elevated, the lower crease should be raised to achieve symmetry. Removing a crescent of skin and muscle above the low crease, with care to make the inferior edge (the new location of the lid crease) symmetric with the opposite crease, lysing any attachments inferior to the new crease location, and closing the ellipse by incorporating several stitches through the levator aponeurosis recreates the new lid crease.[48]

High Lid Creases Successfully lowering an excessively high lid crease is difficult. The adhesions forming the current lid crease must be interrupted and an incision made for the new crease closed by suture bites through the levator aponeurosis and the new incision wound edges. In some cases orbicularis muscle transposition from above can prevent the original skin crease adherence to the underlying fibrous tissue. A fat graft between the orbital septum and levator aponeurosis may be required to prevent adhesions.[82]

Excessive Fat Removal A deep medial concavity or superior sulcus results from aggressive medial fat removal. Injection of autogenous fat or dermal fat grafting has been attempted to augment an excessively hollow superior sulcus. Careful conservative fat excision is warranted to avoid superior sulcus syndrome, especially in males, as creation of a deep sulcus feminizes the eyelid.

Wound Dehiscence Wound dehiscence is best handled by resuturing the eyelid if the area of dehiscence is greater than several millimeters in length. Small areas of dehiscence can be allowed to granulate if granulation does not impair final scar cosmesis. If re-approximation is performed the wound bed should be scraped free of granulation tissue and the edges trimmed to expose fresh tissue prior to the second closure. Surgical closure should include adequate muscular closure to minimize this complication.

Suture Milia Suture milia are small cystic epithelial inclusions occurring at suture entrance points into the skin. Common and temporary, suture milia appear approximately 1 week postoperatively and disappear over the ensuing months. Hot compresses may hasten milia resolution. Alternatively a large bore needle or scissors can be used to create an opening in the cyst to aid in healing.

Postoperative Ptosis Injury to the levator aponeurosis through direct intraoperative trauma or from stretching by postoperative hematoma may result in postoperative ptosis.[83] Recent anatomic dissections evidencing terminal branches of the superior division of the oculomotor nerve far anterior in the levator palpebrae superioris muscle prompted speculation that infiltrating local anesthetics affecting these end branches may induce transient ptosis.[84] Mild postoperative ptosis (2 mm or less) from eyelid edema can be observed for spontaneous resolution. Poor levator function or severe ptosis warrants timely surgical exploration, as the fibrotic phase of healing will complicate repair. Surgical correction of prolonged ptosis can be accomplished with a conjunctival Müllerectomy, or external levator repair in mild cases, and levator aponeurosis advancement in more extensive cases.

Dry Eye Symptoms   Dry eye symptoms are a frequent complication of blepharoplasty due to altered lid function and decreased spontaneous blink rate and magnitude. Topical artificial teardrops and lubricating ointment are often sufficient for symptom control, although punctal occlusion may be warranted in the setting of more severe dry eye symptoms. Punctal occlusion at the time of blepharoplasty in patients with dry eye syndrome may be of some benefit in decreasing postoperative exacerbation of symptoms.[85]

Diplopia   Injury to the superior oblique tendon or trochlea, although uncommon, has been described following upper blepharoplasty with medial fat excision.[86,87] Poor visualization during cautery or dissection was implicated during reported cases.[86,87] Recent anatomic dissections confirm a consistent relationship between the trochlea and superior orbital foramen and the superior oblique tendon and the frontozygomatic suture.[88] Direct visualization during cautery and dissection coupled with familiarity of associated anatomy decreases the risk of tendon or trochlear damage.

Bleeding   Intraoperative and postoperative bleeding can be vision-threatening complications. Patients should be instructed to discontinue aspirin, nonsteroidal anti-inflammatory drugs, and other platelet-impairing medications 1 to 2 weeks preoperatively. Warfarin is generally withheld 4 days preoperatively. Intraoperative bleeding often results from the orbicularis muscle. Recent evidence suggests a prominent arterial branch, which pierces the orbital septum and levator aponeurosis at the upper aspect of the tarsus, may account for excessive bleeding if damaged when the septum is opened for fat excision.[89]

Aside from causing significant ecchymosis, insufficient hemostasis can result in retrobulbar hemorrhage or hematoma and concomitant loss of vision.[90,91] Many patients will describe a small degree of bruising and swelling postoperatively, often beginning after a sneeze, cough, or in the setting of hypertension. Significant pain, proptosis, marked upper lid swelling, restricted extraocular motions, and/or any decrease in vision raises suspicion for a retrobulbar hemorrhage, a true emergency requiring immediate bedside wound release with or without a lateral canthotomy and cantholysis, hyperosmotic agents, and systemic corticosteroids.

Hematoma presents with severe ecchymosis and eyelid edema. Visual compromise may be present if the lids are tense. Since compression of the globe and optic nerve is of concern, intraocular pressure (IOP) should be measured. If no visual deterioration or increase in IOP is found, conservative management with ice-cold compresses can be used. Visual compromise or increased IOP may necessitate a return to the operating room to reopen the incision site, evacuate any clots, and address the source of bleeding.

Vision Loss   Most cases of vision loss after blepharoplasty are due to hemorrhage or hematoma formation with resultant optic nerve damage or central retinal artery occlusion.[90,92] Angle-closure glaucoma following blepharoplasty has also been reported.[93] Instructing patients to monitor their vision and promptly responding to all patient reports of excessive pain best detect these complications.

Complications of Lower Eyelid Blepharoplasty

Lower Eyelid Retraction   Eyelid malposition after lower lid blepharoplasty has several etiologies: excessive anterior lamella removal, scarring of the orbital septum, inadequate treatment of lower eyelid laxity, or hematoma-associated fibrosis. Delayed lower eyelid retraction resulting from scarring of the orbital septum is largely associated with the anterior approach to lower eyelid blepharoplasty. A posterior approach avoiding incision of the orbital septum has been demonstrated to minimize lower eyelid retraction.[94] Lower eyelid retraction is a more frequent complication in patients with shallow orbits and prominent eyes.

Initial treatment of lower eyelid retraction varies with extent and duration of altered lid position. Early identification of retraction warrants conservative treatment such as vigorous upward massage, placement of temporary traction sutures, or a temporary tarsorrhaphy suture.[95] Postoperative edema may contribute to early postoperative retraction, emphasizing the importance of a period of watchful waiting and conservative therapy.

Persistant retraction resistant to conservative measures can be treated with septal scar tissue lysis and lateral canthopexy. Scar lysis is accomplished by dissection between the orbicularis and septum via an incision associated with a lateral canthotomy.[96] Lateral canthopexy is usually performed using the lateral tarsal strip approach as described previously.[73] Temporary suspension of the lower eyelid to the brow has been proposed to provide further upward traction.[96]

Severe lower eyelid retraction may necessitate posterior lamella extension with a hard palate mucosal or ear cartilage graft, often with a horizontal tightening procedure.[96–99] The palpebral conjunctiva and lower eyelid retractors are incised and recessed. Through a palpebral conjunctival incision inferior to the lower tarsal border, the orbicularis is exposed and the graft sutured inferior to the tarsus in the recipient bed.

Lower Eyelid Ectropion Often symptomatic due to drying of the exposed conjunctiva, lower lid ectropion may exist alone or in combination with lower lid retraction. If previously unappreciated lid laxity is present, horizontal tightening is performed as previously described. A deficit of anterior lamella is addressed using a full-thickness skin graft harvested from the upper eyelid or retroauricular area. Grafts must be sized larger than the ideal final size to accommodate postoperative contracture.

Inadequate Fat Removal Further excision of lower eyelid fat should be addressed through a posterior approach to avoid excessive cutaneous scar formation and lower lid malposition. Often the lateral lower eyelid fat pad is implicated.

Excessive Fat Removal A tear trough deformity, the lower lid analog to the upper lid superior sulcus syndrome, describes a prominent inferior orbital rim and nasojugal fold that may result from aggressive lower lid fat removal. Injection of autologous fat into the deformity, particularly directed at the underlying musculature, has been attempted to address the tear trough deformity.[100,101] Eyelid fibrosis with decreased mobility is associated with excessive fat removal and multiple surgical interventions.

Diplopia Diplopia may result after both transcutaneous and transconjunctival lower lid blepharoplasty due to direct and indirect injury of the inferior oblique and inferior rectus.[87,102] Inferior oblique injury should be suspected in patients complaining of vertical diplopia increasing in gaze contralateral to the operated eye. Recent anatomic dissections demonstrate a consistent relationship between the inferior oblique muscle and the inferior orbital rim, infraorbital foramen, and supraorbital notch.[103] Precise anatomic knowledge coupled with avoidance of an excessively inferior conjunctival incision and care when treating prolapsed fat are recommended to avoid extraocular muscle injury.

Bleeding As previously discussed with complications of upper lid blepharoplasty, hemostasis is critical in blepharoplasty to avoid postoperative retrobulbar hemorrhage and hematoma formation.

Vision Loss Causes of vision loss after lower eyelid blepharoplasty are similar to those described with upper eyelid blepharoplasty.

Adjunctive Procedures

Chemical Peeling

Chemical peeling, or chemexfoliation, involves using a chemical agent to wound the epidermis and dermis, thereby evoking an inflammatory healing response that acts to improve skin texture. The level of the peel is dictated by the depth of penetration, nature of destruction, and inflammatory response. A variety of agents may be employed, most commonly trichloroacetic acid (TCA), glycolic acid, or phenol, and the concentration of the chemical agent varies depending on the depth of peel desired.[104] In general more severe rhytids or skin texture problems require a deeper peel to achieve the desired effect. Medium-depth TCA chemexfoliation in conjunction with transconjunctival lower eyelid blepharoplasty has been demonstrated to achieve excellent results in improving lower eyelid skin appearance.[105]

Evaluating a blepharoplasty patient for chemexfoliation requires additional appreciation of skin pigmentation, often using the Fitzpatrick skin pigment type classification, inquiry into history of herpes simplex infection, and knowledge of the patient's need to return to social activities.[47] Previous herpes infections may require prophylaxis with antiviral agents. Patients with higher Fitzpatrick skin types, extensive sun exposure, or diffuse freckling may have unacceptable scarring, hypopigmentation, or noticeable demarcation borders of treated skin and hence should be considered with caution.[106]

Chemexfoliation relies on even application of the peeling agent to the intended treatment area. Pretreatment of the treatment area with retinoic acid can be performed to enhance uptake. Any skin oil or greases will impair even chemical treatment, making careful soap and water skin cleansing and acetone degreasing crucial to a successful peel. Chemical peeling should follow completion of blepharoplasty surgery. The peel is applied to the skin using sturdy cotton-tipped applicators, with care taken to achieve symmetric application, avoid inadvertent corneal application, and treat more lightly those areas with the thinnest skin (ie, medial canthal and pretarsal skin). Initially a white frost becomes apparent after chemical application, which gives way to deep erythema. Cold compresses to the treated area after the skin has dried may decrease discomfort. A bland lubricating ointment should be applied to treated skin prior to the patient leaving the postoperative recovery area. Postoperative care for patients undergoing chemical peel requires twice to four times daily mild soap cleansing, gentle patting to dry, and ointment re-application until all treated skin has reepithelialized. Sun exposure, which may cause skin burning and hyperpigmentation, should be avoided meticulously by wearing a hat and dark sunglasses during the first month. Careful sunscreen application is advised thereafter.

Complications of chemexfoliation include pigmentary change, scarring or other textural changes, corneal damage, lid position abnormalities, infection, prolonged erythema, acne, and cold sensitivity.

Laser Skin Resurfacing

Laser skin resurfacing employs a CO_2 or erbium laser to thermally remove a defined layer of dermal tissue and shrink collagen, prompting improved skin appearance through collagen contraction, new collagen formation, and remodeling and epidermal growth. The number of passes taken determines the depth of treatment. Laser resurfacing is ideal for patients with minimally pigmented skin who seek improvement of skin with photodamage or acne scarring.[107] Adjunctive CO_2 laser resurfacing of the lower eyelid in conjunction with transconjunctival lower lid blepharoplasty has been demonstrated to successfully address lower eyelid wrinkling that may result from transconjunctival blepharoplasty alone.[108] When compared to a phenol chemical peel, CO_2 laser resurfacing was found to be equally as efficacious in diminishing rhytids in thin-skinned facial areas and more effective at improving texture in thicker glandular facial areas.[109] The erbium:yttrium-aluminum-garnet (YAG) laser has been recently introduced as an alternative method of laser skin resurfacing.

History and physical elements to be explored are similar to those described for patients being evaluated for chemexfoliation. Additionally past use of isotretinoin (accutane) should be obtained, as the drug-induced elimination of glandular architecture contraindicates laser resurfacing for the subsequent 1 to 2 years following drug discontinuation.[110] Prior to undergoing laser resurfacing, patients predisposed to hyperpigmentation are typically treated for several weeks with a skin bleaching agent. Prophylactic antivirals and antibiotics are also commonly employed.

Surgical marking plays a critical role in successful laser resurfacing by providing a roadmap to direct treatment application. After carefully marking all significant rhytids, general anesthesia or monitored sedation coupled with proper local or regional nerve block anesthesia is achieved. Resurfacing is performed using laser settings determined by the area of interest. Resurfacing is carried out methodically, taking care to wipe the ablated tissue away prior to re-treatment to avoid excessive heat absorbance in any given location. Generally one or two passes with lower power are performed on periocular skin.[110] Color change indicates depth of treatment, progressing from pink to orange to yellow-orange to yellow-white as more passes are made or more energy is used per pass. Excessive treatment risks hypertrophic scarring. After procedure completion the skin is irrigated, gently patted dry, and a dry occlusive or wet dressing is applied. Many surgeons have abandoned occlusive dressings in favor of simply keeping the face well lubricated with a bland lubricant such as petroleum jelly. Dilute vinegar and water soaks are favored by many for cleansing. Dressings are changed daily with additional lubrication ointment applied until reepithelialization occurs, generally after 10 to 14 days. Antibiotic ointment is occasionally used; however, the risk of inducing allergies to the applied antibiotic has lessened the frequency of this practice. Ice packs are used postoperatively to reduce edema. Complications are similar to chemexfoliation.

References

1. Katzen LB. The history of cosmetic oculoplastic surgery. In: Putterman AM, editor. Cosmetic oculoplastic surgery: eyelid, forehead, and facial techniques. 3rd ed. Philadelphia (PA): W.B. Saunders; 1999. p. 3–10.
2. Albert DM, Edwards DD. The history of ophthalmology. Cambridge (MA): Blackwell Science; 1996.
3. Glogau RG. Physiologic and structural changes associated with aging skin. Dermatol Clin 1997;15:555–9.
4. Flowers RS. Blepharoplasty. In: Courtiss EH, editor. Male aesthetic surgery. St. Louis (MO): Mosby; 1982.
5. Freund RM, Nolan WB 3rd. Correlation between brow lift outcomes and aesthetic ideals for eyebrow height and shape in females. Plast Reconstr Surg 1996;97:1343–8.
6. Lemke BN, Stasior OG. The anatomy of eyebrow ptosis. Arch Ophthalmol 1982;100:981–6.
7. Mitz V, Peyronie M. The superficial musculoaponeurotic system (SMAS) in the parotid and cheek area. Plast Reconstr Surg 1976;58:80–8.
8. Kikkawa DO, Lemke BN, Dortzbach RK. Relations of the superficial musculoaponeurotic system to the orbit and characterization of the orbitomalar ligament. Ophthal Plast Reconstr Surg 1996;12:77–88.
9. Furnas DW. The retaining ligaments of the cheek. Plast Reconstr Surg 1989;83:11–6.
10. Hamra ST. Repositioning the orbicularis oculi muscle in the composite rhytidectomy [comment]. Plast Reconstr Surg 1992;90:14–22.
11. Owsley JQ. Lifting the malar fat pad for correction of prominent nasolabial folds [comment]. Plast Reconstr Surg 1993;91:463–74; discussion 75–6.
12. Lucarelli MJ, Khwarg SI, Lemke BN, et al. The anatomy of midfacial ptosis. Ophthal Plast Reconstr Surg 2000;16:7–22.
13. Ozdemir R, Kilinc H, Unlu RE, et al. Anatomicohistologic study of the retaining ligaments of the face and use in face lift: retaining ligament correction and SMAS plication. Plast Reconstr Surg 2002; 110:1134–47; discussion 1148–9.
14. Pessa JE, Zadoo VP, Mutimer KL, et al. Relative maxillary retrusion as a natural consequence of aging: combining skeletal and soft-tissue changes into an integrated model of midfacial aging. Plast Reconstr Surg 1998;102:205–12.
15. Pessa JE, Desvigne LD, Lambros VS, et al. Changes in ocular globe-to-orbital rim position with age: implications for aesthetic blepharoplasty of the lower eyelids. Aesthet Plast Surg 1999;23:337–42.
16. Jeong S, Lemke BN, Dortzbach RK, et al. The Asian upper eyelid: an anatomical study with comparison to the Caucasian eyelid. Arch Ophthalmol 1999;117:907–12.
17. DeBacker CM, Putterman AM, Zhou L, et al. Age-related changes in type-I collagen synthesis in human eyelid skin. Ophthal Plast Reconstr Surg 1998;14:13–6.
18. van den Bosch WA, Leenders I, Mulder P. Topographic anatomy of the eyelids, and the effects of sex and age. Br J Ophthalmol 1999;83:347–52.
19. Siegel R. Surgical anatomy of the upper eyelid fascia. Ann Plast Surg 1984;13:263–73.
20. Stasior GO, Lemke BN, Wallow IH, Dortzbach RK. Levator aponeurosis elastic fiber

network. Ophthal Plast Reconstr Surg 1993;9:1–10.

21. Cartwright MJ, Kurumety UR, Nelson CC, et al. Measurements of upper eyelid and eyebrow dimensions in healthy white individuals. Am J Ophthalmol 1994;117:231–4.

22. Shorr N, Cohen MS. Cosmetic blepharoplasty. Ophthalmol Clin North Am 1991;4:17–33.

23. Han MH, Kwon ST. A statistical study of upper eyelids of Korean young women. Korean J Plast Surg 1992;19:930–5.

24. Chen WP. Upper blepharoplasty in the Asian patient. In: Putterman AM, editor. Cosmetic oculoplastic surgery: eyelid, forehead, and facial techniques. 3rd ed. Philadelphia (PA): W.B. Saunders; 1999. p. 101–12.

25. Chen WP. Asian blepharoplasty. Update on anatomy and techniques. Ophthal Plast Reconstr Surg 1987;3:135–40.

26. Hawes MJ, Dortzbach RK. The microscopic anatomy of the lower eyelid retractors. Arch Ophthalmol 1982;100:1313–8.

27. Meyer DR, Linberg JV, Wobig JL, McCormick SA. Anatomy of the orbital septum and associated eyelid connective tissues. Implications for ptosis surgery [comment]. Ophthal Plast Reconstr Surg 1991;7:104–13.

28. Wesley RE, McCord CD Jr, Jones NA. Height of the tarsus of the lower eyelid. Am J Ophthalmol 1980; 90:102–5.

29. Anderson RL. Medial canthal tendon branches out. Arch Ophthalmol 1977;95:2051–2.

30. Gionia VM, Linberg JV, McCormick SA. The anatomy of the lateral canthal tendon. Arch Ophthalmol 1987;105:529–32.

31. Whitnall SE. The anatomy of the human orbit and accessory organs of vision. London, England: Oxford University Press; 1932.

32. Whitnall SE. On a ligament acting as a check to the action of the levator palpebrae superioris muscle. J Anat Physiol 1910;14:131.

33. Goldberg RA, Wu JC, Jesmanowicz A, Hyde JS. Eyelid anatomy revisited. Dynamic high-resolution magnetic resonance images of Whitnall's ligament and upper eyelid structures with the use of a surface coil [comment]. Arch Ophthalmol 1992;110:1598–600.

34. Codere F, Tucker NA, Renaldi B. The anatomy of Whitnall ligament. Ophthalmology 1995;102:2016–9.

35. Lucarelli MJ, Dartt DA, Cook BE Jr, et al. The lacrimal system. In: Kaufman PL, editor. Adler's physiology of the eye. 10th ed. St. Louis (MO): Mosby; 2003. p. 723.

36. Putterman AM, Urist MJ. Muller's muscle-conjunctival resection ptosis procedure. Ophthal Surg 1978;9:27–32.

37. Dresner SC. Further modifications of the Muller's muscle-conjunctival resection procedure for blepharoptosis. Ophthal Plast Reconstr Surg 1991;7:114–22.

38. Brown MS, Putterman AM. The effect of upper blepharoplasty on eyelid position when performed concomitantly with Muller muscle-conjunctival resection. Ophthal Plast Reconstr Surg 2000;16:94–100.

39. Sires BS, Lemke BN, Dortzbach RK, Gonnering RS. Characterization of human orbital fat and connective tissue. Ophthal Plast Reconstr Surg 1998;14:403–14.

40. Sutcliffe T, Baylis HI, Fett D. Bleeding in cosmetic blepharoplasty: an anatomical approach. Ophthal Plast Reconstr Surg 1985;1:107–13.

41. Kikkawa DO, Lemke BN. Orbital and eyelid anatomy. In: Dortzbach RK, editor. Ophthalmic plastic surgery: prevention and management of complications. New York (NY): Raven Press; 1994. p. 1–29.

42. Cook BE Jr, Lucarelli MJ, Lemke BN, et al. Eyelid lymphatics I: histochemical comparisons between the monkey and human. Ophthal Plast Reconstr Surg 2002;18:18–23.

43. Cook BE Jr, Lucarelli MJ, Lemke BN, et al. Eyelid lymphatics II: a search for drainage patterns in the monkey and correlations with human lymphatics. Ophthal Plast Reconstr Surg 2002;18:99–106.

44. Knize DM. Muscles that act on glabellar skin: a closer look. Plast Reconstr Surg 2000; 105:350–61.

45. Knize DM. A study of the supraorbital nerve. Plast Reconstr Surg 1995;96:564–9.

46. Tarbet KJ, Lemke BN. Clinical anatomy of the upper face. Int Ophthalmol Clin 1997; 37:11–28.

47. Fitzpatrick TB. The validity and practicality of sun-reactive skin types I through VI. Arch Dermatol 1988;124:869–71.

48. Putterman AM, editor. Cosmetic oculoplastic surgery: eyelid, forehead, and facial techniques. 3rd ed. Philadelphia (PA): W.B. Saunders; 1999.

49. Fante RG, Elner VM. Transcaruncular approach to medial canthal tendon plication for lower eyelid laxity. Ophthal Plast Reconstr Surg 2001;17:16–27.

50. Furnas DW. Festoons, mounds, and bags of the eyelids and cheek. Clin Plast Surg 1993; 20:367–85.

51. van Bijsterveld OP. Diagnostic tests in the Sicca syndrome. Arch Ophthalmol 1969;82:10–4.

52. Hurwitz JJ. The lacrimal system. Philadelphia (PA): Lippincott-Raven; 1996.

53. McKinney P, Byun M. The value of tear film breakup and Schirmer's tests in preoperative blepharoplasty evaluation. Plast Reconstr Surg 1999;104:566–9; discussion 570–3.

54. Tarbet KJ. Ophthalmic evaluation should be a preoperative requirement prior to blepharoplasty [comment]. Arch Otolaryngol Head Neck Surg 2001;127:723.

55. Pastorek N. Preoperative ophthalmic evaluation is a personal choice [comment]. Arch Otolaryngol Head Neck Surg 2001;127:724.

56. Burke AJ, Wang T. Should formal ophthalmologic evaluation be a preoperative requirement prior to blepharoplasty? [comment] Arch Otolaryngol Head Neck Surg 2001; 127:719–22.

57. Murphy PJ, Patel S, Marshall J. The effect of long-term, daily contact lens wear on corneal sensitivity. Cornea 2001;20:264–9.

58. Patel S, Perez-Santonja JJ, Alio JL, Murphy PJ. Corneal sensitivity and some properties of the tear film after laser in situ keratomileusis. J Refract Surg 2001;17:17–24.

59. Chuck RS, Quiros PA, Perez AC, McDonnell PJ. Corneal sensation after laser in situ keratomileusis [comment]. J Cataract Refract Surg 2000;26:337–9.

60. Silver B. Photographing the blepharoplasty patient. In: Putterman AM, editor. Cosmetic oculoplastic surgery eyelid, forehead, and facial techniques. 3rd ed. Philadelphia (PA): W.B. Saunders; 1999. p. 39–46.

61. Steinbrook RA, Hughes N, Fanciullo G, et al. Effects of alkalinization of lidocaine on the pain of skin infiltration and intravenous catheterization. J Clin Anesth 1993;5:456–8.

62. Petrelli RL. The treatment of lacrimal gland prolapse in blepharoplasty. Ophthal Plast Reconstr Surg 1988;4:139–42.

63. Leone CR. Treatment of a prolapsed lacrimal gland. In: Putterman AM, editor. Cosmetic oculoplastic surgery eyelid, forehead, and facial techniques. 3rd ed. Philadelphia (PA): W.B. Saunders; 1999. p. 169–78.

64. Greene D, Koch RJ, Goode RL. Efficacy of octyl-2-cyanoacrylate tissue glue in blepharoplasty. A prospective controlled study of wound-healing characteristics. Arch Facial Plast Surg 1999;1:292–6.

65. Januszkiewicz JS, Nahai F. Transconjunctival upper blepharoplasty [comment]. Plast Reconstr Surg 1999;103:1015–8; discussion 1019.

66. Guerra AB, Berger A 3rd, Black EB 3rd, et al. The bare area of the upper conjunctiva: a closer look at the anatomy of transconjunctival upper blepharoplasty. Plast Reconstr Surg 2003;111:1717–22.

67. Guerra AB, Metzinger SE, Black EB 3rd. Transconjunctival upper blepharoplasty: a safe and effective addition to facial rejuvenation techniques. Ann Plast Surg 2002; 48:528–33.

68. Mikamo M. Plastic operation of the eyelid. J Chugaii Jishimpo 1896;17:1197.

69. Zubiri JS. Correction of the Oriental eyelid. Clin Plast Surg 1981;8:725–37.

70. Kikkawa DO, Kim JW. Asian blepharoplasty. Int Ophthalmol Clin 1997;37:193–204.

71. Weng CJ, Noordhoff MS. Complications of Oriental blepharoplasty. Plast Reconstr Surg 1989;83:622–8.

72. Kikkawa DO, Kim JW. Lower-eyelid blepharoplasty. Int Ophthalmol Clin 1997;37:163–78.

73. Anderson RL, Gordy DD. The tarsal strip procedure. Arch Ophthalmol 1979;97:2192–6.

74. Fagien S. Algorithm for canthoplasty: the lateral retinacular suspension: a simplified suture canthopexy [comment]. Plast Reconstr Surg 1999;103:2042–53; discussion 2054–8.

75. Lemke BN, Cook BE Jr, Lucarelli MJ. Canthus-sparing ectropion repair. Ophthal Plast Reconstr Surg 2001;17:161–8.

76. Nerad JA. The requisites in ophthalmology: oculoplastic surgery. St. Louis (MO): Mosby; 2001.

77. Hamra ST. Arcus marginalis release and orbital fat preservation in midface rejuvenation [comment]. Plast Reconstr Surg 1995; 96:354–62.

78. Goldberg RA. Transconjunctival orbital fat repositioning: transposition of orbital fat pedicles into a subperiosteal pocket. Plast Reconstr Surg 2000;105: 743–8; discussion 749–51.

79. Hester TR, Codner MA, McCord CD, et al. Evolution of technique of the direct trans-blepharoplasty approach for the correction of lower lid and midfacial aging: maximizing results and minimizing complications in a 5-year experience. Plast Reconstr Surg 2000;105:393–406.

80. Freeman MS. Transconjunctival sub-orbicularis oculi fat (SOOF) pad lift blepharoplasty: a new technique for the effacement of nasojugal deformity [comment]. Arch Facial Plast Surg 2000;2:16–21.

81. Steinsapir KD. Aesthetic and restorative midface lifting with hand-carved, expanded polytetrafluoroethylene orbital rim implants. Plast Reconstr Surg 2003;111:1727–37; discussion 1738–41.

82. Shorr N, Christenbury JD, Goldberg RA. Free autogenous "pearl fat" grafts to the eyelids. Ophthal Plast Reconstr Surg 1988;4:37–40.

83. Baylis HI, Sutcliffe T, Fett DR. Levator injury during blepharoplasty. Arch Ophthalmol 1984;102:570–1.

84. Hwang K, Lee DK, Chung IH, Lee SI. Patterns of oculomotor nerve distribution to the levator palpebrae superioris muscle, and correlation to temporary ptosis after blepharoplasty. Ann Plast Surg 2001;47:381–4.

85. Becker BB. Punctal occlusion and blepharoplasty in patients with dry eye syndrome. Arch Otolaryngol Head Neck Surg 1991;117:789–91.

86. Wesley RE, Pollard ZF, McCord CD Jr. Superior oblique paresis after blepharoplasty. Plast Reconstr Surg 1980;66:283–6.

87. Harley RD, Nelson LB, Flanagan JC, Calhoun JH. Ocular motility disturbances following cosmetic blepharoplasty. Arch Ophthalmol 1986;104:542–4.

88. Wilhelmi BJ, Mowlavi A, Neumeister MW. Upper blepharoplasty with bony anatomical landmarks to avoid injury to trochlea and superior oblique muscle tendon with fat resection. Plast Reconstr Surg 2001;108:2137–40; discussion 2141–2.

89. Hwang K, Kim BG, Kim YJ, Chung IH. Lateral septoaponeurotic artery: source of bleeding in blepharoplasty performed in Asians. Ann Plast Surg 2003;50:156–9.

90. Cruz AA, Ando A, Monteiro CA, Elias J Jr. Delayed retrobulbar hematoma after blepharoplasty. Ophthal Plast Reconstr Surg 2001;17:126–30.

91. Mahaffey PJ, Wallace AF. Blindness following cosmetic blepharoplasty: a review. Br J Plast Surg 1986;39:213–21.

92. Kelly PW, May DR. Central retinal artery occlusion following cosmetic blepharoplasty. Br J Ophthalmol 1980;64:918–22.

93. Gayton JL, Ledford JK. Angle closure glaucoma following a combined blepharoplasty and ectropion repair. Ophthal Plast Reconstr Surg 1992;8:176–7.

94. Goldberg RA, Lessner AM, Shorr N, Baylis HI. The transconjunctival approach to the orbital floor and orbital fat. A prospective study. Ophthal Plast Reconstr Surg 1990;6:241–6.

95. Rosenberg GJ. Temporary tarsorrhaphy suture to prevent or treat scleral show and ectropion secondary to laser resurfacing or laser blepharoplasty. Plast Reconstr Surg 2000;106:721–5; discussion 726–7.

96. Baylis HI, Goldberg RA, Groth MJ. Complications of lower blepharoplasty. In: Putterman AM, editor. Cosmetic oculoplastic surgery: eyelid, forehead, and facial techniques. 3rd ed. Philadelphia (PA): W.B. Saunders; 1999. p. 429–56.

97. Cohen MS, Shorr N. Eyelid reconstruction with hard palate mucosa grafts [comment]. Ophthal Plast Reconstr Surg 1992;8:183–95.

98. Patel BC, Patipa M, Anderson RL, McLeish W. Management of postblepharoplasty lower eyelid retraction with hard palate grafts and lateral tarsal strip. Plast Reconstr Surg 1997;99:1251–60.

99. Shorr N, Fallor MK. "Madame Butterfly" procedure: combined cheek and lateral canthal suspension procedure for post-blepharoplasty, "round eye," and lower eyelid retraction. Ophthal Plast Reconstr Surg 1985;1:229–35.

100. Klein AW, Wexler P, Carruthers A, Carruthers J. Treatment of facial furrows and rhytides. Dermatol Clin 1997;15:595–607.

101. Rose JJ Jr, Lemke BN, Lucarelli MJ, et al. Anatomy of facial recipient sites for autologous fat transfer. Am J Cosmet Surg 2003;20:17–25.

102. Ghabrial R, Lisman RD, Kane MA, et al. Diplopia following transconjunctival blepharoplasty. Plast Reconstr Surg 1998;102:1219–25.

103. Mowlavi A, Neumeister MW, Wilhelmi BJ. Lower blepharoplasty using bony anatomical landmarks to identify and avoid injury to the inferior oblique muscle. Plast Reconstr Surg 2002;110:1318–22; discussion 1323–4.

104. Coleman WP 3rd. Dermal peels. Dermatol Clin 2001;19:405–11.

105. Gilbert SE. Transconjunctival blepharoplasty with chemoexfoliation. Ann Plast Surg 1996;37:24–9.

106. Goldberg RA, Joshi AR, McCann JD, Shorr N. Management of severe cicatricial entropion using shared mucosal grafts. Arch Ophthalmol 1999;117:1255–9.

107. Fitzpatrick RE. CO_2 laser resurfacing. Dermatol Clin 2001;19:443–51.

108. Carter SR, Seiff SR, Choo PH, Vallabhanath P. Lower eyelid CO_2 laser rejuvenation: a randomized, prospective clinical study. Ophthalmology 2001;108:437–41.

109. Langsdon PR, Milburn M, Yarber R. Comparison of the laser and phenol chemical peel in facial skin resurfacing. Arch Otolaryngol Head Neck Surg 2000;126:1195–9.

110. Millman AL. Eyelid and facial laser skin resurfacing. In: Putterman AM, editor. Cosmetic oculoplastic surgery: eyelid, forehead, and facial techniques. 3rd ed. Philadelphia (PA): W. B. Saunders; 1999. p. 355–66.

111. Lemke BN, Lucarelli MJ. Anatomy of the ocular adnexa, orbit and related facial structures. In: Nesi FA, Lisman RD, Levine MR, editors. Smith's ophthalmic plastic and reconstructive surgery. St. Louis (MO): Mosby; 1998. p. 3–78.

112. Lemke BN, Della Rocca RC. Surgery of the eyelids and orbit: an anatomical approach. East Norwalk (CT): Appleton & Lange; 1990.

113. Knize DM, editor. The forehead and temporal fossa anatomy and technique. Philadelphia (PA): Lippincott; 2001. p. 39.

CHAPTER 65

Basic Principles of Rhinoplasty

James Koehler, DDS, MD
Peter D. Waite, MPH, DDS, MD

For many cosmetic surgeons rhinoplasty is one of the most challenging surgical procedures. A clear understanding of nasal anatomy is critical in order to provide an esthetic result that does not compromise nasal function. Developing a pattern of analysis of the nose is vital for proper diagnosis and for determining the most appropriate treatment plan. Numerous rhinoplastic techniques have been described. Some surgeons favor an endonasal approach whereas others believe that an external approach is more desirable. Each surgeon must become familiar with all technique options in order to address the wide variety of challenges of rhinoplasty surgery.

The goal of this chapter is to give a broad overview of the diagnosis and treatment of nasal deformities. It is by no means exhaustive since multiple textbook volumes have been written on this subject. The reader should gain an understanding of nasal anatomy and determine how to systematically analyze the nose. Both endonasal and external rhinoplasty will be described.

Nasal Anatomy

A clear understanding of nasal anatomy is important to successfully perform nasal procedures and decrease the incidence of complications.

Surface Anatomy

The terms used to describe the surface anatomy of the nose are important in nasal form analysis and for treatment plan formulation (Table 65-1). For descriptive purposes the spatial relationships are described as cephalic, caudal, dorsal, basal, anterior, posterior, superior, and inferior (Figure 65-1).

Skin and Soft Tissue

The soft tissue that overlies the bone and cartilage may influence the final result of rhinoplasty. The thickness of the skin will determine how it will re-drape after performing a rhinoplasty. The skin thickness varies along the dorsum of the nose. The skin is fairly thick and mobile in the region of the nasion. It quickly thins over the nasal dorsum and is generally thinnest and most mobile in the mid-dorsal region (rhinion). In the distal third of the nose the skin tends to be more thick and adherent and has an increased sebaceous content.

A patient with thin skin will show dramatic changes with alteration of the underlying bone and cartilage, and this limits room for error since little is camouflaged by the thickness of the skin. Conversely for thick-skinned individuals more

Table 65-1   Surface Anatomy of the Nose
Glabella: the most forward projecting point of the forehead in the midline at the level of the supraorbital ridges
Radix: the junction between the frontal bone and the dorsum of the nose
Rhinion: the anterior tip at the end of the suture of the nasal bones
Dorsum: the anterior surface of the nose formed by the nasal bones and the upper lateral cartilages
Supratip break: the slight depression in the nasal profile at the point where the nasal dorsum joins the lobule of the nasal tip
Infratip lobule: the portion of the tip lobule that is found between the tip-defining points and the columellar-lobular angle
Tip-defining points: there are four tip defining points, which include the supratip break, the columellar-lobular angle, and the most projected area on each side of the nasal tip formed by the lower lateral cartilages
Alar sidewall: the rounded eminence forming the lateral nostril wall
Alar-facial junction: the depressed groove formed on the face where the ala joins the face
Columella: the skin that separates the nostrils at the base of the nose

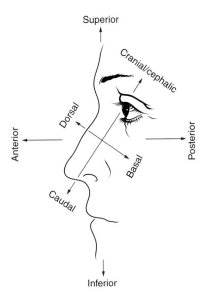

FIGURE 65-1 *Spatial descriptors. In describing the relationship of one anatomic unit to another many terms are used. The standard relationships are anterior, posterior, superior, and inferior. The nose is also described in terms of dorsal, basal, caudal, and cranial (or cephalic) positions. Adapted from Austermann K. Rhinoplasty: planning techniques and complications. In: Booth PW, Hausamen JE, editors. Maxillofacial surgery. New York: Churchill Livingstone; 1999. p. 1378.*

aggressive sculpturing of the nasal skeleton must be performed in order to effect significant changes. Although thick skin may mask imperfections it does not redrape as well and can result in underlying fibrosis and formation of a polybeak deformity (supratip scarring). Better results are possible with thin-skinned patients, however the margin for error is smaller. The surgeon must sometimes modify the technique depending on the type of skin of the patient.

Superficial Musculoaponeurotic System and Nasal Musculature

The muscles of the nose are encased in the nasal superficial musculoaponeurotic system (SMAS). This is a fibromuscular layer that separates the skin and subcutaneous tissue from the nasal cartilage and bone. The SMAS of the nose is in continuity with the SMAS of the face. During rhinoplastic surgery the dissection is performed beneath the SMAS. Violating the SMAS will often result in increased bleeding, scarring, and postoperative edema.

The muscles of the nose can be divided into four categories: the elevators, the depressors, the compressors, and the dilators (Figure 65-2). The muscles of significance are the paired depressor septi nasi. These muscles can result in drooping of the nasal tip during smiling. This added tension on the nasal tip must be recognized preoperatively and addressed by resection in order to achieve a cosmetic result.[1]

Blood Supply

There is a rich blood supply to the subdermal vascular plexus of the nose that arises from branches of both the internal and external carotid arteries. The blood supply from the internal carotid artery that supplies the external nose includes the dorsal nasal artery and the external nasal artery. The dorsal nasal artery is a branch of the ophthalmic artery. The external nasal artery is a branch of the anterior ethmoid artery.

The external nose is also supplied by branches of the facial artery and the internal maxillary artery, which originate from the external carotid artery. The facial artery branches include the angular artery, lateral nasal artery, alar artery, septal artery, and superior labial artery (Figure 65-3).

The internal nose is supplied by the internal and external carotid branches. The ophthalmic artery, a branch of the internal carotid, branches into the anterior and posterior ethmoidal arteries. The anterior ethmoidal artery supplies the anterosuperior part of the septum and the lateral nasal wall. The posterior ethmoid artery supplies the septum, lateral nasal wall, and the superior turbinate.[2]

The internal maxillary artery branches include the sphenopalatine artery and the greater palatine artery. The sphenopalatine artery supplies most of the posterior part of the nasal septum, lateral wall of the

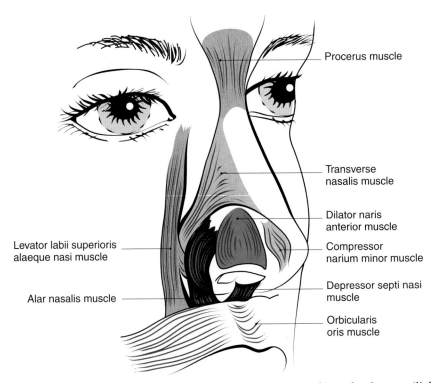

Procerus muscle

Transverse nasalis muscle

Dilator naris anterior muscle

Compressor narium minor muscle

Depressor septi nasi muscle

Orbicularis oris muscle

Levator labii superioris alaeque nasi muscle

Alar nasalis muscle

FIGURE 65-2 *Nasal musculature. The muscles of the nose are grouped into the elevators (light blue), the depressors (dark blue), the compressors (light gray), and the dilators (dark gray). Adapted from Jewett B. Anatomic considerations. In: Baker SR, editor. Principles of nasal reconstruction. St. Louis (MO):Mosby; 2002. p. 17.*

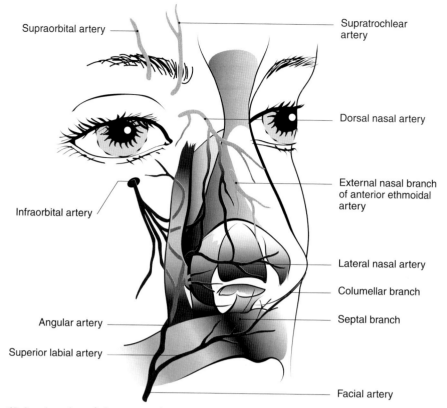

FIGURE 65-3   *Arteries of the external nose. The arterial supply of the external nose comes from branches of the external carotid artery* (dark blue) *and the internal carotid artery* (light blue). *Adapted from Jewett B. Anatomic considerations. In: Baker SR, editor. Principles of nasal reconstruction. St. Louis (MO): Mosby; 2002. p. 18.*

conclusion is that the primary blood supply to the nasal tip comes from the bilateral lateral nasal arteries that course in a plane superficial to the alar cartilages in the subdermal plexus approximately 2 to 3 mm above the alar groove. Thus a columellar incision does not compromise tip blood supply. Also there are no significant veins and minimal lymphatics in the columellar region.[3,4] Some surgeons believe that external rhinoplasty remains more edematous for longer postoperative periods than an endonasal rhinoplasty.

Bone and Cartilage

The structure of the nose consists of the paired nasal bones as well as the frontal process of the maxilla. The bone is thickest near the junction with the frontal bone and tapers as it joins with the upper lateral cartilages.

The upper lateral cartilages are in intimate contact with the nasal bones and underlie the nasal bones for approximately 6 to 8 mm. The connection between the

nose, roof, and part of the nasal floor. The greater palatine artery supplies a portion of the anterior and inferior portion of the nasal septum (Figure 65-4).[2]

The surgically significant area for internal nasal bleeding is known as Kiesselbach's plexus (also termed Little's area). This is the area in the anteroinferior part of the nasal septum which is a common site of expistaxis. It is where the sphenopalatine, greater palatine, superior labial artery, and anterior ethmoid arteries anastamose (Figure 65-5).[2] The venous drainage of the nose is primarily from the facial and ophthalmic veins.

One concern during nasal surgery is the possibility of compromised blood flow to the nasal tip if the surgeon performs an external rhinoplasty. The blood supply to the nasal tip has been analyzed by lymphoscintigraphic studies, cadaver dissections, and histologic sections.[3,4] The

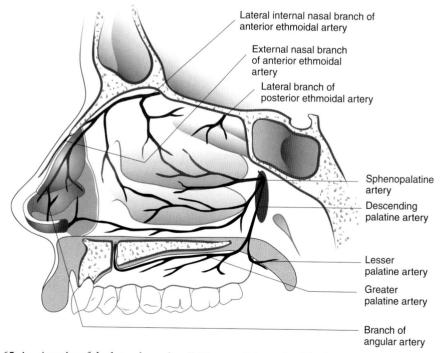

FIGURE 65-4   *Arteries of the lateral nasal wall. The arterial supply of the lateral nasal wall arises from branches of the external carotid artery* (black) *and the internal carotid artery* (blue). *Adapted from Jewett B. Anatomic considerations. In: Baker SR, editor. Principles of nasal reconstruction. St. Louis (MO): Mosby; 2002. p. 23.*

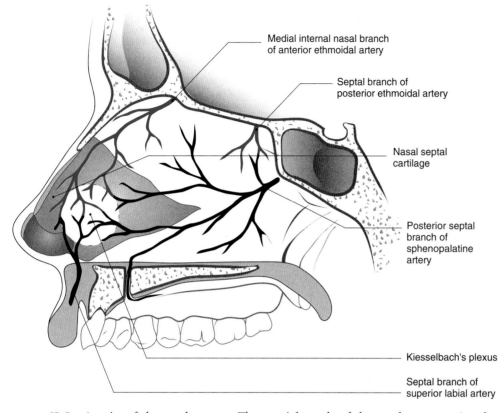

FIGURE **65-5** *Arteries of the nasal septum. The arterial supply of the nasal septum arises from branches of the external carotid artery* (black) *and the internal carotid artery* (blue). *Kiesselbach's plexus is formed by the sphenopalatine artery, greater palatine artery, superior labial artery, and anterior ethmoid arteries. It is a common site of epistaxis. Adapted from Jewett B. Anatomic considerations. In: Baker SR, editor. Principles of nasal reconstruction. St. Louis (MO): Mosby; 2002. p. 23.*

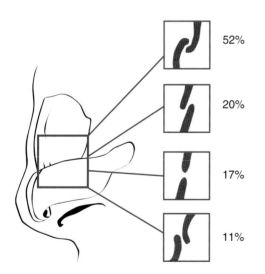

FIGURE **65-6** *Configurations of the scroll. The relationship of the upper lateral and lower lateral cartilages is termed the scroll. Anatomic studies have identified four common configurations: interlocked (52%), overlapping (20%), end to end (17%), and opposed (11%). Adapted from Lam SM and Williams EF III.[5]*

nasal bones and upper lateral cartilages should not be violated since this may disrupt the internal nasal valve causing nasal obstruction and asymmetry. The internal nasal valve is formed by the junction of the upper lateral cartilages and the nasal septum.

The lower lateral cartilages comprise the lower third of the nose and connect to the upper lateral cartilages in a union described as the scroll. There are various configurations of the scroll.[5,6] The scroll is described as interlocked (52%), overlapping (20%), end to end (17%), or opposed (11%) (Figure 65-6). The scroll provides significant support to the nasal tip. When performing an endonasal rhinoplasty this area is violated by the intercartilaginous incision (Figures 65-7–65-9). The lower lateral cartilage is divided into medial and lateral crura. The medial crura are in intimate contact with the nasal septum and

provide tip support. The lateral crura extend superiorly and form dense fibroareolar tissue attachments with the pyriform aperture. The intermediate crus is the diverging of the medial crus before turning to become the lateral crus proper. The highest point of the intermediate crus is an important surgical landmark known as the tip-defining point (Figure 65-10).

The nasal septum is formed by both bone and cartilage. The ethmoid and vomer provide bony support posteriorly. The quadrangular cartilage provides support anteriorly (Figure 65-11).

Support for the nasal tip is classified into major and minor divisions. The major tip support comes from the size, shape, and strength of the lower lateral cartilages, the attachment of the medial crura of the lower lateral cartilage to the caudal septum, and the fibrous attachment of the lower lateral cartilage to the upper lateral cartilage. The minor tip support comes from the nasal spine, the membranous septum, the cartilaginous dorsum, the sesamoid complexes, the interdomal ligaments, and the alar attachments to the skin (Table 65-2).[5]

Nerves

The sensory nerve supply to the skin of the external nose is supplied by the ophthalmic and maxillary divisions of the

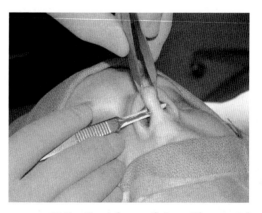

FIGURE **65-7** *Partial transfixion. The partial transfixion incision through the membranous septum and short of the medial crural foot pads.*

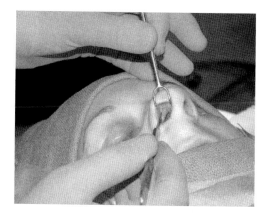

FIGURE **65-8** *Intercartilaginous incision. The intercartilaginous incision, between the upper and lower cartilage, allows access to the nasal dorsum. Note the incision does not violate the nasal valve.*

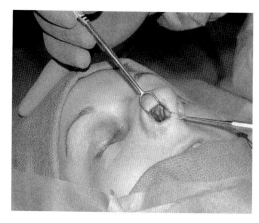

FIGURE **65-9** *Connecting intercartilaginous and partial transfixion incisions. The intercartilaginous incision extends along the upper edge of the lateral crus to connect with the transfixion incision. This will provide access for a septoplasty during internal rhinoplasty.*

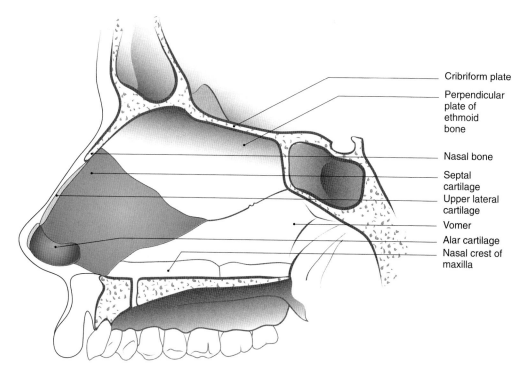

FIGURE **65-11** *Anatomy of the nasal septum. The nasal septum is composed of the perpendicular plate of the ethmoid, the vomer, and the quadrangular cartilage. Adapted from Jewett B. Anatomic considerations. In: Baker SR, editor. Principles of nasal reconstruction. St. Louis (MO): Mosby; 2002. p. 22.*

trigeminal nerve. Branches of the supratrochlear and infratrochlear nerves supply the skin in the region of the radix and rhinion. The lower half of the nose is supplied by the infraorbital nerve and the external nasal branch of the anterior ethmoidal nerve (a branch of the nasociliary nerve that arises from the ophthalmic branch of the trigeminal nerve) (Figure 65-12).

The main sensory nerve supply to the nasal septum comes from the internal nasal nerve (a branch of the anterior ethmoidal nerve) and the nasopalatine nerve (Figure 65-13). The lateral nasal wall sensation is supplied by the anterior ethmoidal nerve, branches of the pterygopalatine ganglion, branches of the greater palatine nerve, the infraorbital nerve, and the anterior superior alveolar nerve.

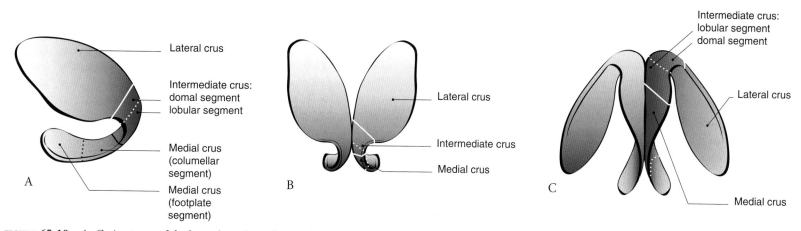

FIGURE **65-10**   A–C, *Anatomy of the lower lateral cartilages. The lower lateral cartilages are often described as having a lateral crus, medial crus, and an intermediate crus. The intermediate crus is the most projected portion of the lower lateral cartilages and these form two of the tip-defining points seen on nasal tip analysis. Adapted from Jewett B. Anatomic considerations. In: Baker SR, editor. Principles of nasal reconstruction. St. Louis (MO):Mosby; 2002. p. 21.*

Table 65-2   Tip Support Mechanisms

The three major tip support mechanisms include
1. The size, shape, and strength of the lower lateral cartilages
2. The attachment of the medial crura to the caudal septum
3. The attachment of the lower lateral cartilages to the upper lateral cartilages

The minor tip support mechanisms include
1. The interdomal ligament
2. The sesamoid complex extending the support of the lateral crura to the piriform aperture
3. The attachment of the alar cartilages to the overlying skin
4. Cartilaginous septal dorsum
5. Nasal spine
6. The membranous septum

Parasympathetic innervation is derived from branches of the pterygopalatine ganglion which are derived from cranial nerve VII. Some sympathetic branches reach the nasal cavity via the nasociliary nerve.[2,7]

Nasal Valve

The airflow through the nose is regulated by the internal and external nasal valves. The external nasal valve is comprised of the lower lateral cartilage and the nasal septum and floor. Collapse of the external nasal valve can sometimes be noted when the nares become occluded on even gentle inspiration. This problem is seen in patients with narrow nostrils, a projecting nasal tip, and thin alar sidewalls. External nasal valve collapse is usually seen in patients who have had previous rhinoplasty surgery and excessive trimming of the cephalic portion of the lower lateral cartilages. It is also seen with increased age and in facial nerve paralysis. The external nasal valve collapse can be corrected by deprojecting the overprojected nose, realigning the lateral crura into a more caudal orientation, and placing alar batten grafts to provide structural support and prevent collapse.[8]

The internal nasal valve is formed by the junction of the septum with the upper lateral cartilages. The angle formed should be a minimum of 10° to 15° to maintain patency. Deviation of the nasal septum or separation of the upper lateral cartilages from the nasal bones can lead to obstruction. This problem is also seen after rhinoplasty if the patient has had weakening of the upper and lower lateral cartilages. These patients often have a pinched appearance in the supra-alar region. The Cottle test is used to evaluate obstruction at the internal valve by using a finger to distract the check and lateral wall of the nose thereby opening the valve. If nasal airflow is dramatically improved, then the internal valve may require correction. These patients often have symptomatic relief by the use of external taping devices. Surgical correction involves the placement of spreader grafts between the septum and upper lateral cartilages to increase the angle at this junction.[8–10]

Cosmetic Evaluation

The cosmetic evaluation begins in the same way as with any examination, by eliciting the chief complaint of the patient. The patient should be given a mirror and cotton-tipped applicator to point out specific cosmetic concerns. Following this a thorough medical history should be obtained. Specific attention should be directed toward

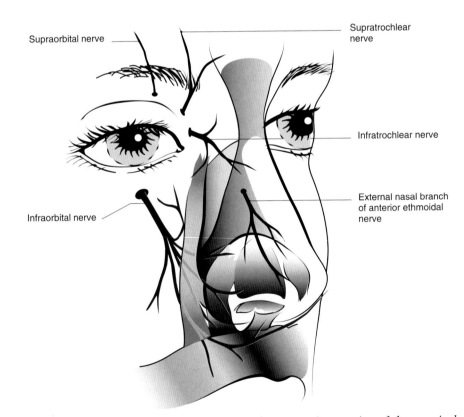

FIGURE **65-12**   *Sensory nerves of the external nose. The sensory innervation of the nose is derived from the V₁ (ophthalmic: colored black) and from V₂ (maxillary: colored blue) divisions of the trigeminal nerve. Adapted from Jewett B. Anatomic considerations. In: Baker SR, editor. Principles of nasal reconstruction. St. Louis (MO): Mosby; 2002. p. 19.*

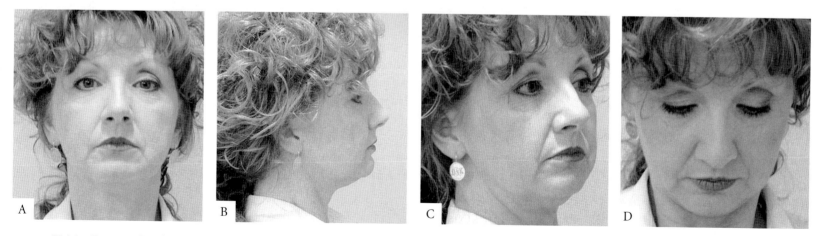

FIGURE 65-13   *Sensory nerves of the nasal septum. The main sensory nerve supply comes from the internal nasal nerve (a branch of the anterior ethmoidal nerve V₁ (black) and the nasopalatine nerve V₂ (blue). Adapted from Jewett B. Anatomic considerations. In: Baker SR, editor. Principles of nasal reconstruction. St. Louis (MO): Mosby; 2002. p. 19.*

Internal nasal
(anterior
ethmoidal)

Medial
posterior
superior

Nasopalatine

and its proportions should be done. Refer to Chapter 54, "Database Acquisition and Treatment Planning," for additional information on facial analysis in orthognathic surgery.

Nasal Analysis

The nasal examination should be performed in a systematic manner so that the proper diagnosis is attained (Figures 65-14 and 65-15).

General Assessment

Skin

The skin should be assessed for its thickness, mobility, and sebaceous gland content. Any pigmentations or scars should also be noted. Thick skin does not redrape well after rhinoplasty.

Symmetry

Any gross asymmetries in all views should be noted.

Lateral View *Nasofrontal Angle* The nasofrontal angle is defined as the angle formed from lines that are tangential to the glabella and the nasal dorsum and intersect through the radix as seen on a profile view. The normal angle is between 125° and 135° (Figure 65-16).

obtaining a history of nasal trauma, nasal obstruction, previous nasal surgery, and medications (including over-the-counter and herbal medications).

Psychiatric Stability

In addition to analyzing the nose the surgeon needs to assess if the patient is psychologically prepared for a cosmetic procedure. Patients should have realistic expectations and motivations. A patient who is internally motivated (eg, wishes to improve their self-esteem) to have the procedure is a better candidate than one who desires the procedure for external reasons (eg, spouse wants them to have it done).[11,12]

The surgeon should beware of patients who are indecisive, rude, uncooperative, depressed, have unrealistic expectations, or have significant personality disorders because they may never be satisfied. Other warning signs of poor patients are those who overly flatter, are talkative, consider themselves to be a very important patient, have minimal or no deformity, are surgeon shoppers, price hagglers, or involved in litigation. Most importantly, do not operate on a patient that you do not like.[11–14]

General Facial Analysis

Prior to performing a specific analysis of the nose, a global assessment of the face

A

B

C

D

FIGURE 65-14   *Preoperative rhinoplasty. A, Preoperative frontal view shows the width of the nose and alar base. B, Preoperative lateral view shows the nasal profile and dorsum in relation to the nasofrontal angle and nasolabial angle. C, Preoperative three-quarter, or oblique view, is most natural and often revealing for harmony of the orbital rims and gull wings that flow into the nasal dorsum. D, Preoperative basal view is either taken from above or below the patient and is a good view of tip and base morphology.*

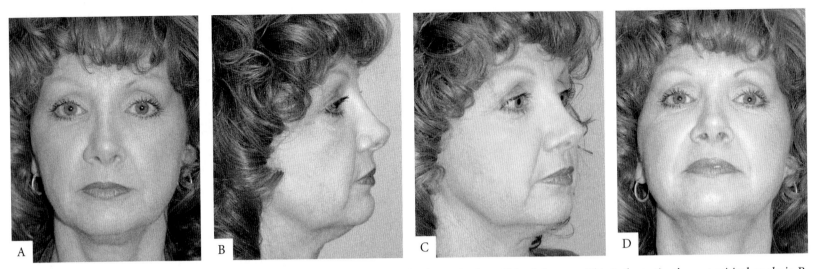

FIGURE 65-15 *Postoperative rhinoplasty. A, Postoperative frontal view shows the change in the width of the nose. This is the patient's most critical analysis. B, Postoperative lateral view shows the change in dorsal reduction and tip position. C, Postoperative three-quarter, or oblique view, demonstrates the symmetry and graceful balance of the nose with the face. D, Postoperative basal view shows the width of the nose and any tip deviation from the dorsal midline.*

The postion of the radix should then be assessed in terms of its anteroposterior and vertical positions from a profile view. The radix should lie in a vertical plane

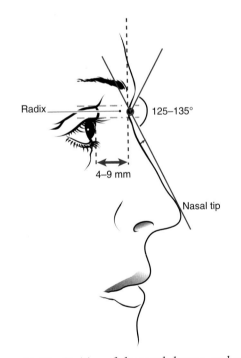

FIGURE 65-16 *Position of the nasal dorsum and radix. The nasal dorsum is typically 2 mm behind a line drawn from the radix to nasal tip in women. In men the nasal dorsum typically lies on this line. The radix should lie between the upper eyelid margin and the supratarsal folds in a vertical plane and approximately 4 to 9 mm anterior to the corneal plane. Adapted from Austermann, K., Rhinoplasty: planning techniques and complications. In: Booth PW, Hausamen JE, editors. Maxillofacial surgery. New York: Churchill Livingstone; 1999. p. 1380.*

somewhere between the lash line and the supratarsal folds. In addition it should be 4 to 9 mm anterior to the corneal plane (see Figure 65-16).

Nasal Dorsum In women the nasal dorsum should lie approximately 2 mm posterior to a line drawn from the radix to the nasal tip. In males the nasal dorsum should lie on this line or slightly in front of it (see Figure 65-16).

The length of the nose (radix to tip) can be measured clinically or on photographs taken during the initial examination. The ideal nasal length should approximate the distance from stomion to menton if the lower facial height is proportionate to the middle facial height (glabella to subnasale). If the lower face height is not proportionate it is best to estimate the nasal length as 0.67 times the middle facial height.

Nasal Tip Definition The nose should have four tip defining points which when drawn on the nose in the frontal view appear as two equilateral triangles (Figure 65-17). These points include the supratip break, the columellar-lobular angle, and the two tip-defining points (the most projected portion of the nasal tip)

Nasal Tip Projection Nasal tip projection can be defined as the distance that the tip (pronasale) projects anterior in the facial plane.[15] Perception of nasal tip projection can be influenced by may factors: upper lip length, nasolabial angle, nasofrontal angle, dorsal hump, and

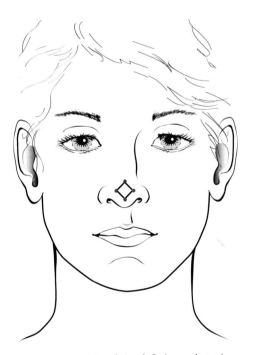

FIGURE 65-17 *Nasal tip-defining points. A nose should have four tip-defining points. These are defined by the supratip, columellar-lobular angle, and the tip-defining points of each intermediate crus of the lower lateral cartilages.*

chin projection. There are several methods to determine if the nasal tip projection is adequate. Most cosmetic rhinoplasty procedures are designed to preserve tip projection.

The simplest method to remember is Simons' method, which states that the lip-to-tip ratio is 1:1. Essentially the length of the upper lip (from subnasale to labrale superioris) should equal the nasal projection (measured from subnasale to pronasale). This method may be invalid because of the wide variation in lip lengths.[16]

The Goode method is another way of determining nasal projection. Using the Goode method a line is drawn from the radix to the nasal tip. A second line is drawn from the radix to the alar columellar junction. A third line is drawn perpendicular to this and passes through the nasal tip. Goode's analysis states that if the nasofacial angle is between 36° and 40°, then the length of the perpendicular line passing through the nasal tip should be 0.55 to 0.6 of the length of the nasal dorsum (Figure 65-18).[16]

Rohrich describes another technique of assessing nasal tip projection. If the nasal dorsal length is appropriate, the tip projection should be 0.67 times the ideal nasal length. The ideal nasal length should be equal to the distance from stomion to menton or 1.6 times the distance from the nasal tip to stomion. The tip projection is measured from the alar facial junction to the nasal tip.[17] This method is subject to a great deal of facial variation.

Additionally a vertical line drawn from the most projected portion of the upper lip should divide the nose in two equal halves between the alar facial groove and the nasal tip. If the anterior portion is greater than 60%, then the nose is likely to be overprojected (Figure 65-19).[17]

Nasal tip Rotation The nasal tip rotation is evaluated by the nasolabial angle and the columellar-lobular angle. Nasolabial angle is defined as the angle formed by lines that are tangential to the columella of the nose

and the philtrum of the lip and intersect at the subnasale. In women this should be approximately 95° to 110°, whereas in men this should be 90° to 95°. Lip position may be dependent on tooth position. The columellar-lobular angle is defined as the angle formed by the intersection of a line tangential to the columella and a line tangential to the infratip lobule. This angle is normally between 30° and 45°.

Tip Support The strength of the cartilage in the tip of the nose is apparent when one presses on the tip. A nose with poor support may require cartilaginous struts to counteract the inherently weakened tip from the rhinoplasty. The effect of facial animation should also be noted. Some patients have overactive depressor septi nasi muscles, which result in a drooping nasal tip on smiling. The columella show on a lateral view should be 3 to 4 mm below the inferior alar rim.[13]

Frontal View *Width of Nasal Dorsum* The width of the nasal body and tip should be approximately 80% of the alar base width. This is assuming that the alar base is in proper anatomic proportions. The alar base width should approximate the intercanthal distance. If the width of the nasal dorsum is significantly greater than 80%, then lateral nasal osteotomies should be considered. The eyebrows should gracefully flow into the nasal dorsum analogous to a gull wing in flight.

The alar rims and columella should also be a gently curving line that appears as a bird in flight.

Alar Width The alar base width should approximate the intercanthal distance. Seldom is the nasal width less than the intercanthal dimension.

Basal View From a basal view the columella-to-lobule ratio should be 2:1. Nostril size and shape should also be noted. An esthetic nostril is teardrop

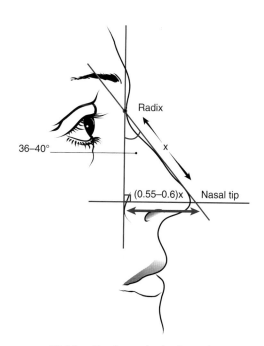

FIGURE **65-18** *Goode method of nasal projection. This method is sometimes used to determine adequacy of nasal projection. If the nasofrontal angle is between 36° to 40°, then the length of a perpendicular line through the nasal tip should be 0.55 to 0.6 the length of the nasal dorsum. x = nasal length. Adapted from Austermann, K., Rhinoplasty: planning techniques and complications. In: Booth PW, Hausamen JE, editors. Maxillofacial surgery. New York: Churchill Livingstone; 1999. p. 1380.*

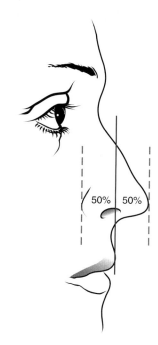

FIGURE **65-19** *Nasal projection. A vertical line through the most projected part of the upper lip should divide the nose into two equal parts. If the nasal tip comprises > 60%, then the nose may be overprojected.*

shaped, but there is a great amount of ethnic variation (Figure 65-20).

Oblique View The oblique view is most natural and sometimes more revealing than standard photographs. It demonstrates the flow of subunits and facial harmony. The three-quarters view is how we usually see each other in routine interaction.

Functional Considerations

Although the patient desires cosmetic correction of their nose, the functional significance of the nose should be closely considered. Nasal airflow through both the internal and external nasal valves should be evaluated. The septum should be evaluated for deviation and perforations. The septum is often a good site for harvesting autogenous cartilage for grafting. The turbinates should be evaluated for hypertrophy. Rhinoscopy with a nasal speculum can be performed both before and after the administration of a topical decongestant.

Photographs

The examination is not complete without standardized facial photographs. The standard facial photographs should include frontal, right, and left lateral views; right and left oblique views; and a high and low basal view. Close-up views are taken if warranted. The photographs are beneficial from a medicolegal standpoint, and they also allow the surgeon to

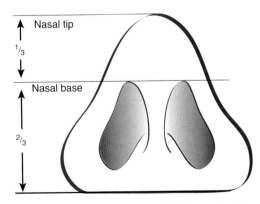

FIGURE 65-20 *Columella-to-lobule ratio. The columella-to-lobule ratio should be 2:1.*

study the nose in more detail and to develop a surgical plan.

Anesthesia

Proper anesthesia of the nose is important to ensure minimal distortion of the tissues as well as to provide adequate hemostasis. Prior to injecting the nose, cottonoids or cotton-tipped applicators soaked in 4% cocaine or oxymetazoline are placed in each nostril to constrict the mucous membranes of the turbinates. If the rhinoplasty is to be performed under sedation, then cocaine is preferred because of its anesthetic properties. If the procedure is performed under general anesthesia, then oxymetazoline is sufficient.

Three cottonoids are placed in each nostril: one along the middle turbinate, one along the superior nasal vault, and one along the inferomedial septum.

Local anesthesia is achieved with 2% lidocaine with 1:100,000 epinephrine. In an endonasal rhinoplasty the following areas are injected:

- 0.5 cc deposited at the junction of each upper and lower lateral cartilage (intercartilaginous area)
- 0.5 cc deposited in the region of each marginal incision
- 3 cc along the nasal dorsum and lateral nasal bones (hugging periosteum)
- 1 cc along the nasal septum
- 0.5 cc at each alar base
- 1 cc at each infraorbital nerve
- 1 cc at the nasal tip

For external rhinoplasty the following additional area is injected:

- 1 cc to the columella

Incisions/Sequencing

There are multiple incision techniques used to gain access to the cartilage and bone support of the nose.

Complete Transfixion

This incision provides access to the caudal septum, medial crura, and nasal spine.

The incision is made with a no. 15 blade, beginning just caudal to the superior caudal end of the nasal septum. The incision extends inferiorly through the membranous septum, following the cephalic margin of the medial crura (see Figures 65-7 and 65-21A). It results in ptosis and deprojection of the nose.

Partial Transfixion

This incision is similar to the complete transfixion incision except that it stops at the level of the medial footpads of the lower lateral cartilages. The advantage of this incision is that the attachments of the medial footpads of the lower lateral cartilages to the caudal septum are not disrupted (see Figures 65-7 and 65-21B).

Hemitransfixion

This incision is a complete transfixion incision that is performed on only one side of the membranous septum. It does not traverse both mucosal surfaces and therefore some attachments of the medial crura to the caudal septum are maintained. Access to the nasal septum is good with this incision; however, delivery of the lower lateral cartilage on the side opposite to the incision is difficult (see Figures 65-7 and 65–21C).

Killian Incision

This incision is seldom used in rhinoplasty. It is a useful incision to gain access to the nasal septum if only a septoplasty is to be performed. The incision is made several millimeters cephalad to the caudal edge of the septum. It can be extended onto the nasal floor if needed.

Intercartilaginous Incision

This incision is made at the junction of the upper and lower lateral cartilages. The nare is elevated superiorly with a double skin hook. A no. 15 blade should pass below the lower lateral cartilage and above the upper lateral cartilages. This incision is typically made after a transfixion incision. The intercartilaginous incision is then

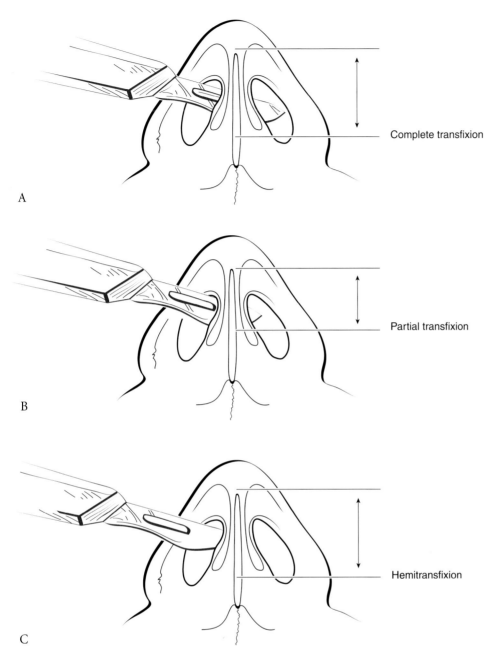

A

B

C

FIGURE **65-21** *Transfixion incisions. A, A complete transfixion incision is made caudal to both the medial crura and through the membranous septum. B, A partial transfixion incision is similar except the incision stops short of the medial foot pads of the medial crura. C, A hemitransfixion incision is a complete transfixion incision that is performed only on one side, therefore the other medial crura and footpad is not violated.*

Complete transfixion

Partial transfixion

Hemitransfixion

connected to the transfixion incision (see Figures 65-8, 65-9, and 65-22).

Intracartilaginous Incision

This incision is made through both the vestibular nasal mucosa and a portion of the lower lateral cartilages. This incision is similar to the intercartilaginous incision except that it is made 3 to 5 mm posterior

to the junction of the upper and lower lateral cartilages. This incision in effect performs a complete cephalic strip of the lower lateral cartilages without the need for delivering the cartilage. The disadvantage is that the lower lateral cartilage is not directly visualized and it may therefore be difficul to achieve symmetry between the right and left sides.

Rim/Marginal Incision

This incision parallels the caudal edges of the lower lateral cartilages. The incision is used in combination with an intercartilaginous incision in an endonasal rhinoplasty. The two incisions allow the lower lateral cartilage to be delivered and visualized. This allows the surgeon to more accurately trim the cartilage if needed. In an open rhinoplasty this incision is combined with a transcolumellar incision in order to gain access to the lower lateral cartilage and nasal dorsum (Figure 65-23).

Transcolumellar Incision

This incision is made through the thinnest portion of the columella at a level just superior to the flaring of the medial crura. The incision can be made with a notched V in the center of the columella or as a "stair step." This will break up the scar and assist in closure. This incision is connected with a marginal incision bilaterally for open rhinoplasty (see Figure 65-23).

The two principle techniques are the endonasal and external rhinoplasty. Each of these techniques will be described in general terms, in the order in which the authors perform them. Other surgeons may perform the sequence in a different order (Tables 65-3 and 65-4).

Septoplasty

In rhinoplasty surgery there are several reasons to access the nasal septum: (1) to correct nasal airflow obstruction, (2) to assist in the correction of asymmetries, and (3) to harvest cartilage for tip grafting.

Access to the nasal septum in an endonasal approach is through a partial-transfixion incision, which is connected to bilateral intercartilaginous incisions. The partial-transfixion incision can be extended to the nasal floor on the side on which the septoplasty is to be performed. After completing the incisions the caudal aspect of the nasal septum is exposed by dissecting the mucoperichondrium from one

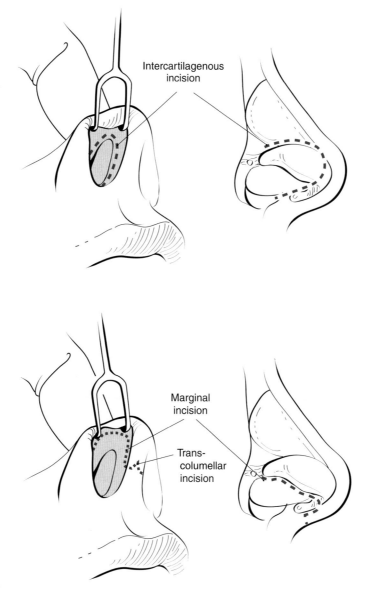

FIGURE **65-22**   *Intercartilaginous incisions. The intercartilaginous incision is made at the junction of the upper and lower lateral cartilages. The blade should pass below the lower lateral and above the upper lateral cartilage. Adapted from Alexander R. Fundamental terms, considerations, and approaches in rhinoplasty. In: Waite PD, editor. Atlas of the oral and maxillofacial surgery clinics of North America: rhinoplasty. Philadelphia (PA): W.B. Saunders; 1995. p. 19.*

FIGURE **65-23**   *Marginal incision. This incision is made parallel to the caudal edge of the lower lateral cartilage. This incision can be combined with bilateral intercartilaginous incisions for a cartilage delivery technique in endonasal rhinoplasty or combined with a transcolumellar incision for an external rhinoplasty. Adapted from Alexander R. Fundamental terms, considerations, and approaches in rhinoplasty. In: Waite PD, editor. Atlas of the oral and maxillofacial surgery clinics of North America: rhinoplasty. Philadelphia (PA): W.B. Saunders; 1995. p. 19.*

Table 65-3   Surgical Sequence for Endonasal Rhinoplasty
The general sequence is
1. Local anesthesia
2. Partial transfixion incision (see Figure 65-7)
3. Intercartilaginous incision (join with partial transfixion) (see Figures 65-8, 65-9, 65-21, and 65-22)
4. Septoplasty (if needed) (see Figures 65-24 and 65-25)
5. Dorsal reduction (see Figures 65-28–65-30)
6. Lateral nasal osteotomies (see Figure 65-31)
7. Marginal incision (see Figure 65-23)
8. Delivery of lower lateral cartilages (see Figure 65-37)
9. Tip modification (ie, cephalic strips/cartilage grafting/suture techniques)
10. Alar base modification (see Figure 65-41)
11. Closure, taping, and splinting

Table 65-4   Surgical Sequence for External Rhinoplasty
The general sequence is
1. Local anesthesia
2. Bilateral marginal incisions (see Figure 65-23)
3. Columellar incision (see Figure 65-23)
4. Skeletonization of upper and lower lateral cartilages and nasal dorsum
5. Dorsal reduction
6. Dome division if access is needed to the septum for septoplasty or graft harvest
7. Septoplasty (if needed)
8. Turbinate reduction
9. Lateral nasal osteotomies
10. Tip modification (ie, cephalic strips/cartilage grafting/ suture techniques)
11. Alar base modification
12. Closure, taping, and splinting

side. Two tunnels will be developed, one superior and the other inferior, which will ultimately be joined so that wide exposure of the septum is obtained.[18] Intially sharp dissection is done with a no. 15 blade or scissors to expose a portion of the caudal septum. The perichondrium is gently scored using a no. 15 blade. A dental amalgam condenser is then used in a sweeping motion to develop a plane between the perichondrium and the nasal septum (Figure 65-24). Once this plane of dissection is started a Freer or Cottle elevator can be used to complete the septal envelope (Figure 65-25). The mucoperichondrium is

tightly bound at the junction of the septum and the maxillary crest.

Once the septum is exposed it can be treated in four ways: (1) resection, (2) morselization, (3) segmental transection, and (4) swinging door flaps.[18] Submucosal resection allows a significant portion of cartilage to be harvested for grafting. At least 1 cm should be maintained superiorly and anteriorly in an L-shaped configuration to provide support for the nose (Figure 65-26). In order to resect the cartilage a Cottle elevator is used to cut the cartilage. Fomon scissors may be used to make the superior and inferior cuts

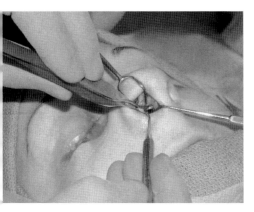

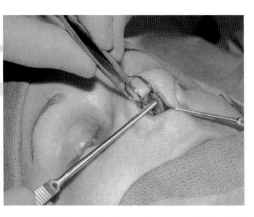

FIGURE **65-24** *Identifying perichondrium. The perichondrium is elevated with a dental amalgam condenser. One will notice a slight blue-gray cartilage and a distinct plane of dissection.*

FIGURE **65-25** *Elevation of mucoperichondrium. The Cottle elevator is specifically designed to elevate the nasal envelope without perforation.*

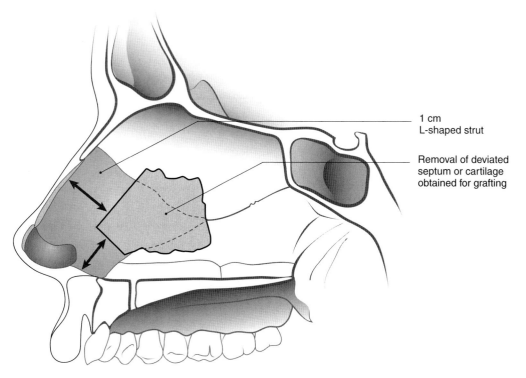

1 cm
L-shaped strut

Removal of deviated
septum or cartilage
obtained for grafting

FIGURE **65-26** *Resection of cartilage/bone from the nasal septum. This may be done to harvest cartilage for grafting procedures or for removal of grossly deviated septum. It is important to maintain 1 cm dorsally and caudally for nasal support.*

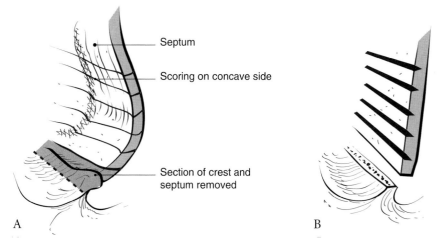

Septum

Scoring on concave side

Section of crest and
septum removed

A

B

FIGURE **65-27** *Septal repositioning. A deviated nasal septum can be repositioned by removing the obstruction inferiorly (A) and cross-hatching the cartilage to allow the deviated portion to be repositioned (B). Adapted from Robinson RC. Functional septorhinoplasty. In: Waite PD, editor. Atlas of the oral and maxillofacial surgery clinics of North America: rhinoplasty. Philadelphia (PA): W.B. Saunders; 1995. p. 35.*

through the bony septum. The cartilage can also be removed with a Ballenger swivel blade. If no cartilage is needed for the rhinoplasty, the resected cartilage can be morselized and replaced. Morselization can be performed in situ. Another technique for aligning the septum is through a segmental transection. In this technique the mucoperichondrium is elevated on one side of the septum. Cross-hatching with a no. 15 blade is performed to weaken the cartilage (Figure 65-27). The mucoperichondrium on the other side of the septum provides support. 4-0 gut mattress sutures can be positioned through the septum to assist in realignment. A septal splint is placed for 1 week. Finally a swinging door type flap can be used to reposition a large segment of flat cartilage

that is improperly angulated. The mucoperichondrium is elevated on one side. Through and through incisions are made on either side of the deviated cartilage. The cartilage is also separated from the maxillary crest so that it can hinge into a more normal position. Septal splints may

be required for 1 week. In all septal procedures a 4-0 gut on a straight needle is routinely used to perform a mattress suture through the septum and mucosa. This decreases the likelihood of a septal hematoma formation and circumvents the need for nasal packs.

Tears in the septal mucosa are not uncommon. However, it is not problematic as long as the tears are only on one side of the septum. Unilateral tears require no elaborate closure. If the tear is through and through, at least one side should be closed. This is best done with a 5-0 chromic gut suture.

Turbinectomy

Although the focus of this chapter is the cosmetic rhinoplasty, some mention needs to be made on maintaining function. Inferior turbinate hypertrophy is a problem that can result in nasal obstruction after cosmetic rhinoplasty, if the problem is not recognized preoperatively. Hypertrophy of the inferior turbinates is the most common cause of nasal airway obstruction.[19,20] Hypertrophy can be caused by numerous factors. Most commonly it is related to allergic symptoms. Hypertrophy caused by allergy should be managed medically with antihistamines and topical corticosteroids. If this fails, then surgical management can be considered.[21] In cases of a deviated nasal septum the turbinate on the side at which the nasal passage is enlarged can become hypertrophic with time. In patients with anatomic enlargement of the turbinate, the problem needs to be recognized so that the nasal passage does not become obstructed when the septum is straightened.

Management of inferior turbinate hypertrophy is controversial and outside the scope of this chapter. The surgical procedures used to treat this problem have included corticosteroid injection, turbinate out-fracture, electrocautery, cryosurgery, laser reduction, partial turbinate resection, total turbinate resection, submucous turbinate resection, and vidian neurectomy.[20–24] Each of these procedures has various advantages and disadvantages and the procedure chosen depends on the patient. The most common complications from turbinate surgery are hemorrhage, atrophic rhinitis, and ozena.

Nasal Dorsum

Reduction

One of the most dramatic changes that can be achieved in rhinoplasty surgery is correction of a dorsal hump. There are many ways to remove the hump. Some surgeons use a scalpel and osteotome, whereas others use rasps, and a few use power rasps. The authors recommend to first incise the cartilaginous convexity below the nasal bones and then to use a Rubin osteotome to remove the bony hump (Figures 65-28–65-31). Care must be taken to keep the osteotome directed superficially, since it can deflect downward and result in over-reduction. After removing the gross hump, sequential rasping can be used for refinement. After removal of any significant dorsal hump, the patient is left with an open roof deformity. This must be closed with lateral nasal osteotomies (see Figure 65-31).

Augmentation

Augmentation is indicated when there has been excessive reduction from previous rhinoplasty or from a post-traumatic defect. Several techniques are used to augment the nasal dorsum.

Autogenous Augmentation In the setting of acute trauma, cranial bone grafts can be used to provide support. These are cantilevered off the frontal bone with a miniplate. The graft must be properly

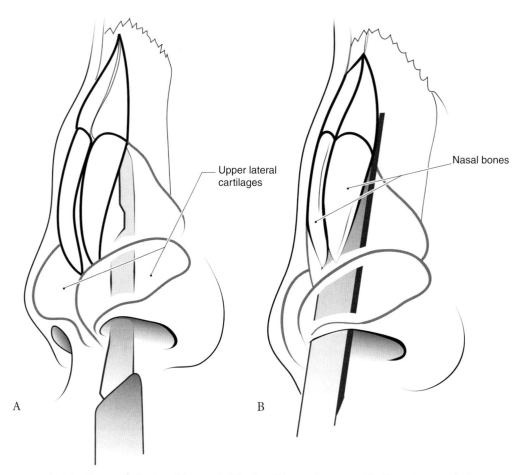

Upper lateral cartilages

Nasal bones

A

B

FIGURE 65-28 *Removal of a dorsal hump. A, The dorsal hump is removed by first using a scalpel to incise through the upper lateral cartilages. B, Next, a Rubin osteotome is used to reduce the bony prominence. Care is needed to keep the osteotome from being directed too far posteriorly thereby over-reducing the dorsum. Adapted from Austermann, K., Rhinoplasty: planning techniques and complications. In: Booth PW, Hausamen JE, editors. Maxillofacial surgery. New York: Churchill Livingstone; 1999. p. 1389.*

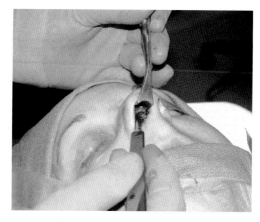

FIGURE **65-29** *Dorsal reduction. An Aufricht retractor lifts the dorsal drape and can protect the skin during hump reduction. A no. 15 blade is used to incise the cartilaginous dorsum. Working through this incision, an osteotome or rasp is used to reduce the bone of the dorsum.*

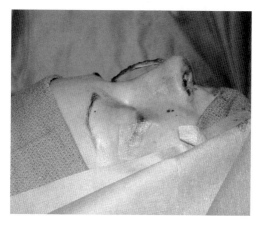

FIGURE **65-30** *Dorsal reduction. The dorsum should be about two-thirds of the cartilage and one-third of the bone.*

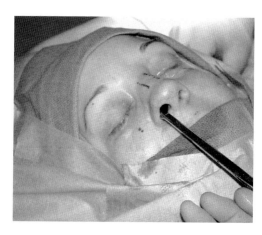

FIGURE **65-31** *Lateral nasal osteotomies. Removal of a large dorsal hump will often leave a flat open roof deformity, and this can be reduced by lateral nasal osteotomies with an invert chisel, saw, or rasp.*

shaped so that it provides support but does not distort the shape of the nose.[25–27] Rib cartilage can also be harvested for augmentation of the nasal dorsum. Silicone sizers can be used to estimate the size and shape of graft needed. Once the graft is harvested, a 0.035 inch K-wire can be placed in the center of the graft to stabilize it. Rib grafts have a tendency to distort with time and the K-wire may help limit this tendency.[28]

For a less aggressive augmentation, autogenous cartilage harvested from the nasal septum can be used. This can be layered and sutured together. It is then placed through traditional rhinoplasty incisions.[29–31]

Alloplastic Augmentation Another technique is to use cadaveric dermis along the nasal dorsum. The advantage here is that no harvesting is required and the material is pliable. However, the resorption of this material is unpredictable. Other implantable materials include silicone and expanded polytetrafluoroethylene (ePTFE) implants. These can be contoured to the appropriate size intraoperatively. The issue with implants is that the grafts can extrude or become infected. Meticulous placement is essential.[31–34]

Osteotomies

Osteotomies are performed after the nasal reduction has been performed. The purposes of lateral nasal osteotomies include reduction of the open nasal roof, correction of deviated nasal bones, and narrowing of a wide nasal base (see Figure 65-31).

There are two principal types of nasal osteotomy: lateral and medial. The lateral nasal osteotomy can be performed at different levels. It typically begins low on the piriform rim and can end either high or low in its relationship to the nasal bones. Thus the osteotomy is often termed as a low-to-low osteotomy or a low-to-high osteotomy. These osteotomies can be performed via an internal or external tech-

nique. Regardless of which technique is used, limited periosteal dissection is favored so that support is provided to the nasal bones. Medial osteotomies are seldom needed but can be used to obtain a controlled fracture in patients with thick nasal bones or when a low-to-low technique is used. Also, regardless of the osteotomy technique, the osteotomies should not be carried above the intercanthal line. The bone above this point becomes much thicker and mobilization becomes difficult. Care should be taken when performing medial osteotomies, since the thicker portion of the nasal bone can be included in the lateral osteotomy segment and result in widening of the upper nasal dorsum. This is termed a rocker deformity.

Lateral nasal osteotomies are not always required to close an open roof deformity after dorsal hump reduction. Some surgeons believe it is better to place spreader grafts in those patients with short nasal bones so that compromise of the internal nasal valve does not occur. If an osteotomy is performed in a patient with shorter nasal bones, then a low-to-high technique is preferred.

Nasal Tip

Understanding the mechanisms of nasal tip support is critical when performing rhinoplasty. The surgeon must understand both the desired and undesired changes that occur from the surgical approach or technique.[35]

The three major tip support mechanisms include the following:

1. The size, shape, and strength of the lower lateral cartilages
2. The attachment of the medial crura to the caudal septum
3. The attachment of the lower lateral cartilages to the upper lateral cartilages

The minor tip support mechanisms include the following:

1. The interdomal ligament
2. The sesamoid complex, extending the support of the lateral crura to the piriform aperture
3. The attachment of the alar cartilages to the overlying skin
4. The cartilaginous septal dorsum
5. The nasal spine
6. The membranous septum[36,37]

Certain surgical procedures can affect tip support. For example a complete transfixion incision will disrupt the fibrous attachments of the caudal septum to the medial crura thus leaving little support for the nasal tip. Suturing techniques and cartilage strut grafts may be necessary to reestablish support if this incision is performed. Intercartilaginous incisions, which are useful to gain access to the nasal dorsum, interrupt the ligamentous connections of the upper and lower lateral cartilages. This can result in cephalic tip rotation, which may or may not be desirable. A cephalic strip procedure creates even further disruption and rotation of the lower lateral cartilages. Most often tip rhinoplasty is designed to refine and decrease the tip lobule while maintaining or even increasing rotation and projection.

The cartilaginous support of the nasal tip is often described in terms of a tripod concept.[38,39] The medial crura of both the lower lateral cartilages together form one strut of the tripod, and each of the lateral crura of the lower lateral cartilages forms a strut. By selectively shortening or lengthening any of these struts, the tip position can be altered.

The tip position changes are referred to in terms of both projection and rotation. Tip projection is the distance from the tip of the nose to the alar-facial junction. Increasing tip projection is one of the most difficult procedures to perform in rhinoplasty surgery. Nasal tip projection can be increased by both grafting and nongrafting techniques.

Tip Projection   *Increasing Tip Projection*   Nongrafting techniques to increase nasal projection include the following:

1. Suturing of divergent medial crura: For this technique to be effective there must be diverging medial crura. Intervening soft tissue may require excision prior to suturing with mattress sutures.[40]
2. Lateral crural steal: The lower lateral cartilage is skeletonized and the lateral crura cartilages are sutured with a mattress suture so that the lateral crura now contributes to the medial crura (Figure 65-32). This results in increased projection and some rotation as well.[41,42]

Grafting techniques to increase projection include the following:

1. Collumellar strut: This technique involves the placement of a strut of septal cartilage between the feet of the medial crura and abutted against the nasal spine. The medial crura are elevated superiorly with double skin hooks and the cartilage strut is sutured to the medial crura via mattress sutures. Only a minor amount of tip projection can be increased with this method.
2. Peck graft: This is an onlay graft in the region of the nasal tip. Layers of cartilage are placed in the domal region to increase projection. The graft material is either conchal or septal cartilage. The cartilage is secured to the dome by sutures. This technique can increase projection by 2 to 6 mm (Figure 65-33).
3. Umbrella graft: This technique involves the creation of a cartilaginous structure that resembles the appearance of an umbrella. It is useful when both tip projection and support of weak medial crura are required. The umbrella graft is constructed from harvested septal, ear, or rib cartilage. It is then sutured in position so that the "handle" of the umbrella is between the medial crura and the "canopy" of the umbrella rests atop the dome. The canopy portion can be modified to incorporate the Peck graft technique by stacking layers of cartilage (Figure 65-34).[43]
4. Shield graft: This graft was first described by Sheen.[30] A piece of septal cartilage is shaped to form a trapezoidal configuration measuring 6 to 8 mm superiorly and 5 mm inferiorly. The graft is usually 10 to 12 mm long and is beveled so that the corners are blunted. The graft is placed in a pocket through an endonasal approach or sutured in position via an open approach. The superior and lateral aspect of the graft forms the tip-defining points (Figure 65-35).[30]

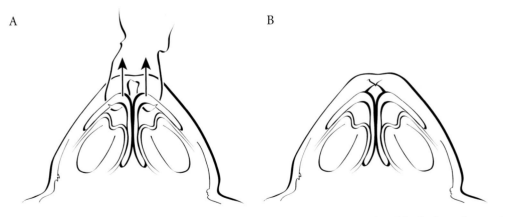

A   B

FIGURE **65-32**   *Lateral crural steal. A, B, A horizontal mattress suture is placed in the lateral crura in order to increase nasal projection and narrow the nasal tip. Adapted from Taylor CO. Surgery of the nasal tip. In: Waite PD, editor. Atlas of the oral and maxillofacial surgery clinics of North America: rhinoplasty. Philadelphia (PA): W.B. Saunders; 1995. p. 61.*

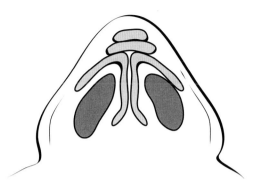

FIGURE **65-33** *Peck graft. This involves the placement of layers of cartilage grafts in the region of the nasal tip to increase nasal projection. Adapted from Taylor CO. Surgery of the nasal tip. In: Waite PD, editor. Atlas of the oral and maxillofacial surgery clinics of North America: rhinoplasty. Philadelphia (PA): W.B. Saunders; 1995. p. 62.*

Decreasing Tip Projection Decreasing tip projection involves reduction of the tip supporting mechanisms. Achieving acceptable results when decreasing projection can be difficult since nasal definition can be lost.[44] If the nasal projection needs to be decreased, be certain to first confirm that the problem is not the result of an optical illusion caused by a low radix position. If the problem is a low radix, then a dorsal radix graft is the appropriate treatment.

Methods to decrease projection include the following:

1. Complete transfixion incision: As discussed above, a complete transfixion incision will decrease tip support. Intercartilaginous incisions or cephalic strips will also weaken the tip support but will increase tip rotation.
2. Lower the septal angle: If the septum is providing significant support for the nasal tip, then the septal angle must be lowered. This is done by excision of a portion of the caudal septum. Additionally the medial crura can be separated from the caudal septum to decrease projection.
3. Crural excision: To dramatically decrease tip projection the medial and lateral crura may need to be sectioned, overlapped, and sutured into a new position with less projection. This technique maintains the natural shape of the tip at the domes (Figure 65-36). Excision of a segment cartilage in the domes and suturing them back together can be done, but it will change the shape of the nasal tip.

Sometimes, after decreasing the nasal projection, the patient may have flaring of the ala and increased infratip columellar show. This can be treated with an alar base resection but should be used judiciously.

Tip Rotation *Increasing Tip Rotation*
Understanding the tripod concept and tip supporting mechanisms is important when determining which of the following methods to use to increase tip rotation.

1. Removal of dorsal hump: A subtle way to increase rotation of the tip is to reduce a dorsal hump if present.
2. Resection of the caudal septum: A small triangular piece of caudal septum can be removed. The base of this triangular shape is at the nasal dorsum.
3. Cephalic strips from lower lateral cartilages: A complete strip of cephalic cartilage from the lower lateral cartilages will result in increased tip rotation. Even an intercartilaginous incision will result in some tip rotation (Figure 65-37).
4. Shorten the lateral crura
5. Shield graft: A shield graft gives the illusion of increased tip rotation.
6. Augmentation of premaxilla: Placement of cartilage or ePTFE in the premaxilla region below the anterior nasal spine will also give the illusion of increased tip rotation.

Decreasing Tip Rotation Decreasing tip rotation is done by two methods:

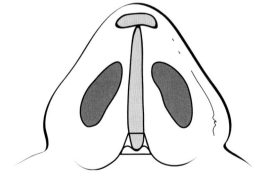

FIGURE **65-34** *Umbrella graft. This is essentially a columellar strut graft placed between the medial crura, combined with a tip graft. This technique improves support of the medial crura as well as increases nasal projection. Adapted from Taylor CO. Surgery of the nasal tip. In: Waite PD, editor. Atlas of the oral and maxillofacial surgery clinics of North America: rhinoplasty. Philadelphia (PA): W.B. Saunders; 1995. p. 61.*

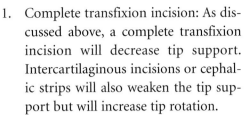

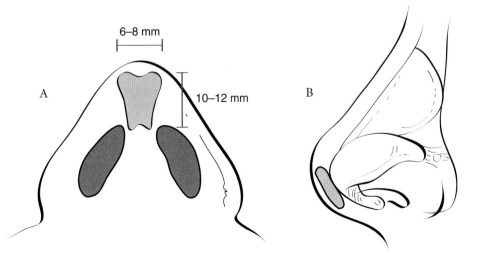

FIGURE **65-35** *Shield graft. A, B, This is a grafting technique used to redefine the tip-defining points of the nose. The graft is typically 6 to 8 mm wide superiorly, 5 mm wide inferiorly, and 10 to 12 mm long. Adapted from Taylor CO. Surgery of the nasal tip. In: Waite PD, editor. Atlas of the oral and maxillofacial surgery clinics of North America: rhinoplasty. Philadelphia (PA): W.B. Saunders; 1995. p. 62.*

1. Trim the caudal septum near the anterior nasal spine
2. Augment the nasal dorsum: this creates the illusion of decreased tip rotation.

Tip Shape   In addition to changing the tip position, the tip shape must also be considered. Historically changes to the nasal tip were performed by selective cartilage excision and reapproximation. The Goldman tip is an example of such a technique. The current trend is to preserve and re-orient existing cartilage and place cartilaginous grafts if required.[45] Excessive grafting can be unpredictable in the long run.

Although cartilage preservation is emphasized there is still sometimes a need to remove cartilage. There are three principal techniques of cartilage excision in the nasal tip region: a complete strip technique, a weakened complete strip technique, and an interrupted strip technique. A greater resection generally results in more dramatic tip narrowing and rotation.

Complete strip techniques involve the removal of a complete piece of cartilage from the cephalic end of the lower lateral cartilages (see Figures 65-37 and 65-38). This procedure is thought to be more stable since it leaves an intact strip of the inferior border of the lower lateral cartilage. Aggressive resection can result in loss of tip support, alar notching, alar retraction, and the appearance of increased collumellar show. Most surgeons feel that a minimum width of 6 mm is required to maintain the structural integrity of the lower lateral cartilage.

The weakened complete strip technique involves the removal of a complete cephalic strip followed by weakening of the cartilage by selective morselization of the medial and lateral crura with a scalpel blade.

An interrupted strip involves division of the lateral crura from the dome (Figure 65-39). This technique provides greater rotation than a complete strip but can also result in complications, including loss of tip support, alar notching, and alar retraction. In addition the nasal tip can develop a pinched appearance. The classic Goldman tip is an example of an interrupted strip technique (Figure 65-40). In this technique the lateral crura are divided lateral to the tip-defining points. The medial segments are sutured together, which results initially in increased tip projection. The lateral crural segments are left alone as independent units. This procedure is no longer commonly used because of problems with tip asymmetry, pinched appearance of the nasal tip, and long-term tip ptosis.

For patients with a broad nasal tip, transdomal suturing techniques are often used to narrow the tip. Volume reduction is performed first if needed by cartilage excision as described above. Next, excision of excessive interdomal soft tissue is performed. A 4-0 polydioxanone transdomal suture is placed in a horizontal mattress fashion to narrow and re-orient the alar cartilages. The advantage of this technique is that the suturing can be done multiple times until the surgeon is satisfied with the result. Additionally the long-term results of this technique have been favorable.[46–48]

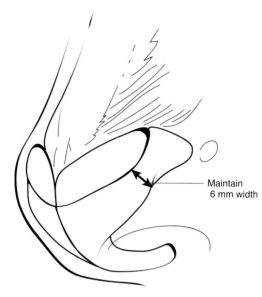

Maintain 6 mm width

FIGURE **65-38**   *Complete strip technique. This involves the excision of a strip of cartilage on the cephalic portion of the lower lateral cartilage. This will result in increased tip rotation. It is important to maintain a minimum of 6 mm width of cartilage for structural support of the nose. Adapted from Taylor CO. Surgery of the nasal tip. In: Waite PD, editor. Atlas of the oral and maxillofacial surgery clinics of North America: rhinoplasty. Philadelphia (PA): W.B. Saunders; 1995. p. 58.*

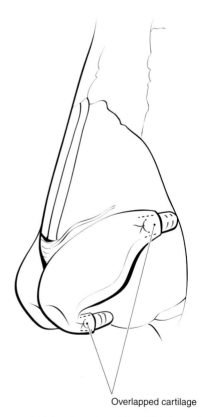

Overlapped cartilage

FIGURE 65-36   *Crural excision. This is used when the nasal tip needs dramatic deprojection. A portion of the lateral crura is excised and the ends are sutured back together.*

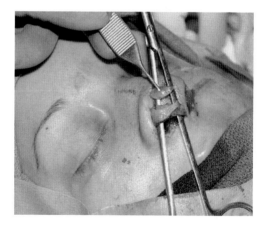

FIGURE **65-37**   *Delivery of lower lateral cartilage. The lower lateral cartilage is best delivered by a marginal incision or exposed through an open rhinoplasty for direct visualization and surgical manipulation. Tip refinement is improved in this case by complete tip reduction to reduce the volume of the tip.*

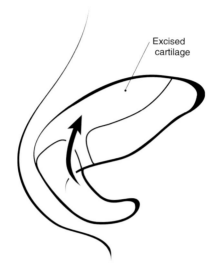

FIGURE **65-39** *Interrupted strip technique. This is similar to the complete strip except the remaining cartilage is also divided in a vertical fashion. This allows for even greater tip rotation, as indicated by the* arrow; *however, it can result in a pinched nasal tip and functional problems. The cartilage can be weakened by scoring it in a vertical fashion and this is termed a weakened complete strip technique. Adapted from Taylor CO. Surgery of the nasal tip. In: Waite PD, editor. Atlas of the oral and maxillofacial surgery clinics of North America: rhinoplasty. Philadelphia (PA): W.B. Saunders; 1995. p. 59.*

Nasal Base Alar Reduction

The alar base should approximate the intercanthal distance and be no more than 1 to 2 mm wider than this. The nostrils should have a symmetric appearance. Asymmetry of the nostril is often due to a deviated nasal septum and this should be reevaluated prior to consideration of an alar base resection.

The primary procedure to reduce the alar base width is an alar base resection. Alar modification is often considered in cases where the nose has to be deprojected or to balance the anatomy in certain ethnic types. It is mandatory to be conservative when performing alar reduction since it is difficult to correct an overreduction. If there is any doubt, the surgeon should delay the alar base reduction until a later date.[49]

The procedure is performed by excising a small wedge of vestibular mucosa

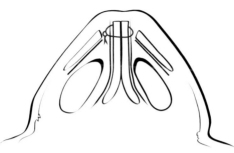

FIGURE **65-40** *Goldman tip. This is an interrupted strip technique in which the lateral crura are divided lateral to the tip-defining points. The medial segments are then sutured together to increase nasal tip projection and to narrow the nasal tip. Adapted from Willis AE, Costa LE. Surgical management of the nasal base. In: Waite PD, editor. Atlas of the oral and maxillofacial surgery clinics of North America: rhinoplasty. Philadelphia (PA): W.B. Saunders; 1995. p. 61.*

and skin. The angulation can be adjusted so that greater reduction of the outer perimeter of the ala is reduced and only limited reduction of the internal perimeter is performed.[49] The excision should be conservative and will rarely be greater than 3 mm in width (Figure 65-41).

Postoperative Management

After performing the rhinoplasty the surgeon must decide whether intranasal stents or packing is necessary. We generally do not place nasal packing. If the septum requires additional support during healing, then silicone stents are placed. These stents are also used if there are mucosal tears or if a turbinectomy was performed. The stents help reduce the incidence of synechiae formation. The stents are secured to each other by a 3-0 silk suture passed through the columella and are typically left in place for 1 week.

Next the nasal dorsum is splinted. Benzoin or mastisol is painted on the nasal dorsum and ¼ inch brown paper tape is applied. After placement of the tape the splint is applied. A metal Denver splint or thermoplastic splint is contoured and applied. Additional paper tape can be placed over the splint.

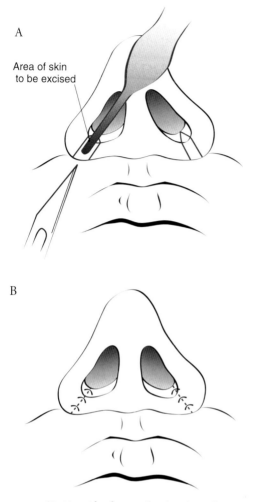

FIGURE **65-41** *Alar base reduction (Weir's excision). A, This is used to narrow an overly wide nostril. B, A small amount of vestibular mucosa and skin is excised and sutured together. The excision is usually 1 to 2 mm wide*

References

1. Rohrich RJ, Huyn B, Muzaffar AR, et al. Importance of the depressor septi nasi muscle in rhinoplasty: anatomic study and clinical application. Plast Reconstr Surg 2000;105:376–83; discussion 384–8.
2. Hollinshead W. Anatomy for surgeons: the head and neck. 3rd ed. Philadelphia (PA): Lippincott-Raven; 1982.
3. Rohrich RJ, Muzaffar AR, Gunter JP. Nasal tip blood supply: confirming the safety of the transcolumellar incision in rhinoplasty. Plast Reconstr Surg 2000;106:1640–1.
4. Toriumi DM, Mueller R, Grosch T, et al. Vascular anatomy of the nose and the external rhinoplasty approach. Arch Otolaryngol Head Neck Surg 1996;122:24–34.
5. Lam SM, Williams LE. Anatomic considerations in aesthetic rhinoplasty. Facial Plast Surg 2002;18:209–14.

6. Dion MC, Jafek BW, Tobin CE. The anatomy of the nose. External support. Arch Otolaryngol 1978;104:145–50.

7. Janfaza P, Nadol JB, Galla R, et al. Surgical anatomy of the head and neck. 1st ed. Philadelphia (PA): Lippincott Williams & Wilkins; 2001. p. 908.

8. Toriumi DM, Josen J, Weinberger M, et al. Use of alar batten grafts for correction of nasal valve collapse. Arch Otolaryngol Head Neck Surg 1997;123:802–8.

9. Sheen JH. Spreader graft: a method of reconstructing the roof of the middle nasal vault following rhinoplasty. Plast Reconstr Surg 1984;73:230–9.

10. Gunter JP, Rohrich DR, William P. Dallas rhinoplasty. 1st ed. Vol 1. St. Louis (MO): Quality Medical Publishing, Inc.; 2002. p. 654–656.

11. Correa AJ, Sykes JM, Ries WR. Considerations before rhinoplasty. Otolaryngol Clin North Am 1999;32:7–14.

12. Meyer L, Jacobsson S. The predictive validity of psychosocial factors for patients' acceptance of rhinoplasty. Ann Plast Surg 1986;17:513–20.

13. Tardy ME Jr, Dayan S, Hecht D. Preoperative rhinoplasty: evaluation and analysis. Otolaryngol Clin North Am 2002;35:1–27,v.

14. Rohrich RJ. The who, what, when, and why of cosmetic surgery: do our patients need a preoperative psychiatric evaluation? Plast Reconstr Surg 2000;106:1605–7.

15. Petroff MA, Mcollough EG, Hom D, et al. Nasal tip projection. Quantitative changes following rhinoplasty. Arch Otolaryngol Head Neck Surg 1991;117:783–8.

16. Crumley RL, Lanser M. Quantitative analysis of nasal tip projection. Laryngoscope 1988;98:202–8.

17. Gunter JP, Rohrich DR, William P. Dallas rhinoplasty. 1st ed. Vol 1. St. Louis (MO): Quality Medical Publishing, Inc.; 2002. p. 65.

18. Gunter JP, Rohrich RJ. Management of the deviated nose. The importance of septal reconstruction. Clin Plast Surg 1988;15:43–55.

19. Courtiss EH, Goldwyn RM, O'Brien JJ. Resection of obstructing inferior nasal turbinates. Plast Reconstr Surg 1978;62:249–57.

20. Pollock RA, Rohrich RJ. Inferior turbinate surgery: an adjunct to successful treatment of nasal obstruction in 408 patients. Plast Reconstr Surg 1984;74:227–36.

21. Jackson LE, Koch RJ. Controversies in the management of inferior turbinate hypertrophy: a comprehensive review. Plast Reconstr Surg 1999;103:300–12.

22. Mabry RL. Intranasal steroids in rhinology: the changing role of intraturbinal injection. Ear Nose Throat J 1994;73:242–6.

23. Rohrich RJ, Kreuger JK, Adams WP Jr, et al. Rationale for submucous resection of hypertrophied inferior turbinates in rhinoplasty: an evolution. Plast Reconstr Surg 2001;108:536–44; discussion 545–6.

24. Elwany S, Harrison R. Inferior turbinectomy: comparison of four techniques. J Laryngol Otol 1990;104:206–9.

25. Posnick JC, Seagle MB, Armstrong D. Nasal reconstruction with full-thickness cranial bone grafts and rigid internal skeleton fixation through a coronal incision. Plast Reconstr Surg 1990;86:894–902; discussion 903–4.

26. Jackson IT, Choi HY, Clay R, et al. Long-term follow-up of cranial bone graft in dorsal nasal augmentation. Plast Reconstr Surg 1998;102:1869–73.

27. Celik M, Tuncer S. Nasal reconstruction using both cranial bone and ear cartilage. Plast Reconstr Surg 2000;105:1624–7.

28. Gunter JP, Clark CP, Friedman RM. Internal stabilization of autogenous rib cartilage grafts in rhinoplasty: a barrier to cartilage warping. Plast Reconstr Surg 1997;100:161–9.

29. Sancho BV, Molina AR. Use of septal cartilage homografts in rhinoplasty. Aesthetic Plast Surg 2000;24:357–63.

30. Sheen JH. Achieving more nasal tip projection by the use of a small autogenous vomer or septal cartilage graft. A preliminary report. Plast Reconstr Surg 1975;56:35–40.

31. Toriumi DM. Autogenous grafts are worth the extra time. Arch Otolaryngol Head Neck Surg 2000;126:562–4.

32. Parker Porter J. Grafts in rhinoplasty: alloplastic vs. autogenous. Arch Otolaryngol Head Neck Surg 2000;126:558–61.

33. Adamson PA. Grafts in rhinoplasty: autogenous grafts are superior to alloplastic. Arch Otolaryngol Head Neck Surg 2000;126:561–2.

34. Romo T 3rd, Sclafani AP, Jacono AA. Nasal reconstruction using porous polyethylene implants. Facial Plast Surg 2000;16:55–61.

35. Adams WP Jr, Rohrich RJ, Hollier LH, et al. Anatomic basis and clinical implications for nasal tip support in open versus closed rhinoplasty. Plast Reconstr Surg 1999;103:255–61; discussion 262–4.

36. Tardy ME Jr, Cheng EY, Jernstrom V. Misadventures in nasal tip surgery. Analysis and repair. Otolaryngol Clin North Am 1987;20:797–823.

37. Thomas JR, Tardy ME Jr. Complications of rhinoplasty. Ear Nose Throat J 1986;65:19–34.

38. McCollough EG, Mangat D. Systematic approach to correction of the nasal tip in rhinoplasty. Arch Otolaryngol 1981;107:12–6.

39. Anderson JR. New approach to rhinoplasty. A five-year reappraisal. Arch Otolaryngol 1971;93:284–91.

40. Tebbetts JB. Shaping and positioning the nasal tip without structural disruption: a new, systematic approach. Plast Reconstr Surg 1994;94:61–77.

41. Foda HM, Kridel RW. Lateral crural steal and lateral crural overlay: an objective evaluation. Arch Otolaryngol Head Neck Surg 1999;125:1365–70.

42. Kridel RW, Konior RJ, Shumrick KA, et al. Advances in nasal tip surgery. The lateral crural steal. Arch Otolaryngol Head Neck Surg 1989;115:1206–12.

43. Mavili ME, Safak T. Use of umbrella graft for nasal tip projection. Aesthetic Plast Surg 1993;17:163–6.

44. Tardy ME Jr, Walter MA, Patt BS. The overprojecting nose: anatomic component analysis and repair. Facial Plast Surg 1993;9:306–16.

45. Tebbetts JB. Rethinking the logic and techniques of primary tip rhinoplasty: a perspective of the evolution of surgery of the nasal tip. Otolaryngol Clin North Am 1999;32:741–54.

46. Tardy ME Jr, Patt BS, Walter MA. Transdomal suture refinement of the nasal tip: long-term outcomes. Facial Plast Surg 1993;9:275–84.

47. Daniel RK. Rhinoplasty: a simplified, three-stitch, open tip suture technique. Part I: primary rhinoplasty. Plast Reconstr Surg 1999;103:1491–502.

48. Daniel RK. Rhinoplasty: a simplified, three-stitch, open tip suture technique. Part II: secondary rhinoplasty. Plast Reconstr Surg 1999;103:1503–12.

49. Tardy ME Jr, Patt BS, Walter MA. Alar reduction and sculpture: anatomic concepts. Facial Plast Surg 1993;9:295–305.

CHAPTER 66

Rhytidectomy

G. E. Ghali, DDS, MD
T. William Evans, DDS, MD

Face-lifting has received significant attention over the past several decades owing to increasing patient demands for a more youthful appearance. The face undergoes harmonious changes in the facial skeleton, deep soft tissue elements, and skin texture during the aging process. Dissection of cadavers has identified facial ligaments, muscle expansions, and dissection planes that give us a better understanding of facial aging and rejuvenation. Perhaps more importantly, it has also been the catalyst for the evolution of a variety of face-lifting techniques. The goal of facial rejuvenation should be to address all components of aging, leaving the patient with a younger-appearing face and a long-lasting result. If this is accomplished, the patient's face and neck will continue to age harmoniously.[1]

Critical evaluation of early techniques and a clear understanding of surgical anatomy have provided insight into the perils and pitfalls of surgical rejuvenation of the face and have resulted in the complexity of various rhytidectomy techniques. Today rhytidectomy is one of the most frequently performed esthetic surgical procedures in the United States.

There are numerous techniques currently used for performing face-lifts but no general agreement as to which of these techniques is most effective[2]; facial esthetic surgeons have discussed the advantages and disadvantages of superficial and deep face-lifts for many years. A clear consensus is difficult because patient variables such as past medical history, anatomy, genetic background, social history (eg, smoking, alcohol), motivation to have esthetic surgery, and environment make it virtually impossible to perform a blinded long-term prospective clinical study. Evaluation of facial esthetic surgery is also difficult because most procedures yield satisfactory results initially, often producing enough improvement to be accepted as a good result.

History

Although doubt still exists as to who performed the first face-lift, most authorities date the procedure to the early part of the twentieth century.[3–13] Historically, rhytidectomy procedures may be divided into three main categories: skin excision, subcutaneous undermining, and superficial musculoaponeurotic system (SMAS) manipulation. Early rhytidectomy procedures were limited to skin excision and wound closure without any appreciable subcutaneous undermining.[3,4,8–10,14] Beginning in the late 1920s, the conventional face-lift operation, consisting of skin dissection with subcutaneous undermining, was established.[13]

The subcutaneous rhytidectomy was the preferred technique for many years. A small amount of subcutaneous tissue is elevated with the skin and is simply redraped, leaving the patient with less redundancy. However, this technique does not address underlying skeletal deformities, ptotic deep soft tissue structures, or changes in skin texture. Therefore, it usually results in a more unnatural look and increases the likelihood of complications, particularly skin slough.

In an attempt to improve the results obtained with the subcutaneous face-lift, several clinicians described techniques to correct platysmal banding and submental lipomatosis.[15–18] The third historic category came with the advent of SMAS manipulation. Multiple surgeons have described various techniques involving the SMAS and platysma to enhance cervicofacial rhytidectomy.[1,19–35] In 1974 Skoog described a procedure based on surgical anatomy.[19] At that time the subdermal plane was accepted by most to be the anatomic limit for face-lifting and rejuvenation. Skoog's technique redraped the skin and platysma together, leaving the patient with a more youthful jaw line.

Subsequently Mitz and Peyronie's description of the SMAS provided an anatomic basis for restoration of the face.[21] Hamra (initially with the deep-plane and later with the composite rhytidectomy) and, later, Owsley (with the multiplanar/multivector approach) modified and improved Skoog's technique by performing a more complete release of the nasolabial fold.[35,36] Ramirez showed that after subperiosteal release, the soft tissues of the cheek, forehead, jowls, lateral canthus, and eyebrows can be restored to their youthful relationship with the underlying skeleton.[37] Finally, Watson and colleagues described a technique similar to that of Owsley but combined it with laser resurfacing.[38] This technique involved a larger plane of subdermal or subcutaneous undermining than that described by Hamra.

Four generations of rhytidectomy techniques are recognized (Table 66-1).[39] Current literature has popularized more complex procedures including the deep-plane and composite rhytidectomies.[1,34,35] These methods have incorporated multiplanar dissections and craniofacial techniques in an attempt to gain better control of the midface soft tissues. Whether these techniques provide longer-lasting results remains to be shown.[1,34,35,39–42] Multiple authors have cautioned that the more complex deep-plane and composite rhytidectomies typically carry increased morbidity.[1,40,41,43–49]

Patient Evaluation

When a rhytidectomy is being contemplated, the treatment requirements of the surgeon must be balanced with the desires of the patient (Table 66-2).[50] These requirements are critical for proper patient selection. The patient evaluation must include general medical and psychological considerations in addition to physical facial features. Neglect of any aspect of the patient evaluation can lead to future problems.[51]

Table 66-1	Generations of Rhytidectomy
I	Subcutaneous dissection only with variable skin undermining
II	Subcutaneous dissection + SMAS plication or imbrication
III	Subcutaneous dissection + SMAS plication or imbrication + deep midface section dissection
IV	Composite dissection
SMAS = superficial musculoaponeurotic system.	

Table 66-2	Rhytidectomy Requirements	
Patient	*Surgeon*
Minimal morbidity risk	Safe and predictably consistent outcomes
Long-lasting results	Reasonable operative time
Quick recovery	Reasonable cost to patients
Affordable	Reasonable postoperative recovery period
Performed on outpatient basis; will be ambulatory	Adaptable for revision procedures
	Teachable to residents and fellows

A thorough medical evaluation must be completed prior to surgery. Medical illnesses such as diabetes, hypertension, hypothyroidism, and asthma must be appropriately treated and controlled preoperatively. Medical evaluation is essential for detecting conditions that may adversely affect a patient's ability to tolerate an anesthetic or that may compromise the final surgical result. Appropriate consultations regarding cardiovascular disease, pulmonary disease, coagulopathies, and other active medical problems should be obtained preoperatively. Current medication profiles should be elicited, including aspirin and aspirin-containing compounds, nonsteroidal anti-inflammatory drugs, and herbal drugs, as well as high doses of vitamin E. Examination of prior surgical incisions, such as those resulting from previous thyroidectomies or parotidectomies, is useful in evaluating the wound-healing capacity.

Tobacco and alcohol use, as well as the use of illicit substances, may increase the incidence of surgical complications. Cigarette smoking, diabetes mellitus, and previous head and neck radiation therapy may also impede healing and should be recognized preoperatively. Patients should be told that cigarette smoking significantly increases the likelihood of skin flap necrosis, poor healing, and unsightly scars.[52,53] Studies have demonstrated a 12-fold greater risk of skin slough in smokers compared with that in nonsmokers.[52,53] Animal studies involving skin flap experiments have also supported this conclusion.[52–57]

A review of the patient's psychological history should focus on motivation for surgery and outcome expectations. Patients seeking surgery based on recent emotional events or with unrealistic expectations should be further counseled and the procedure postponed or cancelled.[58,59]

The goal of face-lifting is to correct anatomic changes to the face and neck that have occurred as a result of the normal aging process. Patients considered for rhytidectomy present with various degrees of age-related alterations to the facial soft tissues. Ideally, face-lift candidates are 45 to 55 years of age, are in good health, are of normal weight, possess a good bone structure, and possess a thin neck and a deep cervicomental angle. Physical examination of the patient includes a detailed regional evaluation of the face. A face-lift is capable of correcting specific anatomic regions, and a complete and detailed description of the patient's physical characteristics is important. A systematic evaluation allows the surgeon to assess the areas that can be improved with an isolated rhytidectomy and to determine whether other ancillary procedures will be beneficial. Additionally, a detailed regional evaluation provides an opportunity for the surgeon and the patient to understand the limitations of the rhytidectomy; the surgeon can refer to the evaluation when explaining the expected outcome.

Evaluation of the upper facial one-third includes the forehead and upper and lower eyelids. In general, these areas are not affected by the standard rhytidectomy and are therefore not addressed in this review. Evaluation of the middle facial one-third includes the face and ears. The quality of the skin should be noted, including thickness, redundancy, previous scarring, fine or coarse rhytids, and the location of the hairline. Patients with significant elastosis or actinic damage do not obtain and retain the same quality of results as do patients possessing good skin quality. Assessment of the ear lobe shape and position is critical, and any deviations from normality should be pointed out to the patient preoperatively. Documentation of the nasolabial folds, including length, depth, and symmetry, as well as an assessment of the degree of jowls should be noted. Presence of perioral rhytids is important because they are not corrected with rhytidectomy procedures.

The evaluation of the lower facial one-third includes the chin, jaw line, and neck. A useful preoperative classification of the neck for cervicofacial rhytidectomy divides the neck profile into six distinct classes (Table 66-3).[60] Using this classification, the clinician can identify each patient's specific abnormality and choose the most appropriate procedure for optimal results (Figure 66-1). Skin redundancy, platysmal banding, cervicomental angle, and submental fat accumulation are important to note in this region. Additionally, the degree of ptosis of the submandibular glands should be assessed and recorded at this time.

Preoperative photographs provide invaluable medicolegal documentation as well as an opportunity to review patient characteristics before and during surgery. The surgeon should obtain the photographs of the full face in repose and smiling, right and left profiles, and right and left three-quarter views. Close-ups of the forehead, eyebrows, and periorbital and perioral regions should be taken, depending on the particular deformity.

An essential component of the patient evaluation includes the preoperative visit.

Table 66-3	Dedo Classification of Facial Profiles
Classification	*Comments*
I. Normal	Well-defined cervicomental angle
	Good muscle tone
	No submental fat
II. Cervical skin laxity	Obtuse cervicomental angle owing to relaxed skin
III. Submental fat accumulation	Requires submental lipectomy
IV. Platysma muscle banding	Requires muscle clipping, plication, or imbrication
V. Retrognathia/microgenia	Requires genioplasty or orthognathic surgery
VI. Low hyoid	Difficult to alter
	Important to inform patient of limitation

Adapted from Dedo DD.[60]

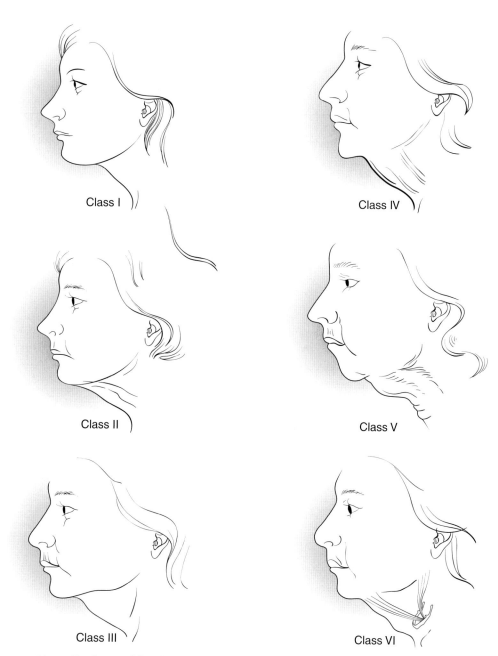

Class I

Class II

Class III

Class IV

Class V

Class VI

FIGURE 66-1   *Six classes of facial profiles by Dedo. Adapted from Dedo DD.*[60]

It is an excellent opportunity to educate the patient regarding various aspects of the procedure, postoperative care, and expectations. It is wise to review any and all patient instructions during the preoperative visit including medications, skin cleaning, and makeup. Patients must discontinue all aspirin-containing compounds, nonsteroidal anti-inflammatory medications, and vitamin E at least 2 weeks prior to surgery. Germicidal shampoo and skin cleaners are used several days before the scheduled date of the procedure to reduce bacterial counts. The patient should wash his or her hair and face and remove all makeup the night before surgery. A written copy of postoperative instructions should be given to and reviewed with the patient (Appendix).

A description of the expected convalescence is appropriate during the preoperative visit. In general, 10 to 14 days is a reasonable time period to wait for ecchymosis to resolve sufficiently to allow camouflage with makeup. Patients should not expect to return to work or social activities before this time. They should be educated regarding expectations in the early postoperative period since those unaware of the slow evolution of results will quickly become frustrated. It should be clearly explained that appearance will continue to improve over a period of several months.

Surgical Technique

Superficial-Plane Rhytidectomy

Once appropriate monitors are placed and the patient is adequately sedated, proposed incision lines and anticipated areas of undermining are marked with a skin marker while the patient is seated in an upright position. The face, neck, and hair are prepped with an appropriate antiseptic surgical scrub. Skin preparations should include the full length of the planned incision and all exposed skin within the surgical field.

Our preference is to perform rhytidectomies under local anesthesia with appropriate sedation and analgesia. Suitable agents include intravenous fentanyl, midazolam, ketamine, and/or propofol. Local anesthesia is provided along the incision line with a 2% lidocaine solution with 1:100,000 epinephrine via a dental syringe. Hydrodissection is performed within the planned plane of dissection with a tumescent anesthetic technique (Figure 66-2).[61–66]

Although multiple techniques exist for mixing the tumescent solution, our preference is to mix 20 mL of a 2% lidocaine with 1:100,000 epinephrine solution with 180 mL of normal saline, creating a solution of 0.2% lidocaine with a 1:1,000,000 epinephrine concentration. This mixture is administered through four trocar sites: temporal, infralobular, mastoid, and submental (Figure 66-3). The solution is deposited subcutaneously in the supra-SMAS plane.

Hydrodissection should extend 1 cm beyond the proposed undermining mark that delineates the anticipated extent of flap

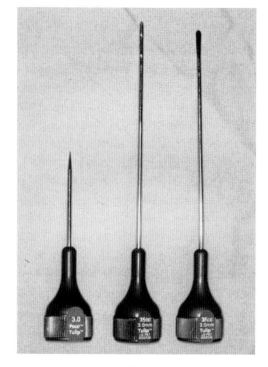

FIGURE **66-2**   From left to right: *procar/trocar, infiltrator, and dissector used for the tumescent technique.*

development. Approximately 75 mL of the tumescent anesthetic solution is deposited per side, with an additional 50 mL deposited

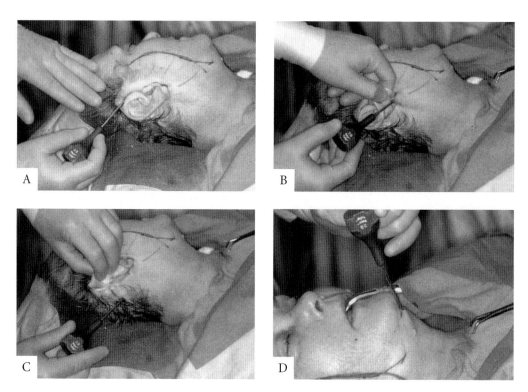

FIGURE **66-3**   *Four trocar sites are typically used:* A, *temporal;* B, *infralobular;* C, *mastoid;* D, *submental.*

in the submental region. The anesthetic is allowed to work for 8 to 10 minutes before proceeding. Typically, the contralateral side is not infiltrated until just prior to initiating closure on the first side.

Following deposition of the anesthetic solution, blunt cannula dissection of the cervicofacial and submental regions is performed. The cervicofacial dissection is generally performed without suction (Figure 66-4), whereas the submental dissection is performed under suction (Figure 66-5). The submental dissection, using the blunt cannula, is accomplished prior to the initiation of the cervicofacial dissection. As previously mentioned, the planned incisions should be marked with the patient seated in an upright position,

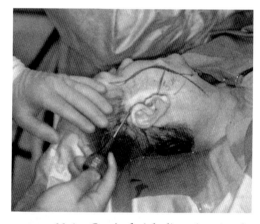

FIGURE **66-4** *Cervicofacial dissection in the supra-SMAS (superficial musculoaponeurotic system) plane without suction.*

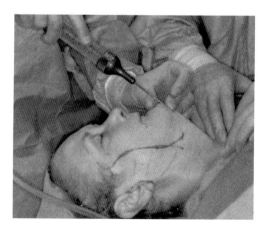

FIGURE **66-5** *Submental dissection in the supraplatysmal plane under suction.*

and prior to administration of the local anesthetic, to prevent distortion of local anatomy. There are numerous modifications of the standard face-lift incision, but several general principles should be followed closely.[67–70]

It is not necessary to shave the hair in the incision area. If necessary, the hair may be braided along the proposed incision, with the temporal extension placed no more than 2 cm within the hair and parallel to the hairline. Some surgeons recommend a pretrichial incision to prevent the posterosuperior migration of the temporal line.

The incision should be extended inferiorly toward the root of the helix, anterior to the curve of the crus helicis, following the margin of the tragus, and proceed anteriorly just above the base of the incisura intertragica (Figure 66-6). Preservation of the incisura helps to prevent distortion of the tragus postoperatively, providing a more esthetic scar. The incision curves inferiorly 1 to 2 mm below the junction of the lobule with the cheek, rising superiorly onto the back of the conchal bowl approximately 3 to 5 mm and reaching the level of the postauricular sulcus or superior crus of the antihelix. The incision is then directed posteroinferiorly approximately 4 to 5 cm into the scalp of the retromastoid region (Figure 66-7).

If significant cervical skin redundancy is noted, the incision may parallel the posterior hairline for several centimeters before being directed into the hair-bearing skin. This maneuver can prevent a step deformity in the posterior hairline when significant cervical skin is excised. Care must be taken to maintain approximately a 90% angle at the reflection of the posterior flap to prevent skin slough at the tip of the flap.

Several considerations for incision design are important in the male patient.[18,71] In the temporal region the planned incision is affected by the patient's hair pattern. Individuals with thick temporal hair can tolerate a standard incision. Those with thinning hair,

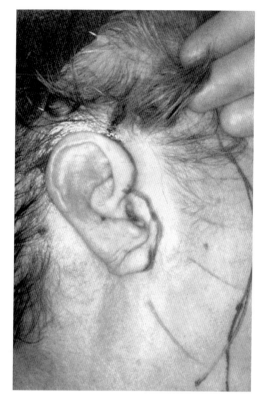

FIGURE **66-6** *Temporal, preauricular, and infralobular components of the typical rhytidectomy incision.*

temporal recession, or significant male pattern baldness require a modification of the incision design.

In the preauricular region, the male sideburn must be taken into consideration and the non–hair-bearing skin anterior to the ear must be left intact to prevent an unnatural appearance. Therefore, the incision should extend in a linear fashion, following a natural skin crease adjacent and parallel to the sideburn. This is in contrast to the curved incision used in female patients.

Last, the posterior extension of the incision is placed along the margin of the postauricular hairline. Although this placement has the potential to be slightly more noticeable, the importance of preventing posterior displacement or a step deformity to the hairline must be taken into account. A final consideration in the male patient is the inevitable transfer of hair-bearing skin into the postauricular region or into the ear canal itself.

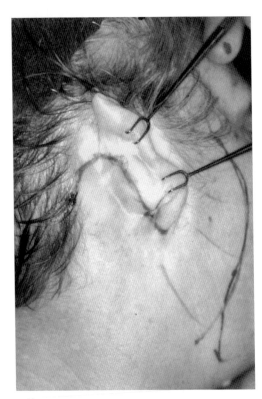

FIGURE **66-7** *Postauricular and mastoid components of the typical rhytidectomy incision.*

Management of the cervical region, if indicated, is begun with the placement of a transverse incision in a submental skin crease as an extension of the submental trocar puncture (Figure 66-8). This incision should not be placed in the dominant crease of the "double-chinned" deformity, as scarring may result during the healing process and accentuate the crease. The incision should be approximately 2 cm in

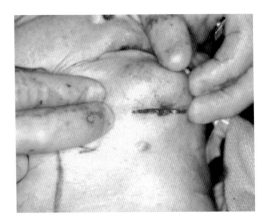

FIGURE **66-8** *Submental incision placed to address platysmal banding.*

length and placed just inferior to the dominant crease.

Dissection in the submental region proceeds in a subcutaneous plane and joins the lateral subcutaneous neck planes subsequent to the submental dissection. Excess subcutaneous fat may be excised with sharp scissors or a cannula, if indicated. Lipectomy in the submental region should be done cautiously. Overly enthusiastic removal of fat in this region can lead to an atrophic appearance of the cervical facial tissues or a "cobra" neck deformity.[17]

Next, the anterior borders of the platysma bands are identified, and excess subcutaneous tissue is removed. The medial borders should be released along their deep surface from the submental region inferiorly to the level of the thyroid cartilage. The medial borders are then repositioned in the midline, and any overlapping tissue is excised. Plication of the medial platysma borders proceeds from the submental region to the level of the thyroid cartilage with a 2-0 slow-resorbing suture (Figure 66-9).

A horizontal myotomy of the inferior aspect of the platysma may be beneficial in accentuating the cervicomental angle and relieving tension along the anterior surface of the neck. Partial horizontal transection is frequently all that is required and can be performed with sharp scissors at the inferior-most aspect of the dissection of the medial borders. If complete transection is indicated, the lateral aspect of the platysma can be excised through the lateral neck face-lift flap.[25,28,72,73]

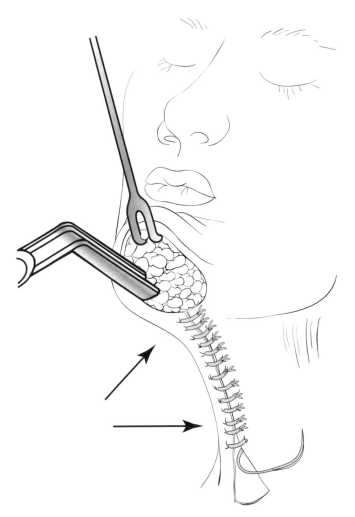

FIGURE **66-9** *Platysmal plication accomplished.*

Flap Development Flap development is initiated by undermining 1 cm along the entire length of the face-lift incision. This is accomplished in a subdermal plane with a blade or sharp scissors, using skin hooks for retraction (Figure 66-10). On the underside of the flap, maintain approximately 3 to 4 mm of subcutaneous fat to preserve the subdermal vasculature.

In the temporal region, the depth of the flap should be carried through the temporoparietal fascia (subgaleal) down to the loose areolar tissue overlying the deep temporal fascia. Dissection in this plane creates a thicker flap, providing increased protection from any ischemic injury that would damage hair follicles and create subsequent alopecia. The temporal dissection is extended in this plane using a combination of blunt and sharp dissection.

Blunt-tipped scissors should be used in a push-cutting motion into the residual tunnels that were developed secondary to the previous blunt cannula dissection (Figure 66-11). Rees T-clamps are used for countertraction and aid in the dissection. Undermining in this plane can be safely carried superiorly to the level of the lateral canthus.

At this point the dissection is carried inferiorly and medially across the cheek in the subcutaneous plane. This zone of transition from the sub-SMAS (deep to the temporoparietal fascia) to the subcutaneous plane of dissection corresponds to

the mesotemporalis that contains the superficial temporal artery and the frontal branch of the facial nerve.[74–76] The facial nerve is located anterior and inferior to the frontal branch of the superficial temporal artery, so preservation of this vessel during dissection helps to protect this important nerve.

The extent of undermining necessary depends on the patient. Younger patients without excessive laxity of the skin require only 4 to 5 cm of undermining, but older patients with redundant tissue and severe jowling may require undermining to within 1 cm of the oral commissure. When platysma banding is present, the cervical dissection is carried inferiorly to the level of the thyroid cartilage and should communicate with the dissection from the contralateral side.

In the postauricular region, the flap should be developed in the subcutaneous plane below the ear lobe to protect the great auricular nerve. This nerve is the one most commonly injured during rhytidectomy procedures (Figure 66-12).[77–79] The great auricular nerve runs just deep to the superficial fascia overlying the sternocleidomastoid muscle and supplies sensation below and behind the ear. With the head turned 45° toward the contralateral side, the great auricular nerve consistently crosses the middle of the sternocleidomastoid muscle at a level 6.5 cm below the caudal edge of the bony external auditory canal (Erb's point).[79] Maintaining subcutaneous dissection below the ear lobe helps protect the great auricular nerve, but above the level of the ear lobe, the greater auricular is not at risk and dissection may be carried deeper.[80] Meticulous hemostasis is then accomplished with bipolar cautery. Overzealous use of electrocautery should be avoided on the skin-flap side to reduce the risk of ischemic injury and flap necrosis.

Next, the underlying SMAS in the cheek region is manipulated. Many of the age-related changes in the facial region are due to ptosis of the underlying fat. Correc-

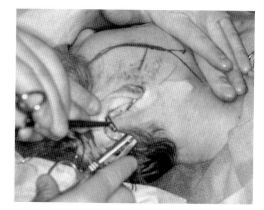

FIGURE **66-11** *Scissors are used in a push-cutting motion with the tips up.*

tion of these changes is best obtained by repositioning this tissue along direction lines (vectors) different from those used for the skin flap. Independent bidirectional suspension of the SMAS and the skin flap reposition the ptotic facial tissues, providing longer-lasting results and reducing an unnatural appearance.

SMAS manipulation can be by plication, imbrication, or a combination of these techniques; there are proponents of each method. *Plication* is a technique whereby the SMAS is folded upon itself to obtain the desired repositioning, and *imbrication* is a technique in which the SMAS is incised or excised so that the distal portion is repositioned to overlap the proximal tissue (Figure 66-13).

SMAS plication is accomplished with a 2-0 slow-resorbing suture on a tapered

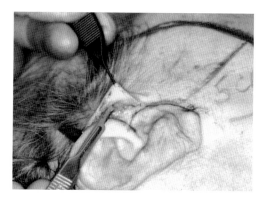

FIGURE **66-10** *Flap development initiated by 1 cm undermining via a blade or sharp dissection scissors.*

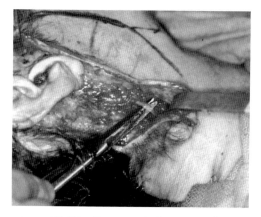

FIGURE **66-12** *Great auricular nerve demonstrated.*

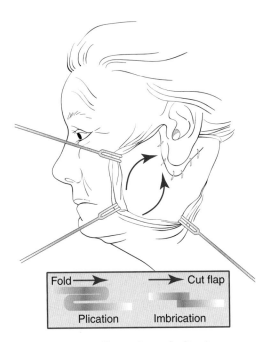

FIGURE **66-13**   *Illustration of plication versus imbrication.*

needle (Figure 66-14). All knots are buried to prevent irritation to the skin flap or palpability. Two key sutures are placed initially, with the first extending from the fascia overlying the angle of the mandible to the fascia immediately inferior to the tragus. The second suture is placed from the fascia lateral to the oral commissure to the fascia immediately superior to the tragus. Several additional sutures may be placed, if needed, in the preauricular and postauricular areas. This suture placement provides a posterosuperior repositioning of the ptotic tissues.

Imbrication requires elevation of a sub-SMAS flap. An incision is made horizontal-ly just inferior to the zygomatic arch and vertically posterior to the angle of the mandible. Landmarks for the incision include the zygomatic arch, tragus, platysma muscle, and the mandible (Figure 66-15). The horizontal incision is made approximately 1 cm below and parallel to the zygomatic arch to prevent damage to the frontal branch of the facial nerve. The middle portion of the tragus may be used as a reference for staying below the zygomatic arch.

The incision is carried forward 2 to 3 cm. The vertical incision descends inferiorly along the posterior border of the platysma several centimeters below the angle of the mandible. It is important to keep the incision posterior to the angle of the mandible to prevent damage to the marginal mandibular branch of the facial nerve. The SMAS is then elevated for 2 to 3 cm in a sub-SMAS plane (Figure 66-16). The flap is redraped posterosuperiorly and sutured using the technique previously described for plication.

Redraping of the skin flap is performed with the patient's head in a neutral position. Extension or flexion of the neck influences the amount of skin excised and may adversely affect the outcome. Key suspension staples or sutures are placed prior to trimming the skin flap. In general, the skin flap is redraped in a posterosuperior direction with an emphasis on the posterior direction. The majority of the needed superior suspension is accomplished by SMAS

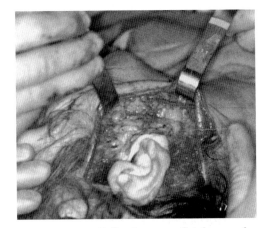

FIGURE **66-16**   *Following superficial musculoaponeurotic system flap elevation, 2-0 resorbable suture on a tapered needle is used for buried knots to secure the imbrication.*

manipulation. Care should be taken to prevent a misdirection of facial rhytids and a distortion of the temporal hairline. Careful assessment of appearance should be made prior to suturing the flap in place.[81]

The first key skin-suspension suture (or staple) is placed in the temporal region just above the ear. The flap is then grasped, and the appropriate vector is determined and held in place while the flap is trimmed and the staple placed. The second staple is placed in the postauricular region at the most posterior and superior aspect of the flap. Careful attention should be given to proper inset of the ear. In a nonoperated ear, the long axis of the ear lobe hangs 10 to 15° posterior to the long axis of the ear proper. This relationship must be maintained to prevent obvious deformities of the ear.

Skin Closure   Trimming of excess skin is performed with a blade or Iris scissors (Figure 66-17). It is important to be aware of the amount of skin to be excised in the temporal region to prevent distortion of the hairline. The distance from the lateral canthus to the anterior margin of the temporal hairline should be recorded preoperatively to serve as a reference for skin excision. Skin closure in the hair-bearing scalp (ie, temporal and mastoid regions) is performed with subdermal 3-0 resorbable sutures. Staples may be

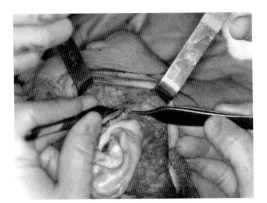

FIGURE **66-14**   *The area of plication is assessed.*

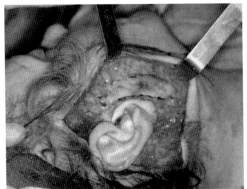

FIGURE **66-15**   *The area of proposed resection in preparation for imbrication is marked.*

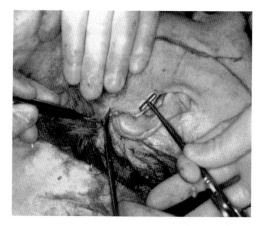

FIGURE **66-17** *Following the placement of key staples, flap trimming is accomplished with a blade or Iris scissors.*

used to approximate skin margins of the temporal and mastoid scalp. Our preference is to provide a layered closure to minimize tension on the most superficial aspect of the skin.[81] The immediate postauricular region is closed with a 4-0 plain gut suture, without the need for deep sutures. In the preauricular region, a 4-0 resorbable suture is placed followed by approximation of the skin edges with a 6-0 or 7-0 nylon running suture. The deep layers of the submental incision are closed with 4-0 resorbable suture, and 6-0 nylon is used for the skin edges.

The decision of whether to place drains must be made on an individual basis, depending on how much oozing or edema is present. In our experience drains are rarely needed. Antibacterial ointment and gauze dressings should be placed along the incision lines. Gauze is also placed preauricularly and postauricularly as well as in the submental region. The entire face should then be wrapped, taking care to prevent excessive tightness of the dressing as it can lead to ischemia of the flaps (Figure 66-18). Additionally, the appropriate positioning of the ears under the dressing should be noted. Dressings should not be manipulated for evaluation until the first postoperative day. Most complications in rhytidectomy occur early in the postoperative period (ie, 24–36 h); close follow-up is therefore essential.[82–85] Some surgeons prefer to use

no dressings postoperatively.[86] The degree of edema and ecchymosis postoperatively is frequently underestimated and can be quite shocking to the patient, despite the surgeon's best attempts to educate him or her. The patient's hair should be gently cleansed and rinsed for additional comfort. Incision lines should be cleansed daily with a 1:1 solution of hydrogen peroxide and water. Antibacterial ointment should be used until all sutures are removed.

The preauricular sutures are removed after 4 to 5 days, as are the staples in the temporal and mastoid regions after 10 days. Patients should be instructed not to wash their hair until all sutures have been removed and then to wash only gently with baby shampoo. Written suggestions for the avoidance of ultraviolet light and high heat from hair dryers and for the use of sunblock and incision massage should be given to the patient and repeated orally in the early postoperative visits. The effects of the procedure are still striking for years after surgery (Figures 66-19 and 66-20).

Deep-Plane Rhytidectomy

After the induction of general anesthesia and intubation, 3 cc of sterile methylene blue is introduced through each parotid duct to stain the parotid glands. This allows for confident and safe dissection and is an excellent teaching aid.

The circle of knowledge and caution (CKC) is then drawn on both cheeks (Figure 66-21). This is a circle of required precise knowledge of facial anatomy needed by both experienced and inexperienced surgeons performing face-lifts. Point A, representing the origin of the zygomaticus major muscle, is measured along a line from the lateral canthus to the tragion, 2 cm posterior and 2.5 cm inferior to the lateral canthus. Point B, representing the perforating branch of the transverse facial artery, is measured 3 cm posterior and 3.5 cm inferior to the lateral canthus. A circle is drawn with point A as the center

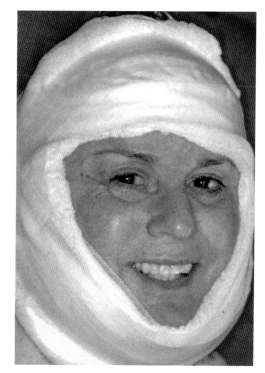

FIGURE **66-18** *Typical face-lift dressing immediately postoperatively.*

and the radius being the distance between points A and B. Obviously, these measurements are not exact in every patient.

The CKC represents the most complex area of anatomy and the most dangerous area in terms of risk in a deeper-plane face-lift procedure. The perforating branch of the transverse facial artery that is accompanied by a small sensory branch of the zygomaticofacial nerve is the "caution sign." If the artery is severed during the sub-SMAS dissection, it gives a bloody warning to the surgeon that the CKC is near; with careful dissection in the known area of this artery, preservation can be accomplished but is not mandatory in nonsmokers. Safe entrance into the CKC is from superior to this perforating branch over the origin of the zygomaticus major muscle through the zygomatic osteocutaneous ligament. If this is followed, the surgeon will never encounter the zygomatic branch of the facial nerve and only occasionally will encounter the branch of the zygomatic branch that enters the deep aspect of the superior third of the zygomaticus major muscle.

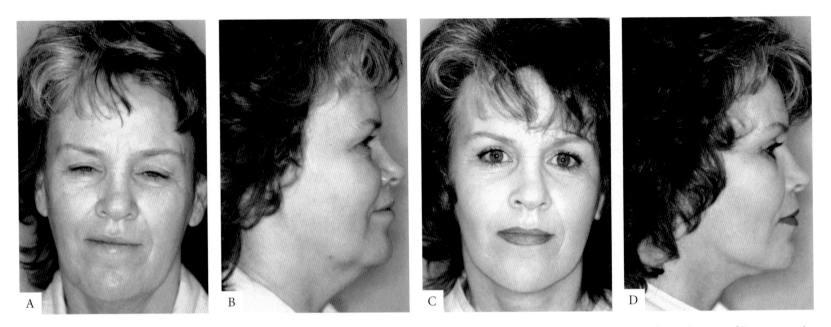

FIGURE 66-19   *Typical result achieved with a superficial-plane rhytidectomy including superficial musculoaponeurotic system imbrication:* A *and* B, *preoperative photographs;* C *and* D, *photographs taken 2 years postoperatively.*

The contents of the CKC are the perforating branch of the transverse facial artery, the zygomatic osteocutaneous ligaments, the infraorbital osteocutaneous ligaments, the superior portion of the masseteric fasciacutaneous ligaments, the origins of the zygomaticus muscles, the inferolateral portion of the orbicularis oculi muscle, the zygomatic branch of the facial nerve and its branch to the deep aspect of the superior third of the zygomaticus major muscle, the occasionally present inferior palpebral branch of the facial nerve to the orbicularis oculi muscle, and possibly the parotid duct.

Xylocaine 2% with epinephrine 1:50,000 is instilled only in the area of the planned incision, not under the skin flap or the SMAS flap. Since an endoscopic brow lift is usually performed simultaneously with this deep-plane technique, an incision, as drawn in Figure 66-22, is usually preferred in both females and males. We prefer the pretragal incision unless a female patient specifically requests a retrotragal incision. Incisions in the sideburn and in the posterior hair edge are significantly beveled to allow hair growth through the resultant scar.

Preauricular subcutaneous dissection is performed to a level superficial to the lateral part of the orbital portion of the orbicularis oculi, which interrupts the fibrous septa in the superficial fat layer that cause crow's-feet rhytids and also interrupts the fibrous septa of the zygomatic osteocutaneous ligaments and masseteric fasciacutaneous ligaments. The subcutaneous dissection proceeds 2 cm posterior to the oral commissure and extends just inferior to the lower border of the mandible, where the previously performed cervical subcutaneous dissection is encountered. This subcutaneous dissection is not taken to the melonasolabial groove to allow the SMAS–malar fat pad–skin complex to remain intact. Postauricular subcutaneous dissection is performed superficial to the sternocleidomastoid-investing fascia to the level of the cricoid cartilage and anterior in the neck to the previously performed cervicoplasty subcutaneous dissection superficial to the investing superficial fascia of the platysma muscle. The posterior border of this dissection is the anterior border of the trapezius muscle (Figure 66-23). The subcutaneous dissection is significantly

reduced in smokers and patients with other microvascular disease, and this may compromise the natural postoperative result. In smokers the perforating branch of the transverse facial artery is not interrupted in either the subcutaneous or sub-SMAS planes and is maintained for perfusion of the skin flap border.

The SMAS incision is marked posterior to anterior along the inferior border of the zygomatic arch until the origin of the posterior border of the superficial head of the masseter muscle is palpated (the zygomatic arch descends to meet zygomatic buttress). The marking is then directed toward the pupil extending over the orbital portion of the orbicularis oculi muscle and fascia to the level of the inferior orbital rim. The preauricular SMAS marking is 1 cm anterior and parallel to the skin incision (Figure 66-24). At the lobule of the ear, the SMAS marking turns posteriorly 10° and extends to the level of the cricoid cartilage (extent of neck dissection) parallel and anterior to the posterior border of the platysma muscle.

The SMAS incision is made through the vascular orbicularis oculi muscle with cautery; then a scalpel is used to

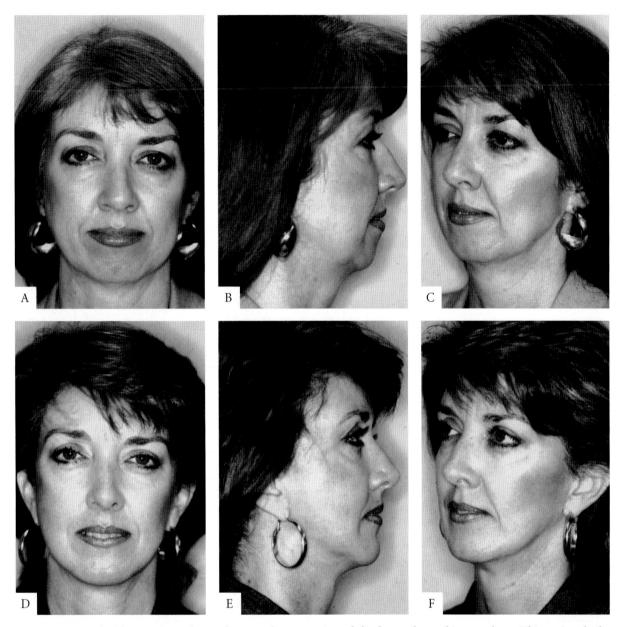

FIGURE **66-20**   *Rhytidectomy procedures often complement various skeletal or orthognathic procedures. This patient had a superficial rhytidectomy, rhinoplasty, and augmentation genioplasty. A–C, Preoperative views; D–F, 2½ years postoperatively.*

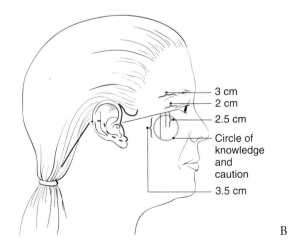

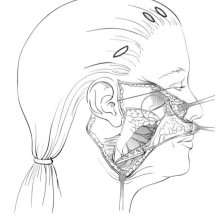

FIGURE **66-21**   A, *The circle of knowledge and caution (CKC) is constructed by measuring 2 cm and 3 cm from the lateral canthus along a line from the lateral canthus to the tragion. From these respective points, 2.5 cm and 3.5 cm inferior is the origin of the zygomaticus major muscle and the perforating branch of the transverse facial artery. The circle is drawn with the origin of the zygomaticus major as the center, and the radius is the distance from this point to the perforating branch of the transverse facial artery. B, CKC transposed over the extended multiplanar multivector face-lift dissection.*

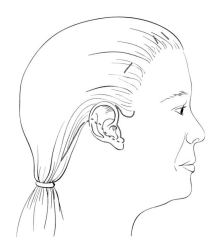

FIGURE 66-22   *Face-lift skin incision (pretragal).*

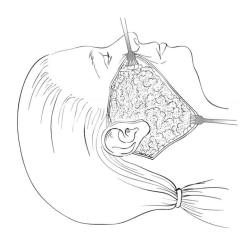

FIGURE 66-23   *Subcutaneous dissection (sideburn and postauricular hair clipped, not shaved).*

continue the incision to approximately 2 cm below the ear lobe. Scissor dissection to protect the great auricular nerve and the external jugular vein completes the SMAS incision in the neck to the level of the cricoid cartilage.

SMAS flap elevation is started with a scalpel at the posterosuperior edge, and sharp dissection exposes the sub-SMAS fat at the superior pole of the parotid gland that protects the frontal branch of the facial nerve. Continued inferior sharp dissection exposes the parotid fascia seen easily because of the blue-stained parotid gland. The CKC area is dissected last, after the rest of the entire SMAS flap is mobilized (Figure 66-25).

As previously described, there is strict adherence between the SMAS aponeurosis and the parotid fascia, and sharp dissection is required to separate the SMAS from the parotid fascia. This same adherence from scarring after SMAS repositioning is what helps give this deeper-plane technique long-term stability. A SMAS incision anterior to the parotid fascia does not give this benefit, and more dependence is placed on the sutures.

Once the anterior edge of the blue-stained parotid gland is seen or the dissection becomes much easier because of fatty/areolar tissue, sharp dissection is stopped. The remainder of the sub-SMAS flap dissection, except for the CKC area, can be achieved with blunt scissor dissection, remaining just deep to the facial SMAS and the neck platysma fascia. The deep fat layer is areolar and more fatty, allowing blunt dissection over the masseteric fascia to or through the masseteric fasciacutaneous ligaments and deep to the platysma fascia in the neck to join the previously performed cervicoplasty dissection. The area over the posterior portion of the submandibular gland is gently bluntly dissected. The only exception to this is in the area of the platysma cutaneous ligaments, where sharp dissection is required. Care is taken around the angle of the mandible to remain just deep to the neck platysma fascia to remain clear of the marginal mandibular branch of the facial nerve, which is rarely seen. Multiple cervical branches of the facial nerve perforating the deep fasciae that penetrate the deep surface of the platysma muscle are visualized in the neck, and vertical blunt scissor dissection preserves them.

The CKC area is next addressed. The caution sign is the perforating branch of the transverse facial artery (Figure 66-26). Once this is encountered, sharp sub-SMAS dissection with scissors is directed superior to this vessel, through the zygomatic ligaments until the origin of the zygomaticus major muscle is visualized (Figure 66-

27). Dissection is continued over and parallel to the zygomaticus muscles deep to the superficial leaf of investing superficial facial fascia (SMAS) of the zygomaticus muscles and deep to the anterior portion of the divided orbicularis oculi muscle and its investing fascia (SMAS) for about half the length of the zygomaticus muscles (Figure 66-28). This dissection is safe if it remains superficial to the zygomaticus muscles and deep to the cut anterior edge

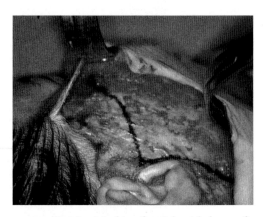

FIGURE 66-24   *Marking for right-sided superficial musculoaponeurotic system incision. The anterosuperior portion of the mark is directed toward the right pupil, not the lateral canthus.*

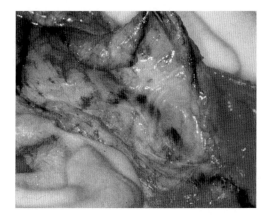

FIGURE 66-25   *The initial sharp dissection of the right-sided superficial musculoaponeurotic system (SMAS) flap, separating the SMAS from sub-SMAS fat superior to the superior pole of the methylene blue–stained parotid gland, and the SMAS from the parotid fascia over the methylene blue–stained parotid gland. The appearance of sub-SMAS fat and the outline of the anterior border of the parotid gland determine the end of sharp dissection and the start of blunt dissection between the SMAS and masseteric fascia.*

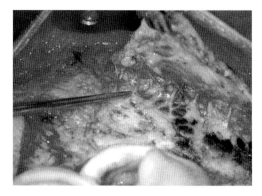

FIGURE **66-26** *Right-sided sub-SMAS (superficial musculoaponeurotic system) dissection with the instrument pointing to the perforating branch of the transverse facial artery—the start of the circle of knowledge and caution.*

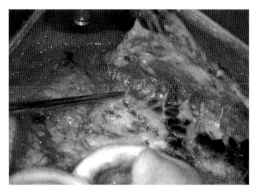

FIGURE **66-27** *Right-sided sub-SMAS (superficial musculoaponeurotic system) dissection with a clamp grasping portions of the zygomatic osteocutaneous ligaments, which will be interrupted to uncover and visualize the origin of the zygomaticus major muscle.*

posterior immobile neck SMAS. Moderate posterior traction is placed on the preauricular SMAS flap, the excess is excised, and the mobile SMAS flap is sutured to the posterior immobile SMAS (Figure 66-31). The SMAS is reapproximated to maintain the integrity of the SMAS/mimetic muscles complex to allow natural animation. Stability is obtained by having the resultant scarring of the SMAS complex in close relationship with the natural facial fascial tissue adherence areas. The vectors of traction are opposite the vectors of aging, with excess SMAS being removed that should be approximately equal to the amount of tissue ptosis present before surgery (Figure 66-32).

Excessive traction on the anterosuperior portion of the SMAS flap will flatten the melonasolabial groove completely giving an unnatural result. Sufficient repositioning of the malar fat pad to rejuvenate, not obliterate, the melonasolabial groove is desired. Rarely, dissection deep to the malar fat pad but superficial to the facial mimetic muscles is required to mobilize the malar fat pad sufficiently, and the malar fat pad is elevated and independently sutured to the SMAS.[87–90] The skin is then redraped along a slightly superoposterior vector, and a cut is made to free the ear lobe. The skin flap is then elevated, and any bleeders are coagulated. The area of surgery is irrigated well

of the orbicularis oculi muscle. Dissection is continued through the zygomatic osteocutaneous ligaments and the infraorbital osteocutaneous ligaments (often to the nose) (Figure 66-29) and carefully through the superior masseteric fasciacutaneous ligaments until the SMAS flap, which includes the ptotic malar fat pad, is freely mobilized (Figure 66-30). If more mobilization is required (rarely occurs), blunt dissection is accomplished cautiously through the masseteric fasciacutaneous ligaments to the anteroinferior insertion of the masseter muscle exposing the buccal fat pad, the peripheral branches of the zygomatic and buccal branches of the facial nerve, and the facial vessels.

Moderate superoposterior traction is placed on the passively mobile SMAS flap, a back cut is made at the superoposterior point, and a key 2-0 slow-resorbing suture is used to fix the SMAS flap to the immobile superoposterior SMAS. The appropriate amount of superior SMAS flap is then excised along with a pie-shaped section of SMAS/orbital portion of the orbicularis oculi muscle. This section is then re–approximated with 2-0 slow-resorbing suture in a superoposterior vector elevating the midface, relocating any prolapsed infraorbital fat, and improving the lower eyelid/cheek junction (along with the pre-

vious interruption of the infraorbital osteocutaneous ligaments). The superior SMAS flap is then sutured with a 2-0 slow-resorbing suture in a vertical vector to elevate the lower face and jowl.

Moderate posterosuperior traction is then placed on the SMAS flap in a direction parallel and slightly superior to the inferior border of the mandible, a back cut is made, and another key 2-0 slow-resorbing suture is placed to fix this SMAS flap to the stout parotid cutaneous ligaments to define the inferior border of the mandible. Mild posterior traction is placed on the neck SMAS (platysma), the excess is excised, and the mobile neck SMAS flap is sutured to the

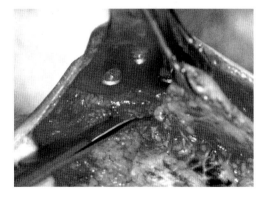

FIGURE **66-28** *Right-sided subsuperficial fascia dissection superficial to the zygomaticus major muscle for approximately half the length of the muscle.*

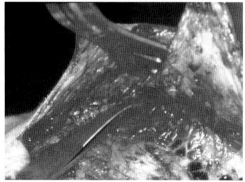

FIGURE **66-29** *Right-sided suborbicularis oculi muscle/SMAS (superficial musculoaponeurotic system) dissection in the suborbicularis oculi fat to interrupt the infraorbital osteocutaneous ligaments, often as far medial as the nose.*

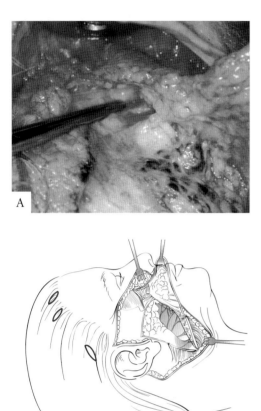

A

B

FIGURE 66-30 *A, Right-sided complete mobilization of superficial musculoaponeurotic system flap. The instrument is pointing to the zygomaticus minor muscle. The cut edge of the orbicularis oculi muscle invested by superficial fascia and fat can be seen. B, Illustration of the anatomy in Figure A.*

with saline, and both the SMAS and the undersurface of the skin flap are dried with sponges. Fibrin glue is sprayed in all areas, and the skin flap is appropriately positioned. Compression without movement is applied for 5 minutes.

Excess skin is carefully excised and closure is performed with 5-0 polyglactin 910 sutures in the subcutaneous layer, dermal adhesive on the preauricular skin incision, and 5-0 fast-absorbing gut suture in the postauricular skin incisions. No drains are used. Cotton is placed over the areas of surgery, and moderate pressure is applied for 8 to 12 hours with facial and occipital pressure bands. The dressing is intended to prevent abnormal facial and neck movement during the first 8 to 12 hours of the postoperative period.

Summary

Over the past two decades, numerous rhytidectomy techniques have been described to improve the results of facial rejuvenation. When contemplating facial rejuvenation surgery, the treatment requirements of the surgeon must be balanced with the desires of the patient. These requirements are critical in defining the advantages of one technique of face-lifting over the other. As we prepare our patients for esthetic

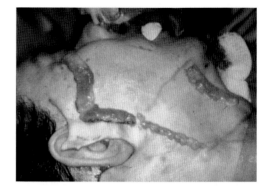

FIGURE 66-32 *The amount of facial and neck superficial musculoaponeurotic system (SMAS; including the central neck SMAS from cervicoplasty) removed in a typical extended multiplanar multivector face-lift. Notice the passive redraping of the skin.*

surgery, we must consider all the variables discussed and individualize each treatment plan. Not all patients should undergo a deep-plane face-lift; however, many will benefit from release of the retaining ligaments and a repositioning of tissues in multiple vectors.

In the realm of oral and maxillofacial surgery, the rhytidectomy procedure finds great application as an adjunct to traditional skeletal surgery. It seeks to reverse the effects of gravity and relaxation of the facial skin and fascia by resuspending the facial units and eliminating excess skin and subcutaneous tissue. Although a wide variety of

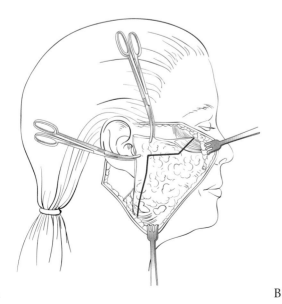

A

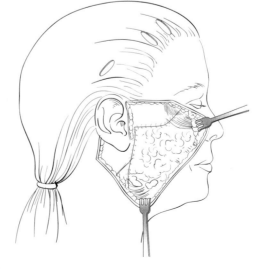

B

FIGURE 66-31 *A and B, Moderate traction is placed on the superficial musculoaponeurotic system (SMAS) flap, the excess SMAS is excised after the superoposterior key suture is placed, and the SMAS flap is sutured in the appropriate vectors to the fixed SMAS.*

techniques are reported for face-lifting, we have attempted to provide a broad overview of the superficial-plane rhytidectomy and deep multiplanar techniques. These techniques are both efficacious and safe. By tailoring the approach to the specific needs of each patient, based on a thorough knowledge of surgical anatomy, the maxillofacial surgeon should achieve consistently good results with minimum morbidity.

References

1. Hamra ST. Composite rhytidectomy. Plast Reconstr Surg 1992;90:1–13.

2. Miller TA. Face-lift: which technique? Plast Reconstr Surg 1997;100:501.

3. Joseph J. Hangewangenplastik (Melomio-plastik). Dtsch Med Wochenschr 1921;47:287.

4. Lexer E. Die Gesamte Wiederherstellungschiurgie. Vol 2. Leipzig: JA Barth; 1931.

5. Rogers BO. A brief history of cosmetic surgery. Surg Clin North Am 1971;51:265–88.

6. Rogers BO. The development of aesthetic plastic surgery: a history. Aesthet Plast Surg 1976;1:3.

7. Rogers BO. A chronologic history of cosmetic surgery. Bull N Y Acad Med 1977;47:265–302.

8. Passot R. La chirirgie esthetique des rides du visage. Presse Med 1919;27:258.

9. Bourguet J. La disparipion chirurgicale des rides et plis du visage. Bull Acad Med (Paris) 1919;82:183.

10. Bettman AG. Plastic and cosmetic surgery of the face. Northwest Med 1920;19:205.

11. Kolle FS. Plastic and cosmetic. New York: Appleton;1911. p. 116–7.

12. Miller CC. Semilunar excision of the skin at the outer canthus for the eradication of crow's feet. Am J Dermatol 1907;11:483.

13. Barnes H. Truth and fallacies of face peeling and face lifting. Med J Reconstr 1927;126:86.

14. Hollander E. Cosmetic surgery. In: Joseph M, editor. Handbuch der Kosmetik. Leipzig: Verlag von Veit; 1912.

15. Aufricht G. Surgery for excess skin of the face and neck. In: Wallace EB, editor. Transaction of the International Society of Plastic Surgeons. Second Congress. London: Livingstone; 1960. p. 495–502.

16. Adamson JE, Horton CE, Crawford HH. The surgical correction of the "turkey gobbler" deformity. Plast Reconstr Surg 1964;34:598–605.

17. Millard DR, Pigott RW, Hedo A. Submandibular lipectomy. Plast Reconstr Surg 1968;41:513–22.

18. Baker TJ, Gordon HL. Rhytidectomy in males. Plast Reconstr Surg 1969;44:219–22.

19. Skoog T. Plastic surgery—new methods and refinements. Philadelphia: WB Saunders; 1974.

20. Guerro-Santos J, Espaillat L, Morales F. Muscular lift in cervical rhytidoplasty. Plast Reconstr Surg 1974;54:127–30.

21. Mitz V, Peyronie M. The superficial musculoaponeurotic system (SMAS) in the parotid and cheek area. Plast Reconstr Surg 1976;58:80–8.

22. Owsley JQ. Platysma-fascial rhytidectomy: a preliminary report. Plast Reconstr Surg 1977;60:843–50.

23. Owsley JQ. SMAS-platysma face lift. Plast Reconstr Surg 1983;71:573–6.

24. Connell BF. Cervical lifts: the value of plastyma muscle flaps. Ann Plast Surg 1978;1:32–43.

25. Connell BF. Contouring the neck in rhytidectomy by lipectomy and a muscle sling. Plast Reconstr Surg 1978;61:376–83.

26. Gerro-Santos J. The role of the platysma muscle in rhytidoplasty. Clin Plast Surg 1978;5:29–49.

27. Guerro-Santos J. Surgical correction of the fatty fallen neck. Ann Plast Surg 1979;2:389–96.

28. Aston SJ. Platysma muscle in rhytidoplasty. Ann Plast Surg 1979;3:529–39.

29. Lemmon ML, Hamra ST. Skoog rhytidectomy: a five year experience with 577 patients. Plast Reconstr Surg 1980;65:283–97.

30. Lemmon ML. Superficial fascia rhytidectomy. A restoration of the SMAS with control of the cervicomental angle. Clin Plast Surg 1983;10:449–78.

31. Kaye BL. The extended neck lift: the "bottom line." Plast Reconstr Surg 1980;65:429–35.

32. Kaye BL. The extended face-lift with ancillary procedures. Ann Plast Surg 1981;6:335–46.

33. Teimourian B. Face and neck suction-assisted lipectomy associated with rhytidectomy. Plast Reconstr Surg 1983;72:627–33.

34. Hamra ST. The tri-plane facelift dissection. Ann Plast Surg 1984;12:268–74.

35. Hamra ST. The deep-plane rhytidectomy. Plast Reconstr Surg 1990;86:51–61.

36. Owsley JQ. Lifting the malar fat pad for correction of prominent nasolabial folds. Plast Reconstr Surg 1993;91:463–74.

37. Ramirez OM. The subperiosteal rhytidectomy: the third-generation facelift. Ann Plast Surg 1998;28:218–32.

38. Watson SW, Stone TL, Sinn DP. The four dimensional rhytidoplasty. Am J Cosmet Surg 2001;18:5–13.

39. Duffy MJ, Friedland JA. The superficial-plane rhytidectomy revisited. Plast Reconstr Surg 1994;93:1392–403.

40. Psillakis JM, Rumley TO, Camargos A. Subperiosteal approach as an improved concept for correction of the aging face. Plast Reconstr Surg 1988;82:383–94.

41. De la Plaza R, Valiente E, Arroyo JM. Supraperiosteal lifting of the upper two-thirds of the face. Br J Plast Surg 1991;44:325–32.

42. Ramirez OM, Maillard GF, Musolas A. The extended subperiosteal facelift: a definitive soft-tissue remodeling for facial rejuvenation. Plast Reconstr Surg 1991;88:227–36.

43. Keller GS. KTP laser rhytidectomy. Facial Plast Surg Clin North Am 1993;1:157.

44. Beeson WH. Extended posterior rhytidectomy. Facial Plast Surg Clin North Am 1993;1:215.

45. Binder WJ. A comprehensive approach for aesthetic contouring of the midface in rhytidectomy. Facial Plast Surg Clin North Am 1993;1:253.

46. Rubin LR, Simpson RL. The new deep plane face lift dissections versus the old superficial techniques: a comparison of neurologic complications [editorial]. Plast Reconstr Surg 1996;97:1461–5.

47. Baker DC. Deep dissection rhytidectomy: a plea for caution [editorial]. Plast Reconstr Surg 1994;93:1498–9.

48. Adamson PA, Moran ML. Complications of cervicofacial rhytidectomy. Facial Plast Surg Clin North Am 1993;1:133–42.

49. Kaye BL. The superficial-plane rhytidectomy revisited [discussion]. Plast Reconstr Surg 1994;93:1404–5.

50. Ghali GE, Smith BR. A case for superficial rhytidectomy. J Oral Maxillofac Surg 1998;56:349–51.

51. Baker TJ. Patient selection and psychological evaluation. Clin Plast Surg 1978;5:3–14.

52. Rees TD, Liverett DM, Guy CL. The effect of cigarette smoking on skin-flap survival in the facelift patient. Plast Reconstr Surg 1984;73:911–3.

53. Webster RC, Kazda G, Hamden US, et al. Cigarette smoking and facelift: conservative versus wide undermining. Plast Reconstr Surg 1986;77:596–604.

54. Lawrence WT, Murphy RC, Robson MC, et al. The detrimental effect of cigarette smoking on flap survival: an experimental study in the rat. Br J Plast Surg 1984;37:216–9.

55. Kaufman T, Eichenlaub EH, Levin M, et al. Tobacco smoking: impairment of the experimental flap survival. Ann Plast Surg 1984;13:468–72.

56. Craig S, Rees TD. The effects of smoking on experimental skin flaps in hamsters. Plast Reconstr Surg 1985;78:842–6.

57. Nolen J, Jenkins RA, Kurihara K, et al. The acute effects of cigarette smoke exposure on experimental skin flaps. Plast Reconstr Surg 1985;75:544–51.

58. Edgerton MT, Webb WL, Slaughter R, et al. Surgical results and psychosocial changes following rhytidectomy. Plast Reconstr Surg 1964;33:503–21.

59. Goin MK, Burgoyne RW, Goin JM, et al. Prospective psychologic study of 50 female facelift patients. Plast Reconstr Surg 1980;65:436–42.

60. Dedo DD. A preoperative classification of the neck for cervicofacial rhytidectomy. Laryngoscope 1980; 90:1894–6.

61. Schoen SA, Taylor CO, Owsley TG. Tumescent technique in cervicofacial rhytidectomy. J Oral Maxillofac Surg 1994;52:344–7.

62. Klein JA. The tumescent technique for liposuction surgery. Am J Cosmet Surg 1987;4:263.

63. Lillis PJ. Liposuction surgery under local anesthesia: limited blood loss and minimal lidocaine absorption. J Dermatol Surg Oncol 1988;14:1145–8.

64. Klein JA. Tumescent technique for regional anesthesia permits lidocaine doses of 35 mg/kg for liposuction: peak plasma lidocaine levels are diminished and delayed 12 hours. J Dermatol Surg Oncol 1990;16:248–63.

65. Klein JA. The tumescent technique anesthesia and modified liposuction technique. Dermatol Clin 1990;8:425–37.

66. Lillis PJ. The tumescent technique for liposuction surgery. Dermatol Clin 1990;8:439–50.

67. Talamas I. A nondeforming rhytidectomy incision. Aesthetic Plast Surg 1999;23:228–32.

68. Stuzin JM, Baker TJ, Baker TM. Refinements in face lifting: enhanced facial contour using Vicryl mesh incorporated into SMAS fixation. Plast Reconstr Surg 2000;105:290–301.

69. Knize DM. Periauricular facelift incisions and the auricular anchor. Plast Reconstr Surg 1999;104:1508–20.

70. Little JW. Hiding the posterior scar in rhytidectomy: the omega incision. Plast Reconstr Surg 1999;104:259–72.

71. Baker DC, Aston SJ, Guy CL, et al. The male rhytidectomy. Plast Reconstr Surg 1977;60:514–22.

72. Peterson R. The role of the platysma muscle in cervical lifts. In: Symposium on surgery of the aging face. St. Louis: Mosby; 1978. p. 115–24.

73. Connell BF. Contouring the neck in rhytidectomy by lipectomy and a muscle sling. Plast Reconstr Surg 1978;61:376–83.

74. Aston SJ. Platysma muscle in rhytidoplasty. Ann Plast Surg 1979;3:529–39.

75. McKinney P, Tresley GE. The "maxi-SMAS": management of the platysma bands in rhytidectomy. Ann Plast Surg 1984;12:260–7.

76. Baker DC, Conley J. Avoiding facial nerve injuries in rhytidectomy. Anatomical variation and pitfalls. Plast Reconstr Surg 1979;64:781–95.

77. Liebman EP, Webster RC, Berger AS, et al. The frontalis nerve in the temporal brow lift. Arch Otolaryngol 1982;108:232–5.

78. Stuzin, JM, Wagstrom L, Kawamoto HK, et al. Anatomy of the frontal branch of the facial nerve: the significance of the temporal fat pad. Plast Reconstr Surg 1989;83:265–71.

79. McKinney P, Katrana DJ. Prevention of injury to the greater auricular nerve during rhytidectomy. Plast Reconstr Surg 1980; 66:675–9.

80. McKinney P, Gottlieb J. The relationship of the great auricular nerve to the superficial musculoaponeurotic system. Ann Plast Surg 1985;14:310–4.

81. Webster RC, Smith RC, Karolow WW, et al. Comparison of SMAS plication with SMAS imbrication in face-lifting. Laryngoscope 1982;92:901–12.

82. Webster R, Smith R, Hall B. Facelift—better results with safer surgery of the head and neck. In: Ward P, Berman W, editors. Plastic and reconstructive surgery of the head and neck. St. Louis: CV Mosby; 1984. p. 321–3.

83. Gordon HL. Rhytidectomy. Clin Plast Surg 1978; 5:97–107.

84. Baker DC. Complications of cervicofacial rhytidectomy. Clin Plast Surg 1983; 10:543–62.

85. Rees TD, Baker DC. Complications of aesthetic facial surgery. In: Conley J, editor. Complications of head and neck surgery. Philadelphia: WB Saunders; 1980.

86. Aston SJ. Problems and complications in platysma-SMAS cervicofacial rhytidectomy. In: Kaye B, Gradinger G, editors. Symposium on problems and complications in aesthetic plastic surgery of the face. St. Louis: CV Mosby; 1983.

87. Owsley JQ. Lifting the malar fat pad correction of prominent nasolabial folds. Plast Reconstr Surg 1994;93:463-74.

88. Owsley JQ. Elevation of the malar fat pad superficial to the orbicularis oculi muscle for correction of prominent nasolabial folds. Clin Plast Surg 1995;22:2.

89. Owsley JQ, Weibel TJ. Multiple vector face-lift: SMAS-platysma rotation flap plus midface malar fat pad suspension, Oper Tech Plast Reconstr Surg 1995;2:99–107.

90. Forrest CR, Phillips JH, Bell A, Gruss JS. The biomechanical effects of deep tissue support as related to brow and facelift procedures. Plast Reconstr Surg 1991;88:427–32.

Appendix   Postoperative Rhytidectomy Instructions

Immediately upon Arriving Home

Head elevation: Lie down with your head and back elevated on two pillows. You must sleep in this position for 1 week.

Dressings: Do not remove bandages. These will be removed at the office on your first postsurgery visit.

Ice packs: Place ice packs (ice in freezer bags or packages of frozen peas) over the cheek areas on and off over a period of 24 hours. *Do not* put ice on after 24 hours unless you are told to do so.

Swelling: Ice packs will keep swelling and bruising to a minimum.

Bruising: Bruising often lasts 7 to 14 days.

Medication: Take pain medication *only if needed* and with food or crackers.

Diet: Upon arriving home from surgery, begin with clear liquids until fully awake; then begin regular food intake with soft foods.

Suture care: Keep all sutures clean with a peroxide-water solution. Keep sutures covered with antibiotic ointment at all times. Clean three to five times per day.

One Day or More after Surgery

Moist heat: Ice packs are to be discontinued 24 hours after surgery. *Wait 12 hours;* then you may begin moist heat. Use a moist washcloth between an electric heating pad and your face. Do not use heat continuously; for example, use for 30 minutes and then off for 30 minutes. *Do not* set the heating pad higher than *medium* at any time, regardless of how cool it feels to you.

Activity: Stay up as much as possible. Avoid bending over or lifting heavy objects for 1 week. Strenuous activities should be limited for 2 to 3 weeks.

Work: Most people plan to return to work in 2 weeks. This depends on how you feel about being seen with bruising. Most of the bruising can be masked with makeup if you prefer to return earlier.

Makeup: Cosmetics may be applied on the sixth day. Ask about special coverup products for bruising. Mint green coverstick followed by a flesh-tone foundation will cover most bruises.

Bathing: You may bathe or shower, but keep the bandages dry. When bandages are removed, gently wash the facial areas.

Hair care: You may wash your hair on the fifth day after surgery. *Do not bend over* to wash your hair; this may cause bleeding or swelling to occur. Use medium heat on your hair dryer. High heat or hot rollers should not be used for 7 to 10 days. You may use color on your hair in 3 weeks.

Diet: Eat regular but soft meals. You will need to take vitamins and minerals to help with the healing. We will be glad to give you vitamin and mineral information.

Sun: Protect your facial skin from excessive sun exposure for 1 month after surgery.

Please report any of the following to our office:

Excessive pain or bleeding
Itching or rash around stitches
Oral temperature > 100°F (37.8°C)
Excessive swelling/bruising, fatigue, or depression

CHAPTER 67

Forehead and Brow Procedures

Angelo Cuzalina, MD, DDS

Upper facial cosmetic surgery has enjoyed an unprecedented increase in popularity over the past decade. The yearning of baby boomers to look and feel rejuvenated has led to new endoscopic techniques aimed at creating a more youthful and natural appearance with shorter recovery periods than existed in past decades.[1–3] The ultimate goal of improving a person's appearance remains unchanged. Society shapes our views of what looks attractive, and no mathematic formula can ever be used to determine an ideal eyebrow position (Figure 67-1). Each individual has his or her own unique perception of facial beauty. For most people the upper face and eyes impart more emotion than does any other part of the human body; it is clear that rejuvenation of this vital area can provide an esthetically pleasing result.

Esthetic concerns of the forehead and brow regions of the face affect a wide range of age groups. Unlike the standard lower face and neck rhytidectomy, which more commonly affects patients after the age of 45 years, cosmetic concerns in the upper third of the face may be evident for patients in their twenties and thirties owing to genetic predisposition. The forehead and brow area must be entirely evaluated for a wide range of interlacing diagnoses. Matching the problem(s) to the ideal rejuvenation technique(s) is essential for maximum esthetic benefits. Thinning skin and laxity owing to age and gravity

encompass only a portion of the forehead and brow dilemmas that must be addressed when planning rejuvenation procedures (Figure 67-2).

The aging process typically leads to forehead and brow ptosis on almost every patient; however, it is important to distinguish whether the ptosis in the forehead and brow region is owing to problems with brow position, upper eyelid laxity, or a combination of the two (Figure 67-3). Other problems such as dynamic lines caused by muscle activity in the glabellar

region, variable hairline patterns, bony abnormalities, and asymmetries, as well as skin texture itself, also must be assessed in relation to each other. Achieving the patient's desired expectation depends not only on sound surgical skill and judgment, it also depends critically on communication between the surgeon and patient. Truthful disclosure of what can reasonably be attained is prudent and helps to prevent patient dissatisfaction.

Rejuvenation of the upper third of the face is one of the most rewarding and

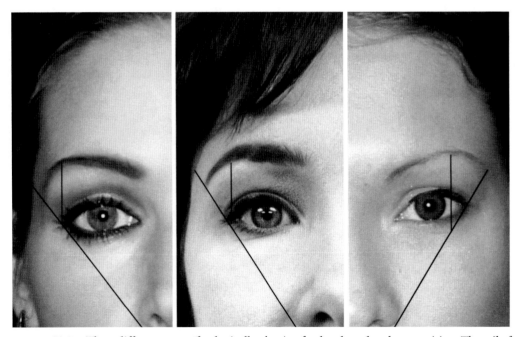

FIGURE **67-1** *Three different types of esthetically pleasing foreheads and eyebrow position. The tail of the eyebrow is located along the alar-canthal line. The greatest brow arch is seen in the lateral third between the lateral limbus and canthus of the eye. The outer half of the brow is "ideally" located 5 to 10 mm above the orbital rim in females.*

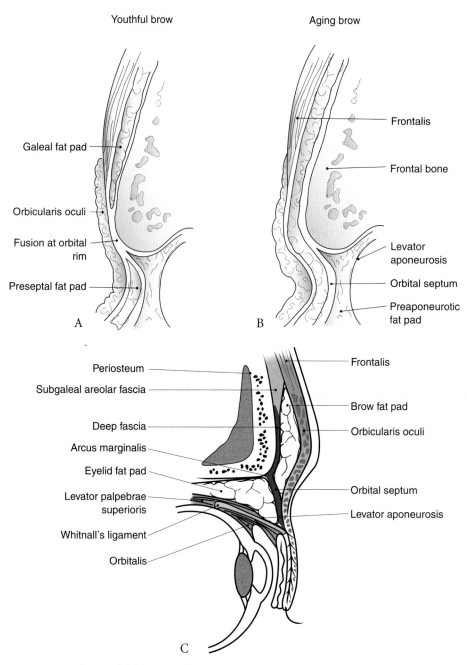

Youthful brow

Galeal fat pad

Orbicularis oculi

Fusion at orbital rim

Preseptal fat pad

A

Aging brow

Frontalis

Frontal bone

Levator aponeurosis

Orbital septum

Preaponeurotic fat pad

B

Periosteum

Subgaleal areolar fascia

Deep fascia

Arcus marginalis

Eyelid fat pad

Levator palpebrae superioris

Whitnall's ligament

Orbitalis

Frontalis

Brow fat pad

Orbicularis oculi

Orbital septum

Levator aponeurosis

C

FIGURE 67-2   A, *The youthful brow is elevated proportionately and has densely adherent periorbital fascia and muscle.* B, *Brow descent owing to aging and the associated loss of fascial integrity, along with orbital fat prolapse.* C, *Crosss-section of the brow near the mid-pupillary position.*

fulfilling procedures a surgeon can offer to select patients. Specific elevation and correction of lateral hooding can be appear natural and still impart a tremendous improvement in the patient's overall beauty and youthful appearance (Figure 67-4). The goal of this chapter is to review the upper third of facial anatomy specific to forehead and brow rejuvenation techniques and to discuss a variety of the most

common techniques for rejuvenating the forehead and brow region.

Anatomic and Esthetic Considerations

It is generally accepted that a youthful forehead is roughly one-third of the overall facial height.[4–9] Essentially, the distance from the hairline to the glabella is equal to the distance from the glabella to the point

at the base of the columella or subnasale (Figure 67-5). A youthful-appearing eyebrow is different for men and women. The female eyebrow should be arched with the highest point of the brow on a sagittal line from the lateral canthus.[10,11] The entire brow itself should be above the orbital rim. In general the medial brow of the female is located ideally 1 to 3 mm above the orbital rim and the lateral third of the brow 5 to 10 mm above the rim.[12] This is in contrast to a typical male eyebrow that should lie at or only slightly above the orbital rim in a more horizontal or uniform arch fashion (Figure 67-6). Elevating the lateral third of the male eyebrow disproportionately more than the remaining brow will create a feminine appearance.

The detailed anatomy of individual areas has been well described in the literature and often relates to the specific procedure being performed.[13–25] Therefore, the following anatomic discussion is simplified by separating the specific regions into bony landmarks, muscle and fascial anatomy, vessel and nerve anatomy, and specific endoscopic anatomy, and each anatomic region is addressed individually as it relates to specific surgical procedures.

Bony Landmarks

Bony landmarks of the forehead and brow region can be focused all around the frontal bone, which makes up the highest percentage of the upper third of the face. The connections (suture lines such as the nasofrontal, zygomaticofrontal, and coronal) are important landmarks because they can be clinically relevant for limits of dissection and can help surgeons determine their location during dissection. For instance, the zygomaticofrontal suture line is an ideal location to end most basic brow lift dissections (Figure 67-7). Additional dissection can be performed if midface lifting is also planned or if the patient desires more elevation at the lateral canthal region. Overaggressive dissection here in many patients can create an unnatural

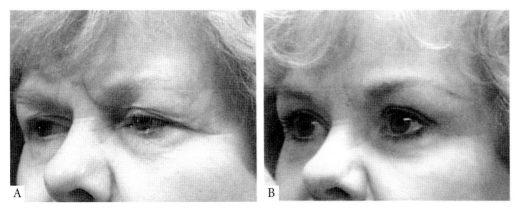

FIGURE **67-3** A, *Rejuvenation of the upper third of the face must address whether the problem is limited to brow ptosis, eyelid ptosis, or a combination of both, as seen in the patient on the left. Skin texture must also be evaluated. B, This photograph was taken 1 month after a coronal brow lift, upper blepharoplasties, and full-face laser resurfacing.*

cat's-eye appearance, particularly if too much tissue is elevated medially along the suture line and lateral canthus. Likewise, the nasofrontal suture line is a nice landmark to note during dissection for a few reasons. First, dissection usually needs to proceed only a few millimeters below this suture level onto the nasal bones for adequate release. Second, the paired procerus muscles can be identified here and transection performed if required. Third, depending on the level of horizontal transection in this area, the nasofrontal angle point of takeoff can be altered slightly if desired. Last, nasal tip rotation can be achieved if wanted, especially with significant dissection below the nasofrontal suture line.

Another general bony landmark is the orbital rim, which limits inferior dissection but must be well visualized and free of periosteal attachments to lift the brow and brow fat pads for long-term results. Important muscle and fascial attachments are also located at the level of the orbital rim medially and laterally. The tenacious temporal fusion line (zone of fixation) that exists along the temporal ridge must be identified during dissection.[26,27] It is also important to know its location preoperatively so that proper incision placement can be made to facilitate a clean dissection under this area that enhances visualization endoscopically (Figure 67-8).

Bony thickness varies in different areas of the skull. In addition, venous lakes present on the inside surface of the skull tend to be more centralized around the sagittal suture line. If bone tunnels or screws are planned for fixation purposes, the midline should be avoided, if possible, because of the sagittal sinus as well as higher-density venous lakes in this area (Figure 67-9). Thickness does increase

posteriorly near the occiput, but screw or bone tunnel fixation here is more challenging and is not required. Caution must be taken also to avoid lateral placement because of thinness of the lateral skull and the middle meningeal arteries. Knowledge of average thickness for a given location and internal anatomy indicates that the safest location for bone tunnels or screws is located along a parasagittal line approximately at the midpupil or lateral limbus line and just anterior to the coronal suture (see Figure 67-9).

Muscle and Fascial Anatomy

Paired muscles of the forehead and brow region are often thought of as elevators and depressors. Although several depressor muscles can pull the brow down or obliquely, the only true elevator of the forehead, the frontalis, moves upward to raise the brow. This movement, along with some static tone, maintains brow position but also can lead to horizontal creases over time. The frontalis originates from the deep galeal plane (galea aponeurotica that

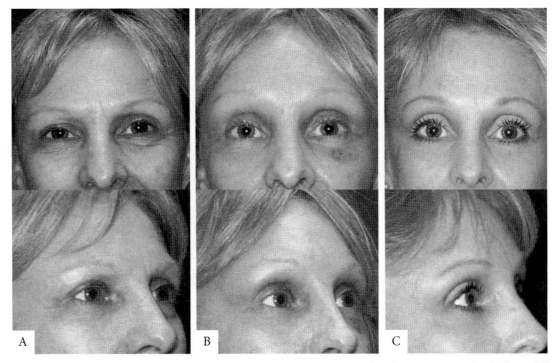

FIGURE **67-4** A, *Preoperative view of patient with classic lateral hooding brow ptosis and only "pseudo" upper eyelid laxity or ptosis. B, One week following endoscopic forehead and brow lift only. (Slight overcorrection is noted in this early period.) C, Correction of lateral hooding with isolated brow lift after 1 month.*

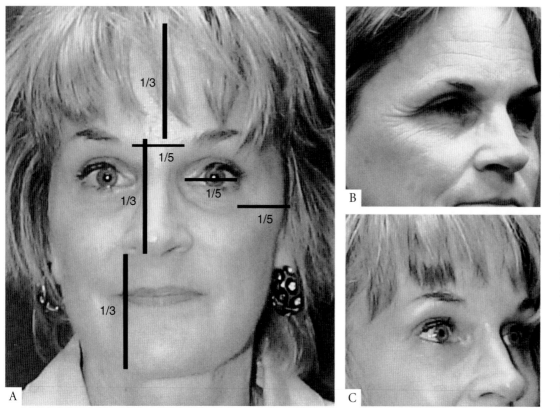

FIGURE **67-5** A, *Example of ideal facial proportions based on vertical facial thirds and horizontal proportions approximately the width of the eye or one-fifth of the facial width. B, Preoperative. C, Six weeks following endoscopic forehead and brow lift along with laser skin resurfacing.*

connects to the occipitalis posteriorly). It inserts into the orbital portion of the orbicularis oculi, which inserts into the dermis immediately below the eyebrow. Its lateral extension fuses into the dense collection of fascia almost 1 cm wide, called the zone of adherence, which extends along the superior temporal line and ends inferiorly just above the zygomaticofrontal suture.

The fascial attachments, known as the orbital ligament (see Figure 67-7), are the inferior termination point of the zone of adherence near the orbital rim where connective tissue fibers of the temporoparietal fascia are fixated to the bone at the superolateral orbital rim (Figure 67-10). Lateral and posterior along a near horizontal line from the orbital ligament is the orbicularis-temporal ligament, which is the transverse fusion zone of fibers from the lateral orbicularis, the temporoparietal fascia, and the tempo-

ralis fascia. These are important clinical anatomic areas because freeing the zones of adherence is necessary to achieve long-term results with lift procedures. However, care is required in this region to avoid overzealous stretching and injury to the facial nerve.

The acronym *SCALP* applies for the standard layers in the forehead: *s*kin, sub*c*utaneous tissue, *a*poneurosis (the thick galeal fascia), *l*oose areolar (subgaleal) plane, and *p*eriosteum[28–30]; however, the galeal fascia fuses into the frontalis muscle and its midline fascial attachments at this level. This allows a sliding movement over the scalp with contraction of the muscle. The frontalis and galea together can also be thought of as an extension of the temporoparietal fascia in the temporal region as well as the superficial musculoaponeurotic system (SMAS) below the level of the zygomatic arch.[31–33] The temporoparietal fascia appears somewhat loose or spongy clinically and houses the temporal nerve within its undersurface.

Many other paired forehead and brow muscles thought of as depressors are present along the brow to facilitate facial expression.[34–41] The two most well known are the procerus and the corrugator supercilii, which are present in the glabella (Figure 67-11). The procerus muscles are paired superiorly but fuse inferiorly into one muscle belly that originates from the nasal bones and cartilage. Superiorly procerus fibers insert into medial frontalis and the overlying dermis. The procerus is responsible for depression and frowning in the midline, which often creates a horizontal crease ("bunny lines") across

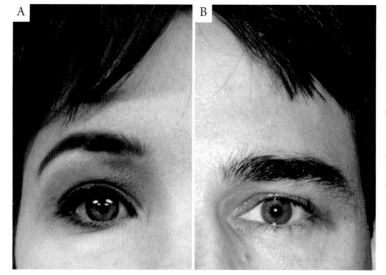

FIGURE **67-6** A, *Female brow shown with a nicely accentuated arch in the lateral third well above the orbital rim. B, The average male brow position is level with the orbital rim with a symmetric arch form.*

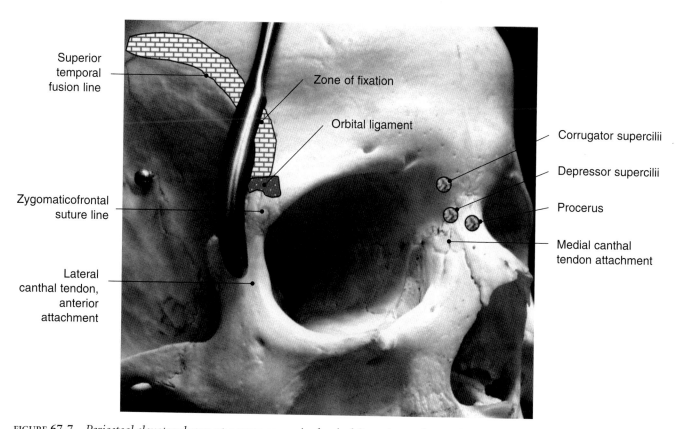

Superior temporal fusion line

Zone of fixation

Orbital ligament

Corrugator supercilii

Depressor supercilii

Procerus

Zygomaticofrontal suture line

Medial canthal tendon attachment

Lateral canthal tendon, anterior attachment

FIGURE **67-7** *Periosteal elevator shown at a more aggressive level of dissection to elevate the lateral canthus slightly, if desired. Fascial and muscle attachments are labeled. Elevation at this level detaches only the superficial layer of the lateral canthal tendon. (The deep portion of the lateral canthus is 5 mm within the orbital rim attached to Whitnall's tubercle.)*

the upper portion of the nose. The corrugator supercilii are depressors that act obliquely across the glabella and produce the classic vertical lines seen when squinting (Figure 67-12). The corrugator originates from the frontal bone just above the nasal bones and inserts in the dermis of the medial brow. The corrugator has two heads, the oblique and the transverse, which act to pull the medial brow in respective locations. Together the paired procerus muscles and corrugator are the main depressors of the medial brow and are the most common muscles treated with botulinum toxin type A to help alleviate frown lines in the glabella. These same two muscles are also most often transected during a brow or forehead lift to achieve a smoother and longer-lasting result (Figure 67-13).

Another depressor muscle of importance is the depressor supercilii, which originates on the frontal process of the

maxilla just below the corrugator supercilii and inserts in the medial frontalis fibers and dermis just above the medial brow. Because it lies superficial to the corrugator, it can be easily paralyzed inadvertently by botulinum toxin. It is also

important to note because it lies behind the corrugator and can be transected by aggressive dissection through the corrugator during a brow lift. Although patients with a very low medial brow position may occasionally benefit from this

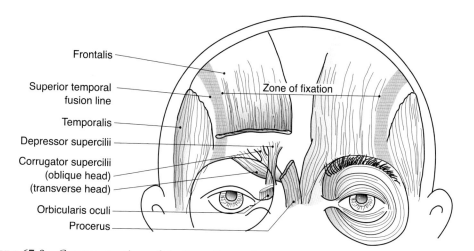

Frontalis

Superior temporal fusion line

Temporalis

Depressor supercilii

Corrugator supercilii (oblique head) (transverse head)

Orbicularis oculi

Procerus

Zone of fixation

FIGURE **67-8** *Cutaway portions of the frontalis muscles, procerus, and orbicularis oculi on one side demonstrate the relationship to the deeper depressors of the brow (corrugator supercilii and depressor supercilii). The zone of fixation (in blue) runs medial to the superior temporal fusion line.*

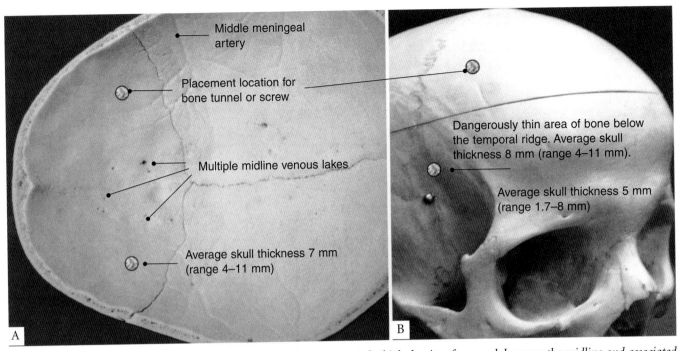

FIGURE 67-9 A, *Inside view of the calvarium of the skull demonstrating the high density of venous lakes near the midline and associated structures. B, Illustration of the ideal location placement for bone screws or tunnels based on ideal vector of lift and anatomic limitations.*

maneuver, it often gives rise to over-elevation of the medial brow following surgery, which causes the patient to look somewhat surprised (Figure 67-14). Superficial to the depressor supercilii is the orbital portion of the orbicularis oculi that inserts into portions of the adjacent depressors, the superficial surface of the inferior frontalis, as well as the dermis below the brow.[42,43] The orbital portion of the orbicularis muscle originates in part from the medial canthal tendon and adjacent bone. Deep to all the depressors is the galeal fat pad, which lies immediately below the transverse head of the corrugator and helps in identification of muscular landmarks.[44] The galeal fat is usually exposed clinically instantly after transection through the periosteum along the orbital rim (Figure 67-15).

Finally, paired temporalis muscles are located in each temporal fossa, where they originate and then insert on the coronoid process of the mandible. The importance of these muscles during upper facial rejuvenation chiefly pertains to their overlying fascia, which can be used to delineate surgical planes and aid in fixation. The spongy temporoparietal fascia is superficial to the dense and shiny white temporalis fascia. The temporalis fascia adheres to the temporalis muscles below and splits into a superficial and deep layer in the lower half of the fossa. For consistency, the superficial layer of deep temporalis fascia (which really describes only that portion of deep temporalis fascia at the level of the split and below) is subsequently referred to simply as temporalis fascia. In essence, this term will be used to describe any of this deep thick fascial layer that is seen clinically from the temporal crest down to the zygomatic arch (Figure 67-16).

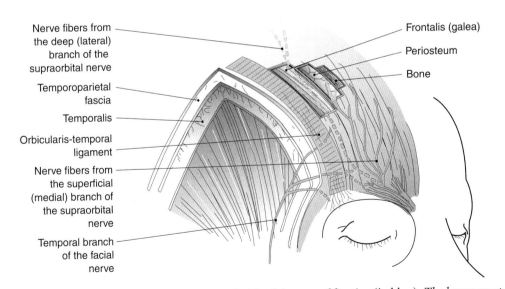

FIGURE 67-10 *Layers of fascia are seen on each side of the zone of fixation (in blue). The layers must be elevated and connected to a uniform sliding plane surgically to achieve pleasing and long-lasting brow lift results, while not damaging the associated motor and sensory nerves.*

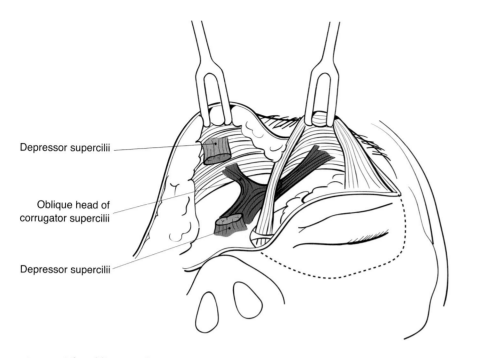

FIGURE **67-11**   *The oblique and transverse heads of the corrugator supercilii are seen behind the stump of the depressor supercilii. Both heads of the corrugator muscles and the orbicularis oculi insert into the dermis below the brow.*

Depressor supercilii

Oblique head of corrugator supercilii

Depressor supercilii

One method of fixation during brow lifting is the use of suture to fixate the temporoparietal fascia from below a skin incision to the dense and adherent temporalis fascia above the incision to elevate the lateral brow. Some surgeons advocate removing a window of temporalis fascia and exposing the underlying temporalis muscle in hopes of creating scarification in this region and improving fixation longevity.[12]

Vessel and Nerve Anatomy

Blood supply to the upper face and scalp is plentiful and comes from multiple sources. Several major vessels of the upper face originate from the external carotid artery including the superficial temporal artery and the facial artery. These give rise to the blood supply in the medial canthal region via the angular artery and in the lateral canthal region by way of the frontal or anterior branch of the superficial temporal artery. The internal carotid artery gives way to the middle meningeal artery and the ophthalmic artery. The ophthalmic artery then gives rise to the supraorbital and supratrochlear arteries, which exit their respective foramina and supply the majority of the forehead and midscalp with blood. The terminal arterial branches of the upper face have major anastomoses with adjacent vessels.

Venous drainage of the upper face follows the respective arterial supply but can be somewhat more variable. However, one particular vein, known as the sentinel vein (medial zygomaticotemporal vein), runs perpendicular through the temporalis fascia connecting the superficial and middle temporal veins (Figure 67-17).[45] The sentinel vein can most often be found approximately 1 cm lateral or posterior to the zygomaticofrontal suture line. It is clinically significant during endoscopic procedures because, if injured, it can result in impaired field visualization and significant bruising.

Nerve supply parallels arterial supply to some degree. The supratrochlear and supraorbital nerves, which are responsible for the majority of sensation in the forehead, exit via the same foramina or general location as do the supraorbital and supratrochlear blood vessels. The sensory nerves originate from the first division of the trigeminal nerve. The supraorbital nerve has two divisions after exiting its foramen: the deep (or lateral) division supplies the more lateral and posterior portion of the forehead and scalp, and the superficial (or medial) division pierces the frontalis and runs superficially to the muscle, supplying sensation to the forehead along the midpupil line (Figure 67-18). The location of the supraorbital nerve's exit is relatively consistent. The supraor-

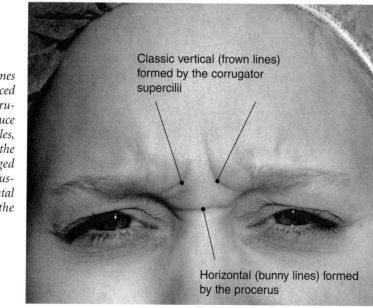

FIGURE 67-12   *Frown lines of the glabella are produced by the actions of the corrugator supercilii to produce the classic vertical wrinkles, whereas the actions of the more vertically arranged fibers of the procerus muscle produce the horizontal wrinkles seen across the bridge of the nose.*

Classic vertical (frown lines) formed by the corrugator supercilii

Horizontal (bunny lines) formed by the procerus

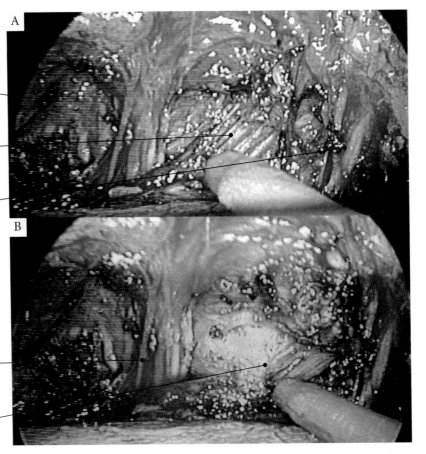

Procerus

Intact corrugator
supercilii

Supraorbital
vessels and nerve

Supratrochlear
vessels and nerve

Transected
corrugator
supercilii

FIGURE 67-13 *Endoscopic views of the right side of the forehead. Location of the corrugator supercilii relative to the supraorbital nerve (A) immediately before it is transected with a needle-tip cautery (B). Following transection through the belly of the corrugator supercilii.*

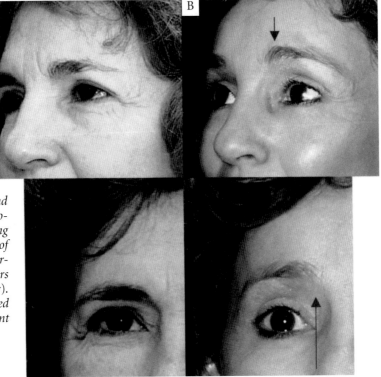

FIGURE 67-14 *Before (A) and after (B) photos following endoscopic forehead and brow lifting demonstrating good elevation of the lateral hooding but over-resection of the medial depressors in the area indicated (arrow). This can result in a surprised look, especially when the patient elevates the brow, as shown.*

bital foramen or notch is typically found within 1 mm of a line drawn in a sagittal plane tangential to the medial limbus (Figure 67-19).[46] The deep division has been known to exit as often as 10% from another foramen that can be as high as 1.5 cm above the orbital rim.

The supratrochlear nerves exit from around the orbital rim at an average of 9 mm medial to the exit of the supraorbital nerve.[46] The nerves supply sensation to the midforehead with some overlap from the supraorbital nerves. Infratrochlear nerves, also from division one of the trigeminal nerve, exit just below the supratrochlear nerves around the medial orbital rim to supply sensation to the upper nose and medial orbit. Zygomaticofrontal and zygomaticotemporal nerves are from the second division of the trigeminal nerve. They exit their respective small foramina and supply sensation to the lateral orbit and temporal regions of the face.

The facial nerve supplies motor innervation to the forehead and glabella.[47–51] The frontal (or temporal) branch of the facial nerve supplies the frontalis muscle, the superior portion of the orbicularis oculi, the superior portion of the procerus, and the transverse head of the corrugator supercilii. The zygomatic branch of the facial nerve supplies the medial head of the orbicularis oculi, the oblique head of the corrugator supercilii, the inferior portion of the procerus, and the depressor supercilii (Figure 67-20).

The auriculotemporal nerve, from the third division of the trigeminal nerve, supplies sensation in front of the ear to the temporal skin above the zygomatic arch and along the course of the superficial artery. It may be confused clinically during a face-lift with the frontal branch of the facial nerve. It can, however, be distinguished from the facial motor nerve because it runs within 1 cm anterior to the tragus of the ear and parallel to the superficial temporal artery. The much more significant frontal branch of the facial nerve

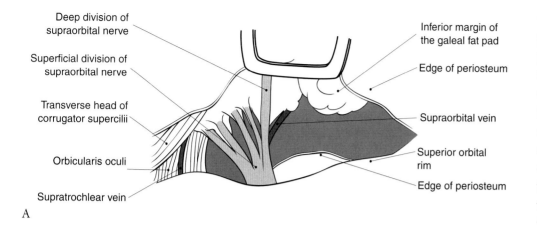

Deep division of
supraorbital nerve

Superficial division of
supraorbital nerve

Transverse head of
corrugator supercilii

Orbicularis oculi

Supratrochlear vein

A

Inferior margin of
the galeal fat pad

Edge of periosteum

Supraorbital vein

Superior orbital
rim

Edge of periosteum

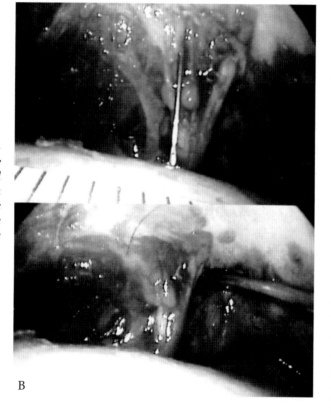

B

FIGURE **67-15** A, *Right-sided forehead landmarks.* B, *Endoscopic view of the right supraorbital nerve and vessels. The first view is seen with a 27-gauge needle over the nerve trunk after it is placed through the skin of the brow level with the patient's medial limbus (iris).*

techniques are highly variable among surgeons.[52–59] I prefer to dissect within a completely subperiosteal plane medially to the temporal crest and in the plane immediately above the temporalis fascia below the temporal line on each side. Subperiosteal dissection in the lateral forehead helps to avoid injury to the deep or lateral division of the supraorbital nerve, which runs in the subgaleal plane near the zone of fixation. Some surgeons begin their dissection in a subgaleal plane in the posterior scalp.[59,60] Regardless, a space is created in the safer posterior areas of the scalp to allow room for placement of an endoscope, which aids dissection in the more risky areas of the forehead.

The first anatomic landmark the surgeon must consider is the zone of fixation along the superior temporal crest. Its inferior edge is found near the superior lateral orbital rim. A convergence of fibers from the periosteum, galea, temporalis, and temporoparietal fascia interlace and fuse to form the zone of adherence, much in the same way the layers of tissue planes come together at the level of the zygomatic arch. The zone of fixation can be elevated bluntly at the hairline level and a couple of centimeters below, but as the surgeon approaches the lateral brow beginning approximately 2 cm above brow level, use of an endoscope aids dissection. At this point the ligament has branches of the temporal nerve within it, and care must be taken to remain against the bone and temporalis fascia below to avoid nerve injury. Another fibrous attachment, the orbicularis-temporal ligament, is also present here and contains motor nerve fibers (see Figure 67-17); it is the decussation of fibers from the temporoparietal fascia and of the temporal fascia that extends laterally from the orbital ligament. The zone of adherence becomes even more tenacious as the orbital ligament (see Figure 67-7) at the orbital rim level is approached. Slow meticulous dissection is required at this point to avoid nerve injury as well as injury to the sentinel

runs an average of 2 cm anterior to the tragus when crossing the zygomatic arch. The temporal branch of the facial nerve crosses the arch at an oblique angle at an average of 2 cm posterior to the orbital rim. The depth of the temporal nerve is just below the SMAS at the arch and below the temporoparietal fascia immediately above the arch. The frontal (temporal) branch usually has divided into two rami at the level of the arch and has at least four branches by the time it reaches the level of the eyebrow.

Endoscopic Anatomy

Initial dissection must be performed to gain adequate space for the endoscopic equipment. This early dissection is performed in the posterior forehead and temporal regions; endoscopy-guided dissection is used for the last 2 cm above the orbital rim and zygomatic arch. Elevation of the deep tissues in this "safe zone" is essentially performed blindly through each of the small scalp incisions. Incisions and specific tissue release and fixation

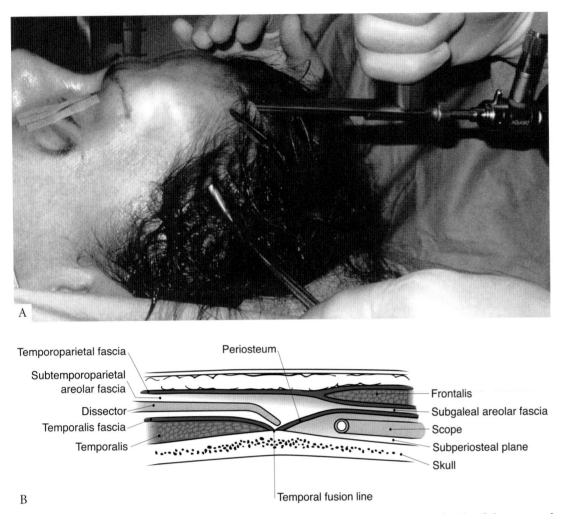

A

Temporoparietal fascia

Subtemporoparietal areolar fascia

Dissector

Temporalis fascia

Temporalis

Periosteum

Frontalis

Subgaleal areolar fascia

Scope

Subperiosteal plane

Skull

B

Temporal fusion line

FIGURE **67-16** *A and B, Endoscopic dissection must connect the tissue planes on each side of the temporal crest. Various approaches may be used as long as the anatomic planes seen above are sufficiently understood to allow proper tissue release, a clean endoscopic view, and protection of the facial nerve.*

behind the supraorbital nerve at the rim level where the deep (or lateral) division of the nerve is closely adherent to periosteum (see Figure 67-15). Preoperatively marking a point on the brow at a level tangential to the medial limbus iris helps the surgeon to easily identify the location of the supraorbital vessels and nerves.[46] Dissection through the periosteum in this region should be performed slowly and superficially to avoid injury to these structures. The transverse head of the corrugator supercilii is seen at the orbital rim level behind the supraorbital vessels and nerves. The corrugator supercilii can be carefully transected or partially excised.[61] Medially, the oblique head of the corrugator is encountered, and by a transection through this portion of muscle, the supratrochlear nerve and depressor supercilii muscle may be seen and protected from injury. Medially, in the glabella, the procerus muscle, which is variable in thickness, is seen. Care should be taken to avoid overaggressive muscle resection in thin patients as this can result in an atrophic defect in the glabella. Deeper dissection toward the skin level under the brow will lead to the orbicularis oculi but is typically not necessary to gain the desired effect (except with regard to the lateral orbicularis, where limited transection may improve lateral brow elevation).[62,63] Also, one or more incisions through the periosteum at higher levels

vein that is located within the orbicularis-temporal ligament approximately 1 cm laterally to the zygomaticofrontal suture. Careful dissection exposes an intact sentinel vein that can be seen piercing through the temporal fascia at a perpendicular angle and entering the temporoparietal fascia above (see Figure 67-17).

Dissection above the orbital rims in the subperiosteal plane should expose the entire superior orbital rim from each zygomaticofrontal suture. The curvature of the rims should be visualized so that transection through the periosteum can be made at the level of the rims. The nasofrontal suture may not always be seen but can be felt by the periosteal elevator used to lift tissue. When transecting through the

periosteum across the entire orbital rim, subgaleal fat is often encountered initially, except when the transection is directly

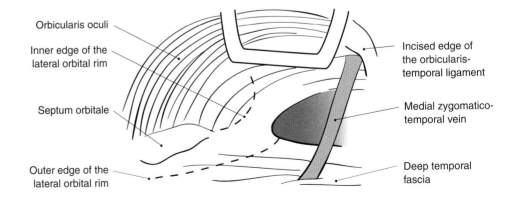

Orbicularis oculi

Inner edge of the lateral orbital rim

Septum orbitale

Outer edge of the lateral orbital rim

Incised edge of the orbicularis-temporal ligament

Medial zygomatico-temporal vein

Deep temporal fascia

FIGURE **67-17** *Dissection below the patient's right temporal crest is shown with release of the orbicularis-temporal ligament. The medial zygomaticotemporal (sentinel) vein seen here pierces the temporalis fascia approximately 1 cm posterior to the zygomaticofrontal suture line.*

under the frontalis muscle in the midline can be performed but is only required if deep horizontal lines are present.[64] It is more important to gain complete release of the retaining lateral ligaments, transection of those muscles causing glabellar lines, and adequate separation of the periosteum along the orbital rim to get the elevation of brow and forehead tissues for the most pleasing and long-term esthetic result.[65–75]

Preoperative Evaluation and Surgical Preparation

Determining whether a patient will benefit from a brow or forehead lift and which procedure will work best is critical to avoid disappointing the patient. Commonly the novice surgeon notices only horizontal forehead lines as an indication for a brow lift. Unfortunately, this is much less of a problem for most patients than is a low lateral brow position (hooding) or glabellar crease (see Figure 67-3). As discussed above, the ideal female brow position is above the orbital rim at a level that varies among individuals. An average distance of 5 to 10 mm of brow elevation above the rim in the lateral third generally looks most pleasing. Men require a straight-up elevation of the entire brow to avoid feminizing their appearance by overelevation of the lateral brow. In addition, men may benefit more from a standard upper blepharoplasty and local transpalpebral brow lift if the brow ptosis is minimal. As with any cosmetic surgery, a decision regarding the risks and benefits must be made and must conform to the patient's desires. Patient education is required so that they know the risks as well as what can *realistically* be achieved (Figure 67-21). Even with fairly aggressive muscle resection and forehead elevation, patients often form new dynamic lines in the upper face following surgery. Lateral crow's-feet owing to the action of the orbicularis oculi when smiling may appear improved following a brow lift since the muscle is unfolded. However,

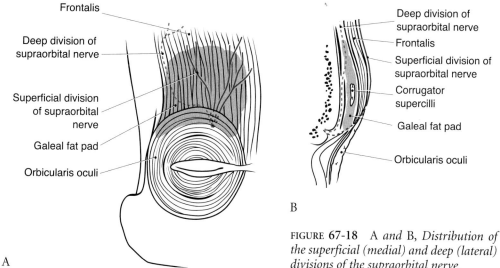

A

B

FIGURE **67-18**   A *and* B, *Distribution of the superficial (medial) and deep (lateral) divisions of the supraorbital nerve.*

they are not completely eliminated by brow lifting alone, and the patient must understand that botulinum toxin therapy may be required to treat these particular lines on an ongoing basis.[76]

In addition to lines on the forehead, lines in the glabella, brow ptosis, and the condition of the patient's skin must also be evaluated. Intrinsic skin and collagen damage from the effects of sun, age, and smoking

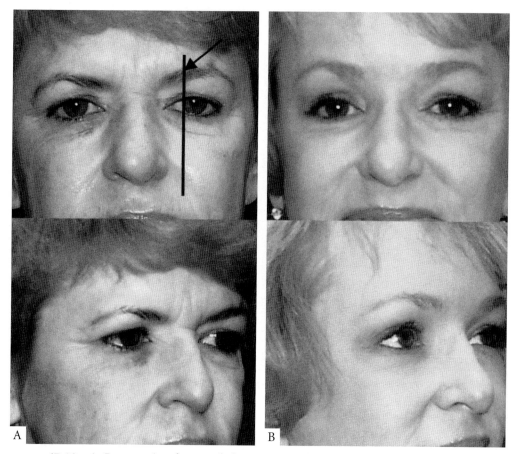

A   B

FIGURE **67-19**   A, *Preoperative photograph demonstrating the location of the supraorbital vessels by a line drawn vertically from the medial iris.* B, *One and a half years following an endoscopic forehead and brow lift. No blepharoplasty was ever performed.*

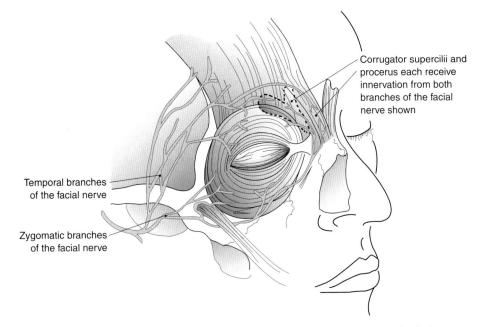

Corrugator supercilii and procerus each receive innervation from both branches of the facial nerve shown

Temporal branches of the facial nerve

Zygomatic branches of the facial nerve

FIGURE **67-20** *Motor nerve supply to the forehead depressor muscle comes from both the temporal and zygomatic branches of the facial nerve.*

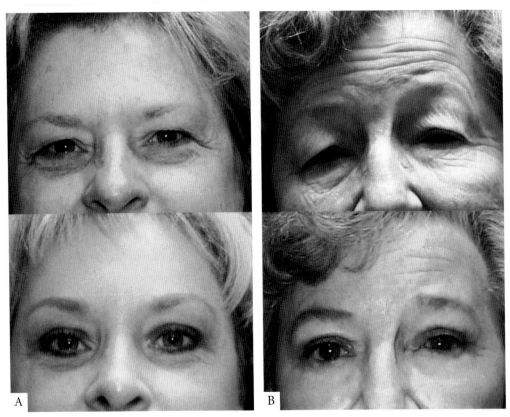

FIGURE **67-21** A, *Because of both brow ptosis and upper eyelid laxity, the patient shown required upper blepharoplasties as well as endoscopic forehead and brow lifting to achieve the results she desired. B, The patient is shown before and after only blepharoplasty and full-face laser skin resurfacing. She has multiple problems including asymmetry of the brows owing to a blepharospasm on the left side, eyelid asymmetry and severe laxity, pseudoelevation of the brows owing to frontalis compensation for severe eyelid ptosis, and severe actinic skin damage. She is not a good candidate for simultaneous brow lifting since a change in brow position will likely occur following the removal of the eyelid ptosis. She is a good candidate for botulinum toxin therapy on her left side.*

are not treated by lifting alone. Topical skin care (eg, retinoic acid, microdermabrasion, pulsed-light therapy, sunblocks) along with possible surgical resurfacing must be considered.[77–79] In general the forehead can be treated safely with chemical peels or laser skin resurfacing into the dermal level simultaneously with brow-lifting procedures, provided the lifting is performed with a subgaleal or subperiosteal technique rather than a subcutaneous one. Finally, bony irregularities or hypertrophic bony orbital rims can be evaluated for treatment by means of a cephalometric radiograph or computed tomography (CT) scan as required. Bony contouring can be performed on a limited basis endoscopically, but a major reduction for significant bone hypertrophy such as a frontal boss is best treated with an open (coronal) approach. The amount of bone reduction is limited by the pneumatization of the frontal sinus, which is best evaluated by CT. Although treatment planning for placement of bone tunnels does not require a preoperative CT, a standard cephalometric radiograph may help to reassure the surgeon regarding the thickness of corticocancellous bone available.

As with any surgical procedure, appropriate preoperative laboratory and other indicated tests must be performed. Written instruction are given to the patient regarding pre- and postoperative care, including instructions for shampooing hair with antibacterial soap or other antiseptic shampoo and avoidance of the use of hair spray or other hair products immediately prior to surgery. The patient should be thoroughly instructed on the critical need to avoid all medications that may cause platelet dysfunction 10 days prior to surgery (including aspirin and other nonsteroidal anti-inflammatory drugs, vitamin E, and many over-the-counter herbal supplements). Endoscopic techniques require a very dry operating field that necessitates strict avoidance of these medications as well as proper preoperative injection of vasoconstrictive agents.

Prior to anesthesia, photos are taken and the patient is marked while awake and sitting up. Following the introduction of general anesthesia or intravenous sedation, the patient is prepped and carefully injected with local anesthetic with epinephrine. I prefer to use a local anesthetic with 1:100,000 epinephrine along the entire orbital rim, and a tumescent anesthesia solution (250 cc of normal saline mixed with 1 cc of 1:1,000 epinephrine and 20 cc of 2% lidocaine) in the remaining upper forehead, temple, and posterior scalp. Careful injection in the desired tissue planes helps to avoid the formation of a hematoma during the injection and allows for a nearly bloodless procedure. Minor shaving of hair along the marked incision lines is performed if desired immediately prior to the final preparation and draping of the area.

Coronal Forehead and Brow Lift

Still one of the most common approaches for forehead and brow lifting, the classic coronal lift involves an incision across the entire forehead from ear to ear, staying well behind the hairline.[80–88] Dissection is typically in the subgaleal or subperiosteal plane and then connects to the subtemporoparietal plane laterally. This gives great exposure of the entire orbital rims for bony osteoplasty, if required, and treatment of muscles that require resection including the depressors (corrugator and procerus) as well as the frontalis. Heavy horizontal forehead creases can be addressed with this technique either by way of midline myotomies or minor midline thinning of the frontalis. Major resection of the frontalis should be avoided to prevent postoperative irregularities and strange facial expressions during frontalis movement. The lateral frontalis should be avoided to prevent nerve damage, ptosis, and other irregularities.

Regrettably, the coronal lift also has the disadvantages of a long incision and a significant elevation of the hairline.

Patients with a high hairline are not good candidates for this technique since a significant amount of scalp excision is required. Many surgeons believe this scalp excision is a reasonable trade-off because they feel that the technique gives a more lasting approach than do newer endoscopic techniques. If performed correctly, the endoscopic technique can be as long lasting and possibly more precise than open brow-lifting techniques. Care must be taken with the coronal lift to avoid elevating the medial brow too much and creating a very high hairline. Roughly, to gain 1 cm of brow elevation, 1.5 to 2 cm of scalp must be excised with this technique. The amount of tissue excised is not a precise determinant of the amount of brow elevation obtained. Scoring of the underlying fascia and muscle resection can cause the tissue to stretch oddly, making prediction of the exact brow elevation difficult.

The benefits of the coronal lift include great exposure and relatively easy dissection. It can also be used to extend the procedure into a deep-plane face-lift by dissection over the zygomatic arches and onto the zygoma and masseter. This much more aggressive lift gives excellent elevation of the midface but greatly increases postoperative edema and the potential for motor nerve damage. The extended technique should only be attempted by an experienced surgeon,[89–93] and careful consideration should be given to alternative treatments. Comparatively, the basic coronal lift is an easier procedure for the novice surgeon. When selecting this tried-and-true method, one should take into account the disadvantages, including the lengthy scar and possible hair loss, significant scalp anesthesia, and a significantly elevated hairline.

Trichophytic or Pretrichial Forehead and Brow Lift

Although trichophytic and pretrichial lifts are sometimes thought to be the same procedure, the *pretrichial* lift actually involves

an incision in front of the hairline. With this procedure, hair does not grow anterior to the incision, leaving a visible scar in front of the hairline. In contrast, in the *trichophytic* lift, although still at the frontal hairline, the incision is placed just behind the hairline. This incision is beveled so that follicles in front of the initial skin incision survive and hair grows anterior to the incision to better camouflage the resulting scar. It should be noted that many surgeons use these terms interchangeably. Even better than the trichophytic lift is the irregular trichophytic hairline, which not only employs a beveled incision but creates a wavy pattern along the hairline for a more natural postoperative appearance compared with a straight-line scar.

Regardless of the specific incision design, the ultimate advantages of the trichophytic forehead and brow lift include great exposure (similar to that with the coronal approach) and the ability to lower a high forehead. Unlike the classic coronal lift, bare forehead skin is excised from the hairline. Also, lateral incisions and dissection are usually limited with this technique unless required. Incision design can even improve hair thinning in the temporoparietal areas by excising the area of hair loss and bringing forward areas of dense hair–bearing scalp. The posterior scalp and hairline can be brought forward to lower a high forehead by almost any amount. The more lowering that is desired, the more posterior is the dissection and release. Limited or no posterior dissection can be performed if the hairline is to remain at the same level.

The forward dissection is the technique that varies the most among surgeons. A totally subperiosteal technique versus a subgaleal technique is an option. A subcutaneous technique has recently become more popular, particularly when the depressors in the lower brow do not require treatment.[94] Staying superficial to the frontalis breaks the dermal insertions that create deep horizontal rhytids. The subcutaneous lift is occasionally combined with deep dissection to treat glabellar lines as well as horizontal lines in the forehead.

Overall, the trichophytic technique of forehead and brow lifting is an invaluable tool for any surgeon performing facial cosmetic surgery. When a patient presents with a high forehead and low brow position, the trichophytic approach is the procedure of choice to correct both problems. The main disadvantage is the potential for a visible incision despite best efforts. All prospective patients considering this technique must be informed of the chance that there may be a visible scar at the hairline. Surprisingly, when presented with the potential problems and given the choice, many patients prefer to undergo an endoscopic approach with a slight elevation in hairline rather than risk a visible hairline scar. Still, the patient with an extremely high hairline is often thrilled with the lower hairline obtainable only with the trichophytic approach. Attention to detail and gentle soft tissue management are essential to attaining a natural hairline and hidden scar with this popular technique.

Endoscopic Forehead and Brow Lift

Early attempts at endoscopic surgery began over a century ago with Nietze's description of a crude cystoscope. A few decades ago endoscopic surgery progressed through use in upper gastrointestinal examinations and then intra-abdominal surgery. However, facial endoscopic cosmetic surgery did not blossom until the early 1990s. Over the past decade the endoscopic forehead and brow lift procedure has been considered by many to be the state-of-the-art technique for upper facial rejuvenation.[95–97] It is versatile and can be combined with many other procedures. The most noted benefits of the endoscopic technique are the smaller scars hidden in the hairline and selective brow elevation without the need for removal of any hair or skin (Figure 67-22).

The technique involves several incisions placed strategically behind the hairline to gain access for early blunt dissection and insertion of the endoscope and tissue retractor. Other incisions can be used as ports for dissecting tools such as periosteal elevators, electrocautery, lasers, tissue graspers, and suction instruments. Among surgeons a variety of incision (port) designs are used. Fixation points are usually placed at these incision sites; therefore, I prefer five separate 2.5 cm long incisions placed for easy access but mostly for ideal fixation placement. Each of the five incisions begins approximately 1 cm posterior to the hairline. One is placed in the midline in the sagittal plane and two in the parasagittal plane tangential to the lateral third of the brow (where maximum lift is typically desired in females). This same incision can be moved slightly medially in male patients to give a more even brow elevation. The midline incision plus the two parasagittal incisions are aligned vertically to avoid unnecessary transection of sensory nerves originating from the supraorbital nerves below. The two parasagittal incisions are placed medial to the temporal crest to gain access to skull bone rather than the more lateral temporalis fascia. Bone is the strongest fixation tissue available and ideally should be used thus.[98–100]

It is important to access the subperiosteal plane easily for a clean future endoscopic view. Accidental placement of the parasagittal incisions too far laterally over the zone of fixation or temporalis muscle makes pocket development difficult and obscures future endoscopic visualization. Moreover, the parasagittal incisions are located in a thick area of the frontal bone where there is a low density of venous lakes. Placing the incision here helps to prevent accidental intracranial injury during bone tunnel creation or placement of bone screws.

Lastly, two temporal incisions are made, one on each side of the head, for direct access to the thick temporal fascia. These incisions are placed perpendicular to the desired elevation vector from the lateral canthal region. Coincidently, the temporal incision parallels the course of the temporal branch of the facial nerve

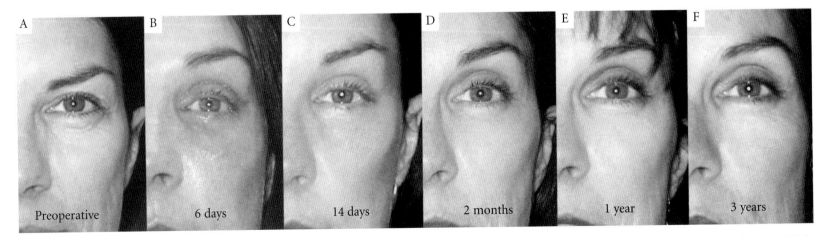

A   Preoperative   B   6 days   C   14 days   D   2 months   E   1 year   F   3 years

FIGURE 67-22   *A to F, Sequential appearance following endoscopic forehead and brow lifting (eyelid and skin resurfacing procedures were also performed). Slight overelevation of the brow is noted for 6 days after surgery, as expected. The brow position remains very stable from 2 weeks to 3 years after the surgery.*

that is located 2 to 3 cm inferior to this incision. It also parallels the superficial temporal artery and vein. Arranging the three medial incisions on a vertical axis and the two temporal incisions in an oblique position to parallel the nerve and blood supply in each area can reduce interference with sensation and vascular supply to the scalp.

Dissection is performed through the above incisions down through periosteum medial to the temporal crest and down to temporalis fascia lateral to the crest. Some surgeons may elect to use a subgaleal rather than subperiosteal placement of the incision medially. Total subperiosteal dissection medial to the temporal lines rather than subgaleal dissection leads to better fixation and long-term stabilization (see Figure 67-22).

Blunt and blind dissection can be carried out after reaching the subperiosteal and subtemporoparietal planes through the five incisions. Finger dissection and long curved endoscopic periosteal elevators are used to lift the tissue anteriorly to a point 2 cm above the orbital rims and zygomatic arch. Posteriorly blunt dissection should elevate the temporal tissues a few centimeters behind the ear, where the temporal fossa becomes self-limiting. The subperiosteal dissection above needs to elevate the scalp at least 10 cm posteriorly but can extend as far back as the lambdoid suture. Once these areas are freed, a connection can be made from the temporal region to the subperiosteal dissection through the upper portion of the zone of fixation at the temporal crest by finger dissection (Figure 67-23). Blind release of the more inferior portion of the temporal line where the facial nerve crosses should be avoided. Endoscope-guided dissection here helps to prevent nerve injury. Using finger dissection the upper zone of fixation is broken through proceeding from the temporal incision toward the medial scalp, rather than vice versa, to prevent creation of a false tunnel in the spongy or foamy temporoparietal fascia. False tunnels along the temporal crest create problems when the endoscope is inserted through the parasagittal port to visualize the lateral forehead; the tunnels force the placement of the endoscope in a more superficial plane within the temporoparietal fascia, which greatly increases the chance of nerve injury. Therefore, it is critical to stay firmly against the periosteum and the temporalis fascia when initially elevating the scalp and forehead.

Following blunt elevation of the scalp from each incision for complete flap elevation, the endoscope is normally inserted through one of the three more medial incisions. Poor initial blunt dissection makes the initial endoscopic dissection feel very tight, and care must be taken not to perforate the skin by excessive retraction. Medial dissection over the nasofrontal suture and orbital rims is per-formed under direct endoscopic vision with a curved and smooth elevator to avoid inadvertent tearing of the periosteum. The periosteum may be thin in some patients, in whom a straighter elevator may be used to transect the periosteum at the level of the rim (arcus marginalis). However, the entire rolled edge of the orbital rim must be visualized before proceeding with periosteal incision (Figure 67-24). Typically the periosteum is more precisely incised with a needle-tip cautery or laser set at low power. The supraorbital nerves and vessels as described earlier are at a level tangential to the medial limbus and are immediately behind (superficial to) the periosteum from the internal endoscopic view.[46,101] This necessitates meticulous cautery dissection here to avoid injury to these structures (see Figure 67-24). Suction placed by an assistant from another port is required to maintain

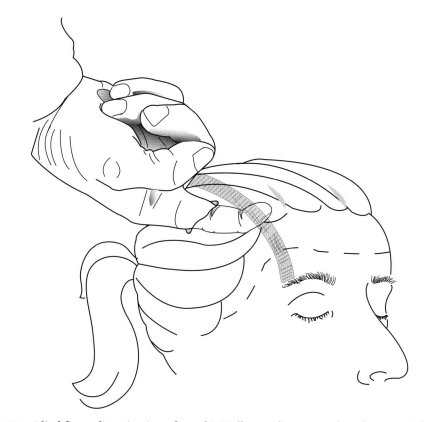

FIGURE **67-23** *Blind finger dissection is performed initially, avoiding overzealous dissection inferiorly. Dissection proceeds from the subtemporoparietal plane laterally to the already elevated subperiosteal plane medially. The opposite direction of elevation (medial to lateral) may produce false tunnels in the temporoparietal tissue, which impair future endoscopic vision.*

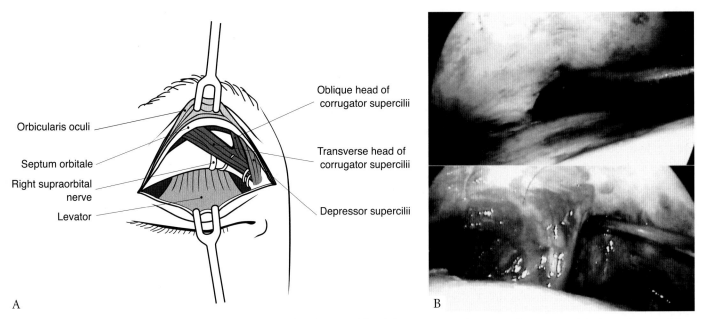

Orbicularis oculi

Septum orbitale

Right supraorbital nerve

Levator

Oblique head of corrugator supercilii

Transverse head of corrugator supercilii

Depressor supercilii

A   B

FIGURE 67-24   A, *This line drawing demonstrates the orbital rim and local depressor muscle as seen from a transblepharoplasty incision.* B, *Endoscopic photographs show the rolled border of orbital rim prior to periosteal release in the first view and the supraorbital nerve and vein in the next view after excising through the periosteum.*

a clear view when using cautery or laser. Temporal incisions work well for suction ports during dissection over the rims since the endoscope and cautery take up most of the room through any of the middle three incision sites. With clear and near blood-less dissection at this point, transection can be performed through the corrugator supercilii and procerus. If unwanted bleeding is encountered and cannot be controlled easily with pinpoint accurate cautery, then pressure should be applied externally over the rim until improved visualization allows for control of bleeding without nerve damage.

Vertical rhytids in the glabella created by the corrugators can be improved greatly by transection through these muscles. Likewise, horizontal glabellar lines are treated by transection of the procerus muscle that creates these particular facial wrinkles. Some surgeons advocate more aggressive surgical avulsion of these muscles with endoscopic biopsy forceps. Aggressive muscle removal may lead to a more permanent treatment of glabellar lines compared with isolated transection only, but should be avoided in most cases owing to an increased risk of significant postoperative

irregularities and abnormal facial expression. As a rule, patients prefer a more natural appearance with some minor return of frown lines to risking a bizarre facial expression and glabellar depression.

Once the periosteum is completely freed across the orbital rims and appropriate muscles have been treated, the cut periosteal edges are spread apart (periosteal elevators work well for this) by at least 1 cm to aid the release at the arcus marginalis. This allows significant and long-term brow elevation. Next the lateral orbital rim must be exposed in the subperiosteal plane after careful release below the zone of fixation and orbital ligament. Dissection along the anterior and inferior aspects of the temporal crest must be performed cautiously to avoid temporal nerve injury. Overzealous retraction of the dense tissue here that contains the nerve can result in nerve damage. Staying snuggly against periosteum and the temporalis fascia helps to prevent nerve damage and produces a much cleaner dissection. Slowly creating a distinct plane of dissection down to the zygomaticofrontal suture line and avoiding excess retraction helps to prevent unwanted bleeding from the sen-

tinel vein (zygomaticotemporal vein), which needs not be sacrificed for a standard endoscopic forehead and brow lift.

Dissection for a standard endoscopic brow lift should not proceed all the way to the zygomatic arch but should stop approximately 1 cm above this level. If an extended midface lift is planned and there is a desire to elevate tissue over the zygomatic arch itself, then dissection must go below the superficial layer of deep temporal fascia just above the arch. Abbreviated midface lifts performed simultaneously with endoscopic brow lifts may simply stay in the subperiosteal plane along the lateral orbital rim and avoid the more risky full-arch release. The beauty of the classic endoscopic brow lift is its versatility and the ease with which additional procedures can be combined simultaneously with this elegant cosmetic surgery. For instance, the temporal incision of an endoscopic forehead lift can easily be extended inferiorly to meet up with the preauricular incision from a standard lower face-lift. Also, midface lifting (with intraoral dissection) can connect the intraoral subperiosteal dissection over the zygoma to the subperiosteal plane from the endoscopic brow lift through a tunnel near the lateral orbital rim (Figure 67-25).

After all dissection is complete, appropriate elevation and fixation is required (Figure 67-26). Many techniques have been described such as tissue suture only, bone screws and plates, resorbable screws, bone tunnels, local skin excision, temporalis muscle exposure for added scarification, tissue glue, and tight head wraps.[102] Regardless of any specific fixation technique, the key to long-term fixation is adequate lower forehead tissue release during endoscopic dissection. Failure to adequately release internal tissue results in a relapse of brow ptosis, even with heavy fixation and the appearance of a "nice" lift during surgery.

Once complete internal release of the forehead is obtained, the specific lifting vectors must be determined for the most pleasing esthetic effect. The lateral third of the female brow is elevated to the greatest extent, which is up to 1 cm above the orbital rim. The medial brow should be only slightly above the rim level and

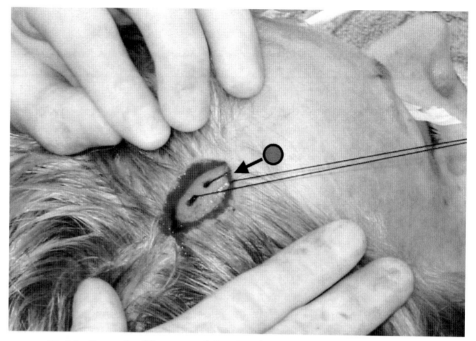

FIGURE **67-26** *Example of bone tunnel fixation shown at the site of the right parasagittal incision. The anterior circle represents the position of suture placement through the galea, which elevates the lateral brow toward the bone tunnel.*

definitely below the middle and lateral brow levels to avoid a surprised or bewildered expression (see Figure 67-14). Typically the glabellar region is elevated on its own without the need for midline fixation, which helps to avoid overelevation medially. The lateral third of the brow is lifted straight up and fixated at the level of the hairline. The galeal tissue is typically secured to bone at this point, while the lateral brow is held at the desired height or 1 to 2 mm above the desired level.[12] Very little relapse occurs with proper technique and averages only 1 to 2 mm after 2 weeks. Measurements can also be made with clear circular templates from the pupil to brow to help improve symmetry. The brow position remains very stable following this early recovery period (see Figure 67-22). A question remains as to the time required for complete fixation of the periosteum. Some animal studies suggest a full 12 weeks are required for what is termed *full histologic periosteal refixation*.[103] However, there is clinical evidence suggesting adequate fixation occurs in as little as 7 days. An example is the common fixation technique used by many surgeons who place a single transcutaneous bone screw at each parasagittal incision, which is removed

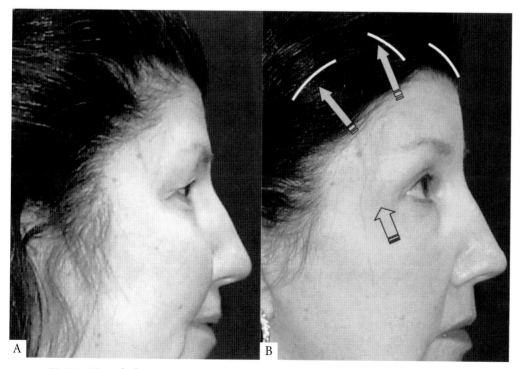

FIGURE **67-25** *Views before (A) and after (B) an endoscopic forehead, brow, and midface lift. Arrows represent vectors of lift. Fixation is performed at the level of the hairline through the temporal and parasagittal incisions shown.*

after only 1 week. The 1-week fixation technique has been used with success for many years. It has been suggested that longer bony fixation may provide longer-term retention and less early relapse that some have considered normal. The key to long-term fixation seems for now to be determined usually by proper tissue dissection and release.

Although there are many fixation techniques, the use of bone tunnels at the parasagittal incisions appears to be one of the best methods for fixating the galea and periosteum near the hairline to a bone tunnel created posteriorly under the incision using a single heavy suture (see Figure 67-26). Fixation of the lateral tail of the brow is performed at each temporal incision, where an isolated heavy suture plicates the temporoparietal fascia in a posterior and superior vector to the thick temporalis fascia. Optional creation of a small window of exposed temporalis muscle in this area may aid in internal scar formation and fixation. The vector of lift at this outer tail of the brow follows a line drawn at an angle from the outer nasal ala that passes just beside the lateral canthus (see Figure 67-25).

Final closure of the hair-bearing scalp incisions can be performed with skin staples only with excellent scar formation since no skin is excised and no pressure exists at the incision sites. Redundant tissue (forehead skin) created by an average of 1 cm of brow elevation is easily distributed evenly over the posterior 15 to 20 cm of elevated scalp, which essentially absorbs or redistributes this excess tissue with few to no signs of bunching. Because of this phenomenon, the endoscopic forehead and brow lift tends to elevate the hairline only a very small amount compared with the open skin excising coronal technique.

Interestingly, in a survey performed in 1998 of American Society of Plastic Surgeons members, of the total 6,951 brow lifts performed by 570 members who returned the questionnaire, 3,534 involved a coronal technique and incision and 3,417 were performed endoscopically. The most noted difference was the higher risk of hair loss with the coronal technique; however, both techniques enjoyed very low overall complication rates.

Direct Brow Lift

The direct brow lift involves excision of an ellipse of skin adjacent to and just above the eyebrow (Figure 67-27). A beveled incision is used to parallel the hair follicles of the brow or so that some follicles remain at the base of the bevel to grow later above the scar. The dissection remains in the subcutaneous plane to avoid muscle or nerve injury.

Advantages of the direct brow lift are that it is a simple procedure (with an easy two-layer closure), it can be performed under local anesthesia, and it can treat brow position asymmetries. It remains a good alternative technique that may be an excellent option for an elderly patient who has severe brow ptosis and heavy wrinkles but cannot tolerate more extensive surgery and would benefit from a short procedure under local anesthesia. The main disadvantage is the potentially visible scar immediately above the brow.

Midforehead and Brow Lift

Incisions made in the middle or upper forehead regions have similar advantages and disadvantages to the direct brow lift.[104–107] The incisions are made on each side of the forehead in an elliptic fashion so that the resulting scar follows a horizontal line already present in the forehead. Although this is probably the least used of all the techniques described, it may be a practical alternative for the elderly patient with thin eyebrows and deep horizontal rhytids who requires a short procedure under local anesthesia.

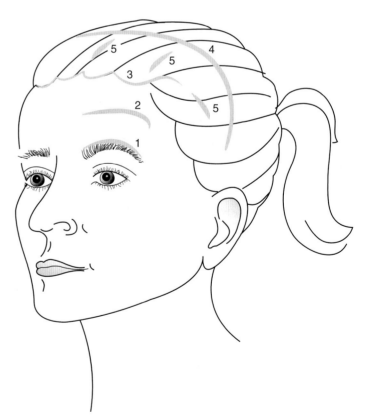

FIGURE **67-27** *Representative incisions for typical brow-lifting procedures: (1) direct brow lift, (2) midforehead lift, (3) trichophytic brow lift, (4) coronal brow lift, and (5) endoscopic brow lift.*

Transpalpebral and Other Local Brow Procedures

There has been a significant increase in the movement toward minimally invasive techniques to perform cosmetic surgery. New techniques for forehead and brow rejuvenation fill the literature and offer potentially exciting methods to gain esthetic improvement with less risk than with current procedures. A few such procedures include lateral brow lifting with temporal incisions only, denervation techniques through small punctures around the brow, and direct approaches through an upper blepharoplasty incision. It should be noted that although procedures such as making small punctures to destroy medial portions of facial nerve innervating medial depressors may seem minimally invasive, they are certainly not without risk.

Many of the "minimally invasive" procedures take advantage of the proximity of the local depressor muscle. For instance, the transpalpebral or transblepharoplasty approach for forehead rejuvenation gains access to the local depressors through an upper eyelid incision.[108] Dissection through this incision involves a short distance to the corrugator supercilii, the procerus, and depressor supercilii of the glabella, which can each be selectively transected from this incision to reduced unwanted wrinkles and elevate the medial brow (see Figure 67-11). Likewise, the orbicularis can be incised and subperiosteal dissection performed above the orbital rim to elevate the lateral brow through this same local incision. Suture plication of the periosteum above the rim may further elevate the lateral brow.

Another adjunctive technique in the upper third of the face is that of fat grafting in areas of age-related fat atrophy. Fat can essentially be grafted anywhere; however, caution is required in the glabellar region where occasional local necrosis can occur from fat infiltration. This also occurs occasionally after collagen injections in the same region.[109] There are a great number of alternative techniques, and each must be evaluated for safety, efficacy, and longevity on an individual basis.

Botulinum Toxin–Assisted Brow Lift

Botulinum toxin has been used for nearly two decades to improve the esthetic appearance of the upper third of the face by reducing wrinkles of the forehead (horizontal lines), glabella (frown and bunny lines), and lateral orbital crow's-feet (laugh lines).[110] More recently it has been used specifically to elevate certain regions of the brow to obtain a "chemical brow lift."[111] The depressor muscles are paralyzed with botulinum toxin not only to reduce the wrinkles they create but also to allow the frontalis muscle to elevate the brow farther because of the decrease in muscular antagonism. By decreasing the tone and downward pull of the orbicularis immediately below the brow, the lateral third of the eyebrow elevates approximately 2 to 4 mm from the result of botulinum toxin placed in the upper crow's-feet area. Such treatment of depressor muscles in the glabellar region can help elevate the medial brow. Of course, as with surgical brow lifting, overcorrection in the medial brow may result in an abnormal facial expression.

Dosages used vary with individuals. Botox comes in a 100-unit vial to be mixed with 1 to 10 cc normal saline. The more dilute solutions (6–10 cc/100 units) begin to loose efficacy and can distort the tissue, whereas high concentration mixtures (1–2 cc/100 units) may be wasteful and imprecise. Regardless of dilution, it is the total dosage in units of botulinum toxin and its proper placement that determine the outcome. For most individuals 5 to 10 units is all that is required for each lateral crow's-foot region. However, the larger muscles of the glabella (procerus and corrugators) require at least 15 units of the toxin and up to 50 units for maximum results. Appropriate dosage in the glabella is the most variable. Treatment of horizontal forehead lines typically requires between 15 and 25 units. It should be noted that simultaneous treatment of horizontal forehead lines from the frontalis may decrease or eliminate brow elevation that otherwise may have been created by botulinum toxin treatment of the depressor muscles. Moreover, excessive toxin treatment of horizontal lines close to the eyebrows (within 1 cm) should often be avoided owing to the risk of true ptosis of the forehead, brow, and upper eyelids.

Botulinum toxin has also been recommended to aid long-term stability of the surgical forehead and brow lift. The theory involved is that control of the downward pull of the depressors (by temporarily paralyzing them chemically) gives the periosteum time to attach securely in an elevated position. The injection can be done during surgery but there is an increased risk of eyelid ptosis and an unwanted delay since botulinum toxin typically takes 3 to 5 days to take full effect. Therefore, ideally botulinum toxin is injected 1 to 2 weeks prior to surgery. Regardless of any benefit this may give to long-term surgical fixation, the resulting reduction in wrinkles of the forehead and glabella and in crow's-feet is almost always popular with patients, even though the results last for only 3 to 6 months.

Adjunctive Procedures: Skin Care and Micropigmentation

A variety of procedures can be used for the superficial treatment of poor skin texture and are covered more completely in Chapter 69, "Skin Rejuvenation Procedures." For complete rejuvenation of the upper third of the face, skin resurfacing techniques may be required to address aging problems, especially those related to sun exposure, that cannot be adequately treated with lifting methods alone.

Prior to any resurfacing procedure such as laser skin resurfacing, chemical peels, or dermabrasion, the patient should be treated with topical skin medications to decrease the risk of scarring and pigment problems. Retinoic acid–type preparations used for ideally 6 weeks prior to resurfacing and 4% hydroquinone for patients with darker skin tones (Fitzpatrick 3 or higher) are two possibilities (see Chapter 69, "Skin Rejuvenation Procedures"). Simultaneous resurfacing procedures can be accomplished with brow lifting provided the surgical plane of dissection is subperiosteal or subgaleal and not subcutaneous.

Another adjunctive procedure growing in popularity is medical micropigmentation. The use of new skin pigments that do not contain iron oxide has improved the appearance of tattoos placed to enhance a thin eyebrow or as permanently applied eyeliner. The ink is relatively permanent but often requires touch-ups owing to some fading over the first 3 to 5 years. Patients who have poor hand motor skills can greatly benefit from this procedure. A certified technician under a doctor's supervision usually performs the micropigmentation. However, consultation with a surgeon prior to micropigmentation is important since placement of a permanent brow tattoo in a more elevated position may create problems if the patient desires a surgical brow lift later. Therefore, if a patient is seeking brow lifting in addition to the micropigmentation, it is advisable to perform the surgical brow lift prior to the permanent makeup if feasible.

Postoperative Care

Following surgical forehead and brow lifting, a compression bandage is applied using a material such as Coban or Coflex. The pressure helps to limit edema and hematoma formation while possibly improving fixation. Typically a drain is not required if a very dry field has been maintained. The patient should be instructed to limit activity and to use cold compresses over the eyes and brows. Head elevation is also recommended for the first several

days. Avoidance of antiplatelet drugs preoperatively, a careful surgical technique, and the immediate postoperative use of cold compresses, elevation, and limited strenuous activity significantly decrease postoperative healing time.

The relatively snug postoperative dressing may be removed on postoperative day 1 to visually inspect the surgical site for any problems. A less constrictive Velcro-type head wrap can then be used to allow patient comfort and easy removal for showering. Patients are allowed to gently shampoo their hair after 24 hours but must be cautioned to avoid water pressure directly over any incision sites. Each incision is then cleaned twice a day with a dilute peroxide solution, and a thin layer of antibiotic ointment is applied for the first week. Staples are removed at the end of 1 week. Chemical treatments of hair such as "perms" should be delayed for at least 2 weeks to avoid possible hair loss as a reaction to the harsh chemicals. Hot curling irons or other similar devices must be used with caution since areas of scalp anesthesia may be present for months and can predispose a patient to an accidental self-inflicted burn.

Complications

Fortunately, major complications are rare with properly performed forehead and brow rejuvenation procedures. Good patient selection, diligent preoperative planning, meticulous surgical technique, and thorough postoperative care are all required to help limit the chance for complications.[112–115] Minor complications can always occur despite a surgeon's best efforts. No matter how minor the problem, the patient must be treated with concern and compassion. Typically patients who undergo cosmetic surgery are expecting to look better as soon as possible and are not always as tolerant of perioperative problems as are trauma patients. Extensive edema and ecchymoses are not normally considered complications but may war-

rant appropriate reassurance and even simple suggestions to hasten recovery when feasible. Suggestions regarding makeup from a well-trained staff member may greatly improve a postoperative patient's mood when shown how to better hide persistent erythema or ecchymosis.

True complications include poor scar appearance, wound dehiscence, hematoma, skin sloughs or perforations, asymmetries, sensory disturbances, facial paralysis, eyelid ptosis, corneal abrasions, dry eye syndrome, hair loss (alopecia), infection, relapse, irregular facial expressions, and contour irregularities. Of all these potential problems, permanent facial paralysis and major tissue loss are the most devastating. Fortunately, these particular complications are rare (< 0.3%, which is less than that for a standard lower face-lift). Regardless, it is critical to know the precise anatomy and to avoid improper or excessive retraction, overzealous cautery, and overthinning of the flaps when transecting the depressors. In addition, hematomas must be diagnosed and treated without delay.

Some problems such as corneal abrasions can be very concerning to the patient owing to the severe pain and can be nearly eliminated by proper technique and perioperative attention to detail. For instance, an eye lubricant should always be used. Also, thought should be given to the placement of temporary tape strips, such as Steri-Strips, over the eyelids or a tarsorrhaphy suture to help prevent inadvertent scratching of the cornea by gauze or tubing, for example, during the procedure (see Figure 67-16). All severe pain requires immediate evaluation, and suspected abrasion should be treated by appropriate ophthalmic drops for pain and patching of the affected eye for 12 to 24 hours. Appropriate ophthalmologic consultation is required for persistent or uncontrollable eye pain, persistent dry-eye symptoms, or unusual changes in vision. Minor blurred vision for the first 12 hours is not unusual owing to chemosis and use of ophthalmic ointments.

Alopecia and sensory disturbances can be bothersome to the patient and often are not permanent. The problem is the inability to predict whether the numbness a patient has will partially, fully, or not go away, and just how soon is might be alleviated. With proper technique, an endoscopic forehead and brow lift has a high rate of sensory nerve recovery, but full recovery may take several months and require patient reassurance. Although exact numbers are not known, empiric observation of the last 150 endoscopic brow lifts that I have performed suggests that sensory disturbances are an occasional early concern but an unusual complaint after 6 to 12 months. Alopecia, on the other hand, is a significant concern, especially if it persists longer than 6 to 12 months. Hair may return after an average 4- to 8-month dormancy period of the hair follicle. However, excessive tension on the flaps, rough handling of wound margins, or excessive use of cautery near follicles may lead to permanent hair loss that requires treatment.[116]

Proper planning, technique, and postoperative care helps to reduce the incidence of complications. Immediate and appropriate treatment along with sincere concern for the patient's well-being should help to reduce the chance of the situation worsening or patient being dissatisfied.

Summary and Conclusions

An explosion in the number of rejuvenation techniques for the upper face in the past decade, lead by the use of endoscopes and botulinum toxin, has revolutionized the treatment of aging in this area. Cosmetic surgery treatment of the upper third of the face is frequently an essential component for complete facial rejuvenation. Procedures are highly variable and can offer improvement to both young and old. Matching the problems to the ideal rejuvenation techniques is essential for maximum esthetic benefits. Even the best surgical technique can result in inadequate or even poor results if improper patient selection or incorrect diagnoses are made; for this reason, the forehead and brow area must be evaluated critically for a wide range of interlacing diagnoses.

Specific skin problems vary with a patient's age and sex, but gravity remains consistent and nonselective; therefore, the only issues regarding the occurrence of brow ptosis are when it will occur and how severe it will be. Wrinkles are also inevitable but may be dynamic or static in nature. Thanks to botulinum toxin, the previously difficult treatment of dynamic upper facial lines can be effected at low risk with a simple injection. The common and consistent finding of brow ptosis, especially in the lateral third of the brow, may now be selectively treated endoscopically to achieve a more youthful appearance. Society's idea of beauty at any one moment in time will ultimately help to guide the patient and surgeon to choose where the brow should be placed as opposed to merely raising it higher. True rejuvenation is likely more complex and involves multiple modalities and even tissue replacement such as fat grafting. Only time and persistence will prove what best restores youth to the upper face.

Facial cosmetic surgery continues to rise in popularity exponentially. The aging population wants to feel and look more youthful but nonetheless demands to remain natural looking. Today's discerning patient is often very knowledgeable on the subject of their cosmetic surgery options and may insist on a specific technique. The advice of a well-trained surgeon and diagnostician may make or break the ultimate result and prevent a cosmetic disaster. It is vital that the surgeon refuse to perform treatment that is not in the best interest of the patient. Cosmetic surgery is a luxury and is an optional procedure, no matter how much of an emergency it seems to the patient. At the end of the day, it is the surgeon's responsibility to provide the patient with the best and safest options available to achieve realistic goals.

References

1. Ramirez OM. Endoscopic techniques in facial rejuvenation. An overview. Part 1. Aesthetic Plast Surg 1994;8:141–147.
2. Isse NG. Endoscopic facial rejuvenation. Endo-forehead, the functional lift. Case reports. Aesthetic Plast Surg 1994;18:21–9.
3. Tessier P. Ridectomie frontale. [Lifting frontale.] Gaz Méd Fr 1968;75:55–65.
4. Becker FF, Johnson CM. Surgical treatment of the upper third of the aging face. In: Cummings CW, Fredrickson JM, Harker LA, editors. Otolaryngology-head and neck surgery. St. Louis: Mosby; 1986. p. 475.
5. Zide BM, Jelks GW. Surgical anatomy of the orbit. New York: Raven Press; 1985.
6. Fagien S. Eyebrow analysis after blepharoplasty in patients with brow ptosis. Ophthal Plast Reconstr Surg 1992;8:210.
7. Ellis DAF, Ward D. The aging face. J Otolaryngol 1986; 15:217–23.
8. Johnson JD, Hadley RC. The aging face. In: Converse JM, editor. Reconstructive plastic surgery. Philadelphia: WB Sanders; 1964. p. 1306–42.
9. Powell H, Humphrieys B. Proportions of the aesthetic face. New York: Thieme-Stratton; 1984.
10. Huntley HE. The divine proportion. New York: Dover; 1970.
11. Rickets RM. Divine proportion of facial aesthetics. Clin Plast Surg 1982;9:401.
12. Evans TW. Browlift. Atlas of Oral Maxillofac Surg Clin North Am 1998;6:111–33.
13. Ellis DAF, Bakala CD. Anatomy of the motor innervation of the corrugator supercilii muscle: clinical significance and development of a new surgical technique for frowning. J Otolaryngol 1998;27:222–7.
14. Larrabee WF, Mahielski KH. Surgical anatomy of the face. New York: Raven Press; 1993.
15. Gonzalez-Ulloa M. Facial wrinkles, integral elimination. Plast Reconstr Surg 1962;29:658.
16. Bostwick J, Eaves F, Nahai F. Endoscopic plastic surgery. St. Louis: Quality Medical Publishers; 1995.
17. Hiatt JL, Gartner LP. In: Gardner J, editor. Textbook of head and neck anatomy. 2nd ed. Baltimore: Williams and Wilkins; 1987. p. 156–245, 373–45.
18. Hamas RS. Reducing the subconscious frown by endoscopic resection of the corrugator muscles. Aesthetic Plast Surg 1995;19:21–5.
19. Salasche SJ, Bernstein G, Senkarik. Surgical anatomy of the skin. Appleton & Lange; 1988.
20. Edwards BF. Bilateral neurotomy for the frontalis hypermotility. Plast Reconstr Surg 1957;19:341–4.

21. Ellis DAF, Masri H. The effect of facial animation on the aging upper half of the face. Arch Otolaryngol Head Neck Surg 1989;115:710–2.

22. Brennan HG. The forehead lift. Otolaryngol Clin North Am 1980;13:209.

23. Rafaty FM, Brennan HG. Current concepts in brow pexy. Arch Otolaryngol Head Neck Surg 1983;109:152.

24. Rafaty FM, Goode RL. The browlift operation in a man. Arch Otolaryngol Head Neck Surg 1978;104:69.

25. Rafaty FM, Goode RL, Fee WE. The browlift operation. Arch Otolaryngol Head Neck Surg 1975;101:467.

26. Knize DM. Reassessment of the coronal incision and subgaleal dissection for foreheadplasty. Plast Reconstr Surg 1998;102:478.

27. Grant JCB, editor. Grant's atlas of anatomy. 6th ed. Baltimore: Williams & Wilkins, 1972.

28. Tolhurst DE, Carstens MH, Greco RJ, et al. The surgical anatomy of the scalp. Plast Reconstr Surg 1991;87:603.

29. Tremolada C, Candiani P, Signorini M, et al. The surgical anatomy of the subcutaneous fascial system of the scalp. Ann Plast Surg 1994;32:8.

30. Carstens MH, Greco RJ, Hurwitz DJ, et al. Clinical applications of the subgaleal fascia. Plast Reconstr Surg 1991;87:615.

31. Waite PD, Cuzalina LA. Rhytidectomy. In: Fonseca RJ, editor. Oral and maxillofacial surgery: cleft/craniofacial/cosmetic surgery. Vol 6. Philadelphia (PA): WB Saunders Co; 1998. p. 365–81.

32. Tobin HA, Cuzalina LA, Tharanon W, Sinn DP. The biplane face lift: an opportunistic approach. J Oral Maxillofac Surg 2000; 58:76–85.

33. Tobin HA, Cuzalina LA. SMAS surgery versus deep-plane rhytidectomy. In: Pensak ML, editor. Controversies in otolaryngology. New York: Thieme; 2001. p. 148–55.

34. Knize DM. Transpalpebral approach to the corrugator supercilii and procerus muscles. Plast Reconstr Surg 1995;95:52–60.

35. Aiache AE. Transblepharoplasty brow-lift. Presented at the American Society of Aesthetic Plastic Surgery; 1995 May; San Francisco, CA.

36. Boyd B, Caminer D, Moon HK. Innervation of the procerus and corrugator muscles and its significance in facial surgery. Paper presented at the annual meeting of the ASPRS; 1997 September; San Francisco, CA.

37. Knize DM. A study of the supraorbital nerve. Plast Reconstr Surg 1997;99:1224.

38. Knize DM. Muscles that act on glabellar skin: a closer look. Plast Reconstr Surg 2000; 105:350.

39. Netter FM. Atlas of human anatomy. Summit (NJ): Ciba-Geigy; 1989.

40. Knize DM. An anatomically based study of the mechanism of eyebrow ptosis. Plast Reconstr Surg 1996;97:1321.

41. De la Plaza R, De la Cruz L. A new concept in blepharoplasty. Aesthet Plast Surg 1996; 20:221.

42. Lemke BN, Stasior OG. The anatomy of eyebrow ptosis. Arch Ophthalmol 1982;100:981.

43. Meyer DR, Linberg JV, Wobig JL, et al. Anatomy of the orbital septum and associated eyelid connective tissues. Ophthal Plast Reconstr Surg 1991;7:104.

44. Aiache AE, Ramirez OM. The suborbicularis oculi fat pads: an anatomic and clinical study. Plast Reconstr Surg 1995;95:37.

45. Trinei FA, Januszkiewicz J, Nahai F. The sentinel vein: an important reference point for surgery in the temporal region. Plast Reconstr Surg 1998;101:27.

46. Cuzalina LA, Holmes J. A simple and reliable landmark for identification of the supraorbital nerve in surgery of the forehead: an in vivo anatomical study. J Oral Maxillofac Surg 2003.[Submitted]

47. Gosain AK, Sewall SR, Yousif NJ. The temporal branch of the temporal nerve: how reliably can we predict its path? Plast Reconstr Surg 1997;99:1224.

48. Ellis E, Zide MF, editors. Surgical approaches to the facial skeleton. Baltimore: Williams & Wilkins; 1995. p. 59–169

49. Liebman E, Webster R, Berger A, et al. The frontalis nerve in the temporal brow lift. Arch Otolaryngol Head Neck Surg 1982; 108:232–35.

50. Furnas DW. Landmarks for the trunk and the temporofacial division of the facial nerve. Br J Surg 1965; 52:694.

51. Correia P, Zani R. Surgical anatomy of the facial nerve as related to ancillary operations in rhytidoplasty. Plast Reconstr Surg 1973;52:549–52.

52. Isse NG. Endoscopic forehead lift. Clin Plast Surg 1995; 22:661.

53. Isse NG. The endoscopic approach to forehead and brow lifting. Aesthetic Plast Surg 1998;18.

54. Vasconez LO, Core GB, Gamboa-Bobadilla M, et al. Endoscopic techniques in coronal brow lifting. Plast Reconstr Surg 1994;94:788.

55. Morselli PG. Fixation for forehead endoscopic lifting: a simple, easy, no-cost procedure. Plast Reconstr Surg 1996 97:1309.

56. Marchac D, Ascherman J, Arnaud E. Fibrin glue fixation in forehead endoscopy: evaluation of our experience with 206 cases. Plast Reconstr Surg 1997;100:704.

57. Hoeing JF. Rigid anchoring of the forehead to the frontal bone in endoscopic facelifting: a new technique. Aesthetic Plast Surg 1996;20:213.

58. De la Fuente A, Santamaria AB. Facial rejuvenation: a combined conventional and endoscopic assisted lift. Aesthetic Plast Surg 1996;20:471.

59. Isse NG. Endoscopic forehead lift, evolution and update. Clin Plast Surg 1995;2:661.

60. Adamson PA, Johnson CM, Anderson JR, et al. The forehead lift: a review. Arch Otolaryngol Head Neck Surg 1985;111:325–9.

61. Liang M, Narayaman K. Endoscopic oblation of the frontalis and corrugator muscles: a clinical study. Plast Surg Forum 1992; XV:54.

62. Su CT. Technique for division and suspension of the orbicularis oculi muscle. Clin Plast Surg 1981;8:673.

63. Byrd HS, Andochick SE. The deep temporal lift: a multiplanar lateral brow, temporal, and upper face lift. Plast Reconstr Surg 1996;97:928.

64. Kerth JD, Triumi DM. Management of the aging forehead. Arch Otolaryngol Head Neck Surg 1990;116:1137–42.

65. Chierici G, Miller A. Experimental study of muscle reattachment following surgical detachment. J Oral Maxillofac Surg 1984;42:485.

66. Ramirez OM. Endoscopic subperiosteal browlift and facelift. Clin Plast Surg 1995; 22:639–60.

67. Tobin HA. The extended subperiosteal coronal lift. Am J Cosmet Surg 1993;10:47–57.

68. Psillakis JM, Rummley TO, Camargos A. Subperiosteal approach in an improved concept for correction of the aging face. Plast Reconstr Surg 1988;82:383–92.

69. Maillard GF, Cornette de St Cyr B, Scheflan M. The subperiosteal bicoronal approach to total face lifting: the SMAS-deep musculoaponeurotic system. Aesthetic Plast Surg 1991;15:285–91.

70. Ramirez OM. Endoscopic techniques in facial rejuvenation: an overview. Aesthetic Plast Surg 1994;18:141–371.

71. Daniel RK, Ramirez OM. Endoscopic assisted aesthetic surgery. Aesthetic Plast Surg 1994;14:18–20.

72. Toledo LS. Facial rejuvenation: technique and rationale. In: Fodar P, Isse N, editors. Endoscopically assisted aesthetic plastic surgery. St. Louis: Mosby; 1996. p. 91–105.

73. Psillakis JM. Subperiosteal approach for surgical rejuvenation of the upper face. In: Psillakis J, editor. Deep face-lifting techniques. New York: Thieme; 1994. p. 51–63.

74. Hinderer UT. The sub SMAS and subperiosteal

rhytidectomy of the forehead and middle third of the face: a new approach to the aging face. Facial Plast Surg Clin North Am 1992;8(1):18–32.

75. Dempsey PD, Oneal RM, Izenberg PH. Subperiosteal brow and midface lifts. Aesthetic Plast Surg 1995; 19:59–68.

76. Blitzer A, Brin MF, Keen MS, et al. Botulinum toxin for the treatment of hyperfunctional lines of the face. Arch Otolaryngol Head Neck Surg 1993;119:1018–22.

77. Ruess WR, Owsley JQ. The anatomy of the skin and fascial layers of the face in aesthetic surgery. Clin Plast Surg 1987;14:677–82.

78. McCollough EG, Langsdon PR. Dermabrasion and chemical peel. New York: Thieme; 1998.

79. Buzzell RA. Effects of solar radiation on the skin. Otolaryngol Clin North Am 1993;26:1–11.

80. Ortiz-Monasterio FG, Olmedo A. The coronal incision in rhytidectomy: the brow lift. Clin Plast Surg 1978;5:167.

81. Ellenbogen R. Transcoronal eyebrow lift with concomitant upper blepharoplasty. Plast Reconstr Surg 1983; 71:490.

82. Wojtanowski MH. Bicoronal forehead lift. Aesthetic Plast Surg 1994;18:33.

83. Abul-Hassan HS, Van Drasek Ascher G, Acland RD. Surgical anatomy and blood supply for the fascial layers of the temporal regions. Plast Reconstr Surg 1986;77:17.

84. Stuzin JM, Wagstrom L, Kawamoto HK, et al. Anatomy of the frontal branch of the facial nerve: the significance of the temporal fat pad. Plast Reconstr Surg 1989;83:265.

85. Savani A. Physiopathology of the aging face. In: Psillakis JM, editor. Deep face-lifting techniques. New York: Thieme; 1994. p. 11–23.

86. De la Plaza R, Valiente E, Arroya JM. Supraperiosteal lifting of the upper two thirds of the face. Br J Plast Surg 1991;4:325–32.

87. Wassef M. Superficial fascial and muscular layers in the face and neck: a histologic study. Aesthetic Plast Surg 1987;11:171.

88. Tirkanits B, Daniel RK. The biplanar forehead lift. Aesthetic Plast Surg 1990;14:111.

89. Ramirex OM, Maillard GF, Musolas A. The extended subperiosteal face lift: a definitive soft-tissue remodeling for facial rejuvenation. Plast Reconstr Surg 1991: 88:227–36.

90. Psillakis JM. Embryology and anatomy review of the superficial fascia or SMAS. In: Psillakis JM, editor. Deep face-lifting techniques. New York: Thieme; 1994. p. 1–11.

91. Bosse JP, Papillon J, editors. Surgical anatomy of the SMAS at the malar region. In: Transactions of the Ninth International Congress of Plastic and Reconstructive Surgery. New York: McGraw-Hill; 1987.

92. Owsley JQ. Aesthetic facial surgery. Philadelphia: WB Saunders; 1994.

93. Yousif NJ, Mendelson BC. Anatomy of the mid-face. Clin Plast Surg 1995;22:227–41.

94. Guyuron B, Davies B. Subcutaneous anterior hairline forehead rhytidectomy. Aesthetic Plast Surg 1988;12:77.

95. Aiache AE. Endoscopic face-lift. Aesthetic Plast Surg 1994;18:275.

96. Ramirez OM. Endoscopic forehead and facelift: step-by-step. Open Tech Plast Reconstr Surg 1995;2:116–26.

97. Matarasso A, Terino EO. Forehead-brow rhytidoplasty: reassessing the goals. Plast Reconstr Surg 1994; 93:1378.

98. Newman JP, LaFerriere KA, Koch RJ, et al. Transcalvarial suture fixation for endoscopic brow and forehead lifts. Arch Otolaryngol Head Neck Surg 1997;123:313.

99. Kim SK. Endoscopic forehead scalp flap fixation with K-wire. Aesthetic Plast Surg 1996;20:217.

100. Pakkanen M, Salisbury AV, Ersek RA. Biodegradable positive fixation for endoscopic browlift. Plast Reconstr Surg 1996;98:1087.

101. Knize DM. A study of the supraorbital nerve. Plast Reconstr Surg 1995;96:564.

102. Loomis MG. Endoscopic brow fixation without bolsters or miniscrews. Plast Reconstr Surg 1996;98:373.

103. Dyer WK, Yung RT. Botulinum toxin-assisted brow lift. In: Larrabee WF, Thomas JR, editors. Facial plastic surgery clinics of North America: rejuvenation of the upper face. Vol 8, Number 3. Pennsylvania: W.B. Saunders Company; 2000. p. 343–54.

104. Brennan HG, Rafty FM. Midforehead incisions in treatment of the aging face. Arch Otolaryngol Head Neck Surg 1982;108:732–4.

105. Johnson CM, Waldman SR. Midforehead lift. Arch Otolaryngol Head Neck Surg 1983;109:155–9.

106. Cook TA, Brownrigg PJ, Wang TD, et al. The versatile midforehead browlift. Arch Otolaryngol Head Neck Surg 1989;115:163.

107. Johnson CM, Walman SR. Midforehead lift. Arch Otolaryngol Head Neck Surg 1983;109:155.

108. Guyuron B, Michelow BJ, Thomas T. Corrugator supercilii muscle resection through a blepharoplasty incision. Plast Reconstr Surg 1995;95:691–6.

109. Stegman SJ, Chu S, Armstrong RC. Adverse reactions to bovine collagen implant: clinical and histologic features. J Dermatol Surg Oncol 1988;14:39–47.

110. Keen MS, Khosh MM. The role of botulinum toxin A in facial plastic surgery. In: Willet JM, editor. Facial plastic surgery. Upper Saddle River (NJ): Prentice Hall; 1997. p. 323–9.

111. Frankel AS, Kamer FM. Chemical browlift. Arch Otolaryngol Head Neck Surg 1998;124:321.

112. Beeson WH, McCollough EG. Complications of the forehead lift. Ear Nose Throat J 1985;64:27.

113. Connell BF, Lambros VS, Neurohr GH. The forehead lift: techniques to avoid complications and produce optimal results. Aesthetic Plast Surg 1989;13:217.

114. Matarasso A. Endoscopic assisted forehead-brow rhytidoplasty: theory and practice. Aesthetic Plast Surg 1995;19:141.

115. Daniel RK, Tirkantis B. Endoscopic forehead lift, aesthetics and analysis. Clin Plast Surg 1995;22:605–18.

116. Mayer TG, Fleming RW. Management of alopecia. In: Cummings CW, Fredrickson JM, Harker LA, et al, editors. Otolaryngology—head neck surgery. St. Louis: Mosby; 1986. p. 429.

CHAPTER 68

Liposculpting Procedures

Milan J. Jugan, DMD

Liposculpting procedures in oral and maxillofacial surgery have been described in the literature since the 1930s; however, since the introduction of blunt cannula liposuction in the late 1970s, the theories, techniques, and indications for fat removal and transfer have evolved tremendously. Excisional techniques of fat removal used for treating most patients with localized submental lipodystrophy yielded variable results, scarring, and high complication rates. In the cervicofacial region the closed liposuction technique has proven to be an excellent technique for the removal of submental fat and, in addition, has provided a simplified technique with relatively few complications. Also, improved techniques for harvesting, preparing, and injecting fat to augment facial defects or create a more youthful appearance have been developed and are demonstrating long-term success. This chapter discusses a wide range of facial liposculpting procedures to include cervicofacial liposuction, autologous fat transfer, and the use of these techniques as adjunctive procedures to facilitate orthognathic, reconstructive, and maxillofacial cosmetic surgery procedures.

Cervicofacial Liposuction

History

Sculpting the body by removing localized fat deposits has been well documented in the literature for almost a century. Early excisional body-sculpting techniques included direct lipectomy and open instrument curettage.[1] These techniques were also used in an attempt to remove fat and sculpt the regions of the face and neck. Maliniak described submental fat removal and neck contouring with the excision of redundant tissue in the early 1930s.[2] Two decades later Davis reported using curettes to remove fat through a small submental incision.[3] Our modern techniques of cervicofacial liposuction in oral and maxillofacial surgery can be traced to the pioneering work of four surgeons. Schrudde introduced a technique called *lipexeresis* in 1972.[4] Modifying a uterine cannula, he described a procedure by which he tunneled in the subcutaneous fat and removed fat particles by suction. In the 1980s Illouz defined several principles for the successful treatment of localized lipodystrophy.[5] His technique of *lipolysis* is accomplished by injecting a mixture of saline and hyaluronidase solution into the surgical site, causing fat cells to rupture. He theorized that this rupturing of fat cells would make their removal by suction cannulas more efficient. Fournier developed the closed syringe technique, using small-diameter cannulas with an attached plastic syringe to generate the necessary negative pressure.[6] Finally, Klein developed the tumescent technique, a safe and effective procedure used by most surgeons today.[7] His technique uses large volumes of dilute epinephrine solution with or without lidocaine. Although the benefit of a large-volume fat removal without creating an electrolyte imbalance is not generally a concern for the oral and maxillofacial surgeon, the reduction in blood loss, decrease in postoperative ecchymosis, and decreased need for compression garment wear all benefit the cervicofacial liposuction patient.

Indications

Cervicofacial suction-assisted lipectomy is mainly used to correct or improve the body-contour irregularities caused by localized fat deposits in the head and neck region. Specifically, those localized fat deposits that tend to be resistant to dieting and exercise tend to respond favorably. In addition to its use as an esthetic procedure, the techniques mastered in cervicofacial liposuction may be used to facilitate flap elevation, defat pedicled flaps, and remove benign lipomas.[8,9]

In the maxillofacial region liposuction is most effective in contouring the submental, submandibular, and jowl regions of the face. These areas tend to be easily accessible to the liposuction cannulas for removal of the fat deposits and are also amenable to compression garment placement to facilitate recontouring of the regions. Various authors have also suggested the use of liposuction to contour and smooth deep nasolabial folds and to remove buccal fat pads to recontour full cheeks.[10,11] In my experience, nasolabial folds are more predictably managed with augmentation procedures (fat injection) than with fat removal. In addition, removal of buccal fat pads may create a hollowing of the buccal region, owing to progressive fat atrophy with aging, and an unnatural noncosmetic-appearing midface.

Patient Evaluation

Successful cervicofacial liposuction requires careful patient selection and a clear diagnosis of the pathologic entity desired to be modified. The patient's skin tone, skeletal configuration, muscular support of the neck, and body habitus should all be evaluated.

The ideal candidate is a woman of average weight and good skin elasticity, who demonstrates localized adipose accumulations that do not correspond to the patient's overall body habitus. If a patient has recently undergone significant weight loss, she should be advised that the ideal time for cervicofacial liposuction procedures is after 6 months of stable weight management. Patients who are generally overweight respond poorly to liposuction procedures and should be treated with caution. If the operating surgeon decides to proceed, these patients should be at the lower end of their usual weight range to obtain maximum benefit from the proposed surgery. In general, women are excellent candidates for cervicofacial liposuction, probably owing to their thinner less sebaceous skin, which tends to contract in a more predictable fashion over the reduced subcutaneous fat.

Skin elasticity should be evaluated in all patients undergoing cervicofacial liposuction. Patients should have sufficient skin elasticity to facilitate smooth and uniform redraping of skin over the recontoured fat and muscle. Those patients with skin excess or extremely lax or inelastic skin may achieve suboptimal results such as postoperative sagging and should be counseled on the benefit of adjunctive skin-tightening procedures to achieve the desired results.[12]

Finally, those patients with obtuse cervicomental angles, in addition to fat accumulation, may require deeper plane procedures to achieve an acceptable cosmetic improvement. Patients with platysmal decussation may benefit from platysmal plication in addition to liposuction to achieve a more youthful-appearing cervicofacial region. In those patients with platysmal ptosis and an obtuse cervicomental angle, liposuction alone leads to less-than-optimal results. These patients are best approached with liposuction in combination with suture suspension to lift the platysma and recreate the cervicomental angle.[13]

Instrumentation

For the most part, relatively little equipment is required to perform cervicofacial liposuction. Various companies manufacture a host of devices; however, the basic equipment remains a suction device and aspiration cannulas.

Cannula design has changed since the description of the procedure by Illouz.[5] A variety of lengths, diameters, and tip designs are available to the surgeon, and the cannula should be chosen according to the procedure being performed. The length of the cannula may vary depending on the specific surgical goal. A short cannula may be chosen to access only the submental region, but a longer cannula or second surgical incision may be needed to work at the angle of the mandible. In general, a 25 to 30 cm length is sufficient for most surgeries in the head and neck region.

Cannula diameter affects the volume of fat removed. It is important to remember that the amount of tissue that can be removed with a pass of the cannula depends on the diameter of the cannula lumen and the suction pressure. Therefore, under an equal amount of pressure, a larger-diameter cannula lumen removes more fat than does a cannula of smaller diameter. If the goal of surgery is to rapidly remove a large amount of excess adipose tissue, then a larger-diameter cannula is chosen. If the goal is to accurately remove a small amount of fat with more control, then a smaller diameter is chosen. A cannula diameter of 2 to 6 mm is generally used in cervicofacial liposuction procedures.

Finally, tip design is evaluated. Most importantly, the cannula should have a smooth tip and aperture opening. Fat is drawn into the cannula lumen through the aperture opening by the vacuum from the suction unit and then avulsed by the back-and-forth movement of the cannula. Neurovascular structures are pushed aside by a blunt smooth tip. Sharp edges will cut and shave, placing surrounding blood vessels and nerves at greater risk for injury. Damage to these structures may result in alterations to sensation, seroma, hematoma, or necrosis of overlying skin. Again, the goals of the surgery are important when choosing a tip design. A narrow cannula with round tips may be used for the precise removal of small fatty deposits. Flat spatula cannulas are more commonly used in open procedures to defat flaps because an effective seal may be maintained with the underlying tissue bed.

In general, cannula design should be selected to facilitate the goal of the surgical procedure, and a variety of designs should be available to provide the patient with an optimum outcome. Figures 68-1 to 68-3 show examples of various cannula designs available for cervicofacial liposculpting procedures.

The suction device provides the vacuum to the aspiration cannula for removal of the fat deposits. This negative pressure may be generated via a hand-held syringe, wall suction, or commercially available suction unit. Hand-held syringe devices are good for use in the head and neck region owing to their low cost, portability, and ease of handling. They provide an efficient technique for precise contouring of

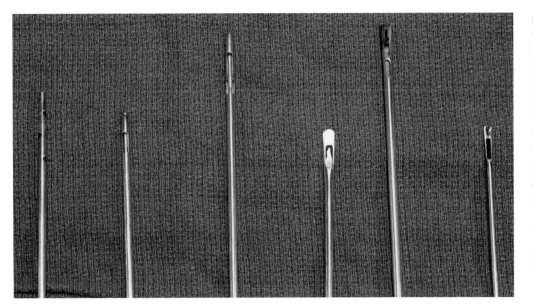

FIGURE **68-1** *Various designs of cannula tip available for syringe liposuction systems.*

irregularities secondary to cervicofacial adiposity.[6] The negative pressure is generated by placing 5 cc of tumescent solution into the cannula-syringe unit, placing the cannula working port beneath the flap, and pulling back on the plunger to create the vacuum. When the plunger is pulled back to the fullest extent, it is possible to obtain 1 atm of negative pressure. Various plunger locks are manufactured to hold the plunger in position during the operation. A disadvantage of this system is the loss of vacuum that occurs if tissue contact is lost.

Wall suction and commercially available suction units are useful for closed and open liposuction techniques. They provide continuous vacuum and are most useful for removing large amounts of fat or defating a flap.

A final consideration for choosing a suction device is the ability to vary the amount of negative pressure through the cannula. Whereas 1 atm of negative pressure is ideal for liposuction procedures, 0.5 atm of negative pressure is more appropriate to harvest fat for fat-injection techniques.

Anesthesia

Liposculpting procedures may be performed in various settings from an office or surgicenter to a main operating room.

Although some patients may desire general anesthesia, the vast majority of cervicofacial procedures may be performed with local anesthesia and intravenous sedation.

The tumescent technique of superficial liposuction, published by Jeffery Klein in 1987,[7] has become the standard against which all other techniques are compared. It is distinct from other liposuction techniques in that the entire procedure can be performed under local anesthesia only if the surgeon so desires. Most importantly for the patient, the tumescent technique provides excellent anesthesia and out-

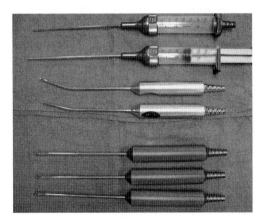

FIGURE **68-2** *Examples of various cannulas available for cervicofacial liposculpting procedures. Note the differences in cannula length, diameter, tip design, and ability for use with a syringe or suction aspiration system.*

standing hemostasis. To understand Klein's tumescent technique, one needs to review the wet technique of Illouz.[5] Illouz injected hypotonic saline, lidocaine, epinephrine, and hyaluronidase into the liposuction site, attempting to cause lysis of fat cells and improve fat extraction. With the wet technique, excessive blood loss remained a significant risk. Large cannulas were used to remove as much fat as possible in the shortest amount of time. Postoperatively, bruising was extensive and patients wore compressive garments for several weeks. Klein's technique for the head and neck advocates the use of a local anesthetic solution containing normal saline, 0.1% lidocaine, epinephrine at a concentration of 1:1,000,000, and bicarbonate. Table 68-1 provides concentration data on several mixtures of tumescent solution that I use. Klein also demonstrated that a large amount of lidocaine could be injected into the superficial fat compartments without a large increase in serum lidocaine levels since aspiration of the infiltrate and fat were being performed.[7] In general, 50 to 100 cc of Klein's solution are used in the cervicofacial region for liposuction procedures.

In 1997 the American Academy of Cosmetic Surgery published its *Guidelines for Liposuction Surgery* and stated, "The tumescent infiltration (technique) has been shown over the last 9 years to be the safest for liposuction and lipocontouring, with the fastest recovery time and least complications for the patient."[14]

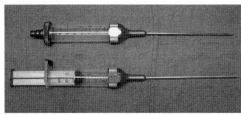

FIGURE **68-3** *Syringe liposuction system set up for standard syringe liposuction and adaptation to a suction aspiration system. This system is particularly useful for collecting harvested fat in the syringe.*

Table 68-1 Tumescent Solution Concentration Data			
Component	*Solution A**	*Solution B†*	*Solution C‡*
Lidocaine (1%)	50 cc (500 mg); 0.05%	100 cc (1,000 mg); 0.1%	150 cc (1,500 mg); 0.15%
Epinephrine (1:1,000)	0.5 cc (0.5 mg); 1:2,000,000	1.0 cc (1.0 mg); 1:1,000,000	1.5 cc (1.5 mg); 1:666,666
Bicarbonate (1 mEq/mL)	10 cc; 10 mEq/L	10 cc; 10 mEq/L	10 cc; 10 mEq/L
Normal saline	1,000 mL	1,000 mL	1,000 mL

*Solution A is used for patients undergoing liposculpting procedures for the first time.
†Solution B is used for revision liposculpting procedures.
‡Solution C is used for liposuction-assisted rhytidectomy procedures and fat harvesting.

Although the tumescent technique will continue to evolve with research and evolution of equipment, it certainly has proven to be a safe and effective therapy for cervicofacial liposuction.

Technique

The goal of cervicofacial liposuction is to create a smooth and regular contour of the head and neck regions by the precise removal of localized fat deposits while minimizing external scaring. To that end, the patient must be educated on the risks and benefits of the procedure. A preoperative consultation should be performed that includes adequate photodocumentation of the patient's preoperative condition. Informed consent for liposuction surgery and sedation must be reviewed and obtained. Appendix A shows a sample consent form for a cervicofacial liposuction procedure. The patient's medical history should be reviewed for any contraindications to surgery and to determine any potentially modifiable factors (eg, use of nonsteroidal anti-inflammatory drugs or herbal medications, and smoking).

On the day of surgery the patient is marked up in the sitting position, and the areas of proposed fat removal are reviewed and verified with the patient. Various other anatomic structures may be marked up depending on the surgeon's preference, but I recommend marking the inferior border of the mandible, sternocleidomastoid muscle, and the top of the thyroid cartilage, as well as the proposed surgical incisions.

All skin incisions should be large enough to accommodate placement of the aspirating cannulas. Incisions that are too large leave an unsightly scar when healed, and incisions that are too small may be damaged by friction from the back-and-forth motion of the cannula. The submental and submandibular areas may be liposuctioned using a single incision in the submental crease. The jowl area may be best approached from an incision in the posterior earlobe crease. A small incision in the nasal vestibule area may allow access to facial adiposity not adequately removed through the previously described incisions.

The patient is placed in a modified semi-Fowler position, monitors are placed, and supplemental oxygen is delivered. Intravenous sedation is then titrated to the level desired by the operating surgeon. Local anesthetic is infiltrated into the incision sites, and an incision is made through the dermis. A small pocket is then created within the superficial fat plane between the dermis and the platysma or superficial musculoaponeurotic system (SMAS). Tumescent liposuction solution is then infiltrated into this space via an infiltrating cannula. Care is taken to remain in the compartment of superficial fat above the platysma muscle. The cannula is advanced in a plane parallel to the skin surface and is easily palpable during the infiltration process. The cannula is advanced in a systematic manner throughout the area to be treated, and the solution is injected as the cannula is being with-

drawn. In the average patient, 100 to 150 cc of solution is deposited in the plane of dissection. The area is then to remain undisturbed by instrumentation for 10 to 15 minutes, allowing for maximum vasoconstriction and providing excellent local anesthesia. Effective placement of the tumescent solution will result in blanching of the overlying skin owing to the vasoconstrictive effects of the solution.

After 10 to 15 minutes, an operating cannula is placed into the incision site, and the process of suction-free pretunneling is begun throughout the surgical site. When the operating cannula is inserted, care must be taken to ensure that the aperture opening is directed away from the skin. If facing the skin, the aperture may cause damage to the subdermal plexus, resulting in an increase in postoperative complications and the potential for postoperative epidermal ridge formation. Pretunneling is performed by systematically passing the cannula back and forth through the fat deposits, with care being taken to remain within the superficial fat compartment. Although not mandatory, pretunneling defines the appropriate surgical plane, breaks up fat cells, and aids in the extraction of fat cell content.

Following pretunneling the cannula is connected to the suction device. Fat is removed from the desired areas by directing the cannula through the pretunneled area in the same systematic manner used initially. Again, care is taken to ensure that the aperture opening is directed away from the skin and that the cannula remains in the proper plane of dissection. A superficial plane may be maintained by tenting the skin away from the deep tissues with the tip of the cannula and by palpating the cannula though the skin using the nonoperating hand. Fat is extracted from the superficial fat compartment until the desired contour is achieved. Once the main area of adiposity is reduced, the cannula is carried slightly beyond the margins of the original dissection to feather out the edges of the operative site and to reduce the potential for contour irregularities. The site should be inspected frequently to avoid overcorrection. Direct palpation is the most accurate method to assess the amount of fat removed. The skin should be pinched and rolled between the thumb and index finger. The skin should feel loose, with a thin layer of adipose tissue remaining on the undersurface of the dermis. In most cases the surgeon removes between 20 and 100 cc of fat in the cervicofacial region. Additional contouring may be required following the submental approach; in this case posterior earlobe crease incisions may by used to overlap the dissection areas. The same sequence of pretunneling, inspection, and fat removal is used to optimize the final contour enhancement for the patient.

Following completion of the liposuction, residual blood, tumescent fluid, and fat particles are expressed from the space. The incision sites are closed using a 5-0 or 6-0 monofilament suture such as nylon or polypropylene. The wounds are then covered with an antibiotic ointment and dressings. A light pressure dressing is placed to reduce tissue edema and to immobilize and reshape the skin over the recontoured area. Although multiple regimens for compression exist, I instruct patients to wear the compression garment continuously for 7 days and then only at night for an additional 7 days. Appendix B shows an example of postoperative instructions for patients undergoing cervicofacial liposuction.

Complications

Postoperative complications associated with cervicofacial liposuction are rare. Since liposuction of the head and neck region usually involves the removal of < 100 cc of fat from a limited area, the complications associated with whole-body liposuction procedures, such as significant blood loss, rapid fluid shifts, hypotension, shock, and death, are not seen.

Infections following cervicofacial liposuction occur in < 0.2% of cases,[15] and a low rate should be expected with adherence to strict sterile procedure. Since cervicofacial liposuction is a sterile procedure, antibiotics are not required. However, literature suggests that they are commonly used as a prophylactic measure by many surgeons.[16]

Hematomas and seromas are rarely seen. Compression garment wear limits the potential for this complication. Small hematomas or seromas are generally managed by needle aspiration and extended wear of a compression garment until completely resolved.

Contour irregularities are probably the most common postoperative complication. They may be treated based on the etiology of formation. Those complications related to excess skin (sagging) should be treated with a skin-tightening procedure. Irregularities of the underlying muscle (platysmal ptosis or platysmal decussation) should be corrected by a procedure designed to correct muscular problems. Both of the above-mentioned complications are the result of poor patient selection and diagnosis. Contour irregularities owing to inadequate fat removal may be corrected with further liposculpting procedures; however, overaggressive removal of fat may be more difficult to correct.

Injuries to the branches of the facial nerve or the greater auricular nerve are rare and may be avoided by adhering to the appropriate technique and ensuring that dissection is in the correct surgical plane. If facial nerve injury does occur, monitoring and early referral to an appropriate specialist is indicated.

Liposuction as an Adjunctive Procedure

Orthognathic Surgery

Orthognathic surgical procedures have long been recognized as a means to manipulate the esthetics of the face. Hard tissues of the facial skeleton are manipulated by osteoplasty, osteotomy, and skeletal implants to modify a patient's appearance. However, the skin and subcutaneous tissues do play a role in determining a portion of facial esthetics, particularly in the cervicomental region. Those orthognathic procedures that affect the position of the mandible also affect the esthetics of the submental and neck region. For instance, a patient undergoing a mandibular setback procedure may have an esthetic cervicomental angle prior to the procedure but have lax submental tissue following the procedure. This modification of an adjacent esthetic subunit of the head and neck underscores the need for a total facial analysis of our orthognathic patients prior to the initiation of surgical treatment. In the case of liposculpting procedures, a patient's submental, jowl, and neck regions may be treated with cervicofacial liposuction in conjunction with orthognathic surgery to better define the inferior border of the mandible, remove unesthetic submental fat deposits, or assist in tightening lax submental tissues to establish an acceptable cervicomental angle. An important limitation to consider with this type of combined treatment is the etiology of the original craniofacial defect being treated. In those patients with severely hypoplastic mandibles, a deficiency in cervicomental skin and muscle may also exist. In such a case cervicofacial liposuction would not be a benefit in recreating an esthetic cervicomental angle. Figure 68-4 demonstrates reconstruction of the cervicomental region in a patient undergoing combined orthognathic and liposculpting procedures.

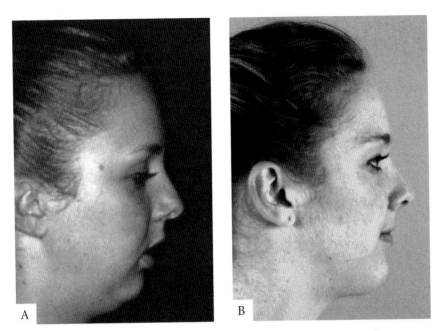

FIGURE **68-4**   *This patient underwent orthognathic surgery consisting of a segmental Le Fort I osteotomy with impaction, bilateral sagittal split ramus osteotomies, advancement genioplasty, and cervicofacial liposuction. A, Preoperative view. B, Postoperative view. Note the esthetic appearance of the cervicomental angle.*

Chin Augmentation   Cervicofacial liposuction may be performed in conjunction with chin augmentation or advancement genioplasty if the patient exhibits a hypoplastic genial process. The combination of procedures enhances the results that the patient would receive from liposuction alone.[17] The advancement genioplasty or chin augmentation improves the final result by accentuating the depth of the cervicomental angle. In many cases a chin implant may be placed using the same incision through which the liposuction was performed by slightly increasing the size of the incision to accommodate the chin implant. Advancement genioplasty may be performed through an intraoral incision, with closure occurring prior to the start of liposuction; this allows the field to be cleared of all contaminated instruments and provides the surgeons with the opportunity to change their gloves.

Liposuction-Assisted Rhytidectomy

Liposuction may be used to enhance the results of rhytidectomy (face-lift) when significant submental adiposity exists. Both open and closed liposuction techniques may be used. Three main areas may be addressed with the liposuction technique. First, the technique of pretunneling may assist the surgeon in elevating the facial flap. The blunt-tipped cannula may be passed easily through the subcutaneous fat layer to assist in the dissection and limit the potential for damage to the subdermal plexus. Second, following elevation of the flap, the spatula cannula may be used to defat the SMAS layer and the posterior aspect of the platysma. This maneuver helps to better identify the surgical plane and to limit the potential for postoperative contour irregularities. Any fat that may be associated with excessive jowls may be eliminated from overlying the SMAS at this time. Finally, liposuction may be used in the neck and submental areas to eliminate fatty deposits and potentiate the appropriate redraping of the neck and facial skin. It is important to remember that liposuction provides only an adjunct to rhytidectomy and that SMAS suspension with skin excision must still be per-

formed. Figure 68-5 illustrates a case in which a patient underwent liposuction-assisted rhytidectomy.

Autologous Fat Transfer

History

Autologous fat transfer for soft tissue augmentation or reconstruction continues to be viewed with guarded acceptance by surgeons throughout the world. Many surgeons are able to obtain predictable results, a fact that has spurred continued interest in the concept of fat transfer. In addition, many practitioners now feel that the loss of fat volume in the face may lead to premature aging and a less-than-cosmetic appearance. As a result, there has been a resurgence in the acceptance of fat-injection techniques. The technique itself was first introduced by Neuber in 1893, when he used a free fat graft from the upper extremity to reconstruct a periorbital defect.[18] His data seemed to suggest that smaller grafts were more successful in that they had a greater chance for long-term survival. Building on this knowledge, Verderame in 1909 advocated overcorrection of defects to the significant amount of graft resorption associated with autologous fat transfer.[19] It is important to realize that these studies involved sharply dissected fat grafts with defined clinical margins for vascular ingrowth and not bluntly dissected fat from liposuction harvest procedures. Research continued into sharply dissected autologous fat grafts with several human studies by Peer in the 1950s.[20,21] He sharply dissected fat from the abdomens of 13 individuals and divided the fat into two equal grafts. One graft was inserted in entirety, whereas the other graft was sharply subdivided into multiple smaller pieces. His studies demonstrated that the greatest damage to the graft occurred at the cut margins and that the grafts that were cut into smaller pieces retained less of their volume. Although this would seem to be contradictory to

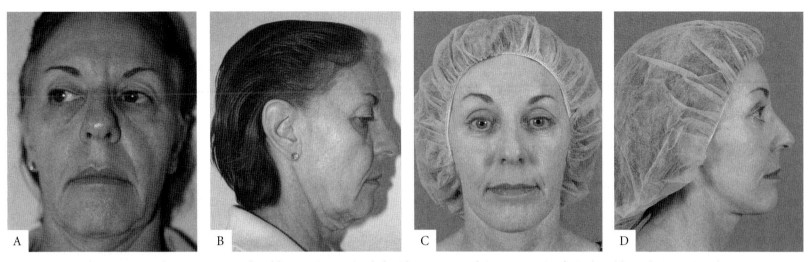

FIGURE **68-5** *This patient underwent a cervicofacial liposuction-assisted rhytidectomy. A and B, Preoperative frontal and lateral views. C and D, Postoperative frontal and lateral views. Note the excellent definition of the inferior border of the mandible and the esthetic appearance of the cervicomental angle.*

earlier research demonstrating greater graft volume survival in smaller grafts, the contradiction relates to the surgical damage created by the sectioning of a larger graft into smaller portions versus the harvesting of a smaller graft initially.

Blunt lipectomy with autologous fat grafting by injection has recently become popular owing to the relative ease of the procedure. Illouz first wrote about the grafting of liposuctioned fat in 1986,[22] and others have published multiple positive reports of the technique based on clinical experience[23–25]; however, little scientific information on the validity of this technique has become available until recently. Fournier and Otteni studied histologically the damage to lipocytes following their extraction by blunt cannula liposuction and noted no damage to the cells.[16] It is important to note that these studies were carried out using large-diameter cannulas, not the smaller-diameter cannulas used today. More recently Carpaneda demonstrated that the aspirated material retrieved following liposuction consists of adipose cells, collagen fibers, vessels, nerves, ruptured cells, inflammatory proteins, proteases, and lipogenic enzymes.[26] Campbell and colleagues studied adipocyte glucose oxidation and lipid synthesis following suction extraction and injection through needles of varying sizes.

Their research showed that the smaller-diameter needles were associated with increasing cell damage.[27] More current research focuses on limiting damage to cells on extraction and providing an appropriate environment for cell survival during transfer. Various techniques involve the use of platelet gel, enriched tissue culture medium, and albumin to promote the survival of fat cells and maintain the volume of the grafted tissue.[28–30]

Autologous Fat Injection

The technique for autologous fat transfer by injection varies with the provider. As demonstrated by the limited literature review previously presented, there are multiple theories and techniques associated with fat transfer. The following technique has been used over a period of years, providing predictable cosmetic results for many patients.

As with cervicofacial liposuction, the appropriate preoperative consultation, medical evaluation, photodocumentation, and informed consent procedures are necessary for all patients. Patients should identify the defect that they desire to be corrected or describe the cosmetic enhancement that they wish to be achieved by autologous fat transfer. Prominent nasolabial or melolabial folds, prominent nasojugal grooving, and atrophic lips are all cosmetic deformi-

ties that lend themselves to correction by autologous fat injection. At the preoperative appointment, a site for fat harvest is chosen. Acceptable sites include the abdomen, lateral thigh, and buttocks.

On the day of surgery, the area to receive fat augmentation is clearly marked and confirmed with the patient. The procedure may be carried out under local anesthesia, but I prefer the use of light conscious sedation and local anesthesia for enhanced patient comfort. The technique previously described for tumescent liposuction is followed for harvesting fat, with one exception. Research indicates that fat cell damage is reduced when lower vacuum pressures are used. In this case 0.5 atm of vacuum pressure is advocated for the harvest of fat to be re-injected. Once the fat is harvested, it is moved to a sterile back table for preparation. The area of harvest is cleaned, excess tumescent solution and debris are expressed, and the wound is closed. The area is then covered with a compressive garment.

At our institution fat to be injected is then processed through a centrifuge at 3400 rpm for 3 minutes to separate viable fat cells from damaged cells and blood products. Following processing, the undesired materials are decanted from the viable fat cells, which are then transferred to an injection syringe.

Fat is transferred into the desired tissue location with a 14-gauge injection cannula and a high-pressure injection device, as demonstrated in Figure 68-6. It is important to remember that the fat should be injected with two to three passes of the cannula in various planes. Theoretically, multiple passes provide an increased surface area for vascular ingrowth leading to increased graft volume survival. Figure 68-7 shows a patient receiving an autologous fat graft to the lips during a rhytidectomy procedure. The grafting cannula is then removed and the area cleaned. There is no need to suture closed the injection sites.

Dermal Fat Grafts

First introduced by Neuber in 1893,[18] dermal fat grafts are used for a variety of reconstructive and cosmetic techniques. In the maxillofacial region a variety of soft tissue deficit reconstructions have been performed using dermal fat grafts, including soft tissue enhancement of hemifacial atrophy patients, reconstruction following radical parotidectomy, repair of gunshot wounds, and various cosmetic augmentation procedures. Peer demonstrated less resorption in dermal fat grafts than with free fat grafting, although he still reported a 50% loss of weight and volume of the grafted fat at 1 year.[20] Research by Longacre and by Neumann,[31,32] who both used pedicled dermal fat grafts for reconstructive procedures, achieved excellent results

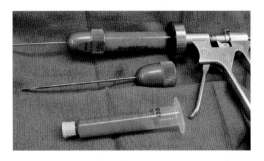

FIGURE **68-6**   *Autologous fat prepared for injection transfer. The high-pressure injection device is loaded with a 10 cc syringe of graft material. Two injection cannulas are available for use.*

with retention of fat and postulated that the pedicled blood supply accounted for the reduction in overall fat resorption. Although these grafts do provide a reliable result, they should only be selected for smaller defects of the maxillofacial region. For larger defects microvascular transfer of skin and muscle provides a more predictable and stable cosmetic result.

The technique for obtaining a dermal fat graft is well described. A site for harvesting the graft is selected that has thick but relatively hairless skin. Two techniques for accessing the dermis and fat are generally accepted. The first employs a split-thickness skin graft (0.036 to 0.041 cm), which is lifted to expose the underlying dermis. Sharp excision of the dermal fat graft with a knife is then performed. Care must be taken to ensure that the fat remains attached to the dermis. Figure 68-8 shows a dermal fat graft harvested for soft tissue reconstruction. Once the graft is removed, local hemorrhage is controlled, and the area is closed. The second newer technique involves de-epithelialization of the skin with a CO_2 laser. This technique is extremely helpful in managing a specific area, as in an island or a pedicled flap, and in facilitating an elliptic area of de-epithelialization to allow for straight-line closure. The CO_2 laser is set at 10 W of power with a 1 to 2 mm spot size, and the area to be de-epithelialized is then systematically lasered. When the area has been completed, the area is débrided with a wet sponge. Often, two or three passes with the laser are needed to completely de-epithelialize the area. Care must be taken to limit the thermal damage to the underlying dermis and fat. Once the de-epithelialization is completed, the dermis and fat are harvested with a knife, local hemorrhage is controlled, and the area is closed.

Complications

As with cervicofacial liposuction, the complications associated with the transfer of autologous fat are limited. Primarily, mis-

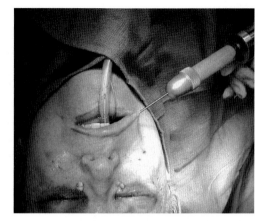

FIGURE **68-7**   *Injection of autologous fat grafts into the lip during a rhytidectomy procedure.*

placement of the graft, infection, and loss of significant graft volume are worthy of mention. Grafts are generally overcontoured to account for the loss of graft volume during the healing phase. Since the location of graft volume loss is difficult to predict, the potential for graft misplacement exists. Should residual fat remain in an area where it is not desired, the remaining graft may be removed by local suction lipectomy with a syringe and a small cannula. Infection of the graft site is possible if meticulous sterile technique is not followed. I advocate the use of prophylactic antibiotics for all patients undergoing autologous fat transfer. Finally, loss of significant fat volume may occur leading to patient dissatisfaction and irregular or unacceptable contour. Since fat-volume retention seems to be related to a number of variables, patients should be counseled concerning the potential need for multiple

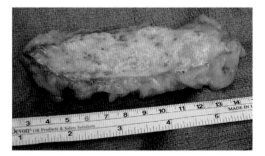

FIGURE **68-8**   *Example of a dermal fat graft harvested for soft tissue reconstruction.*

grafting procedures to achieve the final result. Our experience indicates that most patients achieve their expected results with two or three grafting procedures.

Summary

Liposculpting procedures of the cervicofacial region provide patients with a simple and predictable means for improving their facial esthetics. The procedures have been described in the scientific literature for over 100 years and have been performed safely by many oral and maxillofacial surgeons. Cervicofacial liposculpting techniques can also be used to enhance the results of orthognathic surgery and other more involved maxillofacial cosmetic surgery procedures. With the advent of the tumescent liposuction technique, small-diameter cannulas, and the syringe suction technique, the procedures are easily and safely performed in the modern oral and maxillofacial surgery office environment. Autologous fat-transfer techniques for facial reconstruction and maxillofacial esthetic surgery have also found a place in the contemporary oral and maxillofacial surgery practice.

The views expressed in this chapter are those of the author and do not represent the official policy or position of the Department of the Navy, Department of Defense, or US Government.

References

1. Fischer G. The evolution of liposculpture. Am J Cosmet Surg 1997;14:231–8.
2. Maliniak JW. Is the surgical restoration of the aged face justified? Med J Rec 1932;135:321–2.
3. Davis AD. Obligations in the consideration of myeloplasties. J Int Surg 1955;24:568–73.
4. Schrudde J. Lipexeresis in the correction of local adiposity. In: First Congress of International Society of Aesthetic Plastic Surgery. Rio de Janeiro; 1972.
5. Illouz YG. Body contouring by lipolysis: a 5-year experience with over 3000 cases. Plast Reconstr Surg 1983;72:591–7.
6. Fournier P. Chance and lipoextraction: thoughts and progress in lipoplasty (reduction and augmentation). Am J Cosmet Surg 1988;5:249–51.
7. Klein JA. The tumescent technique for liposuction surgery. Am J Cosmet Surg 1987;4:263–7.
8. Field LM. Adjunctive liposurgical debulking and flap dissection in neck reconstruction. J Dermatol Surg Oncol 1986;12:917–20.
9. Hallock GG. Liposuction for debulking free flaps. J Reconstr Microsurg 1986;2:235–9.
10. Newmann J, Nguyen A, Anderson R. Liposuction of the buccal fat pad. Am J Cosmet Surg 1986;3:1–9.
11. Teimourian B. Suction lipectomy of the face and neck. Facial Plast Surg 1986;4:35–41.
12. Courtiss EH. Suction lipectomy of the neck. Plast Reconstr Surg 1985;76:882–9.
13. Giampapa VC, DiBernardo BE. Neck recontouring with suture suspension and liposuction: an alternative for the early rhytidectomy candidate. Aesthetic Plast Surg 1995;19:217–23.
14. American Academy of Cosmetic Surgery. 1997 guidelines for liposuction surgery. Am J Cosmet Surg 1997;14:387–95.
15. Newman J, Dolsky RL. Evaluation of 5,458 cases of liposuction surgery. Am J Cosmet Surg 1984;1:25–34.
16. Fournier PF, Otteni FM. Lipodissection in body sculpting: the dry procedure. Plast Reconstr Surg 1983;72:598–609.
17. Newman J, Dolsky RL, Mai ST. Submental liposuction extraction with hard chin augmentation. Arch Otolaryngol 1984;110:454–7.
18. Neuber F. Fat grafting. Chir Kongr Verh Dtsch Ges Chir 1893;22:66–71.
19. Verderame H. Uber Fett transplantation bei adharenten knochennarben am orbitalrand. Klin Monatshefte Augenheilkd 1909;47:433–7.
20. Peer LA. Loss of weight and volume in human fat grafts. Plast Reconstr Surg 1950;5:217–30.
21. Peer LA. The neglected free fat graft. Plast Reconstr Surg 1956;18:233–50.
22. Illouz YG. The fat cell "graft": a new technique to fill depressions. Plast Reconstr Surg 1986;78:122–3.
23. Bircoll M, Novak BH. Autologous fat transplantation employing liposuction techniques. Ann Plast Surg 1987;18:327–9.
24. Chajchir A, Benzaquen I. Fat-grafting injection for soft tissue augmentation. Plast Reconstr Surg 1989;12:921–34.
25. Teimourian B. Repair of soft-tissue contour deficit by means of semiliquid fat graft. Plast Reconstr Surg 1986;78:123–4.
26. Carpaneda CA. Study of aspirated adipose tissue. Aesthetic Plast Surg 1996;20:399–402.
27. Campbell GL, Laudenslager N, Newman J. The effect of mechanical stress on adipocyte morphology and metabolism. Am J Cosmet Surg 1987;4:89–97.
28. Fulton JE. Stabilization of fat transfer to the breast with autologous platelet gel. Int J Cosmet Surg 1999;7:6. 273–9.
29. Har-Shai Y, Lindenbaum ES, Gamliel-Lazarovich A, et al. An integrated approach for increasing the survival of autologous fat grafts in the treatment of contour defects. Plast Reconstr Surg 1999;104:945–54.
30. Kaminski MV Jr, Wolosewick JJ, Smith J. Preservation of interstitial colloid: a critical factor in fat transfer. Oral Maxillofac Surg Clin North Am 2000;12:4. 631–9
31. Longacre JJ. Use of local pedicle flaps for reconstruction of breast after subtotal or total mastectomy. Plast Reconstr Surg 1953;11:380–403.
32. Neumann CG. The use of large buried pedicled flaps of dermis and fat, clinical and pathological evaluation of hemiatrophy. Plast Reconstr Surg 1953;11:315–32.

Appendix A

INFORMED CONSENT FOR SUCTION-ASSISTED LIPECTOMY (SURGICAL AND SUCTION-ASSISTED FAT REDUCTION)*

I hereby authorize Dr. _____ and staff to perform the following procedure:

_____

_____

and to administer the anesthetic I have chosen, which is ( ) local anesthetic, ( ) intravenous sedation, ( ) or general anesthetic.

Other treatment options: _____

Please initial each paragraph after reading. If you have any questions, please ask your doctor *before* initialing.

Liposuction

I hereby acknowledge that the following has been explained to me and that I have had an opportunity to ask questions.

_____ 1. Suction-assisted lipectomy is the technique to remove a localized collection of fat beneath the skin.

_____ 2. I understand the purpose of the surgery is to treat and attempt to correct the appearance of localized areas on my body.

_____ 3. I have been completely candid and honest with my surgeon regarding my motivation for undergoing a lipectomy, realizing that a new appearance does not guarantee an improved life.

_____ 4. I understand that if I am an active smoker I must cease smoking at least 2 weeks prior to surgery. Failure to follow this instruction can have dramatic effects on the success of the surgery.

_____ 5. It has been explained to me that suction-assisted lipectomy is not a substitute for weight reduction that can ordinarily be obtained by dieting and exercise and that it is not a cure for obesity. It is a surgical technique suitable for selected patients.

_____ 6. I hereby acknowledge that I have attempted to accurately provide Dr. _____ and/or his staff with an accurate medical history, realizing that withholding certain information may adversely affect my diagnosis and the final result of the surgery.

_____ 7. It has been explained to me that my physical condition may require surgical lipectomy, in which excess skin and fat may be removed instead of or in addition to suction-assisted lipectomy.

Surgical Considerations

_____ 1. The technique of liposuction has been explained to me. I have been told that suction-assisted lipectomy may be performed under local anesthesia or, in selected cases, with the use of intravenous sedation or a general anesthetic. The procedure begins with small incisions approximately 1 cm long. The doctor will then insert a blunt-ended tubular instrument (catheter) into the area of the incision and then, using suction, extract the deposits of fat. I have been advised that additional incisions may be necessary to gain adequate access to all areas of unwanted fat deposits.

Postoperative Considerations

_____ 1. The incisions will be closed with small sutures. Generally, the scars are small. However, I have been advised that in some cases scarring may be unpredictable and a second procedure may be required to reduce the scarring.

_____ 2. Following the surgery I have been told that a snug dressing of elastic gauze may be applied to the entire area to help the skin conform smoothly to the shape of the underlying tissue. This pressure-type bandage is generally worn for about 2 weeks. Some bruising and swelling may persist for several weeks after the operation. Some postoperative pain can be expected, and medication will be prescribed to provide some relief.

_____ 3. I have been advised and acknowledge that there is no guarantee that the procedure will improve my appearance. Patients react differently depending upon age and health. Some individuals have less skin elasticity and may require additional procedures to remove or tighten excess skin. Further, some people have skin that tends to wrinkle more than do others. To assist in healing, strenuous physical activity such as aerobics or physical labor must be avoided during the first week postoperatively.

Risks and Complications

Dr. _____ has explained to me there are certain inherent and potential risks in any treatment plan or procedure and that, in this specific instance, such operative risks include but are not limited to the following:

_____ 1. There is a possibility that a second surgery/procedure will need to be performed in the event the doctor encounters an abundance of excess fat.

_____ 2. Ordinarily, liposuction of the face and neck does not require blood transfusions. However, all patients respond differently. I have been told that there is a possibility that a blood transfusion will be performed, and I have been advised of my rights regarding autologous blood (self and family transfusions).

_____ 3. The surgery will involve areas of certain cranial or facial nerves. Damage to the nerves can result in numbness, which is usually temporary. However, in rare cases the numbness can be permanent. Additionally, there is a risk of damage to nerves that affect motor function. For example, there may be an inability to purse the lips. The condition is usually temporary; however, in rare conditions it can be permanent.

_____ 4. It is possible that after fat removal the overlying skin will not be smooth; rather, it may have a "washboard" appearance. A second liposuction procedure or other cosmetic surgery may be necessary to correct this condition.

_____ 5. In the event that fat is to be removed from the cheek area, I have been advised that a change in facial tone occurs in some cases. The condition is usually temporary; however, on rare occasions this condition can be permanent.

(CONTINUED ON NEXT PAGE)

_____ 6. Any surgery involves the risk of infection requiring antibiotic treatment. Most cases resolve without complication; however, in rare situations treatment of a serious infection may require hospitalization.

_____ 7. There is a possibility of localized collections of blood in areas of fat removal. Secondary procedures to remove the blood may be required.

Anesthesia

In the event that I am to receive intravenous or general anesthesia, I understand and agree that I am not to have had and/or have not had anything to eat or drink for 8 hours before my surgery. *FAILURE TO FOLLOW THIS INSTRUCTION MAY BE LIFE THREATENING!*

_____ 1. I consent to the administration of ( ) local anesthetic, ( ) intravenous sedation, or ( ) general anesthetic, having first had the risks and benefits of each explained to me.

_____ 2. I have been made aware that certain medications, drugs, anesthetics, and prescriptions that I may be given can cause drowsiness, incoordination, and a lack of awareness, which may be worsened by the use of alcohol and other drugs. I have been advised not to operate any vehicle or hazardous machinery and not to return to work while taking such medications, or until I am fully recovered from the effects of the same. I understand this recovery may take up to 24 hours or more after I have taken the last dose of medications. If I am given sedative medication during my surgery, I agree to have a responsible adult drive me home and accompany me until I am fully recovered from the effects of the sedation.

_____ 3. I understand that certain anesthetics can cause bodily injury and death.

No Guarantee of Treatment Results

_____ 1. No guarantee or assurance has been given to me that the proposed treatment will be curative and/or successful to my complete satisfaction. Owing to individual patient differences, there may exist a risk of failure or relapse, my condition may worsen, or selective re-treatment may be required in spite of care provided.

_____ 2. I have had an opportunity to discuss with Dr. _____ my past medical and health history including any serious problems and/or injuries and have fully informed him of the same.

_____ 3. I agree to cooperate fully with the recommendations of Dr. _____ while I am under his care, realizing that any lack of such cooperation can result in less-than-optimal results or may be life threatening.

_____ 4. If any unforeseen condition should arise in the procedure of the operation calling for the doctor's judgment regarding procedures in addition to or different from those now contemplated, I request and authorize the doctor to provide the appropriate service.

Miscellaneous

_____ 1. I request the disposal by authorities of this medical facility of any tissues or parts that it may be necessary to remove.

_____ 2. I understand that photographs and movies may be taken of this operation and that they may be viewed by various personnel undergoing training or indoctrination at this or other facilities. I consent to the taking of such pictures and observation of the operation by authorized personnel, subject to the following conditions:

A. My name and my family's name are not to be used to identify said pictures.

B. Said pictures are to be used only for purposes of medical/dental study or research.

For Female Patients

I have advised Dr. _____ as to whether I am currently using birth control pills. I have been advised and informed that certain antibiotics and some pain medications may neutralize the therapeutic effect of birth control pills allowing for conception and resulting in pregnancy. I agree to consult with my family physician to initiate additional forms of mechanical birth control during the period of my treatment with Dr. _____ and until I am advised by my physician that I can return to using birth control pills exclusively.

I have had an opportunity to have my questions answered, and I certify that I understand the English language.

_____

Patient's (or legal guardian's) signature   Date/Time

_____

Witness's signature   Date

Counseling Physician/Dentist: I have counseled this patient as to the nature of the proposed procedure(s), attendant risks involved, and expected results, as described above.

_____

Counseling physician/dentist's signature

Adapted from a form by the Oral and Maxillofacial Surgery Clinic, Naval Medical Center, San Diego, CA.

Appendix B

POSTOPERATIVE INSTRUCTIONS FOR FACIAL LIPOSUCTION*

Please read your instructions carefully and call us if you have any questions.
Swelling and a large amount of discoloration are normal following liposuction surgery.
The following instructions are designed to help you minimize discomfort after surgery.

Position
Elevate your head and back using several pillows or use a recliner chair with the head at a 45° angle. It is important that you do so for *1 to 2 days* after your surgery. Lay on your back, rather than on your side or stomach.

Ice
Ice may be used over the surgical area for the first *24 hours* around the clock, as directed (leaving it off for eating and performing hygiene).

Activity
During your *first day* after surgery, stay up as much as possible. You should sit, stand, or walk around rather than remain in bed. However, you should rest when you become tired. Avoid bending or lifting more than 2.5 kg during the first week. You may do *passive exercises only!* Stay away from any activity that raises the pressure in your face for *2 weeks* as excessive pressure may cause a severe bleed. Avoid excessive talking and extreme facial movements (which may increase bleeding/bruising).

Diet
- Day of surgery, postoperatively: Start with clear cool fluids when these are tolerated, advance to warm *(not hot!)* fluids and very soft foods only, such as soups, dairy products, and applesauce.
- From the second day after surgery until your next office visit: Eat warm soft foods or cool foods—foods that do not require a lot of chewing. Also, make sure you are drinking lots of fluids during your postoperative recovery, at least eight 250 mL glasses a day for about 3 weeks. *This is very important!*
- One week after surgery: Resume your regular diet.

Medication
Pain medication: Take one dose when you arrive at home, then as needed every *4 to 6 hours* for discomfort or pain.
Caution: Do not drive or operate dangerous machinery while taking narcotic pain medication. Do not drink alcohol while taking pain medication or antibiotics.

Heat
Begin using moist heat on the second postoperative day. A moist towel should be placed between the skin and the heat source. Do not use heat continuously, only for *20 minutes four times per day* for a *2-week period*.

Sun Exposure
Protect the facial skin from excessive sun exposure for 1 month after surgery. Use a sunblock that is SPF 15 or higher. Wear a hat.

Sports
Do not participate in swimming, gym activities, or strenuous activities for *1 week*. Do not dive or ski for *2 months*. Passive exercise such as walking is permitted.

Acetylsalicylic Acid
The use of acetylsalicylic acid (Aspirin or medications containing ASA) should be avoided for *10 days* prior to surgery. Take acetaminophen (Tylenol) for headaches and minor pain.

Smoking
Smoking should be stopped at least *2 weeks* prior to surgery. Smoking impairs circulation, and good circulation is needed for proper healing. An adequate blood supply leads to a good surgical result for you.

Bruising/Swelling
Bruising and swelling are to be expected. Bruising is usually gone in 7 to 10 days. The swelling takes a while longer to subside.

Bleeding
If the dressing or elastic support is quite bloodstained, this should be reported to the doctor *immediately!*

Dressings
A compression dressing must be worn continuously for 1 week; it may be removed for short periods of time and then reapplied. Leave this on *24 hours a day for the first week,* and then mainly wear the support dressing at night.

Bathing
You may bathe in the tub or shower, and shampoo your hair during the *first day* after surgery. Use mild soaps and shampoos to avoid irritation.

Shaving
Resume shaving when swelling subsides and the area is not too tender.

Care of Your Incisions
Supplies needed: bacitracin ointment, 1/2 oz; cotton-tip applicators (eg, Q-Tips)
1. Use cotton-tip applicators and warm water to clean all blood and material from the cuts. *Do not* leave any crusts or blood on the stitched areas. Repeat a minimum of four to five times per day.
2. Cover *all* cuts and abrasions with ointment—do not allow *any* areas to dry out or scab over.
3. Do not apply any bandages or other materials to the surgical area unless otherwise instructed.

Follow-Up Appointments
Please check off postoperative appointments as they are kept:
1 to 2 days _____ 5 days _____ 2 weeks _____
2 months _____ 6 months _____

Final Note
Faithful adherence to the preoperative and postoperative instructions will not only help to minimize swelling, pain, and discomfort, but will also aid in achieving an excellent surgical result. If you do have problems, don't hesitate to contact our office for assistance.

Please report any of the following to our office:
- Excessive bleeding
- Sudden swelling
- Any itching, rash, or reaction to any of the medications
- Temperature above 101°F (38.3°C) (taken orally)

Adapted from a form by the Oral and Maxillofacial Surgery Clinic, Naval Medical Center, San Diego, CA.

CHAPTER 69

Skin Rejuvenation Procedures

Gary D. Monheit, MD

The pursuit of youth and beauty has become a hallmark of the baby-boomer generation, which has now advanced to midlife and beyond. The distinct increase in an older population due to newer medical and technological advancements and career development has brought a larger healthy population interested in cosmetic procedures. This mid-age population has remained active in the workforce and now demands "no downtime" procedures for skin rejuvenation that will maintain their appearance for work and pleasure. This has encouraged the development of new lasers, new fillers, botulinum toxin, cosmoceuticals, and many other innovations that have reduced the downtime and increased the safety of our cosmetic facial rejuvenation procedures. Anyone interested in providing facial cosmetic procedures and surgery needs to become familiar with all the procedures now available.

Aging of the skin is the combined result of both intrinsic factors and extrinsic external influences from the environment. Intrinsic aging is the roles that genetics plays in relation to chronologic age. These include alteration of skeletal mass and proportion, atrophy and redistribution of subcutaneous fat, increased laxity of underlying fascia and musculature, and skin changes characterized by thinning and atrophy. Most intrinsic factors cannot be prevented, but rejuvenative changes can be made with cosmoceutical agents and resurfacing procedures.

Extrinsic factors are preventable environmental influences leading to premature aging of the skin, including ultraviolet (UV) exposure, smoking, chemicals, and gravity. UV exposure is the primary environmental factor, preferentially affecting those with a lighter skin color. The mechanism includes the production of UV-inducing oxygenated fine radiants that have been shown to invite a cascade of molecular events leading to the production of collagen-degrading enzymes. This creates the characteristic features of photoaging, including rough texture, atrophy, fine and coarse wrinkles, and sallow and leathery appearance with dyschromia.[1]

In the evaluation of the patient with photoaging, equal emphasis must be placed on prevention as well as treatment. Agents available range from cosmoceutical topical agents to filling agents that include resurfacing devices such as chemical peels, ablative resurfacing lasers, and dermabrasion. An initial consultation is performed to determine which of these tools is best for the patient based on severity and diversity of the condition.

Methods to evaluate photoaging include the Glogau classification of wrinkles. It classifies patients into one of four groups based on degree of severity (Table 69-1). Category I patients are young, with "no wrinkles" and minimal photoaging and are best managed with cosmoceutical agents and superficial resurfacing procedures such as light chemical peels and microdermabrasion. Category II patients are in their thirties, with early to moderate signs of photoaging and characterized by wrinkles in motion. Category III patients have moderate to advanced photoaging with static wrinkles requiring more significant ablative resurfacing techniques. Category IV patients are the oldest, with more severe photoaging changes and wrinkles

Table 69-1　Glogau's Classification of Photoaging
Group I: Mild (typically age 28–35 years) 　A. Little wrinkling or scarring 　B. No keratoses 　C. Requires little or no makeup
Group II: Moderate (age 35–50 years) 　A. Early wrinkling; mild scarring 　B. Sallow color with early actinic 　　keratoses 　C. Little makeup
Group III: Advanced (age 50–65 years) 　A. Persistent wrinkling or moderate 　　acne scarring 　B. Discoloration with telangiectasias 　　and actinic keratoses 　C. Wears makeup always
Group IV: Severe (age 60–75 years) 　A. Wrinkling: photoaging, gravitational, 　　and dynamic 　B. Actinic keratoses with or without 　　skin cancer or severe acne scars 　C. Wears makeup with poor coverage

significant enough to justify deep resurfacing and other surgical techniques.[2]

Ablative resurfacing injures the skin in a controlled fashion to a specific depth, encouraging the growth of new and improved skin. These methods include chemical peeling, dermabrasion, and laser resurfacing. Skin resurfacing techniques are divided into superficial, medium depth, and deep, relating to the level of injury (Figure 69-1). The deeper procedures are restricted to the face since other body areas do not have the healing capacity to rejuvenate new skin after such an injury. Care must also be taken with the neck, which may scar with medium-depth or deep injury.[3]

Table 69-2 presents a useful classification system for categorizing skin resurfacing methods. It is based on the objective data collected by Stegman, who correlated strengths of trichloroacetic acid (TCA) by biopsy of depth of tissue destruction and then new collagen rejuvenation.[4] Thus superficial, medium depth, and deep resurfacing correlates modalities of peeling, dermabrasion, and laser to common denominators; namely, inflammation and injury.[4]

A useful method of assessing skin-related photoaging is the Monheit-Fulton index (Table 69-3). This system categorizes the visual changes in photoaging skin and quantitates the amount to guide the physician with appropriate therapy. The system combines age-related textural and lesional changes into a numeric system that will predict how aggressive a physician should be in using superficial, medium-depth, and deep resurfacing procedures.[5]

Medical Care of Photoaging Skin

The basis of all rejuvenative therapy involves using sunscreen protection and cosmoceutical preparations that will help reverse photoaging changes. These products include sunscreens, retinoids, hydroxy acids, antioxidants, and bleaching agents as needed.

Ultraviolet damage is caused by both UVB (290 to 320 nm) and UVA (320 to 400 nm). Both the burning rays of UVB and the more deeply penetrant UVA cause problems of photocarcinogenesis and photoaging of the dermis. Most sunscreens provide adequate protection against the burning effects of UVB but deliver only partial protection against UVA. Sunscreens are divided into chemical and physical blockers. The chemical

Table 69-2   Classification of Ablative Skin Resurfacing Methods*
Superficial: Very Light[†]
Low-potency formulations of glycolic acid or other alpha-hydroxy acid
10–20% TCA (weight-to-volume formulation)
Jessner's solution (see Table 69-3)
Tretinoin
Salicylic acid
Microdermabrasion
Superficial: Light[†]
70% glycolic acid
Jessner's solution
25–30% TCA
Solid CO_2 slush
Microdermabrasion
Medium-Depth
88% phenol
35–40% TCA
Jessner's–35% TCA
70% glycolic acid–35% TCA
Solid CO_2–35% TCA
Conservative manual dermasanding
Erbium:YAG laser resurfacing
Conservative CO_2 laser resurfacing
Deep
Unoccluded or occluded Baker-Gordon phenol peel
TCA in concentrations > 50%
Wire brush or diamond fraise dermabrasion
Aggressive manual dermasanding
Manual dermasanding or motorized dermabrasion after a medium-depth peel
Aggressive erbium:YAG laser resurfacing
CO_2 laser resurfacing
Combination erbium:YAG/CO_2 laser resurfacing

CO_2 = carbon dioxide; TCA = trichloroacetic acid; YAG = yttrium-aluminum-garnet.
*Although this classification represents an oversimplification, because the depth of injury actually varies somewhat along a continuum for each different type of resurfacing procedure, it is helpful when discussing the various options with a patient.
[†]Techniques for ablative laser resurfacing of superficial depth have been developed but are probably impractical.

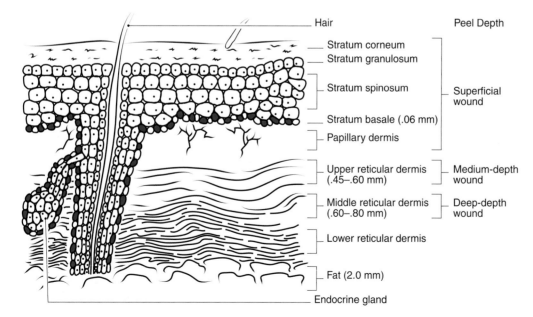

FIGURE **69-1**   *Cross-section of skin with superficial, medium, and deep wound areas.*

Table 69-3   Monheit-Fulton Index of Photoaging Skin

Texture Changes	Points				Score
Wrinkles—dynamic	1	2	3	4	____
(% of potential lines)	< 25%	< 50%	< 75%	< 100%	
Wrinkles—photoaging	1	2	3	4	____
(% of potential lines)	< 25%	< 50%	< 75%	< 100%	
Cross-hatched lines—fine lines	1	2	3	4	____
(% of potential lines)	< 10%	< 20%	< 40%	< 60%	
Sallow color and dyschromia	1	2	3	4	____
	Dull	Yellow	Brown	Black	
Leathery appearance	1	2	3	4	____
Crinkly (thin and parchment)	1	2	3	4	____
Pebbly (deep whitish nodules)	2	4	6	8	____
(% of face)	< 25%	< 50%	< 75%	< 100%	
Pore no. and size	2	4	6	8	____
	< 25%	< 50%	< 75%	< 100%	

Lesions	Points				Score
Freckles—mottled skin	1	2	3	4	____
(no. present)	< 10	< 25	< 50	< 100	
Lentigenes (dark/irregular)	2	4	6	8	____
and SKs (size)	< 5 mm	< 10 mm	< 15 mm	< 20 mm	
Telangiectasias—erythema	1	2	3	4	____
flush (no. present)	< 5	< 10	< 15	> 15	
Actinic keratoses and	2	4	6	8	____
seborrheic keratoses	< 5	< 10	< 15	> 15	
(no. present)					
Skin cancers (no. present—	2	4	6	8	____
now or by history)	1 ca	2 ca	3 ca	> 4 ca	
Senile comedones	1	2	3	4	____
(in cheekbone area)	< 5	< 10	< 20	> 20	

Total Score					____

Corresponding Rejuvenation Program

Score	Needs
1–6	Skin-care program with tretinoin, glycolic acid peels
7–11	Same plus Jessner's peel; pigmented lesion laser and/or vascular laser
12–16	Same plus medium peel—Jessner's–TCA peel; skin fillers and/or botulinum toxin
17 or more	Above plus laser resurfacing

Staff Signature	Date		Patient Signature	Date

screens include oxybenzene, para-aminobenzoic acid, and octyl methoxycinnamate. The physical blockers nowadays are transparent micronized formulations of titanium dioxide and afford more complete UVA and UVB protection.[6]

Topical retinoids have a direct effect on epidermal cell proliferation and dermal collagen growth. They have demonstrated significant effects on photoaging skin including dyschromias, epidermal growths, and fine wrinkle lines. The Federal Drug Administration has approved topical retinoids for the treatment of aging and photodamaged skin in the form of tretinoin cream (0.05% or 0.02%) and most recently tazarotene cream 0.1%. Use of a retinoid with a sunscreen is basic in skin care for photoaging skin problems. It is also used prior to resurfacing procedures to enhance the epidermal and dermal regenerative effect after resurfacing injury.[7]

Hydroxy acids have become a part of skin care programs for their effect on thinning the stratum corneum and decreasing epidermal cell cohesion. This has a regenerative effect on epidermal cell kinetics, giving the skin texture a plumper rejuvenative appearance. There is little definitive evidence that topical alpha-hydroxy acids have an effect on dermal collagen per se.[8]

Topical antioxidants have shown an effect in retarding the reactive oxygen species created by ultraviolet damage. Vitamin C (ascorbic acid) has been shown to be a potent scavenger of free oxygen radials. Topical products have shown activity in the experimental mode but clinical efficacy as of yet is anecdotal. Vitamin E is a lipid-soluble antioxidant that has become popular in topical form, but little true objective data are present to document its effect on photoaging skin.[9]

Chemical Peeling

Chemical peeling remains one of the most popular choices for both patient and physician. In comparison to some of the newer options available, chemical peels have a long-standing safety and efficacy record, are performed with ease, are low in cost, and have a relatively quick recovery time. Various acidic and basic compounds are used to produce a controlled skin injury and are classified as superficial, medium-depth, and deep peeling agents according to their level of penetration, destruction, and inflammation (see Table 69-2). In general superficial peels cause epidermal injury and occasionally extend into the papillary dermis, medium-depth peels cause injury through the papillary dermis to the upper reticular dermis, and deep peels cause injury to the midreticular dermis.[4]

Prior to the application of peeling solutions the surgeon must vigorously cleanse the skin surface to remove residual oils, debris, and excess stratum corneum. The face is initially scrubbed with 4" × 4" gauze pads containing 0.25% Irgasan (Septisol solution; Calgon Vestal Laboratories, St. Louis, MO, USA), then rinsed with water and dried. Because of the defatting and degreasing properties of acetone, gauze pads moistened in an acetone preparation are then used to cleanse the skin even further. The importance of cleansing in the peeling procedure cannot be overemphasized. A thorough and evenly distributed cleansing and degreasing of the face assures uniform penetration of the peeling solution and leads to an even result without skip areas (Figure 69-2).[10]

The effect of a chemical peel is dependent upon the agent used, its concentration, and the techniques employed before and during its application. Each wounding agent used in peels has unique chemical properties and causes a specific pattern of injury to the skin.[3] It is important for the physician using these solutions to be familiar with their cutaneous effects and proper methods of application to ensure correct depth of injury. The marketplace has been flooded with numerous proprietary formulations of these peeling agents, with each product claiming

unique advantages. These products are often expensive and have not been unequivocally shown to be safer or more effective than the conventional solutions. The following sections will therefore focus on the specific chemical agents that are actively responsible for producing the various patterns of injury.

Superficial Chemical Peeling

Superficial chemical peels are indicated in the management of acne and its postinflammatory erythema, mild photoaging (Glogau I and II), epidermal growths such as lentigines and keratoses, as well as melasma and other pigmentary dyschromias. Multiple peels on a repeated basis are usually necessary to obtain optimal results. The frequency of peels and degree of exposure to the peeling agent may be increased gradually as necessary. Results are enhanced by medical or cosmoceutical therapy.[11] All superficial chemical peels share the advantages of only mild stinging and burning during application as well as minimal time needed for recovery. They are a part of office-based procedures.[12]

Superficial chemical peels are divided into two varieties; very light and light (see Table 69-2). With very light peels the injury is usually limited to the stratum corneum and only creates exfoliation, but the injury may extend into the stratum granulosum. The agents used for these peels include low potency formulations of glycolic acid, 10 to 20% TCA, Jessner's solution (Table 69-4), tretinoin, and salicylic acid. Light peels injure the entire epidermis down to the basal layer, stimulating the regeneration of a fresh new epithelium. Agents used for light peels include 70% glycolic acid, 25 to 35% TCA, Jessner's solution, and solid carbon dioxide (CO_2) slush.[13] During the application of superficial peeling agents, there may be mild stinging followed by a level I frosting, defined as the appearance of erythema and streaky whitening on the surface (Figure 69-3).

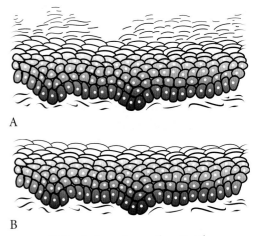

FIGURE 69-2 A, *Irregular surface.* B, *Clean regular surface.*

Alpha-hydroxy acid (AHA) peeling agents have been used widely in skin rejuvenation programs since the early 1990s. The depth of injury is determined by the specific AHA used, its pH, the concentration of free acid, the volume applied to the skin, and the duration of contact or time that the agent is left on the skin before neutralization.[8] In low concentrations (20 to 30%), AHAs have been shown to decrease the cohesion of corneocytes at the junction of the stratum corneum and the stratum granulosum, whereas higher concentrations (up to 70%) are associated with complete epidermolysis. Weekly or biweekly applications of 40 to 70% unbuffered glycolic acid with cotton swabs, a sable brush, or 2" × 2" gauze pads have been used most often for acne, mild photoaging, and melasma.[8] The time of application is critical for glycolic acid, as it must be rinsed off with water or neutralized with 5% sodium bicarbonate after 2 to 4 minutes.

Application of 10 to 20% TCA with either a saturated 2" × 2" gauze pad or

Table 69-4 Jessner's Solution (Combes' Formula)
Resorcinol, 14 g
Salicylic acid, 14 g
85% lactic acid, 14 g
95% ethanol (q.s.a.d.), 100 mL
q.s.a.d. = quantum satis ad ("up to sufficient quantity").

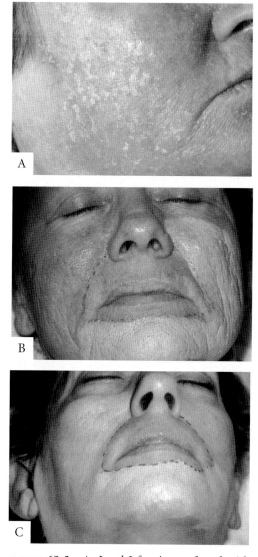

FIGURE **69-3** A, *Level I frosting as found with light chemical peeling; erythema with streaky frosting.* B, *Level II—erythema with diffuse white frosting.* C, *Level III—solid white enamel frosting.*

sable brush produces erythema and a very light frost within 15 to 45 seconds. The depth of penetration of the peeling solution is related to the number of coats applied; thus, deeper penetration and injury can occur with overcoating. Ideally, a level I frosting is obtained with superficial TCA peels. Protein precipitation results and leads to exfoliation without vesiculation. Concentrations of TCA up to 35% can also be used alone as a superficial peeling agent but may create an injury that extends partially into the upper dermis.[13]

Jessner's solution is a combination of keratolytic ingredients that have been used for over 100 years in the treatment of inflammatory and comedonal acne as well as hyperkeratotic skin disorders (see Table 69-4). Jessner's solution has intense keratolytic activity, initially causing loss of corneocyte cohesion within the stratum corneum and subsequently creating intercellular and intracellular edema within the upper epidermis if application is continued.[14] The mode of application for the Jessner's peel is similar to that of the 10 to 20% TCA peel. The clinical end point of treatment is erythema and blotchy frosting. It is a good repetitive peel for photoaging skin because of its inflammatory effects. The peel can be repeated every 2 weeks.

Salicylic acid, a beta-hydroxy acid that is one of the ingredients in Jessner's solution, can also be used alone in superficial chemical peeling.[15] It is a preferred therapy for comedonal acne as it is lipophilic and concentrates in the pilosebaceous apparatus. It is quite effective as an adjunctive therapy for open and closed comedones and resolving post-acne erythema (Figure 69-4). It is also a peel of choice for melasma and pigmentary dyschromia because it has minimal inflammatory action. Used repeatedly it has the least risk of postinflammatory hyperpigmentation. Superficial peeling for abnormal pigmentation is combined with skin care and topical retinoids, a bleaching product (hydroquinone, including 4 to 8%), and an adequate sunscreen.[16]

Prior to the initial treatment with a superficial peel, both patient and physician must understand the limitations, especially on photoaging, to avoid future disappointment. The effect of repetitive superficial chemical peels never approaches the beneficial effect obtained with a single medium-depth or deep peel, in that the improvements in photoaged skin following superficial peels are usually subtle because there is little to no effect on the

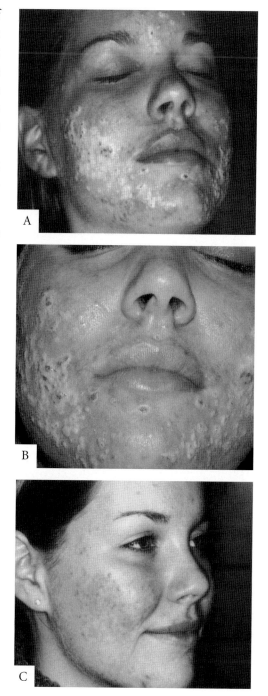

FIGURE **69-4** *Salicylic acid peels are effective for the treatment of acne and comedones. Repetitive treatment over 6 weeks with acne treatment will hasten resolution of the condition.* A, *Pretreatment, active acne.* B, *Perifollicular frosting seen with salicylic acid, a lipophilic chemical.* C, *Posttreatment result 6 weeks later.*

dermis. Nevertheless their ease of use and minimal downtime makes these "lunchtime" peels rewarding for patients with realistic expectations and are a favorite among the busy baby boomers.

Medium-Depth Chemical Peeling

Medium-depth chemical peels consist of controlled damage through the epidermis and papillary dermis, with variable extension to the upper reticular dermis. During the 3 months postoperatively, there is increased collagen production with expansion of the papillary dermis and the development of a mid-dermal band of thick elastic-staining fibers.[4] These changes correlate with continued clinical improvement during this time.

For many years 40 to 50% TCA was the prototypical medium-depth peeling agent because of its ability to ameliorate fine wrinkles, actinic changes, and preneoplasia. TCA as a single agent for medium-depth peeling has fallen out of favor because of the high risk of complications, especially scarring and pigmentary alterations, when used in strengths approaching 50% and higher.[17] Today most medium-depth chemical peels are performed using 35% TCA in combination with either Jessner's solution, 70% glycolic acid, or solid CO_2 as a "priming" agent (Table 69-5). These combination peels have been found to be as effective as 50% TCA alone but with fewer risks. The level of penetration is better controlled with these combination peels, thereby avoiding scarring seen with higher concentrations of TCA.

Brody developed the use of solid CO_2 to freeze the skin prior to the application of 35% TCA.[18] This causes complete epidermal necrosis and significant dermal edema, thereby allowing deeper penetration of the TCA in selected areas.[10] Monheit then described a combination medium-depth peel in which Jessner's solution is applied, followed by 35% TCA.[14] Similarly, Coleman and Futrell have demonstrated the use of 70% glycolic acid prior to the application of 35% TCA for medium-depth peeling.[19] Jessner's solution and glycolic acid both appear to effectively weaken the epidermal barrier and allow deeper, more uniform, and more controlled penetration of the 35% TCA.

Current indications for medium-depth chemical peeling include Glogau level II or moderate photoaging, epidermal lesions such as actinic keratoses, pigmentary dyschromias, and mild acne scarring, as well as blending of the effects of deeper resurfacing procedures. The most popular of the medium-depth peels for facial rejuvenation is the Jessner's–35% TCA peel, with other combination peels being used less frequently. This peel has been widely accepted because of its broad range of uses, the large number of people in whom it is indicated, its ease of modification according to the situation, and its excellent safety profile. It is not a "lunchtime" treatment, however, and should be considered a surgical procedure requiring preoperative consideration and preparation, operative sedation, and aftercare for 1 week or more.

The Jessner's–35% TCA peel is particularly useful for the improvement of mild to moderate photoaging. (Figure 69-5). It freshens sallow atrophic skin and softens fine rhytids with minimal risk of textural or pigmentary complications (see Figure 69-5). Collagen remodeling occurs for as long as 3 to 4 months postoperatively, during which there is continued improvement in texture and rhytids. When used in conjunction with a retinoid, bleaching agent, and sunscreens, a single Jessner's–35% TCA peel lessens pigmentary dyschromias and lentigines more effectively than do repetitive superficial peels (Figure 69-6). Epidermal growths such as actinic keratoses also respond well to this peel. In fact the Jessner's–35% TCA peel has been found to be as effective as topical 5-fluorouracil chemotherapy in removing both grossly visible and clinically undetectable actinic keratoses but has the added advantages of lower morbidity and greater improvement in associated photoaging (Figure 69-7).[20]

This peel is also useful to blend the effects of other resurfacing procedures with the surrounding skin. Patients who undergo laser resurfacing, deep chemical peeling, or dermabrasion to a localized area such as the periorbital or perioral region often develop a sharp line of demarcation between the treated and untreated skin. This is because the surrounding photoaging skin has significant dyschromia and textural aging. The treated skin may appear hypopigmented (also known as pseudohypopigmentation) in comparison to the untreated skin. A Jessner's–35% TCA peel performed on the adjacent untreated skin helps to blend the treated area into its surroundings. For example, a patient with advanced photoaging in the periorbital region and moderate photoaging on the remaining face may desire CO_2 laser resurfacing only around the eyes. In this patient, medium-depth chemical peeling of the areas not treated with the laser would improve the photoaging in these regions and avoid a line of demarcation.[21] It is important to note that when used in combination with other resurfacing procedures such as laser irradiation or dermabrasion, the peel should be performed first, in order to

Table 69-5 Agents Used for Medium-Depth Chemical Peeling	
Agent	*Comment*
40–50% TCA	Not recommended
Combination 35% TCA–solid CO_2 (Brody)	The most potent combination
Combination 35% TCA–Jessner's (Monheit)	The most popular combination
Combination 35% TCA–70% glycolic acid (Coleman)	An effective combination
88% phenol	Rarely used

CO_2 = carbon dioxide; TCA = trichloroacetic acid.

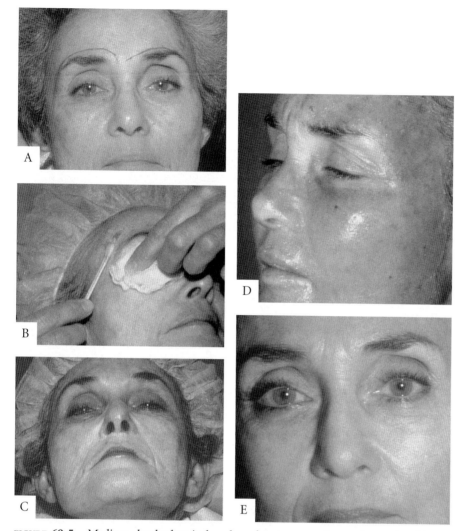

FIGURE **69-5** *Medium-depth chemical peel used to treat moderate photoaging skin. A, Preoperative photograph demonstrating epidermal growths with aging textural changes. B, Application of 35% trichloroacetic acid directly after Jessner's solution. C, White enamel frosting (level III) from 35% trichloroacetic acid. D, Desquamation and inflammation 4 days after peel. E, Final results 6 months later.*

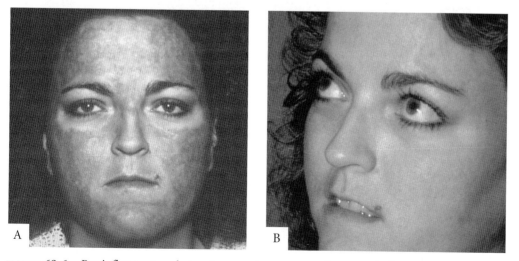

FIGURE **69-6** *Postinflammatory hyperpigmentation unresponsive to topical agents (hydroquinone and tretinoin) and superficial chemical peeling. Full response to medium-depth chemical peel and topical agents. A, Preoperative. B, Six weeks postoperative.*

avoid accidental application of the peeling agent onto previously abraded areas of skin (Figure 69-8).

Using either cotton-tipped applicators or 2″ × 2″ gauze pads, a single even coat of Jessner's solution is applied first to the forehead, followed by the cheeks, nose, and chin, and lastly, the eyelids. Proper application of Jessner's solution causes minimal discomfort and creates a faint frost within a background of mild erythema (level I). After a 1- to 2-minute wait for the Jessner's solution to completely dry, 35% TCA is then applied evenly with one to four cotton-tipped applicators (Figure 69-9). The effectiveness of this peel is directly dependent on the depth of penetration of the peeling solutions, and this depth is a function of the adequacy of degreasing and the amount of both solutions applied. The use of cotton swabs, particularly for the application of TCA, is advantageous because is allows the surgeon to easily vary the amount of solution applied according to the patient's specific needs. The amount of TCA delivered to the skin surface is determined by the number of applicators used, their degree of saturation, the amount of pressure applied to the skin surface, and the duration of their contact with the skin. Four moist cotton-tipped applicators are applied in broad strokes over the forehead and on the medial cheeks. Two mildly soaked cotton-tipped applicators can be used across the lips and chin, and one damp cotton-tipped applicator on the eyelids. The depth of penetration and completion of the peel reaction can be monitored by the level of frosting. A full combination Jessner's–35% TCA peel should obtain a level II to III frosting. One should never overcoat TCA on a level III frosting, as the injury may be pushed to a level that can cause complications (ie, pigmentation or scarring).

Anatomic areas of the face are peeled with TCA sequentially from the forehead to temple to cheeks and finally to the lips

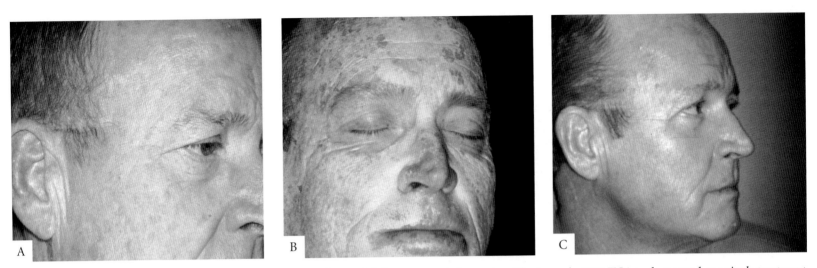

FIGURE **69-7**   *Medium-depth chemical peel for treatment of diffuse actinic keratoses and photoaging. The Jessner's–35% TCA peel was used as a single treatment, with healing in 8 days. A, Preoperative. B, Frosting after trichloroacetic acid. C, One month postoperative.*

and eyelids. Careful feathering of the solution into the hairline and around the rim of the jaw and brow conceals the demarcation line between peeled and nonpeeled skin. Areas of wrinkled skin are stretched taut with the help of an assistant to allow even application of the solution into the folds and troughs. This technique is particularly helpful on the skin of the upper and lower lips. For perioral rhytids, TCA is applied with the wood portion of a cotton-tipped applicator and extended onto the vermilion border (see Figure 69-9D).

Eyelid skin must be treated delicately and carefully to avoid overapplication and to prevent exposure of the eyes to TCA solution.[22] The patient should be positioned with the head elevated at 30 degrees, and excess peel solution on the cotton tip should be squeezed out so that the applicator is semidry. With the eyes closed a single applicator is rolled gently from the periorbital skin onto the upper eyelid skin without going beyond the moveable lid. Another semidry applicator is then rolled onto the lower eyelid skin within 2 to 3 mm of the lid margin while the patient is looking superiorly. Excess peel solution should never be left on the lids because it can roll into the eyes, and tears should be immediately dried with a cotton-tipped applicator

because they may pull the solution into the eye by capillary action.

The white frost from the TCA application appears on the treated area within 30 seconds to 2 minutes (see Figure 69-5C). This response is representative of keratocoagulation and indicates that the TCA's physiologic reaction is complete. TCA

takes longer to frost than phenol preparations but a shorter period of time than the superficial peeling agents. The desired end point in medium-depth peeling is level II to level III frosting (Table 69-6). Level II frosting is defined as a white-coated frosting with a background of erythema (see Figure 69-3B).

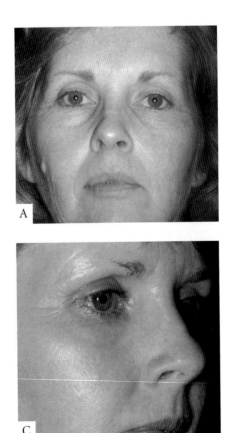

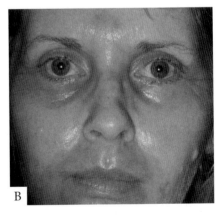

FIGURE **69-8**   *Combination procedure using perioral–periorbital carbon dioxide laser resurfacing with Jessner's–35% TCA peel over the remaining face. The peel will blend color and texture of the laser-treated areas. A, Preoperative: the eyelids and lips need deeper resurfacing than cheeks, which require only medium-depth injury. B, Four days postoperative: note the difference in rate of healing between laser- and peel-treated areas. C, One year postoperative.*

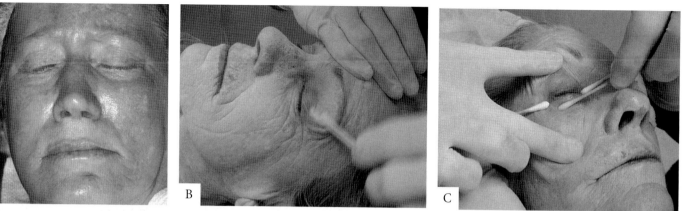

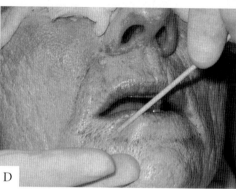

FIGURE **69-9** *Technical aspects of the Jessner's–35% trichloroacetic acid (TCA) peel. A, Appearance of level I frosting after application of Jessner's solution; erythema with blotchy frosting. B, TCA (35%) applied after Jessner's solution dries with an even application using cotton-tipped applicators, one to four. A level III or white enamel frosting is obtained. C, Eyelids are treated with one cotton-tipped applicator moistened with 35% TCA. A dry applicator is used to absorb tears during eyelid peeling. D, Lip rhytids are peeled with saturated cotton-tipped applicators. The wooden shaft is used to rub peel solution further into the lip rhytids.*

Level III frosting, which is associated with penetration to the reticular dermis, is a solid white enamel frosting with no background of erythema (see Figure 69-5C). A deeper level III frosting should be restricted only to areas of thick skin and heavy actinic damage. Most medium-depth chemical peels achieve a level II frosting, and this is especially important over the eyelids and areas of sensitive skin. Areas with a greater tendency to form scars, such as the zygomatic arch, the bony prominences of the jawline, and chin, should receive no greater than level II frosting.

Before re-treating an area with inadequate frosting, the surgeon should wait at least 3 to 4 minutes after the application of TCA to ensure that frosting has reached its peak. Each cosmetic unit is then assessed, and areas of incomplete or uneven frosting are carefully re-treated with a thin application of TCA. Additional applications of TCA increase the depth of penetration as well as the risk of complications, so one should apply more solution only to the underfrosted areas.

Although there is an immediate burning sensation as the peel solution is applied, the discomfort begins to subside as frosting occurs and resolves fully by the time of discharge. This peel can be performed with light sedation such as

- Diazepam 10 mg orally
- Meperidine 50 mg intramuscularly
- Hydroxyzine 25 mg intramuscularly

After the skin is cooled with saline the patient will remain comfortable throughout the postoperative period. Cool saline compresses offer symptomatic relief at the conclusion of the peel. Unlike the compresses in glycolic acid peels, the saline following a TCA peel simply provides relief and does not "neutralize" the acid.

Deep Chemical Peeling

Patients with more extreme photoaging skin may require deep chemical peeling, motorized dermabrasion, or laser resurfac-ing to improve their greater degree of skin damage. As discussed with medium-depth peels, deep chemical peeling leads to production of new collagen and ground substance, down to a level in proportion with the depth of the peel. The peeling agent of choice is the Baker-Gordon phenol peel.

The Baker-Gordon peel uses phenol in a formulation that permits deep penetration into the dermis, deeper than full-strength phenol.[23] The Baker-Gordon formula consists of Septisol solution, croton oil, and tap water added to a solution of phenol, reducing its concentration to 50% or 55% (Table 69-7). The mixture of

Table 69-6	Grades of Frosting with Trichloroacetic Acid Peels
Grade	*Visual Finding*
I	Erythema with streaky frosting
II	White frosting with visible erythema
III	White enamel frosting, no erythema

Table 69-7   The Baker-Gordon Formula
88% liquid phenol (USP), 3 mL
Tap water, 2 mL
Septisol liquid soap, 8 drops
Croton oil, 3 drops
USP = United States Pharmacopeia.

ingredients is freshly prepared and must be stirred vigorously prior to application due to its poor miscibility. The liquid soap, Septisol, is a surfactant that reduces skin tension, allowing a more even penetration. Croton oil is a vesicant epidermolytic agent that enhances phenol absorption. Recent investigations into the effects of this peel using varying concentrations of both phenol and croton oil have suggested that the procedure's efficacy is more related to the amount of croton oil than phenol.[24,25]

There are two main variations in deep chemical peeling with the Baker-Gordon phenol formula: occluded and unoccluded. Occlusion of the peeling solution with tape is thought to increase its penetration and extend the injury into the midreticular dermis. This technique is particularly helpful for deeply lined "weather-beaten" faces but should be used only by experienced surgeons because of the higher risk of complications.[26] The unoccluded technique as modified by McCollough and Langsdon involves a more vigorous cleansing of the skin and the application of more peel solution.[27] This may enhance the efficacy of the solution but without penetration as deeply as in an occluded peel. In the hands of a skilled and knowledgeable surgeon both methods are safe and reliable in rejuvenating advanced to severe photoaged skin. Deep chemical peeling can significantly improve or even eliminate deep furrows as well as other textural and pigmentary irregularities associated with severe photoaging (Figure 69-10). A remarkable degree of improvement is the expected result of deep chemical peeling when performed properly on carefully selected patients.

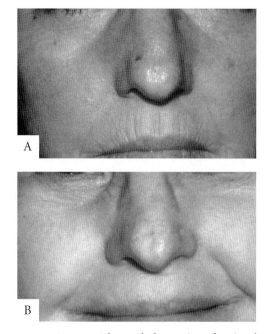

FIGURE **69-10**   *Advanced photoaging of perioral rhytids treated with Baker-Gordon phenol peel. A, Preoperative photograph, demonstrating perioral rhagades, textural and pigmentary changes with epidermal growths. B, Postoperative photograph, 2 years later. Note the phenol peel maintains correction for many years.*

The patient undergoing deep chemical peeling must understand and be willing to accept the significant risk of complications and the increased degree of morbidity. The most notable complications include scarring, textural changes such as "alabaster skin" or "plastic skin," and pigmentary disturbances. It is not uncommon for patients to experience postoperative erythema that can take many months to resolve and that may be followed by variable hypopigmentation (Figure 69-11). Male patients and patients with darker complexions are less favorable candidates for deep chemical peeling since the hypopigmentation is less easily camouflaged. Since phenol is cardiotoxic, preoperative evaluation includes a complete blood count, liver function tests, serum urea nitrogen and creatinine and electrolyte determinations, and a baseline electrocardiogram. Any patient who has a history of cardiac arrhythmias or who is taking a medication known to precipitate

arrhythmias should not undergo a full-face Baker-Gordon phenol peel. Patients with a history of hepatic or renal disease are also poor candidates.

Compared with medium-depth and superficial peeling, the Baker-Gordon phenol peel is a time-consuming procedure and must be performed only in a properly equipped facility. The required waiting period after the treatment of each cosmetic unit limits the rate of cutaneous absorption, thereby preventing the serum levels of phenol from reaching a dangerous peak during the procedure. Intravenous hydration with 1 L of lactated Ringer's solution before the procedure and another liter during the peel also promotes phenol excretion and prevents toxicity. Continuous electrocardiography, pulse oximetry, and blood pressure monitoring are mandatory during the entire perioperative period. Any abnormalities, such as a premature ventricular contraction or premature atrial contraction, necessitate abrupt stoppage of the procedure and careful evaluation for toxicity.[28] Oxygen is supplemented throughout the procedure as some physicians feel that it has a protective effect against cardiac arrhythmias.

After thorough cleansing and degreasing of the skin, the chemical agent is applied sequentially to six esthetic units: forehead, perioral region, right cheek, left cheek, nose, and periorbital region. There is a 15-minute time interval between the

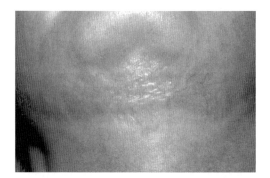

FIGURE **69-11**   *Complications from Baker-Gordon phenol peel with prolonged nonhealing, resulting in hypopigmentation and marbled scarring.*

treatment of each cosmetic area, allowing 60 to 90 minutes for the entire procedure. Cotton-tipped applicators are used with a similar technique as discussed with the medium-depth Jessner's–35% TCA peel, though less solution is used because frosting occurs very rapidly (Figure 69-12). Occlusion of the peel can be accomplished with strips of waterproof zinc oxide tape (eg, 0.5 inch Curity tape) to each cosmetic unit just after the phenol is applied. Care is exercised to extend the peel slightly beyond the mandibular rim to conceal the demarcation between treated and untreated skin. The last esthetic unit, the periorbital skin, is treated cautiously and conservatively to avoid overpenetration which can lead to ectropion or scarring. It is important to remember that diluting a phenol compound with water may increase its penetration, so mineral oil rather than water should be used to flush the eyes if contact occurs.

Application of the peeling agent creates an immediate burning sensation, which lasts for 15 to 20 seconds, subsides for 20 minutes, and then returns for the next 6 to 8 hours. Ice packs may be applied as necessary for patient comfort. Narcotics are usually prescribed on discharge for adequate pain control. Systemic steroids are also administered by some surgeons to lessen the inflammatory response. For untaped peels, petrolatum is applied and a biosynthetic dressing can be used for the first 24 hours.

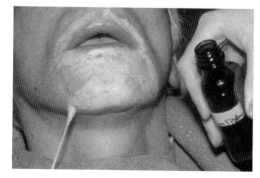

FIGURE **69-12** *Rapid frosting from small amounts of Baker-Gordon phenol solution applied with cotton-tipped applicators.*

Mechanical Resurfacing Procedures

During the past five decades, dermabrasion using a rotating abrasive surface attached to a power-driven hand engine has been considered a premier skin resurfacing procedure for facial scars. It has generally been regarded as a deep resurfacing modality based on its depth of injury and its prolonged healing time. The original descriptions of modern dermabrasion involved the use of a wire brush, which remains in use today.[29,30] In 1957 the diamond fraise was introduced and became the preferred instrument for dermabrasion by some surgeons because it is less aggressive and more forgiving than the wire brush.[31] Recently there has been a resurgence of interest in manual dermasanding which allows for more deliberate and controlled skin planing and microdermabrasion.[32,33]

Microdermabrasion

Microdermabrasion is considered superficial because it removes the stratum corneum and outer epidermis. Its classification as light or very light in comparison to the other superficial resurfacing procedures depends on the techniques and aggressiveness of the operator. The microdermabrasion unit's handpiece is a closed system, which propels aluminum oxide crystals at the skin at high speeds and simultaneously removes them with suction. These units were developed commercially in the mid-1990s and are currently in widespread use in both physicians' offices and nonmedical esthetic spas. Microdermabrasion may be indicated for acneiform conditions, pigmentary dyschromias, and as a "lunchtime" procedure for facial rejuvenation in all skin types.[34,35] Both the patient and physician must understand that the degree of objective improvement with microdermabrasion may be limited. This is a repetitive procedure performed every 2 weeks along with appropriate cosmoceutical agents.

Ideal candidates for microdermabrasion typically are young patients who desire limited facial rejuvenation without "downtime" and thus must have realistic expectations of the limited anticipated results. Patients often report that their skin has a smoother texture and that cosmetics are easier to apply and blend in with their skin more easily (Figure 69-13). Although the role of microdermabrasion in facial rejuvenation has grown dramatically since these units were developed, the scientific data to justify their use has been lacking.

Manual Dermasanding

Manual dermasanding involves abrading the skin by hand using silicon carbide sandpaper or wallscreen commercially available at any hardware store. Its classification as a wounding agent is entirely dependent on the type of paper used, the force applied by the surgeon, and the duration of contact with the skin. Although it can be used to produce a wound as deep as with wire brush dermabrasion or several passes with a pulsed CO_2 laser, manual dermasanding is probably most commonly used as a medium-depth or "minimally deep" resurfacing modality (Table 69-8).

Manual dermasanding is most often used for resurfacing localized regions to minimize the appearance of a scar or to

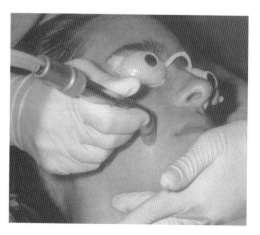

FIGURE **69-13** *Microdermabrasion: aluminum oxide crystals are propelled at high speeds within a closed system and removed with suction.*

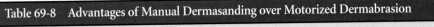

Table 69-8 Advantages of Manual Dermasanding over Motorized Dermabrasion
Greater control over depth of injury, particularly on the lips and orbital rims
Blending of abraded areas into adjacent unabraded areas accomplished more easily and with better results
Lower cost and greater simplicity of instrumentation and set-up
No risk of aerosolizing infectious particles
Possibly lower incidence of postinflammatory hypopigmentation[37,38]

blend or enhance the effects of a medium-depth chemical peel or a combination procedure.[36] It can be used following CO_2 laser resurfacing to feather the transition into hair-bearing areas that are inaccessible to the laser. Manual dermasanding of the eyebrows and hairline and gentle abrasion of the upper neck at the inferior aspect of the laser-irradiated zone are all effective at minimizing lines of demarcation between treated and untreated skin (Figure 69-14). It can also be useful immediately after laser resurfacing for stubborn rhytids, particularly in the perioral region. Manual dermasanding can improve the outcome by producing a slightly greater depth of injury in a controlled fashion where further thermal injury would be risky. It will also remove adherent necrotic debris and thermal damage, thus speeding up the healing process. Similarly a medium-depth chemical peel can be immediately followed by manual dermasanding on the more troublesome areas to enhance the results and also along the borders of the peeled skin to blend the effects. Our clinical

experience suggests that dermasanding after a Jessners–35% TCA peel may yield impressive postoperative results that approach those seen with either motorized dermabrasion or CO_2 laser resurfacing in patients with photoaging skin. (Figure 69-15). This combination is particularly helpful in patients who may not tolerate the greater degree of sedation often necessary with CO_2 laser resurfacing.

The necessary materials for manual dermasanding include silicon carbide sandpaper or wallscreen. Both may be purchased in a variety of grades: fine grade (no. 400), medium grade (nos. 220–320), and coarse grade (no. 180). The sandpaper is easy to use because of its flexibility and is easily cut into smaller pieces, which can be steam autoclaved. A 1.5" × 3" piece of sterilized sandpaper is wrapped around either the barrel of a 3 mL syringe or a rolled-up 2" × 2" gauze pad and moistened with saline or a soap-free cleanser for lubrication. A 1% solution of lidocaine with epinephrine may be used instead if additional anesthesia is necessary. Both back-and-forth and circular motions are used to gradually abrade the skin layer-by-layer until the hills and valleys are softened or adjacent areas are blended to the desired degree. Coarse grades may be used initially for "debulking," followed by finer grades later in the procedure. The fine grade is used to blend delicate areas of skin, such as around the eyelids. At the completion of the procedure the dark-colored silicon carbide particles remaining on the skin surface should be rinsed off because there is a theoretical risk of their becoming implanted.

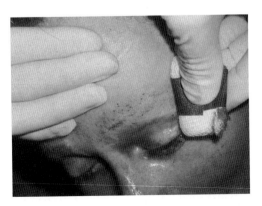

FIGURE 69-14 *Manual dermasanding using 320-grit silicone carbide sandpaper to blend carbon dioxide laser resurfacing into the eyebrow area.*

Motorized Dermabrasion

Some of the units most commonly used today are the Bell hand engine (Bell International, Burlingame, CA), the AEV-12 hand engine (Ellis International, Madison, NJ), and the Osada surgical handpiece (Osada, Inc., Los Angeles, CA). A topical refrigerant spray (Frigiderm, Frigiderm Corp., Costa Mesa, CA) is used to produce anesthesia and to harden the skin as it is abraded. The spray immobilizes the topographic features so that there is no distortion by the pressure of the abrasive instrument.

The two abrasive instruments most often employed with these units are the wire brush and the diamond fraise. The wire brush has numerous small-caliber stainless steel wires that project circumferentially from the curved side of a cylindrical hub. A diamond fraise consists of a stainless steel cylinder to which industrial-grade diamonds are bonded to create the abrasive surface. As compared with wire brush instruments, diamond fraises are manufactured with a greater variety in shape, width of abrasive surface, wheel diameter, and coarseness of grit. The wire brush is more aggressive and cuts more quickly and more deeply into the skin with each stroke, thereby posing a greater risk of injury and requiring more skill to operate. Although the diamond fraise is generally safer and more forgiving, it may not yield the degree of improvement possible with the wire brush, especially for more stubborn conditions such as deep acne scarring (Figure 69-16).

Because dermabrasion with either instrument is highly technique-dependent and its learning curve is steep, there may be considerable variability in the clinical results obtained by different operators. It is very important for beginning dermabraders to attain thorough hands-on instruction from an experienced operator in order to be adequately trained. The proper techniques for motorized

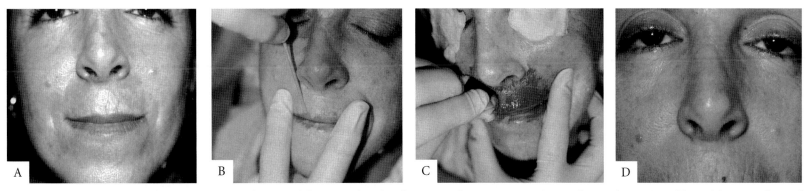

FIGURE **69-15** *Medium-depth chemical peel with manual dermasanding for photoaging skin. A, Preoperative: moderate photoaging of face with more advanced perioral rhagades. B, Jessner's–35% trichloroacetic acid peel applied over face including the perioral area. C, Manual dermasanding to the perioral skin to bloody points. D, One-month postoperative photograph revealing improvement in all areas.*

dermabrasion have also been the subject of comprehensive reviews in the literature.[37–39] Careful evaluation of the depth of injury throughout the procedure is critical to ensure sufficient depth for optimal results without penetrating beyond the desired level and risking scarring. Because of the potential for aerosolization of infectious particles during dermabrasion, appropriate precautions are mandatory to protect the operating room staff.

Moderate to severe acne scarring is the most notable indication for dermabrasion, as laser resurfacing has yielded variable results and chemical peeling is generally disappointing (Table 69-9). Dermabrasion selectively planes off the "hilltops" that surround the atrophic "valleys," whereas chemical peeling and lasers produce an injury of equivalent depth in both areas (Figure 69-17).

The use of CO_2 lasers has revolutionized resurfacing techniques for photoaging skin. Because of the varying properties of lasers, the physician must be thoroughly familiar with the physics, technology, and operating geometry of the laser. Whether or not the laser is pulsed, continuous, or computer scanned impacts the physiologic response. The level of destruction is different for each laser; thus, the physician should be familiar with the laser of choice. For reliable vaporization of skin layers, a pulsed laser with a computer-generated scanner (CPG) makes the procedure safer. Each pass destroys 75 to 100 μm of tissue with a zone of thermal damage below. Thus, two to three passes with an ultrapulse CO_2 laser is maximal for rejuvenation of photodamaged skin—a deep resurfacing technique. The zone of thermal damage causes collagen shrinkage or contraction, which is a unique characteristic for CO_2

laser resurfacing. This gives an added benefit to wrinkle treatment that is not found with either dermabrasion or chemical peeling. This is especially true with perioral and periorbital wrinkled skin.

CO_2 laser resurfacing requires anesthesia: either general operative anesthesia or tumescent local anesthesia for the entire face. Laser safety precautions are needed to prevent laser fire or laser injury to the employees, the unprotected skin, the teeth, or even the endotracheal tube for general anesthesia. These must be protected with appropriate laser-resistant materials: eye shields, teeth guards, and appropriate laser-resistant endotracheal tube wrapping. Using the CPG the operator must remember that the pulse overlap for a chosen pattern size and shape is set so that each pattern is made to touch yet not overlap. The density is an important parameter in determining laser beam intensity. One

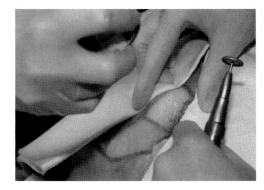

FIGURE **69-16** *Mechanical dermabrasion is performed with a diamond fraise over rigid skin cooled with a topical refrigerant spray.*

Table 69-9 Conditions for Which Motorized Dermabrasion May Be the Preferred Resurfacing Modality
Acne scarring
Surgical or traumatic scars
Benign neoplastic processes (multiple trichoepitheliomas, syringomas, adenoma sebaceum)
Malignant and premalignant neoplastic processes (skin cancer treatment and prevention in basal cell nevus syndrome and xeroderma pigmentosum as well as management of extensive carcinoma in situ)
Extensive epidermal lesions such as epidermal nevi
Decorative or traumatic tattoos unresponsive to the pigmented lesion lasers
Rhinophyma

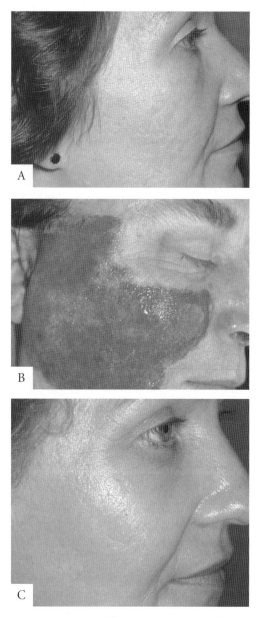

FIGURE **69-17**   *Full-face dermabrasion performed for acne scars. A, Preoperative: shallow and atrophic scars most amenable to dermabrasion. B, Postoperative dermabrasion prior to biosynthetic dressing. C, Three months postoperative.*

should not go above a density of 6 with facial resurfacing. Each pass should cover the face fully, vaporizing the tissue to ash and debris, which is wiped off between each pass. The visual end point is a mauve or slightly yellow discoloration indicating denaturization of dermal collagen. Further passes cause deeper dermal scarring. Special care must be taken over scar-prone areas such as the bony prominences of the chin, jawline, malar ridge, and forehead.

The eyelid is treated more conservatively as collagen can precipitate an ectropion, with or without scar. The lips are treated with two to three passes but not over the vermilion line as this can flatten the lip in an unesthetic manner. Bordered facial creases such as the jawline and neck should be blended with light chemical peeling and minimal dermasanding to soften the demarcations of treated and untreated photoaging neck skin.

Of equal importance to the operative technique is proper postoperative wound care. Partial thickness skin wounds heal fastest when kept at or near 100% humidity or occlusive or semi-occlusive dressings. Nonstick pads and hydrogels are changed daily to remove coagulation debris and necrotic tissue. This is important to prevent secondary wound infection with resultant scarring. My usual postoperative program is 4 to 5 days of biologic hydration, changed daily, followed by 5 days of 0.25% acetic acid soaks (1 teaspoon white vinegar in 1 pint of warm water) four times a day followed by occlusive ointments such as petrolatum ointment or eucerin cream. After 10 days, the patient is usually ready for light cleansers and creams and a mild topical steroid cream for erythematous areas (Table 69-10).

Full makeup can be used with sunscreen after 2 weeks. Sunscreen with strong sun avoidance should be adhered to for 2 to 3 months to prevent postlaser hyperpigmentation.

Herpes simplex infection can occur during the healing period following medium-depth or deep ablative injury. Antiviral prophylaxis should begin during the operative session and continue beyond reepithelialization, 10 to 14 days. If infection occurs, punctate vesicles occur with pain and full treatment therapy should be carried out to prevent scarring.

Delayed wound healing may be a sign of bacterial infection, or resurfacing too deep to heal normally. It should be treated with biologic dressings, appropriate

Table 69-10   Avoiding Complications Postoperatively for Skin Resurfacing
Use proper occlusive wound care, and monitor daily.
Watch for pain; it may indicate herpes simplex virus infection.
Watch and treat early bacterial and fungal infection.
Evaluate closely and follow areas of poor healing.
Treat prolonged erythema or early scarring early and vigorously.

antibiotics, and cortisones as indicated. The diligent physician must watch his or her patients carefully during the postoperative course to catch these complications early and prescribe appropriate treatment. This will prevent the permanent complications of pigmentation changes and scarring.

Conclusions

The general public has a renewed interest in skin rejuvenation. Although there are many techniques presently available, it is up to the cosmetic physician to match the appropriate tool with the patient's needs, to give proper benefit with the least risk. These tools call for special training and experience, and as one gains further knowledge and skill, these procedures generally occupy a rewarding part of one's practice.

References

1. Leyden JJ. Photodamage: an overview. Skin Allergy News 2003;Suppl:3–4.
2. Glogau RG. Chemical peeling and aging skin. J Geriatr Dermatol 1994;2(1):30–5.
3. Monheit GD, Chastain MA. Chemical peels in facial rejuvenation: non-surgical modalities. Facial Plast Surg Clin North Am 2001;9(2):243.
4. Stegman SJ. A comparative histologic study of the effects of three peeling agents and dermabrasion on normal and sun-damaged skin. Aesthetic Plast Surg 1982;6:123–5.
5. Monheit GD. Consultation for photoaging skin, presented at the American Academy of Dermatology Annual Meeting; 1999 March 20; New Orleans, LA.

6. Lowe, NJ. Textbook of facial rejuvenation. London: Martin Danitz; 2002. p. 3–11.

7. Kligman, AM. Topical retinoic acid (tretinoin) for photoaging: conceptions and misperceptions. Cutis 1996;57:142–4.

8. Moy LS, Murad H, Moy RL. Glycolic acid peels for the treatment of wrinkles and photoaging. J Dermatol Surg Oncol 1993; 19:243–6.

9. Draelos, ZD. Topical agents used in association with cosmetic surgery. Semin Cutan Med Surg 1999; 18(2):112–8.

10. Monheit GD. Skin preparation: an essential step before chemical peeling or laser resurfacing. Cosmet Dermatol 1996;9(9):13–4.

11. Rubin M. Manual of chemical peels. Philadelphia (PA): Lippincott; 1995. p. 50–67.

12. Clark CP. Office-based skin care and superficial peels: the scientific rationale. Plast Reconstr Surg 1999; 104:854–64; discussion 65–6.

13. Brody HJ. Chemical peeling. St. Louis (MO): Mosby; 1992. p. 59–60.

14. Monheit GD. The Jessner's + TCA peel: a medium depth chemical peel. J Dermatol Surg Oncol 1989;15:945–50.

15. Kligman D, Kligman AM. Salicylic acid peels for the treatment of photoaging. Dermatol Surg 1998;24:325–8.

16. Monheit, GD. Chemical peeling for pigmentary dyschromias. Cosmet Dermatol 1995;8(5):10–5.

17. Brody HJ, Hailey CW. Medium-depth chemical peeling of the skin: a variation of superficial chemosurgery. J Dermatol Surg Oncol 1986;12:1268–75.

18. Brody HJ. Variations and comparisons in medium depth chemical peeling. J Dermatol Surg Oncol 1989;15:953–63.

19. Coleman WP, Futrell JM. The glycolic acid trichloroacetic acid peel. J Dermatol Surg Oncol 1994;20:76–80.

20. Witheiler DD, Lawrence N, Cox SE, et al. Long-term efficacy and safety of Jessner's solution and 35% trichloroacetic acid vs 5% fluorouracil in the treatment of widespread facial actinic keratoses. Dermatol Surg 1997;23:191–6.

21. Monheit GD. The Jessner's-TCA peel. Facial Plast Surg Clin North Am 1994;2:21–7.

22. Morrow DM. Chemical peeling of eyelids and periorbital area. J Dermatol Surg Oncol 1992;18:102–10.

23. Baker, TS, Gordon HL. Chemical face peeling. In: Surgical rejuvenation of the face. St. Louis (MO): C.V. Mosby; 1986. p. 230–2.

24. Hetter GP. An examination of the phenol-croton oil peel: Part I. Dissecting the formula. Plast Reconstr Surg 2000;105:227–39; discussion 49–51.

25. Hetter GP. An examination of the phenol-croton oil peel: part IV. Face peel results with different concentrations of phenol and croton oil. Plast Reconstr Surg 2000;105:1061–83; discussion 84–7.

26. Alt T. Occluded Baker/Gordon chemical peel. Review and update. J Dermatol Surg Oncol 1989;15:980–93.

27. McCollough EG, Langsdon PR. Chemical peeling with phenol. In: Roenigk H, Roenigk R, editors. Dermatologic surgery: principles and practice. New York (NY): Marcel Dekker; 1989. p. 997–1016.

28. Beeson WH. The importance of cardiac monitoring in superficial and deep chemical peeling. J Dermatol Surg Oncol 1987;13:949–50.

29. Burks JW. Abrasive removal of scars. South Med J 1955;48:452–9.

30. Kurtin A. Corrective surgical planing of the skin. Arch Dermatol Syphil 1953;68:389–97.

31. Alt TH. Facial dermabrasion: advantages of the diamond fraise technique. J Dermatol Surg Oncol 1987;13:618–24.

32. Harris DR, Noodleman FR. Combining manual dermasanding with low strength trichloroacetic acid to improve actinically injured skin. J Dermatol Surg Oncol 1994; 20:436–42.

33. Chiarello SE. Tumescent dermasanding with cryospraying. A new wrinkle on the treatment of rhytids. Dermatol Surg 1996; 22:601–10.

34. Bernard RW, Beran SJ, Rusin L. Microdermabrasion in clinical practice. Clin Plast Surg 2000;27:571–7.

35. Warmuth IP, Echt A, Scarborough DA, Bisaccia E. Microdermabrasion: a new rejuvenation treatment option. Cosmet Dermatol 1999;12:7–10.

36. Zisser M, Kaplan B, Moy RL. Surgical pearl: manual dermabrasion. J Am Acad Dermatol 1995;33:105–6.

37. Yarborough JM. Dermabrasion by wire brush. J Dermatol Surg Oncol 1987;13:610–5.

38. Alt TH. Technical aids for dermabrasion. J Dermatol Surg Oncol 1987;13:638–48.

39. Yarborough JM, Coleman WP, Lawrence N. Wire brush dermabrasion. In: Coleman WP, Lawrence N, editors. Skin resurfacing. Baltimore (MD): Williams & Wilkins; 1998.

CHAPTER 70

Alloplastic Esthetic Facial Augmentation

Bruce N. Epker, DDS, MSD, PhD

Alloplastic esthetic facial augmentation of the chin, mandibular angles and inferior borders, skeletal nasal base, and cheeks is the standard of care, as opposed to autogenous augmentation. A variety of approved alloplastic facial implants are available to the surgeon. In general, marketed implants are proven nontoxic, noncarcinogenic, and nonantigenic, and they are inert in body fluids.[1–3] Moreover, the optimal material is user friendly; it is easily modified, maintains the desired shape, is not mobile, and is cost effective.

No single implant possesses all of these optimal properties, yet some are clearly closer to these ideals than others. The more commonly employed esthetic facial implants, which most closely achieve these ideals, include porous polyethylene, silicone, and polytetrafluoroethylene (PTFE) and high-density polyethylene. It is not the intent of this article to compare and contrast these facial implant materials as they are all approved and acceptable and each is espoused by different surgeons as the preferred material for cosmetic esthetic facial augmentation.

To achieve predictable and successful results with alloplastic esthetic facial augmentation, special attention to the differential diagnoses established via a detailed patient evaluation,[4–11] meticulous surgical technique, proper modification, and placement of the implant are essential. Accordingly, this chapter emphasizes and details these aspects of esthetic facial augmentation.

An additional item discussed herein is still controversial—the use of antibiotics with surgery for alloplastic facial augmentation. A recent survey of surgeons revealed a spectrum of opinions. Approximately 30% of surgeons use no antibiotics or intravenous antibiotics only during surgery. About an additional 30% continue antibiotics for 1 to 3 days postoperatively, and 40% use them for 4 to 7 days postoperatively.[12] Unfortunately, the incidence of infection with the various regimens is not available; however, the overall incidence is very low. I use a single intraoperative dose of intravenous antibiotics at the commencement of surgery; generally, I use cephalosporin regardless of whether an extraoral or intraoral approach is taken.[13,14]

Finally, alloplastic nasal augmentation is not discussed here as, in general, I prefer autogenous materials for this purpose.

The Chin

Alloplastic chin augmentation is generally reserved for the patient who has lax and/or redundant soft tissues or who is undergoing simultaneous neck surgery, such as cervicofacial liposuction, platysma plication, or rhytidoplasty. When this approach is used, special care is directed to evaluating for a tapered chin appearance or "marionette grooves," which frequently exist in the older patient population. Many commercially available alloplastic chin implants *do not* provide adequate lateral augmentation and posterior extension in the parasymphysis regions to correct these problems. Therefore, the modification or selection of a properly sized and shaped alloplastic implant is important.

Preoperative planning consists of a systematic sequential esthetic clinical evaluation and a lateral cephalometric evaluation to determine the specific shape and magnitude of the augmentation.

Chin augmentation has long been an esthetic adjunct to numerous orthognathic, craniofacial, and cosmetic procedures. Various authors have proposed and extolled the advantages of their "modifications" of this basic operation, but, despite its widespread application, its esthetic demands and results are not yet well specified.[15–17]

This procedure is planned to achieve specific esthetic objectives:

- Frontally, a well-defined smooth inferior border of the mandible that separates the lower third of the face from the neck proper is important for good esthetics. A lack of this distinct border detracts from good chin-neck esthetics. A posteriorly well-extended implant and proper inferior placement, at the inferior mandibular border, help to achieve this objective.

- The esthetically attractive chin is balanced in width with the other facial features, especially the bizygomatic and bigonial facial widths. Many individuals with recessed chins also have dolichocephalic facial features, or what has been described as the "pointed chin" or "witch's chin." When this condition exists and is not deliberately modified, augmentation of the chin often results in an accentuation of the existing pointed chin. In persons with this facial structure, augmentation of the chin should be accomplished by *enhanced lateral augmentation*. This is accomplished by modifying standard chin implants as described in the surgical technique discussion to follow.

- The esthetically attractive chin has no evidence of parasymphyseal depressions or grooves. These soft tissue marionette grooves may exist independently of or in concert with the pointed chin. This condition is accentuated in most older individuals. When these grooves exist, special attention is given to lateral or parasymphyseal augmentation, similar to that used to improve the pointed chin.

- The esthetics of anteroposterior chin position is determined by evaluating the cephalometric values: NB:Pog, A:Pog, and subnasale perpendicular. The normal relations of these are as follow: NB:Pog line has the lower incisor tip and bony chin prominence on a 2:1 to 1:1 relationship. Line A:Pog has the tip of the lower incisor on or 1 to 2 mm posteriorly positioned. The soft-tissue chin is 4 mm distal to SN perpendicular. These values are used to determine the optimal relationship of the hard

and soft tissues of the chin relative to lower incisor position, lower lip, and upper lip. Two qualifiers regarding esthetic anteroposterior chin augmentation are important in the context of the proposed cephalometric treatment planning. First, *do not* advance the bony chin beyond the anterior position of the lower incisor as determined by the NB:Pog and A:Pog criteria, even when subnasale perpendicular soft tissue values suggest otherwise. Second, in older individuals, often those undergoing cervicofacial liposuction, rhytidoplasty, or both, anteroposterior augmentation of the chin to its "ideal" hard and soft tissue values generally results in an excessive amount of chin projection *in the eyes of the patient.* This is perhaps because the individual has had the deficient condition for so many years that he or she has become accustomed to it.

In sum, before performing esthetic chin augmentation, consider all of these criteria and *do not* rely primarily on achieving the ideal anteroposterior chin position; otherwise, the esthetic results in a significant number of patients will fall short of the desired results.[18]

This procedure is most often performed under local anesthesia with sedation, along with other procedures such as blepharoplasty, rhinoplasty, cervicofacial liposuction, and rhytidoplasty.

With a surgical marking pen, the true chin and neck midlines are marked to aid subsequently in precise implant positioning; also, the planned submental incision is marked.[19] When this procedure is being performed under local anesthesia with sedation, bilateral inferior alveolar nerve blocks are given with 2% lidocaine with 1:100,000 epinephrine. Next, the submental area where the incision is to be made and the entire area to be undermined subperiosteally are infiltrated with about 7 to 10 cc of local anesthetic with epinephrine.

Seven to 10 minutes are allowed to pass after infiltration of the local anesthetic.

The implant is to be placed through a submental incision of about 5 cm, made just distal to the normal submental crease. When the incision is made in the naturally occurring submental crease, it can accentuate this crease and cause an unesthetic dimpling in that area. The incision is made through the skin and subcutaneous tissue, and hemostasis is obtained with needle-point diathermy. The incision is then carried directly down to the inferior border of the mandible and through the periosteum with diathermy cutting.

After identification and exposure of the inferior border of the mandible, a subperiosteal dissection is completed along the entire inferior aspect of the mandibular symphysis, *well posterior* on each side to the region of the gonial notch. Following exposure of the inferior border, the subperiosteal dissection is carried superiorly beginning anteriorly. Laterally it is extended superiorly only enough to allow the mental neurovascular bundles to be identified and visualized. No attempt is made to expose them extensively because doing so increases the potential for neurosensory defects to the lower lip and chin.

An extended preformed implant is generally selected, one that is configured in such a way that it extends posteriorly into the molar region.[8,17,19] In patients with a tapered (pointed) chin or marionette grooves, the selected implant is modified. The selected implant is 2 to 4 mm greater in the anteroposterior dimension than the desired anteroposterior augmentation.[19] This dimension is reduced at surgery and, in essence, accentuates the parasymphysis augmentation to improve the pointed chin or parasymphysis depressions. These alterations are made to provide a more lateral (parasymphysis) augmentation than is available in most preformed alloplastic chin implants (Figure 70-1).

After trial insertion of the implant, the surgeon determines the need for addition-

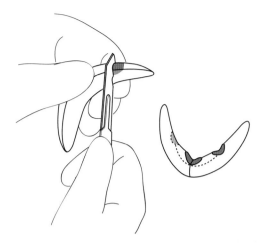

FIGURE **70-1** *Reduction of the anteroposterior thickness effects a rounding of the chin and visibly changes a pointed chin into a more rounded one. Adapted from Epker BN.[19] p. 27.*

al adaptations in either the implant or the subperiosteal dissection to ensure that it *rests passively* on the lateral and inferior borders of the mandible. The mental neurovascular bundles are visualized during the trial insertion to make certain that the implant does not encroach on them. If this does occur, these areas are marked in situ on the implant, and the implant is removed and these areas relieved.

On completion of all adaptations, two holes are drilled through the implant and outer cortex of the underlying bone. The implant midline and marked facial midline are checked, and the implant is then stabilized with titanium screws to prevent inadvertent early postoperative displacement and to avoid mobility of the implant. If the implant is porous, it is vacuum impregnated with an antibiotic solution before it is definitively stabilized into position.

The incision is closed in layers with 4-0 polyglactin 910 platysma muscle sutures, 4-0 chromic gut subcutaneous sutures, and 5-0 braided polyester or monofilament nylon skin sutures. Antibiotic ointment and a perforated film absorbent dressing (Telfa) are placed over the incision, and a multiple-layered 1.25 cm tape dressing is placed to reduce edema and or hematoma formation. The dressing is left in place for 48 hours. When additional neck surgery is done, as is frequently the case with this procedure, a more extensive neck pressure dressing may be placed. Generally, intraoperative antibiotics are used and no postoperative antibiotics given.

Sutures are removed on the fifth postoperative day, and after 7 to 10 days any areas of irregularity caused by edema or hematoma are treated by deep massage and heat. No other special treatment is needed.

Complications that occur with this procedure vary and are generally minimal.[18]

The patient seen in Figure 70-2 is shown before and after alloplastic chin augmentation, emphasizing lateral parasymphysis augmentation to reduce the pointed appearance of the chin and the marionette grooves.

Mandibular Angle and Inferior Border

A well-defined mandibular angle and inferior mandibular border are important to an esthetically pleasing face. Indeed, *proper definition in this region is the very basis of visually separating the face from the neck,* thereby making them distinct from one another. When this area is not well defined, the face and neck become confluent and unattractive. Accordingly, in selected individuals esthetic augmentation of the mandibular angles and inferior mandibular borders is to be considered.[19]

The differential diagnosis of poor definition of the angle and inferior mandibular borders is important; one must consider whether it results from abnormal skeletal support, cervicofacial lipomatosis, soft tissue redundancy, or a combination of these conditions

A routine clinical evaluation via multidirectional observation and palpation can readily allow the surgeon to diagnose cervicofacial lipomatosis and/or soft tissue redundancy. A standard lateral cephalometric evaluation of the mandibular plane angle is used to determine the presence and degree of an underlying skeletal support abnormality. The normal mandibular plane angle (FH:Go-Gn) is 24°. One then draws the normal inferior border line angle. This in essence represents the newly to be constructed inferior mandibular border and allows the surgeon to determine the specifics of vertical and anteroposterior implant design.

The vertical linear distance between the two mandibular planes (the patient's and the constructed normal) in the gonial angle is measured. This distance is the amount of vertical change in the angle that would be indicated to create ideal skeletal support. Generally, the older the patient, the less one augments this area all the way to the ideal. The lateral superior height is measured so that it extends to above the midramus. Anteroposteriorly the mental foramen is generally the limiting extent of the implant. Finally, frontal face esthetics is evaluated to determine the approximate desired lateral width of the implant in the angle-ramus area. In the esthetically pleasing face, the mandibular angle area is medial to the zygomatic area so that the face tapers slightly from the zygomatic area.

When soft tissue conditions coexist with the defined underlying skeletal abnormalities, correction of the skeletal deformity may produce significant improvements in the associated soft tissue conditions. Finally, when identifiable skeletal and major associated soft tissue problems coexist, the skeletal surgery described herein can be done either primarily or simultaneously with liposuction or rhytidoplasty; however, I prefer to perform the face- and neck-lift secondarily.

Once the above data are established, a preformed porous polyethylene implant is selected and appropriately modified at surgery as discussed in the surgical technique section to follow.[20–23]

Surgery can be performed with general anesthesia or intravenous sedation and local anesthesia.[19] Inferior alveolar nerve blocks are given bilaterally. In addition, a 2% local anesthetic containing 1:200,000

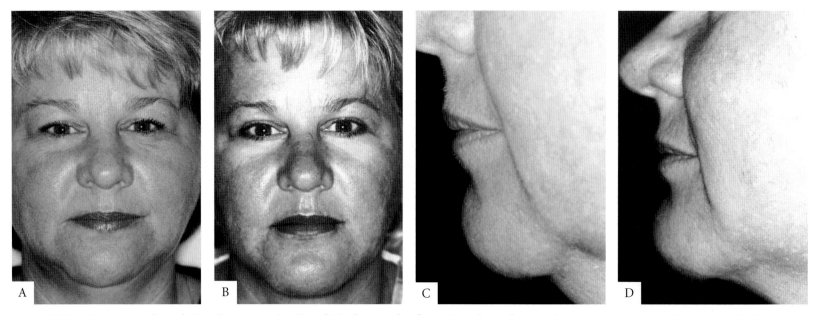

FIGURE **70-2**   *Preoperative (A and C) and postoperative (B and D) photographs of a patient who underwent chin augmentation to reduce a pointed chin appearance illustrating more lateral augmentations.*

epinephrine is infiltrated bilaterally just lateral to the mandible from midramus to the angle and along the entire lateral aspect of the mandibular body to the region of the mental neurovascular bundle. Approximately 10 cc of local anesthetic is infiltrated on each side. The surgical procedure is begun about 7 to 10 minutes after injection of the local anesthetic.

The incision is begun posterolaterally, just anterior to the bulge of the fat pad, midway down to the depth of the sulcus. This incision is made through the mucosa, buccinator, and periosteum, anteriorly to the region of the canine tooth; however, as one proceeds anteriorly into the premolar region, the incision is initially carried only through the mucosa to avoid inadvertently transecting the mental neurovascular bundle.

After the mental neurovascular bundle is exposed, the remainder of the dissection is done entirely in the subperiosteal tissue plane. This begins anteriorly with deliberate mobilization of the tissues around the mental neurovascular bundle, carrying the dissection inferiorly subposteriorly to the inferior border of the mandible. The dissection is next carried posteriorly to the angle of the mandible, while the masseter

muscle is elevated superiorly about half way up the ascending mandibular ramus. No attempt is made to penetrate the periosteum at the inferior and posterior borders of the mandible.

In the region of the mandibular angle and along the posterior border, a J-shaped periosteal elevator is used to complete the subperiosteal dissection (Figure 70-3).

Once the lateral body and ascending ramus of the mandible are exposed in the subperiosteal tissue plane, the periosteum can be opened with finger dissection at the inferior aspect, as necessary for adequate relaxation.

My preferred augmentation material is porous polyethylene, which is available in several preformed sizes and shapes. The approximate size and shape of the implant should be determined previously, as discussed in the previous section. On the basis of the measurements, the preformed implant is modified during the actual surgical procedure. After the initial modifications, before a try-in placement, the implant is vacuum impregnated with an antibiotic solution. This is achieved by placing the implant into a 60 or 90 cc syringe in which the antibiotic solution is present, inserting the plunger of the

syringe and evacuating all air, and repeatedly withdrawing the plunger forcefully while holding a finger over the end of the syringe. This removes the air from the porous implant and replaces it with the concentrated antibiotic solution. The procedure requires considerable effort and pressure, often taking a few minutes. When this process reaches its end point, the implant sinks in the solution.

The initial try-in is then done. Additional modifications are often necessary, such as notching the implant in the region of the mental neurovascular bundle and molding it slightly into a curved

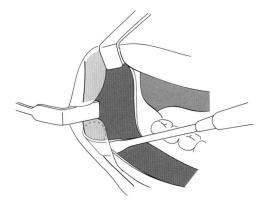

FIGURE **70-3**   *Use of a J-shaped elevator to remove the tenacious angle muscle attachments. Adapted from Epker BN.[19] p. 84.*

configuration to adapt it more precisely to the lateral aspect of the ramus and body of the mandible. To bend the implant, it is placed in sterile hot saline; this removes its original memory and allows it to be readily molded.

The implant is inserted into position. Once inserted and its inferior and posterior aspects "locked" beneath the posterior and inferior borders of the mandible, the implant is inspected for any final adaptations. At this point the implant is removed, placed back into the antibiotic, and the wound packed.

The identical dissection is then completed on the opposite side, and before insertion of the second implant, the same basic modifications are made to a second implant so that the implants are virtual mirror images of one another. This assumes that the patient has a symmetric deformity in this area. When asymmetry exists, it is identified and recorded preoperatively, and the modification of the implants for independent shaping of the right and left sides is done preoperatively.

After completion of the dissection on the second side and the try-in of the second implant, both implants are ready for final insertion. The implants are irrigated free of blood and debris and vacuum impregnated again with the antibiotic solution. One or two monocortical titanium screws are placed to stabilize the implant (Figure 70-4).

The implant is inserted on one side first, and the incision is closed in two layers. The first layer is the periosteal and buccinator muscle, which is closed with 3-0 chromic sutures. Then, with a running 3-0 chromic horizontal mattress suture, the mucosal layer is closed. Interrupted sutures are finally placed as needed to effect a watertight closure of the incision. After completion of closure on one side, the second antibiotic-impregnated implant is placed into the opposite side, and the stabilization and layered closure are completed.

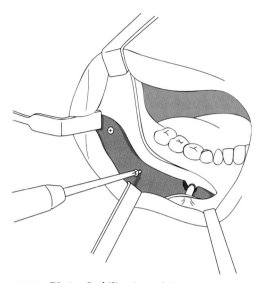

FIGURE **70-4** *Stabilization of the implant with monocortical titanium screws. Adapted from Epker BN.[19] p. 89.*

A multilayered 1.25 cm tape dressing is placed so that the tape extends from the cheek area well inferiorly into the neck, thereby applying primarily lateral pressure to this area to minimize postoperative edema and hematoma. When this dressing is applied, it is placed so that the pressure is directly applied laterally. This dressing is left in place for 48 hours. On removal of the tape dressing, the patient is instructed to use heat to decrease the swelling.

Postoperatively the patient is placed on a clear liquid diet for the first 24 hours and then advanced to a full liquid diet for 4 to 5 days. After this time, he or she may begin a mechanical soft diet for 10 to 14 days until the intraoral incision lines are completely healed. After approximately 2 weeks, the implants are self-stabilized by fibrous soft tissue ingrowth, and the incisions are completely healed; at this time unlimited physical activity is permitted.

At the 2-week period patients generally have some limitation in the range of mandibular motion because of the surgery and its sequelae. Accordingly, they are placed on a regimen of active jaw exercises, three times a day for approximately 5 minutes each. These exercises consist of maximum interincisal opening, protrusion, and clenching. Generally, within 7 to 14 days asymptomatic full range of mandibular motion is obtained.

This procedure is designed to accentuate and normalize the mandibular angle and inferior mandibular border to set the lower third of the face off clearly from the neck, making each into a discrete esthetic unit. Additionally, this procedure effects some tightening of the overlying soft tissues, affecting a "mini face-lift" in individuals who have slight skin laxity and/or mild jowls (Figure 70-5). The procedure is often done in concert with other orthognathic, reconstructive, and cosmetic facial procedures.

Skeletal Nasal Base

The indication for skeletal nasal base augmentation is based on a clinical esthetic facial evaluation in individuals who are not Class III maxillary deficient. This condition is frequently associated with inherent nasal deformities.[19–24] The typical clinical esthetic findings are outlined below.

Frontally the alar base width is highly variable but most often is somewhat narrow, and the upper lip vermilion is often deficient or exhibits a "gullwing" appearance. Moreover, the patient has deficiency in the paranasal areas, as opposed to prominent soft tissue nasolabial folds (Figure 70-6A). In profile, flat to concave paranasal anatomy and a groove ratio of nasal tip–subnasale to subnasale-alar is approximately 1:1 instead of the normal 2:1. In addition, the following most often coexist: a relatively prominent nose, poor nasal tip projection, unesthetic nasal tip rotation (droop), and lack of a supratip break (Figure 70-6B).[25]

Anatomically, the skeletal nasal base is the area that, in part, determines paranasal fullness, alar base position, nasal tip support, *relative* nasal prominence, and internal nasal valve (liminal valve) function. Accordingly, the esthetics of these areas depends on but is not totally determined by the underlying skeletal anatomy.

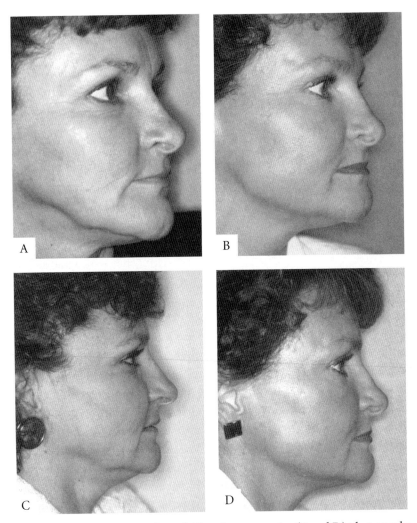

FIGURE 70-5 *Preoperative (A and C) and postoperative (B and D) photographs of a patient who underwent mandibular angle–inferior border augmentation. Note the tightening of soft tissues with a reduction of the laxity, especially in the jowl. Reproduced with permission from Epker BN.[19] p. 94.*

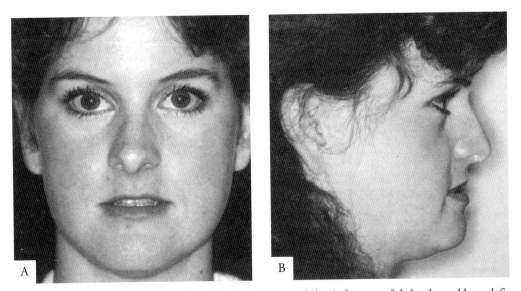

FIGURE 70-6 *A and B, Patient with a Class I occlusion and classic features of skeletal nasal base deficiency. Reproduced with permission from Epker BN.[19] p. 116.*

The cephalometric analysis may or may not exhibit evidence of maxillary deficiency in the presence of a Class I occlusion. This is true because these cephalometric values have traditionally been determined by measures around a point that may not be deficient. However, the piriform rims per se, as well as the immediate adjacent areas of the maxilla, are deficient. Unfortunately, these areas are not amenable to measurement or evaluation with conventional lateral cephalometrics.

Individuals to be considered for skeletal nasal base augmentation are those with *isolated skeletal nasal base deficiency* who possess a functional Class I relationship and are not candidates for orthognathic surgical consideration. In some individuals, in whom a skeletal Class III deformity exists in the mandible and is corrected with an osteotomy to set back the mandible, the skeletal nasal base deficiency can be simultaneously corrected by skeletal nasal base augmentation.[24] Finally, this procedure is indicated in certain individuals who present for rhinoplasty and/or septorhinoplasty.[25]

Two approaches to the surgery are used, depending on the severity of the deficiency as determined by the clinical findings: a limited approach and an extended approach. The limited approach is used when the magnitude of augmentation planned is minimal (2–3 g of hydroxylapatite per side). In such individuals the alar base width is generally normal, and in profile the nasal size, tip projection, and a supratip area are essentially normal. This approach *does not* noticeably affect the upper lip vermilion exposure.

Conversely, the extended approach permits alar base width adjustment and control of upper lip vermilion exposure (increased exposure). Also, since it is used for larger augmentations (4–6 g per side), it effects a relative decrease in nasal size, increasing the tip projection and supratip break.

The procedure can be readily performed under either general or local anesthesia with or without sedation. Before injection of the local anesthetic, the alar base width is measured and an esthetic determination is made as to its most desirable postoperative width. About 10 minutes before initiation of the actual surgery, the infraorbital nerves are blocked bilaterally, and 10 cc of 2% lidocaine with 1:200,000 epinephrine is infiltrated from the zygomatic-alveolar crest area on one side to the same area on the opposite side, up into the region of the frontal process of the maxilla. When the limited augmentation is to be done, about 2 to 3 g of hydroxylapatite are used on each side, as opposed to 4 to 6 g for the extended augmentations.

The limited approach is achieved through two vestibular incisions. On each side a diagonal incision is made from the piriform rim area in the depth of the vestibule down to the level of the attached gingiva in the canine region. This incision is carried directly down to bone. The anterior maxilla is then subperiosteally exposed so that the surgeon can visualize the piriform rim of the nose medially and extended superiorly and laterally by the desired amount (Figure 70-7). The augmentational material is perhaps most easily delivered by means of the syringe technique. About

2 to 3 g of nonresorbable hydroxylapatite is mixed with sterile saline and a collagen hemostatic and placed into a 3 cc syringe that has had the delivery end cut off.[13] Closure is performed with running 3-0 chromic horizontal mattress sutures. No dressings are placed. Gentle external massage is done to ensure symmetry.

For the extended augmentation approach, a standard horizontal incision is made in the depth of the maxillary vestibule from the second premolar area on one side to the same area on the opposite side. This incision is carried directly down to bone, and the entire anterior maxilla is exposed subperiosteally. The exposure *extends posteriorly only to the anterior aspect of the zygomatic alveolar crest,* then superiorly to expose the infraorbital nerve and medially above the nerve onto the infraorbital rim. The lateral and inferior region of the bony piriform rim is exposed including the anterior nasal spine. The periosteum in this region is carefully mobilized over the piriform rim and into the nasal cavity for about 5 mm. In this phase of the subperiosteal dissection, care is exercised not to tear the periosteum and enter the nasal cavity. When this occurs it is best to suture this communication to avoid possible postoperative infection.

Before augmentation, sutures are placed to control the alar base width. A hole is drilled in the anterior nasal spine. Depending on the *predetermined esthetic desires* for alar base width changes, these sutures are variably tightened to control the alar base width at its presurgical width, permit it to widen, or allow it to somewhat narrow. This latter objective is seldom indicated in this condition because the alar base width is most often narrow, and the patient generally benefits from some controlled degree of alar base widening. However, when this area is not controlled with alar base retention sutures as described, *it widens unpredictably* and often excessively. Two separate 2-0 slowly resorbable sutures are placed through a single hole drilled

through the anterior nasal spine region. Next, the upper lip is grasped, and the forefinger is placed facially, precisely over the inferior alar rim while the lip vestibule is retracted with the intraorally placed thumb. With toothed forceps the area in the vestibular incision directly adjacent to the everted alar rim is firmly grasped. This tissue is a combination of the fibroareolar extension of the lower lateral cartilage and the lateral nasalis muscle; occasionally, a small sesamoid accessory of cartilaginous component is noted (Figure 70-8). When *the proper tissue is grasped* and the lip released from the fingers while maintaining the tissue grasped with forceps, the alar base is readily advanced medially toward the columella; the alar base is then observed and measured facially. Sometimes several attempts at grasping the proper tissue with the forceps must be made to identify the tissue that permits virtually unrestricted medial movement of the alar base. For the alar base cinch procedure to be effective, the proper tissue in this area must be identified bilaterally to effect symmetric control of the alar bases.

Once the proper tissue is identified, while it is maintained in the forceps, a Burnell or figure-of-eight tendon-type suture is placed with a 2-0 polyfilament slowly absorbable suture. A separate suture is passed through each side first and the needle left attached to the suture (Figure 70-9). Then each needle is passed

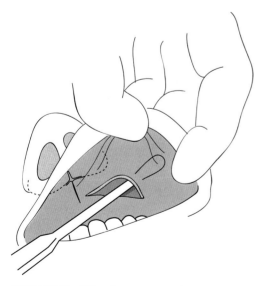

FIGURE 70-7 *When less augmentation is necessary, the limited incision approach is used. Adapted from Epker BN.[19] p. 126.*

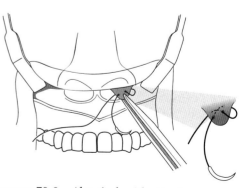

FIGURE 70-8 *Alar cinch with attention to proper tissue selection and suture technique. Adapted from Epker BN.[19] p. 123.*

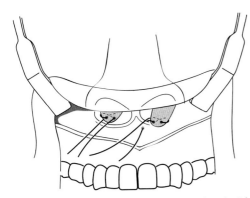

FIGURE 70-9   *Independent suturing of each side to anterior nasal spine. Adapted from Epker BN.*[19] *p. 124.*

through the hole placed in the anterior nasal spine. These sutures are later tied after the actual augmentation.

The skeletal nasal base augmentation is performed with a nonabsorbable mixture of particulate hydroxylapatite and a hemostatic collagen preparation, moistened with sterile saline. Only enough collagen hemostatic material is used to form a dough mass that does not flow.

Generally, between 8 and 12 g of hydroxylapatite are used in the extended approach, depending on the relative severity of the skeletal nasal base deficiency. The mixture is separated into two equal portions so that equal augmentation is attained on both sides. After placement, it is molded with a periosteal elevator to conform it to the underlying bone. Most often this material is extended superiorly to the infraorbital nerve and often more medially to the infraorbital rim. Care is taken not to place much of the material into the region of the frontal process of the maxilla because this unesthetically widens the nose. Once the implants are placed bilaterally, equally and symmetrically adapted, and contoured to create facial symmetry, the incision is closed.

First, the alar base sutures are tied. Each suture is independently hand tied while that side's alar base width is observed (measured) facially. As a general principle, the alar base should be narrowed 2 mm more than desired because some widening tends to occur postopera-

tively. Next, the vestibular incision is closed with deliberate attention to control of the upper lip fullness and the amount of exposed vermilion. Often, after the alar base cinch sutures are tied, the labial mucosa is somewhat tethered superiorly and must be undermined in the region of the alar base cinch suture. This is important to avoid reduction of the upper lip's vermilion exposure with the subsequent vestibular closure.

When there is no desire to alter the preexisting upper lip esthetics, the mucosal portion of the incision is closed in the usual V-Y fashion, with the vertical extent of the Y being about 10 to 15 mm. This basically avoids reduction in exposure of the upper lip vermilion (Figure 70-10).

More often, it is desirable to increase the exposure of the upper lip vermilion, especially when the preoperative lip has gullwing characteristics. In these instances an extended closure is done, requiring extensive undermining of the upper lip mucosa. While the lip is retracted with a single skin hook placed precisely in the midline and with a retractor placed laterally, undermining of the lip mucosa is performed with small scissors. The extent of the mucosal undermining is determined by the desired esthetic changes in the upper lip. When maximal increased exposure of the upper lip vermilion is wanted, as is the case with a gullwing upper lip appearance, extensive undermining is achieved anteriorly almost to the wet line of the lip and an equivalent amount posteriorly. When this undermining is completed, it is critical that the surgeon be able to pass the scissors freely from one side to the other, demonstrating a continuous pocket. Next, the horizontal vestibular limbs are closed with interrupted or continuous 45° angled sutures to reduce tension and further advance the mucosa.

When the extensive mucosal undermining is done with a V-Y closure, a dental cotton roll coated with an antibiotic ointment is inserted into the depth of the

labial vestibule in the midline, and tape is placed tightly over the lip to maintain pressure. The tape is extended inferiorly over the lip mucosa. When this is not done, considerable lymphedema occurs in the midline of the upper lip. The cotton roll and tape dressing are left in place for 48 hours and then removed. Similarly, layered tape dressings are applied to the paranasal regions and maintained for 48 hours. Cold is applied to the face during this time.

After surgery and the removal of the dressing, the patient must maintain a liquid to very soft diet for 7 to 10 days until the vestibular incision is well healed. After 3 to 4 days he or she is instructed to begin forceful lip exercises to further reduce edema. At this time, when the edema is resolving, the surgeon gently palpates the paranasal areas to ensure symmetry. The implanted material can be gently molded for about 5 to 7 days before it assumes a solid state without flow properties.

The limited exposure approach is done primarily to reduce mild paranasal depressions (Figure 70-11). The extended procedure produces esthetic changes consistent with improved frontal face esthetics,

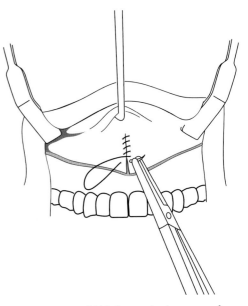

FIGURE 70-10   *V-Y closure is done to enhance exposure of upper lip vermilion. Adapted from Epker BN.*[19] *p. 127.*

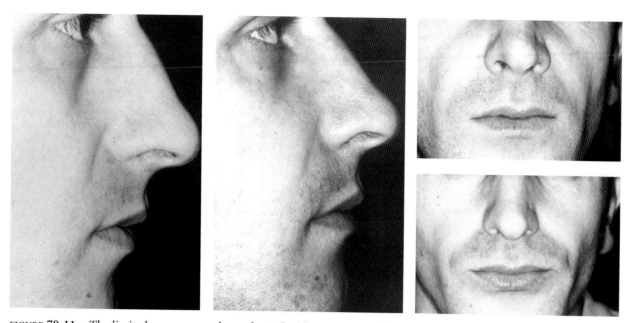

FIGURE 70-11   *The limited exposure can be performed without significant effects on the nose or upper lip.*

including improved upper lip fullness, increased exposure of the upper lip vermilion, improved balance of the alar base width with the remainder of the facial features, and decreased prominence of the nasolabial folds. In profile the concave-to-flat paranasal region becomes normally convex. Prominence of the nose is decreased, nasal tip projection is improved, often with the creation of a supratip break, and some cephalic rotation of the nasal tip is achieved (Figure 70-12). This extended procedure is frequently used with other skeletal/soft tissue cosmetic maxillofacial procedures, especially rhinoplasty.

The Cheek

Esthetic cheek augmentation may be indicated as an isolated esthetic maxillofacial surgical procedure or be performed in concert with other skeletal/soft tissue facial esthetic surgeries.[26–35] As with the other procedures discussed in this chapter, this statement implies that the patient both *possesses* the deformity (albeit to highly variable degrees) and *desires* enhancement. Moreover, it must be appreciated that three patients with the same degree of anatomic deformity may each desire different degrees of augmentation, much the same as occurs with breast augmentation.

Esthetic cheek augmentation is indicated in individuals who frontally exhibit poor lateral cheek projection (bizygomatic width) in relation to the bigonial and bitemporal widths. Many such patients *appear* to exhibit vertically long faces, even though they do not possess any of the

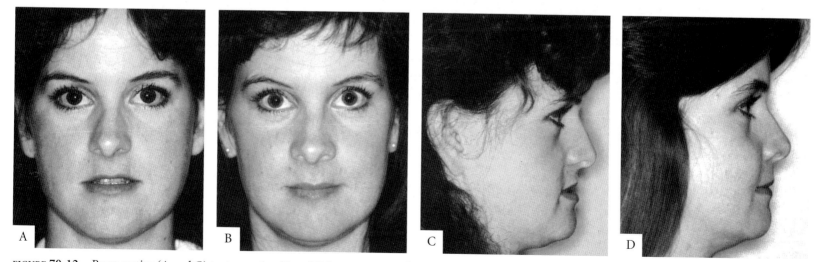

FIGURE 70-12   *Preoperative (A and C) postoperative (B and D) appearances after an extended approach with an alar cinch and a V-Y augmentation of the upper lip. Reproduced with permission from Epker BN.[19] p. 130–1.*

objective criteria of the long-face syndrome. This is because of the abnormal facial length-to-width relationships caused by the abnormal narrow bizygomatic width. Similarly, poor cheek projection is noted in the three-quarter oblique view. In profile these same individuals possess variable degrees of inadequate cheek and/or lateral infraorbital rim projection.[19,25]

A detailed systematic esthetic examination of this area is performed because the evaluation of this area of the face must be multidirectional. Esthetic judgments made exclusively from a single view are incomplete with respect to the specificity of the deficiency.

Frontally the area of maximum cheek prominence is located about 10 mm lateral and 15 mm to 20 mm inferior to the lateral canthus. The cheek prominence is positioned more laterally than the mandibular angle. The bizygomatic width of the esthetically attractive face is the widest dimension of the face, with the bitemporal width and bigonial widths following. Silver has defined a malar prominence triangle, which very closely locates the malar prominence to this same location.[26]

From the profile perspective, the cheek prominence and infraorbital rim in the esthetically attractive individual are situated so that the infraorbital rim is about equally projected with the anteriormost projection of the globe, and the cheek prominence is located several millimeters anterior to the globe. This relationship results in the cheek area being *clearly convex* in its configuration, as opposed to flat or concave.

Most analyses of the malar prominence that have been described in the literature are from the three-quarters view. These include Hinderer's, Wilkinson's, Powell and colleagues', and Prendergast and Schoenrock's methods.[36–39] These methods result in highly variable ideal locations for the malar prominence, both vertically and laterally. Specifically, Hinderer's method is too nonspecific, Wilkin-

son's locates the prominence quite inferiorly, and Prendergast and Schoenrock's locates it medially. Powell and colleagues' analysis is comparable with the frontal view values recommended by the author. In the three-quarters oblique esthetic assessment, the esthetically attractive contralateral cheek prominence extends well beyond a line from the lateral commissure of the mouth to the lateral canthus. Its most prominent location is about 15 to 20 mm beneath the lateral canthus.

The basal view simply supplements the findings from the other perspectives and also reveals both the true lateral and, to a lesser degree, anterior projections of the cheeks. This view is important to best determine the symmetry of the cheeks.

The surgeon must not only evaluate the cheek prominence proper but also the buccal area because excessive fullness in the buccal region can lead the surgeon to the erroneous *impression* that cheek deficiency exists. When cheek deficiency and buccal fullness coexist, the surgeon must exercise caution with respect to whether and how much cheek augmentation versus buccal fat pad reduction is to be performed.

A mark is made on the face in the ideal region of the cheek eminence, 10 mm lateral and 15 to 20 mm inferior to the lateral canthus. This mark aids in the proper superoinferior and lateral positioning of the cheek implant. Similarly, it helps in *predetermining* the desired lateral and anteroposterior thickness of the cheek augmentation. It is important to create a gentle convex surface curvature beginning in the infraorbital area and extending inferiorly 15 to 20 mm. In concert with this marking, a tangent from the soft tissue gonial angle to this region is constructed with a ruler to "estimate" the desired lateral projection as determined by the criteria previously discussed.

The procedure can be readily performed under either general anesthesia supplemented with a local anesthetic with 1:200,000 epinephrine, or local

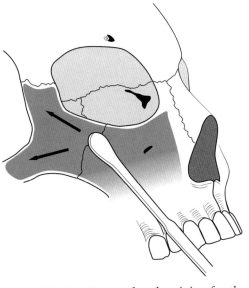

FIGURE 70-13 *Extent of undermining for the placement of a cheek implant. Adapted from Epker BN.[19] p. 147.*

anesthesia and sedation. About 10 minutes before surgery the infraorbital nerves are blocked bilaterally with a few cubic centimeters of 2% lidocaine with 1:200,000 epinephrine. A few minutes later the entire maxillary vestibule is infiltrated transorally with approximately 10 cc of the same agent, from the zygomatic-alveolar crest area on one side to the same area on the opposite side. In addition, the subperiosteal dissection extends laterally along the zygomatic arch.

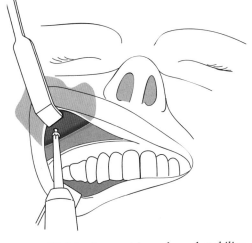

FIGURE 70-14 *Symmetric and good stabilization of the right and left cheek implants is best achieved with screw fixation. Adapted from Epker BN.[19] p. 152.*

A horizontal vestibular incision is made with diathermy in the depth of the vestibule from the canine region distally to that of the molars. This incision is carried tangentially down to bone, and the entire malar area is sequentially exposed subperiosteally. This exposure extends superiorly to the infraorbital nerve and then medially above the nerve to expose the infraorbital rim. Next, the superior and lateral extents of this subperiosteal dissection are completed. Superiorly, lateral to the infraorbital nerve, the lateral infraorbital rim is exposed. The subperiosteal dissection is then extended along the lateral aspect of the zygomatic arch posteriorly. The dissection must be liberal enough to create an adequate "pocket" into which the implant can be placed *passively* (Figure 70-13).

Once the subperiosteal dissection is completed, the predetermined desired size and shape of the implant is adapted for a try-in. Currently a large number of different-shaped cheek implants exist, constructed from various materials. Moreover, variable techniques and even locations for their placement are espoused. I currently prefer porous polyethylene implants because they do not have complete memory, are readily modifiable at surgery, are porous (resulting in tissue ingrowth and self-stabilization), and are able to be optimally molded after heating in sterile hot saline. When porous polyethylene is used, it is vacuum impregnated with an antibiotic as described above. Careful adaptation of the preformed implants is necessary to obtain optimal results.

After initial trial the implant is revised with a surgical blade and/or heating to mold it to the underlying bone. The need for any additional adjustments

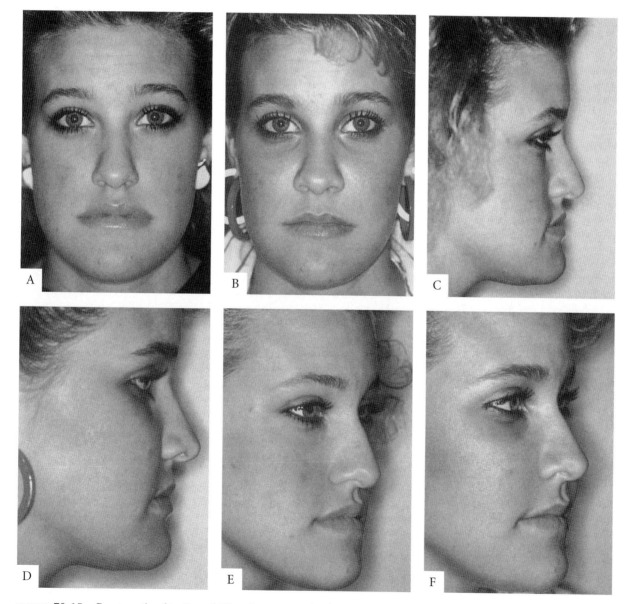

FIGURE **70-15** *Preoperative (A, C, and E) and postoperative (B, D, and F) appearances of a patient who underwent a cheek augmentation. Reproduced with permission from Epker BN.[19] p. 156–7.*

is determined at this time while the implant is held in its proper position, visualized through the incision, and facially palpated.

After the final adjustments are completed on the first side, the contralateral implant is modified to be a mirror image so that perfect right-to-left symmetry is achieved, unless the patient possesses some asymmetry. The identical vestibular incision and subperiosteal dissection is then carried out on the opposite side.

The implants are then both rinsed in the antibiotic solution, placed carefully into their proper location, and stabilized with one or two titanium screws. It is essential that the positioning and stabilization of the right and left cheek implants be precisely symmetric and that they exhibit no tendency to rotate or displace. If either of the latter is evident on one or both sides, a second screw is placed to prevent this movement (Figure 70-14).

Any asymmetry or instability of one or both implants at the termination of surgery will become clinically evident after resolution of the edema following surgery; *this is the most frequent cause for postoperative patient concern after this procedure.*

The vestibular incision is closed with a single-layered 3-0 plain horizontal mattress gut suture. A layered tape dressing is applied for 48 hours. After removal of the dressing the patient maintains a liquid to very soft diet for 7 to 10 days until the vestibular incisions are well healed. After complete healing of the vestibular incisions, the patient is instructed to begin vigorous lip exercises to expedite resolution of residual edema and to improve natural lip motion.

This procedure may be performed independently or in concert with other skeletal/soft tissue esthetic maxillofacial procedures as described in the introductory section of this chapter. The results obtained with this procedure can be predictable and esthetically impressive (Figure 70-15).

Summary

Alloplastic facial augmentation has become a standard of care. Careful preoperative detailed systematic esthetic evaluations permit the various areas of the face to be augmented precisely.

References

1. Yaremchuk MJ, Rubin JP, Posnick JC, et al. Implantable materials in facial aesthetic and reconstructive surgery: biocompatibility and clinical application. J Craniofac Surg 1996;7:473–84.

2. Rubin JP, Yaremchuk MJ. Complications and toxicities of implantable biomaterials used in facial reconstructive and aesthetic surgery; a comprehensive review of the literature. Plast Reconstr Surg 1997;100:1336–45.

3. Silver FH, Maas CS. Biology of synthetic facial implant materials. Facial Plastic Surg Clin North Am 1994;2:241–53.

4. Singh S, Baker JL. Use of expanded tetraflouroethylene in aesthetic surgery of the face. Clin Plast Surg 2000;27:579–93.

5. Levine B, Berman WE. The current status of expanded polytetraflouroethylene (Gore-Tex) in facial plastic surgery. Ear Nose Throat J 1995;74:681–84.

6. Frodel JL, Lee S. The use of high-density polyethylene implants in facial deformities. Arch Otolaryngol Head Neck Surg 1998;124:1219–23.

7. Spector M, Flemming WR, Sauer BW, et al. Early tissue infiltrate in porous polyethylene implants into bone: a scanning EM study. J Biomed Mater Res 1975;9:537–45.

8. Wellisz T, et al. Characteristics of tissue response to MedPor porous polyethylene implants in the human face. J Long-Term Effects MedPor Implant 1993;3:223–35.

9. Karras SC, Wolford LM. Augmentation genioplasty with hard tissue replacement implants. J Oral Maxillofac Surg 1998;56:549–52.

10. Pearson DC, Sherris DA. Resorption beneath Silastic mandibular implants. Arch Otolaryngol Head Neck Surg 1999;1:261–4.

11. Vuyk HD. Augmentation mentoplasty with solid silicone. Clin Otolaryngol 1996;21:106–18.

12. Perrotti JD, Castor SA, Perez PC, Zins JE. Antibiotic use in esthetic surgery: a national survey and literature review. Plast Reconst Surg 2002;15:1685–93.

13. Holz G, Novotny-Lenhard J, Kinzig M, Soergel F. Single dose antibiotic prophylaxis in maxillofacial surgery. Chemotherapy 1994;40:65–9.

14. Sylaidas P. Postoperative infection following clean facial surgery. Clin Plast Surg 1997;39:341–5.

15. Shaber EP. Vertical interpositional augmentation genioplasty with porous polyethylene. Int J Oral Maxillofac Surg 1987;16:678–84.

16. Zeller SD, Hiatt WR, Moore DL, Fain DW. Use of preform hydroxylapatite blocks for grafting in genioplasty procedures. Int J Oral Maxillofac Surg 1986;15:665–8.

17. Choe KS, Stucki-McCormick SV. Chin augmentation. Facial Plastic Surg Clin North Am 2000;16:45–54.

18. Scaccia FJ, Allphine AL, Stepmick DW, et al. Complications of augmentation mentoplasty. A review of 11,095 cases. Int J Aesth Rest Surg 1983;1:3–8.

19. Epker BN. Esthetic maxillofacial surgery. Philadelphia: Lea & Febiger; 1994.

20. Themistocles G, Salvatore MA, Sotereanos GC, et al. Alloplastic augmentation of the mandible angle. J Oral Maxillofac Surg 1996;54:1417–23.

21. Ousterhout DK. Mandibular angle augmentation and reduction. Clin Plast Surg 1991; 18:153–9.

22. Alache AE. Mandibular angle implants. Aesthet Plast Surg 1992;16:349–54.

23. Bikhazi HB, Antwerp RV. The use of Medpor in cosmetic and reconstructive surgery: experimental and clinical evidence. Plast Reconstr Surg 1990;6:271–33.

24. Epker BN, Fish LC, Stella, J, et al. Dentofacial deformities: an integrated orthodontic-surgical approach. St. Louis: D.V. Mosby Co; 1998.

25. Epker BN. Correction of the skeletal nasal base in rhinoplasty. J Oral Maxillofac Surg 1991;49:938–43.

26. Silver WE. The use of alloplastic materials in contouring the face. Facial Plast Surg 1986;3:81–98.

27. Binder WJ. Submalar augmentation. An alternative to face-lift surgery. Arch Otolaryngol Head Neck Surg 1989;115:797–803.

28. Brennan GH. Augmentation malarplasty. Arch Otolaryngol Head Neck Surg 1982; 108:441–5.

29. Giampapa VG. Aesthtic recontouring of the midfacial skeleton: a regional approach. Am J Cosmet Surg 1988;4:583–8.

30. Marble HB Jr, Alexander JM. A precise technique for restoration of bony facial contour deficiencies with silicone rubber implants: report of cases. J Oral Surg 1972;30:737–41.

31. O'Quinn B, Thomas JR. The role of Silastic in malar augmentation. Facial Plast Surg 1986;3:99–105.

32. Tobin HA. Malar augmentation as an adjunct

to facial cosmetic surgery. Am J Cosmet Surg 1986;3:3–13.

33. Whitaker L. Aesthetic augmentation of the malar-midface structures. Plast Reconstr Surg 1987;80:337–44.

34. Mladick RA. Alloplastic cheek augmentation. Clin Plast Surg 1991;18:29–38.

35. Robiony M, Costa F, Demitri V, Politi M. Simultaneous malaroplasty with porous polyethylene implants and orthognathic surgery for correction of malar deficiency. J Oral Maxillofac Surg 1998;56:734–41.

36. Hinderer UT. Malar implants for improvement of facial appearance. Plast Reconstr Surg 1975;56:157–65.

37. Wilkinson TS. Complications in esthetic malar augmentation. Plast Reconstr Surg 1983; 71:643–7.

38. Powell NB, Riley RW, Laub DR. A new approach to evaluation and surgery on the malar complex. Ann Plast Surg 1988;20:206–14.

39. Prendergast M, Schoenrock LD. Malar augmentation. Arch Otolaryngol Head Neck Surg 1989;115:964–9.

CHAPTER 71

Otoplastic Surgery for the Protruding Ear

Todd G. Owsley, DDS, MD

Auricular deformities, in particular prominent or protruding ears, are a common congenital anomaly, affecting nearly 5 % of the Caucasian population.[1] Congenital in nature, children are most likely to suffer the consequences of the deformity in the form of ridicule by their peers. Protruding ears, commonly referred to as prominauris, can be predictably treated for children prior to entering grade school, and thus help the children avoid the emotional trauma caused from the ridicule. Otoplastic surgery is primarily performed on children and can be a valuable service for the patient and satisfying for the surgeon.

It is important for the surgeon to understand the history of various surgical techniques to develop a predictable and successful technique to address the problem of protruding ears. Dieffenbach (1845) is credited with the first otoplastic technique to correct a prominent auricle.[2] Ely, in 1881, authored the first case report describing correction of prominent ears in a 12-year-old boy who was being teased at school.[3] Since that report, over 180 surgical techniques have been described in the literature for the correction of protruding ears.

When clinically evaluating the facial complex, the ears are often overlooked. If protruding ears are present, reduction otoplasty as an adjunctive or isolated procedure can be performed predictably

and often with satisfying results. A thorough understanding of the embryology and development of the human auricle along with the resultant external anatomy of the ear are of paramount importance in developing a predictable and stable technique to deal with the common auricular deformities.

Embryology of the Auricle

Malformations of the auricle are common, occurring in 1 out of 12,500 births.[4] They can occur alone or in combination with a syndrome affecting the head and neck structures. The embryogenesis of the auricle exemplifies in miniature the precise and logical progression so characteristic of the developing human form. The external ear development during the third to twelfth weeks of embryonic life is complex. The precursors to the auricle present in days 36 to 38 of intrauterine life, developing first from the first branchial groove where the first (mandibular) and second (hyoid) branchial arches are present (Figure 71-1). Both arches give rise to the auricular hillocks often referred to as the auricular tubercles of His.[4] Numbers 1, 2, and 3 arise from the caudal border of the mandibular arch, while numbers 4, 5, and 6 are formed from the cephalic border of the hyoid arch. The auricular hillocks present in their most prominent and characteristic form by

intrauterine day 41. During this same stage, the groove between the mandibular and hyoid arches (hyomandibular groove) widens and deepens by the increased growth of the hillocks. This groove eventually forms the external auditory canal and concha. By day 43 to 45, the hillocks have migrated and coalesced to form the auricle.[4] During this union, the mesenchyme of the hyoid arch increases substantially relative to the mandibular arch to contribute 85% of the external adult ear. Hillocks 2 and 3 from the mandibular arch lose their individuality and fuse to form the helical crus. Later, hillocks 4 and 5 from the hyoid arch merge and alter their configuration as they give rise to the helix and antihelical fold. Hillock 1 remains prominent and becomes the tragus, and hillock 6 becomes the antitragus.[4]

Surgical Anatomy

The majority of the growth of the pinna is completed by an early age. The average child has 85% ear development by 3 years of age. The ear is nearly fully grown by the age of 7 to 8 years. The ear height continues to grow into adulthood, but the width and distance of the ear from the scalp changes little after 10 years of age. It is important to note that each individual's ears often vary in size and shape.[5] The average adult ear is approximately 6.5 cm

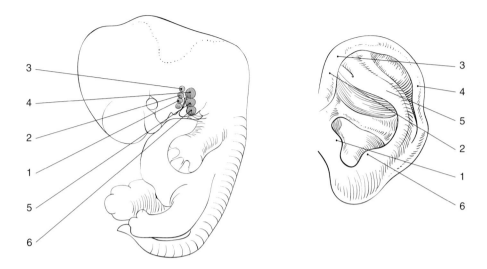

FIGURE 71-1 *Development of the auricle from the first and second branchial arches. The numbers cin the left diagram correspond with the structures in the right diagram. Adapted from Owsley T. Otoplastic surgery for the protruding ear. In: Fonseca RJ, editor. Oral and maxillofacial surgery. Vol. 6. Philadelphia (PA): W.B. Saunders; 2000. p. 408-18.*

in length and 3.5 cm in width. In the normal ear, the auricle lies between horizontal lines drawn from the upper rim of the orbit and the nasal spine. The normal posterior wall of the conchal bowl is set at an angle of approximately 90° to the mastoid.[6] A second 90° angle is formed as the antihelical fold and is called the scapha-conchal angle. These two angles in combination with the curvature of the helix set the auricle adjacent to the scalp at approximately 25 to 35° and is called the auriculocephalic angle (Figure 71-2).[7] In otoplastic surgery, when correcting prominent ears, there are three important anatomical pearls that can be used intraoperatively to assess the final result. The helical rim should be seen just lateral to the most lateral presence of the antihelix from the frontal view. The distance measured between the helical rim and the mastoid area is slightly less than 2 cm. Finally, the distance between the skull and the uppermost aspect of the helix is approximately 1 cm (Figure 71–3A and B).

The auricular cartilage is a unique and delicate structure that is intricately shaped with multiple elevations and depressions providing both skeletal support and form to the adult ear. The cartilage of the auricle is a single piece of yellow (elastic) fibrocartilage with a complicated relief on the anterior, concave side and a smooth, posterior convex side. Cartilage thickness is fairly uniform throughout. The cartilage is covered on both surfaces by a thin, firm, adherent layer of perichondrium. The anterior lateral surface of the cartilage is covered with a fine, thin skin, closely adherent to the cartilaginous framework. Subcutaneous fat is practically nonexistent, but a diffuse subdermal vascular plane exists which supports flap viability.[8] The posterior surface of the cartilage framework is draped with a less adherent skin that contains two layers of fat and a larger subdermal plexus of arteries, veins, and nerves.

A helical border terminates anteriorly in a crus, commonly called the radix, which lies almost horizontally above the external auditory meatus. The antihelix crowning the posterior conchal wall separates and diverges into both a superior and anterior crus enclosing the triangularis fossa. Between the helix and the antihelix lies a long, deep furrow called the scaphoid fossa. The conchal cavity, composed of the cymba (superior) and cavum (inferior) concha, arises from the floor, which is

approximately 8 mm deeper than the overlying tragus and antitragus. The inferior tip of the helical cartilage is referred to as the cauda or tail. Extending from this inferiorly is the lobule, hanging devoid of skeleton (Figure 71-4A and B).

Blood Supply

The arterial blood supply to the ear is derived principally from two main branches of the external carotid artery: superficial temporal artery and posterior auricular artery. The superficial temporal artery emerges from the parotid capsule, 1 cm in front of the ear deep to the veins and below the anterior auricular muscle. It gives off the superior, medial, and inferior branches supplying the anterior and anterolateral surface of the auricle (Figure 71-5A). The posterior surface is dominantly supplied by the posterior auricular artery which travels parallel to the postauricular crease upwards crossing below the great auricular nerve and under the posterior auricular muscle. Awareness of this relationship is important to avoid damage to the artery or nerve during surgery. The posterior auricular artery gives off three

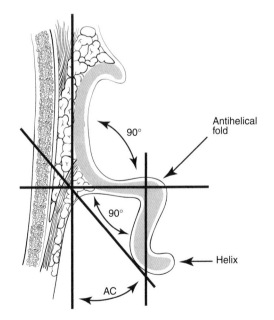

FIGURE 71-2 *An axial section at the level of the helical crus demonstrates the ideal auriculocephalic angle (AC) of 30°. Adapted from Tanzer RC.[20]*

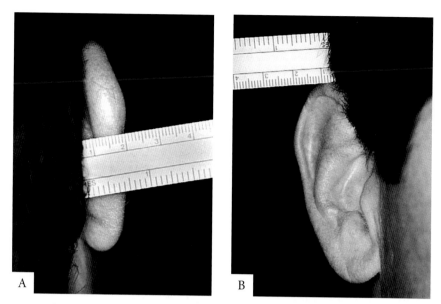

FIGURE 71-3   A, B, *Anatomic "pearls," useful intraoperatively. Reproduced with permission from Owsley T. Otoplastic surgery for the protruding ear. In: Fonseca RJ, editor. Oral and maxillofacial surgery. Vol. 6. Philadelphia (PA): W.B. Saunders; 2000. p. 408–18.*

branches: superior, medial, and inferior, providing a greater volume of blood to the postauricular ear than its anterior counterparts. These same vessels perforate the auricular cartilage over a large surface of the anterior ear and anastomose with the branches of the superficial temporal artery. The external ears have a tremendous blood supply, allowing multiple surgical approaches or salvage of the ear following traumatic avulsion.

Venous drainage of the ear via the complementary veins is into the external jugular vein. Lymphatic drainage is into three surrounding areas via the complex and extensive fine network of lymphatic vessels.

Nerve Supply

The sensory nerve supply is primarily from the anterior and posterior branches of the great auricular nerve. The nerve is an important surgical landmark traveling 8 mm posterior to the postauricular crease. When dissecting in this area, care must be taken to avoid damage to the nerve which can result in near complete anesthesia to the ear. Less important contributions of sensation are made by the auriculotemporal and lesser occipital

nerves to the conchal cavity and external auditory meatus (Figure 71-5B). Regional anesthesia of the auricle is readily accomplished by instilling anesthetic solution along its base anteriorly and posteriorly. Supplemental anesthesia may be needed at the posterior wall of the external auditory meatus supplied by the auricular branches of the vagus nerve (Arnold's nerve).

Deformities

Ear deformities are common and variable due to the complex embryologic

engineering that takes place in the development of the auricle as described previously. Many classification systems of ear deformities have been attempted. Tanzer classifies congenital ear defects, correlating embryologic development with a surgical approach for correction of the deformity.[9] Marx has a well accepted classification system subdividing microtia into three groups according to severity.[10] Rogers simplifies classification of congenital ear defects, dividing them into four groups according to various stages of arrested development: microtia, lop ear, cup ear, and protruding ear.[6] In this chapter addressing the prominent ear, the term *protruding* is used as a general term to refer to any ear that is more prominent than is considered "normal." It is beyond the scope of this chapter to classify other congenital abnormalities and their correction.

Protruding Ear

In patients with protruding ears, there are two major deformities that individually or in combination account for the majority of the abnormalities. There are several lesser deformities seen that can accentuate the abnormality as well. The most common seen is a poorly developed antihelical fold which can involve both the superior and anterior crura. This eliminates a defi-

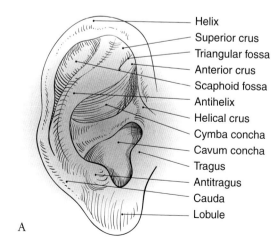

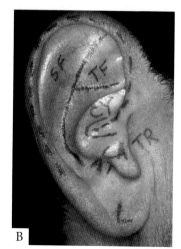

FIGURE 71-4   A, B, *Anatomy of the external ear.*

Labels for Figure 71-4 A:
Helix
Superior crus
Triangular fossa
Anterior crus
Scaphoid fossa
Antihelix
Helical crus
Cymba concha
Cavum concha
Tragus
Antitragus
Cauda
Lobule

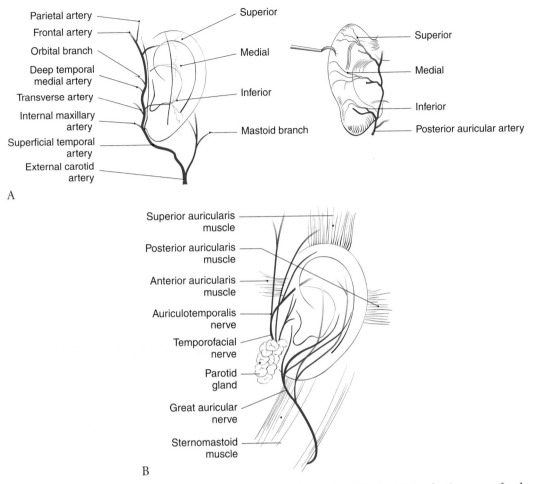

FIGURE 71-5   A, *Arterial blood supply.* B, *Nerve supply. Adapted from Owsley T. Otoplastic surgery for the protruding ear. In: Fonseca RJ, editor. Oral and maxillofacial surgery. Vol. 6. Philadelphia (PA): WB Saunders; 2000. p. 408–18.*

nition between the conchal cavity and scapha resulting in the lateral projection of the upper portion of the helix. The second abnormality seen is the formation of excessive conchal cartilage, in particular the posterior conchal wall. This causes significant protrusion of the auricle. It is not uncommon to recognize some degree of both abnormalities present producing the protruding auricle.

Other potential deformities are a protruding earlobe, irregularities along the helix including an unrolled margin of the helical rim and more recently described an anteriomedially displaced insertion of the postauricular muscle. Of importance, this deformity is often bilateral and can be associated with ossicular deformities and a hearing deficit. [11]

Obviously, precise recognition of the cause or causes of the protruding ear is crucial in formulating the surgical technique to be employed in correction of the abnormality.

Surgical Correction

Perhaps the most important indication for surgical correction of prominent ears is to eliminate the psychosocial effects that the ear defect produces. Macgregor and others have well documented the irreversible social and psychological consequences that facial anomalies, especially the ears, can inflict. [12] The ridicule by peers begins as early as age 4 to 5 years during development, described as the body image concept. This leads to problems with social adjustment, self-image

deficit, and ultimately behavioral disorders. Therefore, most patients present at an early age for surgical correction. Most surgeons agree that surgical correction of the ear can be performed safely between 4 years of age and the beginning of school attendance to avoid the ridicule, becoming one of the most common elective procedures performed in young children. Adults also present to correct a lifelong cosmetic defect.

Surgical Techniques

Many otoplasty techniques described in the surgical literature are similar and have evolved over an 80-year experience. Many techniques only address the conchal hypertrophy without mention of the antihelical fold. The described techniques generally can be subdivided into a "suture-only" technique, cartilage splitting or weakening technique, or a combination of the two.

Furnas (1968) described his suture-only technique for the correction of the prominent ear deformity. [13] This technique consisted of a postauricular approach, removing the skin, connective tissue, and vestigial posterior auricular muscle and its ligament down to the underlying mastoid fascia. A total of 2 to 3 nonresorbable sutures are placed through conchal cartilage and mastoid fascia and tightened to the new desired retracted position of the ears. This remains a commonly used technique to set back the ears in patients with conchal hypertrophy alone. Problems associated with this technique have been relapse secondary to the cartilaginous memory, a shallow conchal bowl, and irregularities created in folding the conchal floor. Another difficult problem seen is displacing the conchal bowl anteriorly, creating narrowing of the external auditory canal.

The Converse-Wood-Smith technique is used to correct and create an antihelical fold using a cartilage cutting and suture method. [14] Several full thickness cuts through cartilage are placed in the scaphoid fossa. The cartilage is then folded on itself, described as "tubing," and permanent horizontal mattress sutures are placed forming the new antihelical fold. Additionally, if excessive conchal cartilage is present, it can be addressed with a cartilage incision added at the rim of the bowl to reduce the bowl and retract the ear. A new antihelical fold is formed, however, typically with sharp cartilaginous ridges seen through the thin anterior auricular skin.

This chapter will describe two techniques that address the two fundamental abnormalities in protruding ears and have produced consistent, satisfying cosmetic results, and have essentially eliminated the fear of relapse. The Davis method addresses the protruding ear caused by a hypertrophic posterior wall of the conchal bowl. The Mustarde method is used to create a new antihelical fold (Figure 71-6).

The refinement of other abnormalities such as the prominent earlobe will also be discussed.

Davis Method

The Davis method, for the correction of conchal hypertrophy, is a cartilage excision technique performed in a step-wise fashion.[8,15]

1. Marking the cartilage excision: Initially, the area of cartilage to be removed is marked on the skin of the anterior surface of the conchal bowl. Methylene blue transfixion tattoos are preferred and demonstrated to mark the posterior surface of the conchal cavity. The line lies just below the lower crus border, carries forward into the cymbal fossa, and continues around as an "arrowhead" to preserve a well-defined, helical radix. The tracing should continue forward against the posterior edge of the external auditory canal. From that location, it curves posteriorly

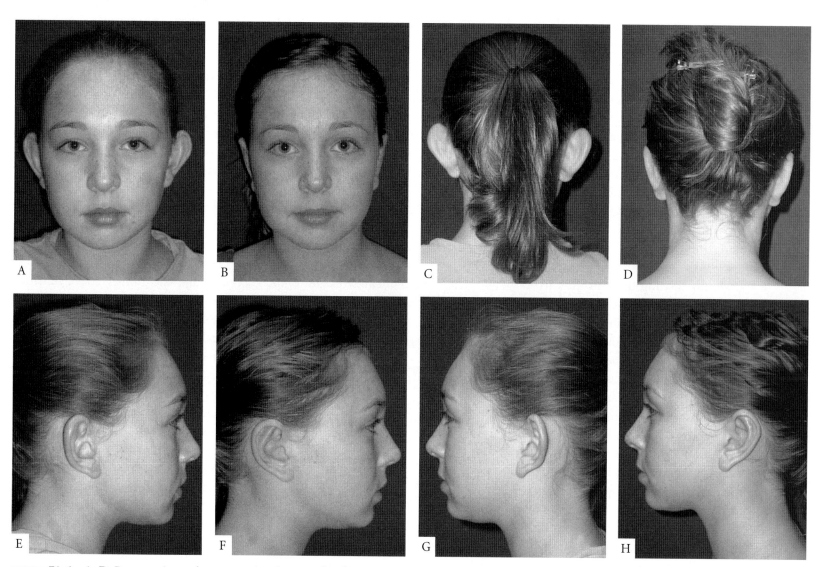

FIGURE 71-6   A–D, *Preoperative and postoperative photographs of an 11-year-old girl who presented for correction of protruding ears. Her diagnosis was a combination of conchal hypertrophy and lack of antihelical fold formation bilaterally. The Davis and Mustarde techniques were used on both ears. E–H, Lateral views of both ears demonstrating a natural-appearing, new antihelical fold and a deepened conchal bowl.*

into the cavum concha, continuing onto the posterior conchal wall, leaving 8 mm of posterior conchal wall height measured from the conchal scaphal junction. This should complete the circle which should appear "kidney bean" shaped including the entire conchal bowl. The exact height of the posterior wall is important and must be measured for each case individually (Figure 71-7A–C).

2. Removal of skin and cartilage: Prior to beginning the actual surgical procedure, local anesthesia is used for hydrodissection of the tightly adhered anterior auricular skin along the conchal bowl. This simplifies the dissection of cartilage from the overlying skin. The concha is exposed through a postauricular elliptical skin excision. The width of the ellipse is only to remove the predicted excess skin that is produced with ear retropositioning. The closure of the incision should be passive. This area is predisposed to hypertrophic or keloidal scarring when closed under tension. Once having removed the postauricular skin, the conchal cartilage is visualized along with the previously placed tattoo marks. The marks are used as a guide for incising through the cartilage, taking care to avoid perforation of the anterior skin. The dissection is then carried onto the anterior conchal cartilage surface subperichondrially. The hydrodissection along with a small, sharp Freer elevator allows separation between the skin and cartilage. The cartilage is then removed which includes the entire conchal bowl with the exception of the 8 mm left along the posterior conchal wall. The ear is then placed passively onto the mastoid surface, and the new projection of the helical rim is observed and carefully measured. Any defective prominence can be revised with further cartilage removal. The postauricular muscle

and underlying connective tissue are removed down to the underlying mastoid fascia to allow for passive skin draping of the conchal floor, producing a natural-appearing, deepened conchal bowl. Any excessive postauricular skin can be removed at this time (Figures 71-7D–F).

3. Ear fixation: The ear is fixed in its new position with 3 to 4 mattress transfixion sutures of 3-0 silk that perforate the skin anteriorly, anchor deeply into the postauricular muscle stump, and pass back through the anterior skin. The mattress sutures are then gently tied over a dental cotton roll, moistened with a triple antibiotic ointment, which has been placed into the cymbal and caval fossa, making sure to place one end of the cotton roll into the external auditory canal to avoid postoperative stenosis. The sutures and cotton roll hold the ear in place during healing, stretch and flatten the skin uniformly over the conchal floor, and give depth to the conchal bowl. The postauricular incision is then closed in a running fashion with a resorbable suture, leaving a small opening inferiorly for drainage. The cotton roll dressing is left in place for a minimum of two weeks for optimal healing (Figures 71-7G–I)

Mustarde Method

The Mustarde method, first described in 1959, is indicated for the prominent ear with a poorly formed or lack of an antihelical fold.[16] This cartilage weakening technique relies on precisely placed horizontal mattress sutures, creating a new antihelical fold. It is rarely performed alone and used commonly in combination with the Davis method described above.

1. Antihelical fold markings: The scapha is folded back against the underlying scalp by applying digital pressure on the superior helical rim,

which creates an antihelical fold. The crest of the fold is marked with a surgical marker. To prepare for placement of the mattress sutures, marks are placed parallel to the crest at least 7 mm apart to avoid creating too narrow of a fold. The lateral marks placed on the skin are transferred to the underlying cartilage with a hypodermic needle dipped in methylene blue (Figures 71-8A and B).

2. Dissection and cartilage weakening: Local anesthetic solution is infiltrated along the scaphal fossa beneath the anterior auricular skin, hydrodissecting the skin from the underlying cartilage. This is to facilitate the anterior dissection and mattress suture placement. The postauricular skin is then removed in an identical fashion as described with the Davis method. Once having identified the marks placed on the posterior surface of the scaphoid cartilage, a Freer elevator is passed through a small horizontal incision created through the cartilage at the most inferior aspect of the new antihelical fold. The anterior auricular skin is then dissected from the underlying cartilage corresponding to the crest of the new antihelical fold. Through the tunnel dissected along the anterior surface of the cartilage, the body of the new antihelical fold is weakened to facilitate folding and remove the inherent memory. Many methods have been described, however cartilage weakening can be performed adequately using a Brown-Adson forceps, a nasal rasp, or a dermabrader with a small diamond fraise (Figures 71-8C–E).

3. Suture placement: Nonresorbable, horizontal mattress sutures (4-0 Mersilene) are placed. The sutures are all placed through the medial perichondrium, cartilage, and lateral perichondrium, being careful not to include the anterior skin. The sutures should be

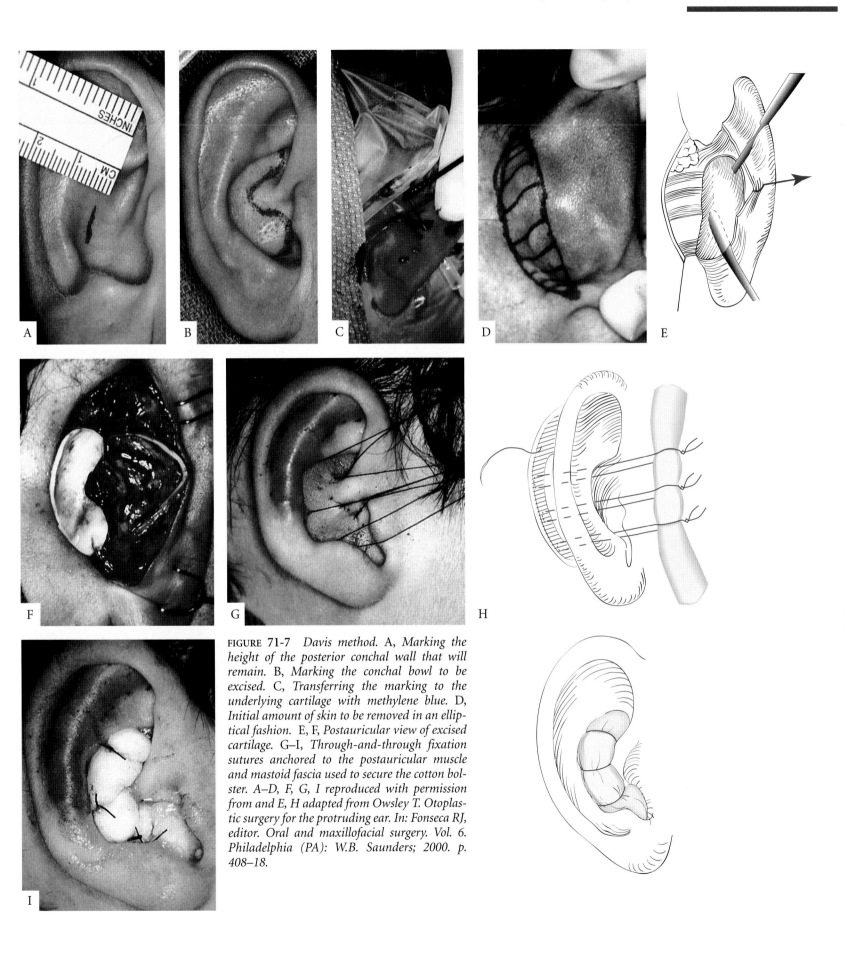

FIGURE 71-7 *Davis method. A, Marking the height of the posterior conchal wall that will remain. B, Marking the conchal bowl to be excised. C, Transferring the marking to the underlying cartilage with methylene blue. D, Initial amount of skin to be removed in an elliptical fashion. E, F, Postauricular view of excised cartilage. G–I, Through-and-through fixation sutures anchored to the postauricular muscle and mastoid fascia used to secure the cotton bolster. A–D, F, G, I reproduced with permission from and E, H adapted from Owsley T. Otoplastic surgery for the protruding ear. In: Fonseca RJ, editor. Oral and maxillofacial surgery. Vol. 6. Philadelphia (PA): W.B. Saunders; 2000. p. 408–18.*

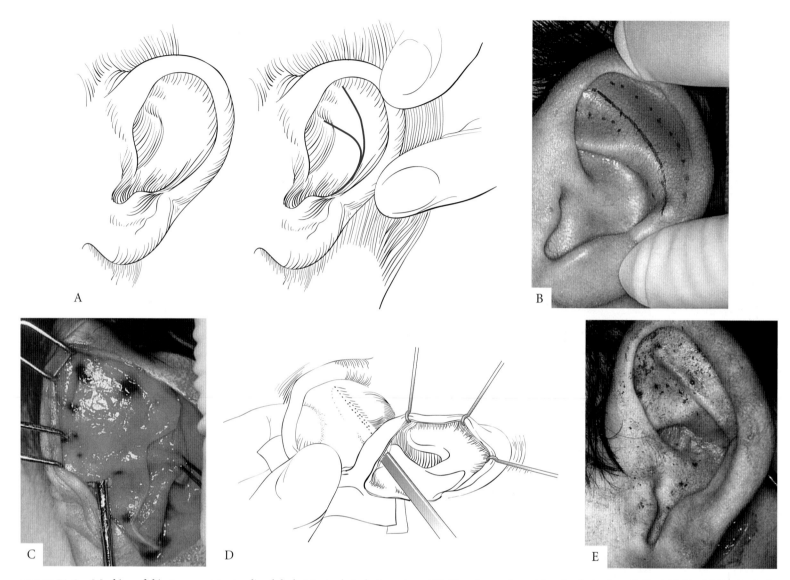

FIGURE 71-8   *Marking of skin to correct protruding lobule Mustarde technique. A and B, Creating and marking the desired antihelical fold by folding back the helix with digital pressure. Lines, parallel to the crest of the fold, are marked and transferred to the underlying cartilage and used for suture placement. C–E, Dissection of the scaphoid fossa beneath the anterior skin for weakening and creation of the desired antihelical fold.* (CONTINUED ON NEXT PAGE)

placed perpendicularly across the antihelical fold, so that upon tightening, a well-rounded, antihelical fold will be created. The sutures are tightened under direct observation and adjusted accordingly to form the new antihelical fold (Figures 71-8F and G).

4. Dressing: The dressing is important and is placed to provide adequate pressure to obliterate dead space and avoid a postoperative hematoma formation. A carefully layered dressing is placed over the anterior and opposing posterior surfaces of the scaphoid region with a quarter-inch petrolatum gauze, followed by 4 x 4 inch fluffs, held secure with a pressure-type facial dressing (Figures 71-8H and I).

Correction of the Protruding Earlobe

A protruding earlobe often accompanies a protruding ear. If so, it must be identified and corrected simultaneously. If the lobule of the ear protrudes, an extension of the posterior auricular incision is drawn with a surgical marker in the shape of a **V** onto the earlobe. Finger pressure on the freshly marked lobe, compressing it to the mas-

toid skin, produces a mirror image imprint forming a **W**-shaped (fish tail) portion of skin to be excised. After this portion is excised and hemostasis achieved, closure is accomplished with a 4-0 plain gut suture. The two **V**-shaped incisions are brought together reducing the protruded state of the lobule (Figure 71-9A and B).[14]

Complications

The incidence of complications after reduction otoplasty is quite low.[17] The major complications to be avoided are infection and keloid formation. Immediate

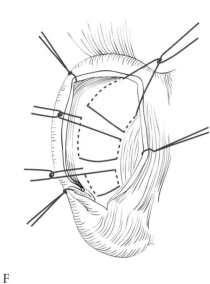

F

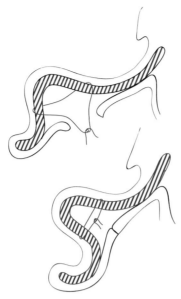

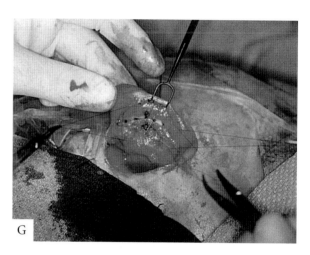

G

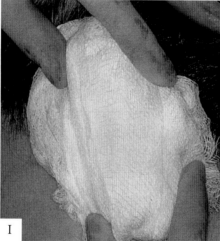

H

I

FIGURE **71-8** (CONTINUED) F and G, *Placement of the horizontal mattress sutures to create a new antihelical fold.* H and I, *Placement of petrolatum gauze and fluffs as an important pressure dressing. B, C, E, G–I reproduced with permission from and A, D, F adapted from Owsley T. Otoplastic surgery for the protruding ear. In: Fonseca RJ, editor. Oral and maxillofacial surgery. Vol. 6. Philadelphia (PA): W.B. Saunders; 2000. p. 408–18.*

complications include pressure necrosis from an overly tight dressing and hematoma formation. Delayed or long term complications include hypertrophic or keloid scar formation, recurrence of the ear deformity, neurosensory deficits, and unesthetic results.

Hematoma

Postoperative hematoma formation, with an incidence of 2 to 4 %, is the most common problem that requires immediate and aggressive intervention.[17] It is most often related to inadequate hemostasis achieved at the time of surgery. Other factors in hematoma formation include an overly tight wound closure without drainage at the base of the wound, postoperative trauma, hypertension, and a preexisting bleeding dyscrasia. Persistent pain beneath the dressing or significant bleeding through and around the dressing suggests hematoma formation and demands prompt inspection. The presence of a hematoma is indicated by a tense and bluish swelling beneath the auricular skin, most often in the retroauricular space. Management includes suture removal, blood clot evacuation, hemostasis, and reclosure of the wound with a large pressure dressing reapplied. Large doses of antibiotics are advisable to prevent perichondritis. If this problem remains untreated, it can result in fibrosis, perichondritis, and cauliflower ear deformity.

Perichondritis

Wound infection in otoplasty occurs in the early postoperative period and is usually a sequela to an undetected or inadequately treated hematoma. Symptoms include pain, erythema, fever, and discharge that may or may not be present. Treatment includes high doses of antibiotics following appropriate wound cultures. Common bacteria include *Staphylococcus aureus*, *Escherichia coli*, and *Pseudomonas aeruginosa*. Adequate drainage is achieved by opening all sutures and carefully irrigating necrotic debris from the wound. All correction sutures must be removed and the cosmetic deformity addressed at a later

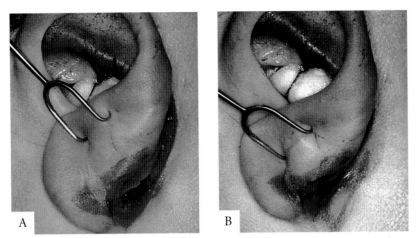

FIGURE 71-9   A, B *Marking of skin to correct protruding lobule. Areas marked are excised in "fishtail" fashion and closed. Reproduced with permission from Owsley T. Otoplastic surgery for the protruding ear. In: Fonseca RJ, editor. Oral and maxillofacial surgery. Vol. 6. Philadelphia (PA): W.B. Saunders; 2000. p. 408–18.*

date. The complication can be devastating, causing massive cartilage destruction with a severe deformity resulting, even with aggressive therapy. Prophylactic antibiotics have not been scientifically proven to be beneficial, but are often used in the preoperative and postoperative period to avoid this devastating complication.

Keloid and Hypertrophic Scar Formation

The closure line of the skin incision in the postauricular region is susceptible to scar formation, especially closed under tension. It is most commonly seen in younger patients and patients with deeply pigmented skin. Keloid formation, one of the most frustrating of all postoperative complications, requires aggressive therapy. In the early stages of keloid formation, intralesional triamcinolone acetonide is injected weekly until regression or significant improvement is evident. Most hypertrophic scars improve with steroid infiltration, but some keloids can progress into significant unesthetic lesions. Low dose radiation, although potentially dangerous, may provide the only effective means of control of some keloids. The more advanced lesions require surgical excision combined with radiation and delayed skin grafting of the irradiated area, with final

aid from intralesional triamcinolone. The risk can be minimized by ensuring that the skin incision is closed passively.

Esthetic Complications

Inadequate correction of the ear deformity is the most common untoward result of otoplasty, often more obvious to the surgeon than to the patient. Calder and Nassan described at least one complication or residual deformity in 16.6% of all the patients who underwent otoplasty using all techniques.[18] Recurrence of the ear deformity is a more common complication of reduction otoplasty, but is less likely to happen after excising a portion of the cartilage as well as a segment of skin, as described in the Davis method. Depending on sutures alone for achieving correction carries a greater risk of recurrence.

Telephone Ear Deformity

Telephone ear deformity occurs when the root of the helix and the ear lobule remain protruded while the middle half, or third, of the ear is set back against the head. This is more common in a large ear with a wide scapha. The incidence has been reported to be 3%.[19] Reverse telephone ear reveals a pronounced conchal bowl with respect to the lower and upper poles. These deformi-

ties can be avoided by carefully checking the position of the helical root, the upper helical rim, and the lobule at the completion of surgery.

Scapha Buckling

Scapha buckling or a transverse fold can develop in the Mustarde technique. This deformity can be avoided by placing the horizontal mattress sutures closer together where the scapha is widest, combined with adequate anterior scoring or weakening.

Narrowed Meatus

A constricted external auditory meatus can occur if the conchal bowl is rotated anteriorly in setting the ear back in any technique in which the conchal bowl is not excised. This problem is eliminated in the Davis method in which the floor of the conchal bowl is excised. Care must also be taken in placing the inferior end of the cotton roll bolster dressing into the external auditory canal to avoid stenosis.

Summary

Reduction otoplasty carries few complications and can provide satisfying results for both the patient and surgeon in the majority of cases. As in all cosmetic procedures, proper patient selection is imperative. Accurate preoperative assessment of the individual deformities and the appropriate choice of a surgical correction will minimize unfavorable esthetic results. The single greatest cause of an unfavorable result in this procedure is inaccurate diagnosis.

The surgeon must understand the normal external anatomy of the ear and learn to recognize the pathological characteristics of the abnormal ear. Having accurately assessed the deformity, the surgeon needs to be familiar with the various surgical approaches available to correct them. Finally, it is important to have a working knowledge of the potential complications of otoplasty and their prevention and treatment.

References

1. Ellis DA, Keohone JD. A simplified approach to otoplasty. J Otolaryngol 1992;21:66.

2. Deiffenbach JF. Die operative chirurgie. Leipzig (FA): Brockhaus; 1845. Cited by Tanzer RC. Deformities of the auricle. In: Converse JM, editor. Plastic and reconstructive surgery. 2nd ed. Philadelphia (PA): W.B. Saunders; 1997. p. 1710.

3. Ely ET. An operation for prominence of the auricles. Arch Opthalmol Otolaryngol 1881;10:97.

4. Karmody CS, Annino DJ Jr. Embryology and anomalies of the external ear. Facial Plast Surg 1995;11:251–6.

5. Strenstrom SJ. Cosmetic deformities of the ears. In: Grabb W, Smith JW, editors. Plastic surgery. Boston (MA): Little Brown and Co.; 1968. p. 595.

6. Rogers BO. Microtic, lop, cup and protruding ears: four directly inheritable deformities? Plast Reconstr Surg 1968;41:208.

7. Allison GR. Anatomy of the external ear. Clin Plast Surg 1978;5:419–22.

8. Davis JE. Aesthetics and reconstructive otoplasty. New York (NY): Springer-Verlag; 1987. p. 77–87.

9. Tanzer RC. Congenital deformities. Deformities of the auricle. In: Converse JM, editor. Reconstructive plastic surgery. 2nd ed. Philadelphia (PA): W.B. Saunders; 1997. p. 1671.

10. Marx H. Die Missbildungen des Ohres. Sekundare Ohrmissbildungen. In: Handke F, Lubarsch O, editors. Hanbush der speziellen pathologischen Anatomie und Histologie. Vol 12. Berlin: Springer-Verlag; 1926. p. 697.

11. Guyuron B, DeLuca L. Ear projection and the posterior auricular muscle insertion. Plast Reconstr Surg 1997;100:457–60.

12. Macgregor FC. Ear deformities: social and psychological implications. Clin Plast Surg 1978;5(3).

13. Furnas DW. Correction of prominent ears by concha-mastoid sutures. Plast Reconst Surg 1968;42:189–93.

14. Converse SM, Wood-Smith D. Corrective and reconstructive surgery in deformities of the auricle. In: Papasella MM, Shumrick DA, editors. Otolaryngology. Vol 3: head and neck. Philadelphia (PA): W.B. Saunders Co.; 1973. p. 500–27.

15. Davis JE. Prominent ears. Clin Plast Surg 1978;5(3).

16. Mustarde JC. The correction of prominent ears using simple mattress sutures. Br J Plast Surg 1963;5:170.

17. Adamson PA, Strecker HD. Otoplasty techniques. Facial Plast Surg 1995;11:284–300.

18. Calder JC, Nassan A. Morbidity of otoplasty: a review of 562 consecutive cases. Br J Plast Surg 1994; 47:170–4.

19. Lavy J, Sterns M. Otoplasty: techniques, results and complications – a review. Clin Otolaryngol 1997;22: 390–3.

20. Tanzer RC. Congenital deformities. In: Converse J, editor. Reconstructive plastic surgery. Vol 4. 2nd ed. Philadelphia (PA): WB Saunders; 1977.

21. Davis JE. Anatomy of the ear. In: Stark R, editor. Surgery of the head and neck. New York (NY): Churchill Livingston; 1987.

INDEX